AF213010

Handbook of Experimental Pharmacology

Continuation of Handbuch der experimentellen Pharmakologie

Vol. XXV Supplement

Editorial Board

G.V.R. Born, Cambridge · A. Farah, Rensselaer, New York
H. Herken, Berlin · A.D. Welch, Memphis, Tennessee

Advisory Board

S. Ebashi · E. G. Erdös · V. Erspamer · U. S. von Euler · W. S. Feldberg
G. B. Koelle · O. Krayer · M. Rocha e Silva · J. R. Vane · P. G. Waser
W. Wilbrandt

Bradykinin, Kallidin and Kallikrein

Supplement

Contributors

K. D. Bhoola · W. G. Clark · R. W. Colman · E. G. Erdös
F. Fiedler · T. L. Goodfriend · L. M. Greenbaum
A. R. Johnson · M. Lemon · A. P. Levitskiy
H. S. Margolius · R. Matthews · I. H. Mills · H. Z. Movat
C. E. Odya · T. S. Paskhina · J. J. Pisano
J. M. Stewart · R. C. Talamo · A. Terragno
N. A. Terragno · R. Vogel · P. E. Ward · P. Y. Wong

Editor

E. G. Erdös

Springer-Verlag Berlin Heidelberg GmbH 1979

Professor Dr. ERVIN G. ERDÖS, Departments of Pharmacology, and Internal Medicine. The University of Texas, Southwestern Medical School, 5323 Harry Hines Blvd., Dallas TX 75235/ USA

With 83 Figures

This volume completes „Handbuch der experimentellen Pharmakologie, Vol. XXV", published in 1970.

ISBN 978-3-642-67303-0 ISBN 978-3-642-67301-6 (eBook)
DOI 10.1007/978-3-642-67301-6

This work is subject to copyright. All rights are reserved, whether the whole or part of the material is concerned specifically those of translation, reprinting, re-use of illustrations, broadcasting, reproduction by photocopying machine or similar means, and storage in data banks. Under § 54 of the German Copyright Law where copies are made for other than private use, a fee is payable to the publisher, the amount of the fee to be determined by agreement with the publisher.

© by Springer-Verlag Berlin Heidelberg 1979
Originally published by Springer-Verlag Berlin Heidelberg New York in 1979
Softcover reprint of the hardcover 1st edition 1979

The use of registered names, trademarks, etc. in this publication does not imply, even in the absence of a specific statement, that such names are exempt from the relevant protective laws and regulations and therefore free for general use.

Typesetting, printing, and bookbinding: Brühlsche Universitätsdruckerei, Lahn-Gießen. 2122/3130-543210

Preface

Volume XXV of the Handbook of Experimental Pharmacology series entitled "Bradykinin, Kallidin, and Kallikrein" was published in 1970. My aim in editing this volume of the series is not to replace, but to update the 1970 edition. During the decade preceding the publication of Vol. XXV, the existence of kinins and kallikreins gained acceptance, the protein components of the system were purified and characterized and the peptides were synthesized. Even after these accomplishments, interest in the subject has not abated, but has increased substantially. We have learned a great deal about the role that components of the kallikrein–kinin system play in other systems and about the immensely complex and intricate interactions in blood. Directly or indirectly, kallikrein and kinins affect the coagulation of blood, the activation of complement, and the generation of angiotensin. Kinins release or modulate the actions of other agents, including prostaglandins, histamine, and catecholamines. Inhibitors of kallikrein or kininase II are employed, for example, in extracorporeal circulation or in hypertension. Kallikrein, kinins, and kininases, present in urine, were described first in 1925 and 1954, but have been ignored for decades. These substances are now studied extensively because of their possible role in blood pressure regulation. The evidence that kinins have a metabolic function is also increasing. The abundance of active components of the system in genital organs suggests a role in the fertilization process.

The book is organized into chapters which bear upon these issues. The first four chapters discuss kininogenases, the enzymes which release kinins and their inhibitors. Plasma kallikrein, its substrates and its inhibitors and the interrelationships with other blood-borne systems are reviewed in the first chapter. This is followed by a discussion of kininogenases in blood cells including acid kininogenases which form an alternate kinin system.

Reviews of the extensive studies on the structure of glandular kallikreins and their inhibitors are next, summarizing the achievements of a very enlightening period of protein research.

The next section deals with kinins. Structure-activity studies on peptides of the kinin system and on bradykinin potentiators have lead to the synthesis of effective kininase II inhibitors and hopefully, in the future, will lead to the development of specific kinin antagonists. Free, naturally occurring bradykinin and related peptides are next. If we wish to understand the actions of kinins, we must learn about their sites of action and we must be able to assay them accurately and in minute quantities. Chapters on bradykinin receptors and on radioimmunoassay contribute an up-to-date review of these problems. The actions of kinins and kallikrein in the central nervous system and other tissues are described next. Some of the investigations described here may be only initial observations, but might later open new areas of research. Among the most intriguing aspects of research on kinins are studies of their indirect actions, especially their interrelationships with prostaglandins (Chap. XI). Kinins are not stable in the organism; they are rapidly inactivated in blood and kininases in tissues limit their actions. The functioning of kininase I as an anaphylatoxin inactivator and kininase II as the angiotensin I converting enzyme emphasizes the importance of these proteins.

Glandular kallikrein and urinary kallikrein have been scrutinized by many researchers since excretion of the latter seems to be connected with hypertension. Chapters XIII, XIV, and XV describe the results of experimental work on glandular, renal, and urinary kallikrein in laboratory animals and man. Kinins may have a more important role in pathological than in physiological processes, as surveyed in Chap. XVI. The final chapter summarizes the extensive literature published in Russian because it is not easily accessible to readers outside of the U.S.S.R.

In 1966 I wrote in a review (Adv. Pharmacol. *4*, 1–90) "... the status of kinins somewhat resembles that of acetylcholine or histamine. Bradykinin may never become a therapeutically important agent. Nevertheless, if kinins play a significant role in some physiological or pathological conditions, agents which block the effects or inhibit their enzymic metabolism would be of prime importance." Since half of the second prediction seems to be fulfilled by the development of kininase II inhibitors, we may look forward to finding kininase I inhibitors that work in the whole organism, and to the development of active kinin blocking agents.

Finally, I mention with deep regret that Professor EUGEN WERLE is no longer with us; thus he can not witness the exciting developments in the field where he achieved so much, so early, and so far ahead of others.

Dallas, June 1979 E. G. ERDÖS

Contents

II. Kininogenases of Blood Cells (Alternate Kinin Generating Systems).
L. M. GREEN-BAUM. With 4 Figures

III. Enzymology of Glandular Kallikreins. F. FIEDLER. With 1 Figure

VI. Kinins in Nature. J.J. PISANO

VII. Bradykinin Receptors. C.E. ODYA and T.L. GOODFRIEND

VIII. Bradykinin Radioimmunoassay. R.C. TALAMO and T.L. GOODFRIEND

IX. Kinins and the Peripheral and Central Nervous Systems. W.G. CLARK

XIV. Renal and Urinary Kallikreins. P. E. WARD and H. S. MARGOLIUS. With 1 Figure

XV. Renal Kallikrein and Regulation of Blood Pressure in Man. I. H. MILLS. With 3 Figures

XVI. Kallikrein-Kinin System in Pathologic Conditions. R. W. COLMAN and P. Y. WONG. With 1 Figure

XVII. Bradykinin, Kallidin, and Kallikreins. T. S. PASKHINA and A. P. LEVITSKIY. (Survey of the Russian literature). With 6 Figures

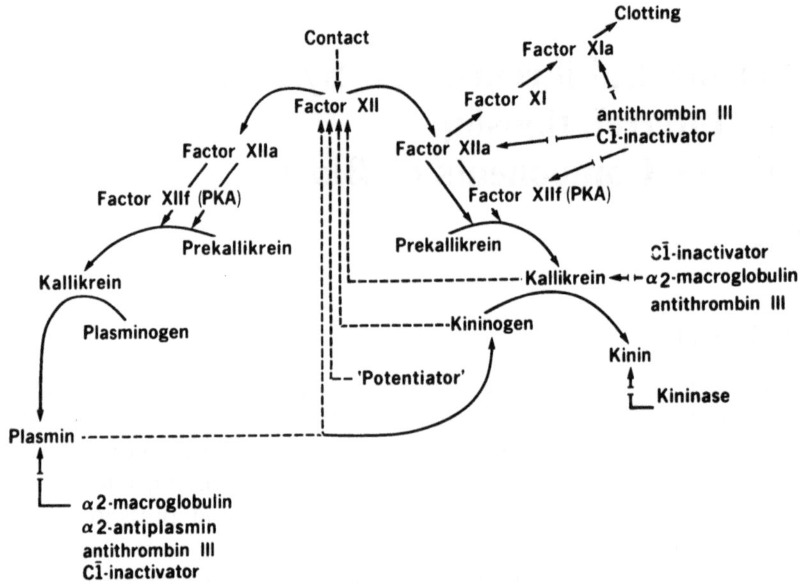

Fig. 1. Schematic representation of the plasma kinin system, its relation to fibrinolysis and the initial stage of the intrinsic clotting system. Inhibitors are represented by interrupted arrows. (From MOVAT, 1978b)

illustrates the interrelationship of the kinin system with the contact phase of blood coagulation and fibrinolysis, as well as the homeostasis maintained by various inhibitors.

This review will describe first the recognition of the kinin system, its components and their interaction with components of the clotting and fibrinolytic systems. It will also describe briefly the interaction between the kinin system and blood cells and its inhibition. Inhibitors of enzymes are described in another chapter of this volume, whereas inhibitors of kinins were reviewed in volume XXV of this series (ERDÖS and YANG, 1970) and more recently (ERDÖS et al., 1977).

B. Initiation of Kinin Formation and Its Relation to Blood Clotting – Early Views and Concepts

I. Permeability Globulin PF/dil, and Its Relation to the Contact Phase of Blood Coagulation and to Kinin Formation

A series of experiments were reported between 1953 and 1958 by MILES and coworkers on a *permeability globulin*, obtained by diluting serum of various species in glass vessels. The vascular permeability-enhancing substance was designated *PF/dil* (permeability factor/dilute) and its properties reviewed in 1964 by MILES (for further details see EISEN and VOGT, 1970; MOVAT, 1978a). PF/dil was visualized to be present in plasma as pro-PF/dil, i.e., in inactive or precursor form and to become activated upon dilution with saline. However, already in 1957 Spector demonstrated that PF/dil is formed only when the dilution is carried out in glass vessels and not in siliconized or plastic tubes. Glass beads activated the serum placed into plastic tubes and generated a kinin-like peptide (reviewed by MARGOLIS, 1963). As pointed out by MILES and co-workers, plasma contained a natural inhibitor of PF/dil. The nature of PF/dil is discussed below and the various plasma proteinase inhibitors in another section. From these data it would appear that the inhibitor was identical with C$\bar{1}$-inactivator and perhaps to some extent with antithrombin III (see below).

PF/dil has been isolated in partially purified form by BECKER and co-worker (KAGEN et al., 1963; BECKER and KAGEN, 1964). It was adsorbed on DEAE cellulose (thereby separated from plasma kallikrein), migrated as a β-globulin and had a sedimentation coefficient of 5.2–6.6 *S*.

MILES and colleagues first believed that PF/dil acted directly on the microcirculation, but subsequently demonstrated liberation of kinin from plasma. When added to either fresh or heated (60 °C for 60 min) plasma, kallikrein released kinin; it is therefore a kinin-forming enzyme or kininogenase. However, PF/dil could liberate kinin only when added to fresh plasma (MASON and MILES, 1962). In heated plasma, factor XII and prekallikrein are inactivated and kallikrein added to such plasma can act only on kininogens. MASON and MILES believed that PF/dil acted as an intermediate step or activator, i.e., converting kallikreinogen (prekallikrein) to kallikrein.

Independently, ARMSTRONG et al. (1955, 1957) and MARGOLIS (1957, 1958) demonstrated a relationship between a pain-producing substance, kinin formation, and the contact phase of blood coagulation. Based on the above data of MILES and co-workers and of MARGOLIS and with the aid of a highly purified preparation of factor XII a (RATNOFF and DAVIE, 1962), RATNOFF and MILES (1964) attempted to elucidate the function of PF/dil. The factor XII used by RATNOFF and MILES was not fully activated but (as found later) contained mixtures of unactivated and activated factor XII in varying proportions. The clotting activity of this mixture could be increased by exposure to kaolin or by adding ellagic acid. It was calculated in retrospect that only about 8% of the factor XII was present in active form. Activated factor XII (factor XII a) was shown to induce bluing, i.e., enhanced vascular permeability when injected into guinea pig skin. RATNOFF and MILES chose a subthreshold dose of factor XII a, i.e., a dose which by itself caused no bluing. When this small amount of factor XII a was added to diluted plasma it induced formation of a permeability factor (PF). Certain anticoagulants, such as protamine sulfate, liquoid or hexadimethrine bromide, inhibited factor XII a from initiating blood coagulation and formation of PF. It had been shown earlier that hexadimethrine bromide inhibits the generation of kinin in plasma induced by glass activation (ARMSTRONG and STEWART, 1962; EISEN, 1964). Other inhibitors, namely soybean trypsin inhibitor (SBTI), diisopropylfluorophosphate (DFP) and the so-called natural inhibitor of PF/dil, inhibited the permeability effect of the PF once it had been generated in plasma. It was shown furthermore, that the formation of PF in plasma by addition of factor XII a was optimal at 37 °C, delayed at 24 °C and non was formed in the cold, during incubation for 18 min. Most pro-PF was present in plasma which was soluble at $^{1}/_{3}$ but insoluble at half saturation with ammonium sulfate. Having shown that factor XII a induces formation of PF in normal plasma in siliconized vessels, the authors concluded that: "the time and concentration relations of this induction indicate that activated Hageman factor in this respect behaves like an enzyme, whose substrate is a precursor of the PF. The precursor was located in a crude globulin fraction. Except for a slightly greater lability on storage, its properties were largely those of the pro-PF postulated as the precursor of the PF/dil. Moreover the properties of the PF formed by activated Hageman factor were in essential those of the PF/dil activated by holding dilute plasma in glass vessels." As indicated above, MILES and co-workers first postulated that PF/dil acted directly on the microcirculation. RATNOFF and MILES proposed a hypothesis which was in keeping with the observations of ARMSTRONG and co-workers, of MARGOLIS, and of MASON and MILES. They wrote: "The sequence of events after the activation of PF/dil is controversial. In our view, from a study of guinea pig and human plasma (MASON and MILES, 1962, and unpublished), the PF activates a kininogenase which in turn produces kinins from the appropriate kininogens of the plasma." Neither RATNOFF and MILES (1964), nor BECKER et al. who carried out studies on PF/dil more or less simultaneously (KAGEN et al., 1963; BECKER and KAGEN, 1964) studied the clot-promoting effect of their partially purified PF/dil, particularly not on factor XII-deficient plasma.

All the components of the kinin system are present in whole diluted plasma. Thus, when RATNOFF and MILES added partially activated factor XII to plasma, prekallikrein was probably converted to kallikrein (see below), which in turn cleaved kininogens to bradykinin. Kinins are rapidly inactivated in plasma by kininases (ERDÖS and YANG, 1970; ERDÖS et al., (1977). The amount of XIIa or fragmented factor XII (XIIf) in the factor XII preparation probably was sufficient to activate some of the prekallikrein to kallikrein, which in turn activated more factor XII by the later-described feedback mechanism (COCHRANE et al., 1973). Factor XIIa can also activate the intrinsic fibrinolytic system and plasmin can cleave factor XII to XIIf (KAPLAN et al., 1971; BURROWES et al., 1971). Judging from the elution pattern of the serum chromatographed on DEAE-cellulose, the PF/dil described by BECKER and KAGEN (1964) probably contained plasminogen and/or plasmin and factor XII (XIIa and XIIf). Factor XIIf has been shown to be potent in inducing enhancement of vascular permeability when injected into guinea pig skin (MOVAT et al., 1969a, b, 1970, 1971a).

Studies using immunoabsorption conducted by KELLERMEYER and RATNOFF (1967) indicated that factor XII and PF/dil were not related. When normal human plasma was treated with rabbit antifactor XII (absorbed with XII-deficient plasma) before dilution it prevented the generation of PF/dil, whereas treatment of plasma after dilution (once the PF had been generated) did not prevent the vascular permeability-enhancing activity. The findings contradict the recent ones of JOHNSTON et al. (1974) described below. In view of recent work there are several ways to interpret the findings of KELLERMEYER and RATNOFF. Anti-enzymes (CINADER, 1965), including antiproteases (ARNON, 1971), act primarily by steric hindrance. It is conceivable that the antibody of KELLERMEYER and RATNOFF was not directed against the active center of factor XII and that such antibodies could block activation of factor XII in whole plasma by sterically inhibiting contact with glass. Another possibility is that addition of anti-XII after PF/dil had been generated seemingly had no effect because the plasma diluted in glass contained, in addition to activated factor XII, plasma kallikrein and plasmin (activated through activation of XII) which induce enhanced vascular permeability (see Sects. D and F). Thus anti-factor XII added before dilution could have prevented the formation of all permeability factors by inhibiting XII, but such antibody added after activation of the plasma would be ineffective against kallikrein. Since the microcirculation of a given area has a limited capability to respond to permeability-enhancing substances, the simple and insensitive method used by KELLERMEYER and RATNOFF may not have detected the differences under their experimental conditions.

Evidence that PF/dil is primarily factor XIIa was furnished by JOHNSTON et al. (1974), who removed PF/dil activity with insolubilized antibody against factor XII, but not by normal γ-globulin linked to Sepharose 4B or by antibody against prekallikrein. Kallikrein was essential for the generation of PF/dil activity, since prekallikrein deficient plasma failed to develop vascular permeability-enhancing activity but addition of purified prekallikrein reconstituted this capacity.

The early observations of ARMSTRONG et al. (1955, 1957) and of MARGOLIS (1957, 1958) describing the relationship of a pain-producing substance, the contact phase of blood coagulation, and kinin-formation have already been mentioned. MARGOLIS recognized the complex nature of the kinin-forming system. In 1963 he stated that: "We must remember that in the main we are dealing with functional entities. Each of these factors may prove to be complex systems and what now looks like a complete identity of two factors may turn out to be only a partial overlap of two systems. Eventually, these entities will be characterized chemically, but before the chemist can supply the answers the physiologist must arrange the data in the form of legitimate questions." (MARGOLIS, 1963). It may be stated that after 15 years the functional components described by MARGOLIS (which, when first described, must have seemed to be quite a puzzle to both the uninitiated and to the investigators working in the field) are well characterized physicochemically. When describing the observations of MARGOLIS and in using his functional terms, the presently accepted chemical entities will be given in parenthesis.

MARGOLIS (1958) found that kinin formation in plasma by glass contact required factor XII (Fig. 2). Factor XII became adsorbed onto the glass or another surface and, following its activation, activated another factor referred to as "component A" (plasma kallikrein). Component A was shown to remain in the plasma (i.e., the fluid phase) where it could generate kinin from kininogen. Surface contact could not consume all the kininogen in plasma. MARGOLIS first exposed plasma to glass powder for 5–10 min. After separation of the glass and standing at room temperature for 3–4 h both component A (i.e., the kinin-forming activity) and kinin had decayed (as we now know, due to the action of certain inhibitors). New exposures of this plasma for 2–4 min to glass induced more kinin-forming activity, but no kinin could be generated. The kinin-forming activity (component A, plasma kallikrein) could be demonstrated in plasma after separation from the glass beads by incubating it with noncontacted plasma as a source of substrate. The inability to generate kinin upon a second exposure of plasma to glass was not due to a lack of kininogen, since salivary and urinary kallikreins could generate kinin (kallidin) from such plasma (KEELE, 1960). It was therefore postulated by MARGOLIS (1960) that the first exposure of plasma to glass depleted it of a substance designated "component B" (HMW kininogen). (As will be described later HMW kininogen, in contrast to LMW kininogen, is rapidly cleaved by plasma kallikrein). Several investigators including MARGOLIS (1966) believed that component A was plasma kallikrein and more recent studies substantiated this, as described below. VOGT (1966) first equated it with an activator

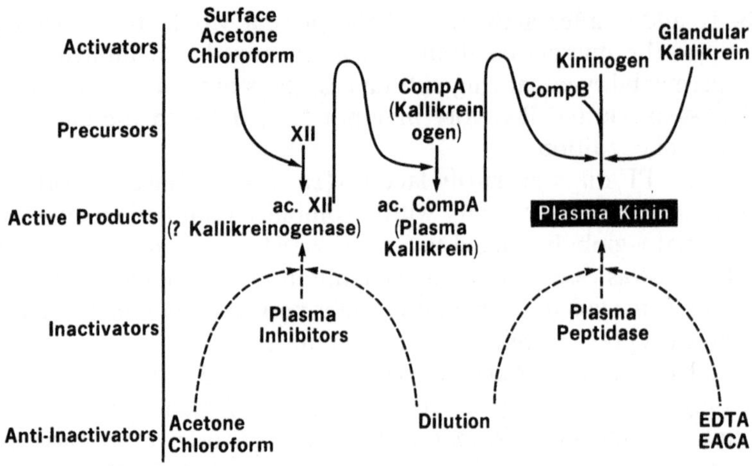

Fig. 2. Schematic representation of the kinin system according to MARGOLIS (1963)

or intermediate enzyme. However, the nature of component B remained obscure for some time. Although it should be stated that among the several possibilities put forward, EISEN (1963) suggested that it may be a portion of the substrate (for further details, see EISEN and VOGT, 1970). As shown in Fig. 2 the concept of MARGOLIS (1963), although incomplete does not differ markedly from the present one.

A recent study (OH-ISHI and WEBSTER, 1975) further confirms that the main component in PF/dil responsible for the vascular permeability enhancing activity is activated factor XII (both XIIa and XIIf). The enhanced vascular permeability, as detected by RATNOFF and MILES (1964), was compared to the prekallikrein activation by diluting the plasma. When the reciprocal of plasma dilution was plotted, the permeability (PF/dil) and prekallikrein-activating activities overlapped. Preparative polyacrylamide electrophoresis of 1:200 plasma diluted in glass tubes showed prekallikrein activating activity in the β-globulin and the albumin regions (i.e., corresponding to XIIa and XIIf) as described under Sect. C. Studies with various deficient plasmas indicated that factor XII (Hageman factor) and prekallikrein (Fletcher factor) were required for maximal activation of plasma and generation of PF/dil. Plasma deficient in $C\bar{1}$-inactivator generated considerably more PF/dil than normal plasma. A number of inhibitors of factor XII inhibited generation of PF/dil. It was interesting that some highly basic substances (e.g., cytochrome c, hexadimethrine bromide) inhibited the activation of factor XII without affecting activated factor XII, whereas others (polylysines) inhibited both activities.

II. The Concept of Two Kinin Systems

As described later, plasma of several species contains two kininogens and when activated plasma or serum is chromatographed two peaks of kinin-forming activity are recovered. VOGT (VOGT, 1965, 1966; VOGT et al., 1967, 1968) postulated the existence of two kinin-forming systems on the basis of some experiments, which were triggered mainly by some unexplained observations of MARGOLIS (1958, 1960, 1963). MARGOLIS had noted that plasma depleted of compound B (HMW kininogen) by glass-contact still contained kininogen from which kinin could be released by glandular kallikreins or trypsin. However, component A (plasma kallikrein) which is present in B-depleted plasma could not act on this kininogen, or had a negligible effect. (The rate of kinin-formation from HMW and LMW kininogens by plasma kallikrein will be described later). At this point it should be noted that MARGOLIS, as described above, on reincubating B-depleted (HMW kininogen-depleted) plasma with glass used a short incubation period. Because the kininogenase and the kininogen present in extensively contacted plasma do not react with each other, VOGT postulated that the two reactants belong to different kinin-forming systems. The kininogenase in the extensively contacted plasma (designated kininogenase II) was believed to require a different kininogen (kininogen II). This kininogen II was thought to be present in fresh plasma, but consumed during surface activation.

Kininogen I, remaining in plasma after surface activation (and susceptible to glandular kallikreins and trypsin) was described as attacked only by another enzyme (kininogenase I), which becomes rapidly inactivated after surface exposure of plasma. Thus, kininogenase I could not be detected in glass-treated plasma. VOGT tried to explain the reasons for the presence in glass-contacted plasma of enzyme II and kininogen I and the absence of enzyme I and kininogen II as follows: After glass exposure kininogenase I was inactivated very rapidly, having no time to act sufficiently on kininogen I. Because kininogenase II was inactivated more slowly, it could act on and totally consume kininogen II. In fact, some kininogenase II activity was still demonstrable after substrate II had been consumed. Later findings of VOGT and DUGAL (1976) explain the earlier findings of two kininogenases acting differently on the substrates of whole plasma. However, these newer findings, described in detail in Sect. D (dealing with prekallikrein and kallikrein), do not quite agree with the earlier concept. Furthermore, VOGT's equation of his enzymes and substrates with those of MARGOLIS do not fit the newer concepts, if the writer's interpretation of MARGOLIS is correct. If MARGOLIS' component B is HMW kininogen and VOGT equates it with his kininogen II then it should be acted on primarily by free plasma kallikrein (see Sect. D), which according to VOGT and DUGAL (1976) is rapidly inactivated in whole plasma. Yet the enzyme rapidly inactivated in VOGT's old concept is kininogenase I. VOGT (1966) has in fact equated kininogenase I with plasma kallikrein. Furthermore, kininogen I was thought to be functionally identical with the kininogen isolated from bovine plasma by HABERMANN and ROSENBUSCH (1962, 1963), which is LMW kininogen, i.e., a poor substrate for plasma kallikrein, as was reported later by several investigators, including VOGT and DUGAL (1976). The main difficulty in reconciling VOGT's (1966) early concepts with those of MARGOLIS (1963) and his own later findings (WENDEL et al., 1972; VOGT and DUGAL 1976; VOGT, 1976) is the fact that there are indeed two kininogens in plasma but only one kininogenase, i.e., plasma kallikrein, which may be free or bound in complexes. This is discussed in Sect. D which deals with kallikrein and prekallikrein.

C. Factor XII (Hageman Factor)

Factor XII deficiency was discovered by RATNOFF (RATNOFF, 1954; RATNOFF and COLOPY, 1955). "We owe our knowledge of the existence of Hageman factor to Mr. John Hageman, a freight switchman on the New York Central Railroad." (RATNOFF,

1966). Coagulation of plasma is enhanced when it is exposed to glass or similar substances, e.g., quartz, kaolin or diatomaceous earth. Mr. Hageman was admitted to hospital in 1953 to be operated for a peptic ulcer. "To everyone's surprise," writes RATNOFF (1966), "his clotting time was greatly prolonged. Mr. Hageman was unaware of any bleeding tendency, nor did he have a family history of bleeding. Suitable studies soon demonstrated that the defect in Mr. Hageman's plasma could not be identified with any of the clotting abnormalities known at that time. Crude experiments demonstrated that his plasma behaved as if it were deficient in a specific clotting factor, found in all other plasmas tested. This substance was therefore named Hageman factor, and its absence designated Hageman trait." The clinical and laboratory findings were described by RATNOFF and co-workers and confirmed by others (see RATNOFF, 1966). These studies included the demonstration that in Hageman trait there is a lack of factor XII, as shown by immunologic techniques (SMINK et al., 1967).

I. Isolation and Purification

Factor XII or Hageman factor was first identified by MARGOLIS (1958) as a definite substance which plays a role in both kinin formation and in intrinsic blood coagulation. Early studies were done with factor XII adsorbed to surfaces such as glass ballotini or crushed glass, as described in Sect. B.

Modern preparative procedure for the isolation of *human factor XII* were first applied by SCHIFFMAN et al. (1960) and by RATNOFF et al. (1961). SCHIFFMAN and co-workers separated factor XII from factor XI on a column of DEAE-cellulose, whereas RATNOFF et al., after adsorbing and heating factor XI-deficient plasma to eliminate several clotting factors, obtained a crude factor XII preparation by batch adsorption with CM-cellulose. However, a highly purified preparation of factor XII was obtained soon thereafter (RATNOFF and DAVIE, 1962). Pooled citrated plasma (1200 ml) was first adsorbed with aluminum hydroxide and then with Filter-Cel. $Al(OH)_3$ adsorbs factors IX, X, V, II, and a portion of XI and Filter-Cel the residual XI. Unlike Hyflo Super-Cel and Celite-512, which activate and fragment factor XII, as described below, adsorption and activation of factor XII by Filter-Cel is negligible (ÖZGE-ANWAR et al., 1972). As in an earlier study (RATNOFF et al., 1961), RATNOFF and DAVIE subjected the adsorbed plasma to batch fractionation with CM-cellulose equilibrated with 0.075 *M* Na-acetate-acetic acid, pH 5.2. After washing with the equilibrating buffer, the crude factor XII was desorbed with 0.6 *M* acetate. The desorbed eluates were precipitated with ammonium sulfate at 60% saturation. After redissolving the precipitates and dialysing against 0.025 *M* barbital buffer (pH 7.45), aliquots were chromatographed on columns of DEAE-cellulose, with a linear gradient, the limiting barbital buffer containing 0.25 *M* NaCl. The final step was column chromatography on CM-cellulose (acetate, pH 5.2, 0.025–0.6 *M*). The final yield was 13% and factor XII had been purified over 5000-fold. However, no evidence of homogeneity was presented. The preparation was pure with respect to other clotting factors but it was not functionally pure with respect to the fibrinolytic system. The untreated preparation did not have fibrinolytic activity, but when streptokinase was added a positive clot lysis time was demonstrated. This finding is compatible with newer ones in which the elution of plasminogen from CM-Sephadex was monitored by immunodiffusion (CHAN and MOVAT, 1976). Once dissolved, factor XII was unstable for long periods and since this was attributed to the low protein concentration it was made up in barbital-saline buffer containing 1% bovine serum albumin. RATNOFF and DAVIE considered their factor XII to be in active form, i.e., XIIa. However, as discussed in Sect. B, in studies with PF/dil (RATNOFF and MILES, 1964) it was found that the factor XII prepared by RATNOFF and DAVIE consisted almost exclusively of unactivated factor XII. Furthermore, this factor XII preparation was not susceptible to inhibition by DFP, indicating that it was in zymogen form, factor XIIa being readily inhibited by DFP (COCHRANE et al., 1976). The factor XII isolated by RATNOFF and DAVIE was probably the best human factor XII preparation available for about 10 years and served in a number of studies and for the preparation of antibody.

A highly purified activated factor XII was isolated from human plasma also by SPEER et al. (1965), but it consisted probably of a mixture of unactivated factor XII, the activated (XIIa), and the fragmented form (XIIf). The main reason for this was probably the initial exposure of the plasma to Hyflo-Super-Cel, which brings about activation and cleavage (presumably enzymatic) of factor XII, as described below. The celite eluates were further purified by isoelectric precipitation, ammonium sulfate precipitation (40%–50% saturation), CM-Sephadex chromatography (ammonium acetate of increasing ionic strength and pH). The purification factor achieved was similar to that of RATNOFF and DAVIE and the recovery was estimated at 25%.

Although factor XII has been implicated in the activation of the kinin system since the studies of MARGOLIS (1958, 1963), the demonstration of a highly anionic low molecular weight activator of the system in guinea pig (MOVAT et al., 1968, 1969b; TRELOAR et al., 1970, 1972), rabbit (TUCKER and WUEPPER, 1969; LAWRENCE et al., 1970), and human serum or plasma (EISEN and GLANVILLE, 1969; KAPLAN and AUSTEN, 1970, 1971; MOVAT et al., 1970, 1971a), but particularly the demonstration that this activator probably derives from factor XII (KAPLAN and AUSTEN, 1970), led to new attempts at isolating factor XII in pure form.

COCHRANE and co-workers reported two methods by which highly purified factor XII was recovered (COCHRANE and WUEPPER, 1971b; REVAK et al., 1974). In the earlier described method normal human or rabbit plasma containing hexadimethrine bromide (50 μg/ml) and EDTA (0.001 *M*) were used, without adsorbing prothrombin or other clotting factors. Proteins soluble at 25%, but precipitable at 55% saturation of ammonium sulfate were redissolved, and chromatographed on DEAE-Sephadex A-50. The equilibrating buffer was 0.01 *M* Na-phosphate, pH 8.0, and elution was performed with a linear gradient to 0.3 *M* NaCl. The anion exchanger had been rinsed in the phosphate buffer containing hexadimethrine bromide (the highly basic hexadimethrine bromide is excluded in such columns). The factor XII-containing fractions (referred to as precursor of prekallikrein activator) were precipitated at 60% saturation of ammonium sulfate, redissolved and rechromatographed on DEAE-Sephadex, elution being carried out by raising the NaCl concentration and lowering the pH. Much of the non-factor XII protein was eluted in this step and the partially purified preparation thus obtained was subjected to gel filtration on Sephadex G-200; here the activity overlapped with the major protein peak, several smaller ones being eliminated. The remaining three contaminants (as visualized by disc gel electrophoresis), were removed by chromatography on CM-Sephadex C-50.

The buffer was citric acid-Na phosphate; the starting buffer had a pH of 5.85 and the limiting buffer 7.4 and contained 0.3 *M* NaCl. When concentration of protein was not carried out by precipitation with ammonium sulfate, positive pressure ultrafiltration was used, the membranes having been rinsed in hexadimethrine bromide. Factor XII obtained in this manner was homogeneous by alkaline disc gel electrophoresis. However, when BAGDASARIAN et al. (1973b) attempted to use this method they found on acrylamide gels a major band with β-mobility and two minor ones with α-mobility. Elution from the gels gave a single band, the activity corresponding to the one with β-mobility. In the second method (REVAK et al., 1974), ammonium sulfate precipitation of plasma and gel filtration were omitted, the procedure consisting of three steps. The first step consisted of DEAE-Sephadex chromatography with a linear gradient of eluting buffer, but the buffer contained hexadimethrine bromide and the limiting buffer 0.6 *M* NaCl. In the second step, the same type of ion exchange was used again with an increasing ionic strength (0.25 *M* NaCl) and a decreasing pH (from 8.1 to 4.6). The third step consisted of chromatography on CM-Sephadex (0.01 *M* phosphate, pH 6.5) with a linear gradient to 0.5 *M* NaCl. With the newer procedure the yield was increased 25–50-fold. From 40.0 mg of factor XII in 1600 ml of plasma, 14–16 mg were recovered. Specific activity for the total material recovered was not given, but the activity in the peak was purified 2500-fold.

The approach used by KAPLAN et al. consisted first (1971) of chromatography of unadsorbed plasma on QAE-Sephadex (0.01 *M* phosphate buffer, pH 7.8, and linear elution to 0.3 *M* NaCl), SE-Sephadex (0.01 *M* phosphate, pH 6.0, and linear elution to 0.5 *M* NaCl) and Sephadex G-100. Subsequently this procedure was improved (WEISS et al., 1974; KAPLAN et al., 1976a). A less steep gradient was used for the QAE-Sephadex and the cation exchanger (SP-Sephadex). After gel filtration on a long column (2.5 × 150 cm) of Sephadex G-150, the proteins were rechromatographed on QAE-Sephadex (0.003 *M* phosphate, pH 8.0, linear elution to 0.2 *M* NaCl). A single band was demonstrable by alkaline disc gel electrophoresis. No recoveries and specific activities were given.

A multistep procedure used by MOVAT and ÖZGE-ANWAR (1974) gave a high degree of purification but poor yield. Starting material was 10 liters of ACD plasma adsorbed on $Al(OH)_3$. It was chromatographed sequentially through QAE-Sephadex (steps), lysine-Sepharose, QAE-Sephadex (steps), Sephadex G-200, CM-Sephadex (gradient), Sephadex G-200, QAE-Sephadex (gradient), and adsorption to and desorption from celite. The first QAE-Sephadex and first gel filtration were carried out in a 37 × 30 cm (KS/370) column. The QAE-Sephadex was equilibrated with 0.1 *M* Tris-HCl (pH 8.0) and when eluted stepwise, factor XII always emerged with 0.11 *M* NaCl. For CM-Sephadex the procedure of RATNOFF and DAVIE (1962) was followed, but in order to achieve a better separation a shallower gradient was used (0.12–0.6 *M* acetate). In the final chromatographic step a very shallow gradient was applied to a QAE-Sephadex column (0.08–0.13 *M* NaCl). However, homogeneity was only achieved when the highly purified factor XII was adsorbed to celite and after thorough washing was desorbed from it. Earlier it has been observed that celite (Hyflo Super-Cel) activates and cleaves factor XII when added to whole plasma (ÖZGE-ANWAR et al., 1972) or to partially purified factor XII (SOLTAY et al., 1971). The interesting observation was made that highly purified factor XII adsorbs to celite and when it is desorbed little or none is in the activated (XIIa) form. In the

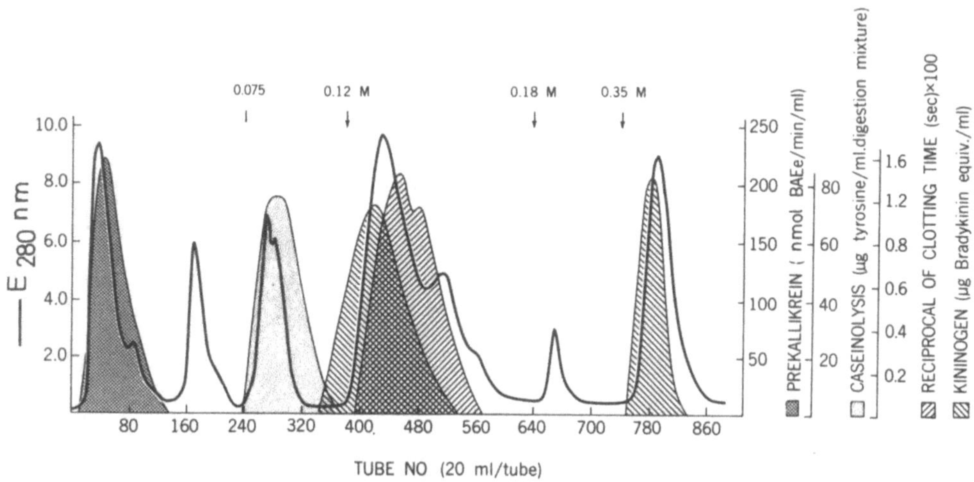

Fig. 3. Elution pattern of components of the kinin system on QAE-Sephadex at pH 8. Prekallikrein elutes in the excluded peak, plasminogen (caseinolysis) when the NaCl is raised to 0.075 *M*, followed by factor XII (clotting) and LMW kininogen (with 0.12 *M* NaCl) and finally HMW kininogen (with 0.35 *M* NaCl). (From HABAL and MOVAT, 1976a)

absence of kaolin it does not correct the clotting abnormality of factor XII-deficient plasma. However, in the presence of kaolin (or celite) and certain plasma factors (discussed below) activation occurs.

During anion exchange chromatography on QAE-Sephadex at pH 8.0 a good initial separation of the various components of the kinin system was achieved (Fig. 3). When elution is carried out by increasing the concentration of NaCl stepwise, this permits the use of very large quantities of plasma, essential for the isolation of trace proteins. Prekallikrein emerges in the excluded peak, plasminogen elutes when the concentration of NaCl is raised to 0.075 *M*, factor XII and LMW kininogen elute at 0.12 *M* and HMW kininogen elutes only after the salt has been raised above 0.3 *M*.

In the above described studies (MOVAT and ÖZGE-ANWAR, 1974), in addition to LMW kininogen, the proteinase inhibitors α_1-antitrypsin, antithrombin III, and α_2-macroglobulin were present in the crude factor XII preparation. Of these, the last was eliminated during gel filtration and the other two in the excluded peak during CM-Sephadex chromatography. It should be pointed out however, that α_2-macroglobulin also emerges in the excluded peak during CM-Sephadex chromatography if gel filtration is omitted. It should be also noted that despite earlier elution of plasminogen, factor XII cannot be recovered by anion exchange chromatography free of plasminogen (and activated plasminogen, i.e., plasmin is known to cleave factor XII) (KAPLAN and AUSTEN, 1971; BURROWES et al., 1971). These observations and the search for a simplified preparative procedure for factor XII led to another study.

CHAN and MOVAT (1976), after adding hexadimethrine bromide (50 µg/ml) and SBTI (10 µg/ml), adsorbed the plasma with $Al(OH)_3$ mainly to remove prothrombin which can interfere with clotting tests. The volume was reduced and some protein eliminated by precipitation at pH 7.4 with polyethylene glycol. The precipitate formed with 4% (final concentration) polyethylene glycol was discarded and the

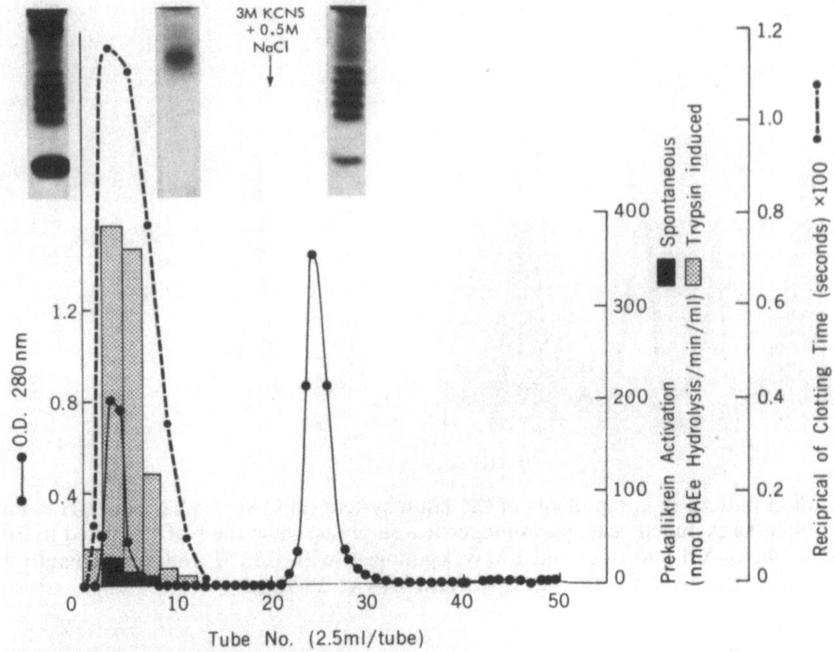

Fig. 4. Purification of factor XII by an indirect immunoabsorbent column with antibody against contaminants. Factor is excluded and the contaminants retained, as shown by the alkaline disc gels. The first gel represents the material applied to the column. The antibody was prepared against proteins eluting with 0.12 *M* NaCl from a QAE-Sephadex column (see Fig. 2), to which factor XII-deficient plasma had been applied. (From CHANand MOVAT, 1976)

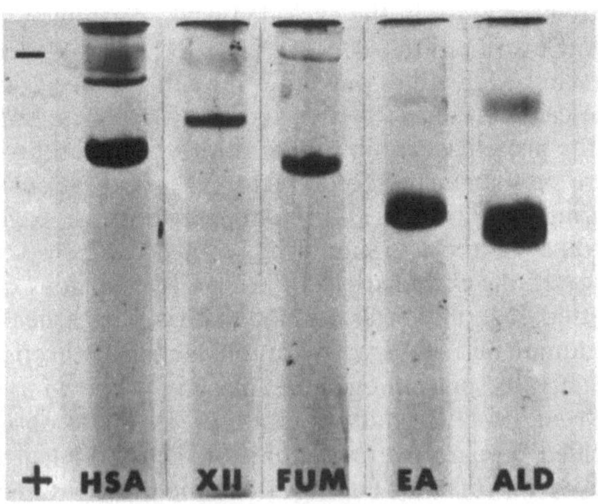

Fig. 5. SDS-disc gel electrophoresis of factor XII, together with the marker proteins of human serum albumin (HSA; MW 69,000), fumarase (FUM; MW 49,000), egg albumin (EA; MW 43,000), and aldolase (ALD; MW 40,000). The second higher MW band of HSA represents the dimer (MW 138,000). (From CHAN and MOVAT, 1976)

supernatant reprecipitated by raising the polyethylene glycol to 16% (see SCHULTZE and HEREMANS, 1966). The redissolved globulins, free of fibrinogen and containing about 30% of the plasma albumin were chromatographed on QAE-Sephadex as shown in Fig. 3. All buffers contained 10 μg/ml of SBTI, the bulk of which eluted with the factor XII-containing fractions, the elution being monitored immunochemically. The CM-Sephadex column was equilibrated with 0.05 *M* citrate buffer, pH 5.8, containing SBTI. NaCl was then added to the buffer, first with SBTI and then without. All the plasminogen was eliminated in this step. The cation exchange chromatography was followed by either gel filtration on Sephadex G-200 (2.5 × 165 cm column) or an "indirect" immunoabsorbent column. The antibody linked to Sepharose 4B in this column was prepared by immunizing rabbits against a fraction of factor XII-deficient plasma. The fraction consisted of the proteins eluting with 0.12 *M* NaCl from QAE-Sephadex (see Fig. 3). From the immunoabsorbent column factor XII eluted as the effluent, whereas the contaminating proteins adsorbed to the column (Fig. 4). Figure 5 shows the homogeneity of the factor XII preparation. In subsequent studies when larger quantities (up to 5 liters) of plasma constituted the starting material and considerably larger CM-Sephadex columns had to be used it was found that the cation exchange step had to be repeated because of carry over of plasminogen. Furthermore, it was found that Sephadex G-200 gave a better separation than Sephadex G-100 (CHAN et al., 1976).

GRIFFIN and COCHRANE (1976a) modified earlier described procedures. They used five preparative steps. No absorption to remove the prothrombin complex and other clotting factors was used. However, they defibrinated the plasma (containing EDTA and hexadimethrine bromide) by heating to 56 °C for 30 min, during which time prekallikrein was also precipitated and removed by centrifugation. Step 2 consisted of DEAE-Sephadex chromatography (Tris-Succinic acid, pH 8.4). Traces of plasminogen were removed by lysine-Sepharose. Step 4 was again DEAE-Sephadex, but with a decreasing pH, instead of a salt gradient. The final step was CM-Sephadex (acetate buffer, pH 5.3) with an increasing NaCl gradient. The yield of factor XII was 25%, the preparation contained more than 95% factor XII, of which less than 2% was in activated form.

Factor XII has been isolated also from *animal plasmas*. SCHOENMAKERS et al. (1965) obtained a homogeneous preparation, purified about 7000-fold from bovine plasma. The plasma was adsorbed with $Al(OH)_3$ and passed through a column packed with glass powder. The adsorbed factor XII was eluted with glycine buffer (pH 9.6), followed by ethanol precipitation to a final concentration of 25%, the pH adjusted to 6.9 with acetic acid and kept overnight in the cold. The formed precipitates (Cohn fractions II and III) were discarded. Zinc acetate (0.25 *M*, pH 5.5) in 25% ethanol was added to the supernatant to a final concentration of 20 m*M* Zn^{2+}. The precipitate which had formed overnight in the cold was dissolved in 0.1 *M* EDTA and the Zn-EDTA separated from the protein on Sephadex G-25. The protein was passed through two consecutive columns of CM-Sephadex; first steps (0.15 *M* acetate, pH 5.2, with increasing NaCl), followed by a gradient (0.3–1.0 *M* NaCl). The final step was anion exchange chromatography on DEAE-Sephadex (0.05 *M* Tris-HCl, pH 7.5, linear gradient to 0.4 *M* NaCl). Recovery was 4.9%. Interestingly, unlike the human material, bovine factor XIIa had arginine esterase activity, the specific activity of which increased in parallel with the clotting activity.

Using essentially the same procedure, Temme et al. (1969) obtained similar results and their bovine factor XIIa, in addition to the esterase and clotting activity, released kinin from human, rat, and dog plasmas and when mixed with a partially purified prekallikrein it enhanced vascular permeability when injected into rabbit skin. Factor XIIa did not enhance vascular permeability when injected directly into rabbit skin. However, in the rabbit there is an unexplained lag phase of about 1.5–2.5 h before enhanced vascular permeability can be demonstrated after injection of activated factor XII (Graham et al., 1965) or activated serum (Movat, 1967).

The preparation isolated by Grammens et al. (1971) seems to have consisted mainly of factor XI since it was excluded during anion exchange chromatography and had a MW (142,000) closer to that of factor XI. The isolation and properties of this factor XII substrate are discussed briefly at the end of Sect. C.

Komiya et al. (1972) used defibrinated euglobulin from 15 liters of plasma which they passed consecutively through CM-Sephadex, DEAE-Sephadex, and CM-Sephadex. For the cation exchange chromatographies, 0.1 *M* acetate buffer, pH 5.0, was used, the proteins being eluted with a gradient of 0.35–0.8 *M* NaCl. For DEAE-Sephadex, an NaCl gradient of 0.07–0.35 *M* in 0.02 *M* Tris HCl buffer, pH 8.5, was employed. The TAMe hydrolytic activity and prekallikrein-activating activities overlapped with the protein peak in the second CM-Sephadex column. However, the addition of elagic acid did not enhance considerably the prekallikrein activating activity for factor XII, indicating that some of it was present in the activated form. The curious observation was made that the end product gave a single main band by analytical disc gel electrophoresis, but when the material was kept frozen for one year and then subjected to electrophoresis multiple bands were detected, including a prealbumin band (XIIf) and elution showed a spread of the clotting activity and an anodal shift of the prekallikrein activating activity.

The isolation used for rabbit plasma by Cochrane and co-workers was essentially the same as used for human plasma (Cochrane and Wuepper, 1971; Cochrane et al., 1972a). In fact most of the early studies of these investigators were done with factor XII obtained from rabbit plasma.

II. Physico-Chemical Properties

The physicochemical properties of unactivated factor XII will be discussed here and those of the activated forms in the next subsection, dealing with activation (Table 1).

The properties of human factor XII have been studied by a number of investigators. Early experiments indicated that factor XII is a β-globulin with an isoelectric point of 6.0–6.5. By gel filtration, a MW of 110,000–120,000 was estimated and the data on sedimentation coefficient varied between 4.5–5.5 *S* (Donaldson and Ratnoff, 1965; Cochrane and Wuepper, 1971; Kaplan et al., 1971; Soltay et al., 1971). Subsequent findings based on SDS disc gel electrophoresis (Cochrane et al., 1972a; Bagdasarian et al., 1973b) and on the sedimentation coefficient, partial specific volume, and diffusion coefficient (Movat et al., 1973a) indicated a MW of about 90,000. More recent studies using SDS disc gel electrophoresis indicate a still lower MW, i.e., 80,000 (Revak et al., 1974) and 76,000–78,000 (Chan and Movat, 1976) respectively. Repeated runs of both human and rabbit factor XII were reported by Cochrane and co-workers to sediment always with the human serum albumin and thus to have an *S*-value of 4.5 (COCHRANE et al., 1976). In their first report COCHRANE and WUEPPER found an inhibitor in the 4.0–4.5 *S* region, which gave false values with crude factor XII, i.e., 6.0–7.0 *S* (see bovine factor XII, described below). Nevertheless, in the writer's laboratory highly purified factor XII (CHAN and MOVAT, 1976) was consistently found to sediment as a 5.0–5.1 *S* protein (CHAN, 1975) (see also Fig. 8). This discrepancy may be due to the MW designation of the cocentrifuged marker proteins. The inhibitor referred to by COCHRANE and WUEPPER (1971) is probably antithrombin III which has an *S*-value and MW slightly smaller than factor XII (ROSENBERG and DAMUS, 1973; BURROWES and MOVAT, 1977) and inhibits activated factor XII (STEAD et al., 1976; CHAN et al., 1977a).

The amino acid composition of factor XII showed a reasonable degree of similarity in experiments carried out in two different laboratories (REVAK et al., 1974; MCMILLIN et al., 1974). The data obtained earlier (SPEER et al., 1965) varied somewhat, but as already indicated the material in these studies probably consisted of unactivated factor XII, XIIa, XIIf, and intermediate forms described under activation in the next subsection.

The concentration of factor XII in human plasma has been estimated to be 29 μg/ml (range: 15–47 μg/ml in 17 subjects), as determined by quantitative radial immunodiffusion (REVAK et al., 1974). With a radioimmunoassay, using iodinated factor XII, similar results were reported (SAITO et al., 1974a). Although the results were expressed in units, it was calculated that the concentration in a pool of normal plasma was 30–40 μg/ml (SPRAGG, 1977).

SCHOENMAKERS et al. (1965) found the $S^0_{20,w}$ of bovine factor XII to be 7.0, the diffusion constant 7.14×10^{-7} cm^2/sec and the MW based on the first two data was estimated to be 82,000. The extinction coefficient was 12.0. The composition was estimated as polypeptide moiety 86.3%, hexoses 5.9%, hexosamines 4.8%, and sialic acid 4.4%. Thus, bovine factor XII is a glycoprotein. KOMIYA et al. (1972) had estimated a molecular weight of 95,000 from gel filtration and about 89,000 was calculated from data based on sucrose density ultracentrifugation, although the *S*-value was not given.

The recent studies of FUJIKAWA et al. (1977) indicate that bovine factor XII is a glycoprotein with a MW of 74,000, containing 13.5% carbohydrate, including 3.4% hexose, 4.7% N-acetylhexosamine and 5.4% N-acetylneuraminic acid. It consists of a single polypeptide chain, with an NH_2-terminal end homologous to the reactive site of a number of protease inhibitors. The amino sequence of the C-terminal was found homologous with the active site of several serine proteases.

The properties of purified factor XII of rabbit plasma (COCHRANE and WUEPPER, 1971b; COCHRANE et al., 1972a) and of partially purified guinea pig plasma (TAKEUCHI and MOVAT, 1972) were found to be essentially similar to human factor XII.

III. Activation of Factor XII

1. Mechanism of Activation

Factor XII can be activated enzymatically by adding a protease, such as trypsin, to factor XII or by contact with negatively charged surfaces. The two mechanisms have been referred to as fluid phase and solid phase activation (COCHRANE et al., 1973).

In early studies, activation of factor XII was studied functionally in whole plasma or serum which was subjected to gel filtration following activation. In such studies, factor XII was found to have a MW of about 110,000 and the smallest fragments 30,000–40,000 (MOVAT et al., 1969b; 1970; 1971a; KAPLAN and AUSTEN, 1970, 1971; KAPLAN et al., 1971; ÖZGE-ANWAR et al., 1972). These same investigators, as well as BAGDASARIAN et al. (1973a, b), found intermediate fragments with prekallikrein-activating activity. However, COCHRANE and co-workers (summarized in COCHRANE et al., 1976) detected activity only in the intact molecule and in the fragmented portion and not in the intermediates. Because the experiments of COCHRANE et al. were done with purified factor XII and their findings are clearer they will be described first. The nature of the intermediate fragments is, as yet, not fully understood and an attempt at their interpretation will be discussed subsequently.

In early studies TUCKER and WUEPPER (1969) exposed rabbit plasma to diatomaceous earth and obtained prekininogenase activator (PKA) by elution with NaCl. PKA was referred to as prekininogenase activator (COCHRANE and WUEPPER, 1971a), as prekallikrein activator (KAPLAN and AUSTEN, 1970; MOVAT et al., 1971a; COCHRANE and WUEPPER, 1971b), as Hageman factor fragments (KAPLAN and AUSTEN, 1971) and as factor or fragment XIIf (ÖZGE-ANWAR et al., 1972). When COCHRANE and WUEPPER (1971b) attempted to use this procedure with purified factor XII they had difficulty in eluting the active material. They therefore treated factor XII with trypsin and inactivated the latter with ovomucoid trypsin inhibitor. In this process factor XII was converted from a protein with a MW of 110,000 and a sedimentation rate of 4.6 *S* to a fragment which possessed PKA activity, had a MW of 32,000 and sedimented at 2.6 *S*. The PKA possessed only 2% of the clot-promoting activity of the intact factor XII molecule. Further studies (COCHRANE et al., 1972a) indicated that trypsinization of rabbit factor XII yields three major subunits of approximately 30,000 MW each. Reduction and alkylation of ^{125}I-labeled factor XII, subjected to SDS disc gel electrophoresis also yielded three subunits of equal size. However, these did not possess PKA activity or clot-promoting activity. It was therefore postulated that rabbit and human factor XII consist of three peptide chains of equal size and charge, held together by *S-S* linkages. Evidence was presented that kallikrein and plasmin can activate factor XII, but that no cleavage occurred under these conditions. In a subsequent publication (COCHRANE et al., 1973) it was shown that on a negatively charged surface, factor XII becomes activated (presumably by conformational changes) but retains its native MW. Such conformational change has subsequently been demonstrated by MCMILLIN et al. (1974) in the circular dichroism spectrum. In fluid phase COCHRANE et al. (1973) could not demonstrated cleavage of rabbit factor XII with kallikrein or plasmin, although activation did occur. However, in preliminary results with human factor XII they demonstrated cleavage into fragments of MW 52,000, 40,000, and 28,000 with trypsin, kallikrein or plasmin. These preliminary observations were then extended and the PKA activity was found exclusively in the 28,000 MW fragment (REVAK et al., 1974). Figure 6 illustrates the proposed sites of cleavage and Fig. 7 demonstrates the cleavage of factor XII by trypsin, factor XII having been radiolabeled and subjected to SDS disc gel electrophoresis. Subsequent studies by REVAK and COCHRANE (1976) defined more precisely the mechanisms underlying cleavage of highly purified factor XII by trypsin, plasmin, or kallikrein and the association of enzymatic and binding activities with separate

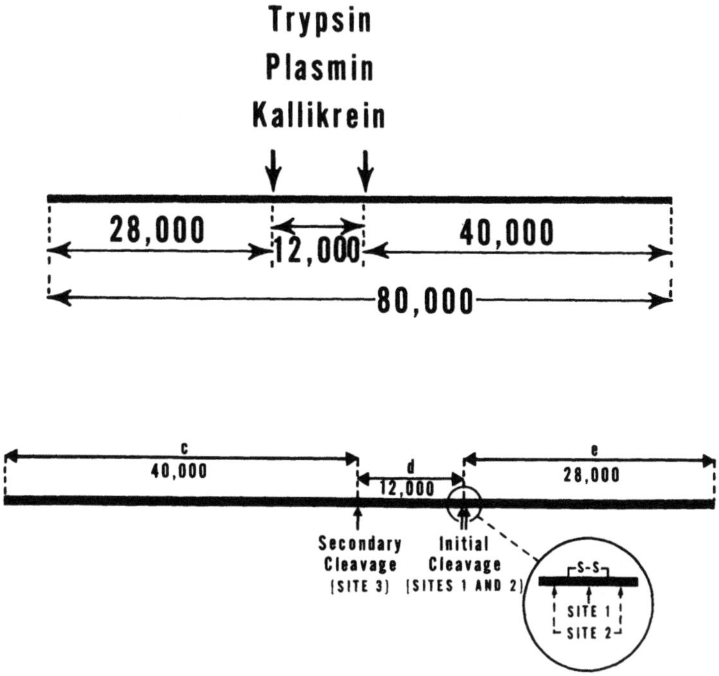

Fig. 6. Diagrammatic representation of cleavage of factor XII by proteases. The lower half shows the possible cleavages giving rise to a free 28,000 MW fragment or one that remains attached to the molecule by an S-S bond described in the text. (From REVAK et al., 1974; and from REVAK et al., 1977)

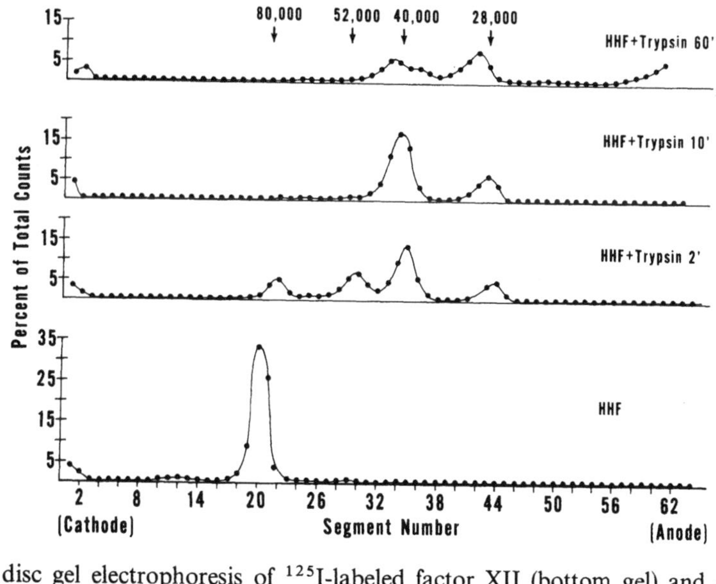

Fig. 7. SDS disc gel electrophoresis of ^{125}I-labeled factor XII (bottom gel) and of factor XII treated with trypsin for 2, 10, and 60 min (upper three gels). The gels were cut into segments and the radioactivity of each segment counted. MW are shown by arrows. (From REVAK et al., 1974)

regions of the factor XII molecule. Advantage was taken of the fact that fragment XIIf (PKA) does not bind to kaolin. Trypsin-treated ^{125}I-labeled factor XII was adsorbed to kaolin. When the supernatant was subjected to SDS disc gel electrophoresis a radioactive peak with a MW of 28,000 was detected. The washed kaolin suspension subjected to electrophoresis revealed peaks of MW 52,000 and 40,000. When labeled factor XII was adsorbed to kaolin and incubated for one hour with kaolin, the 28,000 peak was again recovered in the supernatant. Most of the material remaining adsorbed to kaolin was detected in the 80,000 MW position of intact factor XII together with two small peaks of 52,000 and 40,000 respectively. The XIIf fragment (28 K) migrated in the albumin region by electrophoresis and immunoelectrophoresis in agarose. When mixed with normal plasma the precipitin band of fragment XIIf was more cathodally located, interconnecting with a smaller cathodal arc. This was not observed with $C\bar{1}$-inactivator deficient (anioneurotic edema) plasma. In agarose, factor XII remains near the origin, migrating as a β-globulin. As indicated, REVAK and COCHRANE adsorbed trypsin treated (i.e., fragmented) factor XII with kaolin. By incubating, in turn, anti-factor XII with the fraction adsorbing to and the fraction not adsorbing to kaolin, they prepared two non-cross-reacting antibodies. With the aid of these antibodies they could identify the various fragments by immunoelectrophoresis. These reached from the well (origin) to the albumin region. According to REVAK and COCHRANE the 28,000 MW XIIf fragment (e-region) which does not bind to kaolin is the only part of the molecule responsible for enzymic activity (prekallikrein activation). The 40,000 MW fragment (c-region) has the capacity to bind to negatively charged surfaces. The fragment (d-region) of 12,000 daltons lying between the former two has not been detected as a freely existing polypeptide. While this manuscript was being prepared REVAK and co-workers (1977) treated factor XII bound to a surface with normal plasma and with plasmas deficient in factor XI, prekallikrein, or HMW kininogen. In contrast to normal or factor XI-deficient plasma, which cleaved the factor XII into 52,000 and 28,000 MW fragments rapidly, the cleavage by prekallikrein deficient plasma was slow and that by HMW deficient plasma even slower. In these new studies REVAK et al. postulated fragmentation of the factor XII molecule at two closely situated sites, one of which was within a disulfide loop (Fig. 6, bottom). Cleavage at the site external to the disulfide bond resulted in the release from the surface of the 28,000 MW fragment, containing the enzymatically active site (it subsequently complexed with $C\bar{1}$-inactivator). Cleavage at the site within the disulfide loop resulted in the formation of a 28,000 MW fragment which remained surface-bound, presumably by virtue of the disulfide linkage to the larger fragment.

Studies by other investigators indicate a series of biologically active cleavage products. KAPLAN and AUSTEN (1970) were the first to propose that fragment XIIf may be derived from factor XII. They fractionated human serum and plasma on DEAE-cellulose. With the serum (in contrast to plasma) five bradykinin-generating peaks were eluted when these were mixed with fresh plasma. The first peak was kallikrein since it released kinin also from heated plasma. The remaining four peaks were eluted by increasing the NaCl concentration. Peaks 2 and 3 shortened the partial thromboblastin times (PTT) of factor XII-deficient plasma. Peaks 2–5 were designated activators of prekallikrein and the most anionic peaks with prealbumin bands in alkaline disc gels were estimated to have a MW of 30,000–40,000. On rechromatography of either peak 2 or 3 it eluted in a more anionic position corresponding to peak 5.

POON (1970) estimated by gel filtration the MWs of fractions of human serum, eluted with increasing ionic strength from QAE-Sephadex. That of factor XII was about 125,000 and more anionic fractions were approximately 75,000, 60,000, and 37,000. Factor XII corrected the clotting deficiency in factor XII-deficient plasma, but clotting assays with the more anionic fractions were hampered by the presence of thrombin. However, the most anionic fractions generated kinin from fresh plasma most readily. Only kallikrein (excluded during the anion exchange chromatography) and an "anionic kallikrein" (eluting with macroglobulins during gel filtration) cleaved kinin from heated plasma or a partially purified HMW kininogen, but not from LMW kininogen prepared by the method of JACOBSEN (1966a). The most anionic LMW fraction was subsequently further purified and characterized as PKA or XIIf in whole plasma (MOVAT et al., 1971a) and in celite eluates (ÖZGE-ANWAR et al., 1972). The difficulty with the active intermediate fragments is that they are unstable, having the tendency to gradually convert to the fully fragmented XIIf, a process observed upon repeated chromatography.

KAPLAN and AUSTEN (1971) further examined the above-mentioned "peak 2" (corresponding to factor XII), but used plasma instead of serum and found that following concentration by positive pressure ultrafiltration, rechromatography on DEAE-cellulose, and examination by disc gel electrophoresis, the peak 2 material (containing unactivated factor XII, prekallikrein, plasminogen, and plasmin) had converted to the peaks 3, 4, and 5 obtained by chromatography of serum. They noted "a progressive decrease in size, increase in net negative charge, increased prekallikrein-activating activity, and decreased ability to correct Hageman factor deficiency."

BAGDASARIAN et al. (1973a) isolated a prekallikrein activator from plasma which they first thought not to be related to factor XII. Subsequently, its origin from factor XII was demonstrated (BAGDASARIAN et al., 1973b). It had a MW of 70,000 and the mobility of an α-globulin and was reported to have the tendency to dimerize (MW 135,000; β-globulin). When purified factor XII was treated with plasmin, 22% of the activator activity was attributed to this intermediate. Further treatment did not break down this activator to small (XIIf) fragments. In trypsin-treated factor XII, 10% of the activity was attributed to the 70,000 dalton activator. Kallikrein treatment of factor XII failed to produce the large activator, but did yield LMW activators. The findings of WEBSTER et al. (1973) are in agreement with some of these observations.

Factor XII subjected to sucrose density gradient ultracentrifugation sedimented, based on the markers used, as 5.1 *S* protein, when assayed by the PTT of factor XII-deficient plasma. Extended incubation with plasmin caused a decrease in the clot-promoting activity which sedimented in the original 5.1 *S* and a 4.1 *S* peak (Fig. 8). Prekallikrein activation was detected in three peaks sedimenting at 5.1, 3.7, and 2.7 *S*. Corresponding to the last two, gel filtration in aqueous buffer indicated molecular weights of 60,000 and 30,000, respectively. The latter was 27,500 by gel filtration in guanidine-Sepharose (CHAN, 1975).

Thus, there are these conflicting views. The much better documented studies of COCHRANE and co-workers implicate a single 28,000 MW active fragment, following

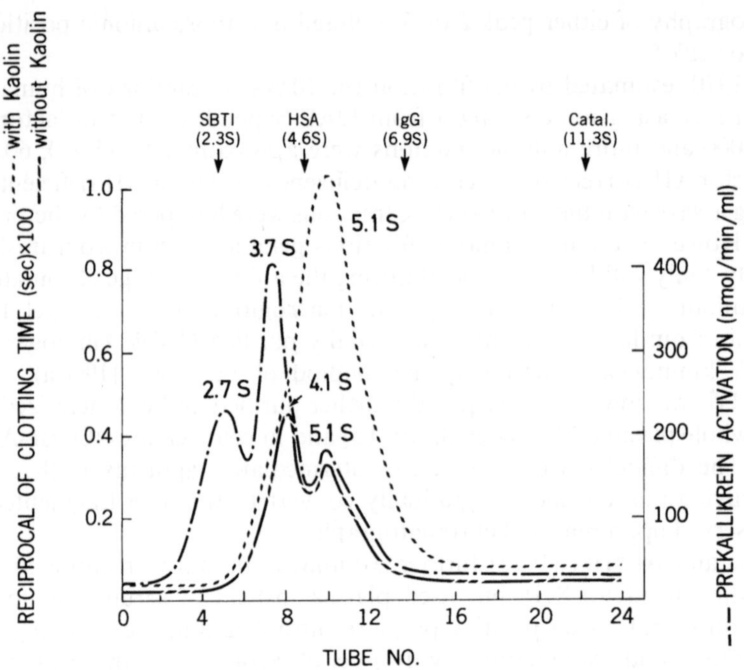

Fig. 8. Sucrose density gradient ultracentrifugation of untreated factor XII (5.1 *S*) and of plasmin treated factor XII (2.7–5.1 *S*). The fragments were assessed in the same way as the untreated factor XII by clotting of factor XII-deficient plasma (the unactivated factor XII with kaolin the plasmin treated factor XII without kaolin) and by their effect on prekallikrein (esterolysis). The slowest sedimenting (2.7 *S*) fragment had effect on prekallikrein, but did not enhance the clotting. (From CHAN, 1975)

cleavage of factor XII at two sites. However, most of these data are based on the behaviour of radiolabeled factor XII fragments. On the other hand, there are findings with less well purified fractions (but based on functional assays) which indicate a gradual cleavage of factor XII with formation of more and more anionic and correspondingly smaller and smaller fragments.

Despite these differences there is good agreement about the physicochemical and biologic properties of the smallest fragment, the PKA or fragment XIIf (MOVAT et al., 1969b; KAPLAN and AUSTEN, 1970; COCHRANE and WUEPPER, 1971a, b; KAPLAN et al., 1971; MOVAT et al., 1971a; WUEPPER and COCHRANE, 1971; ÖZGE-ANWAR et al., 1972; TRELOAR et al., 1972; COCHRANE et al., 1973; VENNERÖD and LAAKE, 1974) (Table 1). It is a highly anionic protein, with an isoelectric point of 4.3–4.6, migrating in the albumin region in agarose or starch block and as prealbumin in alkaline polyacrylamide gel electrophoresis (Fig. 9). It is the smallest of all known proteins of the kinin system with a sedimentation coefficient of 2.6–2.8 *S* and an estimated MW of 28,000–30,000. Fragment XIIf enhances vascular permeability when injected intradermally into guinea pigs, generates kinin from fresh plasma but not from heated plasma nor from purified kininogens. The kinin generation in fresh plasma occurs indirectly through activation of prekallikrein to kallikrein, a process probably responsible for its vascular permeability enhancing activity. When added to prekallikrein it converts it to kallikrein (Fig. 10).

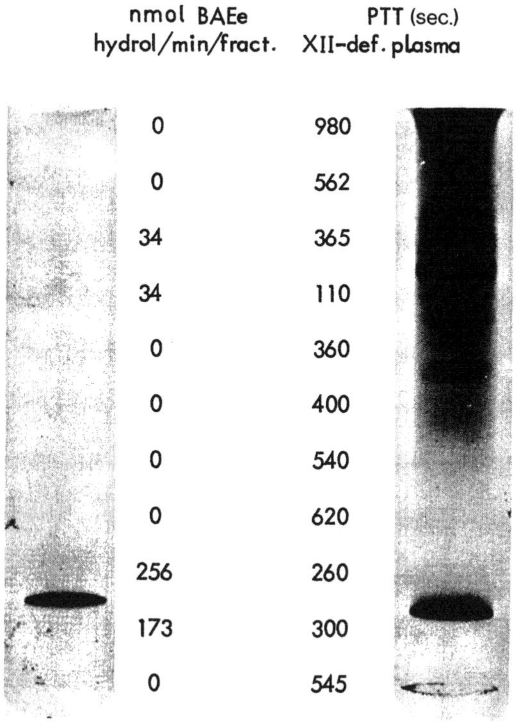

Fig. 9. Preparative disc gel electrophoresis. The stained gel on the right represents partially purified celite eluates and the one on the left the isolated purified fragment XIIf. The two columns show prekallikrein activation (BAEe hydrolysis) and clotting of factor XII deficient plasma of replicate gel slices from gels similar to the one shown on the right

Fig. 10. Kymograph tracing of contraction of a rat uterus suspended in de Jalon solution. The numerals represent contraction by 0.3–0.5 ng/ml of synthetic bradykinin. *A* represents a mixture of fragment XIIf, prekallikrein and kininogen. At *B* and *C* the prekallikrein and fragment XIIf, respectively, were omitted from the reaction mixture. (From Movat et al., 1971a)

2. Activators of Factor XII

Factor XII can be activated in fluid and in solid phase (COCHRANE et al., 1973). Plasma enzymes play an essential role in this, even in solid phase activation and also certain potentiating substances play a role as discussed in the next subsection.

Many of the substances, mostly with a definite negative charge can activate factor XII. The most common ones used in the laboratory include glass, quartz, kaolin, and celite (MARGOLIS, 1963; RATNOFF, 1966). A frequently used activator is elagic acid (RATNOFF and CRUM, 1964). Factor XII can be activated by substances such as cellulose sulfate or carrageenan (KELLERMEYER and KELLERMEYER, 1969; SCHWARTZ and KELLERMEYER, 1969), but more important biologically are condroitin sulfate and articular cartilage (MOSKOWITZ et al., 1970). Other substances of biological significance are components of connective tissue, all present in vessel walls, i.e., collagen, elastin, and basement membrane (NIEWIAROWSKI et al., 1965; WILNER et al., 1968; COCHRANE and WUEPPER, 1971a; HARPEL, 1972). Also of in vivo significance may be substances such as uric acid crystals (KELLERMEYER and BRECKENRIDGE, 1965), L-homocystine (RATNOFF, 1968) and bacterial lipopolysaccharides (PETTINGER and YOUNG, 1970; KIMBALL et al., 1972; MORRISON and COCHRANE, 1974).

Antigen-antibody complexes and aggregated γ-globulin were believed to activate factor XII (DAVIES and LOWE, 1960, 1962; MOVAT, 1967; EISEN and SMITH, 1970; KAPLAN et al., 1971). However, as shown by COCHRANE et al. (1972b) the only preparations of immunoglobulins capable of activating factor XII were those contaminated by bacteria. Since most of the studies with immune complexes were done with serum rather than plasma, and although siliconized vessels were used, it is conceivable that merely the clotting, associated with activation of a number of enzymes, induced activation of factor XII in these studies. It has been shown that chromatography of human serum on DEAE-cellulose is associated with formation of the fragment XIIf prealbumin band KAPLAN and AUSTEN (1970) observed also in the so-called immune complex-activated guinea pig serum (MOVAT et al., 1968). Furthermore, the active material isolated from guinea pig serum was highly anionic (unlike anaphylatoxin) and had an estimated MW of about 30,000, i.e., considerably higher than anaphylatoxin (TRELOAR et al., 1972). It is true that despite antihistamine treatment, the vascular permeability effects of the crude eluates of the immune complexes could have been due in part to anaphylatoxin since the effects of this substance are mainly direct, i.e., not histamine dependent (BODAMER and VOGT, 1970a, b). However, the activation of prekallikrein and the generation of kinin must be attributed to PKA or fragment XIIf (MOVAT et al., 1971a; TRELOAR et al., 1972).

An unsolved problem is the activation of the kinin system in the cold. When plasma is kept at low temperature for extended periods of time, it loses its kinin-forming ability (ARMSTRONG et al., 1967); i.e., less kinin can be generated by trypsin from plasma kept at 4 °C than from plasma kept at room temperature or 37 °C. Factor XII has been implicated indirectly in this process. Hexadimethrine bromide, which prevents activation of factor XII, has a diminished protective effect at 4 °C (ARMSTRONG, 1968). ARMSTRONG postulated that $C\bar{1}$-inactivator may play a role in this process. Indeed JACOBSEN (1966a) found that the initial fractionation of plasma to obtain HMW kininogen had to be done at room temperature. A finding confirmed by HABAL et al. (1974). $C\bar{1}$-inactivator is the principal inhibitor of activated factor XII (FORBES et al., 1970).

Enzymes as activators have already been mentioned repeatedly. It is important in this respect to define "activation." Factor XIIa is referred to as the activated clotting factor XII. COCHRANE et al. (1971b) used trypsin for the activation of factor XII and measured the ability of factor XIIa to activate prekallikrein and correct the clotting defect in factor XII-deficient plasma. Trypsin does indeed cleave factor XII to XIIf, as shown by COCHRANE et al. However, trypsin induces two measurable changes in the factor XII molecule: As the amount of trypsin incubated with factor XII is increased there is simultaneously an increase in prekallikrein activation and a decrease in the PTT with factor XII-deficient plasma (SOLTAY et al., 1971).

Plasmin likewise cleaves factor XII, inducing the formation of prekallikrein activating activity, associated with prealbumin bands (KAPLAN and AUSTEN, 1971). However, plasmin, like trypsin, produces simultaneously both prekallikrein activation and a decrease in clot-promoting activity (BURROWES et al., 1971). Thus, it would appear that contact activation associated with conformational changes of the intact factor XII molecule or limited proteolysis will induce maximum "activation" for clotting of factor XII-deficient plasma, whereas that associated with cleavage will induce maximum "activation" of prekallikrein. However, the enzymatic activity does reside in the fragment XIIf, since the fragment is capable of activating not only prekallikrein, but also factor XI (as discussed below).

Kallikrein is another enzyme which plays an important role in the activation of factor XII (COCHRANE et al., 1973). Its function will be discussed below.

3. Contact Activation

When purified factor XII is exposed to celite, little activation occurs, and the eluates contain mostly unactivated factor XII (MOVAT and ÖZGE-ANWAR, 1974). In contrast, exposure of whole plasma to celite is associated with activation and fragmentation of factor XII (ÖZGE-ANWAR et al., 1972). Thus, additional plasma factors are required for the activation of factor XII. The discovery of certain deficiencies in recent years has led to a better understanding of these factors. One of these is Fletcher factor or prekallikrein, described in Sect. D. A deficiency in HMW kininogen has been described independently under several names (SAITO et al., 1975; COLMAN et al., 1975; WUEPPER et al., 1975a, b; DONALDSON et al., 1976; WEBSTER et al., 1976), the name of the factor referring to the particular patient in which the deficiency was found (FITZGERALD, WILLIAMS, FAUJEAC). These are described in Sect. E. As will be discussed in Sect. F, activation of the fibrinolytic system depends on the activation of factor XII: a measure of fibrinolysis (just as for prekallikrein activation) is an indirect measure of the activation of factor XII. Figure 11 illustrates this. The figure shows that with normal plasma, full activity is reached within 5–10 min, that with factor XII (Hageman factor) deficiency and HMW kininogen (Williams factor) deficiency there is little or no activation of factor XII and consequently of the fibrinolytic system. It shows furthermore that in prekallikrein (Fletcher factor) deficiency, the activation is markedly delayed. The illustration also shows the PTTs of the various deficient plasmas and of normal plasma.

Independent studies showed that a substance referred to as "contact activation cofator" is required for the rapid and full activation of factor XI by factor XIIa (SCHIFFMAN and LEE, 1974, 1975). This substance has later been identified with Fitzgerald factor (SCHIFFMAN et al., 1975) and thus with HMW kininogen.

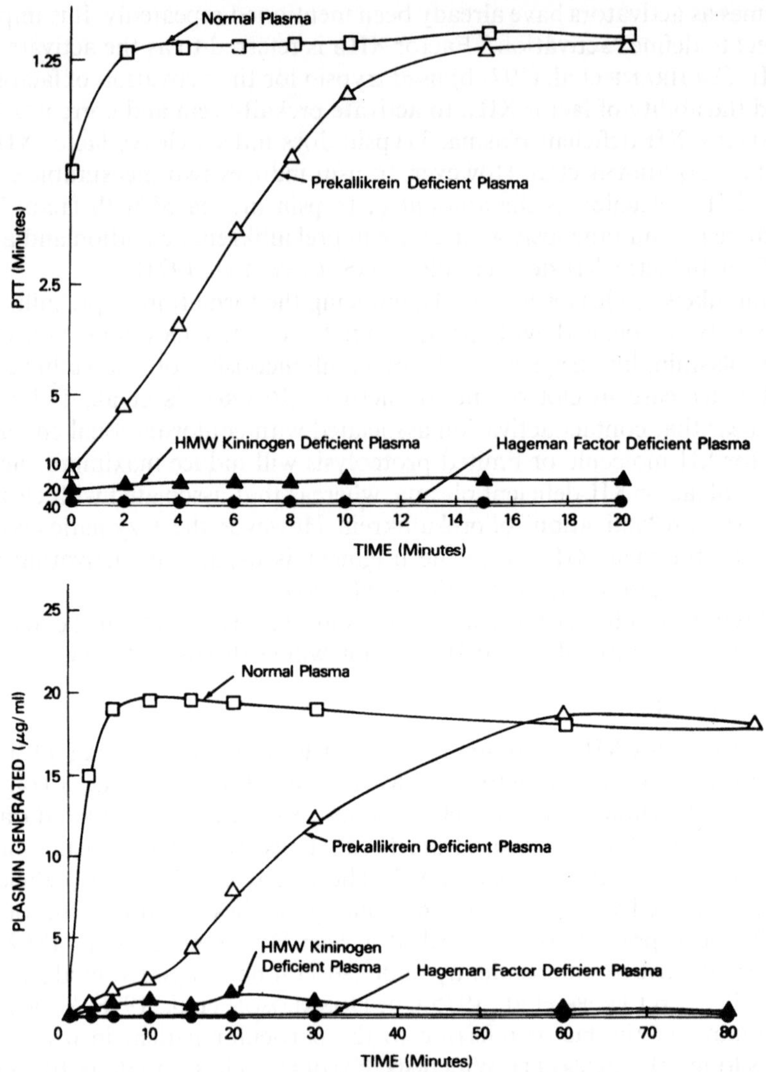

Fig. 11. Partial thromboplastin time in minutes (top) and generation of plasmin in µg/ml (bottom) with normal plasma and plasmas deficient in factor XII, HMW kininogen or prekallikrein. (From MEIER et al., 1977)

Studies were subsequently carried out with isolated components (KAPLAN et al., 1976; GRIFFIN and COCHRANE, 1976b; GRIFFIN et al., 1976; CHAN et al., 1976, 1978; WEBSTER et al., 1976; MEIER et al., 1977). Surface-bound factor XII requires the addition of HMW kininogen for subsequent activation of prekallikrein to kallikrein (KAPLAN et al., 1976) (Fig. 12). The rate of activation of factor XII and of prekallikrein conversion are dose dependent. Increasing (stoichiometric) amounts of HMW kininogen yield a proportionate increase in the amount of prekallikrein that is activated to kallikrein (CHAN et al., 1976, 1977b). Similar observations were made

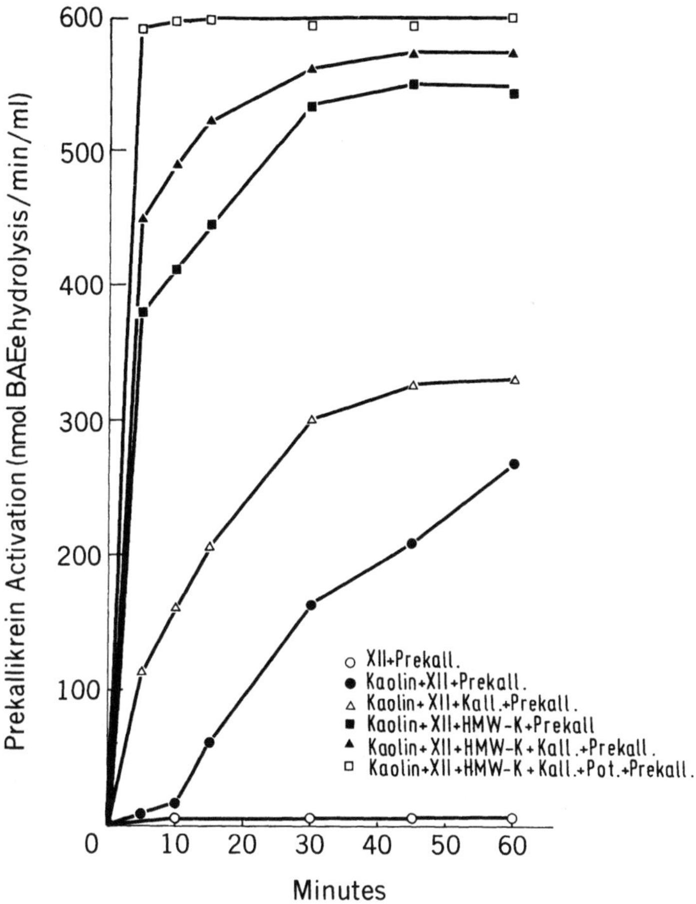

Fig. 12. Rate of activation of prekallikrein by surface-bound factor XII. Factor XII was incubated for 2 min with kaolin followed by another incubation for 10 min with the other reactants shown in the illustration, except prekallikrein. Prekallikrein was then added and the entire mixture incubated for the times indicated. The kallikrein generated from prekallikrein was assayed with BAEe as substrate. Abbreviations: Prekall. = prekallikrein; Kall = kallikrein; HMW – K = high molecular weight kininogen; Pot = potentiator (for further details see CHAN et al., 1976 and 1977b). (From MOVAT, 1978b)

with activation of factor XI (SCHIFFMAN and LEE, 1975; SCHIFFMAN et al., 1977; GRIFFIN and COCHRANE, 1976b; GRIFFIN et al., 1976; SAITO, 1977). GRIFFIN and co-workers further demonstrated that in the presence of HMW kininogen, the cleavage of kaolin-bound ^{125}I-labeled factor XII by kallikrein is increased 11-fold. According to GRIFFIN et al. (1976) HMW kininogen had a dual effect with respect to the kinin system. It enhanced activation of surface-bound factor XII by kallikrein and it enhanced the activation of prekallikrein by surface-bound factor XIIa. However, the latter activity is due to the initial effect of HMW kininogen on the surface-bound factor XII, i.e., probably opening up additional active sites on the factor XII molecule and thus activating prekallikrein more readily. Data of CHAN et al. (1976) indicate that HMW kininogen, while enhancing activation of kaolin-bound factor

XII, does not enhance the conversion of prekallikrein to kallikrein. GRIFFIN et al. (1976) proposed a model in which factor XII and HMW kininogen form a complex on a negatively charged surface, placing factor XII into a conformation which is highly susceptible to proteolytic cleavage. As soon a kallikrein is generated, more factor XII is activated. What remains unanswered is how the process is initiated when all components are unactivated. The fact that mere exposure to a negatively charged surface can bring about configurational changes in the factor XII molecule (McMILLIN et al., 1974) may be the answer, but not a definite one since McMILLIN et al. did not delineate completely the function of the surface bound factor XII. In fact recent findings of MEIER et al. (1977) indicate that mere exposure of factor XII to a surface (Supercel) does not bring about incorporation of [^{3}H]-DFP. Of the various substances added to the surface-bound factor XII, a mixture of factor XII and kallikrein almost doubled the background counts, whereas a mixture of factor XII, kallikrein, and HMW kininogen induced a fourfold increase in the counts. Similar observations were made by GRIFFIN (1977) using kaolin exposed to various reactants followed by SDS disc gel electrophoresis. Factor XII exposed to kaolin took up negligible amounts of [^{3}H]-DFP whereas trypsin-treated factor XII and factor XII exposed to kallikrein in the presence of HMW kininogen took up the label in the 28,000 MW fragment. Thus, the initiation of factor XII activation remains an open question. When activation is demonstrated in the absence of kallikrein, there are probably traces of factor XIIa in the factor XII preparation to convert prekallikrein to kallikrein, which then can activate more factor XII. Conversely there may be traces of kallikrein in prekallikrein, sufficient to spark activation of traces of factor XII and thus initiate the vicious circle. There is of course a negative feedback from a fragment of HMW kininogen, as described below, which may slow down or even inhibit the activation of factor XII. After completion of this manuscript a paper appeared by FRIAR et al. (1977), in which it was described that activation of factor XII by elagic acid (in the absence of kallikrein or factor XIa) may involve a conformational change in which at least some of its hydrophobic regions, previously buried, are exposed to the surrounding environment. The fluorescent probe, 1,6-diphenyl-1,3,5-hexatriene, when added to a solution of elagic acid-activated factor XII, displayed substantially more fluorescence, compared to solutions of the probe and the unactivated form of the protein.

In the described functions of HMW kininogen, the molecule has to be intact. It was first believed that so-called kinin-free kininogen can augment the activation of factor XII (COLMAN et al., 1975; KAPLAN et al., 1976; WEBSTER et al., 1976; SCHIFFMAN et al., 1977). WEBSTER et al. demonstrated that increasing concentrations of kallikrein yielded from HMW kininogen increasing amounts of bradykinin, but the capacity of the HMW kininogen (which was cleaved by this process) was not affected with respect to factor XII (and prekallikrein) activation. On the other hand, WALDMANN et al. (1976) showed that bovine kinin-free HMW kininogen had 30% of the capacity of the intact kininogen molecule to correct the coagulation (PTT) and fibrinolytic (kaolin-activated euglobulin lysis time) abnormalities in HMW kininogen (Fitzgerald)-deficient plasma. Using either trypsin, plasmin, or plasma kallikrein to cleave HMW kininogen, CHAN et al. (1976, 1978) presented evidence that kinin-free HMW kininogen can not enhance the activation of factor XII. Furthermore, with increasing amounts of kallikrein incubated with the HMW kininogen, there was an inverse relationship between the amount of kinin generation and prekallikrein activation by the activated factor XII. Independently, MATHESON et al. (1976) tested the bovine HMW kininogen fragments (KATO et al., 1976a) on HMW-kininogen-deficient (Flaujeac) plasma and found tathat only the intact kininogen and not the fragments could correct the deficiency. (These fragments are described in detail in Sect. E.)

There is some controversy with respect to the activity of the HMW kininogen fragments (IWANAGA et al., 1977). OH-ISHI et al. (1977a, b) reported that fragment 1–2, which is released when bovine HMW kininogen is cleaved by plasma kallikrein, showed negligible kinin-like activity (smooth muscle contraction, hypotension, and increase in vascular permeability). However, both fragment 1–2 and fragment 2 (histidine-rich peptide) strongly inhibited kinin formation in bovine plasma exposed to glass balotini and prolonged the PTT of citrated rat plasma, similar to hexadimethrine bromide. The peptide also inhibited the activation of factor XII by kaolin. On a molar basis, fragment 1–2 was three times more potent than fragment 2. The fragment did not inhibit already activated factor XII, nor the esterolytic activity of plasma kallikrein or plasmin. The findings were interpreted to represent a negative feedback (in contrast to kallikrein, plasmin, and intact HMW kininogen) for the contact activation of factor XII.

Contrary to these findings, MATHESON together with the same Japanese investigators reported in a later submitted but earlier published paper (MATHESON et al., 1976), that peptide 1–2 induced a very rapid and very transient increase in vascular permeability in rabbits and guinea pigs. The peptide was intermediate in potency between bradykinin and histamine and had a synergistic effect when injected together with bradykinin. In a further study MATHESON et al. (1977) incubated peptide 1–2 with plasma kallikrein. The peptide was cleaved slowly into fragment 1 which contained carbohydrate and the histidine-rich fragment 2. The vascular permeability was induced by the C-terminal (approximately 4500 daltons), fragment 2, which on a molar basis was identical to the intact fragment 1–2. Fragment 1 was inactive. Both fragments 1–2 and 2 had a high affinity for glass surfaces. C-terminal arginine was essential for biologic activity because incubation with carboxypeptidase B or N abrogated the ability to enhance vascular permeability.

In addition to HMW kininogen another, as yet unidentified, plasma protein has an enhancing or potentiating effect on the activation of factor XII (Fig. 12). This occurs in a dose-dependent fashion (CHAN et al., 1977b). The potentiator enhanced the activation of factor XII with respect to both prekallikrein activation and activation of factor XI. The activity was found accidentally while studying the inhibition of activated factor XII by antithrombin III (CHAN et al., 1977a). It eluted in the excluded peak when a partially purified preparation of antithrombin III was passed through a heparin-Sepharose 4B column (BURROWES and MOVAT, 1977). The potentiator did not correct the deficiency in factor XII, factor XI, HMW kininogen (Fitzgerald, Williams), and prekallikrein-deficient plasmas. Its estimated MW by gel filtration was about 75,000. This observation of another potentiator may not be new, since WEBSTER et al. (1976) noted that activation of factor XII was more marked when a crude rather than a pure factor XII preparation was used in the assays (activation of prekallikrein) and postulated that the crude preparation may contain an additional factor required for the full activation of factor XII.

IV. Substrates of Factor XII

Factor XII, when activated, can act on *prekallikrein* and convert it to kallikrein. This substrate is described in detail under Sect. D. Factor XII may activate plasminogen proactivator (prekallikrein) to plasminogen activator (kallikrein) as will be discussed in Sect. F. The oldest known substrate of factor XII is factor XI. This substrate has no direct effect on the kinin system, but there is some indication that it may act as a positive feedback in the activation of factor XII (COCHRANE et al., 1973) and its properties will be described here briefly.

Factor XI (Plasma Thromboplastin Antecedent, PTA): An inherited deficiency of factor XI was identified by ROSENTHAL and co-workers (1953). An early preparative study took advantage of its behaviour during anion exchange chromatography and separation from factor XII was achieved (SCHIFFMAN et al., 1960). RATNOFF and co-workers used a partially purified factor XI, prepared from factor XII-deficient plasma to study the enzymic activation of factor XI by activated factor XII (RATNOFF et al., 1961). More highly purified preparations did not become available until the early 1970s, when functional purity was obtained by taking advantage of the fact that factor XI is separable from prekallikrein. On the basis of its MW, and although eluting together with prekallikrein and IgG during anion exchange chromatography, its separation occurred readily during cation exchange chromatography on either SP-Sephadex (KAPLAN and AUSTEN, 1972; MOVAT et al., 1972) or on CM-Sephadex (WUEPPER, 1972) (see Fig. 13). The preparation of WUEPPER seemingly still contained some prekallikrein since trypsin-activateable arginine esterase was present in the preparation and factor XI was measured by this property. More highly purified preparations obtained subsequently were free of such esterase activity (SAITO et al., 1973; HECK and KAPLAN, 1974; MOVAT and ÖZGE-ANWAR, 1974; SCHIFFMAN and LEE, 1974, 1975). HECK and KAPLAN removed traces of IgG with an anti-IgG immunoabsorbent column. MOVAT and ÖZGE-ANWAR recovered a 700-fold, SAITO et al. a 2300-fold, and SCHIFFMAN and LEE a 2800-fold purified factor XI. SCHIFFMAN and LEE took advantage of the adsorption of factor XI to Dicalite 4200. Their method consisted of DEAE-cellulose chromatography of hexadimethrine bromide-containing plasma, followed by two adsorptions to, and elutions from $BaSO_4$, SP-Sephadex, Dicalite 4200, and finally Sephadex G-200. To stabilize factor XI, albumin was added during the Dicalite step and this increased the recovery from 25% to 75%. The most recent attempt to purify factor XI from human plasma was made by BOUMA and GRIFFIN (1977). BOUMA and GRIFFIN used four chromatographic steps for chromatography of 800 ml of plasma, first DEAE-Sephadex (0.04 *M* Tris, 0.01 *M* succinic acid buffer, pH 8.34) from which factor XI was excluded. This was followed by QAE-Sephadex, with a starting buffer of 0.02 *M* asparagine, containing 0.06 *M* NaCl, pH 10.5. Gradient elution was achieved with the same buffer, the limiting pH being 9.0. This partially separated factor XI from the bulk of the protein (IgG). Good separation was obtained using SP-Sephadex at pH 8.1 (0.02 *M* Tris, 0.01–0.15 *M* NaCl) and further purification using SP-Sephadex at pH 5.3 (0.1 *M* acetate, 0.15 *M* NaCl as the starting buffer and 0.35 *M* NaCl as the limiting buffer). When traces of IgG remained (5–25%), the protein was passed through Concanavalin A-Sepharose which adsorbed factor XI. The end product was homogeneous. After the fourth step (Sephadex at pH 5.3) recovery was 19%. After the Concanavalin A-Sepharose the purification was 12,000 fold but the recovery was not given. However, the protein was homogeneous by disc gel electrophoresis. Its concentration in plasma was estimated to be 4 µg/ml.

The *properties* of factor XI and XIa were described by a number of investigators. The MW of factor XI and XIa estimated by gel filtration was given variously as 160,000–180,000 and the isoelectric point as about 9.0 (KAPLAN et al., 1971; WUEPPER and COCHRANE, 1971; WUEPPER, 1972; HECK and KAPLAN, 1974; MOVAT and ÖZGE-ANWAR, 1974). By SDS disc gel electrophoresis, WUEPPER (1972) described a MW of 158,000 in unreduced samples and reduction and alkylation revealed a single band of 80,000. Similar values were reported by HECK and KAPLAN, who reported a MW of 163,000. By reduction and alkylation KAPLAN et al. (1976) likewise found a MW of 80,000–82,000. They noted that reduction of the active molecule yielded 50,000 and 30,000 MW chains. WUEPPER (1972) previously reported values of 46,000 and 27,000. A more recent publication (BOUMA and GRIFFIN, 1977) reported 160,000 for factor XI and 83,000 for reduced factor XI. Activated factor XI had also 160,000 MW but when reduced, two chains were noted of 50,000 and 33,000 MW respectively.

Activation was achieved with trypsin by WUEPPER (1972) and SAITO et al. (1973), with fragment XIIf by KAPLAN and HECK (1974) and by MOVAT and ÖZGE-ANWAR (1974). BOUMA cleaved radiolabeled factor XI with a mixture of factor XII, prekallikrein and HMW kininogen. ^{125}I-labeled factor XI could be also cleaved by normal plasma. Thus, factor XI is cleaved by limited proteolysis either by activated factor XII or by whole plasma. It was by studying activation of factor XI that SCHIFFMAN and LEE (1974) described a substance required for this activation which they named contact activation cofactor and which proved to be HMW kininogen. SAITO (1977) showed recently that HMW kininogen was absolutely required for activation of factor XI by factor XII and ellagic acid. The yield of activated factor XI (XIa) was proportional to the amount of factor XII, HMW kininogen, and factor XI in the mixture, suggesting that to activate factor XI the proteins may form a complex in the presence of ellagic acid. No fragmented factor XII was found under these conditions. However, SAITO confirmed the earlier observations of KAPLAN and HECK (1974) and of MOVAT and ÖZGE-ANWAR (1974) that fragment XIIf activates factor XI and he showed that HMW kininogen was not required for this activation.

V. Inhibition of Factor XII

According to RATNOFF(1966), only impure preparations of factor XIIa are inhibited by DFP. BECKER (1960) was the first to describe inhibition of activated factor XII by DFP. Such a preparation, however, by RATNOFF'S (1966) criteria was impure. Functionally pure factor XIIa, free of other DFP-sensitive enzymes is inhibited by DFP (for a review, see COCHRANE et al., 1976). It is difficult to test inhibition of activated factor XII by SBTI because this agent acts on the substances activated by factor XII. Factor XII has been reported to be susceptible to inhibition by LBTI (SCHOENMAKERS et al., 1965). Since LBTI does not affect kallikrein, the inhibition of activated factor XII by this agent could also be used in studies dealing with prekallikrein activation (WUEPPER, 1972).

More important from a physiologic and pathophysiologic point of view are natural proteinase inhibitors. The first to present evidence of inhibition of factor XIIa (and XIa) by C$\bar{1}$-inactivator were FORBES et al. (1970). When the inhibitor was added to activated XII in increasing concentrations, 4 units of inhibitor induced 50% inhibition in 10 min and 75% in 20 min. Complete inhibition was noted in 20 min with 32 units of inhibitor. SCHREIBER et al. (1973a) using different units (see GIGLI et al., 1970) or quantitating by immunodiffusion, demonstrated the inhibition of fragment XIIf by C$\bar{1}$-inactivator. Since activation of prekallikrein by the XIIf was measured and the inhibitor readily inhibits kallikrein (see Sect. D), C$\bar{1}$-inactivator was added to XIIf at various times before mixing with prekallikrein. The generated kallikrein was measured by the release of bradykinin in fresh plasma. When 500 ng/ml of bradykinin was generated from fresh plasma, the inhibitor (1000 units) induced a progressive decrease with increasing time of incubation, inhibiting completely within 30 min. Of the various proteinase inhibitors tested by CHAN et al. (1977a), only C$\bar{1}$-inactivator and antithrombin III inhibited activated factor XII; α_2-macroglobulin and α_1-antitrypsin in high concentration had no effect. STEAD et al. (1976) studied in detail the inhibition of activated factor XII by antithrombin III. The inhibitor was found to be a progressive, time-dependent inhibition of both XIIa and XIIf. Heparin accelerated the rates of these interactions. SDS disc gels indicated that antithrombin III formed an undissociable complex with factor XII, representing a 1:1 stoichiometric combination. By SDS acrylamide electrophoresis, factor XIIa had an estimated MW of 75,000, antithrombin of 61,500 and the complexes 117,000. Complete conversion into the 117,000 complexed form could not be demonstrated in the absence of heparin, but heparin markedly enhanced the complex formation. Complexing with fragment XIIf could be demonstrated only by radiolabeling the fragment. In this system, the fragment XIIf was estimated to have a MW of 28,000, the inhibitor 58,000 and the complex 85,000.

CHAN et al. (1977a) had found marked enhancement of the inhibition of kallikrein in the presence of heparin by antithrombin III, but heparin had only a moderate effect in the inhibition of activated factor XII. STEAD et al. (1976) on the other hand detected a marked enhancement of the inhibition of factor XII by heparin. However, the system of CHAN et al. varied from that of STEAD et al. in that the reaction took place on a surface (kaolin).

D. Prekallikrein and Kallikrein

I. Isolation and Purification

The early observations of FREY and co-workers that urine contains a substance which in small doses causes hypotension and that a similar substance is present in the blood and in the pancreas led to the belief that kallikrein originated in the pancreas, circulated in the blood and was excreted in the urine (FREY and KRAUT, 1928; KRAUT et al., 1928). This was reviewed by EISEN and VOGT (1970). These authors also reviewed the literature until 1970, pointing out the physicochemical and biologic differences among the various kallikreins.

Plasma kallikrein, the subject of this section, circulates in the blood as a precursor, earlier referred to as kallikreinogen and now as prekallikrein. It can be activated by acetone, alcohol or other organic solvents, by dilution of plasma, acidification and reneutralization, by addition of casein to plasma, or by exposure of plasma to glass for an extended period (for details see EISEN and VOGT, 1970).

Perhaps the first to obtain *human plasma kallikrein* from serum free of other components of the kinin system were BECKER and co-workers (KAGAN et al., 1963; BECKER and KAGAN, 1963) who passed the serum through DEAE-cellulose; the plasma kallikrein appeared in the excluded peak. Similar observations were made by WEBSTER and PIERCE (1967). A further improvement was made by passing the kallikrein obtained by anion exchange chromatography through Sephadex G-200 followed by preparative electrophoresis in order to eliminate the bulk of immunoglobulin G (MOVAT et al., 1970, 1971a). The kallikrein thus obtained had a MW of about 100,000 and migrated as a fast γ-globulin by starch block electrophoresis. It was inhibited much more readily by heat and DFP than fragment XIIf. It was also inhibited by SBTI and Trasylol. COLMAN and co-workers (1969) had prepared human plasma kallikrein by alcohol fractionation, isoelectric precipitation and chromatography on CM- and DEAE-cellulose. Three kallikreins were obtained. Of these, the most cationic was excluded during anion exchange chromatography and seems to correspond to that described by BECKER et al., WEBSTER and PIERCE, and MOVAT et al. having a MW of about 100,000 and a sedimentation coefficient of 5.7 *S*. It was designated kallikrein I. Kallikrein II was slightly more acidic (fast γ-globulin) with a MW of 163,000. Kallikrein III migrated as an α-globulin. Kallikreins I and II were thought to be "closely related if not interconvertible," whereas enzyme III was not susceptible to certain inhibitors tested (SBTI, pancreatic trypsin inhibitor, Trasylol). By gel filtration its MW was estimated to be 124,000. Enzyme I was relatively pure, having been purified 586-fold. More recent studies, in which a high degree of purification was achieved, deal with prekallikrein but some attempts have also been made to purify human plasma kallikrein. FRITZ et al. (1972a) improved on the procedure reported earlier by HABERMANN and KLETT (1966) for the purification of acetone-treated porcine plasma kallikrein. Following activation with casein, the precipitates were redissolved and either subjected directly to affinity chromatography or to ammonium sulfate precipitation, isoelectric precipitation and DEAE-cellulose chromatography. The affinity chromatography column consisted of SBTI linked to CM-cellulose. The enzyme was eluted with 2 *M* urea or 0.05 *M* benzamidine and then passed through Sephadex G-100 or Biogel P-2. A 350-fold purification was achieved with a yield of 60–90%. SAMPAIO et al. (1974) used Cohn fraction IV-1 as starting material, which was acidified and reneutralized to convert prekallikrein to kallikrein, followed by successive use of affinity chromatography on SBTI-Sepharose and aminobenzamidine-Sepharose. The kallikrein was homogeneous by alkaline disc gel electrophoresis. It had an estimated MW of 95,000 by gel filtration. In contrast to the native state, several bands were seen in SDS-gels, presumably reduced and alkylated, although this was not stated in the text (see prekallikrein below). A 1200-fold purification was obtained.

Human plasma prekallikrein was likewise obtained first in a functionally pure form (i.e., devoid of other components of the plasma kinin system) by passing plasma collected in EDTA and containing hexadimethrine bromide through QAE-Sephadex (MOVAT et al., 1971a). This procedure was improved by further passage of the anion exchange excluded peak through Sephadex G-150 and SE-Sephadex (KAPLAN et al.,

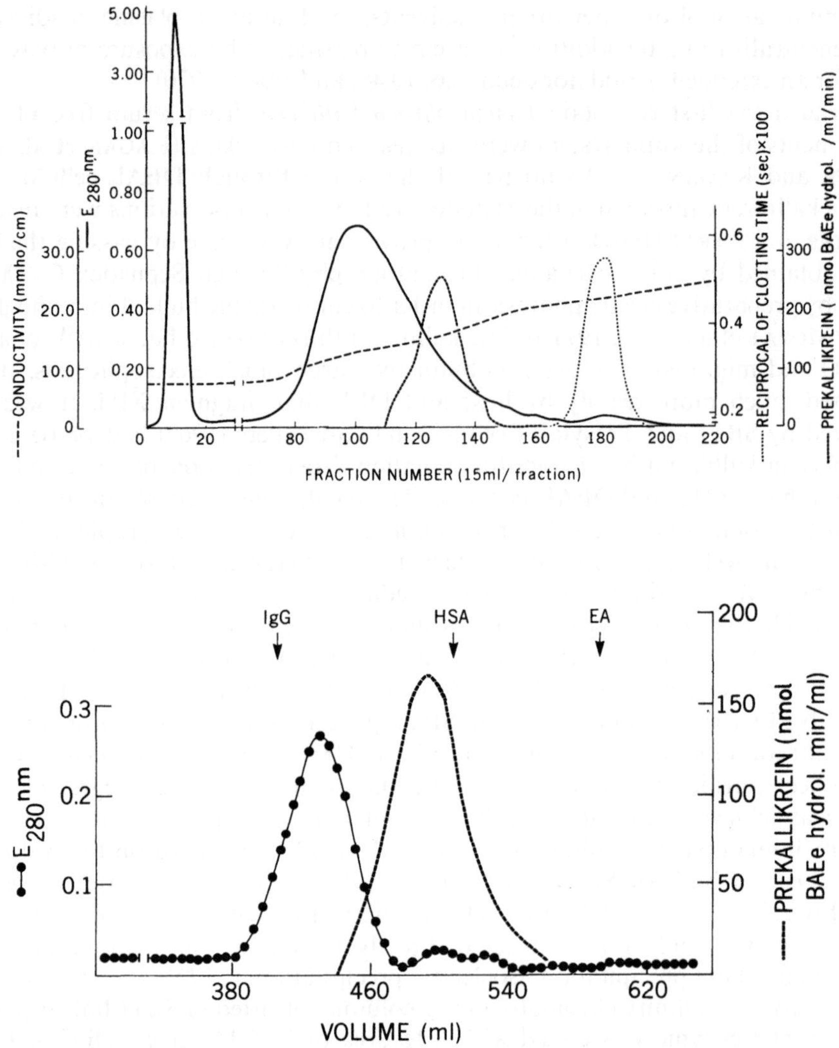

Fig. 13. Chromatography of the excluded peak from a QAE-Sephadex column (see Fig. 3) on a column of SP-Sephadex, equilibrated with 0.01 *M* phosphate buffer, pH 6.0. Prekallikrein eluted after the bulk of the protein, with 0.15 *M* NaCl (upper panel). Rechromatography of prekallikrein on Sephadex G-200 (lower panel)

1971) or Sephadex G-200 and SP-Sephadex (MOVAT et al., 1972) (Fig. 13). Homogeneous preparations were obtained by using affinity chromatography (Fig. 14), i.e., the prekallikrein recovered from QAE-Sephadex was recycled through two interconnected columns of 1 meter each packed with Sephadex G-200 superfine. This step removed the bulk of the IgG. Traces of IgG were then removed by an immunoabsorbent column prepared with antibody against IgG that was free of prekallikrein (obtained by SP-Sephadex). Alternatively, instead of anti-IgG-Sepharose, arginine-

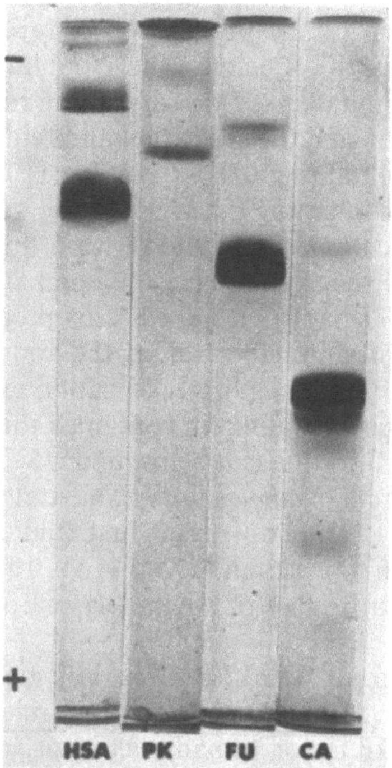

Fig. 14. SDS disc gel electrophoresis of prekallikrein (PK), together with the marker proteins human serum albumin, monomer, and dimer (HSA), fumarase (FU), and carbonic anhydrase (CA) (see Fig. 5). (From MOVAT, 1978b)

Sepharose was used (HABAL et al., 1974). The prekallikrein prepared with the anti-IgG immunoabsorbent column was not entirely homogeneous, but a homogeneous preparation was recovered from the arginine-Sepharose column. This preparation, however, contained 15–30% active enzyme after standing at 4 °C or repeated freezing and thawing and gradually converted entirely to kallikrein. WUEPPER (1972) applied the method described below for rabbit plasma (COCHRANE and WUEPPER, 1972b) and obtained a highly purified preparation which varied in its physicochemical properties from rabbit prekallikrein as will be described. This prekallikrein, together with rabbit prekallikrein, was used in later studies of these investigators dealing with activation of factor XII (COCHRANE et al., 1973). LAAKE and VENERÖD (1973, 1974) purified prekallikrein by subjecting plasma to chromatography on DEAE-Sephadex, followed by further chromatography of the excluded peak on CM-Sephadex, hydroxyapatite, and Sephadex G-100 superfine. The high degree of purity of this preparation was clearly demonstrated in a more recent publication (VENNERÖD et al., 1976), dealing with the interaction between kallikrein (prepared by activating the prekallikrein with factor XIIf) and antithrombin III. KAPLAN and coworkers improved their preparative procedure for obtaining a highly purified preparation of prekallikrein by using QAE-Sephadex, SP-Sephadex, Sephadex G-150 and then an immunoabsorbent prepared with sheep antiserum to human IgG and β_2-glycoprotein I, or by removing the latter with the aid of a Concanavalin-A-Sepharose column (WEISS et al., 1974; KAPLAN et al., 1976, 1977).

REVAK and co-workers (REVAK et al., 1974; REVAK and COCHRANE, 1976) modified the method used earlier for the purification of rabbit prekallikrein (WUEPPER and COCHRANE, 1972b), described below. The globulin soluble in 25% saturated ammonium sulfate was precipitated at 55% saturation, redissolved, dialysed, applied to a DEAE-Sephadex column and the crude prekallikrein eluted in a single step with 0.01 *M* phosphate buffer containing 0.06 *M* NaCl, pH 7.7. After redialysis against 0.01 *M* phosphate, pH 6.0, containing 0.1 *M* NaCl the protein solution was applied to a similarly equilibrated column and eluted with a linear gradient of 0.1–0.25 *M* NaCl. To remove traces of kallikrein, the prekallikrein was passed over Sepharose 4B to which SBTI had been linked. This preparation still contained β_2-glycoprotein and some γ-globulin. However, as the above-mentioned studies using SP-Sephadex indicate, factor XI binds firmly to cation exchangers and REVAK et al. did not indicate whether their prekallikrein contained this clotting factor, which can be readily eliminated by gel filtration (see below under Sect. C).

Prekallikrein and kallikrein of *animal plasmas* have also been studied.

In bovine plasma, SUZUKI and co-workers first studied kallikrein activated with glass (NAGASAWA et al., 1967) or casein (YANO et al., 1970) and more recently they isolated and described the properties of bovine plasma prekallikrein (TAKAHASHI et al., 1972a, b).

The casein-activated serum kallikrein was investigated in detail. DEAE-Sephadex chromatography gave three peaks with kinin-releasing and arginine esterase activity, similar to the kallikreins of human plasma or serum (COLMAN et al., 1969; MOVAT et al., 1970, 1971a). The "anionic kallikreins" seem to represent "cationic," i.e., unbound kallikrein complexed to an unknown α-globulin (WENDEL et al., 1972) and to α_2-macroglobulin (VOGT, 1976, 1977; VOGT and DUGAL, 1976), respectively. However, YANO et al. (1970) investigated only the first eluting peak or cationic kallikrein, using $(NH_4)_2SO_4$ precipitation, batch-adsorption and elution from DEAE-Sephadex and CM-Sephadex, chromatography on CM-Sephadex, and gel filtration on Sephadex G-150. The estimated MW by gel filtration was about 95,000. The enzyme released kinin rapidly from bovine kininogen-I (HMW) but only little from kininogen-II (LMW). The pH optimum was 8.8. It was inhibited by DFP, SBTI, Trasylol, benzamidine, and tosyl lysine chloromethyl ketone (TLCK), but not by lima bean (LBTI) and egg white trypsin inhibitors.

While the kallikrein described above was not homogeneous, TAKAHASHI et al. (1972a, b) succeeded in isolating prekallikrein from bovine plasma in homogeneous form, using the same procedures as for the isolation of kallikrein with the addition of affinity chromatography on arginine-Sepharose 4B. A 1300-fold purification was achieved. It is worth noting that similarly to prekallikrein of rabbit plasma, but not to human prekallikrein, bovine prekallikrein was adsorbed to DEAE-Sephadex at pH 8.0. Corresponding to this, its isoelectric point was about 7.0, i.e., lower than that of human plasma prekallikrein. The prekallikrein was stable in 0.1 *M* NaCl, but gradually lost activity as the ionic strength was decreased. It was stable between pH 6 and 9, but quite unstable below pH 5 and above 10. The proenzyme was stable at 51 °C for 1 h, but at 60 °C some loss occurred. At 62 °C, less than 20% of the activity was recovered after 30 min incubation. Interestingly, a "spontaneous" activation of prekallikrein to kallikrein was not seen under any of these conditions. On the other hand (as described above), while highly purified human plasma prekallikrein prepared by the writer and co-workers (HABAL et al., 1974) with an anti-IgG immunoabsorbent column (to remove traces of IgG) was stable, prekallikrein prepared from human plasma with an arginine-Sepharose column gradually converted to kallikrein.

Using six to seven preparative steps, HABERMANN and KLETT obtained a highly purified preparation of hog serum kallikrein activated with casein (see EISEN and VOGT, 1970). This kallikrein had physicochemical properties which were essentially similar to those of kallikrein isolated from other plasmas. FRITZ et al. (1972a) simplified and improved the procedure by carrying out, after the ammonium sulfate precipitation and anion exchange chromatography, affinity chromatography with SBTI linked to CM-cellulose. After washing out the contaminating proteins, the kallikrein was eluted from the affinity column with 2 *M* urea or 0.05 *M* benzamidine. Both hog and human serum kallikrein were inhibited by a large number of inhibitors, including SBTI, BPTI, and peanut trypsin inhibitor (WUNDERER et al., 1972), as well as by α_1-antitrypsin and C$\bar{1}$-inactivator (FRITZ et al., 1972b). The finding with α_1-antitrypsin does not agree with findings reported above (HABAL et al., 1976).

The most thorough study of prekallikrein was carried out by WUEPPER and COCHRANE (1972b) on rabbit plasma. Plasma was collected in the presence of hexadimethrine bromide and EDTA and salted out with ammonium sulfate. The globulin fraction soluble at 30% saturation and precipitated at 50% saturation was thoroughly dialysed (0.0075 *M* phosphate, pH 8.0) and applied to a DEAE-Sephadex A-50 column. Unlike human plasma kallikrein, rabbit plasma kallikrein did not elute in the excluded peak but in the early part of a linear NaCl gradient. Prekallikrein elution was monitored by converting the prekallikrein to kallikrein with trypsin, neutralizing the trypsin with LBTI and measuring the arginine esterase (BAEe) activity of the generated kallikrein. Pooled fractions containing predikallikrein were precipitated at 60% saturation with ammonium sulfate, rechromatographed on the anion exchanger at pH 6.6, and chromatographed on CM-Sephadex C-50 (citrate-phosphate buffer, pH 6.0). The final purification step was electrophoresis in Pevikon. When the pooled fractions were not concentrated by salting out, they were concentrated by positive pressure ultrafiltration where the membranes were prerinsed in hexadimethrine bromide. After the last step, the specific activity increased to 81 BAEe units/mg protein. A 6000-fold purification was achieved and the segment number containing the bulk of the prekallikrein was homogeneous by disc gel electrophoresis.

II. Physicochemical Properties

While there are some variations among the findings of various investigators, the MW of *human* plasma prekallikrein or kallikrein by gel filtration is approximately 100,000. The lowest value reported by this method is 90,000 (ÖZGE-ANWAR et al., 1972) and the highest 130,000 (KAPLAN et al., 1971). By SDS disc gel electrophoresis, the MW has been estimated to be about 108,000 (WUEPPER, 1972; KAPLAN et al., 1976, 1977). Human prekallikrein and kallikrein have a fast γ- or slow β-electrophoretic mobility in starch block (MOVAT et al., 1971) or agarose (WUEPPER, 1972). The sedimentation coefficient of prekallikrein is 5.2 *S*. Its isoelectric point has been variously reported to be between 8 and 9. MOVAT et al. (1971a) reported a microhetero-

Table 1. Properties of principal components of the kinin-system of human plasma

Substance							
Properties	Factor XII and XIIa	Fragment XIIf (PKA)	Prekallikrein and kallikrein	Plasminogen	Plasmin	LMW Kininogen	HMW Kininogen
Electrophoretic mobility (acetate)	β	Albumin	γ	β	β	α	α
Isoelectric point (pH)	6.0–6.5	4.4–4.6	7.7–9.4	6.2–8.3	6.2–8.3	4.7	4.5
Sedimentation coefficient	4.8–5.2	2.8	5.2	4.4–5.1	4.3	3.85–4.0	4.2
Molecular weight							
Gel filtration (aqueous buffer)	110,000	30,000	100,000–110,000	82,000–92,000[a]	74,500–81,000[a]	55,000 60,000	200,000 220,000
SDS gel electrophoresis or guanidine-Sepharose	76,000–78,000	28,000	108,000			52,000	108,000–110,000
Concentration in plasma (μg/ml)	30			464		[b]	[b]
Activity in kinin system	Activation of prekallikrein and factor XI	Activation of prekallikrein and factor XI	Cleavage of kininogens; activation of factor XII		Cleavage of kininogens; cleavage of factor XII	Source of kinins	Source of kinins; cofactor in contact activation of factor XII

[a] Based on sedimentation coefficient, partial specific volume, and diffusion coefficient.
[b] Total plasma kininogen 675 μg/ml.

geneity, isoelectric focusing occurring between pH 7.6 and 8.8. However, the microheterogeneity was clearly described by WENDEL et al. (1972) and by LAAKE and VENNERÖD (1974), by demonstrating five to six peaks between pH 7.7 and 9.4 when subjected to isoelectric focusing at pH 8–10; the arginine esterase and kinin-forming activities overlapping (Table 1).

The physicochemical properties of *rabbit* prekallikrein have been studied in detail by WUEPPER and COCHRANE (1972). The zymogen had fast γ to slow β mobility. Its sedimentation coefficient by sucrose density gradient was 4.5 and the diffusion coefficient 4.46. The MW was determined by three methods. With an assumed partial specific volume of 0.73, a MW of about 100,000 was calculated from the diffusion coefficient and the *S*-value. A similar MW was estimated by SDS disc gel electrophoresis, whereas by gel filtration in aqueous solution the calculated MW was 102,000. The isoelectric point was 5.9, i.e., considerably lower than human plasma prekallikrein, which is in good agreement with findings during anion exchange chromatography. Even if a DEAE or QAE-Sephadex column is equilibrated with a very low ionic strength buffer, human prekallikrein is excluded from the gel, whereas rabbit prekallikrein (as WUEPPER and COCHRANE have shown) adsorbs to such columns, eluting in the first part of a salt gradient.

Bovine prekallikrein was estimated to have a MW of about 100,000 by gel filtration and 90,000 by both SDS disc gel electrophoresis and by equilibrium ultracentrifugation, assuming a partial specific volume of 0.72. Based on sucrose density gradient ultracentrifugation data, a MW of 80,000 was calculated. Its isoelectric point was about 7.0, i.e., lower than that of human prekallikrein but higher than that of rabbit (TAKAHASHI et al., 1972a).

III. Activation of Prekallikrein to Kallikrein

Activation of human prekallikrein to kallikrein seems to involve limited proteolysis. There is no clear cut difference in the MW, sedimentation coefficient, or isoelectric point between the zymogen and the active enzyme. As already noted, the MW of prekallikrein or kallikrein by SDS disc gel electrophoresis is about 108,000. Reduction and alkylation does not alter this value. However, when kallikrein is reduced and alkylated one finds in the 108,000 MW starting material, two fragments of 65,000 and 36,000 (Fig. 15), suggesting that activation by factor XIIf involves limited proteolytic cleavage; the fragments are linked by disulfide bonds (KAPLAN et al., 1976, 1977). This is in keeping with some of the earlier observations made with bovine (TAKAHASHI et al., 1972b) and rabbit (WUEPPER, 1972) prekallikrein and kallikrein. Recent data indicate that the active center of kallikrein may be in the light chain (MANDLE and KAPLAN, 1977a).

Highly purified prekallikrein was labeled with ^{125}I and kallikrein with ^{131}I. Both had the same mobility in SDS gels (MW about 100,000). When kallikrein was inactivated with [^{3}H]-DFP, reduced and examined in SDS gels, a heavy chain of 56,000 and a light chain of 33,000 were observed and the [^{3}H]-DFP was incorporated into the light chain. Fragments of kallikrein have been observed also in celite eluates (ÖZGE-ANWAR et al., 1972). In addition to factor XII, a number of plasma proteins adsorb to celite, including prekallikrein and factor XI. These are recovered from the eluates in activated form. When the excluded peak recovered by anion exchange

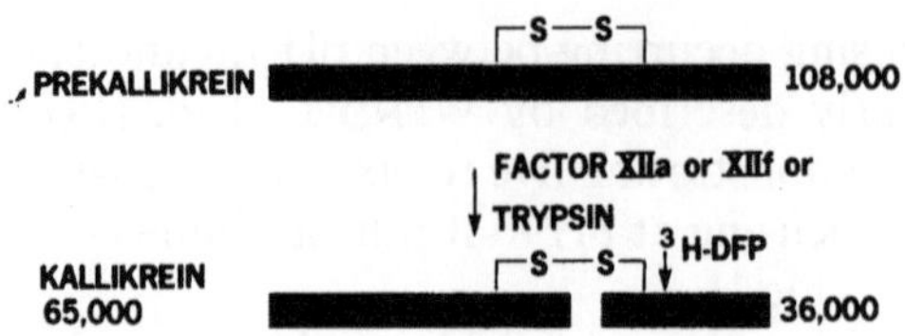

Fig. 15. Gross structure of prekallikrein and kallikrein. The zymogen can be activated by factor XIIa, fragment XIIf, or trypsin, giving rise to two chains. Of those, the 36,000 MW chain seems to contain the active center since it binds labeled DFP. (From MOVAT, 1978b)

chromatography was subjected to gel filtration, the bulk of the kallikrein eluted with an estimated MW of 90,000–96,000. In both species a smaller peak was recovered which was estimated to have a MW of 34,000 and migrated ahead of the main kallikrein band during alkaline disc gel electrophoresis. It was described to be a fragment of kallikrein which contained the active center. Since a series of enzymes become activated upon exposure of whole plasma to celite, it is conceivable that plasmin may have induced the cleavage of kallikrein in the celite eluates as a consequence of factor XII activation (see below).

When rabbit prekallikrein is converted to kallikrein by factor XIIf, a 10,000–11,000 MW fragment is cleaved from the prekallikrein and other changes in the molecule take place (WUEPPER and COCHRANE, 1972). The sedimentation coefficient changes from 4.5 to 4.0 *S*, the diffusion coefficient from 4.46 to 4.59 and the pI from 5.9 to 5.4, i.e., kallikrein becomes smaller and more acidic than prekallikrein. These changes have not been encountered in other species and seemingly no other investigators attempted to repeat these experiments. WUEPPER (1972) subsequently confirmed these findings and demonstrated by SDS disc gel electrophoresis that (in the absence of reduction) the 90,000 MW rabbit prekallikrein when converted to kallikrein consisted of two fragments of 80,000 and 10,000 daltons. However, he noted further proteolytic cleavage during activation, because after reduction and alkylation he recovered fragments of 56,000, 26,000, and 10,000 MW and concluded that there must be two sites of cleavage, of which one must lie between a disulfide bridge.

When bovine prekallikrein was subjected to SDS disc gel electrophoresis, a single band was seen whether the prekallikrein was reduced or not. The same band was detected with kallikrein when the enzyme was unreduced, but in the presence of mercaptoethanol the original kallikrein band disappeared and new faster migrating bands were detected. Exact MW determinations were not done (TAKAHASHI et al., 1972b). Further evidence of limited proteolysis was presented. Kallikrein and prekallikrein treated with activated factor XII were radiolabeled with ^{3}H and after acid hydrolysis the tritiated proteins were separated, identified, and counted. From these findings it was concluded that activation of prekallikrein to kallikrein is accompanied by a specific cleavage of prekallikrein, probably of a single arginyl peptide bond.

In addition to factors XIIa and XIIf, prekallikrein can be converted to kallikrein by trypsin, but not chymotrypsin, thrombin, and $C\bar{1}$ esterase (WUEPPER and COCHRANE, 1972). Plasmin activates prekallikrein indirectly. VOGT (1964) reported that prekallikrein can be converted to kallikrein by plasmin. However, this process occurs through activation and fragmentation of factor XII, which then acts on prekallikrein. Direct conversion of prekallikrein to kallikrein by plasmin could not be demonstrated (KAPLAN and AUSTEN, 1971; BURROWES et al., 1971; MOVAT et al., 1973a). However, plasmin gradually destroys the activity of kallikrein (BURROWES et al., 1973). In this process, enzymatically active fragments of kallikrein of MW of 30,000–40,000 are cleaved; this was also observed in celite eluates of human plasma (ÖZGE-ANWAR et al., 1972) and of guinea pig plasma (TRELOAR et al., 1972). (See also data with SDS disc gels of reduced kallikrein described above.) However, prolonged incubation of kallikrein with plasmin completely inactivates kallikrein. The studies of SEIDEL et al. (1971, 1973) were carried out when some investigators believed that plasma contains two kininogens as well as two corresponding kininogenases. This misconception was solved later mainly by VOGT and co-workers (see below). SEIDEL and co-workers did not work with functionally purified preparations, but with whole plasma or variously treated plasma (e.g., glass exposed). The fact that streptokinase-treated plasma formed kinin must be interpreted that plasmin generates prekallikrein activator activity by activating and cleaving factor XII (XIIa and XIIf) which then converts prekallikrein to kallikrein.

Quite recently ANDREENKO and SUVAROV (1976) again presented some data claiming that prekallikrein can be converted to kallikrein by plasmin in rat plasma. These investigators showed that BAEe hydrolysing activity of prekallikrein can be induced with plasmin and that this was dependent on time and enzyme (plasmin) concentration. As evidence against the hypothesis of activation via factor XII (PKA, XIIf) they showed that their prekallikrein preparation did not correct the deficiency in factor XII-deficient plasma. However, ANDREENKO and SUVAROV did not examine their plasminogen for factor XII activity. In fact, they had to use quite large qunatities of plasmin to obtain activation of prekallikrein. It is more likely that a plasminogen, rather than a prekallikrein preparation contains traces of factor XII. Thus, when streptokinase was added to the plasminogen, the generated plasmin could have acted on the factor XII present in the plasminogen preparation, generating fragment XIIf and thus activating the prekallikrein.

IV. Assays of Prekallikrein and Kallikrein

It has become common practice to measure kallikrein and prekallikrein, when present in a large number of samples (e.g., while monitoring elution during chromatography), by hydrolysis of synthetic arginine esters[1]. Prekallikrein is first converted to kallikrein with a small amount of trypsin and the trypsin neutralized with equimolar amounts, or a slight excess, of LBTI or OMTI which does not inhibit the generated kallikrein. Bioassay or radioimmunoassay is done on the kinin generated from kininogen. However, these procedures are usually only used to determine the kinin-forming capacity of kallikrein in the pools of chromatographed samples. Some investigators determine the kinin-generating ability only in the final product of purification.

In earlier studies, plasma heated to 60–61 °C for 1–2 h was used as a source of kininogen. In such plasma, prekallikrein and factor XII are inactivated but the kininogens can readily be cleaved by kininogenases, including plasma kallikrein. Howev-

1 Recently chromogenic substrates have become available for the assay of several enzymes. These are available from Pentapharm (Basel). The substrate for plasma kallikrein is Chromozyme PK (Bz-Pro-Phe-Arg-pNA HCl).

er, the presence of other kininogenases in heated plasma (e.g., plasmin) has not been ruled out with certainty in each preparation. Therefore, in recent years, more and more investigators in this field have isolated kininogens for use in kinin-generating assays. These will be described in detail in another subheading. At this point it is sufficient to mention briefly that the plasma of probably all mammals contains two kininogens; LMW and a HMW kininogen. As described elsewhere, these kininogens are distinct physicochemically but they also differ functionally since both LMW and HMW kininogens are good substrates for a number of kininogenases (including trypsin, plasmin, glandular, and urinary kallikreins) but only the HMW kininogen is the preferred substrate for plasma kallikrein. For a review see Habal and Movat (1976a) and Sect. E in this publication.

V. Complexing of Prekallikrein and Kallikrein in Plasma

The early belief that kallikrein is formed in the pancreas, circulates in the blood, and is excreted in the urine proved not to be correct. Plasma kallikrein is entirely different from glandular kallikrein. Recent data indicate that plasma *prekallikrein circulates in plasma complexed with another protein.* Human prekallikrein was recovered during gel filtration of plasma or the pseudoglobulin fraction of plasma as a complex with an approximate MW of 300,000. The complex had a pI of 4.3. During anion exchange chromatography prekallikrein with a MW of 98,000 and a pI of 8.0 was separated from the complex. When prekallikrein was added to an acidic fraction, i.e., a protein which adsorbed firmly to DEAE-cellulose (eluting with 0.3 *M* NaCl) a 180,000 MW rather than the 300,000 MW complex formed and was eluted (Nagasawa and Nakayasu, 1973). Recently, Mandle et al. (1976) obtained similar data with whole normal or factor XII-deficient plasma, but could demonstrate both *prekallikrein and HMW kininogen* in the 285,000 MW complex. Molecular sieve chromatography of HMW kininogen-deficient plasma was carried out and the prekallikrein eluted with a molecular weight of 115,000, whereas HMW kininogen eluted with a MW of about 200,000 from prekallikrein-deficient plasma. When the last two deficient plasmas were mixed and subjected to gel filtration, the 285,000 MW complex was again detected. This complex was recovered from plasmas purified both at 4 °C and at 37 °C. When ^{125}I-radiolabeled prekallikrein was added to prekallikrein-deficient plasma, incubated briefly and subjected to gel filtration, a large 285,000 MW peak and a smaller 115,000 MW radioactive peak were recovered. Similar data were obtained with HMW-deficient plasma, reconstituted with HMW kininogen, and incubated with ^{125}I-labeled prekallikrein. Two peaks were noted also when the ^{125}I-labeled prekallikrein was mixed only with HMW kininogen and then subjected to gel filtration. However, functional assay revealed virtually all the activity in the 285,000 MW peak. It was assumed that the smaller peak corresponded to denatured radiolabeled prekallikrein or to a labeled contaminant. Nevertheless, the studies clearly demonstrate the complexing of prekallikrein with HMW kininogen. During ion exchange chromatography the alkaline (prekallikrein) and the acid (kininogen) components dissociate, thus, it is reasonable to assume that they are noncovalently linked, representing a charge interaction. The observation of Nagasawa and Nakayasu (1973) and of Mandle et al. (1976) were discussed at length because they explain the difficulty encountered by many investigators in isolating HMW kininogen. When gel filtration is used as the first purification step, the recovery of HMW kininogen varies considerably from one run to another and it is conceivable that partial activation of the prekallikrein would rapidly bring about the "disappearance" of the HMW kininogen (HABAL, 1975). On the other hand, the intimate association of the components of the complex is of interest, since they must interact to liberate the vasoactive peptide, bradykinin, and on surfaces they enhance the activation of factor XII.

Earlier data indicate that *kallikrein* can also form a *complex with HMW kininogen*. Under these circumstances, the HMW kininogen would be "kinin-free" and in whole plasma the peptide would be inactivated by kininases. However, the activity of kallikrein persists and can be demonstrated. Interestingly, the link between kallikrein and HMW kininogen seems firmer than that with prekallikrein since it persists (at least in part) during a single passage through an anion exchanger at a moderately low ionic strength. This observation may explain the existence of two kininogenases (VOGT, 1966; VOGT et al., 1967; for details see EISEN and VOGT, 1970). Kininogenase activity in acidic HMW fractions was detected first in guinea pig (MOVAT et al., 1968, 1969a) and then in human serum (MOVAT et al., 1970, 1971a). While the size of the complexes in the guinea pig serum was not determined precisely, two separate runs of the same material gave identical results with human serum, one complex eluting in the void volume (MW > 800,000; see below) and another with a MW of about 240,000 (TAMe esterase, kinin generation, and vascular permeability). In this procedure (recycling through Sephadex G-200) the kininogenase in the void volume was well separated from the 240,000 MW peak and the latter in turn from fragment XIIf, which had no kininogenase activity. By starch block electrophoresis, the fragment XIIf migrated in the α_1-albumin region and generated kinin only from fresh plasma. Of the other two which showed kininogenase activity, the > 800,000 MW fraction migrated as a γ-globulin (similar to plasma kallikrein) and the ~240,000 MW fraction as an α-globulin. Some of these findings are in keeping with those of VOGT and co-workers (WENDEL et al., 1972; VOGT and DUGAL, 1976) who examined these phenomena in detail.

In the first experiment, human plasma was exposed to quartz and after washing, the adsorbed protein was eluted with 1 *M* NaCl. When subjected to isoelectric focusing, the arginine esterase and kinin-forming activities paralleled each other and focused in two peaks. One peak, focusing between pH 4.0 and 5.7 (albumin, α-, and β-globulins), made up 50–65% of the total activity. A smaller peak focused between pH 7.5 and 10 (γ-globulins). The acidic fraction, which had a MW of about 180,000 (see NAGASAWA and TAKAYASU above) was precipitated with ammonium sulfate at 50% saturation, redissolved, again subjected to focusing and its pI was still between 4.25–5.0, peaking at 4.7. Human HMW kininogen has a pI of 4.5 (HABAL and MOVAT, 1976a). After anion exchange chromatography (where almost all the activity was excluded), the isoelectric focusing showed activity between pH 7.8 and 9.1. The mobility in cellulose acetate at pH 8.6 was that of a fast γ and the MW after gel filtration was 97,000. Thus, the acidic fraction had properties similar to the cationic kallikrein described under the subheading dealing with the physicochemical properties of prekallikrein and kallikrein. Some of this material was already obtained in the initial isoelectric focusing of the starting material. With respect to inhibitors, the kininogenase resembled classical plasma kallikrein. Thus, VOGT and co-workers

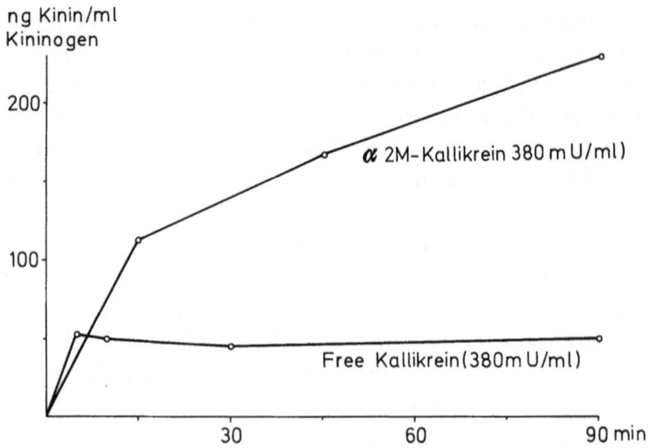

Fig. 16. Release of kinin from plasma by isolated free plasma kallikrein and by kallikrein complexed to α_2-macroglobulin (α_2M-kallikrein) and thus protected from inhibitors. (From VOGT and DUGAL, 1976)

have demonstrated that plasma kallikrein may be associated with a noninhibitory α-globulin from which it is separated during passage through DEAE-cellulose equilibrated with a buffer of very low ionic strength. It is conceivable, despite some discrepancy in MWs, that the anionic kininogenase isolated by MOVAT et al. (1970, 1971a) and that of WENDEL et al. (1972) represent kallikrein complexed with HMW kininogen, as described for prekallikrein by NAGASAWA and NAKAYASU (1973) and MANDLE et al. (1976). The larger prekallikrein HMW kininogen complexes probably represent intact zymogen and kininogen. On the other hand, in the complexes formed with kallikrein the kininogen may be partially fragmented, as will be discussed under the subheading dealing with kininogens (KATO et al., 1976a). Furthermore, WENDEL et al. (1972) dealt with eluates from quartz, which probably contained little HMW kininogen, whereas MOVAT et al. (1970, 1971a) observed the presumed complex in whole serum. These differences may account also for some of the differences between the findings of NAGASAWA and NAKAYASU (1973) and of MANDEL et al. (1976).

As noted above, chromatography of "activated" human serum (MOVAT et al., 1970, 1971a) gave rise to kininogenase and arginine esterase activity eluting between the void volume and the marker apoferritin, i.e., in the macroglobulin peak. HARPEL (1970b) had shown that the kinin-forming (i.e., proteolytic activity) of kallikrein is inhibited by α_2-macroglobulin, whereby its esterolytic activity is only partially inhibited. Similar observations had been made before with other enzymes. HARPEL (1970b, 1973, 1977) also showed that α_2-macroglobulin forms definite complexes with kallikrein. Recently, VOGT and DUGAL (1976) demonstrated that the kallikrein-α_2-macroglobulin complexes have kininogenase activity. When citrated human plasma was treated with acetone, most of the arginine and kinin-forming activity was recovered in the enzyme-inhibitor complex which during gel filtration or anion exchange chromatography eluted in the α_2-position (similar to free kallikrein that complexed with α_2-macroglobulin and released kinin more efficiently from HMW than from LMW kininogen) though its kininogenase activity in the complexed form was lower than that of kallikrein. However, in whole plasma, the efficiencies change. Free plasma kallikrein is rapidly inactivated by plasma proteinase inhibitors, whereas the complex, being protected from further inactivation, is also capable of releasing kinin slowly from LMW kininogen after the HMW kininogen has been consumed (Fig. 16). The finding of WENDEL et al. (1972) partly explain the postulated existence of a second kininogenase in plasma. The action of the kallikrein-α_2-macroglobulin complex explains these early observations further and the effect of the complexes in whole plasma stresses their possible in vivo significance.

VI. Prekallikrein Deficiency

As shown with factor XII deficiency and HMW kininogen deficiency, and several other deficiencies of the blood clotting system and of the complement system, these deficiency states provide excellent tools for the analysis of the lacking protein. In 1965 HATHAWAY et al. described an abnormality of the intrinsic coagulation pathway, in which the PTT was prolonged. Upon prolonged incubation with kaolin the clotting time (HATTERSLEY and HAYSE, 1970), the fibrinolytic and the factor XII activating activities (WEISS et al., 1974; KAPLAN et al., 1976, 1977) are progressively corrected. The factor in normal plasma which corrects the prolonged PTT was designated "Fletcher factor" (HATHAWAY and ALSEVER, 1970), but its recognition as prekallikrein followed 2 years later (WUEPPER, 1972, 1973) and this finding was soon confirmed (WEISS et al., 1974). The observations of WUEPPER were preceded by another one in which it was demonstrated that in a partial thromboplastin test, with rabbit plasma as substrate, there was a moderate but definite enhanced clot-promoting activity when kallikrein was added to such plasma (WUEPPER and COCHRANE, 1972a). WUEPPER's subsequent studies showed that the clotting defect of Fletcher factor-deficient plasma could be corrected by 2% normal, factor XII or factor XI-deficient plasmas. The deficiency was also reconstituted by highly purified human or rabbit prekallikrein. Prekallikrein also corrected the ability of the deficient plasma to generate kinins upon exposure to kaolin. Fibrinolysis (ability to generate plasmin in acidified plasma incubated with kaolin) was likewise abnormal and was normalized by addition of prekallikrein. Similarly, the permeability-inducing effect of diluted glass-contacted plasma was lacking in Fletcher factor-deficient plasma. Finally, as shown by WEISS et al. (1974), Fletcher trait plasma had a diminished rate of factor XII activation and reduced chemotactic activity. The abnormality is due to a lack of prekallikrein, as shown by immunodiffusion, rather than to a functionally altered prekallikrein.

VII. Inhibition of Kallikrein

Natural proteinase inhibitors are discussed in another section of this chapter. Here only the effect of natural plasma proteinase inhibitors on kallikrein will be mentioned briefly. The effect of α_2-macroglobulin has already been discussed. The inhibitor present in highest concentration in plasma, α_1-antitrypsin, was believed to have inhibitory effect (MCCONNELL, 1972), particularly after prolonged exposure (FRITZ et al., 1972b). However, as shown recently antithrombin III is an inhibitor of plasma kallikrein (LAHIRI et al., 1974; BURROWES et al., 1975; VENNERÖD and LAAKE, 1975; VENNERÖD et al., 1976; LAHIRI et al., 1976; HABAL et al., 1976) and antithrombin III is difficult to separate from α_1-antitrypsin (BURROWES and MOVAT, 1976). It is therefore likely that the apparent weak inhibition of kallikrein by α_1-antitrypsin was due to traces of antithrombin III. It may be stated briefly that in their second publication VENNERÖD and LAAKE (1976) clearly demonstrated a complex formation between antithrombin III and kallikrein, using SDS disc gel eleftrophoresis. The principal inhibitor of kallikrein in plasma is $C\bar{1}$-inactivator or C′1 esterase inhibitor (GIGLI et al., 1970; FRITZ et al., 1972b; HARPEL, 1977). It too forms demonstrable complexes with the enzyme.

VIII. Functions of Kallikrein

Known functions of kallikrein include (1) generation of bradykinin from kininogens as discussed here, (2) activation of factor XII (COCHRANE et al., 1973), and (3) chemotactic activity towards neutrophil leukocytes (KAPLAN et al., 1972). Whether kallikrein or a specific plasminogen activator plays a role in the intrinsic, factor XII-dependent fibrinolysis will be discussed in the section dealing with fibrinolysis and the role of plasmin in the kinin system. That kallikrein posses chemotactic activity has not been confirmed in other laboratories. However, the chemotactic effect of factor XII in rabbit ear chambers indirectly supports the view that kallikrein is chemotactic (GRAHAM et al., 1965).

E. Kininogens

I. Isolation and Purification

Kininogens are the substrates in plasma from which the vasoactive kinins are liberated by kinin-forming enzymes or kininogenases, derived from plasma (kallikrein, plasmin), glandular tissues (e.g., pancreas) or blood cells.

In early studies whole plasma was heated to at least 60 °C for 1–3 h, a process which inactivates prekallikrein and factor XII and probably most inhibitors. The plasma can be heated up to 100 °C and despite denaturation, kininogenases can still cleave kinins from the kininogens present in such precipitated plasma. Although a crude procedure by present standards, heated plasma served well in functional studies and is still being used occasionally today.

1. Low Molecular Weight Kininogen of Human Plasma

As will become apparent, purification of bovine LMW kininogen progressed very rapidly in the early and mid 1960s, but *human LMW kininogen* was not obtained in highly purified form until fairly recently. Probably the first attempt to obtain a partially purified preparation of LMW kininogen is attributable to WEBSTER and PIERCE (1963), who first used DEAE-cellulose and calcium hydroxyapatite. The material isolated represented about 15% of that present in the original plasma. These investigators subsequently purified two LMW kininogens, by repeated chromatography on DEAE-cellulose, followed by Sephadex G-200 and hydroxyapatite (PIERCE and WEBSTER, 1966). The two substrates had about the same MW of approximately 50,000 (by gel filtration on Bio-Gel G-200 in the presence of 8 *M* urea and by analytical ultracentrifugation). On a hydroxyapatite column, the earlier eluting kininogen was designated I (32% of total in plasma) and the more firmly binding one kininogen II (68% of total). Because the kinin-forming activity associated with substrate I was abolished by treatment with high doses of carboxypeptidase B, whereas substrate II was unaffected, the authors postulated that kininogen I had the kinin moiety at the C-terminus, whereas in kininogen II this moiety was buried within the molecule.

BROCKLEHURST and MAWR (1966) desalted plasma on Sephadex G-50, passing it directly onto a DEAE-Sephadex column and eluting the proteins by a stepwise increase in NaCl concentration. The kininogen-containing fractions were subjected to gel filtration on Sephadex G-200, which indicated a MW of about 100,000, although a minor peak was detected with a MW of about 200,000. However, this latter peak was considered to be an artefact which had developed during purification. After subtracting the 10% free kinin (believed to have been generated by contaminating plasma kallikrein), the purified preparation yielded 6.0 μg bradykinin equivalents from 1.0 mg of protein.

SPRAGG and co-workers carried out extensive studies (SPRAGG et al., 1970; SPRAGG and AUSTEN, 1971, 1974). In their first study the plasma was precipitated with ammonium sulfate at 45% saturation and this material eluted stepwise from DEAE-cellulose. A single kininogen was recovered, emerging when the NaCl concentration was raised to 0.12 *M*. It was further purified on Sephadex G-100. Trypsin released about three times more kinin than did plasma kallikrein. In later experiments, to avoid activation of prekallikrein to kallikrein and consumption of kininogen, the ammonium sulfate precipitation of plasma was omitted. Hexadimethrine bromide, an inhibitor of factor XII activation (ARMSTRONG and STEWART, 1962; EISEN, 1964; RATNOFF and MILES, 1964) was used in all preparative steps. Instead of stepwise elution, a gradient was applied to the anion exchange column. The substrate recovered was equally susceptible to both plasma kallikrein and trypsin. The MW of the kininogen was estimated to be 70,000 and the isoelectric point 4.6, which upon treatment with neuraminidase changed to 5.4. The functional and physicochemical studies were carried out with a partially purified preparation. To obtain kininogen that was homogeneous by disc gel electrophoresis, the protein was eluted from such gels. This kininogen still yielded kinin upon incubation with trypsin, but plasma kallikrein was no longer capable of releasing kinin from it (SPRAGG and AUSTEN, 1974). It is conceivable in view of the properties of HMW kininogen that the partially purified preparation of SPRAGG and AUSTEN, like that of BROCKLEHURST and MAWR and perhaps even the seemingly homogeneous preparation obtained by COCHRANE and WUEPPER (1971a) from rabbit or human plasma (see below), contained varying quantities of HMW kininogen. Hence the MW between 70,000 and 100,000. This will become more apparent from the discussion of the findings of PIERCE and GUIMĂRAES (1977).

Commencing with JACOBSEN (1966a), several investigators recovered two kininogens of varying purity from human plasma. Isolation of LMW kininogens will be discussed briefly here. In his first attempt, JACOBSEN (1966a) merely separated human plasma into a LMW and a HMW variety by gel filtration. Subsequently, JACOBSEN and KRIZ (1967), working at room temperature as before, employed first DEAE-Sephadex (in which the LMW kininogen bound less firmly than the HMW kininogen), followed by Sephadex G-200 and preparative polyacrylamide electrophoresis. The MW of the LMW kininogen (approx. 57,000) fell into the range obtained in later studies, dealing with human plasma and the earlier data with bovine LMW kininogen (see below). One mg of LMW kininogen recovered by JACOBSEN and KRIZ yielded 3.75 μg bradykinin equivalents. HABAL and MOVAT (1972) first used QAE-Sephadex followed by Sephadex G-200 and CM-Sephadex, all at room temperature. To this was subsequently added to step of ammonium sulfate precipitation after the anion exchange chromatography, followed by chromatography on SP-Sephadex at pH 3.5 (i.e., below the isoelectric point) as the final step (1974). Although this procedure eliminated proteinase inhibitors and the chromatography on SP-Sephadex removed the remaining traces of albumin, it was later found advisable to use instead anion exchange chromatography at pH 9.0, and at pH 7.4 (HABAL and MOVAT, 1976b). In later experiments, only the first two steps, i.e., anion exchange chromatography and the salting out, were done at room temperature and the remainder at 4 °C. However, it was essential to carry out the initial procedures at room temperature. Several attempts at carrying out the entire preparative procedure in the cold resulted in a marked decrease in the recovery of HMW kininogen, but did not affect LMW kininogen.

A highly purified preparation of LMW kininogen was obtained recently by HAMBERG et al. (1975), without recovering any HMW kininogen. The starting material was pooled plasma which was precipitated, with ammonium sulfate at 1.9 *M*, followed by Sephadex G-200, batchwise chromatography on DEAE-cellulose, DEAE-Sephadex with a linear NaCl gradient and Sephadex G-100. The kininogen thus obtained had a high specific activity, an isoelectric point of 4.7, an *S*-value of 3.95 and an estimated MW of 50,000. This material still had traces of albumin and α_2-HS glycoprotein, which were removed by appropriate antibodies.

2. High Molecular Weight Kininogen of Human Plasma

As already indicated, two forms, i.e., a LMW and a HMW kininogen were first reported in human plasma by JACOBSEN (1966a). It was also pointed out in Sect. B that MARGOLIS (1963), without recognizing it as HMW kininogen, showed that one kinin-yielding substance, designated "component *B*" is rapidly consumed following contact with glass (see Fig. 2). From such B-depleted plasma, kinin could still be released by glandular kallikrein or trypsin. Component B is interpreted to represent the currently recognized HMW kininogen and the residual kininogen in B-depleted plasma must represent LMW kininogen.

JACOBSEN and KRIZ (1967), using the above-described preparative procedure succeeded in separating and isolating the two kininogens and estimated the HMW kininogen to have a MW of 197,000. From one mg HMW kininogen they could release 4.0 μg bradykinin equivalents. The ratio of HMW: LMW kininogens according to these investigators is 1:4.

PIERCE (1968) subsequently showed a line of identity between the two kininogens with antibody against the LMW kininogen. Upon treatment with 8 *M* urea, the kinin-yielding capacity of HMW kininogen doubled and its electrophoretic mobility was similar to the LMW kininogen. Furthermore, gel filtration of HMW kininogen in 8 *M* urea on Bio-Gel P-200 revealed a kinin-yielding protein, eluting similar to the LMW kininogens described earlier by PIERCE and WEBSTER (1966).

By gel filtration on Sephadex-200, SEIDEL (1973) confirmed the early findings of JACOBSEN (1966a, b) of two kininogens, except that the estimated MW of HMW kininogen was 110,000. The latter was readily cleaved by trypsin, pancreatic kallikrein, and by a glass-activated kininogenase (presumably plasma kallikrein). The retarded kininogen (MW 50,000) was a poor substrate for the glass-activated kininogenase. On the other and, when plasma was incubated with urokinase (assuming that it generated plasmin) kinin was released and chromatography revealed the disappearance of the LMW kininogen, whereas the HMW substrate was still detectable. This is surprising, since in highly purified form both kininogens are good substrates for plasmin (see Fig. 18).

The isolation procedures used by HABAL et al. were described above. The LMW kininogen was eluted from QAE-Sephadex with 0.12 *M* NaCl (Fig. 3), together with most of the albumin and the proteinase inhibitors, α_1-antitrypsin, α_2-macroglobulin, and antithrombin III. The same fraction contained factor XII. After an intermediate step (0.18 *M*) the concentration of NaCl was raised to 0.35 *M*, which eluted the HMW kininogen in a sharp peak. A similar clear-cut separation was observed on Sephadex G-200 and while the LMW kininogen was excluded during CM-Sephadex chromatography, the HMW substrate was retarded and also separated from $C\bar{1}$-inactivator and inter-α-trypsin inhibitor. Elution from disc gels likewise showed a definite separation of the two substrates (Fig. 17). The difference in susceptibility to plasma kallikrein was striking (Fig. 18). When equipotent kininogen preparations were used and incubated with plasma kallikrein for 10 min, 60 times more kallikrein was needed to release the same amount of peptide from the LMW kininogen as from HMW kininogen (HABAL et al., 1974; HABAL and MOVAT, 1976c). Differences in susceptibility to kallikrein were reported also by VOGT and DUGAL (1976). The two kininogens were subjected to gel filtration in aqueous buffer through Sephadex G-200 and through Sepharose 4B in the dissociating agent, 4.0 *M* guanidine HCl at pH 4.2 (HABAL et al., 1975; HABAL and MOVAT, 1977). The MW of LMW kininogen did not change appreciably, being about 59,000 in aqueous buffer and 52,000 in guanidine HCl, both reduced and unreduced. However, the MW of HMW kininogen was estimated to be about 210,000 in aqueous buffer, 108,000 in guanidine HCl, and when reduced and alkylated two peaks were detected (70,000 and 55,000). Earlier studies using immunodiffusion (HABAL and MOVAT, 1972), indicated that the two kininogens were related antigenically and this was confirmed by demonstrating that antibody against one kininogen inhibited kinin-formation from both kininogens (HABAL et al., 1975). The observation that HMW kininogen was unstable in some preparations after ammonium sulfate precipitation, which was done after the QAE-Sephadex step and separates most of the $C\bar{1}$-inactivator, led to a rapid purification method (HABAL and MOVAT, 1976a). When the $C\bar{1}$-inactivator free precipitates obtained with salting out are dissolved in acetate buffer at pH 5.8–6.0 the kininogen is stable. At neutral pH there is gradual consumption due to an unidentified kininogenase, that can be inhibited by SBTI, $C\bar{1}$-inactivator, or DFP (HABAL and MOVAT, 1976a). This kininogenase is separated from the kininogen on the subsequent CM-Sephadex chromatography using a shallow gradient between 0.25 and 0.4 *M* NaCl.

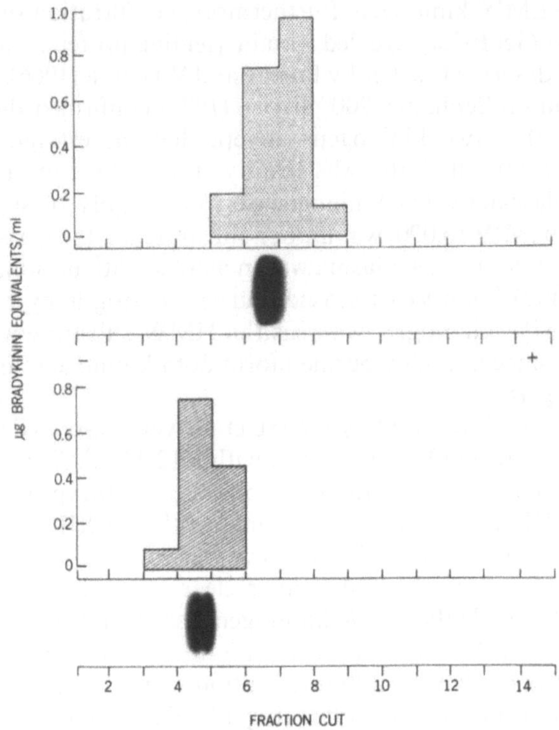

Fig. 17. Preparative polyacrylamide disc gel electrophoresis of LMW (top) and HMW (bottom) kininogens. Fractional cuts from five gels each were extracted, concentrated, and assayed on the estrous rat uterus after incubation with trypsin. Replicate gels were stained. (From HABAL et al., 1974)

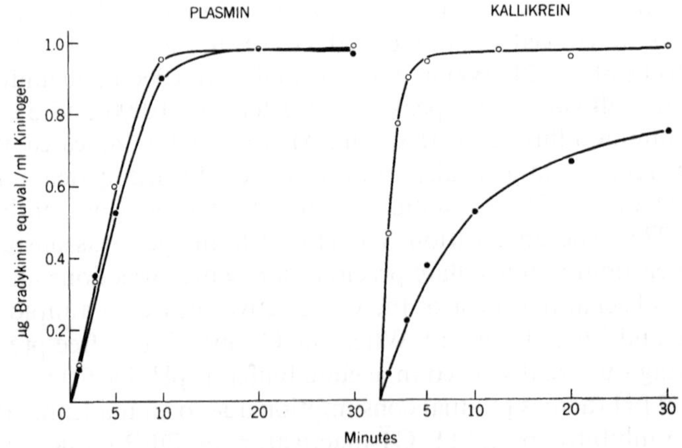

Fig. 18. Cleavage of kinin from HMW kininogen (open circles) and from LMW kininogen (closed circles) by plasmin and by plasma kallikrein. (From HABAL et al., 1976)

The QAE-Sephadex step and the salting out were done at room temperature, but the CM-Sephadex chromatography was carried out at 4 °C.

Recently, multiple forms of kininogens were detected in human plasma (PIERCE and GUIMÃRAES, 1977). Following batch adsorption at room temperature of hexadimethrine bromide-containing, diluted plasma on DEAE-cellulose (pH 6.0) and thorough washing of the anion exchanger with 0.01 *M* phosphate buffer (pH 6.0), proteins were eluted with 0.4 *M* Tris-HCl at pH 6.0. This eluate was passed through a bed of antikininogen-agarose. The antibody was monospecific and obtained by immunization with LMW kininogen (PIERCE and WEBSTER, 1966). Elution from the antikininogen-Sepharose was carried out with 8.0 *M* guanidine HCl. This material was functionally pure, i.e., contained no kininase, aminopeptidase or kininogenase inhibitor activities. The preparation thus obtained was applied to a column of DEAE-cellulose and eluted with a linear gradient between 0.05 and 0.3 *M* phosphate, pH 6.0, at room temperature. The peaks were designated B 1, B 2, B 3.1, B 3.2, and B 4. B 1 eluting first, was the least binding, i.e., the most cationic, and B 4 the firmest binding or most anionic. By gel filtration on a long column of Bio-Gel A-0.5 m, three "classes" designated α, β, and γ were recovered, corresponding to MWs of about 80,000, 150,000, and 225,000, respectively. Peaks B 1 to B 3 were made up of two classes (80,000 and 150,000) whereas peak B 4 contained all three classes. No kininogen of MW 50,000, as described previously (PIERCE and WEBSTER, 1966), was detected. Polyacrylamide disc gel electrophoresis showed three major mobility classes corresponding more or less to the three gel filtration classes. PIERCE and GUIMÃRAES explained the four to five forms of human kininogen revealed by the gradient elution, but not observed by others, by the fact that they used much higher sample loads than other investigators. They further attributed their findings to the use of a gradient instead of stepwise elution. In the writer's opinion, peaks obtained by steps should still reflect the variation in MW when subjected to gel filtration, which was not the experience with either human plasma (HABAL et al., 1974) or bovine plasma described below (KOMIYA et al., 1974a, c). It seems more plausible that with a gradient, the early eluting fractions (80,000 MW) correspond to LMW kininogen and the last eluting ones (225,000 MW) to HMW kininogen. Between these two extremes there are mixtures of varying proportions. In studying the kinetics of various enzymes with two of the kininogens, one representing LMW kininogen (B 2α) and one HMW kininogen (B 4β), these investigators confirmed "quantitatively what JACOBSEN and later HABAL and MOVAT had found qualitatively. That one form of human kininogen is a much better substrate for plasma kallikrein than the other form or forms and that glandular kallikreins, such as human urinary kallikrein, do not discriminate among the various forms." (see Fig. 18).

With a slight modification of the method described by HABAL et al., NAGASAWA and NAKAYASU (1977) isolated from human plasma both kininogens. By disc gel electrophoresis the LMW kininogen had an estimated MW of 78,000 and the HMW substrate of about 120,000. The findings of VOGT and DUGAL (1976) have already been mentioned.

Whereas a few years ago the existence of a HMW kininogen as a native protein, rather than an artefact was still being debated, today, mainly due to the discovery of a deficiency state (described below) it is no longer questioned.

3. Kininogens of Animal Plasmas

Kininogens of *bovine plasma* have been investigated more thoroughly than those of human plasma, probably mainly because of the availability of large quantities of starting material for purification.

The preparative procedure for the isolation of LMW kininogen was described by HABERMANN and ROSENBUSCH (1962, 1963) and by HABERMANN (1963) and the entire subject reviewed by HABERMANN (1970). The properties, described below, were essentially identical to those reported by Japanese investigators (SUZUKI et al., 1966; NAGASAWA et al., 1966; YANO et al., 1967a). HABERMANN did detect a second kininogen, which could be separated by gel filtration but this "– HMW kininogen was characterized as an artefact, very probably a dimer, originating during preparation. It does not appear when the temperature is kept low and the pH above 5.0" (HABERMANN, 1970). It is not surprising that HABERMANN could not detect HMW kininogen, since the starting material was bovine serum collected in glass and it had been demonstrated already by MARGOLIS (1958, 1963) that glass contact consumes component B, i.e., HMW kininogen.

A more recently described preparative procedure yielded a homogeneous preparation of LMW kininogen (KOMIYA et al., 1974c). The same plasma was used for the isolation of HMW kininogen (KOMIYA et al., 1974a), as described below. The plasma was first batch fractionated on DEAE-Sephadex. In the CM-Sephadex chromatography which followed, the LMW kininogen was present in the excluded peak and the HMW kininogen adsorbed to the cation exchanger. The crude LMW kininogen was mixed with DEAE-Sephadex equilibrated with 0.02 *M* Tris-HCl (pH 7.5) containing 0.1 *M* NaCl and poured into a column. After washing with the equilibrating buffer, the LMW kininogen was eluted with 0.4 *M* NaCl. Next the kininogen was applied to a CM-cellulose column equilibrated with 0.005 *M* sodium acetate, from which it was excluded. Batches of this material were passed twice through long columns of Sephadex G-100. The kininogen-containing fractions were dialysed against 0.01 *M* phosphate buffer (pH 8.0) and applied to a column of DEAE-Sephadex and eluted with a linear gradient of 0.01 *M* phosphate with 0.05 *M* NaCl in the mixing vessel and 0.4 *M* NaCl in the reservoir. The procedure was repeated and the end product was homogeneous by disc gel electrophoresis.

Unlike the LMW kininogen of bovine plasma, which had been thoroughly investigated in the last decade, bovine HMW kininogen was studied in considerable detail only in the past 7–8 years. As with human plasma, the impetus came with JACOBSEN's demonstration of two kininogens in the plasma of several species (1966a, b). However, SUZUKI et al. (1967) reported independently, at an international symposium in 1966, on the existence of two kininogens in bovine plasma. Following two early publications (YANO et al., 1967b, 1971) in which heating of the plasma was used (a necessary step required at that time to prevent cleavage of the kininogen by kininogenase of plasma) a simple preparative procedure was described (KOMIYA et al., 1974a). The earlier procedure consisted of four steps: DEAE-Sephadex A-50 (batch), heat treatment (70 °C for 30 min), CM-Sephadex C-50 (batch), and CM-Sephadex C-50 (column). Despite the heat treatment there seemed to be no remarkable denaturation of proteins, or at least of HMW kininogen, since the end product resembled that obtained subsequently without heat treatment. In the later publication (KOMIYA et al., 1974a), the specific activity of the end product was considerably higher despite the simpler preparative procedures. It consisted of batchwise fractionation on DEAE-Sephadex A-50 at pH 7.5 (containing 0.1 *M* NaCl). The supernatant was aspirated, the gel washed (after pouring into a column) with Tris-HCl-NaCl buffer and the crude HMW kininogen eluted from the column with 0.2 *M* acetate buffer (pH 6.2) containing 0.6 *M* NaCl. Hexadimethrine bromide was then added (40 mg/liter), as stated, to prevent activation of prekallikrein and after dialysis and adjustment of the pH to 6.5, the protein solution was mixed with CM-Sephadex C-50, equilibrated with 0.05 *M* acetate (pH 6.2), containing 0.25 *M* NaCl and hexadimethrine bromide. While the batch adsorption and elution with the anion exchanger was done at room temperature, the cation exchange chromatography was carried out at 4 °C. After washing with the equilibrating buffer, the HMW kininogen was eluted with a linear gradient between 0.25 and 0.8 *M* NaCl. The first half of the kininogen peak contained free kinin and was discarded. The second half was further purified first by rechromatography on a column of CM-Sephadex in the presence of DFP and then on Biogel P-300, also in acetate buffer (pH 6.2), containing 0.2 *M* NaCl. The end product gave a symmetrical pattern on ultracentrifugal analysis, a single arc on immunoelectrophoresis and "appeared to be nearly homogeneous when examined by SDS gel electrophoresis." Disc gel electrophoresis at alkaline pH in the absence of SDS showed two close protein bands, similar to those of human HMW kininogen described above. On treatment with plasma kallikrein, instead of the two close bands, a single faster migrating band was detected. This still cross reacted with the anti-HMW-kininogen antiserum. "The results therefore suggest that the two components detected on the gel should be regarded as of the same HMW kininogen species, the only difference being in the charge distribution in their kininogen molecules." The two components were designated HMW kininogen a and b.

This microheterogeneity was further investigated (KOMIYA et al., 1974b). HMW kininogens a and b were partially separated on a long column of CM-Sephadex (conditions as above). Each was found to have a MW of about 80,000. Their tryptic peptide maps and amino acid composition were similar and the difference between the two was attributed to a few peptide bond cleavages along the polypeptide chain of the molecule. The MW of kininogen b, the faster moving band, did not change after reduction, whereas that of kininogen a decreased after cleavage of disulfide bridges. The N-terminal amino acid could not be recovered from the HMW kininogens, indicating that it was in a masked form. The C-terminal end was leucine. On treatment of the two kininogens with cyanogen bromide kininogen a gave rise to lysyl-bradykinin (kallidin) in addition to a fragment from which lysyl-bradykinin was released by trypsin, whereas kininogen b yielded only the fragment containing the lysyl-bradykinin. KOMIYA and co-workers concluded that kininogen b was made up of a single intact polypeptide chain with a C-terminal leucine and a masked N-terminal, whereas kininogen a consisted of two proteins, one with a kinin moiety in the interior and one at the C-terminal. They postulated that "these microheterogeneous kininogens are ... derived from kininogen b by cleavage of a few peptide bonds within polypeptide chains bridged through a disulfide linkage." Further properties are described below.

Kininogens have been isolated also from *other animal* plasmas. From rabbit serum PASHKINA and ERGOVA (1966) isolated a partially purified kininogen, using

Cohn fraction IV-I as the starting step, followed by DEAE-Sephadex A-50. A 140-fold purification was achieved. From the native substrate, kinin was released by both trypsin and kallikrein, but when heat-denatured it was susceptible only to trypsin. It contained a trypsin inhibitor. The kininogen was an α_1-glycoprotein, with an isoelectric point of 3.15–3.50, a sedimentation coefficient of 3.3 *S* and an estimated MW of 48,000. Since the starting material was serum it is not surprising that only LMW kininogen was recovered. A highly purified kininogen, homogeneous by disc gel electrophoresis was isolated from rabbit plasma by Cochrane and Wuepper (1971a). The rabbit plasma (containing EDTA and hexadimethrine bromide) was fractionated with ammonium sulfate, to yield a globulin fraction that was soluble at 25%, but precipitated at 50% saturation. This protein was chromatographed on DEAE-Sephadex, followed by CM-Sephadex, Sephadex G-200, and preparative disc gel electrophoresis. The kininogen had an isoelectric point of 5.1, sedimented at 3.8 *S* and had an estimated MW of 90,000–100,000. In another publication Wuepper and Cochrane (1971) describe passage of the redissolved ammonium sulfate precipitate twice through DEAE-Sephadex (0.05 *M* phosphate buffer first at pH 8.0 and then at 6.6) using a gradient to 0.25 *M* NaCl. This was followed by CM-Sephadex (0.01 *M* phosphate, pH 6.0), in which the kininogen was excluded. The final two steps consisted of Sephadex G-200 and electrophoresis in Pevikon. This preparation too was homogeneous by disc gel electrophoresis and the MW was calculated to be 79,000. The fact that the rabbit kininogen was excluded during CM-Sephadex chromatography indicates that Wuepper and Cochrane were dealing with LMW kininogen (see human and bovine kininogens described above).

Henriques et al. (1967), omitting an earlier-used acidification step, succeeded in isolating a HMW and a LMW kininogen from horse plasma by DEAE-cellulose chromatography.

Recently, HMW kininogen was isolated also from rabbit plasma (Ergova et al., 1976). By alkaline disc gel electrophoresis it migrated as a single band in the α_2-region. The MW by Sephadex G-200 in aqueous buffer was estimated to be 140,000, in analytical ultracentrifugation the sedimentation coefficient was 7.6 *S*. Reduction and alkylation gave rise to two fragments of 80,000 and 30,000, the kinin-containing portion being in the lower MW fragment. Trypsin released 10 μg bradykinin from 1 mg HMW kininogen. Kinin release with human plasma kallikrein from HMW kininogen was very rapid, whereas from LMW kininogen no kinin was released. With rabbit plasma kallikrein, kinin release was demonstrated from both kininogens, but the rate of release from HMW kininogen was faster. However, the rate of release from HMW kininogen was considerably slower with rabbit than with human plasma kallikrein. The rate of cleavage from both kininogens was fastest with human salivary kallikrein.

II. Physicochemical Properties

Some of the properties of the kininogens have already been partially described in conjunction with their isolation (Table 1).

Human LMW kininogen is a single polypeptide chain, the MW given in the recent literature ranging between 50,000 or 52,000 (Hamberg et al., 1975; Habal and Movat, 1976), and 78,000 (Nagasawa and Nakayasu, 1977). The isoelectric point is

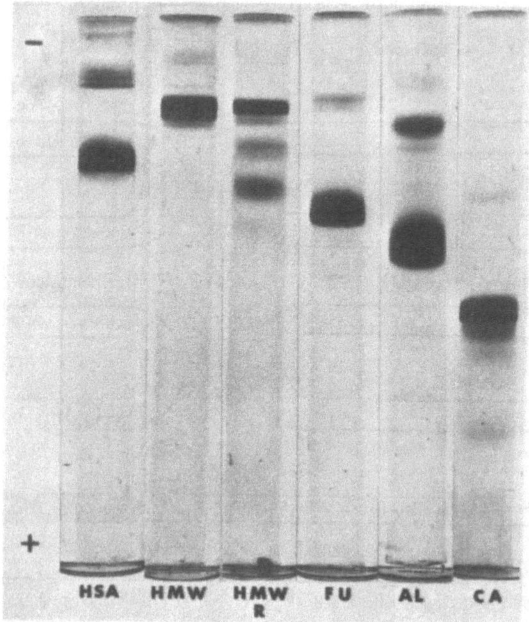

Fig. 19. SDS disc gel electrophoresis of HMW kininogen prepared by the two step procedure of HABAL and MOVAT (1976b). The gel marked HMW-R was reduced and alkylated. Marker Proteins: human serum albumin, fumarase, aldolase, egg albumin (see Fig. 5). (From MOVAT, 1978b)

4.7, binding moderately well to an anion exchanger at alkaline pH and not binding or binding minimally only to a cation exchanger at pH 6.0 but firmly at pH 3.5 (HABAL et al., 1974). It migrates as an α-globulin in alkaline disc gels. The sedimentation coefficient was estimated to be about 4.0 *S* by analytical ultracentrifugation (HAMBERG et al., 1975) and 3.85 *S* by sucrose density gradient ultracentrifugation (HABAL and MOVAT, 1976a). Human LMW kininogen is a glycoprotein.

Human HMW kininogen has been estimated to have a MW of 108,000 by guanidine-Sepharose 4B (HABAL et al., 1975), and 120,000 (NAGASAWA and NAKAYASU, 1977) by SDS-disc gel electrophoresis (Fig. 19). Its sedimentation coefficient is 4.2 *S*. HMW kininogen binds very firmly to both anion exchangers at pH 8.0 and to CM-Sephadex at pH 6.0. It migrates as a β-globulin in alkaline disc gels. Its isoelectric point is 4.5. It has not been examined for carbohydrate content, but it gives a positive reaction with the period acid Schiff reagent, characteristic of glycoproteins.

Bovine kininogens are much better characterized physicochemically (SUZUKI and KATO, 1977). With respect to ion exchangers they behave like the human kininogens. LMW kininogen has a MW of 48,000 and a sedimentation coefficient of 3.66. The diffusion coefficient is 6.16, the partial specific volume 0.688, the intrinsic viscosity 0.063, the extinction coefficient 6.7 and the isoelectric point 3.3. The last finding is not in good agreement with its behaviour on ion exchangers compared to HMW kininogen. The N-terminal amino acid is serine and the C-terminal alanine. Bovine

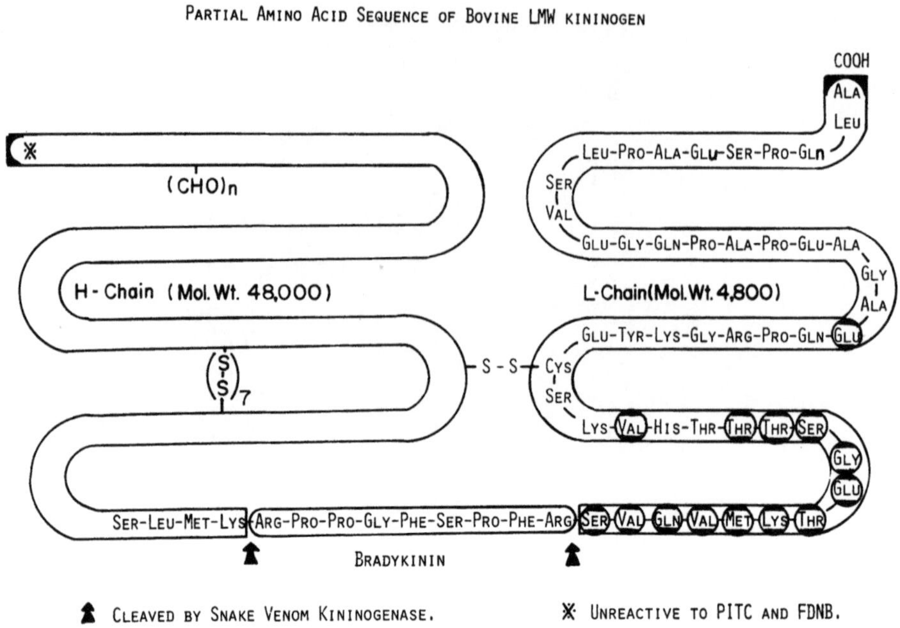

Fig. 20. Structure and partial amino acid sequence of bovine LMW kininogen (courtesy Dr. S. IWANAGA)

LMW kininogen has a total of 373 amino acid residues and 19.8% carbohydrate (Fig. 20).

Bovine HMW kininogen is considerably smaller than human kininogen, the MW having been estimated to be about 76,000 by sedimentation equilibrium and about 80,000 by gel filtration through Sephadex 4B equilibrated with guanidine HCl. The *S*-value is 3.8, the partial specific volume 0.718, the extinction coefficient 7.4, and the isoelectric point 4.5. While the N-terminal is masked, the C-terminal is leucine. It has a total of 581 amino acid residues and a carbohydrate content of 12.6% (Fig. 21) (IWANAGA, 1977).

III. Cleavage of Kininogens

The understanding of the gross structure of HMW kininogen is essential for the understanding of its cleavage. This structure is known only in bovine HMW kininogen. As indicated above, bovine HMW kininogen is a single 76,000–80,000 MW glycopeptide. Two species have been described, HMW kininogen a and b. These have the same number of peptides on tryptic digestion, but differ by one proteolytic cleavage at the C-terminal end of the bradykinin moiety, without loss of bradykinin or any of the fragments to be described. Only a few peptide bonds have been lost in kininogen b, which derives from kininogen a. Thus, limited proteolytic cleavage has occurred in kininogen b. Bradykinin and a peptide designated 1–2 or 1.2 are located within the intrachain disulfide loop (KOMIYA et al., 1974b; HAN et al., 1975, b; 1976a, b, c; KATO et al., 1976a, b). The C-terminal of bradykinin is connected with the N-terminal end of peptide 1–2 within the loop of the HMW kininogen (Fig. 21).

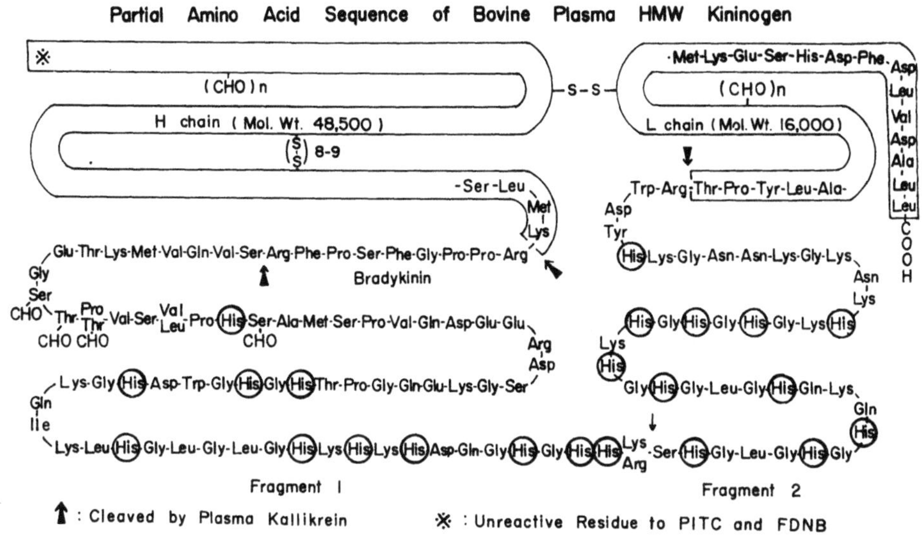

Fig. 21. Structure and partial amino acid sequence of bovine HMW kininogen (courtesy Dr. S. Iwanaga)

When HMW kininogen is incubated with bovine plasma kallikrein, in addition to bradykinin, fragments 1 and 2 are produced. The release of the fragments was monitored by SDS disc gel electrophoresis (Kato et al., 1976a). Fragment 2 is a 4584 MW histidine-rich peptide (Han et al., 1975b). Fragment 1 is a 8000 MW glycopeptide (Han et al., 1976a). At the beginning of the incubation electrophoresis in SDS gel showed mainly the HMW kininogen, with traces of fragment 1–2, fragment 1, and fragment 2. Within 15 min, fragment 1–2 and 1 were intense and fragment 2, although not as intense, was clearly visible. With increasing incubation times fragment 1–2 gradually disappeared and fragments 1 and 2 increased. Additional bands designated X and Y were noted but not identified. Fragment 1–2 increased in parallel to bradykinin, but while the fragment converted into 1 and 2, the amount of bradykinin remained constant. Fragment 1–2 could be isolated and upon incubation with plasma kallikrein yielded fragments 1 and 2. With other kininogenases no such fragmentation was demonstrable. When the digested HMW kininogen was chromatographed on a long column of Sephadex G-75, kinin-free kininogen appeared in the void volume and fragment 1–2 was retarded. Upon reduction and alkylation the kinin-free kininogen (MW 66,000) gave rise to two bands, suggesting that it consists of two polypeptide chains held together by a disulfide bond. The two were separated, consisting of a heavy chain of MW 48,000 and a light chain of 16,000 (Kato et al., 1976a, b).

The hydrolysis of bovine LMW kininogen has also been studied, but not in such detail as that of HMW kininogen (Kato et al., 1976a, b). Because LMW kininogen is not a good substrate for plasma kallikrein, the enzyme used for the cleavage of this substrate was snake venom kininogenase of *Agkistrodon halys blomhoffi*. There was no change in the mobility of LMW kininogen upon incubation with the kininogenase, nor were there any fragments. Upon reduction the main band became slightly faster and another very fast migrating band appeared. By gel filtration on Sephadex

G-75 a large peak, corresponding to the heavy chain (main band by SDS) and a small peak corresponding to the light chain (faint faster band by SDS), were detected. The H-chain consists of 344 amino acid residues and the L-chain of 47 residues. The N-terminal end is Ser and the C-terminal Ala. The C-terminal amino acid of the H-chain is Lys. There is a structural similarity between the H-chains of HMW and of LMW kininogens and the two kininogens cross-react immunologically. While HMW kininogen has a carbohydrate content of 12.6%, that of LMW kininogen is 19.3%. The MW of the H-chain of LMW kininogen is 48,000, i.e., similar to that of HMW kininogen. However, whereas the MW of the L-chain of HMW kininogen is 16,000, that of LMW kininogen is only 4800. The results indicate that the main structural differences between the two kininogens lie in the C-terminal portion next to the bradykinin moiety along the polypeptide chain.

IV. Kininogen Deficiency

Abnormal levels of prekallikrein, plasminogen proactivator, and kininogen were first reported by COLMAN and co-workers at an international symposium in 1974 which was published considerably later (COLMAN et al., 1977) and described subsequently in more detail (COLMAN et al., 1975). The deficiency was referred to as Williams trait. The entity, named first Flaujeac trait by WUEPPER et al. (1975a) and then described in detail (1975b) is a deficiency in HMW kininogen. Earlier a clotting deficiency (Fitzgerald trait) had been recognized (WALDMANN and ABRAHAM, 1974; SAITO et al., 1974b), which was later found also to be an abnormality of fibrinolysis, of kinin generation and of PF/dil activity (SAITO et al., 1975). A fourth patient (Washington) also had HMW kininogen deficiency (DONALDSON et al., 1976) and had abnormal laboratory findings similar to Fitzgerald trait. A fifth case, referred to as Reid trait, was described recently in abstract form (LUTCHER, 1976). Independently, SCHIFFMAN and LEE (1974) recognized a factor referred to as contact activation cofactor. This material was obtained in purified form and found to be identical to Fitzgerald factor (SCHIFFMAN et al., 1975). With the exception of the Fitzgerald trait, which lacks only HMW kininogen, all others have a deficiency in both kininogens. Apart from the inability to generate kinin in these kininogen-deficient plasmas, there is an inability to adequately initiate the activation of the kinin-forming system and consequently of the activation of prekallikrein, of factor XI, and the intrinsic activation of plasminogen. This is caused by the lack of complexing with factor XII and by the lack of enhancement of the activation of the factor. Kininogen is missing and cannot be demonstrated antigenically; thus, it is not an abnormal (inactive) protein. These deficiencies provided final proof for the existence of a second, functionally, and physicochemically distinct kininogen and ended the debate which existed some 6–7 years ago (for a detail, see HABAL, 1975; HABAL and MOVAT, 1976a).

F. The Fibrinolytic System

I. Activation

The enzyme of the fibrinolytic system is plasmin, its zymogen being plasminogen. In older literature the terms fibrinolysin and profibrinolysin are often encountered. A number of extraneous substances, particularly ones of bacterial origin (kinases) such as streptokinase, and cell-derived activators (urokinase) can activate plasminogen and the fibrinolytic system. Trypsin is another enzyme besides urokinase which can activate plasminogen. Recently, a plasminogen activator was isolated from macrophages (UNKELESS et al., 1974) and PMN-leukocytes (GRANELLI-PIPERNO et al., 1977).

This section is concerned with the intrinsic (plasma) fibrinolytic system, which is factor XII dependent. The dependence on factor XII was recognized almost 20 years ago by NIEWIAROWSKI and PROU-WARTELLE (1959) and also described by IATRIDES and FERGUSON (1961). These investigators demonstrated that upon contact of factor XII-deficient plasma, the fibrinolytic system is not activated. An activator of plasma has been demonstrated long before (SCHMITZ, 1936; LEWIS and FERGUSON, 1951; MÜLERTZ, 1953). However, factor XII does not activate plasminogen directly, i.e., it is not the direct activator (RATNOFF and DAVIE, 1962; SCHOENMAKERS et al., 1963) and it has been proposed that factor XII may induce the formation of plasminogen activator from a precursor (IATRIDES and FERGUSON, 1962). This intrinsic activation of the fibrinolytic system can be demonstrated by incubating plasma with kaolin, at acid pH (4.8) in dilute buffer for 1 h. Following centrifugation, plasmin is found in the euglobulin precipitates which are redissolved in neutral physiologic saline.

During the last 7–8 years attempts have been made to isolate and identify the factor XII-dependent activator of plasminogen. OGSTON et al. (1969) demonstrated that plasma adsorbed on glass, which still contained factor XII and plasminogen, no longer contained a factor required for the activation of plasminogen to plasmin. This factor was tentatively called Hageman factor-cofactor. It was present in the non-euglobulin fraction of normal or factor XII-deficient plasma and restored the fibrinolytic activity of glass-treated plasma. It could be recovered also from celite eluates of plasma. The factor was not identical with the substrates of factor XII (prekallikrein or factor XI). That it was not prekallikrein/or kallikrein was shown by inhibition studies since, unlike kallikrein, it was not inhibited by C$\bar{1}$-inactivator. Furthermore, it was not factor XI since it could be recovered from factor XI-deficient plasma. It should be stressed however, that it eluted from anion exchange columns together with factor XIa and kallikrein. The material derived from celite eluate had an estimated MW of 165,000 by gel filtration. Next, KAPLAN and AUSTEN (1972) reported to have succeeded in the isolation of a plasminogen proactovator. The proactivator was excluded from anion exchangers at alkaline pH together with IgG, prekallikrein, and "prePTA" (factor XI, unactivated). During cation exchange chromatography (pH 6.0), the proactivator separated from the bulk of Ig, overlapping with prekallikrein and partially with factor XI. Two Sephadex G-150 gel filtrations of early and late eluting fractions from the cation exchanger resulted in a partial separation from prekallikrein and a complete separation of the plasminogen proactivator from factor XI. The plasminogen proactivator had an isoelectric point of 8.9, showing a single slow migrating band in alkaline disc gel electrophoresis, free of any known functional protein of the fibrinolytic, clotting, or kinin system. The activator was activated by factor XIIa or XIIf and in its activated form converted plasminogen to plasmin, detectable by the fibrin plate assay but not by caseinolysis. The activated form of plasminogen activator was seemingly not susceptible to inhibition by C$\bar{1}$-inactivator, thus being distinguished from kallikrein and factor XIa. Although it was inhibited by DFP, which did not affect the zymogen, neither ROBBINS

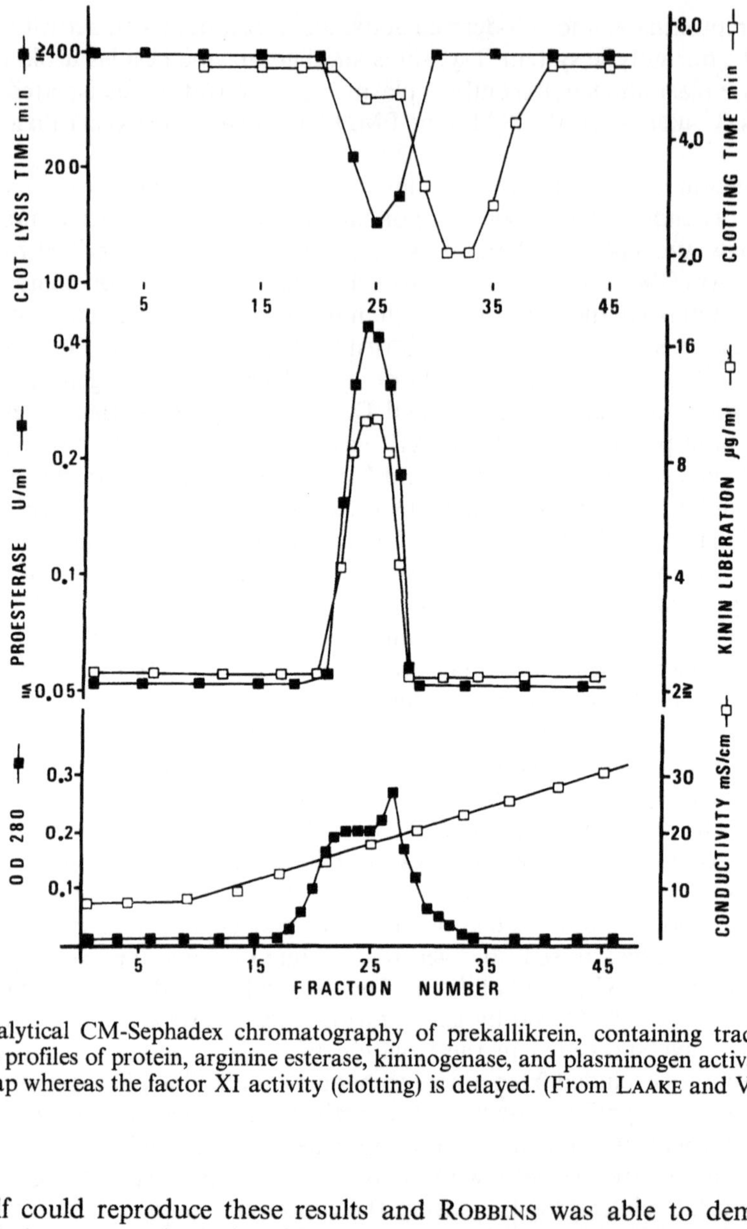

Fig. 22. Analytical CM-Sephadex chromatography of prekallikrein, containing traces of factor XI. The profiles of protein, arginine esterase, kininogenase, and plasminogen activation (clot lysis) overlap whereas the factor XI activity (clotting) is delayed. (From Laake and Venneröd, 1974)

nor myself could reproduce these results and Robbins was able to demonstrate fibrinolysis, but not caseinolysis, with the material isolated by Kaplan (see Movat, 1978a). Kaplan later showed two peaks of plasminogen proactivator activity, one overlapping with prekallikrein (MW 95,000) and the second one with factor XI (MW 180,000) (Kaplan et al., 1977). The peak with the MW of factor XI was believed to represent a dimer. Interestingly, in prekallikrein-deficient (Fletcher trait) plasma only the 180,000 MW plasminogen activator was recovered (65–70% of normal plasma). Laake and Venneröd (1974) could detect only one plasminogen proactivator which completely overlapped in all chromatographic steps with prekallikrein (Fig. 22). Apart from these findings, prekallikrein exhibited microheterogeneity (see

Sect. D) which paralleled the plasminogen proactivator activity. A column of C$\bar{1}$-inactivator coupled to Sepharose 4B was prepared and when kallikrein was passed through it both kallikrein and plasminogen activator were adsorbed to the column. A highly purified homogeneous preparation of kallikrein also possessed plasminogen activator activity. The authors concluded "that plasma prekallikrein may be a mediator of the factor XII-dependent fibrinolytic pathway of human plasma." Subsequently, VENNERÖD and LAAKE (1976) presented evidence that prekallikrein-deficient plasma is devoid of plasminogen proactivator activity. Recently, KAPLAN and coworkers conceded that at least some of the plasminogen proactivator, that of MW 95,000, seems undistinguishable from prekallikrein. The 180,000 MW portion could be identical to factor XI (MANDLE and KAPLAN, 1977b; KAPLAN, 1977). Further investigations are required to ascertain (a) that the plasminogen proactivator of MW ~ 100,000 is prekallikrein and (b) the nature of the proactivator with MW ~180,000. However, in closing this section it should be mentioned that in 1969 COLMAN had already presented some data to show that kallikrein can activate plasminogen (COLMAN, 1969).

II. Plasminogen and Plasmin

The plasminogen activator described above acts on the zymogen plasminogen, converting it to the enzyme plasmin.

1. Isolation and Purification

In the past, plasminogen was prepared from euglobulin precipitates of plasma or from Cohn fraction III, followed by a series of preparative procedures (ROBBINS and SUMMARIA, 1970). After the description of affinity chromatography by DEUTSCH and MERTZ, this method became that of choice for the isolation of plasminogen (DEUTSCH and MERTZ, 1970; LIU and MERTZ, 1971; SODETZ et al., 1972; SUMMARIA et al., 1972; WALLÉN and WIMAN, 1972; HABAL et al., 1976). ROBBINS and SUMMARIA (1976) described affinity chromatography of plasminogen using Cohn fraction III or $III_{2,3}$ or plasma as the original source. They applied one liter of plasma or Cohn fraction at 2 °C to a 9.0 × 30.0 cm column packed with L-lysine-substituted Sepharose 4B equilibrated with 0.1 *M* phosphate buffer, pH 7.4, followed by a wash with the same buffer until the effluent absorbed less than 0.1 at 280 nm. The temperature of the column was then raised to 16 °C and washed with 0.3 *M* phosphate, pH 7.4, to elute adsorbed protein which was not plasminogen. After washing again with 0.1 *M* phosphate and lowering the temperature to 2 °C, the plasminogen was eluted at 2 °C with 0.2 *M* epsilon-aminocaproic acid in 0.1 *M* phosphate at pH 7.4. Depending on the purity, when necessary further fractionation was carried out at 2 °C on DEAE-Sephadex (0.05 *M* Tris and 0.02 *M* lysine, pH 9.0, as the starting buffer and the same buffer containing 0.1 *M* NaCl as the limiting buffer) and/or on Sephadex G-150 columns. WALLÉN and WIMAN (1972) and BURROWES et al. (1972) also found that affinity chromatography was not sufficient. BURROWES used citrated plasma as starting material. The plasminogen eluted in a stepwise procedure with 0.1 *M* Tris HCl (pH 8.0) containing 0.075 *M* NaCl from a QAE-Sephadex column (see Fig. 3). After

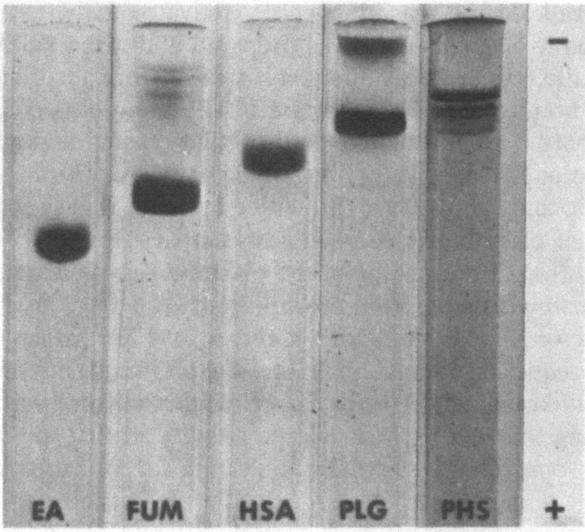

Fig. 23. SDS disc gel electrophoresis of plasminogen (PLG) and of the markers egg albumin (EA), fumarase (FUM), human serum albumin (HSA), and phosphorylase (PHS; MW 94,000). (From HABAL et al., 1976)

the lysine-Sepharose step, the plasminogen was passed through Sephadex G-200, yielding a homogeneous preparation by SDS-disc gel electrophoresis (HABAL et al., 1976) (Fig. 23). Occasionally, some plasmin can be detected. This is probably why ROBBINS and SUMMARIA suggest the addition of 10^{-2} *M* DFP. DFP decays, but if the preparation is to be used immediately it can be removed by dialysis.

2. Physicochemical Properties

Human plasminogen is a single chain monomeric plasma protein which has multiple forms when isolated by isoelectric focusing. It migrates as a fast γ or slow β globulin in agarose and as multiple bands in alkaline disc gels in the presence of epsilon-aminocaproic acid. The molecular forms which focus between pH 6.2 and 6.6 can be prepared from plasma or Cohn fraction III and have glutamic acid at the N-terminal end (RICKLI and CUENDET, 1971; WALLÉN and WIMAN, 1972; SUMMARIA et al., 1973a). Those forms focusing between pH 7.2 and 8.3 could be prepared from Cohn fraction $III_{2,3}$ and had an N-terminal lysine residue (SUMMARIA et al., 1972, 1973a). The two forms are referred to as Glu-plasminogen and Lys-plasminogen, respectively. According to ROBBINS et al. (1975), the sedimentation coefficient of Glu-plasminogen is 5.0 *S* and of Lys-plasminogen 4.4 *S*, the MWs are 83,800 and 82,400, the partial specific volumes 0.706 and 0.709, and the frictional coefficients 1.54 and 1.63, respectively. In contrast, Swedish investigators found slightly different values, i.e., 5.1 *S* and 4.8 *S*; 92,000 and 90,000; 0.706 and 0.709; 1.50 and 1.56, respectively, for Glu-plasminogen and Lys-plasminogen (SJÖHOLM et al., 1973). Gel electrophoresis in SDS indicated a MW of 77,000 (HABAL et al., 1976). Carbohydrate content is less than 2.0%. Both groups of investigators found the *S*-value of plasmin to be 4.3,

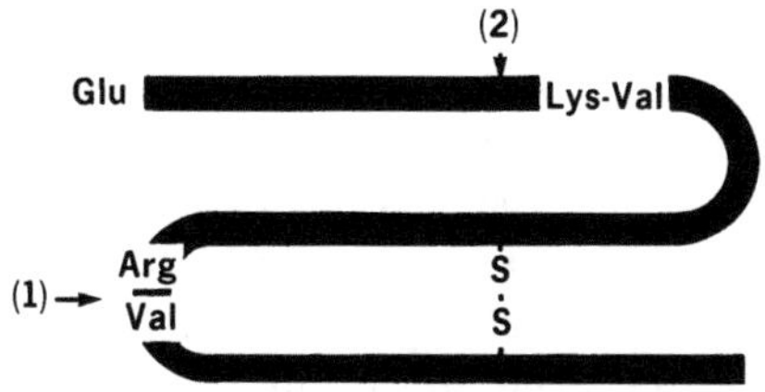

Fig. 24. The gross structure of plasminogen and the sites of cleavage during activation to plasmin (based on KOSOW, 1976)

but the calculated MWs were 76,500 and 81,000, respectively. The partial specific volume, 0.714–0.713 and the frictional coefficient 1.64 and 1.55, respectively. Plasmin consists of a heavy or A chain (MW 48,800) and a light or B chain (MW 25,700) (Fig. 24). By radioimmunoassay the concentration of plasminogen in plasma was estimated to be 206 ± 35 μg/ml (RABINER et al., 1969), and by radial immunodiffusion 464 ± 75 μg/ml (MAGOON et al., 1974) (Table 1).

3. Activation of Plasminogen to Plasmin

It has been known for some time that conversion of plasminogen to plasmin is associated with cleavage of an arginyl-valine bond (ROBBINS et al., 1967) (Fig. 24). However, there is some controversy whether release of a small peptide is a prerequisite for the activation of plasminogen (KOSOW, 1976). Several investigators have demonstrated that a small peptide of about 8000 MW is lost from the N-terminal end during activation (see Fig. 24) (WIMAN and WALLÉN, 1973; WALTHER et al., 1975). However, SODETZ et al. (1974) isolated plasmin with an amino terminal end and MW identical to that of plasminogen by activating it with urokinase in the presence of bovine trypsin inhibitor. The latter prevented the possible autocatalytic action of plasmin, which could have induced the cleavage of the N-terminal peptide.

In addition to enzymatic activation (urokinase), on which the above data are based, plasminogen can be activated by streptokinase which is not an enzyme. Although several mechanisms have been proposed, the most likely is that streptokinase forms a complex with plasminogen (plasmin) and this complex acts as a "plasminogen activator," which is capable of hydrolysing the arginyl-valine bond (KOSOW, 1976). It has not been investigated how the factor XII-dependent activation occurs but since kallikrein is now believed to be the activator, and it is an enzyme, it may act similarly to urokinase.

4. Effect on the Kinin System

As shown in Fig. 1, plasmin induces a positive feedback by activating and cleaving factor XII. The effect of plasmin on factor XII was described in Sect. C, where the fragmentation of factor XII was discussed (see Fig. 8).

Although it was believed that plasmin can activate prekallikrein to kallikrein evidence was presented that this effect is indirect and proceeds via activation of factor XII (see Sect. D).

Some investigators believe that plasmin can act directly on kininogen by cleaving kinin (LEWIS, 1958; EISEN, 1963; BACK and STEGER, 1965; HAMBERG, 1968; GAPANHUK and HENRIQUES, 1970). Others were not able to release kinin by adding partially purified kininogen (BHOOLA et al., 1960; VOGT, 1964; BULUK and MALOFIEJEW, 1965; HAUSTEIN and MARQUART, 1966). The effect of highly purified plasmin on kininogens has not been examined until recently. Older data, from partially purified preparations, indicated that plasmin generates kinin at a much slower rate than plasma kallikrein (EISEN and VOGT, 1970). When preparations of plasmin and kallikrein were used which were approximately equipotent with respect to esterolysis, kallikrein was found to cleave HMW kininogen more rapidly than plasmin. Plasmin acted equally well on both kininogens. Contrary to the findings of GAPANHUK and HENRIQUES (1970), who detected mostly Met-Lys-bradykinin, the peptide recovered when kininogens were cleaved by plasmin was bradykinin (HABAL et al., 1976).

III. Inhibition of Plasmin

The activator of plasminogen present in precursor form in plasma was first believed to be inhibited only by α_2-macroglobulin (SCHREIBER et al., 1973b). However, as discussed above, the plasminogen activator is in fact kallikrein and therefore susceptible to the inhibitors described in Sect. D.

Plasmin is inhibited by DFP, EACA, SBTI, LBTI, TLCK, Trasylol, and by the natural proteinase inhibitors, α_2-macroglobulin, antithrombin III (HIGHSMITH and ROSENBERG, 1974; HABAL et al., 1976), and $C\bar{1}$-inactivator (HARPEL, 1970a). α_1-antitrypsin was found to be a weak inhibitor of plasmin (HABAL et al., 1976). In the older literature one encounters reference to "slow" and "fast" inhibitors of plasmin in plasma (VOGEL et al., 1966). It now seems well established that the recently described α_2-antiplasmin (COLLEN, 1976; MAROI and AOKI, 1976; MÜLLERTZ and CLEMENSEN, 1976) is the fast inhibitor, whereas α_2-macroglobulin, antithrombin III, and $C\bar{1}$-inactivator are the slow inhibitors.

IV. Plasminogen-Independent Fibrinolysis

The factor XII-dependent intrinsic activation of the fibrinolytic system was described in the first part of this section. A factor XII-independent system was described by SCHREIBER and AUSTEN (1974). However, this system was believed to be plasminogen dependent, as well as complement dependent, since clot lysis was abnormal in the plasma of two patients with acquired C3 deficiency and plasma depleted of C3 by zymosan or cobra venom factor.

MOROZ and GILMORE (1976a, b) detected fibrinolysis by a sensitive ^{125}I-labeled fibrin solid phase assay (MOROZ and GILMORE, 1975) in plasmas depleted of plasminogen by affinity chromatography. Various inhibitors (EACA, DFP, SBTI, LBTI) did not inhibit the fibrinolytic activity of the depleted plasma at concentrations at which inhibition of plasmin and urokinase-activated plasma readily occurs. The fibrinolytic activity was factor XII-independent since it was not affected by contact or by hexadimethrine bromide. However, heating to 56 °C for 30 min and treatment with zymozan induced partial inhibition. An increase in fibrinolytic activity was associated with a reciprocal decrease in the activity of the classic and alternative pathways of complement. The authors concluded that normal plasma fibrinolytic activity was relatively independent of plasmin as the ultimate fibrinolytic enzyme, that factor XII-dependent pathways are of minor importance, and that the fibrinolytic activity they demonstrated may include proteinases involved in complement activation as well as other non-plasmin proteinases. These observations remain to be repeated in other laboratories.

G. Kinin Generation by Neutrophil Leukocytes

Most of the studies concerned with kinin generation have dealt in the past with enzymes (kallikreins) derived from tissues (e.g., pancreas) or from plasma (kallikrein, plasmin). A third source of kininogenases are the lysosomal enzymes of neutrophil leukocytes. The lysosomal enzymes are released whenever these cells phagocytose.

The kininogenases of blood cells are described in detail by L.M. GREENBAUM in another chapter of this volume which deals with the leukokinin-forming system. The text which follows deals with the neutral proteases of human neutrophils and the peptides they cleave from purified plasma kininogens.

I. Mechanisms of Lysosomal Enzyme Release From Neutrophils

The release of lysosomal enzymes by neutrophil leukocytes following phagocytosis was reviewed recently by the writer (MOVAT, 1976). Although preformed antigen-antibody or immune precipitates represent the best phagocytic stimulus, immune complexes formed in situ on the cell surface represent an even better stimulus (SAJNANI, 1974; SAJNANI et al., 1974a, 1976). These immune complexes form on the surface of the cell and are eventually taken up by the cell. However, phagocytosis can be prevented by cytochalasin B. It would appear that stimulation of Fc receptors on the cell surface and perhaps within digestive vacuoles (which derive from invaginated cell membrane) is the most important event in the triggering of lysosomal enzyme release. In fact, the presence of IgG is a sine qua non for lysosomal secretion. When latex particles are phagocytozed by neutrophils, enzymes are released only when the beads are coated with IgG (RANADIVE et al., 1973). The mechanism of release is still controversial although all investigators in the field agree that it is an active energy requiring process. Release of lysosomal enzymes is therefore referred to as secretion in order to distinguish it from passive release, such as in cytotoxic release (WEISSMANN et al., 1971, 1973; HENSON, 1971a, b; WRIGHT and MALAVISTA, 1972; BECKER and HENSON, 1973; ZURIER et al., 1974). However, it cannot be denied that release does occur in dying and disintegrating cells (METCHNIKOFF, 1891). The mechanisms proposed for secretion included the process referred to as "regurgitation during feeding," reversed endocytosis and "perturbation" of the cell membrane (WEISSMANN et al., 1971; HAWKINS, 1971; HENSON, 1971a; DAVIES et al., 1973; ZURIER et al., 1973). That release can occur by surface stimulation without ingestion was demonstrated with the aid of immune complexes bound along or incorporated into a nonphagocytozable membrane (HAWKINS, 1971; HENSON, 1971a). The chemical mechanisms during secretion and the modulation of the release process from neutrophils has been studied extensively (WRIGHT and MALAVISTA, 1972; WEISSMANN et al., 1973; HAWKINS, 1973, 1974; HENSON and OADES, 1973; RANADIVE et al., 1973; IGNARO et al., 1974; SAJNANI et al., 1974b; ZURIER et al., 1974) and, as already indicated, resembles secretion and in this respect resembles the release or secretion of chemical mediators during anaphylaxis (AUSTEN, 1974; AUSTEN et al., 1976), although some differences exist (HAWKINS, 1974). Briefly, it has been shown that release is inhibited by inhibitors of anaerobic glycolysis (2-deoxyglucose, iodoacetic acid) but not by an uncoupler of oxidative phosphorylation (2,4-dinitrophenol). A common requirement for secretory processes, calcium, is essential for the release. The role of colchicine, which impairs microtubule function, is not fully ascertained. Most investigators have observed inhibition, but some (HAWKINS, 1974) have observed little effect unless high concentrations were used. An agent which favours microtubule assembly, deuterium oxide, enhances release and was also found to reverse the effect of colchicine. Cytochalasin B, which favours microtubule assembly, enhances release. Of the lysosomal stabilizers, hydrocortisone was an effective inhibitor whereas salicylates did not inhibit release of hydrolases. Exogenous cyclic AMP and compounds which increase cellular levels of AMP inhibit, whereas compounds which increase cellular cyclic GMP enhanced release of lysosomal enzymes (IGNARRO et al., 1974; ZURIER et al., 1974). HAWKINS (1974) found that dibutyril cyclic AMP and theophylline definitively inhibited release, but β-adrenergic agents, disodium chromoglycate and diethylcarbamazine did not.

2. Proteases of Neutrophil Leukocyte Lysosomes

A large number of proteolytic enzymes are present in neutrophil lysosomes (METCHNIKOFF, 1891; OPIE, 1922; GROB, 1949). The neutral proteases of human neutrophils have been reviewed by JANOFF (1972b) but several have been added since then. In experimental animals, the granules contain mainly acid cathepsins, some of which can generate kinin at low pH (GREENBAUM and KIM, 1967; CHANG et al., 1972; GREENBAUM et al., 1973; GREENBAUM, 1977). A cartilage degrading enzyme and a histonase acting at neutral pH have also been demonstrated (WEISSMANN and SPIELBERG, 1968; DAVIES et al., 1971), although some degree of nonspecific proteolytic activity at neutral pH is present in the lysosomes of rabbit neutrophils (WASI et al., 1966).

The best studied protease in human neutrophils is an *elastase-like enzyme* (JANOFF and SCHERER, 1968; JANOFF, 1970, 1972a, 1973; OHLSSON and OLSSON, 1974a; SCHMIDT and HAVEMANN, 1974; FEINSTEIN and JANOFF, 1975b; TAYLOR and CRAWFORD, 1975; BAUGH and TRAVIS, 1976; KRUZE et al., 1976; MOVAT et al., 1976a). Elastases have also been demonstrated in neutrophils of horse (DUBIN et al., 1976; KOJ et al., 1976), pig (KOPITAR and LEBEZ, 1975) and of dog blood (DELSHAMMAR and OHLSON, 1976; ARDELT et al., 1976). The elastase isolated from human spleens is identical to the elastase of neutrophils (STARKEY and BARRETT, 1976). The elastase-like protease of neutrophils is a highly basic protein consisting of three to five charge isomers. Its isoelectric point ranges between pH 10.0 and 11.8 (MOVAT et al., 1976a) and its MW has been found by most investigators, who used SDS disc gel electrophoresis, to be just under 30,000 (26,000–28,000), although OHLSSON and OHLSSON (1974a) and FEINSTEIN and JANOFF (1975b) reported 33,000–35,000. By gel filtration in aqueous buffer the MW was estimated to be only 20,000–23,000. The *S*-value is 2.7. Although referred to as elastase, this neutral protease has a weak elastinolytic activity but it readily degrades cartilage chondromucoprotein (JANOFF and BLONDIN, 1970; IGNARO et al., 1973; MALEMUD and JANOFF, 1975; JANOFF et al., 1976; KEISER et al., 1976). On chondromucoprotein it probably acts in conjunction with the chymotrypsin-like enzyme described below. The elastase-like protease is readily inhibited by DFP and to a lesser degree by SBTI and Trasylol. A series of chloromethyl ketone inhibitors inhibit elastase (TUHY and POWERS, 1975). Of these, some are more specific than others. For elastase, the most specific is MeO-Suc-Ala-Ala-Pro-Val-CH_2Cl (POWERS et al., 1977; POWERS, 1977). Of the natural proteinase inhibitors, the elastase-like enzyme is inhibited by α_1-antitrypsin, α_2-macroglobulin, and antithrombin III (OHLSSON, 1971; JANOFF, 1972a; OHLSSON and OLSSON, 1974b; MOVAT et al., 1976a).

The second well characterized neutral protease of human neutrophil lysosomes is a *chymotrypsin-like enzyme* (RINDLER et al., 1973, 1974; RINDER-LUDWIG et al., 1974; SCHMIDT and HAVEMANN, 1974; GERBER et al., 1974; RINDLER-LUDWIG and BRAUNSTEINER, 1975; FEINSTEIN and JANOFF, 1975a). The same enzyme isolated from spleen has been referred to as *cathepsin G* (BARRETT, 1975). The MW has been estimated to be 20,000–23,000. By cationic disc gel electrophoresis, some investigators (SCHMIDT and HAVEMANN, 1974; RINDLER-LUDWIG and BRAUNSTEINER, 1975) demonstrated three isozymes, of which two migrated faster than lysozyme, others observed a single band (FEINSTEIN and JANOFF, 1975a). An interesting observation was made by RINDLER-LUDWIG and co-workers, that cathepsin G is only slightly soluble at physiologic NaCl concentration, but soluble at 1.0 *M* NaCl. This is useful for the separation from elastase. The enzyme is inhibited by some of the above mentioned chloromethyl ketone inhibitors, of which Z-Gly-Leu-Phe-CH_2Cl is the most specific (POWERS, 1977). The plasma proteinase inhibitors, α_1-antitrypsin, and α_2-macroglobulin, as well as α_1-antichymotrypsin inhibit cathepsin G (OHLSSON and ÅKESSON, 1976).

Collagenase, a metalloproteinase, was detected by LAZARUS and colleagues in granulocyte lysosomes (LAZARUS et al., 1968, 1972). The cleavage of collagen monomers was inhibited by EDTA, but not by serum. The monomers were cleaved into $^1/_3$ and $^1/_4$ length fragments, the cleavage point being probably $^1/_4$ of the length from the C-terminal and of the collagen molecule. The specific cleavage products induced by the collagenase could be further degraded by a nonspecific protease present in lysosomal lysates. This latter enzyme was inhibited by serum. More recently, two collagenases, antigenically related, have been obtained in highly purified form (OHLSSON and OLSSON, 1973). Both enzymes had a sedimentation coefficient of 4.5 *S* and a molecular weight of 76,000, being composed of two subunits of MWs 42,000 and 33,000, respectively. The collagenases were susceptible to inhibition by α_1-antitrypsin and α_2-macroglobulin. The two collagenases differed in their migration in disc gels due to differences in a few residues. The collagenases also degraded proteoglycans and fibrinogen. Since collagenase is metal-dependent (zinc, calcium) it is readily inhibited by chelating agents such as EDTA, 1,10-phenanthroline and by thiol compounds.

The localization of enzymes in the granules or lysosomes of the neutrophil has been studied by zonal sedimentation and isopicnic equilibration in sucrose gradients. By this procedure the lysosomes can be separated into azurophil granules which have an average density of 1.23 and specific granules, whose average density is 1.19 (BAINTON et al., 1971; BRETZ and BAGGIOLINI, 1974). Application of this method to the above three enzymes lead to the localization of the elastase-like enzyme and of cathepsin G (chymotrypsin-like) to the azurophil granules (DEWALD et al., 1975; VIESCHER et al., 1976) and of the collagenase to the specific granules (MURPHY et al., 1977).

Cathepsins A–E are according to BARRETT (1975), a heterogeneous group of peptide hydrolases, which are all cell derived and have an acid pH optimum. Of these, cathepsins B_1, D, and E are endopeptidases and A, B_2, and C are exopeptidases. The latter enzymes comprise the aminopeptidases cleaving single amino acids at the N-terminal and carboxypeptidases cleaving at the C-terminal of a protein.

An *aminopeptidase* of neutrophil leukocytes capable of cleaving the amino acids lysine and methionine from the kinin peptides, lysyl-bradykinin or methionyl-lysyl-bradykinin was described in the writer's laboratory. The enzyme has a neutral pH optimum, an isoelectric point of 4.5, and by gel filtration an estimated MW of 200,000 (PASS et al., 1977). The aminopeptidase has been localized in granules distinct from those which contain the elastin- and chymotrypsin-like activity (azurophils), i.e., derived from the specific granules (FOLDS et al., 1972).

3. Interaction Between Neutrophil Proteases and Plasma Substrates

Acid proteases or cathepsins B, D, or E can cleave kinins from crude kininogen at acid pH (GREENBAUM and KIM, 1967; CHANG et al., 1972; GREENBAUM, 1972), but the substrate has been subsequently shown to be distinct from the kininogen (GREENBAUM et al., 1973; GREENBAUM, 1976), which is the source of the three known vasoactive kinins. The peptides recovered by GREENBAUM are referred to as "leukokinins" and are distinct from the plasma kinins.

The formation of leukokinins is a relatively slow process occurring at acid pH and, thus, peptide generation in vivo is difficult to visualize. A rapid kinin-forming activity was described by MELMON and CLINE (1967) in experiments in which intact neutrophils were incubated with whole plasma or a crude kininogen preparation. The model with the human neutrophils is a complex system and attempts to repeat the original experiment were unsuccessful (WEBSTER, 1973). The availability of highly purified kininogens (HABAL and MOVAT, 1972; HABAL et al., 1974) and the fact that human neutrophils contain neutral proteases, led the writer and co-workers to study the possibility that proteases of neutrophils release kinin from kininogen (MOVAT et al., 1973b). The release occurred rapidly at neutral pH and amounted to about 20% of the peptide releasable (expressed as bradykinin equivalents) by trypsin from the same kininogen preparation. With LMW kininogen it was essential that the substrate be free of α_1-antitrypsin, α_2-macroglobulin, and kininase. When the fragmented neutrophils were subjected to differential centrifugation, the kinin-forming activity was detected in the granule or lysosomal fraction whereas the cell sap or cytosol fraction contained a kinin-inactivating enzyme or kininase which was inhibited by heavy metals. The kinin-forming enzyme was subsequently purified, characterized and found to be similar to the above described elastase-like enzyme (MOVAT et al., 1976a). Yet more recent data indicate that the enzyme is distinct and merely cochromatographed with elastase (WASI et al., 1978). With the whole lysosomal lysate (which contains also the kinin-converting aminopeptidase; PASS et al., 1977), the generated peptide behaved like bradykinin when chromatographed on CM-cellulose (MOVAT et al., 1976a) using the method of HABERMANN and BLENEMANN (1964). When the purified protease was used, the peptide eluted in an intermediate position between bradykinin and Met-Lys-bradykinin, though closer to the undecapeptide (MOVAT et al., 1976b). The peptide generated was not bradykinin but could be converted to it, as demonstrated pharmacologically. When the generated peptide was treated with trypsin or the above described neutrophil-derived aminopeptidase (PASS et al., 1977) its potency increased when tested on the rat uterus.

OLSSON and co-workers described and isolated highly cationic proteins of leukemic myeloid cells (OLSSON and VENGE, 1972, 1974). Of the seven proteins demonstrated by electrophoresis in agarose at acid pH, the four most cationic ones hydrolysed tyrosine esters, indicating a chymotrypsin-like activity (ODEBERG et al., 1975). The chymotrypsin-like proteins induced conversion of the complement components C1s, C4, C3, and C5 upon incubation with these components (VENGE and OLSSON, 1975). Of these, C3 and C5 gave rise to chemotactic activity which, however, disappeared upon prolonged incubation. The chemotactic activity was not very marked, about half that of positive controls and only about twice that of C3 or C5 by itself. Furthermore, C3a, a fragment of C3, is believed not to be chemotactic (MÜLLER-EBERHARD, 1976). Unlike C5a, which shows cross tachyphylaxis with classical anaphylatoxin, C3a is a substance with anaphylatoxin-like, but distinct properties (VOGT, 1974). C3 cleavage products, generated by the kinin-generating neutrophil protease, enhance vascular permeability and generate a spasmogen upon short incubation (MOVAT et al., 1976c; WASI et al., 1978). The cleavage products were demonstrated by acid disc gel electrophoresis and sucrose density gradient ultracentrifugation of radiolabeled C3. The conversion of C3 was also obvious from immunoelectrophoretic analysis. JOHNSON et al. (1976) also demonstrated by immunoelectrophoresis conversion of C3 and C5 upon treatment with the elastase-like enzyme.

H. Plasma Proteinase Inhibitors

The inhibition of the various enzymes of the kinin system was discussed briefly when these enzymes were described. This subheading will be an overview of the properties of the plasma proteinase inhibitors which act on the plasma kinin system. Unlike synthetic and plant inhibitors that are often used in the laboratory, the natural proteinase inhibitors of plasma have in vivo significance since they keep the kinin and related systems in homeostatic balance. Pathologic states usually arise from activation of the kinin system but lack of an inhibitor may also lead to abnormal function and disease states, e.g., angio-edema, due to a lack of $C\bar{1}$-inactivator.

On a weight basis, α_1-antitrypsin and α_2-macroglobulin are in the highest concentration in plasma, but on a molar basis α_1-antitrypsin is by far the most abundant inhibitor. The combining ratios have also to be taken into consideration (HEIMBURGER et al., 1971; HEIMBURGER, 1975).

If plasma is contact-activated most of the kallikrein becomes inactivated by $C\bar{1}$-inactivator, antithrombin III and α_2-macroglobulin, but some remains active. In fact, the α_2-macroglobulin forms complexes with various enzymes in which the active center is not blocked (SHULMAN, 1955; MEYERS and BURDON, 1956; HAVERBACK et al., 1962; JAMES et al., 1966; DYCE et al., 1967). In these complexes the enzymes are "protected" from inhibition by other inhibitors. The catalytic sites of enzymes complexed with α_2-macroglobulin are still capable of acting on small MW substrates and to a lesser degree on higher substrates. The latter are probably excluded by steric hindrance. This type of inhibition is explained by the "trap" mechanism of BARRETT and STARKEY (1973), which requires the attack of α_2-macroglobulin by a proteolytic enzyme resulting in a conformation change entrapping the protease. Although the residual activity is lower than of the original enzyme, the complex has catalytic effect when the α_2-macroglobulin has interacted with either plasmin (HARPEL and MOSESSON, 1973) or kallikrein (VOGT, 1976a, b; VOGT and DUGAL, 1976). The effect of the kallikrein-α_2-macroglobulin complex on kininogen is shown in Fig. 16. Other enzymes inactivated when plasma is contact-activated are plasmin and activated factor XII, both of which are inhibited by the same inhibitors as kallikrein (see Fig. 1).

The mode of action of plasma proteinase inhibitors is not fully understood. A constant feature of the inhibition of trypsin by non-plasma-derived inhibitors (e.g., SBTI or LBTI) is the hydrolysis of a peptide bond (cleavage of a single lysine or arginine residue) located within the disulfide loop of the inhibitor molecule (LASKOWSKI, 1972). From this finding it was postulated that other proteinase inhibitors may have a similar susceptible peptide bond and hydrolysis of the peptide bond may be essential for the enzyme complex formation and the inhibition (LASKOVSKI and SEALOCK, 1971). When proteases interact with the plasma inhibitors the latter undergo cleavage. This has been observed when plasmin or plasma kallikrein interact with α_2-macroglobulin or C$\bar{1}$-inactivator (HARPEL, 1973; HARPEL and COOPER, 1975; HARPEL et al., 1975) and when neutrophil leukocyte protease (elastase) interacts with α_2-macroglobulin or antithrombin III (MOVAT et al., 1976a).

α_1-antitrypsin has little effect on the plasma kinin-system, since it does not inhibit activated factor XII and plasma kallikrein and has little effect on plasmin (HABAL et al., 1976), earlier reports of slow inactivation of kallikrein (FRITZ et al., 1972b), being probably attributable to traces of antithrombin III (BURROWES and MOVAT, 1977). However, α_1-antitrypsin rapidly inactivates neutrophil elastase (OHLSSON, 1971; JANOFF, 1972a; OHLSSON and OLSSON, 1974b; MOVAT et al., 1976a). The antitryptic activity of plasma was first reported in 1894 by FERNI and PERNOSSI. About 90% of the antitryptic activity is confined to the α_1-globulin zone and the bulk of this is due to α_1-antitrypsin. The inhibitor migrates in the α_1-zone by paper, acetate or agarose electrophoresis, but in the albumin region by alkaline disc gel electrophoresis. Its sedimentation coefficient is 3.8 *S*, the diffusion coefficient 5.2, the partial specific volume 0.646, the extinction coefficient 5.3, and the isoelectric point 4.9. It is a glycoprotein, containing 12.2% carbohydrate. Early data indicated a MW of 45,000, but all recent ones obtained by various methods suggest 53,000–54,000 (HERCZ, 1973; LIENER et al., 1973; CROWFORD, 1973; PANNELL et al., 1974; HEIMBURGER, 1975; BURROWES and MOVAT, 1977). Earlier, based on the fact that α_1-antitrypsin forms 1:1 complexes with SBTI and that SBTI binds threefold its weight, an approximate MW of 60,000 was calculated for the inhibitor (VOGEL et al., 1966). The concentration in plasma is 2000–4000 μg/ml (HEIMBURGER, 1975).

α_1-antichymotrypsin has no effect on any of the components of the plasmakinin system but it inhibits cathepsin G, the chymotrypsin-like protease of neutrophils (OHLSSON and ÅKESSON, 1976). Antichymotrypsin has a MW of 69,000, a sedimentation coefficient of 3.9 and a carbohydrate content of 24.6%.

α_2*-macroglobulin*, first isolated by SCHULTZE et al. (1955), has a sedimentation coefficient of 19.6 *S* (BAUMSTARK, 1970) or 18.0 *S* (JONES et al., 1972; HAMBERG et al., 1973), a diffusion coefficient of 2.41, a partial specific volume of 0.735 (HEIMBURGER et al., 1971) and an isoelectric point of 5.3–5.4 (HAMBERG et al., 1973). In the older literature, the MW is cited as 820,000 (SCHULTZE and HEREMANS, 1966), but more recent findings indicate a MW of 725,000 (JONES et al., 1972) or even as low as 650,000 (SAUNDERS et al., 1971). These later findings are in good agreement with the subunit structure of the inhibitor (JONES et al., 1972; HARPEL, 1973). The carbohydrate content is 7.7% (HEIMBURGER, 1975). Its mode of action is described above. The concentration in plasma is 1500–3500 μg/ml in men and 1750–4200 μg/ml in women (HEIMBURGER, 1975).

C$\bar{1}$-inactivator was discovered by RATNOFF and LEPOW (1957) as an inhibitor of the activated first component of complement, as the original designation "C'1 esterase inhibitor" implies. It was purified by PENSKY et al. (1961) and shown later (PENSKY and SCHWICK, 1969) to be identical to the earlier described α_2-neurominoglycoprotein (SCHULTZE et al., 1962). The sedimentation coefficient was estimated to be 3.67 *S* (SCHULTZE et al., 1962; HAUPT et al., 1970) or 4.2 *S* (PENSKY and LEPOW, 1970). The MW of 139,000 by gel filtration (PENSKY and LEPOW, 1970) is too high, presumably due to the high (34.7%) carbohydrate content. The value of 104,000 given by HEIMBURGER (1971, 1975) is in good agreement with data obtained by SDS disc gel electrophoresis (HARPEL and COOPER, 1975; HARPEL et al., 1975). By this method a major band (MW 105,000) and a minor band (MW 96,000) are detected. They show a reaction of identity by immunodiffusion. Reduction and alkylation do not change the MW, indicating a single polypeptide chain. Complexes with plasmin have a MW of 180,000 and 170,000, respectively, but those with plasma kallikrein, although demonstrated with radiolabeled material, have not been determined. As shown in Fig. 1, C$\bar{1}$-inactivator acts on several enzymes of the kinin system.

Antithrombin III is one of the two inhibitors of thrombin; the second one is α_2-macroglobulin (LANCHANTIN et al., 1966; STEINBUCH et al., 1968). Antithrombin activity of human plasma was first observed in 1905 by MORAWITZ. BRINKHOUS et al. in 1939 noted that heparin was effective as an anticoagulant only in the presence of a plasma factor. Later an intimate relationship between the antithrombin activity of plasma and heparin was observed, heparin enhancing up to 100-fold the thrombin neutralizing activity of antithrombin. Recently, purified preparations of antithrombin III have been prepared (ABILDGAARD, 1968; ROSENBERG and DAMUS, 1973; DAMUS and WALLACE, 1974; MILLER-ANDERSON et al., 1974; BURROWES and MOVAT, 1977). HEIMBURGER used $Ca_3 (PO_4)_2$ and ROSENBERG and DAMUS $Al(OH)_3$ to adsorb the antithrombin from plasma. The desorbed antithrombin III was passed by all investigators through a series of chromatographic steps, including affinity chromatography on heparin-Sepharose 4B. ROSENBERG and DAMUS (1973) used isoelectric focusing as the final step to obtain a homogeneous preparation. BURROWES and MOVAT found that α_1-antitrypsin, having a similar charge and MW, cochromatographed with the antithrombin, but could be separated on QAE-Sephadex at pH 7.4. The inhibitor has an α_2-electrophoretic mobility, a sedimentation coefficient of 3.8 *S*, an isoelectric point of 5.1 and a MW of 63,000–65,000. It forms complexes of MW 110,000, 123,000, and 139,000 with plasma kallikrein (VENNERÖD et al., 1976). With plasmin the complex formed has a MW of 142,000 (HIGHSMITH and ROSENBERG, 1974). Complexes with activated factor XII have also been described. Their MW was estimated to be 117,000 (STEAD et al., 1976).

Alpha$_2$-plasmin inhibitor was described recently by three groups of investigators (COLLEN, 1976; MOROI and AOKI, 1976; MÜLLERTZ and CLEMMENSEN, 1976). These studies have subsequently been further extended (WIMAN and COLLEN, 1977; HIGHSMITH et al., 1977; EDY and COLLEN, 1977; MOROI and AOKI, 1977; HARPEL, 1977; AOKI and MOROI, 1978; TEGER-NILSON et al., 1978).

The MW of the inhibitor (often referred to as α_2-antiplasmin or fast inhibitor of plasmin) has been estimated to be about 70,000. It is a single chain polypeptide with an estimated carbohydrate content of 14%. Its sedimentation constant is 3.45 *S*. Its charge and MW indicated that it elutes with other inhibitors (α_1-antitrypsin, antithrombin III). However, affinity chromatography on plasminogen-Sepharose, in addition to other steps, yielded a homogeneous preparation. WIMAN and COLLEN (1977) suggested a procedure in which Cohn fraction I was depleted of plasminogen (lysine-Sepharose), followed by plasminogen-Sepharose and this in turn by DEAE-Sephadex and finally concanavalin A-Sepharose.

The main characteristic of the inhibitor is that it inactivates plasmin instantaneously. The inhibitor has been compared to other known inhibitors of plasmin. HARPEL (1977) reported that when the α_2-antiplasmin was allowed to compete with α_2-macroglobulin, almost as much plasmin was bound to α_2-antiplasmin in mixtures containing a large excess of α_2-macroglobulin (relative to plasmin or α_2-antiplasmin) as was bound in mixtures not containing α_2-macroglobulin. HIGHSMITH et al. (1977) used trace amounts of ^{125}I-labeled plasminogen and studied its distribution amongst the various proteinase inhibitors in whole plasma, after activation to plasmin by urokinase or streptokinase. At 37 °C about 90% of the labeled plasmin was bound to α_2-antiplasmin and about 7% to α_2-macroglobulin. More plasmin was bound to α_2-macroglobulin at 22 °C.

I. Concluding Remarks

The kinin system of blood plasma is complex. The central role is played by factor XII. Through its activation three cascading systems are set into motion: the intrinsic clotting, the fibrinolytic, and the kinin-forming. The three are interrelated not only because factor XII initiates the activation of all three systems, but also because components of one system can interact with components of another. Deficiency of a component of one system affects also the other two. For example, plasmin is the principal enzyme of the fibrinolytic system whose main function is fibrinolysis but it can also act on kininogen to generate kinin. Furthermore, plasmin has a positive feedback; by acting on factor XII it can cause its activation and fragmentation. Prekallikrein is the zymogen of kallikrein (the main kinin-forming enzyme) and exerts a positive feedback on factor XII which is even more significant than that of plasmin. In prekallikrein deficiency, because there is inadequate feedback, there is a clotting abnormality and inadequate intrinsic activation of the fibrinolytic system. In fact, newer data indicate that prekallikrein is probably identical to the plasminogen activator (see Fig. 1).

To date, no physiologic role has been attributed with certainty to kinins. However, they are believed to play a role in pathologic mechanisms. They have been implicated as pharmacologic mediators of the vascular phenomena of acute inflammation and of systemic shock. A direct role of kinins in the inflammatory process has not been demonstrated. However, this is also true of most other mediators. Kinins do fulfill the criteria of a potential pharmacologic mediator (MOVAT, 1978a), i.e., kinins or the precursors leading to their formation are (a) widely distributed in various tissues and in higher species, (b) are readily available and activatable, (c) can induce the vascular phenomena of inflammation when injected, (d) have been isolated from inflammatory lesions and (e) their effect can be suppressed by inhibitors. The final criterion; inhibition of its action by depletion has not been demonstrated adequately.

A number of activators have been listed, which could play a role in vivo. However, potent inhibitors acting at all levels (see Fig. 1) have been described. Therefore, pathologic states could arise from excess activation, which would be only partially counterbalanced by the inhibitors. Alternatively, the homeostatic balance could be tipped by inadequate inhibition. Inhibition can be visualized as inadequate in circumscribed areas. It is therefore possible that in inflammation, enzymes with kininogenase activity, derived from neutrophils, play an essential role.

All these questions remain unanswered and all the knowledge acquired from in vitro studies should be applied to in vivo experiments in order to ascertain the possible role of the kinin system in physiologic or pathophysiologic conditions.

References

Abelous, J. E., Bradier, E.: Action hypertensive de l'urine humaine normale. C.R. Soc. Biol. (Paris) *66*, 511 (1909)

Abildgaard, U.: Highly purified antithrombin 3 with heparin cofactor activity prepared by disc electrophoresis. Scand. J. Clin. Lab. Invest. *21*, 89 (1968)

Andreenko, G. V., Suvorov, A. V.: Effect of plasmin on kallikreinogen. Biochemistry (Biokhimia) *41*, 460 (1976)

Aoki, N., Moroi, M., Tachiya, K.: Effects of α_2-plasmin inhibitor on fibrin clot lysis. Its comparison with α_2-macroglobulin. Thromb. Haemost. *39*, 22–31 (1978)

Ardelt, W., Tomczak, Z., Ksiezny, S., Dudeh-Wojciechowska, G.: Neutral elastolytic proteinase from canine leukocytes, purification, and characterization. Biochim. Biophys. Acta. *445*, 683 (1976)

Armstrong, D.: The effects of temperature on the response of human plasma kinin-forming system to promoting and inhibiting agents. Br. J. Pharmacol. *34*, 670 (1968)

Armstrong, D., Jepson, J. B., Keele, C. A., Stewart, J. W.: Activation by glass of pharmacologically active agents in blood of various species. J. Physiol. (Lond.) *129*, 80 (1955)

Armstrong, D., Jepson, J. B., Keele, C. A., Stewart, J. W.: Pain producing substance in human inflammatory exudates and plasma. J. Physiol. (Lond.) *135*, 350 (1957)

Armstrong, D., Mills, G. L., Stewart, J. W.: Thermally-induced effects on the kinin-forming system of native human plasma, 37 °–0 °C and 37 °–50 °C. In: International symposium on vaso-active polypeptides: bradykinin and related kinins. Rocha e Silva, M., Rothschild, H. A. (eds.), p. 167. Sao Paulo: Soc. Bras. Farmacol. Ther. Exp. 1967

Armstrong, D. A. J., Stewart, J. W.: Anti-heparin agents as inhibitors of plasmin kinin formation. Nature *196*, 689 (1962)

Arnon, R.: Antibodies to enzymes – a tool in the study of antigenic specificity determinants. Curr. Top. Microbiol. Immunol. *54*, 47 (1971)

Austen, K. F.: Reaction mechanisms in the release of mediators of immediate hypersensitivity from human lung tissue. Fed. Proc. *33*, 2256 (1974)

Austen, K.F., Wasserman, S.I., Goetz, E.J.: Mast cell-derived mediators: structural and functional diversity and regulation of expression. In: Molecular and biological aspects of the acute allergic reactions. Nobel Foundation Symposium 33. Johansson, S.G.O., Strandberg, K., Uvnäs, B. (eds.), p. 293. New York, London: Plenum Press 1976

Back, N., Steger, R.: Activation of bovine bradykininogen by human plasma. Life Sci. *4*, 153 (1965)

Bagdasarian, A., Talamo, R.C., Colman, R.W.: Isolation of high molecular weight activators of human plasma kallikrein. J. Biol. Chem. *248*, 3456 (1973a)

Bagdasarian, A., Lahiri, B., Colman, R.W.: Origin of the high molecular weight activator of prekallikrein. J. Biol. Chem. *248*, 7742 (1973b)

Bainton, D.F., Ullyot, J.L., Farquhar, M.G.: The development of neutrophilic polymorphonuclear leukocytes in human bone marrow. J. Exp. Med. *134*, 907 (1971)

Barrett, A.J.: Lysosomal and related proteinases. In: Proteases and biological control. Reich, E., Rifkin, D.B., Shaw, E. (eds.), p. 467. Cold Spring Harbor Laboratory 1975

Barrett, A.J., Starkey, P.M.: The interaction of α_2-macroglobulin with proteinases. Biochem. J. *133*, 709 (1973)

Baugh, R.J., Travis, J.: Human leukocyte granule elastase: rapid isolation and characterization. Biochemistry *15*, 836 (1976)

Baumstark, J.S.: Studies on the elastase-serum protein interaction. II. On the digestion of human α_2-macroglobulin, an elastase inhibitor by elastase. Biochim. Biophys. Acta *207*, 318 (1970)

Becker, E.L.: Inactivation of Hageman factor by diisopropylfluorophosphate (DFP). J. Lab. Clin. Med. *56*, 136 (1960)

Becker, E.L., Kagen, L.: The permeability globulins of human serum and the biochemical mechanism of hereditary angioneurotic edema. N.Y. Acad. Sci. *116*, 866 (1964)

Bhoola, K.D., Calle, E.J.D., Schachter, M.: The effect of bradykinin, serum kallikrein and other endogenous substances on capillary permeability in the guinea pig. J. Physiol. (Lond.) *152*, 75 (1960)

Bodamer, G., Vogt, W.: Beeinflussung der Capillarpermeabilität in der Meerschweinchenhaut durch Anaphylatoxin (AT). Naunyn Schmiedebergs Arch. Pharmacol. *266*, 255 (1970a)

Bodamer, G., Vogt, W.: Contraction of the guinea-pig ileum induced by anaphylatoxin independent of histamine release. Int. Arch. Allergy *39*, 648 (1970b)

Boissonnas, R.A., Guttmann, St., Jaquenod, P.-A.: Synthèse de la L-arginyl-L-propyl-glycyl-L-phenylalanyl-L-seryl-L-propyl-L-phenylalanyl-L-arginine, une nonapeptide présentant les properiétés de la bradykinine. Helv. Chim. Acta *43*, 1349 (1960)

Bouma, B.N., Griffin, J.H.: Human blood coagulation factor XI. Purification, properties, and mechanism of activation by activated factor XII. J. Biol. Chem. *252*, 432 (1977)

Bretz, U., Baggiolini, M.: Biochemical and morphological characterization of azurophil and specific granules of human neutrophilic polymorphonuclear leukocytes. J. Cell Biol. *63*, 251 (1974)

Brinkhaus, K., Smith, H.P., Warner, E.D., Seegers, W.H.: Inhibition of blood-clotting: unidentified substance which acts in conjunction with heparin to prevent conversion of prothrombin into thrombin. Am. J. Physiol. *125*, 683 (1939)

Brocklehurst, W.E., Mawr, G.E.: The purification of a kininogen from human plasma. Br. J. Pharmacol. *27*, 256 (1966)

Buluk, K., Malofiejew, M.: Urokinase-induced activation of kallikreinogen and the release of plasma kinins in renal blood. Acta Med. Pol. *6*, 405 (1965)

Burrowes, C.E., Movat, H.Z.: Isolation of human antithrombin III – its separation from α_1-antitrypsin. Biochem. Biophys. Res. Commun. *74*, 140 (1977)

Burrowes, C.E., Movat, H.Z., Soltay, M.J.: The kinin system of human plasma. IV. The action of plasmin. Proc. Soc. Exp. Biol. Med. *138*, 959 (1971)

Burrowes, C.E., Movat, H.Z., Soltay, M.J.: The role of plasmin in the activation of the kininsystem. In: Vasopeptides, chemistry, pharmacology, and pathophysiology. Back, N., Sicuteri, F. (eds.), p. 129. New York, London: Plenum Press 1972

Burrowes, C.E., Movat, H.Z., Habal, F.M.: unpublished observations (1973)

Burrowes, C.E., Habal, F.M., Movat, H.Z.: Inhibition of human plasma kallikrein by antithrombin III. Thromb. Res. *7*, 175 (1975)

Chan, J.Y.C.: Studies on factor XII (Hageman factor). Dissertation, University of Toronto 1975

Chan, J.Y.C., Movat, H.Z.: Purification of factor XII (Hageman factor) from human plasma. Thromb. Res. *8*, 337 (1976)
Chan, J.Y.C., Habal, F.M., Burrowes, C.E., Movat, H.Z.: Interaction between factor XII (Hageman factor), high molecular weight kininogen and prekallikrein. Thromb. Res. *9*, 423 (1976)
Chan, J.Y.C., Burrowes, C.E., Habal, F.M., Movat, H.Z.: The inhibition of activated factor XII (Hageman factor) by antithrombin III; the effect of other plasma proteinase inhibitors. Biochem. Biophys. Res. Commun. *74*, 150 (1977a)
Chan, J.Y.C., Burrowes, C.E., Movat, H.Z.: Activation of factor XII (Hageman factor): enhancing effect of a potentiator. Thromb. Res. *10*, 309 (1977b)
Chan, J.Y.C., Burrowes, C.E., Movat, H.Z.: Surface activation of factor XII (Hageman factor) – Critical role of high molecular weight kininogen and another potentiator. Agents Actions (1978)
Chang, J., Freer, R., Stella, R., Greenbaum, L.M.: Studies on the formation, partial amino acid sequence chemical properties of leukokinins M and PMN. Biochem. Pharmacol. *21*, 3107 (1972)
Cinader, B.: Antibodies to enzymes – a discussion of the mechanism of inhibition and activation. In: Antibodies to biologically active molecules. Cinader, B. (ed.), Vol. 1, p. 85. New York: Pergamon Press 1965
Cochrane, C.G., Wuepper, K.D.: The kinin-forming system: delineation and activation. In: Immunopathology. Miescher, P. (ed.), Vol. VI, p. 222. Basel, Stuttgart: Schwabe 1971a
Cochrane, C.G., Wuepper, K.D.: The first component of the kinin-forming system in human and rabbit plasma. Its relationship to clotting factor XII (Hageman factor). J. Exp. Med. *134*, 986 (1971b)
Cochrane, C.G., Revak, S.D., Aikin, B.S., Wuepper, K.D.: The structural characterization and activation of Hageman factor. In: Inflammation, mechanisms and control. Lepow, I.H., Ward, P.A. (eds.), p. 119. New York, London: Academic Press 1972a
Cochrane, C.G., Wuepper, K.D., Aikin, B.S., Revak, S.D., Spiegelberg, H.L.: The interaction of Hageman factor with immune complexes. J. Clin. Invest. *51*, 2736 (1972b)
Cochrane, C.G., Revak, S.D., Wuepper, K.D.: Activation of Hageman factor in solid and fluid phases. A critical role of kallikrein. J. Exp. Med. *138*, 1564 (1973)
Cochrane, C.G., Revak, S.D., Ulevitch, R., Johnston, A., Morrison, D.: Hageman factor: characterization and mechanism of action. In: Chemistry and biology of the kallikrein-kinin system in health and disease. Fogarty Internat. Center Proc. No. 27. Pisano, J.J., Austen, K.F. (eds.), p. 17. Washington: U.S. Gov. Printing Office 1977
Colman, R.W.: Activation of plasminogen by plasma kallikrein. Biochem. Biophys. Res. Commun. *35*, 273 (1969)
Colman, R.W., Mattler, L., Sherry, S.: Studies on the prekallikrein (kallikreinogen)-kallikrein enzyme system of human plasma. I. Isolation and purification of plasma kallikrein. J. Clin. Invest. *48*, 11 (1969)
Colman, R.W., Bagdasarian, A., Talamo, R.C., Scott, C.F., Seavey, M., Guimarães, J.A., Pierce, J.V., Kaplan, A.P.: Williams trait. Human kininogen deficiency with diminished levels of plasminogen proactivator and prekallikrein associated with abnormalities of the Hageman factor-dependent pathways. J. Clin. Invest. *56*, 1650 (1975)
Colman, R.W., Bagdasarian, A., Talamo, R.C., Kaplan, A.P.: Williams trait: a new deficiency with abnormal levels of prekallikrein, plasminogen proactivator, and kininogen. In: Chemistry and biology of the kallikrein-kinin system in health and disease. Fogarty Internat. Center Proc. No. 27. Pisano, J.J., Austen, K.F. (eds.), p. 65. Washington: U.S. Gov. Printing Office 1977
Crowford, I.P.: Purification and properties of normal human α_1-antitrypsin. Arch. Biochem. Biophys. *156*, 215 (1973)
Damus, P.S., Wallace, G.A.: Purification of canine antithrombin III – heparin cofactor using affinity chromatography. Biochem. Biophys. Res. Comm. *61*, 1147 (1974)
Davies, G.E., Lowe, J.S.: A permeability factor released from guinea pig serum by antigen-antibody precipitates. Br. J. Exp. Pathol. *41*, 335 (1960)
Davies, G.E., Lowe, J.S.: Further studies on a permeability factor released from guinea pig serum by antigen-antibody precipitations. Relationship to serum complement. Int. Arch. Allergy *20*, 235 (1962)

Davies, P., Rita, G., Krakauer, K., Weissmann, G.: Characterization of a neutral protease from lysosomes of rabbit polymorphonuclear leucocytes. Biochem. J. *123*, 559 (1971)
Davies, P., Fox, R.I., Polyonis, M., Allison, A.C., Haswell, A.D.: The inhibition of phagocytosis and facilitation of exocytosis in rabbit polymorphonuclear leukocytes by cytochalasin B. Lab. Invest. *28*, 16 (1973)
Delshammar, M., Ohlsson, K.: Isolation and partial characterization of elastase from dog granulocytes. Eur. J. Biochem. *69*, 125 (1976)
Deutsch, D.G., Mertz, E.T.: Plasminogen: purification from human plasma by affinity chromatography. Science *170*, 1095 (1970)
Dewald, B., Rindler-Ludwig, R., Bretz, U., Baggiolini, M.: Subcellular localization and heterogeneity of neutral proteases in neutrophilic polymorphonuclear leukocytes. J. Exp. Med. *141*, 709 (1975)
Donaldson, V.H., Ratnoff, O.D.: Hageman factor: alterations in physical properties during activation. Science *150*, 754 (1965)
Donaldson, V.H., Glueck, H.I., Miller, M.A., Habal, F.M., Movat, H.Z.: Kininogen deficiency in Fitzgerald trait: role of high molecular weight kininogen in clotting and fibrinolysis. J. Lab. Clin. Med. *87*, 327 (1976)
Dubin, A., Koj, A., Chudzik, J.: Isolation and some molecular parameters of elastase-like neutral proteinase from horse blood leucocytes. Biochem. J. *153*, 389 (1976)
Dyce, B.J., Wong, T., Adham, N., Mehl, J., Haveback, B.J.: Human plasma kallikrein esterase associated with alpha-2-macroglobulin binding protein. Clin. Res. *15*, 101 (Abstract) (1967)
Edy, J., Collen, D.: The interaction in human plasma of antiplasmin, the fast-reacting inhibitor, with plasmin, thrombin, trypsin, and chymotrypsin. Biochim. Biophys. Acta *484*, 423 (1977)
Eisen, V.: Kinin formation and fibrinolysis in human plasma. J. Physiol. (Lond.) *166*, 514 (1963)
Eisen, V.: Effect of hexadimethrine bromide on plasma kinin formation, hydrolysis of p-tosyl-L-arginine methyl ester and fibrinolysis. Br. J. Pharmacol. *22*, 87 (1964)
Eisen, V., Glanville, K.L.A.: Separation of kinin-forming factors in human plasma. Br. J. Exp. Pathol. *50*, 427 (1969)
Eisen, V., Smith, H.G.: Plasma kinin formation by complexes of aggregated γ-globulin and serum proteins. Br. J. Exp. Pathol. *51*, 328 (1970)
Eisen, V., Vogt, W.: Plasma kininogenases and their activators. In: Handbook of experimental pharmacology. Erdös, E.G. (ed.), Vol. XXV, p. 82. Berlin, Heidelberg, New York: Springer 1970
Elliott, D.F., Lewis, G.P.: Methionyl-lysyl-bradykinin, a new kinin from ox blood. Biochem. J. *95*, 437 (1965)
Erdös, E.G., Yang, H.Y.T.: Kininases. In: Handbook of experimental pharmacology. Erdös, E.G. (ed.), Vol. XXV, p. 289. Berlin, Heidelberg, New York: Springer 1970
Erdös, E.G., Nakajima, T., Oshima, G., Gecse, A., Kato, J.: Kininases and their interactions with other systems. In: Chemistry and biology of the kallikrein-kinin system in health and disease. Fogarty Internat. Center Proc. No. 27. Pisano, J.J., Austen, K.F. (eds.), p. 27. Washington; U.S. Gov. Printing Office 1977
Ergova, T.P., Rossinskaya, E.G., Pashkina, T.S.: Purification and properties of high molecular-weight rabbit kininogen. Biokhimia *41*, 1052 (1976)
Feinstein, G., Janoff, A.: A rapid method of purification of human granulocyte cationic neutral proteases: purification and characterization of human granulocyte chymotrypsin-like enzyme. Biochim. Biophys. Acta *403*, 477 (1975a)
Feinstein, G., Janoff, A.: A rapid method of purification of human granulocyte cationic neutral proteases: purification and further characterization of human granulocyte elastase. Biochim. Biophys. Acta *403*, 493 (1975b)
Ferni, C., Pernossi, L.: Über die Enzyme. Z. Hyg. *18*, 83 (1894)
Folds, J.D., Welsh, I.R.H., Spitznagel, J.K.: Neutral proteases confined to one class of lysosomes of human polymorphonuclear leukocytes. Proc. Soc. Exp. Biol. Med. *139*, 461 (1972)
Forbes, O.D., Pensky, J., Ratnoff, O.D.: Inhibition of activated Hageman factor and activated plasma thromboplastin antecedent by purified $C\bar{1}$ inactivator. J. Lab. Clin. Med. *76*, 809 (1970)
Frair, B.D., Saito, S., Ratnoff, O.D., Rippon, W.B.: Detection by fluorescence of structural changes accompanying the activation of Hageman factor (factor XII). Proc. Soc. Exp. Biol. Med. *155*, 199 (1977)

Frey, E.K., Kraut, H.: Ein neues Kreislaufhormon und seine Wirkung. Arch. Exp. Pathol. Pharmakol. *133*, 1 (1928)
Fritz, H., Wunderer, G., Dittmann, B.: Zur Isolierung von Schweine- und Human-Serumkallikrein durch Affinitätschromatographie. Hoppe Seylers Z. Physiol. Chem. *353*, 893 (1972a)
Fritz, H., Wunderer, G., Kummer, K., Heimburger, N., Werle, E.: α_1-Antitrypsin und C$\bar{1}$-Inaktivator: Progressiv-Inhibitoren für Serumkallikrein von Mensch und Schwein. Hoppe Seylers Z. Physiol. Chem. *353*, 906 (1972b)
Fujikawa, K., Walsh, K.A., Davie, E.W.: Isolation and characterization of bovine factor XII (Hageman factor). Biochemistry *16*, 2270–2278 (1977)
Gapanhuk, E., Henriques, O.B.: Kinins released from horse heat-acid-denatured plasma by plasmin, plasma kallikrein, trypsin, and botrops kininogenase. Biochem. Pharmacol. *19*, 1091 (1970)
Gerber, A., Carsen, J.H., Hadorn, B.: Partial purification and characterization of a chymotrypsin-like enzyme from human neutrophil leucocytes. Biochim. Biophys. Acta *364*, 103 (1974)
Gigli, I., Mason, J.W., Colman, R.W., Austen, K.F.: Interaction of plasma kallikrein with C$\bar{1}$-inactivator. J. Immunol. *104*, 574 (1970)
Graham, R.C., Ebert, R.H., Ratnoff, O.D., Moses, J.M.: Pathogenesis of inflammation II. In vivo observations on the inflammatory effect of activated Hageman factor and bradykinin. J. Exp. Med. *121*, 807 (1965)
Grammens, G.L., Prasad, A.S., Mammen, E.F., Barnhard, M.I.: Physico-chemical and immunological properties of bovine Hageman factor. Thromb. Diath. Haemorrh. *25*, 405 (1970)
Granelli-Piperno, A.G., Vassalli, J.-D., Reich, E.: Secretion of plasminogen activator by human polynuclear leukocytes. Modulation by glucocorticoids and other factors. J. Exp. Med. *146*, 1693 (1977)
Greenbaum, L.M.: Leukocyte kininogenases and leukokinins from normal and malignant cells. Am. J. Pathol. *68*, 613 (1972)
Greenbaum, L.M.: Leukokinins and cellular kininogenases. In: Chemistry and biology of the kallikrein-kinin system in health and disease. Fogarty Internat. Center Proc. No. 27. Pisano, J.J., Austen, K.F. (eds.), p. 455. Washington: U.S. Gov. Printing Office 1977
Greenbaum, L.M., Kim, K.S.: The kinin-forming activities of rabbit polymorphonuclear leucocytes. Br. J. Pharmacol. *29*, 238 (1967)
Greenbaum, L.M., Prakash, A., Semente, G., Johnston, M.: The leukokinin system; its role in fluid accumulation in malignancy and inflammation. Agents Actions *3*, 332 (1973)
Griffin, J.H.: Molecular mechanism of surface-dependent activation of Hageman factor. (HF) (coagulation factor XII). Fed. Proc. *36*, 329 (Abstract) (1977)
Griffin, J.H., Cochrane, C.G.: Human factor XII (Hageman factor). In: Methods in enzymology. Vol. XXV/B: Proteolytic enzymes. Lorand, L. (ed.), p. 56. New York: Academic Press 1976a
Griffin, J.H., Cochrane, C.G.: Mechanisms for the involvement of high molecular weight kininogen in surface-dependent reactions of Hageman factor. Proc. Natl. Acad. Sci. (USA) *73*, 2554 (1976b)
Griffin, J.H., Revak, S.D., Cochrane, C.G.: The Hageman factor system: mechanism of contact activation. In: Molecular and biological aspects of the acute allergic reactions. Nobel Foundation Symposium 33. Johansson, S.G.O., Strandberg, K., Uvnäs, B. (eds.), p. 371. New York, London: Plenum Press 1976
Grob, D.: Proteolytic enzymes. III. Further studies on protein polypeptide, and other inhibitors of serum proteinase, leucoproteinase, trypsin, and papain. J. Gen. Physiol. *33*, 103 (1949)
Habal, F.M.: The kinin system. Isolation of human plasma kininogens, their separation from proteinase inhibitors and their interaction with kininogenases. Dissertation. University of Toronto 1975
Habal, F.M., Burrowes, C.E., Movat, H.Z.: Generation of kinin by plasma kallikrein and plasmin and the effect of α_1-antitrypsin and antithrombin III on the kininogenases. In: Kinins, pharmacodynamics and biological role. Sicuteri, F., Back, N., Haberland, G.L. (eds.), p. 23. New York, London: Plenum Press 1976
Habal, F.M., Movat, H.Z.: Kininogens of human plasma. Res. Commun. Chem. Pathol. Pharmacol. *4*, 477 (1972)
Habal, F.M., Movat, H.Z.: Kininogens of human plasma. Semin. Thromb. Haemostas. *3*, 27 (1976a)

Habal, F.M., Movat, H.Z.: Rapid purification of high molecular weight kininogen. Agents Actions *6*, 565 (1976b)
Habal, F.M., Movat, H.Z.: Some physicochemical and functional differences between low and high molecular weight kininogens of human plasma. In: Chemistry and biology of the kallikrein-kinin system in health and disease. Fogarty Internat. Center Proc. No. 27. Pisano, J.J., Austen, K.F. (eds.), p. 129. Washington: U.S. Gov. Printing Office 1977
Habal, F.M., Movat, H.Z., Burrowes, C.E.: Isolation of two functionally different kininogens from human plasma – separation from proteinase inhibitors and interaction with plasma kallikrein. Biochem. Pharmacol. *23*, 2291 (1974)
Habal, F.M., Underdown, B.J., Movat, H.Z.: Further characterization of human plasma kininogens. Biochem. Pharmacol. *24*, 1241 (1975)
Habermann, E.: Über pH-bedingte Modifikationen des kininliefernden α-Globulins (Kininogen) aus Rinderserum und das Molekulargewicht von Kininogen I. Biochem. Z. *337*, 440 (1963)
Habermann, E.: Kininogens. In: Handbook of experimental pharmacology. Erdös, E.G. (ed.), Vol. XXV, p. 250. Berlin, Heidelberg, New York: Springer 1970
Habermann, E., Blennemann, G.: Über Substrate und Reaktionsprodukte der kininbildenden Enzyme Trypsin, Serum- und Pankreaskallikrein sowie von Crolalusgift. Naunyn Schmiedebergs Arch. Exerc. Pathol. Pharmacol. *249*, 357 (1964)
Habermann, E., Klett, W.: Reinigung und einige Eigenschaften eines Kallikreins aus Rinderblut. Biochem. Z. *346*, 133 (1966)
Habermann, E., Rosenbusch, G.: Reinigung und Spaltung von Kininogen aus Rinderblut. Naunyn Schmiedebergs Arch. Exp. Pathol. Pharmacol. *243*, 357 (1962)
Habermann, E., Rosenbusch, G.: Partielle Reinigung und einige Eigenschaften eines Kininogens aus Rinderblut. Hoppe Seylers Z. Physiol. Chem. *332*, 121 (1963)
Hamberg, U.: Plasma protease and kinin release with special reference to plasmin. Ann. N.Y. Acad. Sci. *146*, 517 (1968)
Hamberg, U., Elg, P., Nissinen, E., Stelwagen, P.: Purification and heterogeneity of human kininogen. Use of DEAE-chromatography, molecular sieving and antibody specific immunoabsorbents. Int. J. Pept. Protein Res. *7*, 261 (1975)
Hamberg, U., Stelwagen, P., Ervast, H.S.: Human α_2-macroglobulin, characterization and trypsin binding. Purification methods, trypsin and plasmin complex formation. Eur. J. Biochem. *40*, 439 (1973)
Han, Y.N., Komiya, M., Kato, H., Iwanaga, S., Suzuki, T.: Primary structure of bovine high molecular weight kininogen: chemical composition of kinin-free kininogen and peptide fragments released by plasma kallikrein. F.E.B.S. Lett. *57*, 254 (1975a)
Han, Y.N., Komiya, M., Iwanaga, S., Suzuki, T.: Studies on the primary structure of bovine high-molecular weight kininogen. Amino acid sequence of a fragment ("histidine-rich peptide") released by plasma kallikrein. J. Biochem. (Tokyo) *77*, 55 (1975b)
Han, Y.N., Kato, H., Iwanaga, S., Suzuki, T.: Bovine high molecular weight kininogen: the amino acid sequence of fragment 1 (glycopeptide) released by the action of plasma kallikrein and its location in the precursor protein. F.E.B.S. Lett. *63*, 197 (1976a)
Han, Y.H., Kato, H., Iwanaga, S.: Identification of Ser-Leu-Meth-Lys-bradykinin isolated from chemically modified high molecular-weight bovine kininogen. F.E.B.S. Lett. *71*, 45 (1976b)
Han, Y.N., Kato, H., Iwanaga, S., Suzuki, T.: Primary structure of bovine plasma high-molecular weight kininogen. The amino acid sequence of a glycopeptide (fragment 1) following the C-terminus of the bradykinin moiety. J. Biochem. (Tokyo) *79*, 1201 (1976c)
Harpel, P.C.: C$\bar{1}$-inactivator inhibition by plasmin. J. Clin. Invest. *49*, 568 (1970a)
Harpel, P.C.: Human plasma alpha 2-macroglobulin. An inhibitor of plasma kallikrein. J. Exp. Med. *132*, 329 (1970b)
Harpel, P.C.: Studies on the interaction between collagen and a plasma kallikrein-like activity. Evidence for a surface-active enzyme system. J. Clin. Invest. *51*, 1813 (1972)
Harpel, P.C.: Studies on human plasma α_2-macroglobulin-enzyme interactions. Evidence for proteolytic modification of the subunit chain structure. J. Exp. Med. *138*, 508 (1973)
Harpel, P.C.: Circulating inhibitors of human plasma, kallikrein. In: Chemistry and biology of the kallikrein-kinin system in health and disease. Fogarty Internat. Center Proc. No. 27. Pisano, J.J., Austen, K.F. (eds.), p. 169. Washington: U.S. Gov. Printing Office 1977
Harpel, P.C.: Plasmin inhibitor interactions. The effectiveness of α_2-plasmin inhibitor in the presence of α_2-macroglobulin. J. Exp. Med. *146*, 1033–1040 (1977)

Harpel, P.C., Cooper, N.R.: Studies on human plasma C$\bar{1}$-inactivator-enzyme interactions. I. Mechanisms of interaction with C$1\bar{s}$, plasmin and trypsin. J. Clin. Invest. *55*, 593 (1975)
Harpel, P.C., Mosesson, M.W.: Degradation of human fibrinogen by plasma α_2-macroglobulin-enzyme complexes. J. Clin. Invest. *52*, 2175 (1973)
Harpel, P.C., Mosesson, M.W., Cooper, N.R.: Studies on the structure and function of α_2-macroglobulin and C$\bar{1}$-inactivator. In: Proteases and biological control. Reich, E., Rifkin, D.B., Shaw, E. (eds.), p. 387. Cold Spring Harbor Laboratory 1975
Hathaway, W.E., Alsever, J.: The relation of "Fletcher factor" to factors XI and XII. Br. J. Haematol. *18*, 161 (1970)
Hathaway, W.E., Belhasen, L.P., Hathaway, H.S.: Evidence for a new plasma thrombplastin factor. I. Case report, coagulation studies and physicochemical properties. Blood *26*, 521 (1965)
Hattersley, P.G., Hayse, D.: Fletcher factor deficiency: a report of three unrelated cases. Br. J. Haematol. *18*, 411 (1970)
Haustein, K.O., Marquardt, F.: Untersuchungen über die Gerinnungs- und Fibrinolysevorgänge im menschlichen Blut. Acta Biol. Ger. *16*, 658 (1966)
Haverback, B.J., Dyce, B., Bundy, H.F., Wirtschafter, S.K., Edmondson, H.A.: Protein binding of pancreatic proteolytic enzymes. J. Clin. Invest. *41*, 972 (1962)
Hawkins, D.: Biopolymer membrane. A model system for the study of the neutrophilic leukocyte response to immune complexes. J. Immunol. *107*, 344 (1971)
Hawkins, D.: Neutrophilic leukocytes in immunologic reactions in vitro. Effect of cytochalasin B. J. Immunol. *110*, 294 (1973)
Hawkins, D.: Neutrophilic leukocytes in immunologic reactions in vitro. III. Pharmacologic modulation of lysosomal constituent release. Clin. Immunol. Immunopathol. *2*, 141 (1974)
Heck, L.W., Kaplan, A.P.: Substrates of Hageman factor. I. Isolation and characterization of human factor XI (PTA) and inhibition of the activated enzyme by α_1-antitrypsin. J. Exp. Med. *140*, 1615 (1974)
Heimburger, N.: Proteinase inhibitors of human plasma – their properties and control function. In: Proteases and biological control. Reich, E., Rifkin, D.B., Shaw, E. (eds.), p. 367. Cold Spring Harbor Laboratory 1975
Heimburger, N., Haupt, H., Schwick, H.G.: Proteinase inhibitors of human plasma. In: Proceedings of the international research conference on proteinase inhibitors. Fritz, H., Tschesche, H. (eds.), p. 1. Berlin, New York: Walter de Gruyter 1971
Henriques, O.B., Kawritscheva, N., Kuznetsova, V., Astraken, M.: Substrates of kinin-releasing enzymes isolated from horse plasma. Nature *215*, 1200 (1967)
Henson, P.M.: The immunologic release of constituents from neutrophil leukocytes. I. The role of antibody and complement on nonphagocytosable surfaces or phagocytosable particles. J. Immunol. *107*, 1535 (1971 a)
Henson, P.M.: The immunologic release of constituents from neutrophil leukocytes. II. The mechanism or release during phagocytosis and adherence to nonphagocytosable surfaces. J. Immunol. *107*, 1547 (1971 b)
Henson, P.M., Oades, Z.G.: Enhancement of immunologically induced granule exocytosis from neutrophils by cytochalasin B. J. Immunol. *110*, 290 (1973)
Hercz, A.: The inhibition of proteinases by human α_1-antitrypsin. Eur. J. Biochem. *49*, 287 (1973)
Highsmith, R.F., Rosenberg, R.D.: The inhibition of plasmin by human antithrombin-heparin cofactor. J. Biol. Chem. *249*, 4335 (1974)
Highsmith, R.F., Weirich, C.J., Burnett, C.J.: Protease inhibitors of human plasmin: interaction in a whole plasma system. Biochem. Biophys. Res. Commun. *79*, 648–656 (1977)
Iatridis, S.G., Ferguson, J.H.: Effect of surface and Hageman factor on the endogenous or spontaneous activation of the fibrinolytic system. Thromb. Diath. Haemorrh. *6*, 411 (1961)
Iatridis, S.G., Ferguson, J.H.: Active Hageman factor: a plasma lysokinase of the human fibrinolytic system. J. Clin. Invest. *41*, 1277 (1962)
Ignarro, L.J., Oronsky, A.L., Perper, R.J.: Breakdown of noncollagenous chondromucoprotein matrix by leukocyte lysosome granule lysates from guinea pig, rabbit, and human. Clin. Immunol. Immunopathol. *2*, 36 (1973)
Ignarro, L.J., Flint, T.F., George, W.J.: Hormonal control of lysosomal enzyme release from human neutrophils. Effects of autonomic agents on enzyme release, phagocytosis, and cyclic nucleotide levels. J. Exp. Med. *139*, 1395 (1974)

Iwanaga, S.: Personal communication (1977)
Iwanaga, S., Komiya, M., Han, Y.N., Suzuki, T.: Amino acid sequence and biological activity of a histidine-rich peptide released from high molecular weight bovine kininogen by plasma kallikrein. In: Chemistry and biology of the kallikrein-kinin system in health and disease. Fogarty Internat. Center Proc. No. 27. Pisano, J.J., Austen, K.F. (eds.), p. 145. Washington; U.S. Gov. Printing Office 1977
Jacobsen, S.: Substrates for plasma kinin-forming enzymes in human, dog, and rabbit plasma. Br. J. Pharmacol. *26*, 403 (1966a)
Jacobsen, S.: Substrates for plasma kinin-forming enzymes in rat and guinea pig plasma. Br. J. Pharmacol. *28*, 64 (1966b)
Jacobsen, S., Kriz, M.: Some data on two purified kininogens from human plasma. Br. J. Pharmacol. *29*, 25 (1967)
James, K., Taylor, F.B., Jr., Fudenberg, H.H.: Trypsin stabilizers in human serum. The role of α_2-macroglobulin. Clin. Chim. Acta *13*, 359 (1966)
Janoff, A.: Mediators of tissue damage in leukocyte lysosomes. X. Further studies on human granulocyte elastase. Lab. Invest. *22*, 228 (1970)
Janoff, A.: Human granulocyte elastase. Am. J. Pathol. *68*, 579 (1972a)
Janoff, A.: Neutrophil proteases in inflammation. Annu. Rev. Med. *23*, 177 (1972b)
Janoff, A.: Purification of human granulocyte elastase by affinity chromatography. Lab. Invest. *29*, 458 (1973)
Janoff, A., Blondin, J.: Depletion of cartilage matrix by a neutral protease fraction of human leukocyte lysosomes. Proc. Soc. Exp. Biol. Med. *135*, 302 (1970)
Janoff, A., Scherer, J.: Mediators of inflammation in leukocyte lysosomes. IX. Elastinolytic activity in granules of human polymorphonuclear leukocytes. J. Exp. Med. *128*, 1137 (1968)
Janoff, A., Feinstein, G., Malemud, C.J., Elias, J.M.: Degradation of cartilage proteoglycan by human leukocyte granule neutral proteases – a model of joint injury. J. Clin. Invest. *57*, 615 (1976)
Johnson, U., Ohlsson, K., Olsson, I.: Effect of granulocyte neutral proteases on complement components. Scand. J. Immunol. *5*, 421 (1976)
Johnston, A.R., Cochrane, C.G., Revak, S.D.: The relationship between Pf/dil and activated Hageman factor. J. Immunol. *113*, 103 (1974)
Jones, J.M., Creeth, J.M., Kekwick, R.A.: Thiol reduction of human α_2-macroglobulin. The subunit structure. Biochem. J. *127*, 187 (1972)
Kagen, L.J., Leddy, J.S., Becker, E.L.: The presence of two permeability globulins in human serum. J. Clin. Invest. *42*, 1353 (1963)
Kaplan, A.P.: Personal communication (1977)
Kaplan, A.P., Austen, K.F.: A prealbumin activator of prekallikrein. J. Immunol. *105*, 802 (1970)
Kaplan, A.P., Austen, K.F.: A prealbumin activator of prekallikrein. II. Derivation of activators of prekallikrein from active Hageman factor by digestion with plasmin. J. Exp. Med. *133*, 696 (1971)
Kaplan, A.P., Austen, K.F.: The fibrinolytic pathway of human plasma. Isolation and characterization of the plasminogen proactivator. J. Exp. Med. *136*, 1378 (1972)
Kaplan, A.P., Spragg, J., Austen, K.F.: The bradykinin-forming pathway in human plasma. In: Biochemistry of the acute allergic reaction. Austen, K.F., Becker, E.L. (eds.), p. 279. Oxford: Blackwell 1971
Kaplan, A.P., Kay, A.B., Austen, K.F.: A prealbumin activator of prekallikrein. III. Appearance of chemotactic activity for human neutrophils by conversion of human prekallikrein and kallikrein. J. Exp. Med. *135*, 81 (1972)
Kaplan, A.P., Meyer, H.L., Mandle, R.: The Hageman factor dependent pathways of coagulation, fibrinolysis, and kinin-generation. Semin. Thromb. Hemost. *3*, 1 (1976)
Kaplan, A.P., Meyer, H.L., Yecies, L.D., Heck, L.W.: Hageman factor and its substrates: the role of factor XI (PTA), prekallikrein, and plasminogen activator in coagulation, fibrinolysis and kinin generation. In: Chemistry and biology of the kallikrein-kinin system in health and disease. Fogarty Internat. Center Proc. No. 27. Pisano, J.J., Austen, K.F. (eds.), p. 237. Washington: U.S. Gov. Printing Office 1977
Kato, H., Han, Y.N., Iwanaga, S., Suzuki, T., Komiya, M.: Bovine HMW- and LMW-kininogens: isolation and characterization of the polypeptide fragments produced by plasma and tissue kallikrein. In: Kinins, pharmacodynamics, and biological role. Sicuteri, F., Back, N., Haberland, G.L. (eds.), p. 135. New York, London: Plenum Press 1976a

Kato, H., Han, Y.N., Iwanaga, S., Suzuki, T., Komiya, M.: Bovine plasma HMW and LMW-kininogens. Structural differences between heavy and light chains derived from kinin-free proteins. J. Biochem. (Tokyo) *80*, 1299 (1976b)
Keele, C.A.: Formation of pain-producing polypeptide (PPS) from plasma. In: Polypeptides which affect smooth muscles and blood vessels. Schachter, M. (ed.), p. 253. London: Pergamon Press 1960
Keiser, H., Greenwald, R.A., Feinstein, G., Janoff, A.: Degradation of cartilage proteoglycan by human leukocyte granule neutral proteases – a model of joint injury. III. Degradation of isolated cartilage proteoglycan. J. Clin. Invest. *57*, 625 (1976)
Kellermeyer, R.W., Breckenridge, R.T.: The inflammatory process in gouty arthritis. I. Activation of Hageman factor by sodium urate crystals. J. Lab. Clin. Med. *65*, 307 (1965)
Kellermeyer, W.F., Jr., Kellermeyer, R.W.: Hageman factor activation and kinin-formation in human plasma induced by cellulose sulfate solutions. Proc. Soc. Exp. Biol. Med. *130*, 1310 (1969)
Kellermeyer, R.W., Ratnoff, O.D.: Abolition of the permeability-enhancing properties of Hageman factor by specific antiserum. J. Lab. Clin. Med. *70*, 365 (1967)
Kimball, H.R., Melmon, K.L., Wolff, S.M.: Endotoxin-induced kinin-formation in man. Proc. Soc. Exp. Biol. Med. *139*, 1078 (1972)
Koj, A., Chudzik, J., Dubin, A.: Substrate specificity and modification of the active centre of elastase-like neutral proteinases from horse blood leucocytes. Biochem. J. *153*, 397 (1976)
Komiya, M., Nagasawa, S., Suzuki, T.: Bovine prekallikrein activator with functional activity as Hageman factor. J. Biochem. (Tokyo) *72*, 1205 (1972)
Komiya, M., Kato, H., Suzuki, T.: Bovine kininogens. I. Further purification of high molecular weight kininogen and its physicochemical properties. J. Biochem. (Tokyo) *76*, 811 (1974a)
Komiya, M., Kato, H., Suzuki, T.: Bovine kininogens. II. Microheterogeneities of high molecular weight kininogens and their structural relationships. J. Biochem. (Tokyo) *76*, 823 (1974b)
Komiya, M., Kato, H., Suzuki, T.: Bovine kininogens. III. Structural comparison of high molecular weight and low molecular weight kininogens. J. Biochem. (Tokyo) *76*, 833 (1974c)
Kopitar, M., Lebez, D.: Intracellular distribution of neutral proteinases and inhibitors in pig leucocytes. Eur. J. Biochem. *56*, 571 (1975)
Kosow, D.P.: The activation mechanism of plasminogen. Int. J. Biochem. *7*, 249 (1976)
Kraut, H., Werle, E.: Der Nachweis eines Kreislaufhormons in der Pankreasdrüse. IV. Mitt. über dieses Kreislaufhormon. Hoppe Seylers Z. Physiol. Chem. *189*, 97 (1930)
Kraut, H., Frey, E.K., Bauer, E.: Über ein neues Kreislaufhormon. II. Mitt. Hoppe Seylers Z. Physiol. Chem. *175*, 97 (1928)
Kruze, D., Menninger, H., Fehr, K., Böni, A.: Purification and some properties of a neutral protease from human leukocyte granules and its comparison with pancreatic elastase. Biochim. Biophys. Acta *438*, 503 (1976)
Laake, K., Venneröd, A.M.: Determination of factor XII in human plasma with arginine proesterase (prekallikrein). I. Preparation and properties of the substrate. Thromb. Res. *2*, 393 (1973)
Laake, K., Venneröd, A.M.: Factor XII induced fibrinolysis: studies on the separation of prekallikrein, plasminogen proactivator, and factor XI in human plasma. Thromb. Res. *4*, 285 (1974)
Lahiri, B., Rosenberg, R., Talamo, R.C., Mitchell, B., Bagdasarian, A., Colman, R.W.: Antithrombin III. An inhibitor of human kallikrein. Fed. Proc. *33*, 642 (Abstract) (1974)
Lanchantin, G.F., Plesset, M.L., Friedmann, J.A., Hart, D.W.: Dissociation of esterolytic and clotting activities of thrombin by trypsin-binding macroglobulin. Proc. Soc. Exp. Biol. Med. *121*, 444 (1966)
Laskovski, M. Jr.: Interactions of proteinases with protein proteinase inhibitors. In: Pulmonary emphysema and proteolysis. Mittman, C. (ed.), p. 311. New York: Academic Press 1972
Laskovski, M. Jr., Sealock, R.W.: Protein-proteinase inhibitors – molecular aspects. In: The enzymes. Boyer, P.D. (ed.), Vol. 3, p. 375. New York: Academic Press 1971
Lawrence, T.G., Cochrane, C.G., Tucker, III., E.S.: Activation of prokininogenase activator (PKA) by clot-promoting factor (CPF) in rabbit plasma. Fed. Proc. *29*, 576 (Abstract) (1970)
Lazarus, G.S., Daniels, J.R., Brown, R.S., Bladen, H.A., Fullmer, H.M.: Degradation of collagen by a human granulocyte collagenolytic system. J. Clin. Invest. *47*, 2622 (1968)
Lazarus, G.S., Daniels, J.R., Liam, J.: Granulocyte collagenase. Mechanism of collagen degradation. Am. J. Pathol. *68*, 656 (1972)

Lewis, G.P.: Formation of plasma kinins by plasmin. J. Physiol. (Lond.) *140*, 285 (1958)
Lewis, J.H., Ferguson, J.H.: Studies on a proteolytic enzyme system of blood. IV. Activation of profibrinolysis by serum fibrinolysokinase. Proc. Soc. Exp. Pathol. Med. *78*, 184 (1951)
Liener, I.E., Garrison, O.R., Pravda, Z.: Purification of α_1-antitrypsin by affinity chromatography on Concanavalin A. Biochem. Biophys. Res. Comm. *51*, 436 (1973)
Liu, T.H., Mertz, E.T.: Studies on plasminogen. IX. Purification of human plasminogen from Cohn fraction III by affinity chromatography. Can. J. Biochem. *49*, 1055 (1971)
Lutcher, C.L.: Reid trait: A new expression of high molecular weight kininogen (HMW-kininogen) deficiency. Clin. Res. *24*, 47 A (Abstract) (1976)
Magoon, E.H., Austen, K.F., Spragg, J.: Immunoelectrophoretic analysis and radial immunodiffusion assay using plasminogen purified from fresh human plasma. Clin. Exp. Immunol. *17*, 345 (1974)
Malemud, C.J., Janoff, A.: Identification of neutral proteases in human neutrophil granules that degrade articular cartilage proteoglycan. Arthritis Rheum. *18*, 361 (1975)
Mandle, R., Jr., Kaplan, A.P.: Hageman factor substrates. Human plasma prekallikrein: mechanism of activation by Hageman factor and participation in Hageman factor-dependent fibrinolysis. J. Biol. Chem. *252*, 6097 (1977 a)
Mandle, R. Jr., Kaplan, A.P.: Plasminogen proactivators of human plasma: relationship to prekallikrein. Fed. Proc. *36*, 329 (Abstract) (1977 b)
Mandle, R., Jr., Colman, R.W., Kaplan, A.P.: Identification of prekallikrein and high molecular weight kininogen as a complex in human plasma. Proc. Natl. Acad. Sci. U.S.A. *73*, 4179 (1976)
Margolis, J.: Plasma pain-producing substance and blood-clotting. Nature *180*, 1464 (1957)
Margolis, J.: Activation of plasma by contact with glass: Evidence for a common reaction which releases plasma kinins and initiates coagulation. J. Physiol. (Lond.) *144*, 1 (1958)
Margolis, J.: The mode of action of Hageman factor in the release of plasma kinin. J. Physiol. (Lond.) *151*, 238 (1960)
Margolis, J.: The interrelationship of coagulation of plasma and release of peptides. Ann. N.Y. Acad. Sci. *104*, 133 (1963)
Margolis, J.: Quantitative studies of kinin-releasing enzymes in plasma. In: Hypotensive peptides. Erdös, E.G., Back, N., Sicuteri, F. (eds.)., p. 198. Berlin, Heidelberg, New York: Springer 1966
Mason, B., Miles, A.A.: Globulin permeability factors without kininogenase activity. Nature *196*, 587 (1962)
Matheson, R.T., Miller, D.R., Lacombe, M.-J., Han, Y.N., Iwanaga, S., Kato, H., Wuepper, K.D.: Flaujeac factor deficiency. Reconstitution with highly purified bovine high molecular weight-kininogen and delineation of a new permeability-enhancing peptide released by plasma kallikrein from bovine high molecular weight kininogen. J. Clin. Invest. *58*, 1395 (1976)
Matheson, R.T., Kato, H., Wuepper, K.D.: Further characterization and inactivation of the permeability-enhancing fragment (Peptide 1-2) of bovine HMW-kininogen. Fed. Proc. *36*, 1064 (Abstract) (1977)
McConnell, D.J.: Inhibitors of kallikrein in human plasma. J. Clin. Invest. *51*, 1611 (1972)
McMillin, C.R., Saito, H., Ratnoff, O.D., Walton, A.G.: The secondary structure of human Hageman factor (factor XII) and its alteration by activating agents. J. Clin. Invest. *54*, 1312 (1974)
Meier, H.L., Pierce, J.V., Colman, R.W., Kaplan, A.P.: Activation and function of human Hageman factor: the role of high molecular weight kininogen and prekallikrein. J. Clin. Invest. *60*, 18 (1977)
Melmon, K.L., Cline, M.J.: Interaction of plasma kinins and granulocytes. Nature *213*, 90 (1967)
Metchnikoff, E.: Lectures on the comparative pathology of inflammation (delivered at the Pasteur Institute, 1891), p. 224. New York: Dover 1968
Meyers, W.M., Burdon, K.L.: Proteolytic activity of whole human serum activated by streptokinase. Arch. Biochem. *62*, 6 (1956)
Miles, A.A.: Large molecular substances as mediators of the inflammatory reaction. Ann. N.Y. Acad. Sci. *116*, 855 (1964)

Miller-Anderson, M., Borg, H., Andersson, L.-O.: Purification of antithrombin III by affinity chromatography. Thromb. Res. *5*, 439 (1974)
Morawitz, P.: Die Chemie der Blutgerinnung. Ergeb. Physiol. *4*, 307 (1905)
Moroi, M., Aoki, N.: Isolation and characterization of α_2-plasmin inhibitor from human plasma. A novel proteinase inhibitor which inhibits activator-induced clot lysis. J. Biol. Chem. *251*, 5956 (1976)
Moroi, M., Aoki, N.: On the interaction of α_2-plasmin inhibitor and proteases. Evidence for the formation of a covalent crosslinkage and non-covalent weak bondings between the inhibitor and proteases. Biochim. Biophys. Acta *482*, 412 (1977)
Moroz, L., Gilmore, N.J.: A rapid and sensitive ^{125}I-fibrin solid phase fibrinolytic assay for plasmin. Blood *46*, 543 (1975)
Moroz, L., Gilmore, N.J.: Fibrinolysis in normal plasma and blood: evidence for significant mechanisms independent of the plasminogen-plasmin system. Blood *48*, 531 (1976a)
Moroz, L., Gilmore, N.J.: Mechanisms involved in enhancement of plasma fibrinolytic activity by chloroform. Blood *48*, 777 (1976b)
Morrison, D.C., Cochrane, C.G.: Direct evidence for Hageman factor (factor XII) activation by bacterial lipopolysaccharides (endotoxin). J. Exp. Med. *140*, 797 (1974)
Moskowitz, R.W., Schwartz, H.J., Michel, B., Ratnoff, O.D., Astrup, T.: Generation of kinin-like agents by chondroitin sulfate, heparin, chitin sulfate, and human articular cartilage: possible pathophysiologic implications. J. Lab. Clin. Med. *76*, 790 (1970)
Movat, H.Z.: Activation of the kinin system by antigen-antibody complexes. In: International symposium on vasoactive polypeptides: bradykinin and related kinins. Rocha e Silva, M., Rothschild, H.A. (eds.), p. 177. Sao Paulo: Soc. Bras. Farmacol. Ther. Exp. 1967
Movat, H.Z.: Pathways to allergic inflammation: the sequelae of antigen-antibody complex formation. Fed. Proc. *35*, 2435 (1976)
Movat, H.Z.: The acute inflammatory reaction. In: Inflammation, immunity, and hypersensitivity. Molecular and cellular mechanisms, 2nd ed. Movat, H.Z. (ed.), p. 1. New York: Harper and Row 1978a
Movat, H.Z.: The kinin-system: its relation to blood coagulation, fibrinolysis, and the formed elements of the blood. In: Reviews of physiology, biochemistry, and pharmacology. *48*, 143 (1978b)
Movat, H.Z., Özge-Anwar, A.H.: The contact phase of blood-coagulation clotting factors XI and XII, their isolation and interaction. J. Lab. Clin. Med. *84*, 861 (1974)
Movat, H.Z., DiLorenzo, N.L., Treloar, M.P.: Activation of the plasma kinin system by antigen-antibody aggregates. II. Isolation of permeability-enhancing and kinin-releasing fractions from activated guinea pig serum. Lab. Invest. *19*, 201 (1968)
Movat, H.Z., Treloar, M.P., DiLorenzo, N.L., Robertson, J.W., Sender, H.B.: The demonstration of permeability factors and two kinin-forming enzymes in plasma. In: Cellular and humoral mechanisms in anaphylaxis and allergy. Movat, H.Z. (ed.), p. 215. Basel, New York: Karger 1969a
Movat, H.Z., Treloar, M.P., Takeuchi, Y.: A small molecular weight permeability factor in guinea pig serum: adsorption to antigen-antibody aggregates. J. Immunol. *103*, 875 (1969b)
Movat, H.Z., Sender, H.B., Treloar, M.P., Takeuchi, Y.: The isolation of and partial characterization of kinin-forming enzymes and other active components of human plasma. In: Bradykinin and related kinins. Back, N., Rocha e Silva, M., Sicuteri, F. (eds.), p. 123. New York, London: Plenum Press 1970
Movat, H.Z., Poon, M.-C., Takeuchi, Y.: The kinin system of human plasma. I. Isolation of a low molecular weight activator of prekallikrein. Int. Arch. Allergy *40*, 89 (1971a)
Movat, H.Z., Uriuhara, T., Takeuchi, Y., Macmorine, D.R.L.: The role of PMN-leukocyte lysosomes in tissue injury, inflammation, and hypersensitivity. VII. Liberation of vascular permeability factors from PMN-leukocytes during in vitro phagocytosis. Int. Arch. Allergy *40*, 197 (1971b)
Movat, H.Z., Soltay, M.J., Fuller, P.J., Özge-Anwar, A.H.: The relationship between the plasma kinin-system and the contact phase of blood coagulation in man. In: Vasopeptides, chemistry, pharmacology, and pathophysiology. Back, N., Sicuteri, F. (eds.), p. 109. New York, London: Plenum Press 1972

Movat, H.Z., Burrowes, C.E., Soltay, M.J., Takeuchi, Y., Habal, F.M., Özge-Anwar, A.H.: The interrelationship between the clotting, fibrinolytic and kinin systems of human plasma. In: Protides of the biological fluids – 20th Colloquium. Peeters, H. (ed.), p. 315. Oxford, New York: Pergamon Press 1973a

Movat, H.Z., Steinberg, S.G., Habal, F.M., Ranadive, N.S.: Demonstration of a kinin-generating enzyme in the lysosomes of human polymorphonuclear leukocytes. Lab. Invest. *29*, 669 (1973b)

Movat, H.Z., Habal, F.M., Macmorine, D.R.L.: Neutral proteases of human PMN-leukocytes with kininogenase activity. Int. Arch. Allergy Appl. Immunol. *50*, 257 (1976a)

Movat, H.Z., Habal, F.M., Macmorine, D.R.L.: The cleavage of a methionyl-lysyl-bradykinin-like peptide from kininogen by a protease of neutrophil leukocyte lysosomes. In: Kinin, pharmacodynamics, and biological roles. Sicuteri, F., Back, N., Haberland, G.L. (eds.), p. 345. New York, London: Plenum Press 1976b

Movat, H.Z., Minta, J.O., Saya, M.J., Habal, F.M., Burrowes, C.E., Wasi, S., Pass, E.: Neutrophil generation of permeability enhancing peptides from plasma substrates. In: Molecular and biological aspects of the acute allergic reactions. Nobel Foundation Symposium 33. Johansson, S.G.O., Strandberg, K., Uvnäs, B. (eds.), p. 391. New York, London: Plenum Press 1976c

Müller-Eberhard, H.J.: The anaphylatoxins: formation, structure, function, and control. In: Molecular and biological aspects of the acute allergic reaction. Nobel Foundation Symposium 33. Johansson, S.G.O., Strandberg, K., Uvnäs, B. (eds.), p. 339. New York, London: Plenum Press 1976

Müllertz, S.: A plasminogen activator in spontaneously active human blood. Proc. Soc. Exp. Biol. Med. *82*, 291 (1953)

Müllertz, S., Clemmensen, I.: The primary inhibitor of plasmin in human plasma. Biochem. J. *159*, 545 (1976)

Murphy, G., Reynolds, J.J., Bretz, U., Baggilioni, M.: Collagenase is a component of specific granules of human neutrophil leucocytes. Biochem. J. *162*, 195 (1977)

Nagasawa, S., Nakaysu, T.: Human plasma prekallikrein as a protein complex. J. Biochem. (Tokyo) *74*, 401 (1973)

Nagasawa, S., Nakayasu, T.: Enzymatic and chemical cleavages of human kininogens. In: Chemistry and biology of the kallikrein-kinin system in health and disease. Fogarty Internat. Center Proc. No. 27. Pisano, J.J., Austen, K.F. (eds.), p. 139. Washington: U.S. Gov. Printing Office 1977

Nagasawa, S., Mizushima, Y., Sato, T., Iwanaga, S., Suzuki, T.: Studies on the chemical nature of bovine bradykininogen. Determination of amino acid, carbohydrate, amino and carboxyl terminals. J. Biochem. (Tokyo) *60*, 643 (1966)

Nagasawa, S., Horiuchi, K., Yano, M., Suzuki, T.: Partial purification of bovine plasma kallikrein activated by contact with glass. J. Biochem. (Tokyo) *62*, 398 (1967)

Niewiarowski, S., Prou-Wartelle, O.: Rôle du facteur contact (Hageman factor) dans la fibrinolyse. Thromb. Diath. Haemorrh. *3*, 426 (1959)

Niewiarowski, S., Bankowski, E., Rogowicka, J.: Studies on the adsorption and activation of Hageman factor (factor XII) by collagen and elastin. Thromb. Diath. Haemorrh. *14*, 387 (1965)

Odeberg, H., Olsson, I., Venge, P.: Cationic proteins of human granulocytes. IV. Esterase activity. Lab. Invest. *32*, 86 (1975)

Ogston, D., Ogston, C.M., Ratnoff, O.D., Forbes, C.D.: Studies on a complex mechanism for the activation of plasminogen by kaolin and by chloroform: the participation of Hageman factor and additional cofactors. J. Clin. Invest. *48*, 1786 (1969)

Oh-ishi, S., Webster, M.E.: Vascular permeability factors (PF/Nat) and Pf/Dil – their relationship to Hageman factor and the kallikrein-kinin system. Biochem. Pharmacol. *24*, 591 (1975)

Oh-ishi, S., Katori, M., Han, Y.N., Iwanaga, S., Kato, H., Suzuki, T.: Possible physiological role of new peptide fragments released from bovine high molecular weight kininogen by plasma kallikrein. Biochem. Pharmacol. *26*, 115 (1977a)

Oh-ishi, S., Tanaka, K., Katori, M., Han, Y.N., Kato, H., Iwanaga, S.: Further studies on biological activities of new peptide fragments derived from high molecular weight kininogen: an enhancement of vascular permeability increase of the fragments by prostaglandin E_2. Life Sci. *20*, 695–700 (1977b)

Ohlsson, K.: Neutral leucocyte proteases and elastase inhibited by plasma alpha$_1$-antitrypsin. Scand. J. Clin. Lab. Invest. *28*, 251 (1971)
Ohlsson, K., Åkesson, U.: α_1-Antichymotrypsin interaction with cationic proteins from granulocytes. Clin. Chim. Acta *73*, 285 (1976)
Ohlsson, K., Olsson, I.: The neutral proteases of human granulocytes. Isolation and partial characterization of two granulocyte collagenases. Eur. J. Biochem. *36*, 473 (1973)
Ohlsson, K., Olsson, I.: The neutral proteases of human granulocytes. Isolation and partial characterization of granulocyte elastase. Eur. J. Biochem. *42*, 519 (1974a)
Ohlsson, K., Olsson, I.: Neutral proteases of human granulocytes. III. Interaction between human granulocyte elastase and plasma protease inhibitors. Scan. J. Lab. Clin. Med. *34*, 349 (1974b)
Olsson, I., Venge, P.: Cationic proteins of human granulocytes. I. Isolation of the cationic proteins from the granules of leukemic myeloid cells. Scan. J. Haematol. *9*, 204 (1972)
Olsson, I., Venge, P.: Cationic proteins of human granulocytes. II. Separation of the cationic proteins of the granules of leukemic myeloid cells. Blood *44*, 235 (1974)
Opie, E.: Intracellular digestion. The enzymes and anti-enzymes concerned. Physiol. Rev. *2*, 552 (1922)
Özge-Anwar, A.H., Movat, H.Z., Scott, J.G.: The kinin system of human plasma. IV. The interrelationship between the contact phase of blood-coagulation and the plasma kinin system in man. Thromb. Diath. Hemorrh. *27*, 141 (1972)
Pannell, R., Johnson, D., Travis, J.: Isolation and properties of human plasma α-1-proteinase inhibitor. Biochemistry *13*, 5439 (1974)
Pashkina, T.S., Ergova, T.P.: Purification and properties of kininogen (bradykininogen) from rabbit serum. Biokhimiia *31*, 468 (1966)
Pass, E., Movat, H.Z., Wasi, S.: An aminopeptidase of human neutrophil leukocytes – its possible role in enhanced vascular permeability. Agents Actions *8*, 91 (1978)
Pensky, J.: Personal communication (1970)
Pensky, J., Levy, R., Lepow, T.H.: Partial purification of serum inhibitor of C′1 esterase. J. Biol. Chem. *236*, 1674 (1961)
Pettinger, W.A., Young, R.: Endotoxin-induced kinin (bradykinin) formation: activation of Hageman factor and plasma kallikrein in human plasma. Life Sci. *9*, 313 (1970)
Pierce, J.V.: Structural features of plasma kinins and kininogens. Fed. Proc. *27*, 52 (1968)
Pierce, J.V., Guimarães, J.A.: Further characterization of highly purified human plasma kininogens. In: Chemistry and biology the kallikrein-kinin system in health and disease. Fogarty Internat. Center Proc. No. 27. Pisano, J.J., Austen, K.F. (eds.), p. 113. Washington: U.S. Gov. Printing Office 1977
Pierce, J.V., Webster, M.E.: The purification and some properties of two different kallidinogens from human plasma. In: Hypotensive peptides. Erdös, E.G., Back, N., Sicuteri, F., Wilder, A.F. (eds.), p. 130. New York: Springer 1966
Poon, M.-C.: The kinin system of human plasma. Dissertation. University of Toronto 1970
Powers, J.C.: Personal communication (1977)
Powers, J.C., Gupton, B.F., Harley, D.A., Nishino, N., Whitley, R.J.: Specificity of porcine pancreatic elastase, human leukocyte elastase and cathepsin G. Inhibition with peptide chloromethyl ketones. Biochim. Biophys. Acta *485*, 156 (1977)
Rabiner, S.F., Goldfine, I.D., Hart, A., Summaria, L., Robbins, K.C.: Radioimmunoassay of human plasminogen and plasmin. J. lab. Clin. Med. *74*, 265 (1969)
Ranadive, N.S., Sajnani, A.N., Alimurka, K., Movat, H.Z.: Release of basic proteins and lysosomal enzymes from neutrophil leukocytes of the rabbit. Int. Arch. Allergy *45*, 880 (1973)
Ratnoff, O.D.: A familial trait characterized by deficiency of a clot-promoting fraction in plasma. J. Lab. Clin. Med. *44*, 915 (1954)
Ratnoff, O.D.: The biology and pathology of the initial stages of blood-coagulation. Prog. Hematol. *5*, 204 (1966)
Ratnoff, O.D.: Activation of Hageman factor by l-homocystine. Science *162*, 1007 (1968)
Ratnoff, O.D., Colopy, J.E.: A familial hemorrhagic trait associated with a deficiency of a clot-promoting fraction of plasma. J. Clin. Invest. *34*, 602 (1955)
Ratnoff, O.D., Crum, J.D.: Activation of Hageman factor by solutions of ellagic acid. J. lab. Clin. Med. *63*, 359 (1964)

Ratnoff, O.D., Davie, E.W.: The purification of activated Hageman factor (activated factor XII). Biochemistry *1*, 967 (1962)
Ratnoff, O.D., Miles, A.A.: The induction of permeability-increasing activity in human plasma by activated Hageman factor. Br. J. Exp. Pathol. *45*, 328 (1964)
Ratnoff, O.D., Davie, E.W., Mallet, D.L.: Studies on the action of Hageman factor: evidence that activated Hageman factor in turn activates plasma thromboplastin antecedent. J. Clin. Invest. *40*, 803 (1961)
Ratnoff, O.D., Lepow, I.H.: Some properties of an esterase derived from preparation of the first component of complement. J. Exp. Med. *106*, 327 (1957)
Revak, S.D., Cochrane, C.G.: The relationship of structure and function in human Hageman factor. The association of enzymatic and binding activities with separate regions of the molecule. J. Clin. Invest. *57*, 852 (1976)
Revak, S.D., Cochrane, C.G., Johnston, A.R., Hugli, T.E.: Structural changes accompanying enzymatic activation of human Hageman factor. J. Clin. Invest. *54*, 619 (1974)
Revak, S.D., Cochrane, C.G., Griffin, J.H.: The binding and cleavage characteristics of human Hageman factor during contact activation. A comparison of normal plasma with plasmas deficient in factor XI, prekallikrein, or high molecular weight kininogen. J. Clin. Invest. *59*, 1167 (1977)
Rickli, E.E., Cuendet, P.A.: Isolation of plasmin-free plasminogen with N-terminal glutamic acid. Biochem. Biophys. Acta *250*, 447 (1971)
Rindler, R., Hörtnagel, H., Schmalzl, F., Braunsteiner, H.: Hydrolysis of a chymotrypsin substrate and of naphthol AS-D acetate by human leukocyte granules. Blut *26*, 239 (1973)
Rindler, R., Schmalzl, F., Braunsteiner, H.: Isolierung und Charakterisierung einer chymotrypsinähnlichen Protease aus neutrophilen Granulozyten des Menschen. Schweiz. Med. Wochenschr. *104*, 132 (1974)
Rindler-Ludwig, R., Braunsteiner, H.: Cationic proteins from human neutrophil granulocytes; evidence for their chymotrypsin-like properties. Biochim. Biophys. Acta *379*, 606 (1975)
Rindler-Ludwig, R., Schmalzel, F., Braunsteiner, H.: Esterases in human neutrophil granulocytes: evidence of their protease nature. Br. J. Haematol. *27*, 57 (1974)
Robbins, K.C., Summaria, L.: Human plasminogen and plasmin. In: Methods in enzymology. Perlmann, G.E., Lorand, L. (eds.), Vol. XIX, p. 184. New York, London: Academic Press 1970
Robbins, K.C., Summaria, L.: Plasminogen and plasmin. In: Methods in enzymology. Lorand, L. (ed.), Vol. XLV/B, p. 257. New York, London: Academic Press 1976
Robbins, K.C., Summaria, L., Hsieh, B., Shar, R.J.: The peptide chains of human plasmin. Mechanism of activation of human plasminogen to plasmin. J. Biol. Chem. *242*, 233 (1967)
Robbins, K.C., Bernabe, P., Arzadon, L., Summaria, L.: NH_2-terminal sequence of mammalian plasminogens and plasmin S-carboxymethyl heavy (A) and light (B) chain derivatives. J. Biol. Chem. *248*, 7242 (1973)
Robbins, K.C., Boreisha, I.G., Arzadon, L., Summaria, L., Barlow, G.H.: Physical and chemical properties of the NH2-terminal glutamic acid and lysine forms of human plasminogen and their derived plasmins with an NH2-terminal lysine heavy (A) chain. J. Biol. Chem. *250*, 4044 (1975)
Rocha e Silva, M., Beraldo, W.T., Rosenfeld, G.: Bradykinin a hypotensive and smooth muscle stimulating factor released from plasma globulin by snake venom and by trypsin. Am. J. Physiol. *156*, 261 (1949)
Rosenberg, R.D., Damus, P.S.: The purification and mechanism of action of human antithrombin-heparin cofactor. J. Biol. Chem. *281*, 6490 (1973)
Rosenthal, R.L., Dreskin, O.H., Rosenthal, N.: A new hemophilia-like disease caused by deficiency of a third plasma thromboplastin factor. Proc. Soc. Exp. Biol. Med. *82*, 171 (1953)
Saito, H.: Purification of high molecular weight kininogen and the role of this agent in blood coagulation. J. Clin. Invest. *60*, 584 (1977)
Saito, H., Ratnoff, O.D., Marshall, J.S., Pensky, J.: Partial purification of plasma thromboplastin antecedent (factor XI) and its activation by trypsin. J. Clin. Invest. *52*, 850 (1973)
Saito, H., Ratnoff, O.D., Pensky, J.: Radioimmunoassay of human Hageman factor (HF, factor-XII) (Abstract). Fed. Proc. *33*, 226 (1974a)
Saito, H., Ratnoff, O.D., Donaldson, V.H.: Defective activation of clotting, fibrinolytic and permeability-enhancing systems in human Fletcher trait plasma. Circ. Res. *34*, 641 (1974b)

Saito, H., Ratnoff, O.D., Waldmann, R., Abraham, J.P.: Impaired Hageman factor (factor XII) mediated reactions in "Fitzgerald trait." Blood J. Hematol. *44*, 934 (Abstract) (1974c)
Saito, H., Ratnoff, O.D., Waldmann, R., Abraham, J.P.: Fitzgerald trait. Deficiency of a hitherto unrecognized agent, Fitzgerald factor, participating in surface-mediated reactions of clotting, fibrinolysis, generation of kinins, and the property of diluted plasma enhancing vascular permeability (PF/Dil). J. Clin. Invest. *55*, 1082 (1975)
Sajnani, A.N.: The mechanism of release of lysosomal material from polymorphonuclear leukocytes. Dissertation. Univ. of Toronto 1974
Sajnani, A.N., Ranadive, N.S., Movat, H.Z.: The visualization of receptors for the Fc portion of the IgG molecule on human neutrophil leukocytes. Life Sci. *14*, 2427 (1974a)
Sajnani, A.N., Ranadive, N.S., Movat, H.Z.: Mobilization and release of cationic protein B_2 from rabbit PMN-leukocytes. Tex. Rep. Biol. Med. *32*, 2 (1974b)
Sajnani, A.N., Ranadive, N.S., Movat, H.Z.: Redistribution of immunoglobulin receptors on human neutrophils and its relationship to the release of lysosomal enzymes. Lab. Invest. *35*, 143 (1976)
Sampaio, C., Wong, S.-C., Shaw, E.: Human plasma kallikrein. Purification and preliminary characterization. Arch. Biochem. Biophys. *165*, 133 (1974)
Saunders, R., Dyce, B.J., Vannier, W.E., Haverback, B.J.: The separation of alpha-2-macroglobulin into five components with differing electrophoretic and enzyme binding properties. J. Clin. Invest. *50*, 2376 (1971)
Schiffman, S., Lee, P.: Preparation, characterization, and activation of a highly purified factor XI: evidence that a hitherto unrecognized plasma activity participates in the interaction of factors XI and XII. Br. J. Haematol. *27*, 101 (1974)
Schiffman, S., Lee, P.: Partial purification and characterization of contact activation cofactor. J. Clin. Invest. *56*, 1082 (1975)
Schiffman, S., Rapaport, S.T., Ware, A.G., Mehl, J.W.: Separation of plasma thromboplastin antecedent (PTA) and Hageman factor (HF) from human plasma. Proc. Soc. Exp. Biol. Med. *105*, 453 (1960)
Schiffman, S., Lee, P., Waldmann, R.: Identity of contact activation cofactor and Fitzgerald factor. Thromb. Res. *6*, 451 (1975)
Schiffman, S., Lee, P., Feinstein, D.I., Pecci, R.: Relationship of contact activation cofactor (CAC) procoagulant activity to kininogen. Blood *49*, 935 (1977)
Schmidt, W., Havemann, K.: Isolation of elastase-like and chymotrypsin-like neutral proteases from human granulocytes. Hoppe Seylers Z. Physiol. Chem. *335*, 1077 (1974)
Schmitz, A.: Über die Proteinase des Fibrins. Z. Physiol. Chem. *244*, 89 (1936)
Schoenmakers, J.G., Kurstjens, R.M., Haanen, C., Zilliken, F.: Purification of activated bovine Hageman factor. Thromb. Diath. Haemorrh. *9*, 546 (1963)
Schoenmakers, J.G.G., Matze, R., Haanen, C., Zilliken, F.: Hageman factor, a novel sialoglycoprotein with esterase activity. Biochim. Biophys. Acta *101*, 166 (1965)
Schreiber, A.D., Austen, K.F.: Hageman factor-independent fibrinolytic pathway. Clin. Exp. Immunol. *17*, 587 (1974)
Schreiber, A.D., Kaplan, A.P., Austen, K.F.: Inhibition by $C\bar{1}INA$ of Hageman factor fragment activation of coagulation, fibrinolysis, and kinin generation. J. Clin. Invest. *52*, 1402 (1973a)
Schreiber, A.D., Kaplan, A.P., Austen, K.F.: Plasma inhibitors of the components of the fibrinolytic pathway in man. J. Clin. Invest. *52*, 1394 (1973b)
Schwartz, H.J., Kellermeyer, R.W.: Carrageenan and delayed hypersensitivity. II. Activation of Hageman factor by carrageenan and its possible significance. Proc. Soc. Exp. Biol. Med. *132*, 1021 (1969)
Seidel, G.: Two functionally different kininogens in human plasma. Agents Actions *3*, 12 (1973)
Seidel, G., Stücker, H.-U., Vogt, W.: Significance of direct and indirect kinin formation by plasmin in human plasma. Biochem. Pharmacol. *20*, 1859 (1971)
Seidel, G., Wendel, U., Schaeger, M.: Activation of a specific plasma kininogenase with trypsin and plasmin. Biochem. Pharmacol. *22*, 929 (1973)
Shulman, N.R.: Proteolytic inhibitor with anti-coagulant activity separated from human urine and plasma. J. Biol. Chem. *213*, 655 (1955)
Sjöholm, I., Wiman, B., Wallén, P.: Studies on the conformational changes of plasminogen induced during activation to plasmin and by 6-aminohexanoic acid. Eur. J. Biochem. *39*, 471 (1973)

Smink, M., Daniel, T.M., Ratnoff, O.D., Stvitsky, A.B.: Immunologic demonstration of a deficiency of Hageman factor-like material in Hageman trait. J. Lab. Clin. Med. *69*, 819 (1967)
Sodetz, J.M., Brockway, W.J., Castellino, F.J.: Multiplicity of rabbit plasminogen. Physical characterization. Biochemistry *11*, 4451 (1972)
Sodetz, J.M., Brockway, W.J., Mann, K.G., Castellino, F.J.: The mechanism of activation of rabbit plasminogen by urokinase. Lack of a preactivation peptide. Biochem. Biophys. Res. Commun. *70*, 729 (1974)
Soltay, M.J., Movat, H.Z., Özge-Anwar, A.H.: The kinin system of human plasma. V. The probable derivation of prekallikrein activator from activated Hageman factor (XIIa). Proc. Soc. Exp. Biol. Med. *138*, 952 (1971)
Speer, R.J., Ridgeway, H., Hill, J.M.: Activated Hageman factor (XII). Thrombos. Diath. Haemorrh. *14*, 1 (1965)
Spragg, J.: Immunological assays for components of the human plasma kinin-forming system. In: Chemistry and biology of the kallikrein-kinin system in health and disease. Fogarty Internat. Center Proc. No. 27. Pisano, J.J., Austen, K.F. (eds.), p. 175. Washington: U.S. Gov. Printing Office 1977
Spragg, J., Austen, K.F.: The preparation of human kininogen. II. Further characterization of human kininogen. J. Immunol. *107*, 1512 (1971)
Spragg, J., Austen, K.F.: The preparation of human kininogen. III. Enzymatic digestion and modification. Biochem. Pharmacol. *23*, 781 (1974)
Spragg, J., Haber, E., Austen, K.F.: The preparation of human kininogen and the elicitation of antibody for use in a radial immunodiffusion assay. J. Immunol. *104*, 1348 (1970)
Starkey, P.M., Barrett, A.J.: Neutral proteases of human spleen. Purification and criteria for homogeneity of elastase and cathepsin G. Biochem. J. *155*, 255 (1976)
Stead, N., Kaplan, A.P., Rosenberg, R.D.: Inhibition of activated factor XII by antithrombin-heparin cofactor. J. Biol. Chem. *251*, 6481 (1976)
Steinbuch, M., Blatrix, C., Josso, F.L.: Action anti-protéase de l'α_2-macroglobuline II. Son rôle d'antithrombine progressive. Rev. Franc. Etud. Clin. Biol. *13*, 179 (1968)
Summaria, L., Arzadon, L., Bernabe, P., Robbins, K.C., Barlow, G.H.: Studies on the isolation of the multiple molecular forms of human plasminogen and plasmin by isoelectric focusing methods. J. Biol. Chem. *247*, 4691 (1972)
Summaria, L., Arzadon, P., Bernabe, P., Robbins, K.C., Barlow, G.H.: Characterization of the NH_2-terminal lysine forms of human plasminogen isolated by affinity chromatography and isoelectric focusing methods. J. Biol. Chem. *248*, 2984 (1973a)
Summaria, L., Arzadon, P., Bernabe, P., Robbins, K.C.: Isolation, characterization, and comparison of the S-carboxymethyl heavy (A) and light (B) chain derivatives of cat, dog, rabbit, and bovine plasmins. J. Biol. Chem. *248*, 6522 (1973b)
Suzuki, T., Kato, H.: Protein components of the bovine kallikrein-kinin system. In: Chemistry and biology of the kallikrein kinin system in health and disease. Fogarty Internat. Center Proc. No. 27. Pisano, J.J., Austen, K.F. (eds.), p. 107. Washington: U.S. Gov. Printing Office 1977
Suzuki, T., Iwanaga, G., Nagasawa, S., Saito, T.: Purification and properties of bradykininogen and of bradykinin-releasing and destroying enzymes in snake venom. In: Hypotensive peptides. Erdös, E.G., Back, N., Sicuteri, F., Wilder, A.F. (eds.), p. 149. Berlin, Heidelberg, New York: Springer 1966
Suzuki, T., Iwanaga, S., Kato, T., Nagasawa, S., Kato, H., Yano, M., Horiuchi, K.: Biochemical properties of kininogens and kinin-releasing enzymes. In: International symposium on vasoactive polypeptides: bradykinin and related kinins. Rocha e Silva, M., Rothschild, H.A. (eds.), p. 27. Sao Paulo: Soc. Braz. Farmacol. Ther. Exp. 1967
Takahashi, H., Nagasawa, S., Suzuki, T.: Studies of prekallikrein of bovine plasma. I. Purification and properties. J. Biochem. (Tokyo) *71*, 471 (1972a)
Takahashi, H., Nagasawa, S., Suzuki, T.: Conversion of bovine prekallikrein to kallikrein. Evidence of limited proteolysis of prekallikrein by bovine Hageman factor (factor XII). F.E.B.S. Letters *24*, 98 (1972b)
Takeuchi, Y., Movat, H.Z.: Conversion of Hageman factor (factor XII) of the guinea pig to prekallikrein activator and inhibition of the formed kallikrein by a natural plasma inhibitor. Eur. J. Immunol. *2*, 345 (1972)

Taylor, J.C., Crawford, I.P.: Purification and preliminary characterization of human granulocyte elastase. Arch. Biochem. Biophys. *169*, 91 (1975)
Teger-Nilsson, A.-C., Friberger, P., Gyzander, E.: Antiplasmin determination by means of a chromogenic dipeptide substrate. In: Progress in chemical fibrinolysis and thrombolysis. Davidson, J.F., Rowan, R.M., Samama, M.M., Desnoyers, P.C. (eds.), Vol. 3, p. 305. New York: Raven Press 1978
Temme, H., Jahreiss, R., Habermann, E., Zilliken, F.: Aktivierung von Gerinnungs- und Kininsystem durch eine Plasmaesterase (Hageman-Faktor). Reinigung und Wirkungsbedingungen. Hoppe Seylers Z. Physiol. Chem. *350*, 519 (1969)
Treloar, M.P.: The plasma kinin system in the guinea pig. Dissertation. University of Toronto 1970
Treloar, M.P., Pyle, H.A., Özge-Anwar, A.H., Takeuchi, Y., Movat, H.Z.: Isolation of prekallikrein activator from guiniea pig serum or plasma adsorbed to immune precipitates or celite: possible relationship to Hageman factor. Eur. J. Immunol. *2*, 338 (1972)
Tucker, III., E.S., Wuepper, K.D.: Contact factor (CF) activation of rabbit kininogenase. Fed. Proc. *28*, 363 (Abstract) (1969)
Tuhy, P.M., Powers, J.C.: Inhibition of human elastase by peptide chloromethyl ketones. F.E.B.S. Letters *50*, 359 (1975)
Unkeless, J., Gordon, S., Reich, E.: Secretion of plasminogen activator by stimulated macrophages. J. Exp. Med. *139*, 834 (1974a)
Venge, P., Olsson, I.: Cationic proteins of human granulocytes. VI. Effects on the complement system and mediation of chemotactic activity. J. Immunol. *115*, 1505 (1975)
Venneröd, A.M., Laake, K.: Isolation and characterization of a prealbumin activator of prekallikrein from acetone-activated human plasma. Thromb. Res. *4*, 103 (1974)
Venneröd, A.M., Laake, K.: Inhibition of purified plasma kallikrein by antithrombin III and heparin. Thromb. Res. 7, 223 (1975)
Venneröd, A.M., Laake, K.: Prekallikrein and plasminogen proactivator: absence of plasminogen proactivator in Fletcher factor deficient plasma. Thromb. Res. *8*, 519 (1976)
Venneröd, A.M., Laake, K., Solberg, A.K., Strömland, S.: Inactivation and binding of human plasma kallikrein by antithrombin III and heparin. Thromb. Res. *9*, 457 (1976)
Viescher, T.L., Bretz, U., Baggiolini, M.: In vitro stimulation of lymphocytes by neutral proteinases from human polymorphonuclear leukocyte granules. J. Exp. Med. *144*, 863 (1976)
Vogel, R., Trautschold, I., Werle, E.: Natürliche Proteinaseinhibitoren. Stuttgart: Thieme 1966
Vogt, W.: Kinin formation by plasmin: an indirect process mediated by activation of kallikrein. J. Physiol. (Lond.) *170*, 153 (1964)
Vogt, W.: Ein komplettes zweites kininbildendes System in menschlichem Plasma. Naunyn Schmiedebergs Arch. Exp. Pathol. Pharmakol. *251*, 186 (1965)
Vogt, W.: Demonstration of the presence of two separate kinin-forming systems in human and other plasmas. In: Hypotensive peptides. Erdös, E.G., Back, N., Sicuteri, F. (eds.), p. 185. Berlin, Heidelberg, New York: Springer 1966
Vogt, W.: An active kallikrein-α_2-macroglobulin complex generated by treatment of human plasma with acetone. In: Kinins, pharmacodynamics and biological roles. Sicuteri, F., Back, N., Haberland, G.L. (eds.), p. 281. New York, London: Plenum Press 1976a
Vogt, W.: Formation of kininogenase-α_2-macroglobulin complex during activation of human plasma with acetone. In: Chemistry and biology of the kallikrein-kinin system in health and disease. Fogarty Internat. Center Proc. No. 27. Pisano, J.J., Austen, K.F. (eds.), p. 75. Washington: U.S. Gov. Printing Office 1977
Vogt, W., Dugal, B.: Generation of an esterolytic and kinin-forming kallikrein-α_2-macroglobulin complex in human serum treated with acetone. Naunyn Schmiedebergs Arch. Pharmacol. *294*, 75 (1976)
Vogt, W., Wawretschek, W.: Weitere Untersuchungen zur Existenz zweier kininbildender Systeme in menschlichem Plasma. Naunyn Schmiedebergs Arch. Exp. Pathol. Pharmakol. *260*, 223 (1968)
Vogt, W., Garbe, G., Schmidt, G.: Untersuchungen zur Existenz zweier verschiedener kininbildender System in menschlichem Plasma. Naunyn Schmiedebergs Arch. Exp. Pathol. Pharmakol. *256*, 127 (1967)

Waldmann, R., Abraham, J.P.: Fitzgerald factor: A heretofor unrecognized coagulation factor. Blood J. Hematol. *44*, 934 (Abstract) (1974)
Waldmann, R., Scili, A.G., McGregor, R.K., Carretero, O.A., Abraham, J.P., Kato, H., Han, Y.N., Iwanaga, S.: Effect of bovine HMW-kininogen and its fragments on Fitzgerald trait plasma. Thromb. Res. *8*, 785 (1976)
Wallén, P., Wiman, B.: Characterization of human plasminogen. II. Separation and partial characterization of different molecular forms of human plasminogen. Biochem. Biophys. Acta *257*, 122 (1972)
Walther, P.J., Hill, R.L., McKee, P.A.: The importance of the preactivation peptide in the two stage mechanism of human plasminogen activation. J. Biol. Chem. *250*, 5926 (1975)
Wasi, S., Murray, R.K., Macmorine, D.R.L., Movat, H.Z.: The role of PMN-leukocyte lysosomes in tissue injury, inflammation and hypersensitivity. II. Studies on the proteolytic activity of PMN-leukocyte lysosomes of the rabbit. Br. J. Exp. Pathol. *42*, 411 (1966)
Wasi, S., Movat, H.Z., Pass, E., Chan, J.Y.C.: Production, conversion and destruction of kinins by human neutrophil leukocyte proteases. In: International symposium on neutral proteases of human polymorphonuclear leucocytes; biochemistry, physiology, and clinical significance. Havemann, K., Janoff, A. (eds.). Munich, Baltimore: Urban and Schwarzenberg 1978
Webster, M.E.: Personal communication (1973)
Webster, M.E., Pierce, J.V.: The nature of kallidins released from human plasma by kallikreins and other enzymes. Ann. N.Y. Acad. Sci. *104*, 91 (1963)
Webster, M.E., Pierce, J.V.: Studies on the enzymes involved in the activation of human plasma kallikreins. In: International Symposium on vasoactive polypeptides: bradykinin and related kinins. Rocha e Silva, M., Rothschild, H.A. (eds.), p. 155. Sao Paulo: Soc. Braz. Farmacol. Ther. Exp. 1967
Webster, M.E., Beaven, V.H., Nagal, Y., Oh-ishi, S., Pierce, J.V.: Interaction of Hageman factor, prekallikrein activator and plasmin. Life Sci. *13*, 1201 (1973)
Webster, M.E., Guimarães, J.A., Kaplan, A.P., Colman, R.W., Pierce, J.V.: Activation of surface-bound Hageman factor: pre-eminent role of high molecular weight kininogen and evidence for a new factor. In: Kinins, pharmacodynamics, and biological roles. Sicuteri, F., Back, N., Haberland, G.L. (eds.), p. 285. New York, London: Plenum Press 1976
Weiss, A.S., Gallin, J.I., Kaplan, A.P.: Fletcher factor deficiency. A diminished rate of Hageman factor activation caused by absence of prekallikrein with abnormalities of coagulation, fibrinolysis, chemotactic activity, and kinin-generation. J. Clin. Invest. *53*, 622 (1974)
Weissmann, G., Spielberg, I.: Breakdown of cartilage proteinpolysaccharide by lysosomes. Arthritis Rheum. *11*, 162 (1968)
Weissmann, G., Zurier, R.B., Spieler, P., Goldstein, I.: Mechanisms of lysosomal enzyme release from leucocytes exposed to immune complexes and other particles. J. Exp. Med. *134*, 149s (1971)
Weissmann, G., Zurier, R.B., Hoffstein, S.: Leukocytes as secretory organs of inflammation. Agents Actions *3*, 370 (1973)
Wendel, U., Vogt, W., Seidel, G.: Purification and some properties of a kininogenase from human plasma activated by surface contact. Hoppe Seylers Z. Physiol. Chem. *353*, 1591 (1972)
Werle, E., Götze, W., Keppler, A.: Über die Wirkung des Kallikreins auf den isolierten Darm und über eine neue dermakontrahierende Substanz. Biochem. Zfschr. *289*, 217 (1937)
Wilner, G.D., Nossel, H.L., Leroy, E.C.: Activation of Hageman factor by collagen. J. Clin. Invest. *47*, 2608 (1968)
Wiman, B., Collen, D.: Purification and characterization of human antiplasmin, the fast-acting plasmin inhibitor in plasma. Eur. J. Biochem. *78*, 19–26 (1977)
Wiman, B., Wallén, P.: Activation of human plasminogen by an insoluble derivative of urokinase. Eur. J. Biochem. *36*, 25 (1973)
Wright, D.G., Malawista, S.E.: The mobilization and extracellular release of granular enzymes from leukocytes during phagocytosis. J. Cell Biol. *53*, 788 (1972)
Wuepper, K.D.: Biochemistry and biology of components of the plasma kinin-forming system. In: Inflammation, mechanisms, and control. Lepow, I.H., Ward, P.A. (eds.), p. 93. New York, London: Academic Press 1972
Wuepper, K.D.: Prekallikrein deficiency in man. J. Exp. Med. *138*, 1345 (1973)

Wuepper, K.D., Cochrane, C.G.: Isolation and mechanism of activation of components of the plasma kinin-forming system. In: Biochemistry of the acute allergic reactions. Austen, K.F., Becker, E.L. (eds.), p. 299. Oxford, London, Edinburgh, Melbourne: Blackwell 1971

Wuepper, K.D., Cochrane, C.G.: Effect of kallikrein on coagulation in vitro. Proc. Soc. Exp. Biol. Med. *141*, 271 (1972a)

Wuepper, K.D., Cochrane, C.G.: Plasma prekallikrein: isolation, characterization, and mechanism of action. J. Exp. Med. *135*, 1 (1972b)

Wuepper, K.D., Miller, D.R., Lacombe, M.-J.: Flaujeac trait: deficiency of kininogen in man. Fed. Proc. *34*, 859 (Abstract) (1975a)

Wuepper, K.D., Miller, D.R., Lacombe, M.J.: Flaujeac trait: deficiency of human plasma kininogen. J. Clin. Invest. *56*, 1663 (1975b)

Wunderer, G., Kummer, K., Fritz, H.: Charakterisierung des Schweine- und Human-Serumkallikreins durch die Hemmbarkeit mit Protein-Proteinase-Inhibitoren. Hoppe Seylers Z. Physiol. Chem. *353*, 1646 (1972)

Yano, M., Kato, H., Nagasawa, S., Suzuki, T.: An improved method for the purification of kininogen II from bovine plasma. J. Biochem. (Tokyo) *62*, 386 (1967a)

Yano, M., Nagasawa, S., Horiuchi, K., Suzuki, T.: Separation of a new substrate kininogen-I from plasma kallikrein in bovine plasma. J. Biochem. (Tokyo) *62*, 504 (1967b)

Yano, M., Nagasawa, S., Suzuki, T.: Purification and properties of bovine serum kallikrein activated with casein. J. Biochem. (Tokyo) *67*, 713 (1970)

Yano, M., Nagasawa, S., Suzuki, T.: Partial purification and some properties of high molecular weight kininogen, bovine kininogen-I. J. Biochem. (Tokyo) *69*, 471 (1971)

Zurier, R.B., Hoffstein, S., Weissmann, G.: Cytochalasin B: effect on lysosomal enzyme release from human leukocytes. Proc. Natl. Acad. Sci. U.S.A. *70*, 844 (1973)

Zurier, R.B., Weissmann, G., Hoffstein, S., Kammerman, S., Tai, H.H.: Mechanisms of lysosomal enzyme release from human leukocytes. II. Effects of cAMP and cGMP, autonomic agonists, and agents which affect microtubule function. J. Clin. Invest. *53*, 297 (1974)

Kininogenases of Blood Cells (Alternate Kinin Generating Systems)

L. M. GREENBAUM

A. Introduction

It is now clear that the plasma kallikrein-kinin generating system, once thought of as the sole mechanism of kinin generation, is now part of a group of kinin generating systems that are present in the body. The generating systems include a variety of normal and pathological tissues and fluids. Because of the involvement with the coagulation system, the plasma system will generate kinins very rapidly upon injury or disease and still must be considered the major kinin generating system in the body. It is also clear, however, that in the absence of plasma HMW kininogen, as for example in the blood disorder known as Williams Trait (COLMAN et al., 1977), kinin generation still occurs. This must be in part the result of the liberation of kinin from "alternate" kinin generation systems. Table 1 lists these alternate kinins generating systems which will now be described and compared to the kallikrein-kinin generating system of plasma.

B. The Leukokinin Generating System

Leukokinins are pharmacologically active peptides of 21–25 amino acids which are formed by an acid protease of cells and tissues acting on a protein substrate known as leukokininogen. The leukokininogen is present in extracellular fluid but not in cells. The term leukokinin is derived from the fact that the acid protease was discovered in leukocytes as well as in murine leukemic cells. The leukokinin generating system specifically differs from the kallikrein-kinin generating system in its formation in that:

a) The enzyme catalyzing leukokinin formation is bound in a cell rather than present in blood as a zymogen; b) the enzyme must be released from the cell to act on

Table 1. Alternative kinin generating systems

Release of leukokinin forming enzymes from leukocytes and neoplastic cells (GREENBAUM et al., 1969)
Release of kallikrein from human PMN cells following ingestion of immune complexes (MOVAT et al., 1973)
Release of kallikrein from human basophils by antigen in the presence of IgE (NEWBALL et al., 1975)
Release of kallikrein from rat peritoneal cells by catecholamines (ROTHSCHILD and CASTANIA, 1974)
Release of leukokinin-forming enzymes from fibroblasts (BACK and STEGER, 1970)

the substrate; c) the enzyme differs from plasma kallikrein but clearly resembles cathepsin D; d) the substrate, leukokininogen, differs from HMW bradykininogen (normal substrate for plasma kallikrein) and LMW kininogen (a substrate for glandular kallikrein).

I. Chemistry of the Leukokinins

Four leukokinins known respectively as leukokinin A, H, M, and PMN, have been isolated. The abbreviations represent the *source* of enzyme which catalyzed their formation. Table 2 identifies the source of enzyme and substrate as well as some of the known physical and chemical properties of the leukokinins.

The leukokinins have an amino acid composition of 21–25 amino acids. In this regard, they are different from bradykinin, lysyl-bradykinin or methionyl-lysyl-bradykinin which have 9–11 amino acids, respectively. Table 3 describes the amino acid composition of the leukokinin molecules and compares them with bradykinin. One of the outstanding features of the leukokinins is that each contains only one phenylalanine moiety as contrasted with bradykinin which has two. Thus the leukokinin molecule does not contain bradykinin per se. It is possible that a substitution for phenylalanine may occur and a bradykinin analog may be found when the leukokinins are eventually sequenced.

Two of the leukokinins, H and A, may be considered endogenous products of ascites fluids in human ovarian carcinoma and murine ascites (L-1210 cells) since both the substrate and the enzyme producing leukokinin A and H are found in the respective ascites fluids (JOHNSTON and GREENBAUM, 1973; GREBOW et al., 1977). In this regard, they are of more interest than the leukokinins PMN and M produced in vitro.

End group analysis of the leukokinins indicates that of the three partially sequenced ones, none have a common sequence (Table 3).

While further sequencing of the molecules may clarify this apparent paradox, the best current explanation is that the substrate protein from which they are produced may differ from species to species.

II. Pharmacologic Properties of Leukokinins

Leukokinins are most active on a molar basis in increasing the vascular permeability of guinea pig and rabbit skin (see Table 4). Similar to bradykinin and its analogs, the leukoki-

Table 2. Sources and amino acid composition of leukokinins

Leukokinin	Amino acids	MW	Source of enzyme	Source of substrate	N-Terminal	Reference
A	23	2762	Ascites fluid (murine)	Ascites fluid (murine)	Pyr-Glu	JOHNSTON (1973)
H	24	2770	Ascites fluid (human)	Ascites fluid (human)	Leu-Ala-Tyr-Thr	GREBOW et al. (1977)
PMN	21	2416	Polymorph cells (rabbit)	Plasma (human)	–	FREER et al. (1972)
M	25	2826	Macrophage (rabbit)	Plasma (human)	Arg-Ala-Ser	CHANG et al. (1972)

Table 3. Amino acid residues of leukokinins

Amino acid	PMN	M	A	H	Bradykinin
Alanine	1	2	1	1	–
Arginine	2	3	4	2	2
Aspartic acid	1	1	1	–	–
Cystine 1/2	–	–	–	–	–
Glutamic acid	1	2	1	2	–
Glycine	2	2	2	–	1
Histidine	1	1	1	–	–
Isoleucine	–	–	–	–	–
Leucine	1	1	1	3	–
Lysine	2	3	3	1	–
Methionine	–	–	–	–	–
Phenylalaine	1	1	1	1	2
Proline	3	3	3	2	3
Serine	2	2	1	2	1
Threonine	1	1	1	4	–
Tryosine	2	1	1	2	–
Valine	1	2	1	4	–
Total amino acids	21	25	23[a]	24	9

The abbreviations represent the source of enzyme which catalyzed the formation of peptide. PMN-polymorphonuclear leukocyte (rabbit) (CHANG et al.; FREER et al., 1972); M-alveolar macrophage (rabbit), A-ascites fluid, mastocytoma (mouse); JOHNSTON and GREENBAUM (1973); H-ascites fluid, ovarian carcinoma (human) (GREBOW et al., 1978).

[a] Includes one residue of tryptophan. PMN, M, and H leukokinins were not analyzed for tryptophan.

Table 4. Comparison of activities of leukokinin and bradykinin[a]

Permeability	H	A	PMN	M
Rabbit	0.20	0.37	1.3	4.5
Guinea pig	0.30	–	1.3	–
Blood pressure depression				
Rat	0.09	–	10.0	–
Rabbit	0.05	0.22	3.5	1.0
Rat uterus contraction	0.03	0.15	0.00	0.26
Guinea pig Ileum	0.001	0.08	0.80	0.08

[a] Bradykinin is equal to 1.0; A lower number indicates lesser activity than bradykinin; A higher number indicates greater activity than bradykinin.

nins are vasoactive and depress blood pressure probably by relaxing arteriolar smooth muscle as demonstrated by the ability of leukokinin H to increase femoral and coronary flow in the dog (PRAKASH et al., 1977). Of isolated tissues, leukokinins contract the rat uterus and only weakly the guinea pig ileum. Leukokinins relax the rat duodenum.

When measured against bradykinin in these assay systems, the leukokinins have a potency of 20% (leukokinin H)–500% (leukokinin M) of the potency of bradykinin in increasing vascular permeability, thus demonstrating that leukokinins are effective permeability producing agents. Some leukokinins (H and A) are much weaker in causing depression of blood pressure than is bradykinin. On the other hand; leukokinins PMN and M are as potent or more potent than bradykinin in this regard. Leukokinins are much less active than bradykinin in contracting the rat uterus and have almost no activity on the guinea pig ileum.

When compared with one another, leukokinins PMN and M are more potent vasodepressors than leukokinins H and A, the leukokinins produced by neoplastic cells. Leukokinins PMN and M are also more potent on a molar basis in increasing vascular permeability than leukokinins H and A. Thus, overall, the white cell mediated leukokinins are more impressive on a molar basis than the leukokinins derived from neoplastic cells in terms of their potency.

III. Leukokinin Forming Enzyme

1. Overall Properties

The leukokinin-forming enzyme is currently considered to be very similar to, or the same as, cathepsin D. The evidence for this is the acid pH optima and the striking inhibition of leukokinin-forming activity by pepstatin. Cathepsin D is a lysosomal enzyme. The cellular location of the leukokinin-forming enzyme indicates, however, that it is bound to the nuclear membrane fraction as well as to other cellular fractions. Since cathepsin D had been postulated by BARRETT (1975) to be secreted within the cell, its location in many parts of the cell may be an artifact of this secretion during isolation.

2. Measurement of Activity of Leukokinin-Forming Enzyme

Two methods are currently in use to assay cells and tissues for leukokinin forming activity:

(a) Direct formation of leukokinin; in this procedure, cell homogenates are incubated for 16 h in the presence of a kininogen purified from human blood. The resulting kinin is assayed on the rat uterus in estrus (FREER et al., 1972);

(b) Hydrolysis of tritiated hemoglobin at pH 4.0 in the presence and absence of pepstatin; this procedure takes advantage of the cathepsin D like activity of the enzyme. Cell fractions are incubated with tritiated hemoglobin 15–120 min. The activity of the enzyme after precipitation with trichloroacetic is determined (GRAYZEL et al., 1975) by the tritiated peptides released. Since the leukokinin-forming enzyme is completely inhibited by pepstatin, a pepstatin-treated fraction serves as a control to further identify the enzyme. The method has been described by ROFFMAN, LERNER and GREENBAUM (1978).

3. Sources of Leukokinin-Forming Enzyme

Some of the sources of leukokinin-forming enzyme are listed below (see also Tables 5 and 6).

Table 5. Neoplastic cell kinogenases

Cell type	Species	pH Optimum	Product	Inhibitor	Reference
Leukemic (L-1210)	Murine	Acid	Leukokinin	Pepstatin	GREENBAUM et al. (1969, 1972)
Lymphosarcoma	Murine	Acid	Leukokinin	Pepstatin	GREENBAUM et al. (1969, 1972)
Mastocytoma	Murine	Acid	Leukokinin	Pepstatin	GREENBAUM et al. (1969, 1972)
Fibroblast	Rat	Acid	Leukokinin	Phenylpyruvate	BACK et al. (1975)
Ascites fluid (mastocytoma)	Murine	Acid	Leukokinin	Pepstatin	JOHNSTON and GREENBAUM (1973)
Ascites fluid (ovarian carcinoma)	Human	Acid and neutral	Leukokinin Bradykinin	Pepstatin Trasylol	GREBOW, PRAKASH and GREENBAUM (1978)
Lymphosarcoma	Rat	Neutral and acid	Bradykinin Leukokinin	Trasylol Phenylpyruvate	BACK et al. (1970)

Table 6. Cell derived kinogenases

Cell type	Species	Remarks or pH optimum	Product	Inhibitor	Reference
Polymorphonuclear leukocyte	Rabbit	Acid	Leukokinin	Pepstatin	GREENBAUM and KIM (1967) GREENBAUM et al. (1969) FREER et al. (1972)
Macrophage	Rabbit	Acid	Leukokinin	Pepstatin	CHANG et al. (1972)
Lymphocyte	Human	Acid	Leukokinin	Pepstatin	ENGLEMAN and GREENBAUM (1971)
Spleen	Bovine	Acid I, II[a]	Met-lys-bradykinin (?)	Diazo-nor leucine	YAMAFUJI and TAKEISHI (1975)
Polymorphonuclear leukocyte	Human	Neutral	Met-lys-bradykinin (?)	α-anti trypsin	MOVAT et al. (1975) MELMON and CLINE (1967)
Mast cell	Rat	Catechole amine activated	Bradykinin	Aspirin	ROTHSCHILD et al. (1974a)
Basophil	Human	Anti-IgE Antigen E	Bradykinin	2-Deoxy-glucose, EDTA	NEWBALL et al. (1975)

[a] Two enzymes have been isolated termed "Acid I and II". Acid II is thiol activated

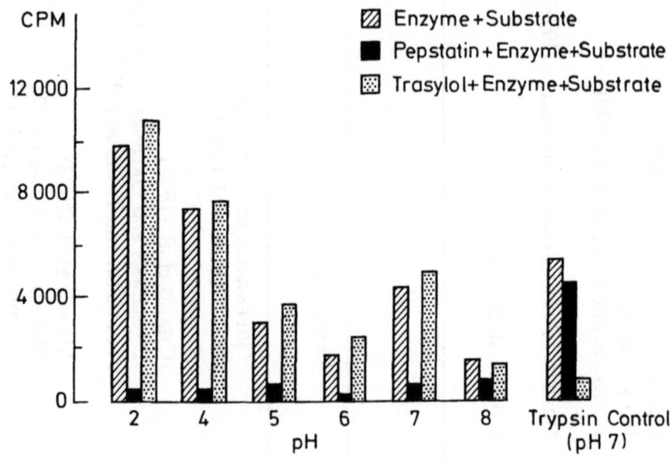

Fig. 1. pH Profile of hydrolytic activity of murine tumor cells on tritiated hemoglobin. Note that the activity is found in the physiologic pH range. This activity presumably is the same as that which forms leukokinins since it is inhibited by pepstatin. Note that trasylol is not effective against this enzyme although it does inhibit trypsin (ROFFMAN et al., 1977)

White Cells:

Polymorphonuclear leukocytes (rabbits and humans)
Macrophages (rabbit)
  alveolar
  peritoneal
Lymphocytes (human)

Neoplastic Cells and Related Fluids:

Leukemic (L-1210, murine)
Lymphosarcoma (murine and rat)
Fibroblast (rat)
Ascites fluid (murine)
  mastocytoma
  L-1210
Ascites fluid (human ovarian carcinoma)
Adenocarcinoma

Tissues:

Spleen (bovine, dog)

4. pH Optima of the Leukokinin-Forming Enzyme

Figure 1 demonstrates that the enzyme is most active in the acid range. It may also be noted that enzyme activity is present at neutral pH although it has about half the optimal activity. *Thus, the formation of leukokinin will proceed at normal body pH as well as in the acid range.*

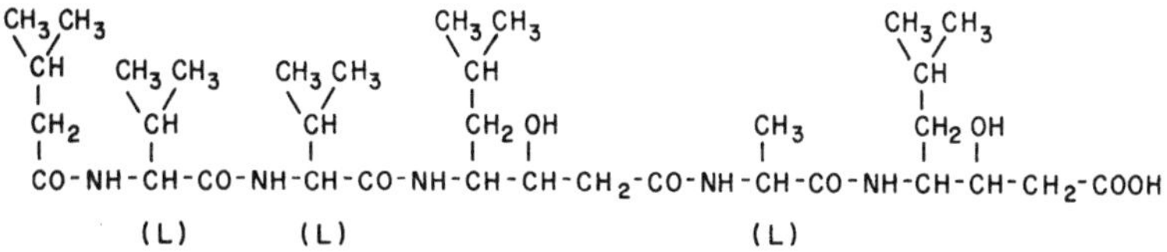

Fig. 2. Structure of pepstatin (isovaleryl): Iso-valeryl-L-valyl-L-valyl-4-amino-3-hydroxy-6-methylheptanoyl-L-alanyl-4-amino-3-hydroxy-6-methylheptanoic acid

5. Inhibitors of Leukokinin-Forming Enzyme and its Differentiation From Plasma Kallikrein

Figure 1 demonstrates that pepstatin inhibits leukokinin-forming enzyme over the entire pH range. On the other hand, the kallikrein inhibitor, aprotinin (Trasylol), does not inhibit the leukokinin-forming enzyme. Thus, by the use of pepstatin in biologic or pathologic systems (see below), the contribution of the leukokinin system to peptide release may be differentiated from bradykinin generation by kallikrein. Inhibition of in vitro leukokinin formation by pepstatin occurs in the concentration of 10^{-6}–10^{-9} M (GREENBAUM et al., 1975). In vivo inhibition of leukokinin generation and subsequently inhibition of ascites fluid formation in tumor-bearing mice was carried out using doses of 80 mg/kg parenterally administered (GREENBAUM and SEMENTE, 1977).

6. Pepstatin

Pepstatin (Fig. 2) is an antibiotic and peptide-like molecule which was first isolated by UMEZAWA and his colleagues from actinomycetes (1970). It is an inhibitor of renin, cathepsin D, leukokinin-forming enzyme, and pepsin. BARRETT (1975) and AOYAGI (1975) have described the kinetics of its inhibition of human cathepsin D. It has a molecular weight of 620. It is difficult to dissolve in water but a 2 mg/ml solution (1.6×10^{-3} M) may be prepared by dissolving it at pH 9–11 and continuously adding NaOH to maintain this pH until dissolved.

7. Leukokininogen

The substrate protein containing leukokinin H, human leukokininogen, has recently been purified by ROFFMAN and GREENBAUM (1978). The source of the protein was ascites fluid from a patient with ovarian carcinoma. Purification of leukokininogen was achieved following ammonium sulfate fractionation, chromatography on Sephadex G-200 and DEAE-Sepharose CL-6 B, and preparative isoelectric focusing in a flat bed of Sephadex G-75. Disc polyacrylamide gel electrophoresis of leukokininogen, in the presence of sodium dodecylsulfate, resulted in the detection of a single protein band with a molecular weight of about 41,000 daltons. The isoelectric pH of this protein was 4.5–4.7 (ROFFMAN and GREENBAUM, 1978). Leukokininogen was a substrate for the leukokinin-forming acid protease and trypsin, but not for plasma kallikrein. In this regard, leukokininogen is similar to LMW kininogen, a plasma protein containing bradykinin, which releases bradykinin after incubation with trypsin but not with plasma kallikrein. HMW kininogen, by contrast, does release brady-

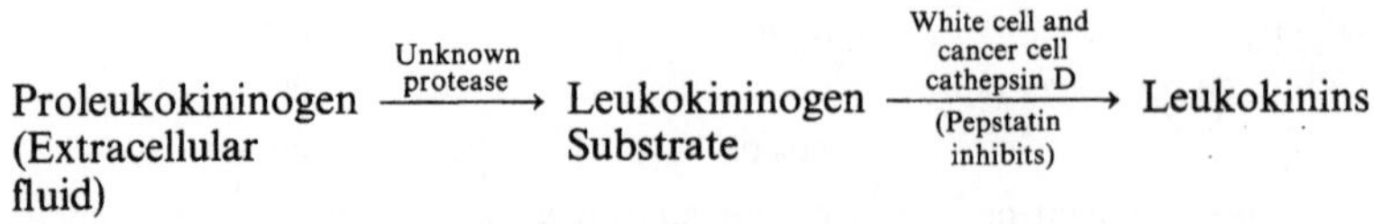

Fig. 3. Current concept of leukokininogen formation as a substrate for the acid protease which catalyzes the formation of leukokinins

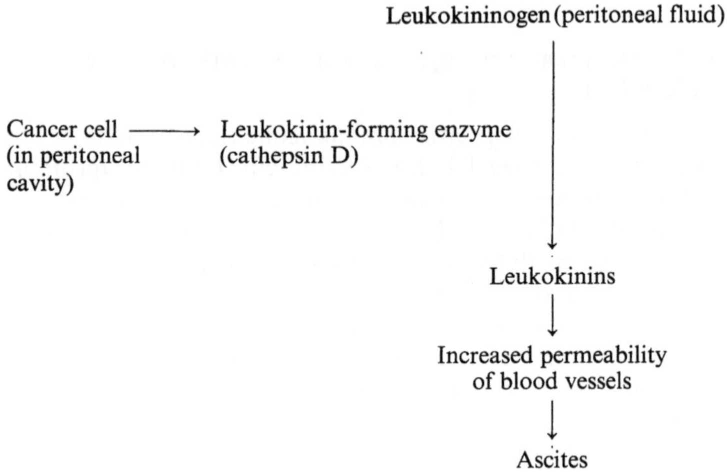

Fig. 4. Relationship of leukokinin formation to ascites fluid formation in neoplastic disease (ovarian carcinoma)

kinin after treatment with both plasma kallikrein and trypsin (PIERCE, 1970). Leukokininogen does not cross react with antisera against LMW kininogen, however, and has a different amino acid content from both that of human and bovine LMW kininogen. Leukokininogen, therefore, is a separate and distinct "kininogen" from those previously isolated.

Leukokininogen unlike HMW bradykininogen is probably not in normal circulating plasma. The evidence indicates that it is formed from a precursor protein (proleukokininogen) by a protease which is (aprotinin Trasylol) sensitive during pathologic events such as neoplastic disease (see Fig. 3). The conversion of normally circulating proleukokininogen can be induced in normal plasma by warming to 57 °C for 30 min (GREENBAUM, 1972).

8. Role of Leukokinins in Inflammation and Neoplastic Disease

The presence of leukokinin-forming enzymes in white cells obviously points to the potential formation of leukokinins as potent inflammatory agents especially in terms of increasing vascular permeability.

The finding of all the components of the leukokinin generating system in ascites of tumor bearing mice (JOHNSTON and GREENBAUM, 1973) gave impetus to experiments to determine whether leukokinin formation was involved in the mechanism of ascites fluid accumulation.

Strong evidence for this was obtained (GREENBAUM et al., 1975) when it was found that administration of pepstatin to mice bearing ascites tumors dramatically inhibited ascites formation although it had little effect on the growth of the cancer cells themselves. Subsequently it was also found that human ascites carried the leukokinin generating system which was inhibited by pepstatin in vitro. The mechanism by which leukokinin formation may induce ascites accumulation is seen in Fig. 4. The use of inhibitors of acid proteases to retard ascites formation in neoplastic disease may have significant importance for therapeutic use (GREENBAUM and SEMENTE, 1977).

C. Human Basophil Kinin Generating System

Human leukocyte preparations from allergic donors when challenged with appropriate antigens release several chemical mediators which include histamine, slow reacting substance of anaphylaxis, eosinophil chemotatic factor of anaphylaxis and platelet activating factor. NEWBALL et al. (1975) have demonstrated that an arginine esterase which generates kinin from kininogen is also released following interaction of antigen or anti-IgE with cell bound IgE. In this regard, the mechanism of release of basophil kallikrein of anaphylaxis is similar to the release of histamine and other mediators of the allergic response.

I. Characteristics of the Kallikrein of Anaphylaxis

Kallikrein is known to hydrolyze N-α-tosylarginine methyl ester (TAMe) and generates bradykinin from citrated human plasma without activating prekallikrein. It also generates bradykinin from highly purified bradykininogen. The release of the enzyme is calcium dependent and is inhibited by EDTA. 2-Deoxyglucose also inhibits this release indicating the need for energy for the process.

The kallikrein of human basophil cells is inhibited partially by soybean trypsin inhibitor (SBTI), completely by di-isopropylfluorophosphate (DFP). Aprotinin inhibits the activity 50% in concentrations of 100 KU/ml.

The release of this enzyme in parallel with histamine and other mediators of anaphylaxis provides a significant link of the kinin generating system with the primary immune reaction and immediate hypersensitivity or allergic reactions.

D. Human Neutrophil Kininogenase

As discussed above, leukocytes from rabbit and human sources contain an acid protease which form leukokinins. MOVAT and associates (1973) discovered that human polymorphonuclear leukocytes following ingestion of immune complexes release a neutral protease which catalyzes the formation of methionyl-lysyl-bradykinin or a similar product from HMW kininogen, the substrate which kallikrein hydrolyzes. The protease had a sedimentation coefficient of 2.75 and a MW of 20,000. Further details of this enzyme and its product may be found in another section. The neutral kininogenase is probably the same as the one first reported by CLINE and MELMON (1966) and MELMON and CLINE (1967) from human PMN cells (see review MILLER et al., 1973).

E. Mast Cell Kininogenase

Mast cells have long been known to be a storage site for histamine, slow reacting substance of anaphylaxis, and other mediators. ROTHSCHILD et al. (1974a) and ROTHSCHILD and CASTANIA (1974) showed that catecholamines can release kininogenase activity from these cells (rat). Kininogenase release is blocked by aspirin as well as α-adrenergic and β-adrenergic blocking agents. The effect of aspirin on kininogenase release may indicate other pathways of the action of aspirin in addition to its actions on prostaglandin synthesis.

F. Neoplastic Cell Kininogenase

Table 5 lists the kininogenases found in neoplastic cells and their properties. GREENBAUM et al. (1969) described first the presence of kinin generating enzymes in murine tumor cells and demonstrated that the enzyme was an acid protease that formed leukokinins (see above). BACK et al. (1973) confirmed the presence of this enzyme or one similar to the leukokinin-forming enzyme in rat fibroblasts. The latter was inhibited by a high concentration of phenylpyruvate. LE BLANC and BACK (1975) have reported that ascites fluid and ascites tumor cells of murine Ehrlich ascites tumors contain components of kinin generating systems. Kallikrein was present as prekallikrein in ascites fluid at levels similar to plasma. It was not active unless treated with acetone.

G. Splenic Kininogenase

YAMAFUJI and TAKEISHI (1975) have further developed the early observations (GREENBAUM and YAMAFUJI, 1966) that catheptic enzymes can catalyze the formation of kinins from plasma substrates (see Table 6). Two enzyme fractions from bovine spleen have been shown to form what presumably is identified as methionyl-lysyl-bradykinin. One of the enzymes is named acid kininogenase II; it is activated by thiol compounds. This is the only known thiol-activated kininogenase. A second kininogenase, acid kininogenase I, does not require thiol activation. These observations add to the list of enzymes contained in tissues which release kinins during injury to tissues or during chronic disease states of organs such as the spleen, but which are different from kallikreins.

Summary

The number of kininogenases aside from plasma kallikrein is impressive in terms of the possibilities of their release following allergic reactions (basophil and PMN cells kininogenases), in neoplastic states (leukokinin-forming kininogenase), following infection and white cell migration (leukokinin-kininogenase) and following injury to tissues (acid proteases). The variety of pharmacologic actions of the kinins released, which include changes in permeability, pain, and blood pressure as well as the potential to release other mediators such as prostaglandins, makes continued research in this area extremely important. The finding that inhibitors of these systems such as pepstatin are effective (GREENBAUM et al., 1975) in ameliorating their effects in vivo provides exciting new therapeutic possibilities.

References

Aoyagi, T., Umezawa, H.: Structures and activities of protease inhibitors of microbial origin. In: Proteases and biological control. Cold Spring Harbor Conference on Cell Proliferation. Reich, E., Rifkin, D.B., Shaw, E. (eds.), pp. 429–454. Cold Spring, N.Y.: Cold Spring Harbor Laboratory 1975

Back, N., Steger, R.: Characterization of pre-kallikrein activity in developing transplanted mammalian tumors. In: Bradykinin and related kinins. Sicuteri, F., Rocha e Silva, M., Back, N. (eds.), pp. 225–237. New York, London: Plenum Press 1970

Back, N., Steger, R.: Kinin-forming activity of cultured mouse fibroblasts L-929. Proc. Soc. Exp. Biol. Med. *143*, 769–774 (1973)

Barrett, A.J.: Lysosomal and related proteinases. In: Proteases and biological control. Cold Spring Harbor Conference on cell proliferation. Reich, E., Rifkin, D.B., Shaw, E. (eds.), pp. 467–493. Cold Spring, N.Y.: Cold Spring Harbor Laboratory 1975

Chang, J., Freer, R., Stella, R., Greenbaum, L.M.: Studies on leukokinins. II: formation and amino acid sequence and chemical properties. Biochem. Pharmacol. *21*, 2095–3106 (1972)

Cline, M.J., Melmon, K.L.: Plasma kinins and cortisol: a possible explanation of the anti-inflammatory action of cortisol. Science *153*, 1135–1138 (1966)

Colman, R.W., Bagdasarian, A., Talamo, R.C., Kaplan, A.P.: Williams trait: a new deficiency with abnormal levels of pre-kallikrein, plasminogen proactivator and kininogen. In: Chemistry and biology of the kallikrein-kinin system in health and diseases. Pisano, J., Austen, F. (eds.), pp. 65–72. Fogerty Internat. Center Proc. No. 27. Washington: U.S. Gov. Printing Office 1977

Engleman, E., Greenbaum, L.M.: The kinin-forming activity of human lymphocytes. Biochem. Pharmacol. *21*, 922 (1971)

Freer, R., Chang, J., Greenbaum, L.M.: Studies on leukokinins III: pharmacological activities. Biochem. Pharmacol. *21*, 3107–3110 (1972)

Grayzel, A.I., Hatcher, V.S., Lazarus, G.S.: Protease activity of normal and PHA stimulated human lymphocytes. Cell Immunol. *18*, 210–219 (1975)

Grebow, P., Prakash, A., Greenbaum, L.M.: The isolation of leukokinin-H from human ascites fluid. Agents Actions 1978, in press

Greenbaum, L.M., Yamafuji, K.: The in vitro inactivation and formation of plasma kinins by beef spleen cathepsins. Br. J. Pharmacol. Chemother. *27*, 230–238 (1966)

Greenbaum, L.M., Freer, R., Chang, J., Semente, G., Yamafuji, K.: PMN-kinin and kinin metabolizing enzymes in normal and malignant leucocytes. Br. J. Pharmacol. *36*, 623–634 (1969)

Greenbaum, L.M., Kim, K.S.: The kinin forming and kininase activities of rabbit PMN cells. Br. J. Pharmacol. *29*, 238–247 (1967)

Greenbaum, L.M.: Leukocyte kininogenases and leukokinins from normal and malignant cells. Am. J. Pathol. *68*, 613–623 (1972)

Greenbaum, L.M., Grebow, P., Johnston, M., Prakash, A., Semente, G.: Pepstatin – an inhibitor of leukokinin formation and ascitic fluid accumulation. Cancer Res. *35*, 706–710 (1975)

Greenbaum, L.M., Semente, G.: Pepstatin – an ascites retardant of L-1210 tumor-bearing mice. J. Natl. Cancer Inst. *59*, 259–262 (1977)

Johnston, M., Greenbaum, L.M.: Leukokinin-forming system in the ascitic fluid of a murine mastocytoma. Biochem. Pharmacol. *27*, 1386–1389 (1973)

Le Blanc, P., Back, N.: Proteases during the growth of Erlich ascites tumor. II: the kallikrein-kinin system. J. Natl. Cancer Inst. *54*, 1107–1114 (1975)

Melmon, K.L., Cline, M.J.: Interaction of plasma kinins and granulocytes. Nature (Lond.) *213*, 90–92 (1967)

Miller, R.L., Reichgott, M.J., Melmon, K.L.: Biochemical mechanisms of generation of bradykinin by endotoxin. J. Infect. Dis. *128*, 144–156 (1973)

Movat, H., Steinberg, S., Habal, F., Randive, N.: Demonstration of a kinin-generating enzyme in the lysosomes of human polymorphonuclear leukocytes. Lab. Invest. *29*, 669 (1973)
Newball, H.H., Talamo, R.C., Lichtenstein, L.M.: Release of leukocyte kallikrein mediated by IgE. Nature (Lond.) *254*, 635–636 (1975)
Pierce, J.V.: Purification of mammalian kallikreins, kininogens, and kinins. In: Handbook of experimental pharmacology. Vol. XXV: Bradykinin, kallidin, and kallikrein. Erdös, E.G. (ed.), pp. 21–51. Berlin, Heidelberg, New York: Springer 1970
Roffman, S., Lerner, S., Greenbaum, L.M.: pH-dependent activity of cathepsin D from neoplastic cells using a sensitive H^3-hemoglobin substrate. In: Acid proteases, structure-function, and biology. Oklahoma Medical Research Foundation (1978) (in publication)
Roffman, S., Greenbaum, L.M.: The properties of leukokininogen isolated from human neoplastic ascites. Biochem. Pharmacol. 1978, in press
Rothschild, A.M., Castania, A.: Lowering of kininogens in rat blood by adrenaline and its inhibition by sympatholytic agents, heparin, and aspirin. Br. J. Pharmacol. *50*, 375–389 (1974)
Rothschild, A.M., Castania, A., Cordeiro, R.S.B.: Consumption of kininogen, formation of kinin and inactivation of arginine ester hydrolase in rat plasma by rat peritoneal fluid cells in the presence of L-adrenaline. Naunyn Schmiedebergs Arch. Pharmakol. *285*, 243–256 (1974a)
Umezawa, M., Aoyagi, T., Morishima, H., Matsuzaki, M., Hamada, M., Takeuchi, T.: Pepstatin – a new inhibitor produced by actinomycetes. J. Antibiot. (Tokyo) *23*, 259–262 (1970)
Yamafuji, K., Takeishi, M.: Bovine spleen acid kininogenases. Life Sci. *16*, 822 (1975)

Enzymology of Glandular Kallikreins

F. FIEDLER

A. Introduction

Even today we call two totally different groups of enzymes kallikrein (EC 3.4.21.8): the glandular, tissue, or organ kallikreins on one hand and the plasma or serum kallikreins on the other. The relationships between these two groups of kallikreins appear to be not closer than, e.g., those between trypsin and thrombin.

Glandular kallikreins occur mainly in pancreas, pancreatic juice, salivary glands, and saliva. The kallikrein found in urine is closely related to these enzymes, a fact to be remembered for nomenclature. Other kallikreins, such as those in human sweat and guinea-pig coagulating gland, probably also belong to this group. This might also be true for the kallikreins found in the venom of snakes and lizards (SUZUKI and IWANAGA, 1970; MEBS, 1969a, b; COHEN et al., 1970).

The central action of a kallikrein is the ability to liberate a kinin peptide from kininogen. Many proteinases can release peptides with kinin activity (PRADO, 1970). One of the enzymes that was recently shown to possess kininogenase activity is the sperm proteinase, acrosin (PALM and FRITZ, 1975). This enzyme does not seem to belong to glandular kallikreins, but it is a trypsin-like enzyme. Problems in the detection and identification of a glandular kallikrein have been discussed by WEBSTER (1970). The most important criterion seems to be the ability to lower the blood pressure of an animal of the same species from which the enzyme has been isolated when a small quantity is injected i.v. In Sect. G I try to describe the general properties of glandular kallikreins from the limited amount of information available.

The present article is limited to glandular kallikreins of mammalian origin. Only investigations involving more or less highly purified preparations are cited. Previous work has been reviewed by WEBSTER (1970). Extensive comments on the purification of glandular kallikreins have been published by PIERCE in 1970. A more recent review was written by NUSTAD et al. (1976).

B. Assay of Glandular Kallikreins

Only work with purified glandular kallikreins is reviewed here. Problems of determination of these enzymes in tissues or body fluids will not be discussed. The assay based on liberation of kinins from kininogen is very sensitive but difficulties were encountered even with partially purified kallikrein samples (MORIWAKI et al., 1974a). The main problem in the determination of glandular kallikreins is the specificity, which has not been solved even with synthetic substrates. Convenient and sensitive assay procedures, however, are based on the enzymic hydrolysis of esters of α-N-acylated arginine and can be monitored in several ways (TRAUTSCHOLD, 1970). Among those methods, spectrophotometric or titrimetric procedures with continuous recording of the course of the reaction are preferred. Only such a technique will allow recognition of possible perturbations and will reveal unusual phenomena such as the time-dependence of the activity observed with porcine glandular kallikreins (FRITZ et al., 1977).

Among the spectrophotometric methods, the assay of SCHWERT and TAKENAKA (1955) based on the direct monitoring of Bz-ArgOEt (BAEe) hydrolysis at 253 nm, as adopted for kallikrein determinations by TRAUTSCHOLD and WERLE (1961), appears to be the method of choice. Due to the high absorbance of the substrate, however, one is limited to substrate concentrations not much higher than 0.5 m*M*. This value is not high when compared to K_m values for most glandular kallikreins, and consequently only a limited extent of hydrolysis can be allowed without undue reduction of reaction rate because of depletion of substrate. WORTHINGTON and CUSCHIERI (1974) elaborated optimum conditions for the determination of pig pancreatic kallikrein. A small activating effect of EDTA (0.1 or 0.8 m*M*) or cysteine (1 m*M*) was observed. Optimal triethanolamine concentration was 10–50 m*M*, and optimal pH, 8.5–9. Concerning optimal pH, however, one should consider that too high a pH value will lead to notable nonenzymic hydrolysis of ester substrate and that the majority of the investigations reported were performed at pH 8; valid comparisons can be made only when identical assay conditions have been used.

Much more indirect and thus subject to more interference is the assay system based on using BAEe as substrate and on measurement of the ethanol liberated via the formation of NADH (TRAUTSCHOLD and WERLE, 1961; TRAUTSCHOLD, 1970). Nevertheless, this method should be used when one needs a spectrophotometric assay that also works in the presence of UV absorbing impurities. Proportionality to the amount of porcine pancreatic kallikrein present has been found only within a certain limited range (FRITZ et al., 1967). WORTHINGTON and CUSCHIERI (1974) proposed 15 min preincubation of the premixed reagents in order to minimize interference by an initial increase in absorbance, according to the original method of TRAUTSCHOLD and WERLE (1961). A total preincubation time of 7 min (FRITZ et al., 1967), however, appears to be sufficient (EICHNER et al., 1976).

For precise determinations of the activity of kallikrein preparations, a titrimetric assay easily performed on an autotitrator appears to be the method of choice. BAEe (10 m*M*) in a volume of 20 ml, 0.1 *M* NaCl and a 0.25 ml burette were used to minimize changes in substrate concentration due to hydrolysis or dilution by the titrating agent. Addition of 0.1 m*M* thioglycolic acid (EDTA gives identical results) eliminated problems with heavy metal ions and 0.1 *M* NaOH was used as titrating agent. The pH was 8.0 and the temperature was 25.0 °C to reduce nonenzymic substrate hydrolysis and possible interference from the uptake of CO_2 that was also counteracted by flushing the reaction vessel with moist CO_2-free nitrogen (FIEDLER et al., 1971; FIEDLER, 1976). A very similar assay system, substituting soybean trypsin inhibitor (SBTI) for thioglycolic acid to allow measurements also in the presence of trypsin and using a borate – KCl buffer, or 0.25 *M* KCl and 0.1 m*M* EDTA, was adopted as F.I.P. (Fédération Internationale Pharmaceutique) method for the standardization of pig pancreatic kallikrein (ARENS and HABERLAND, 1973; International Commission on Pharmaceutical Enzymes, 1974), while ZUBER and SACHE (1974) used 20 m*M* BAEe, 18–20 m*M* $CaCl_2$, and 1.5 m*M* borate buffer in 1 ml, titrating with 0.01 *N* NaOH.

Sensitivity and possibly also specificity of assays using BAEe might be increased by the use of Z-ArgOEt or Ac-Phe-ArgOEt, as esters of this type are better substrates of some glandular kallikreins (NUSTAD and PIERCE, 1974; FIEDLER, 1977).

For the standardization of human urinary kallikrein, 20 m*M* Tos-ArgOMe (TAMe) in 2.5 ml, 0.1 *M* KCl, 2 m*M* Tris-HCl, pH 8.0, 30 °C, titrated with 0.01 M NaOH, has been proposed (BEAVEN et al., 1971; IMANARI et al., 1977). Other methods used for following the hydrolysis of TAMe by kallikrein are based on the determination of methanol and thus should be applicable to other methyl esters. The colorimetric determination of methanol with chromotropic acid (MORIWAKI et al., 1971) was simple to handle and was 10 times more sensitive than the hydroxamate method (WEBSTER and PIERCE, 1961). Still 10 times more sensitive is the determination of the methanol released with 3-methyl-2-benzothiazolone hydrazone (MORIYA et al., 1971), and a fluorimetric assay brought even an additional factor of 10 (MATSUDA et al., 1976b). High sensitivity is also obtained by the use of TAMe with a tritiated alcohol moiety. Either excess of substrate is bound to an ion exchange column (BEAVEN et al., 1971) or the methanol released is separated by extraction with scintillation cocktail and directly counted (IMANARI et al., 1977).

Z-Tyr-p-nitrophenylester, an unspecific kallikrein substrate but highly activated ester, has been applied in an assay of human urinary kallikrein (HIAL et al., 1974).

For the determination of pig pancreatic kallikrein, Bz-DL-Arg-p-nitroanilide (BANA) has been used (GERATZ, 1969; GERATZ et al., 1973), though it is hydrolyzed only very slowly. Higher sensitivity is achieved by the application of more extended p-nitroanilides as Bz-Pro-Phe-Arg-p-nitroanilide (GERATZ et al., 1976) or Bz-Phe-Val-Arg-p-nitroanilide (HALABI and BACK, 1977). The principal advantage of these compounds is the convenience of the assays based on their use.

A BAEe-formazane staining system for the detection of kallikreins on gel electrophoretic media has been described by FUJIMOTO et al. (1972).

C. Glandular Kallikreins of the Pig

I. Porcine Pancreatic Prekallikrein

In porcine pancreas, kallikrein occurs mainly as enzymically inactive prekallikrein. From pancreatic homogenates prepared in the presence of SBTI, only about 10% of the potential kallikrein activity is eluted in an active form after adsorption on DEAE-cellulose (FIEDLER and WERLE, 1967; FIEDLER et al., 1970a). Because of the very easy activation of prekallikrein, even this amount might have been formed during the isolation. The total kallikrein content of porcine pancreas is about 60 mg/kg fresh organ (KUTZBACH and SCHMIDT-KASTNER, 1972). A zymogen representing, most probably, prekallikrein has also been enriched fivefold by means of gel filtration on Sephadex G-75 from porcine pancreatic juice (GREENE et al., 1968).

One of the two forms of prekallikrein observed to occur in porcine pancreas, prekallikrein B (FIEDLER and WERLE, 1967), has been partially purified (FIEDLER et al., 1970a) (Table 1). Only in continuous presence of SBTI was it possible to suppress "spontaneous" activation, most probably due to the action of some other pancreas proteinase, even in the purest preparation obtained. Prekallikrein is very rapidly converted to active enzyme by trypsin, much faster than trypsinogen, as already observed by GREENE et al. (1968).

After activation with bovine trypsin, the specific activity (4 mM BAEe) of the preparation after CM-cellulose purification amounted to about 35% of that of pancreatic kallikrein. On rechromatography on DEAE-cellulose, the activity of several fractions increased up to 70% of pancreatic kallikrein. Prolonged treatment with trypsin did not influence activity. α-Chymotrypsin did not activate prekallikrein. Dialysis and lyophilization led to severe losses of potential activity. The residual potential activity remained stable on storage at −20 °C for several weeks.

Disc electrophoresis also revealed that complete purity had not been achieved. By gel filtration, the molecular weight (MW) of prekallikrein B was found to be similar to that of pancreatic kallikrein. Isoelectric focusing yielded essentially a single peak with an isoelectric point of 4.55, higher than that of kallikrein (FIEDLER et al., 1970a).

II. Porcine Pancreatic Kallikrein B′

During the isolation of prekallikrein, some spontaneously activated kallikrein was separated by the second DEAE-cellulose step (FIEDLER et al., 1970a). This kallikrein differed distinctly from kallikrein isolated by the usual technique from autolyzed porcine pancreas (Table 1) by its higher isoelectric point (main fraction, 4.32; minor one, 4.19). A further difference was observed in the hydrolysis of BAEe: 4 mM substrate (pH 7.8; 25 °C) was hydrolyzed about three times faster by this kallikrein than by kallikrein B from autolyzed pancreas when compared to the rate of BAEe hydrolysis under the conditions of the alcohol dehydrogenase-linked assay (0.5 mM; pH 8.7; 25 °C). In this respect, the new form of kallikrein, named kallikrein B′, resembles porcine submandibular or urinary kallikreins (FRITZ et al., 1977). Kallikrein formed by activation of prekallikrein B with bovine trypsin had properties similar to those of kallikrein B′. The rate of inhibition of kallikrein B′ by diisopropyl phosphofluoridate (DFP) was indistinguishable from that of kallikrein B. The enzyme was also not inhibited by SBTI, but by aprotinin (BPTI). Most probably, kallikrein B′ represents a single-chain form of porcine pancreatic kallikrein, for which the name of α-kallikrein has been proposed (FIEDLER et al., 1977b).

III. Kallikrein From Autolyzed Porcine Pancreas

1. Isolation

All other investigations reported in the literature have been performed with kallikrein isolated from porcine pancreas after some autolytic step during which the prekallikrein is converted to active enzyme. Detailed directions based on the procedures of MORIYA et al. (1965, 1969) starting with fresh pancreas were given by WEBSTER and PRADO (1970). Initial steps of an industrial process consisting of autolysis at 25 °C, precipitation with heavy metal salts, and elution of the precipitate were outlined by KUTZBACH and SCHMIDT-KASTNER (1973). The newer purification procedures compiled in Table 1 start from some industrially preprocessed material and allow the isolation of kallikrein in two distinct forms. Affinity chromatography has

Table 1. Isolation of pancreatic prekallikrein and kallikrein of the pig

	Prekallikrein	Kallikrein							
	FIEDLER et al. (1970a)	TAKAMI (1969b)		KUTZBACH and SCHMIDT-KASTNER (1972, 1973)		ZUBER and SACHE (1974)		FIEDLER (1976)	
Purification steps: 1.	0.1 M acetic acid homogenate	DEAE-Sephadex		DEAE-Sephadex		Ammonium sulfate precipitation		Hydroxyapatite-cellulose	
2.	Ammonium sulfate fractionation	DEAE-Sephadex		SE-Sephadex		Calcium phosphate gel		Hydroxyapatite-cellulose	
3.	SE-Sephadex	Bio-Gel P-30		DEAE-Sephadex		Sephadex G-100		DEAE-cellulose	
4.	DEAE-cellulose	Bio-Gel P-200		DEAE-Sephadex		DEAE-cellulose		DEAE-cellulose	
5.	ECTEOLA-cellulose					DEAE-cellulose			
6.	Sephadex G-75								
7.	CM-cellulose								
8.	DEAE-cellulose								
Forms isolated:	B	A	B	A	B	d_1	d_2	A	B
Specific activity:									
Biologic (dog; KU):		1000/mg	1240/mg	1410/mg glycoprotein					
BAEe (μmol/min):		(10 mM; pH 8.0; 40 °C) 888/mg		(10 mM; pH 8.0; 25 °C)	212/mg glycoprotein	(20 mM; pH 8.0; 25 °C) 109 ± 4.3/mg protein	134 ± 6.9/mg protein	(10 mM; pH 8.0; 25 °C) 230–282/mg protein	282 ± 6/mg protein
Molecular weight:									
Gel filtration:	35,000–39,000	34,000	34,000			34,500	31,000		
Ultracentrifugation:				26,200		32,725	30,643		
Isoelectric point:	4.55					3.75; 3.82; 3.92; 3.97; 4.11	3.93; 4.01; 4.11	3.64; 3.71; 3.85; 3.95; 4.05	

also been investigated (FRITZ et al., 1969) and resulted in a 49-fold purification in a single step (FRITZ and FÖRG-BREY, 1972). With preparative disc electrophoresis, about ninefold purification and a yield of 42% has been achieved (HOJIMA et al., 1975b).

Pig pancreatic kallikrein has been crystallized by KUTZBACH and SCHMIDT-KASTNER (1972).

2. Heterogeneity

As was first observed by HABERMANN (1962), pig pancreatic kallikrein is separated on starch gel or membrane electrophoresis at pH 8.6–8.7 into two forms designated as kallikreins A (higher anodic mobility) and B, discernible also by membrane electrophoresis at pH 7 (FRITZ et al., 1967) and by disc gel electrophoresis in pH 8.9 buffer (KUTZBACH and SCHMIDT-KASTNER, 1972). Kallikreins A and B can be separated on a preparative scale by chromatography on a DEAE ion exchanger, a procedure first devised by SCHMIDT-KASTNER (quoted in FIEDLER and WERLE, 1967). These two preparations also differ in mobility, but yield only a single band in membrane (FIEDLER and WERLE, 1967) or in acrylamide gel electrophoresis (TAKAMI, 1969b; KUTZBACH and SCHMIDT-KASTNER, 1972; FIEDLER et al., 1975) at pH values of 8–9. Two components called kallikreins d_1 and d_2, isolated by ZUBER and SACHE (1974), behaved in an analogous way and probably represent kallikreins B and A, respectively. These authors observed, in addition, small amounts of a third form, d_3, with the highest mobility towards the anode. Kallikrein C, recently isolated by KUTZBACH and SCHMIDT-KASTNER (quoted in FRITZ et al., 1977), is probably identical with this form. FUJIMOTO et al. (1972), however, reported the appearance of as many as five bands staining with their BAEe-formazane procedure, a reaction not inhibited by SBTI, on acrylamide electrophoresis of kallikrein in pH 9.2 buffer.

An additional microheterogeneity of pig pancreatic kallikrein was observed by FRITZ et al. (1967). The enzyme was separated into four or five enzymically active bands on membrane electrophoresis at pH 4–5. After treatment of the kallikrein preparation with neuraminidase, which removed the bound sialic acid residues but did not influence specific activity, only two bands (besides traces of a third one) with slowest anodic mobility remained. Separated kallikreins A or B (not treated with neuraminidase) also showed four bands each with varying staining intensity.

Isoelectric focusing of kallikreins A or B also revealed the presence of a number of components (FIEDLER et al., 1970a). The pattern observed differed somewhat for different enzyme preparations, but within the reproducibility of about ± 0.05 pH units both forms of kallikrein displayed the same components with isoelectric points in the acid region (Table 1). On extensive treatment with neuraminidase, only the component with pI 4.05 was present in both kallikreins A and B (FIEDLER et al., 1970a, 1975). Probably, the fractions with increasingly lower isoelectric points represent kallikrein molecules containing an increasing number of bound sialic acid residues. Treatment with neuraminidase does not, however, influence the electrophoretic differences between kallikreins A and B observable at pH 7–9 (FRITZ et al., 1967; KUTZBACH and SCHMIDT-KASTNER, 1972; ZUBER and SACHE, 1974), i.e., at pH values that do not allow the discrimination of the kallikrein species with varying sialic acid content.

Multiple forms of kallikreins d_1 and d_2 were also observed on isoelectric focusing by ZUBER and SACHE (1974) (Table 1). HOJIMA et al. (1975a, b) obtained up to six peaks with isoelectric points between 4.23 and 3.68 with different preparations of pig pancreatic kallikrein. Gel isoelectrofocusing resolved still more components.

3. Optical Properties

Absorption spectra of unresolved kallikrein and of neuraminidase-treated kallikrein B have been reported. The absorption maximum has been found at 282 nm (FRITZ et al., 1967) or 281 nm (KUTZBACH and SCHMIDT-KASTNER, 1972). $A_{1\,cm}^{0.1\%}$ has been determined as 1.80 at 282 nm for unresolved kallikrein (FRITZ et al., 1967), as 2.00 ± 0.05 at 280 nm for kallikreins A and B on a protein basis (FIEDLER et al., 1975), as 1.66 ± 0.08 for sialic acid-free kallikrein B on a glycoprotein basis (KUTZBACH and SCHMIDT-KASTNER, 1972; recalculated to 1.88 ± 0.09 on a protein basis, FIEDLER, 1976) and as 1.58 on a weight basis (HOJIMA et al., 1975b).

The circular dichroism spectrum at pH 6.4 showed maxima at 203, 235, and 283 nm and was interpreted as kallikrein having a predominantly unordered conformation (KUTZBACH and SCHMIDT-KASTNER, 1972).

4. Molecular Weight

The reported MW and related constants for pig pancreatic kallikrein were compiled by FIEDLER (1976). Recently, HOJIMA et al. (1975b) obtained a MW of 31,000 by gel filtration in agreement with older values of 31,000–35,000 determined with this technique. It is known, however, that glycoproteins tend to give misleadingly high MWs in gel filtration (ANDREWS, 1970). The same is true for SDS electrophoresis, by which a MW of 34,600 was found as a sum of the two chains of kallikrein B (FRITZ et al., 1977) or values of 35,000 and 31,500 as sums of three chains of kallikreins d_1 and d_2, respectively (ZUBER and SACHE, 1974).

The above-mentioned effect will also influence the ultracentrifugation results of the latter authors (Table 1) because Stokes radii from gel filtration experiments were used in the calculations. Taking the correct value of 0.722 for the partial specific volume of the enzyme (KUTZBACH and SCHMIDT-KASTNER, 1972) which is in excellent agreement with values of 0.723 (ZUBER and SACHE, 1974) and 0.721 (FIEDLER et al., 1972b) calculated from the composition, previous ultracentrifugation data are recalculated to the lower MWs of 26,200 and 29,700 (see FIEDLER, 1976). A recent determination (FRITZ et al., 1977) resulted in a MW of $28{,}000 \pm 1000$ for neuraminidase-treated kallikrein B ($s_{20,\,w} = 2.4$–2.5; $D_{20,\,w} = 7.8 \times 10^{-7}\ cm^2\ s^{-1}$).

This value is in excellent agreement with the results of recent determinations from amino acid and average carbohydrate composition; 28,900 for kallikrein B and 27,100 for kallikrein A (both without sialic acid) and 25,600 for the protein part of both forms of the enzyme (FIEDLER et al., 1977b). MWs of 32,566 (d_1) and 33,280 (d_2) were calculated from the amino acid analysis by ZUBER and SACHE (1974) by a procedure that requires extreme precision of the analytical data.

5. Amino Acid and Carbohydrate Composition

Analytical results obtained on pancreatic kallikrein are compiled in Table 2. The amino acid data of FRITZ et al. (1967) and ZUBER and SACHE (1974) were based on

Table 2. Amino acid and carbohydrate composition of porcine glandular kallikreins (residues per molecule)

	Pancreatic A+B	Pancreatic		Pancreatic		Submandibular	Urinary
		d_1	d_2	A	B		
	FRITZ et al. (1967)	ZUBER and SACHE (1974)		FIEDLER et al. (1975, 1977b)		FRITZ et al. (1977)	FRITZ et al. (1977)
Asp	33	33	33–34	28		28	28
Thr	18	19	18	15		16	(15)
Ser	17	18	18	14		14	(12)
Glu	28	29	29	23		23	23
Pro	20	20	21	16		15–16	16
Gly	27	27	28	22		22	22
Ala	16	17	16	13		13	14
Cys/2	10	12	12	10		10	(10)
Val	13	13	13	10		10	11
Met	5	5	5	4		4	4
Ile	14	14	14	12		11	(≧10)
Leu	24	23	24	20		21	21
Tyr	9	10	9	7		7	7
Phe	13	13	12	10		10	10
Lys	13	12	12	10		11	11
His	10	9	9	8		9	8–9
Arg	4	5–6	5	3		3	3
Trp	9	9	9	7		7	
Hexose:	7–8	3.3	2.8				
Mannose	ca. 4			3.6; 2.9	6.0; 5.3		
Galactose	ca. 1			0.80; 0.70	1.6; 1.4		
Fucose	ca. 2			0.51	1.23; 0.95		
Hexosamine:		4.3	2.4				
Glucosamine (gas chromatograph)				4.1; 3.5	9.6; 9.8		
Glucosamine (amino acid analyser)	6–7			3.9	9.2; 9.05		
Sialic acid:	0.9	0.04	0.016				

estimating the MW too high. They are in satisfactory agreement with the composition, backed by the results of sequence determination, when recalculated using the correct MW (FIEDLER et al., 1975). No significant difference between the amino acid composition of kallikreins A and B has been found.

The carbohydrate composition of a mixture of kallikreins A and B obtained by FRITZ et al. (1967) correlates well qualitatively and quantitatively with the data of FIEDLER et al. (1975) (Table 2). Kallikrein B differs from kallikrein A only by containing roughly double the amount of each carbohydrate component (total, 11.5% versus 5.6% of weight). Kallikrein C contains even less carbohydrate than kallikrein A (FRITZ et al., 1977). A higher content of hexosamine was also found by ZUBER and SACHE (1974) in kallikrein d_1 which is probably identical with kallikrein B. Absolute values reported by these workers are, however, also much lower for neutral hexoses.

The average sialic acid content determined by FRITZ et al. (1967) fits well the presumed composition of kallikrein from species containing from zero to three residues per molecule. A possible source of error in the analyses of ZUBER and SACHE (1974) is discussed by FIEDLER et al. (1975).

6. End Groups and Composition From Polypeptide Chains

Pig pancreatic kallikreins A and B isolated from pancreas autolyzates contain one residue each of alanine (as also observed by TAKAMI, 1969b) and of isoleucine at the amino terminals. One proline and about half a residue each of leucine and of serine were found at the carboxyl-terminal end (FIEDLER et al., 1975).

In accordance with these observations, two protein subunits were obtained on SDS electrophoresis of reduced kallikrein B (FRITZ et al., 1977). Two main subunits, named A- and B-chains, were also isolated by gel filtration from reduced and carboxymethylated or aminoethylated kallikrein B (TSCHESCHE et al., 1976a). The name of β-kallikrein has been proposed for the form of kallikrein consisting of two polypeptide chains (FIEDLER et al., 1977b).

In the preparation of kallikrein B investigated, about 10–20% of the B-chain was cleaved at about the middle of the chain (TSCHESCHE et al., 1976a). The name of γ-kallikrein has been suggested for the form of kallikrein containing two cleavage sites (FIEDLER et al., 1977b). The two fragments of the B-chain have approximately the size of the A-chain of kallikrein.

This finding hardly offers an explanation for the observations of ZUBER and SACHE (1974) who found three protein components of different MW during SDS electrophoresis of reduced kallikreins d_1 and d_2. These preparations had only about half the specific activity of the kallikrein B studied by TSCHESCHE et al. (1976a) and FIEDLER et al. (1977b).

7. Amino Acid Sequence

The amino acid sequence of pig pancreatic β-kallikrein B consisting of 232 amino acids has been elucidated with the exception of a single gap of 34 residues in the B-chain (Fig. 1). 44% of the amino acid residues are identical to those found in equivalent positions in porcine trypsin (HERMODSON et al., 1973). This clearly demonstrates that this kallikrein is another pancreatic serine proteinase apart from trypsin, chymotrypsin, and elastase.

A-chain:
16 17 18 19 20 21 22 23 24 25 26 27 28 29 30 31 32 33
Ile-Ile-Gly-Gly-Arg-Glu-Cys-Glu-Lys-Asn-Ser-His-Pro-Trp-Gln-Val-Ala-Ile-
34 37 38 39 40 41 41A 42 43 44 45 46 47 48 49 50 51 52
-Tyr-His-Tyr-Ser-Ser-Phe-Gln-Cys-Gly-Gly-Val-Leu-Val-Asn-Pro-Lys-Trp-Val-
53 54 55 56 57 58 59 60 61 62 63 64 65 65A 66 69 70
-Leu-Thr-Ala-Ala-His-Cys-Lys-Asn-Asp-Asn-Tyr-Glu-Val-Gly-Trp-Leu-Arg-
71 72 73 74 75 76 77 78 79 80 81 82 83 84 85 86 87
-His-Asn-Leu-Phe-Glu-Asn-Glu-Asn-Thr-Ala-Gln-Phe-Phe-Gly-Val-Thr-Ala-
88 89 90 91 92 93 94 95 95A 95B
-Asp-Phe-Pro-His-Pro-Gly-Phe-Asn-Leu-Ser

B-chain:
95Y 95Z 96 97 98 99 100 101 102 103 104 105 106 107 108 109 110
Ala-Asp-Gly-Lys-Asp-Tyr-Ser-His-Asp-Leu-Met-Leu-Leu-Arg-Leu-Gln-Ser-
111 112 113 114 115 116 117 118 119 120 121 122 123 124 125 127 128
-Pro-Ala-Lys-Ile-Thr-Asp-Ala-Val-Lys-Val-Leu-Glu-Leu-Pro-Thr-Gln-Glu-
129 130 132 133 134 135 136 137 138 139 140 141 142
Pro-Glu-Leu-Gly-Ser-Thr-Cys-Gln-Ala-Ser-Gly-Trp-Gly-

B-chain, ctd:
175 176 177 178 179 180 181 182 183 184 184A 185 186 187 188 188A 189
-Lys-Val-Thr-Glu-Ser-Met-Leu-Cys-Ala-Gly-Tyr-Leu-Pro-Gly-Gly-Lys-Asp-
190 191 192 193 194 195 196 197 198 199 200 201 202 203 204 209 210
-Thr-Cys-Met-Gly-Asp-Ser-Gly-Gly-Pro-Leu-Ile-Cys-Asn-Gly-Met-Trp-Gln
211 212 213 214 215 216 217 218 219 220 221 221A 222 223 224 225 226 227
-Gly-Ile-Thr-Ser-Trp-Gly-His-Thr-Pro-Cys-Gly-Ser-Ala-Asn-Lys-Pro-Ser-Ile-
228 229 230 231 232 233 234 235 236 237 238 239 240 241 242 243 244 245
-Tyr-Thr-Lys-Leu-Ile-Phe-Tyr-Leu-Asp-Trp-Ile(Asx,Asx)Thr-Ile-Thr-Glu-Asn-
246
-Pro

Fig. 1. The primary structure of pig pancreatic β-kallikrein B (TSCHESCHE et al., 1976a; FIEDLER et al., 1977b). The numbering is that of chymotrypsinogen (HARTLEY, 1964)

Kallikrein evidently has the same catalytically active charge relay system [i.e., aspartic acid (102), histidine (57), serine (195)] as other serine proteinases. The sequence around the single serine residue reacting with DFP is most probably -Asp-Ser-Gly- (FIEDLER et al., 1971), a result confirming that serine (195) is the active-site serine. The ion pair, isoleucine (16) – aspartic acid (194), stabilizing the structure of other serine proteinases could also be formed in kallikrein. The eight half-cystine residues of kallikrein shown in Fig. 1, as well as those two located in the part not yet sequenced, are in positions equivalent to 10 of the 12 half-cystines of trypsin (FIEDLER et al., 1977b) and are thus able to form five of the six disulfide bridges of trypsin. Kallikrein contains no free sulfhydryl groups (ZUBER and SACHE, 1974). One of the five possible bridges otherwise only occurs in trypsin, an indication of a closer relationship between these two enzymes. Another point of resemblance is the presence of aspartic acid (189), responsible for the specificity of trypsin for basic amino acids. The similarity, however, is not too close. Trypsins of different species are much more closely related, as exemplified by the 82% identity in amino acids of bovine and porcine trypsins (HERMODSON et al., 1973), than are porcine trypsin and kallikrein (44%).

Carbohydrate is most probably bound to asparagine residues in positions 95 (A-chain) and 239 (B-chain) (FIEDLER et al., 1977b). The site of cleavage between the A- and B-chains of kallikrein is not homologous to splits observed in other pancreatic serine proteinases and neither is the second one at positions 174 or 175 that was found in 10–20% of the enzyme preparation. Serine (95B) occurred in only about half of the A-chains, an indication of further degradation at the cleavage site. There is preliminary indirect evidence that even several amino acid residues were removed

(FIEDLER et al., 1977b; FRITZ et al., 1977). Special properties of kallikrein are the additional C-terminal proline residue (246) and the extended kallikrein loop around the site of cleavage between the A- and B-chains, in a region that is probably important for the binding of substrate.

8. Stability

Activity losses of at most 5% were observed during lyophilization of kallikrein solutions (KUTZBACH and SCHMIDT-KASTNER, 1972; FIEDLER et al., 1975). Storage for one year did not result in appreciable loss of activity (ZUBER and SACHE, 1974). Solutions of 0.5 mg/ml could be stored unchanged at 4 °C, pH 8, for at least 12 weeks (ZUBER and SACHE, 1974). Above pH 4.5 or 5, kallikrein solutions are stable at 25 °C (KUTZBACH and SCHMIDT-KASTNER, 1972; WORTHINGTON and CUSCHIERI, 1974; ZUBER and SACHE, 1974). Sialic acid-free kallikrein resembled the native compound in stability (FRITZ et al., 1967). High stability of kallikreins d_1 and d_2 was also observed in heat inactivation experiments. Activity losses began at 58 °C but appreciable activity survived 10 min even at 100 °C (ZUBER and SACHE, 1974).

After 48 h in 8 *M* urea, about 50% activity was recovered (KUTZBACH and SCHMIDT-KASTNER, 1972), while complete inactivation occurred in 8 *M* guanidine HCl after 5 min at 37 °C (ZUBER and SACHE, 1974). Several of the disulfide bridges of kallikrein could be reduced with sodium borohydride, without severe activity losses (ZUBER and SACHE, 1974).

9. Hydrolysis of Amino Acid Esters

Esters of arginine are by far most rapidly hydrolyzed by pig pancreatic kallikrein. At high concentrations, esters of other protected amino acids are also attacked at a notable rate (TAKAMI, 1969a; FIEDLER et al., 1973; ZUBER and SACHE, 1974). As seen from the specificity constants k_{cat}/K_m (BENDER and KÉZDY, 1965) compiled in Table 3, compounds such as the typical chymotrypsin substrate, Ac-TyrOEt, are several orders of magnitude less active than arginine esters as substrates for kallikrein; this is also true for trypsin. [A compilation of corresponding constants for bovine trypsin was published by FIEDLER et al. (1973).] This does not preclude that Z-Phe-p-nitrophenylester with a favourable group in position P_2 and a very good leaving group is also hydrolyzed by this kallikrein (ZUBER and SACHE, 1974), as is Z-Tyr-p-nitrophenylester by trypsin (MARTIN et al., 1959). In contrast to trypsin, kallikrein discriminates strongly between esters of arginine and of lysine (Table 3).

There are notable discrepancies in the Michaelis constants (K_m) in the reports of various investigators. In part, this might be due to differences in reaction conditions. Probably, the various forms of pancreatic kallikrein, differing in the extent of intrachain cleavage suffered during isolation, will have different kinetic constants. Furthermore, at higher substrate concentrations deviations from Michaelis-Menten kinetics have been observed. BAEe exhibits substrate activation at pH 7 and substrate inhibition at pH 9 (FIEDLER and WERLE, 1968), and the latter phenomenon was also observed at pH 8 with concentrations higher than 30 m*M* (ZUBER and SACHE, 1974). TAMe shows especially pronounced substrate activation at concentrations higher than 1 m*M* (FIEDLER and WERLE, 1968; FIEDLER et al., 1975; ZUBER and SACHE, 1974) similar to that observed with trypsin (TROWBRIDGE et al., 1963).

Table 3. Kinetic constants for the hydrolysis of amino acid esters by pig pancreatic kallikrein (pH 8.0, 25 °C, if not stated otherwise)

Substrate	K_m (mM)	k_{cat} (s^{-1})	k_{cat}/K_m (mM^{-1} s^{-1})	Ref.
TAMe	0.33 (40 °C)	(32 μmol/min/mg)		TAKAMI (1969a)
	0.031 ± 0.008	2.7 ± 0.33	150	FIEDLER et al. (1973)
	0.81	3.4	4.2	ZUBER and SACHE (1974)
BAEe	0.27			TRAUTSCHOLD and WERLE (1961)
	0.37 (pH 7)			CHAMBERS et al. (1963)
	1.1 (40 °C)	(433 μmol/min/mg)		TAKAMI (1969a)
	0.104 ± 0.008	123 ± 8	1,180	FIEDLER et al. (1973)
	0.105			WORTHINGTON and CUSCHIERI (1974)
	0.5 (d_1)	74	150	ZUBER and SACHE (1974)
	0.5 (d_2)	100	200	ZUBER and SACHE (1974)
BAMe	0.18 (pH 7)			CHAMBERS et al. (1963)
	0.125 ± 0.020	154 ± 13	1,230	FIEDLER et al. (1973)
Ac-Phe-ArgOMe	0.045	900	20,000	FIEDLER (1976a)
Z-LysOMe	3.8 (40 °C)	(134 μmol/min/mg)		TAKAMI (1969a)
Bz-LysOMe	0.93 (40 °C)	(17 μmol/min/mg)		TAKAMI (1969a)
	2.00 ± 0.28	15.5 ± 1.4	7.75	FIEDLER et al. (1973)
Bz-OrnOMe	2.44 ± 0.30	1.80 ± 0.25	0.74	FIEDLER et al. (1973)
Bz-CitrOMe	12.3 ± 1.4	8.64 ± 0.81	0.70	FIEDLER et al. (1973)
ATEe	50 ± 14	11.2 ± 2.2	0.22	FIEDLER et al. (1973)
Bz-DL-MetOMe	ca. 20	ca. 1.5	0.07	FIEDLER (1968)

The nature of the acyl substituent of the α-amino group is of paramount importance for the rate of amino acid ester hydrolysis by kallikrein. 10 mM ArgOMe (AMe) is hydrolyzed at only 3.5% the rate of BAEe (TAKAMI, 1969a). The specificity constant for the hydrolysis of TAMe is at most $^1/_8$ that of the benzoylated ester, though the K_m is surprisingly low according to the measurements of FIEDLER et al. (1973). Consequently, TAMe is an inhibitor of BAEe hydrolysis (TAKAMI, 1969a). A similarly low K_m, but the highest k_{cat} observed so far for any kallikrein substrate, characterize Ac-Phe-ArgOMe (Table 3). The phenylalanine residue in position P_2 strongly enhances hydrolysis by kallikrein.

Similar observations were made with a series of lysine esters. The rates quoted are relative to BAEe hydrolysis. LysOMe (1.7%), Tos-LysOMe (1.3%), and Ac-LysOMe (5.6%), are worse substrates than Bz-LysOMe (8%). Extension of the acyl substituent (Ac-Gly-LysOMe, 26.5%) and introduction in P_2 of a carbobenzoxy group bearing strong resemblance in its structure to a phenylalanine residue (Z-

LysOMe, 33.5–39%) lead to much better kallikrein substrates (TAKAMI, 1969a; ZUBER and SACHE, 1974).

The influence of the alcohol leaving group is discussed below with the mechanism of catalysis.

10. Protein and Peptide Hydrolysis

Most authors agree that pure pig pancreatic kallikrein has only a very limited ability, if any, to act as a general proteinase. Thus, casein is hydrolyzed by kallikrein 200-times slower than by trypsin (HABERMANN, 1962; SACH et al., 1971; ZUBER and SACHE, 1974). TAKAMI (1969b) reported that casein is hydrolysed faster than polylysine. This observation might indicate contamination by a caseinolytic enzyme. The reported hydrolysis of poor substrates might have actually been due to this contaminating enzyme and not to kallikrein. Hence all the results on the hydrolysis of comparatively poor kallikrein substrates reported in that paper have to be regarded with reservation. This also holds for reports on the cleavage of a peptide from κ-casein by a kallikrein preparation of 870 U (KU?)/mg (JOLLÉS et al., 1963), on caseinolysis and fibrin clot lysis by kallikrein of 11 KU/mg (CHAMBERS et al., 1963), and on the digestion of allergens by kallikrein of 1 (or 10) KU/mg that also hydrolyzed bovine serum albumin (BSA) (BERRENS, 1968).

Highly purified preparations of pig pancreatic kallikrein (1100–1200 KU/mg protein or 1180 KU/mg, respectively) were able to activate procollagenase (EECKHOUT and VAES, 1974) via the activation of a proactivator (EECKHOUT and VAES, 1977) and to release an acid-stable proteinase inhibitor from human inter-α-trypsin inhibitor (BRETZEL and HOCHSTRASSER, 1976).

Polypeptides rich in basic amino acids are cleaved by kallikrein. This is true for clupein, salmin, polyarginine, polylysine, and polyhomoarginine, but not for polyornithine (TAKAMI, 1969b; KATO and SUZUKI, 1970; SACH et al., 1971).

The rate of kinin release from crude bovine kininogen (pH 7.5, 30 °C) has been determined as up to 160 µg bradykinin equivalent/min/mg (MORIWAKI et al., 1974a). Pig pancreatic kallikrein releases from bovine kininogen the dekapeptide kallidin (HABERMANN and BLENNEMANN, 1964) besides traces of bradykinin (HABERMANN and MÜLLER, 1966). Methionyl-kallidin (Met-Lys-bradykinin) is not an intermediate of this reaction and is not cleaved by kallikrein. The only peptide fragment identified in fingerprints of kininogen treated with this kallikrein was kallidin, and the only aminoterminal amino acids detected by Edman degradation were lysine (from kallidin) and serine (following kinin in kininogen) (HABERMANN, 1966). Kallidin relase was possible only from native bovine kininogen II (LMW) or from kininogen denatured with 8 *M* urea or reduced and then reoxidized with air, but not from reduced, carboxymethylated, or performic acid oxidized kininogen (KATO and SUZUKI, 1970). Kallidin was also liberated from bovine HMW kininogen I (YANO et al., 1971). There was observed, in addition, a slow release of two larger peptide fragments (KATO et al., 1976; IWANAGA et al., 1977). Kinin liberation by pancreatic kallikrein was significantly slower when the HMW kininogen had been reduced and carboxymethylated, while the reaction with trypsin was less impaired by this modification. From HMW kininogen in which the lysyl residues had been blocked by citraconylation, the kallikrein also released kallidin at a rate comparable to kinin liberation by trypsin. Oxidation of the methionine residues of the citraconylated preparation nearly completely blocked the attack by kallikrein or by trypsin (IWANAGA et al., 1977).

Extensive treatment of reduced, carboxymethylated and citraconylated bovine HMW kininogen in which all methionine residues had been oxidized with porcine pancreatic kallikrein released a peptide of the sequence Ser-Leu-Met-Lys-bradykinin (HAN et al., 1976). This result contradicts a previous report by HOCHSTRASSER and WERLE (1967) that the kininogen sequences yielding kinin are Ser- and Gly-Arg-Met-Lys-bradykinin. Common to all these structures is the Met-Lys bond that has to be cleaved by kallikrein if kallidin is to be released. From the kininogen fragments isolated by HOCHSTRASSER and WERLE (1967), Met-Lys-bradykinin and either Gly-Arg or Ser-Arg were obtained on cleavage by pig pancreatic kallikrein, in accordance with the predominant arginine specificity of the enzyme. Also, synthetic Gly-Arg-Met-Lys-bradykinin was slowly cleaved by this kallikrein to 80% at the Arg-Met and to 20% at the Lys-Arg bond, but not at the Met-Lys bond (FIEDLER, 1977). The slow rate of attack at the arginyl bond, allowing also some cleavage of the lysyl bond, is presumably caused by the preceding residue being glycine and by the position of the bond cleaved near the amino-terminus of the peptide. There is some inconsistency with the report by HOCHSTRASSER and WERLE (1967) that the kininogen fragment was hydrolyzed quite rapidly.

Pig pancreatic kallikrein evidently is able to hydrolyze methionyl bonds, not only in kininogen but also in smaller peptides, in spite of its inability to attack simple α-N-acylated esters of methionine at a notable rate (FIEDLER, 1968; TAKAMI, 1969a; KATO and SUZUKI, 1970; FIEDLER et al., 1973; ZUBER and SACHE, 1974): Ser-Leu-Met-Lys-bradykinin is cleaved with formation of kallidin (IWANAGA et al., 1977). A special conformation of the kininogen molecule might be necessary for a high hydrolytic rate, but is evidently not essential for the cleavage to take place. Possibly the attack by kallikrein at the methionyl bond is directed by the preceding bulky leucine residue in position P_2 of the substrate (see below). In bovine kininogen, the sequences Gln-Met-Lys and Val-Met-Lys are not cleaved by pancreatic kallikrein (IWANAGA et al., 1977).

The cleavage of the bond at the C-terminus of kinin in kininogen is in accordance with the predominant arginine specificity of pig pancreatic kallikrein as established from experiments with synthetic substrates. HABERMANN (1966) determined the sequence of a kinin-yielding peptic fragment of bovine kininogen as Met-Lys-bradykinyl-Ser-Val-Gln, that was hydrolyzed to Met-kallidin and Ser-Val-Gln. The structure of the fragment was verified by synthesis, and the synthetic peptide had similar kinin activity after treatment with kallikrein (SCHRÖDER and LEHMANN, 1969). A cyanogen bromide peptide from bovine kininogen with the sequence Lys-bradykinyl-Ser-Val-Gln-Val-Hser is hydrolyzed by kallikrein only at the Arg-Ser bond (HABERMANN and HELBIG, 1967; KATO and SUZUKI, 1970).

Other synthetic peptides hydrolyzed by pig pancreatic kallikrein are tetra- and pentalysine and β^{1-24}-corticotropin (SACH et al., 1971). Among a number of arginine-containing peptides, most were either not hydrolyzed at all or at only a very low rate (up to 0.42 μmol/min/mg enzyme protein). Only two of the peptides studied, Pro-Phe-Arg-Ser-Val-Gln and Phe-Ser-Pro-Phe-Arg-Ser-Val-Gln, representing partial sequences of kininogen, were hydrolyzed at a rate amounting to about 10% of the rate of tryptic hydrolysis. The pH-dependence of the cleavage demonstrated, that

Table 4. Preliminary data for the hydrolysis of peptides by pig pancreatic kallikrein B (pH 9.0; 25 °C) (FIEDLER, 1977)

	K_m (mM)	k_{cat} (s^{-1})	k_{cat}/K_m (mM^{-1} s^{-1})
Bradykinyl-Ser-Val-Gln	0.075	7	93
Phe-Ser-Pro-Phe-Arg-Ser-Val-Gln	0.064	6.4	100
Pro-Phe-Arg-Ser-Val-Gln	0.058	5.1	88
Ac-Phe-Arg-Ser-Val-Gln	0.18	6.8	38
Phe-Arg-Ser-Val-Gln	6	8	1.3
Ac-Phe-Arg-Ser-NH_2	0.2	1.8	9
Ac-Gly-Arg-Ser-Val-Gln	15	0.5	0.03

the Arg-Ser bond in these synthetic peptides was indeed a peptide and not an ester bond (WERLE et al., 1973). Kinetic constants for the hydrolysis of these and similar peptides by kallikrein are compiled in Table 4. Shortening of the peptides in the kinin part of the molecule does not notably influence hydrolysis by kallikrein, unless the proline residue is also removed. This drastically raises the K_m. Acetylation of the aminoterminal phenylalanine nearly restores the favourable low value of K_m, whereas k_{cat} is not notably influenced by all these manipulations. Shortening of the latter peptide by two residues at the C-terminus leads to a four-fold lowering of k_{cat} even when the carboxyl group of the terminal serine residue is amidated. The active site of kallikrein evidently is able to interact with at least five succeeding amino acid residues of a peptide substrate.

Substitution of the phenylalanine residue in P_2 of the acetylated peptide by a glycine residue (a change not involving amino acids at the bond hydrolyzed) has a tremendous negative influence on the cleavage of the peptide by kallikrein (Table 4) but not by bovine trypsin. This strong secondary specificity of pig pancreatic kallikrein for a phenylalanine residue in P_2 as it occurs in the natural substrate, kininogen, is striking.

It may be possible, however, that the presence of a phenylalanine residue in P_2 is not specifically necessary for good substrates of kallikrein, but that the bulk of the amino acid side chain in this position is the salient feature. A bulky leucine residue improves the inhibitory properties of peptidyl lysine chloromethyl ketones (see below). In an octacosapeptide (VIP) containing two arginine and three lysine residues, only the arginyl bond in the sequence -Leu-Arg-Lys- was hydrolyzed by kallikrein, but not that in a -Thr-Arg-Leu- sequence (BODANSKY et al., 1974). This same bond was hydrolyzed in a cyanogen bromide fragment of that peptide, a reaction used in the determination of the sequence (MUTT and SAID, 1974). The leucine residue in P_2 of the kininogen peptide Ser-Leu-Met-Lys-bradykinin of IWANAGA et al. (1977) might even be responsible for directing the attack of kallikrein to the methionyl bond.

The nature of the leaving group is also of importance in peptide hydrolysis by pig pancreatic kallikrein. Substitution of serine in a peptide of the type shown in Table 4 by an isosteric α-aminobutyric acid residue notably lowers the rate of hydrolysis

(F. FIEDLER and G. LEYSATH, unpublished result). In bovine HMW kininogen, the only two other bonds (besides those linking the kinin moiety to the kininogen) cleaved by pancreatic kallikrein to any extent are one His-Arg(or Lys?)+Ser and one Trp-Arg+Thr bond (IWANAGA et al., 1977; KATO et al., 1977), distinguished by good β-hydroxy amino acid leaving groups in addition to bulky residues in P_2.

The hydrolysis of nonpeptide amides of arginine by porcine pancreatic kallikrein is very slow. A rate of 0.052 µmol/min/mg was found for Bz-ArgNH_2 (9 m*M*, pH 8, 40 °C) with an enzyme preparation also exhibiting notable casein hydrolysis, but Tos-ArgNH_2 was not hydrolyzed (TAKAMI, 1969b). In that paper, the rate of hydrolysis of BANA (0.9 m*M*) is given as 0.129 µmol/min/mg, while WERLE et al. (1973) reported it as 0.005 µmol/min/mg protein (0.1 m*M*, pH 9, 25 °C) and HOJIMA et al. (1975b) as 0.006. The K_m for this compound is of the order of 0.8 m*M* (GERATZ et al., 1976), while that of Bz-Pro-Phe-Arg-p-nitroanilide was 0.275 m*M* (pH 8.1, 37 °C). The hydrolytic rate of the latter compound was more than 60 times greater than that of BANA (GERATZ et al., 1976) and is reported as either zero or 4.5 µmol/min/mg (0.18 m*M*, pH 8, 25 °C) by AMUNDSEN et al. (1976). K_m for Bz-Phe-Val-Arg-p-nitroanilide was 0.22 m*M* (HALABI and BACK, 1977).

11. Low Molecular Weight Reversible Inhibitors and Activators

Increasing NaCl concentrations up to 0.05 *M* led to some increase in the rate of ester hydrolysis in titration experiments and caused no further change up to 0.5 *M* (FIEDLER and WERLE, 1968). A small stimulation by 0.1 *M* NaCl was also observed by TAKAMI (1969a), while WORTHINGTON and CUSCHIERI (1974) reported a decrease of activity with increasing NaCl concentrations in the presence of triethanolamine. While 1 m*M* $CaCl_2$ had no effect (FIEDLER and WERLE, 1968), 0.1 *M* reduced the rate of hydrolysis to 48% (TAKAMI, 1969a), though 1 *M* was reported to increase activity by 15–20% (ZUBER and SACHE, 1974).

Pig pancreatic kallikrein is inhibited by heavy metal ions (FIEDLER and WERLE, 1968; TAKAMI, 1969a; ZUBER and SACHE, 1974). The inhibition by Zn^{2+} or Hg^{2+} can be reversed by EDTA or thioglycolic acid. These and other chelating agents or sulfhydryl compounds increased somewhat the rate of BAEe hydrolysis by kallikrein, probably by blocking the inhibition by contaminating heavy metal ions (FIEDLER and WERLE, 1968). ZUBER and SACHE (1974) did not observe such an effect. At low triethanolamine buffer concentrations, activation by EDTA or cysteine has also been noted by WORTHINGTON and CUSCHIERI (1974). Possibly, at higher concentrations of triethanolamine, that in itself had some inhibitory effect, or Tris (TAKAMI, 1969a), the complexing capacities of these compounds suffice for abolition of heavy metal inhibition. This might also be the explanation for the slight enhancement by ammonium ions or amino acids such as observed with tryptophan (TAKAMI, 1969a). In Tris buffer, no activation by tryptophan was found. The activation by high concentrations of Tos-LysCh_2Cl (TAKAMI, 1969a), however, might be related to substrate activation by, e.g., TAMe, another possible explanation for the activating effects of positively charged molecules. Some activation of kallikrein by SBTI has also been reported (ARENS and HABERLAND, 1973).

Other reversible inhibitors of kallikrein are dealt with in this volume in the chapter by VOGEL.

12. Active-Site Directed Reagents

The rate of inhibition of pig pancreatic kallikrein B by DFP has been determined as $8 \pm 1\,M^{-1}\,\text{min}^{-1}$ at pH 7.2 and as $13.2\,M^{-1}\,\text{min}^{-1}$ at optimum pH (FIEDLER et al., 1969). This is much lower than the rate of inhibition of other serine proteinases. A single serine residue, most probably located in a sequence -Asp-Ser-Gly- (FIEDLER et al., 1971), reacted with the inhibitor. MARKWARDT et al. (1971) report a rate of $3\,M^{-1}\,\text{min}^{-1}$. Determination of the velocity constants of inhibition by 1 mM DFP at pH 7.2, 25 °C, resulted in identical values of $(9.4 \pm 2.0) \times 10^{-3}\,\text{min}^{-1}$ for kallikrein A and of $(8.6 \pm 2.2) \times 10^{-3}\,\text{min}^{-1}$ for kallikrein B (FIEDLER et al., 1970b). Calculated from the data of ZUBER and SACHE (1974), the corresponding value for kallikrein d_1 at pH 7.4 is $2.5 \times 10^{-3}\,\text{min}^{-1}$.

The latter authors determined the kinetic constants for the inhibition by phenylmethanesulfonyl fluoride (pH 8, 25 °C) as $K_i = 4.6$ mM, $k_2 = 0.03\,\text{min}^{-1}$. Other sulfonyl fluorides for which kinetic constants were reported (pH 8.1, 37 °C), are p-[m(m-fluorosulfonyl-phenylureido)phenoxyethoxy]benzamidine ($K_i = 0.0043$ mM; $k_2 = 0.0425\,\text{min}^{-1}$; GERATZ, 1972) and N-($\beta$-pyridyl-methyl)-3,4-dichlorophenoxyacetamide-p-fluorosulfonylacetanilide bromide ($K_i = 0.031$ mM; $k_2 = 0.0431\,\text{min}^{-1}$; GERATZ and FOX, 1973). A number of further compounds of this class have been investigated by MARKWARD et al. (1971).

Diphenylcarbamylchloride also proved to be an irreversible kallikrein inhibitor with $k_2 = 12.2\,M^{-1}\,\text{min}^{-1}$ (pH 8, 25 °C; ZUBER and SACHE, 1964). Like other serine proteinases, the enzyme is inhibited by halomethylated derivatives of dihydrocoumarins (BÉCHET et al., 1977).

Cinnamoyl imidazole ($k_{ac} = 130 \pm 8$ or $119 \pm 6\,M^{-1}\,\text{s}^{-1}$ at pH 5.2, 25 °C, $k_{deac} = 3.4 \times 10^{-3}\,\text{s}^{-1}$ at pH 8.8 for kallikrein A; 116 ± 2 and 3.5×10^{-3}, respectively, for kallikrein B) and indoleacryloyl imidazole ($260\,M^{-1}\,\text{s}^{-1}$ and $1.2 \times 10^{-3}\,\text{s}^{-1}$ for kallikrein A; 230 and 1.1×10^{-3} for kallikrein B) react indiscriminantly with either form of the enzyme. The resulting cinnamoyl-kallikreins A and B have identical spectra that resemble most closely that of the corresponding trypsin derivative, and the same holds for the indoleacryloyl-enzymes, indicating a very similar architecture of the active site of these serine proteinases (FIEDLER et al., 1972a).

p-Nitrophenyl p′-guanidinobenzoate ($K_s = 81 \pm 56\,\mu M$; $K_m = 79 \pm 63\,nM$; $k_2 = 18 \pm 7\,\text{s}^{-1}$; $k_{deac} = (1.76 \pm 0.06) \times 10^{-2}\,\text{s}^{-1}$ for kallikrein B at pH 8.3, 25 °C (FIEDLER et al., 1972b); $k_{deac} = 1.2 \times 10^{-2}\,\text{s}^{-1}$ for kallikrein d_1 and similar for d_2 (ZUBER and SACHE, 1974)) is useful as an active site titration reagent for pancreatic kallikrein, though the rate of deacylation – identical for kallikreins A and B – is much higher than with trypsin. The method has been used for a determination of the MW of the protein part of the enzyme (FIEDLER et al., 1972b).

The irreversible trypsin inhibitor Tos-LysCH_2Cl does not inhibit pancreatic kallikrein (MARES-GUIA and DINIZ, 1967; FIEDLER, 1968; TAKAMI, 1969a; ZUBER and SACHE, 1974), $t_{1/2}$ being > 600 min even at 5 mM inhibitor concentration (pH 7, 25 °C; FIEDLER et al., 1977a). Under these conditions, Phe-Ala-LysCH_2Cl did not inhibit either. With increasing size of the residue in position P_2 the $t_{1/2}$ of inhibition decreased from 121 ± 13 min with Ala-Val-LysCH_2Cl to 5.9 ± 0.4 min with Ala-Leu-LysCH_2Cl. Kinetic constants were determined as $K_i = 1.04 \pm 0.12$ mM and $k_2 = (2.32 \pm 0.10) \times 10^{-3}\,\text{s}^{-1}$ for the inhibition by Ala-Leu-LysCH_2Cl, and

$K_i = 0.37 \pm 0.05$ mM and $k_2 = (7.8 \pm 0.3) \times 10^{-3}$ s^{-1} for Gly-Val-ArgCH_2Cl, again indicating the predominant arginine specificity of this kallikrein (FIEDLER et al., 1977a). Even Z-PheCH_2Cl with the favourable carbobenzoxy residue in P_2 was observed to inhibit, though with the very high $t_{1/2}$ of 133 h (ZUBER and SACHE, 1974).

13. Mechanism of Catalysis

The catalytically active charge-relay system of the serine proteinases [aspartic acid (102), histidine (57), serine (195)] is located in pig pancreatic kallikrein in equivalent positions. The reaction with DFP and the acylation reactions just mentioned indicate the acylation of the active site serine residue. The irreversible inhibition by chloromethyl ketones suggest the participation of a histidine residue.

Further evidence for the participation of such a residue comes from the pH dependence of reactions catalyzed by kallikrein. The inhibition by DFP is determined by a group with pK_a 6.85 (FIEDLER et al., 1969). A group with pK_a 6.9 in the enzyme-substrate complex and one with pK_a 7.9 in the free enzyme were shown with BAEe as substrate (FIEDLER and WERLE, 1968). This was confirmed by WORTHINGTON and CUSCHIERI (1974) who found values of 7.07 and 7.9, respectively. The possible presence of an additional group with pK_a 5.7 was, however, not corroborated. The activity decreased little even at pH 12. According to TAKAMI (1969a) and ZUBER and SACHE (1974) the pK_a of the group in the enzyme-substrate complex that must be dissociated for development of enzyme activity is 6.5. The group in question with pK_a 6.5–7.07 is generally regarded as the imidazole group of the active side histidine residue in serine proteinases.

The biphasic course of the reaction of p-nitrophenyl p′-guanidinobenzoate with kallikrein, a stoichiometric burst of nitrophenol followed by a slow constant nitrophenol release, directly indicates the functioning of an acyl-enzyme mechanism in the hydrolysis of this ester (FIEDLER et al., 1972b; ZUBER and SACHE, 1974). In the hydrolysis of a number of esters of benzoylated or tosylated arginine with different alcohols, however, k_{cat} was not constant, but paralleled the rate of hydroxyl ion catalyzed hydrolysis (FIEDLER et al., 1973). V_{max} for the hydrolysis of Z-LysOMe also reached only 41% of V_{max} for the corresponding benzyl ester (TAKAMI, 1969a). These observations suggest that with these esters the acylation reaction is rate-limiting.

Activation energies for BAEe hydrolysis have been determined as 10,703 cal/mol for kallikrein d_1 and as 8200 cal/mol for kallikrein d_2 (ZUBER and SACHE, 1974).

IV. Porcine Submandibular Kallikrein

1. Isolation and Molecular Aspects

A new isolation procedure for porcine submandibular kallikrein was developed after preliminary studies on the application of affinity chromatography to this purpose (FRITZ et al., 1969; FRITZ and FÖRG-BREY, 1972) by LEMON et al. (1976) (Table 5). Elution from the BPTI column was achieved with 0.5 M benzamidine and 0.4 M NaCl in pH 6.45 buffer. The preparation obtained migrated on disc electrophoresis as a single but diffuse band, probably because of a heterogeneous carbohydrate moiety. On SDS electrophoresis after reduction, there was a main component called B, and a minor one, A, was found in an overlapping zone of somewhat lower

Table 5. Purification and properties of submandibular and urinary kallikreins of the pig

	Submandibular kallikrein (LEMON et al., 1976; FRITZ et al., 1977)	Urinary kallikrein (TSCHESCHE et al., 1976b; FRITZ et al., 1977)
Assay used in isolation:	BAEe	BAEe
Purification steps: 1.	0.1 *M* acetic acid homogenate	Acetone fractionation
2.	Acetone fractionation	Sephadex G-75
3.	DEAE-cellulose	DEAE-Sephadex
4.	BPTI-Sepharose	BPTI-Sepharose
5.	Gel filtration	Sephadex G-75
6.	DEAE-Sephadex	(DEAE-Sephadex)
Specific activity:		
BAEe	(10 m*M*; pH 8; 25 °C)	(10 m*M*; pH 8; 25 °C)
(μmol/min):	$166/A_{280}$	$168/A_{280}$
	312/mg protein	
Molecular weight:		
Ultracentrifugation:	$38{,}000 \pm 1{,}000$	$40{,}000 \pm 1{,}500$
($\bar{v}=0.722$; B-forms)		
SDS electrophoresis:	35,900 (A)	36,100 (A)
	39,600 (B)	39,600 (B)

apparent MW (Table 5). By DEAE-Sephadex chromatography, the two components were only partially resolved. Fractions containing varying amounts of the two forms of the enzyme showed comparable specific activities (FRITZ et al., 1977).

From the MW of the reduced enzyme it may be concluded that porcine submandibular kallikrein consists of a single polypeptide chain. The MW determined by SDS electrophoresis is probably somewhat higher than the true one, and this is presumably also the case for the value determined by ultracentrifugation. As a more reliable value was not available, the partial specific volume $\bar{v}$ used for the calculation of the latter result was that determined for porcine pancreatic kallikrein (KUTZBACH and SCHMIDT-KASTNER, 1972). There are indications that submandibular kallikrein contains more carbohydrate which would lower $\bar{v}$ and consequently also the calculated MW. A preparation of porcine submandibular kallikrein was resolved by electrofocusing into eight enzymically active components with isoelectric points of 3.29, 3.48, 3.61, 3.80, 3.90, 4.05, 4.19, and 4.37 (FIEDLER et al., 1970b).

The amino acid composition of submandibular kallikrein is given in Table 2. It is very similar to that of the pancreatic enzyme. The first 28 amino-terminal residues of submandibular kallikrein were found to be identical to the corresponding amino acids in the sequence of the A-chain of pancreatic kallikrein. Submandibular and pancreatic (as well as urinary) kallikreins showed immunologic identity (FRITZ et al., 1977).

The molar absorbance at 280 nm has been determined as 48.8×10^3 M^{-1} cm^{-1}, and the ratio $A_{280\,nm}/A_{260\,nm}$ as 1.76 ± 0.02 (FRITZ et al., 1977).

2. Catalytic Properties

The course of hydrolysis of BAEe by porcine submandibular kallikrein has a strange time-dependence. The initial rate of the reaction gradually slows down until a constant rate of hydrolysis is reached. The extent of the decrease in velocity, as well as the time for attainment of a constant rate (e.g., about 5 min with 0.2 mM substrate) depend on substrate concentration. The effect is not due to depletion of the substrate or to product inhibition and is not abolished by the presence of Bz-ArgNH_2. After depletion of the ester, a new addition of BAEe has the same effect. Several other ester substrates show more or less a similar phenomenon. The same behaviour has been observed with porcine urinary kallikrein but never with pancreatic β-kallikrein (FRITZ et al., 1977).

The most probable cause of this initial loss of activity is a substrate-induced rearrangement in the structure of the enzyme. As a consequence, two different Michaelis constants and maximum catalytic rates for the hydrolysis of BAEe can be derived: $K_{m1}=0.15\pm0.01$ mM, $k_{cat1}=138\pm6\ s^{-1}$ at the start of the reaction, and $K_{m2}=0.69\pm0.04$ mM, $k_{cat2}=154\pm6\ s^{-1}$ at the steady-state part of the progress curve (pH 8, 25 °C) (FRITZ et al., 1977). This fact offers an explanation, why LEMON et al. (1976) obtained a K_m of 0.114 mM, whereas TRAUTSCHOLD and WERLE (1961) determined K_m as 0.60 mM.

Thus, the specific activity determined for preparations of porcine submandibular kallikrein (and other porcine single-chain glandular kallikreins) will also strongly depend on the assay conditions used. With 10 mM BAEe on the autotitrator (FIEDLER, 1976b), a specific activity of 312 μmol/min/mg protein has been determined for the stationary phase of the reaction. In the assays that monitor BAEe hydrolysis, either at 253 nm or via NADH formed from the ethanol liberated, both using substrate concentrations of 0.5 mM (TRAUTSCHOLD and WERLE, 1961), only 48% or 33%, respectively, of the above specific activity were obtained. These differences were much smaller in the case of pancreatic β-kallikrein with its low, time-independent K_m (FRITZ et al., 1977). The relative efficiencies of porcine glandular kallikreins in lowering dog blood pressure (TRAUTSCHOLD and WERLE, 1961; LEMON et al., 1976) should be reinvestigated in the light of these findings.

TAMe is hydrolyzed by submandibular kallikrein at a much lower rate than is the benzoylated compound, similar to the rate observed with pancreatic kallikrein. This similarity exists also for the hydrolysis of ATEe and Bz-MetOMe, that are even worse substrates. However, 1 mM Bz-LysOMe is attacked by submandibular kallikrein at a substantially lower rate than by pancreatic kallikrein, possibly because of a higher K_m value. Ac-PheArgOMe (1 mM) is hydrolyzed at nearly four-fold the rate of BAEe, an indication for a secondary specificity for a phenylalanine residue in position P_2 of submandibular kallikrein (FRITZ et al., 1977).

Secondary specificity for a bulky amino acid residue in P_2 is also expressed in the irreversible inhibition of submandibular kallikrein by peptide chloromethyl ketones (FIEDLER et al., 1977a). 5 mM Tos-LysCH_2Cl or Phe-Ala-LysCH_2Cl did not notably inhibit this enzyme, but Ala-Val-LysCH_2Cl was distinctly inhibitory and Ala-Leu-LysCH_2Cl was much more inhibitory. Ala-Leu-LysCH_2Cl ($K_i=1.95$ mM; $k_2=3.62\times10^{-3}\ s^{-1}$ at pH 7, 25 °C) and also Gly-Val-ArgCH_2Cl ($K_i=0.74$ mM; $k_2=16.2\times10^{-3}\ s^{-1}$) proved to be inhibitors of similar efficiency as with pancreatic β-kallikrein. The rate of inhibition by 1 mM DFP [$(6.9\pm0.9)\times10^{-3}$ or $(8.8\pm2.0)\times10^{-3}\ min^{-1}$, measured for two different preparations at pH 7.2, 25 °C] was indistinguishable from that of the inhibition of pancreatic kallikrein (FIEDLER et al., 1970b).

V. Porcine Urinary Kallikrein

1. Isolation and Molecular Aspects

TSCHESCHE et al. (1976b) described a new isolation procedure for porcine urinary kallikrein using an affinity chromatography step (Table 5). Preliminary experiments with the latter technique were conducted earlier (FRITZ et al., 1969; FRITZ and FÖRG-BREY, 1972). On DEAE-Sephadex chromatography, the enzyme preparation was resolved into a double peak. Two forms distinguished as A and B, separated more distinctly than those of submandibular kallikrein, were also observed on SDS gel electrophoresis (FRITZ et al., 1977). On gel isoelectric focusing, numerous bands were observed in the region of pH 3–5 (TSCHESCHE et al., 1976b).

MWs determined for this kallikrein (Table 5) were similar to that of porcine submandibular kallikrein (see above). Evidently, urinary kallikrein is also a single-chain enzyme. Preliminary results on the amino acid composition, that is very similar to that of the other porcine glandular kallikreins, are given in Table 2. Urinary kallikrein had immunologic identity with porcine submandibular and pancreatic kallikreins (FRITZ et al., 1977).

2. Catalytic Properties

The time-dependence of the rate of BAEe hydrolysis was the same as for porcine submandibular kallikrein, as were the relative rates of BAEe hydrolysis under different conditions and the catalysis of the hydrolysis of various amino acid esters. For BAEe hydrolysis, $K_{m1} = 0.19 \pm 0.02$ mM and $V_{max1} = 172 \pm 6$ µmol/min/A_{280}, and $K_{m1} = 0.61 \pm 0.03$ mM and $V_{max2} = 173 \pm 3$ µmol/min/A_{280} have been determined, identical within experimental limits to the constants of submandibular kallikrein (FRITZ et al., 1977). Results of TSCHESCHE et al. (1976b) ($K_m = 0.125$ mM at pH 7.8) and TRAUTSCHOLD and WERLE (1961) ($K_m = 0.44$ mM) can thus be reconciled.

5 mM Tos-LysCH_2Cl or Phe-Ala-LysCH_2Cl did not inhibit this kallikrein either. Inhibitors with a larger residue in P_2, Ala-Val-LysCH_2Cl and Ala-Leu-LysCH_2Cl ($K_i = 1.97$, $k_2 = 3.85 \times 10^{-3}$ s^{-1}), as well as Gly-Val-ArgCH_2Cl ($K_i = 0.63$, $k_2 = 17.1 \times 10^{-3}$ s^{-1}) behaved the same way as against submandibular kallikrein (FIEDLER et al., 1977a). DFP at 1 mM inhibited porcine urinary ($K_i = (7.0 \pm 1.5) \times 10^{-3}$ min^{-1}), submandibular and pancreatic kallikreins at practically the same rates (FIEDLER et al., 1970b).

VI. Relationships of the Porcine Glandular Kallikreins

1. Various Forms of Pancreatic Kallikrein

The two principal forms of kallikrein isolated from autolyzed bovine pancreas, kallikreins A and B, have identical amino acid compositions and end groups. No difference in any catalytic property has been found so far (see also FIEDLER, 1976). Kallikreins A and B, as well as the minor form C, are immunologically identical (FRITZ et al., 1977). All three forms of kallikrein thus appear to contain the same protein part. Evidently the only difference among these forms of the enzyme is their carbohydrate moieties. The differences in the amounts of neutral and amino sugars they contain (Table 2) are sufficient to account for the observed differences in chromatographic and electrophoretic behaviour. The existence of multiple forms of glycoproteins due to carbohydrate heterogeneity is a well-known phenomenon, as is the microheterogeneity based on a varying content of sialic acid residues (MONTGOMERY, 1972), that becomes evident during electrophoresis of kallikreins A or B at a pH near the isoelectric point.

The occurrence of two forms of prekallikrein, A and B, in pancreas strongly argues in favour of kallikreins A and B being distinct products of biosynthesis and not of degradation during the isolation. It is not known in which form kallikrein, respectively prekallikrein, is secreted into the pancreatic juice. The forms with a lower carbohydrate content may represent only biosynthetic intermediates.

Prekallikrein, similar to the proenzymes of other pancreatic serine proteinases, is probably synthesized as a molecule consisting of a single protein chain. Tryptic activation presumably leads to a form of active enzyme, α-kallikrein, which also consists of a single polypeptide chain, exemplified in all probability by kallikrein B′. The autolysis of pancreas homogenates included in most isolation procedures for this enzyme, offers ample opportunity for an attack by endo- and exopeptidases. The single intrachain split found in the major form of kallikrein isolated in this way, β-kallikrein (existing in forms A as well as B), is certainly introduced during this step. Exopeptidases are probably responsible for some of the heterogeneity of the protein part of this enzyme that is caused by removal of several amino acid residues at the cleavage site. Further degradation yields another form of kallikrein with a second site of cleavage. Thus, γ-kallikrein is composed of three polypeptide chains in which some heterogeneity at the additional site of cleavage also exists. Whether this form of kallikrein is catalytically active, and whether β- or γ-kallikreins occur in vivo in significant amounts and participate in the physiologic function of kallikrein, are still open questions.

2. Pancreatic, Submandibular, and Urinary Kallikreins

The esterolytic activities of porcine submandibular and urinary kallikreins are indistinguishable even in the unique time-dependence of the hydrolysis of several of the substrates, as are their reactions with active-site directed reagents. The same is true for HMW inhibitors (FRITZ et al., 1977). These data suggest a very great similarity, if not identity, of the protein structures of these two enzymes. This is corroborated by the similarity of their amino acid compositions, their immunologic identity, and their structure as single-chain molecules. Both kallikreins occur in two forms, A and B, with similar MW. The latter observation suggests that even the carbohydrate portions of the two enzymes might be very similar. There were, however, some differences in the resolution of the two forms in SDS electrophoresis and also some minor differences in electrophoretic mobility in immune-electrophoresis.

Porcine pancreatic kallikrein is immunologically identical with submandibular and urinary kallikrein. The amino acid composition of this enzyme is also very similar. The sequence of the first 28 amino-terminal amino acids of submandibular kallikrein is identical with that of pancreatic kallikrein. The small differences in catalytic properties of submandibular and urinary kallikreins on one hand and the pancreatic enzyme on the other, are easily explained by the isolation of pancreatic kallikrein from autolyzed pancreas mainly as the β-form with an intrachain split. Differences in catalytic behaviour between, e.g., single-chain bovine β-trypsin and α-trypsin carrying an intrachain split have been observed before (ROBERTS and ELMORE, 1974; FOUCAULT et al., 1974). There are indications that the esterase activity of kallikrein B′, which is probably the single-chain α-form of porcine pancreatic kallikrein, closely resembles that of the single-chain submandibular and urinary enzymes.

It thus appears almost certain that the rigidly gene-coded protein parts of all three porcine glandular kallikreins are identical. Differences in the carbohydrate part may be expected to exist in glycoproteins synthesized in different organs. It is surprising that the MWs of the A and the B forms of submandibular and urinary kallikreins are so similar. Marginal differences in electrophoretic behaviour might have been caused by some degradation of carbohydrate. Elucidation of the structure of the carbohydrate moieties of these enzymes might give a hint to the origin of porcine urinary kallikrein.

D. Glandular Kallikreins of Man

I. Human Pancreatic Kallikrein

Human pancreatic kallikrein has been prepared by MORIYA et al. (1963) (Table 6). On gel electrophoresis at pH 8.7, a main protein band migrating towards the anode, somewhat slower than human urinary kallikrein, and a faint band of higher mobility were observed. The enzyme hydrolyzed TAMe with the same ratio of esterolytic versus biologic (dog vasodilator) activity as kallikrein from human urine.

FEINSTEIN et al. (1974) isolated several proteinases from extracts of human pancreas, applying as a first step affinity chromatography on lima-bean trypsin inhibitor (LBTI)-Sepharose. These authors mention preliminary evidence of kallikrein in low concentrations in some fractions subsequently eluted from SE-Sephadex. It appears questionable whether a glandular kallikrein would behave that way. The proteins passing through the affinity column were devoid of TAMe hydrolyzing activity. A small amount of esterase activity, though, would have been hardly detectable by a UV spectrophotometric assay in the presence of a large amount of protein.

FIGARELLA et al. (1975) stated that the two human anionic trypsinogens isolated by them constitute all of the potential BAEe esterase activity in human pancreatic juice. Both of the trypsins hydrolyzed casein and were inhibited by Tos-LysCH$_2$Cl and human pancreatic secretory trypsin inhibitor. However, in a recent paper MANIVET and FIGARELLA (1977) report on the purification of a kallikrein from human pancreatic juice.

II. Human Salivary Kallikrein

1. Isolation and Molecular Aspects

After DEAE-cellulose chromatography of human saliva, at least 10 peaks with TAMe esterase activity were detected. All but the main kallikrein peak accounting for 70% of the total were inhibited by a mixture of SBTI and LBTI (IMANARI et al., 1977). Several newer procedures compiled in Table 6 have been described for the isolation of this kallikrein. MODÉER (1977b) used affinity chromatography for this

Table 6. Isolation and properties of human pancreatic and salivary kallikreins

	Pancreatic kallikrein	Salivary kallikrein			
	MORIYA et al. (1963)	FUJIMOTO et al. (1973a, b)	HOJIMA et al. (1975a)	MORIWAKI et al. (1974a)	MODÉER (1977a, b)
Assay method used in purification:	Dog blood flow	Dog blood flow	Dog?		BAEe, TAMe
Purification steps: 1.	0.05 M acetic acid extract	Acetone powder	Acetone powder		Ultrafiltration
2.	DEAE-cellulose (batchwise)	DEAE-cellulose (batchwise)	DEAE-cellulose (batchwise)		SBTI-Sepharose
3.	Acetone fractionation	Hydroxyapatite gel	Sephadex G-100		BPTI-Sepharose
4.	Ammonium sulfate fractionation	DEAE-Sephadex A-50	Electrofocusing		
5.	Sephadex G-75	Sephadex G-100	Sephadex G-25		
6.	DEAE-Sephadex	Sephadex G-200			
Purification factor:	15,000	2280	1480		610
Yield:	15%	35%	29%		34%
Specific activity:					
Biologic (dog, KU):	$440/A_{280}$ 550/mg	$1117/A_{280}$	$554/A_{280}$	$365/A_{280}$	
Kinin release (μg BK/min):		(crude bovine kininogen) $14.6/A_{280}$		(crude bovine kininogen) $36.1/A_{280}$	(heated dog plasma) 11.2/mg (V_{max})
BAEe (μmol/min):		(1 mM; pH 8; 25 °C) $5.8/A_{280}$	(1 mM; pH 8; 25 °C) $4.6/A_{280}$	(1 mM; pH 8; 30 °C) $6.0/A_{280}$	(1 mM; pH 8.1; 25 °C) $5.5/A_{280}$
K_m (mM):		0.41			0.40 (pH 8.5)
TAMe (μmol/min):		(1 mM; pH 8; 25 °C) $7.7/A_{280}$	(1 mM; pH 8; 25 °C) $5.2/A_{280}$	(33 mM; pH 8.5; 30 °C) $18.3–21.0/A_{280}$	(1 mM; pH 8; 25 °C) $2.6/A_{280}$
K_m (mM):		0.57			0.55 (pH 8.5)
Molecular weight:					
Gel filtration:		28,000			38,000
Ultracentrifuge:		23,500			
Isoelectric point:		4.0	4.17		4.3

Table 7. Amino acid composition of human salivary and urinary kallikreins

	Salivary kallikrein		Urinary kallikrein			
	FUJIMOTO et al. (1973b)		HIAL et al. (1974)		PORCELLI et al. (1974a)	
	Residues	mol-%	Residues	mol-%	Residues	mol-%
Asp	14	9.66	40	10.01	25	7.72
Thr	8	5.52	25	6.20	20	6.17
Ser	13	8.73	36	9.00	25	7.72
Glu	17	11.85	50	12.61	38	11.73
Pro	7	4.82	48	12.01	25	7.72
Gly	13	8.78	44	11.01	30	9.26
Ala	13	8.78	22	5.40	30	9.26
Cys/2	2	1.36	10	2.60	4	1.23
Val	10	7.02	21	5.20	20	6.17
Met	2	1.32	2	0.60	4	1.23
Ile	4–5	3.07	10	2.60	14	4.32
Leu	11	7.46	19	4.80	20	6.17
Tyr	4	2.63	14	3.60	8	2.47
Phe	5	3.51	14	3.60	14	4.32
Lys	11	7.46	15	3.80	27	8.33
His	4	2.63	8	2.00	12	3.70
Arg	5	3.51	18	4.40	8	2.47
Trp	3	1.88	2	0.55		
Total	146–147		398		324	
Glucosamine					7	

purpose. "Trypsin-like" enzymes were first removed by adsorption on SBTI-Sepharose. 77% of the BAEe esterase and 73% of the TAMe esterase activities were not bound. Elution of kallikrein from the subsequent BPTI-Sepharose affinity column was performed with a pH 3.6 buffer, about 0.2 *M*. Yield and specific activity of this material were comparable to those obtained with more conventional techniques.

Human salivary kallikrein behaved as a homogeneous protein in the ultracentrifuge. It showed a single protein band that was stained with a BAEe-formazane reagent in gel electrophoresis with pH 8.6 or 9.2 buffers (FUJIMOTO et al., 1973b; HOJIMA et al., 1975a). In a similar range of acid pH only a single enzymically active peak was observed in isoelectric focusing by several authors (Table 6). Results of the MW determinations by gel filtration, however, differed widely and the value calculated from sedimentation equilibrium analysis was much lower (Table 6). Absorbance of the enzyme at 280 nm has been determined as 2.1/mg (FUJIMOTO et al., 1973b). The results of an amino acid analysis (recovery of amino acids, 86% by weight) are given in Table 7.

FUJIMOTO et al. (1973a) found human salivary kallikrein to be stable in a pH 8 buffer in the frozen state for at least half a month. Repeated freezing and thawing caused a rapid loss of activity. Only about 40% of activity was recovered after lyophilization. In pH 8 buffer, about 80% of the enzyme's activity remained even after treatment at 60 °C for 1 h, but 10 min at 75 °C inactivated most of the enzyme. Stability up to 60 °C was also reported by MODÉER (1977b). His kallikrein preparation could be stored at 4 °C, pH 8, for several weeks without significant loss of activity. On incubation for 30 min at 25 °C, the enzyme was stable at pH 7–9. At pH 9.5, there was a small loss of activity. About 70 and 80% of activity survived at pH 2.5 and 4, respectively (MODÉER, 1977b).

2. Catalytic Properties

Human salivary kallikrein was a vasodilator in the dog and released kinin from kininogen (Table 6). In the presence of 2% BSA, the enzyme had a leucotactic effect on rat neutropil leucocytes (MODÉER, 1977a). This kallikrein had negligible caseinolytic and no kininase activity (FUJIMOTO et al., 1973a).

Specific activities and Michaelis constants determined with BAEe and TAMe are compiled in Table 6. The data reported by different authors are remarkably similar, with the notable exception of the slower hydrolysis of TAMe observed by MODÉER. The optimum pH for the hydrolysis of TAMe is about 8 (FUJIMOTO et al., 1973a) or 8.6, a value also found with BAEe (MODÉER, 1977b). BANA was hydrolyzed at only 0.2% the rate of BAEe, and no hydrolysis of Ac-TyrOEt or Lys-p-nitroanilide by human salivary kallikrein has been observed (MODÉER, 1977b).

Ca^{2+}, Mg^{2+}, and Ni^{2+} ions, in concentrations up to 1 mM, did not influence BAEe esterase activity, Mn^{2+} and Cd^{2+} were marginal inhibitors, while Co^{2+}, Cu^{2+}, Zn^{2+}, Fe^{2+}, and Hg^{2+}, as well as p-chloromercuribenzoic acid, cysteine, iodobenzoic acid, and p-amino-benzamidine inhibited. Marginal inhibition was seen with EDTA, Tos-PheCH$_2$Cl, and Tos-LysCH$_2$Cl (MODÉER, 1977b). PASKHINA et al. (1968) did not observe inhibition of a crude preparation of salivary kallikrein by Tos-LysCH$_2$Cl.

III. Human Urinary Kallikrein

1. Isolation and Molecular Aspects

Results on human urinary kallikrein obtained by various workers differ in part appreciably. For example, PIERCE and NUSTAD (1972) stated that at least 95% of the TAMe esterase activity of human urine is due to the kallikrein isolated by them, while HIAL et al. (1974) write: "that no kinin-releasing activity was detected that could be associated with any significant level of TAMe esterase activity in the urine samples." At least one other arginine esterase, urokinase, is known to occur in human urine. As several of the preparations of human urinary kallikrein hitherto obtained (Table 8) have been characterized only insufficiently, it is possible that different enzymes have been isolated as kallikrein, possibly even in a single preparation.

It is generally agreed that multiple forms of human urinary kallikrein are resolved by electrofocusing. Three to six components with isoelectric points in a similar acid region of pH were invariably observed (Table 8).

PIERCE and NUSTAD (1972) mention in their abstract the TAMe esterase and the biologic activity of their enzyme preparations. Three human kallikrein types, A, B, and the most common AB, were revealed by hydroxyapatite chromatography of individual urine samples in the presence of 3 M NaCl. Even single components isolated by electrofocusing of the type B material had the same pattern of three protein bands on electrophoresis in 16% polyacrylamide gels. SDS electrophoresis of the pI 4.13 peak also gave three bands of different MWs (Table 8).

The human urinary kallikrein isolated by MORIYA and co-workers (a preparation of 180 KU/mg and 5 TAMe units/mg) had eight protein bands migrating towards the anode. Three of them reacted positively with a BAEe-formazane staining in the presence of SBTI (FUJIMOTO et al., 1972). The preparation described by HOJIMA et al. (1975a), of much lower specific activity (Table 8), displayed one main protein band and some slower additional components on disc electrophoresis. MORIYA et al. (1963) demonstrated only a single protein zone migrating to the anode. Three components (1–3) isolated by means of electrofocusing by MATSUDA et al. (1976a) each yielded a single protein band on gel electrophoresis at pH 8.

The kallikrein isolated by SPRAGG and AUSTEN (1974) "showed two prealbumin bands, an albumin band and a faint β contaminant upon alkaline disc gel electrophoresis."

The preparation of HIAL et al. (1974) displayed a single component on polyacrylamide (7.5%) electrophoresis in pH 8.2 buffer. In cellogel electrophoresis at pH 9.5, additional minor components also staining as glycoprotein were detected.

Vastly different MWs were determined with different methods for the various preparations of human urinary kallikrein (Table 8). The amino acid composition of two different samples is given in Table 7. PORCELLI et al. (1974a) found glucosamine in their enzyme preparation. The glycoprotein nature of their material was demonstrated by HIAL et al. (1974) by PAS staining.

Human urinary kallikrein liberated virtually only kallidin and no further peptide fragment from bovine HMW kininogen (IWANAGA et al., 1977).

2. Catalytic Properties of the Preparations of MORIYA and Co-Workers

The vasodilatory activity in the dog and the kininogenase activity characterize the preparations obtained by MORIYA and co-workers as a kallikrein. The specific activity decreased to nearly one half on lyophilization of partially purified urinary kallikrein (HOJIMA et al., 1975a).

Of the three components of similar MWs separated by electrofocusing by MATSUDA et al. (1976a), fractions 2 and 3 showed specific activities reduced to a comparable extent in all the assay systems used (Table 8). This could indicate that these two components were less pure. Certain other differences were also reported, though it is difficult to judge whether these should be regarded as significant. K_m values were slightly different (Table 8), also for BAMe (0.33, 0.19, and 0.23 mM), and the optimum pH for TAMe hydrolysis were 8.0, 8.3, and 7.5 respectively. Activation energies of this reaction were 11.7 and 14.5 kcal/mol for components 1 and 3, whereas a notably different value of 5.1 was obtained for component 2. Activity losses up to 50%, higher after 10 min than after 1 h, were observed on heating at pH 8.0 at temperatures up to 75 °C. Component 1 was the most and 3 the least stable. In inactivation experiments with urea and with guanidinium hydrochloride, component 2 was the most stable one, the other two behaved similarly to each other. In the isolation procedure applied, a step of heat treatment at 60 °C for 10 h was included, and this might have influenced the specific activities of the more heat-labile components 2 and 3 more than that of component 1.

Table 8. Isolation and properties of human urinary kallikrein

	(MORIYA et al., 1963; PIERCE, 1970; WEBSTER and PRADO, 1970)	PIERCE and NUSTAD (1972)	(MORIYA et al., 1973; MATSUDA et al., 1976a)
Assay method used in purification:	Dog blood flow	(TAMe)	Esterolysis Dog vasodilation
Purification steps: 1.	Dialysis	Pressure dialysis	Crude powder
2.	Amberlite IRC 50 (batchwise)	DEAE-Sephadex	DEAE-cellulose
3.	DEAE-cellulose (batchwise)	Hydroxyapatite	Acetone fractionation
4.	Acetone fractionation	Electrofocusing	Sephadex G-100
5.	Ammonium sulfate fractionation		DEAE-Sephadex
6.	Sephadex G-75		Electrofocusing
7.	DEAE-Sephadex		Sephadex G-75
Purification factor:	5700 (650 based on non-dialyzable solids)		200 (step 5)
Yield:	6%		40% (step 5) (4–6%, each component)
Components:			1 2 3
Specific activity:			
Biologic (dog, KU):	430/mg		200 122 $115/A_{28}$
Kinin release (µg BK/min):			(partially purified bovine kininogen) 27 19 $17/A_{280}$
BAEe (µmol/min):			(1 mM; pH 8; 25 °C) 2.8 1.7 $1.4/A_{280}$
K_m (mM):			0.56 0.38 0.48
TAMe (µmol/min):	($11.5/A_{280}$)		(1 mM; pH 8; 25 °C) 3.1 1.9 $1.6/A_{280}$
K_m (mM):			0.75 0.49 0.33
			(33 mM; pH 8; 30 °C) 9.9 5.3 $4.6/A_{280}$
Molecular weight:			
Gel filtration:			27,000 27,000 29,000
SDS electrophoresis:		23,800; 29,300; 36,400 (all from pI 4.13 peak)	
Ultracentrifugation:	40,500		
Composition:			
Isoelectric point:		3.84–4.33 (six peaks) (main peaks, 4.04; 4.06; 4.13)	3.9 4.0–4.04 4.12–4.20

With all three components of human urinary kallikrein, the rate of hydrolysis of 1 mM BAEe was slightly lower than that of 1 mM TAMe (Table 8). Incidentally, the specific activity of components 2 and 3 with BAEe is comparable to that of the kallikrein preparation of PORCELLI et al. (1974a). The use of 33 mM TAMe at 30 °C resulted in about a three-fold higher rate of hydrolysis than at a concentration of 1 mM at 25 °C, possibly an indication of substrate activation. K_m values determined for BAEe hydrolysis (Table 8) are comparable to a previous value of 0.57 mM of TRAUTSCHOLD and WERLE (1961).

3. Catalytic Properties of the Preparation of HIAL et al.

Though evidently isolated in a high degree of purity, the preparation of human urinary kallikrein obtained by HIAL et al. (1974) is conspicuous by its low esterase activity. Intravenous application of 0.14 mg of this enzyme caused an appreciable lowering of arterial blood pressure in the rat, and a kinin was readily liberated from

ɪɪᴍᴀ et al. (1975a)	Sᴘʀᴀɢɢ and Aᴜsᴛᴇɴ (1974)	Pᴏʀᴄᴇʟʟɪ et al. (1974a)	Hɪᴀʟ et al. (1974)	Oʟᴇᴍᴏɪʏᴏɪ et al. (1977)
ɔg vasodilation)	Kinin liberation	BAEe	Kinin liberation	Kinin liberation
ıde powder AE-cellulose ıhadex G-100 droxyapatite ıhadex G-75	Ultrafiltration DEAE-cellulose Sephadex G-100	Benzoic acid precipitation DEAE-cellulose Sephadex G-100 Hydroxyapatite Neocel 5% Gel electrophoresis Sephadex G-100	Sephadex G-25 DEAE-Sephadex Sephadex G-150 Sephadex G-150	Ultrafiltration DEAE-cellulose DEAE-cellulose Sephadex G-100
		(64 from step 2)	25	500
		0.8%	43.5%	
5/A_{280} .5/mg after lyophilization)	(human kininogen) 20/mg		(partially purified dog kininogen) 12.5/mg (V_{max})	(heated plasma) 230/mg protein
mM: pH 8: 25 °C) .4/mg		(1 mM: pH 8: 25 °C) 1.5/mg	(pH 8: 25 °C) 0.34/mg (V_{max}) 1.34	
mM: pH 8: 25 °C) ·0/mg	(10/mg)		(pH 8; 25 °C) 0.37/mg (V_{max}) 1.14	
	25,000–30,000	37,000	43,600	27,000–43,000
		35,400	42,666	
7; 3.90; 4.04; 4.12; 4.28			3.80; 3.95; 4.06	3.8–4.4

dog kininogen, a reaction inhibited by BPTI. These criteria indicate the kallikrein nature of this preparation.

BAEe and TAMe were hydrolyzed only comparatively slowly, but at similar rates (Table 8). K_m values for both substrates were two to three times higher than those reported by other authors, except the 2.6 mM obtained for TAMe by Bᴇᴀᴠᴇɴ et al. (1971). With higher concentrations of TAMe, a pronounced substrate activation was observed. Neither BANA, nor p-nitrophenyl or ethyl p-guanidinobenzoate, nor Ac-TyrOMe were hydrolyzed, but Z-Tyr-p-nitrophenyl ester was cleaved at a relatively fast rate ($K_m = 0.19$ mM; $V_{max} = 2.0$ µmol/min/mg). The hydrolysis of this highly activated amino acid ester does not seem to be a conspicuous property.

Benzamidine competitively inhibited ($K_i = 6.42$ mM) with TAMe as substrate, whereas 9 mM had no effect on kinin release and 2 mM none on Z-Tyr-p-nitrophenyl ester hydrolysis. The latter determination was performed in the presence of dioxane, that was also a competitive inhibitor ($K_i = 0.2$ M). Previously, 9% inhibition of kinin release by about 0.9 m*M* benzamidine had been reported under conditions, where horse urinary kallikrein was inhibited by 29% (DINIZ et al., 1965).

Among active site directed irreversible inhibitors, only DFP showed a slow inhibition (17%, 8 h, 3 m*M* inhibitor, pH 8.1, 25 °C) of esterase and kinin-releasing activities, whereas Tos-LysCH_2Cl had no effect. Lack of inhibition of a crude preparation of human urinary kallikrein by Tos-LysCH_2Cl has been described earlier by PASKHINA et al. (1968).

Incubation with 25 m*M* iodoacetamide also failed to inactivate the enzyme. This observation is highly interesting, as HIAL et al. (1974) found the presence of four easily accessible SH groups per molecule of their enzyme. These are evidently not essential for enzyme activity. Free sulfhydryl groups have not been observed before in native pancreatic serine proteinases, a class of enzymes to which glandular kallikreins appear to belong. In bovine trypsin, reduction and alkylation of a single disulfide bridge led to a form of enzyme that had much lower capacity to hydrolyze BAEe, both k_{cat} and K_m being involved. Also, affinity for benzamidine decreased by two orders of magnitude (KNIGHTS and LIGHT, 1976). In the kallikrein preparation of HIAL et al., reduction of disulfide bridges might have occurred in vivo or in vitro, and this modification could explain the different properties of this material.

IV. Comparison of the Three Human Glandular Kallikreins

The ratio of the hydrolysis rate of 33 m*M* versus 1 m*M* TAMe by human urinary and by salivary kallikreins are similar, as are K_m values for BAEe as well as TAMe (Tables 6 and 8). The ratios of vasodilatory, kinin releasing, TAMe and BAEe esterase activities of human salivary kallikrein have been determined as 17.4:1.72:1:0.29. Under identical conditions, the corresponding activity ratios were 20.2:2.72:1:0.28 for human urinary kallikrein (MORIWAKI et al., 1974a). Within the limits of experimental errors, these ratios can be regarded as identical. Nevertheless, the specific activities of the preparations, e.g., 9.9 TAMe units/A_{280} for urinary and 21 U/A_{280} for submandibular kallikrein, the highest specific activities reported for these enzymes (Tables 6 and 8), are distinctly different. The most probable explanation, is a lower degree of purity of the urinary enzyme preparation. The possibility of heat denaturation has already been mentioned.

MWs reported for these enzymes vary between 23,500 and 43,600 and are therefore of little use for comparative purposes. It is, however, striking that isoelectric focusing of salivary kallikrein has always demonstrated a single peak with an isoelectric point between 4.0 and 4.3 (Table 6), in a region of pH where the fraction with the highest isoelectric point among the multiple forms of urinary kallikrein has been observed (Table 8). From what we learned about porcine pancreatic kallikrein, one may advance the working hypothesis that salivary kallikrein as well as the above mentioned component of urinary kallikrein are sialic acid-free derivatives of otherwise similar enzymes.

For human pancreatic kallikrein, the least well characterized of these enzymes, the same ratio of biologic versus TAMe esterase activity has been observed as for human urinary kallikrein (MORIYA et al., 1963).

These few indications of a high degree of similarity of the three human glandular kallikreins are strongly supported by the immunologic identity. Antibody to human urinary kallikrein forms a line of identity with human salivary or pancreatic kallikrein or the kallikrein from sweat (IMANARI et al., 1977). [A kallikrein from human sweat has been partially purified by FRÄKI et al. (1970).] Antibody to human urinary kallikrein cross-reacts with human saliva and pancreatic juice (MANN and GEIGER, 1977). Antiserum to human pancreas recognized human urinary kallikrein. This ability was lost after treatment with submaxillary or kidney tissue (OLEMOIYOI et al., 1977).

An apparent contradiction against identity might be seen in the vastly different amino acid compositions reported for human salivary and urinary kallikreins (Table 7). The MW bases chosen for expression of the results are evidently highly uncertain. If one recalculates the data to a mol % basis there remain conspicuous differences even between the two reports on urinary kallikrein. The preparation of PORCELLI et al. (1974a) had a yield of only 0.8% – this might conceivably indicate that it represents only a minor component of urine – and was not characterized as a kallikrein by depressor or kininogenase activities. Only a single amino acid analysis has been conducted with this preparation. FUJIMOTO et al. (1973a) regard their result on salivary kallikrein as preliminary. These data should be confirmed before accepted as evidence for the nonidentity of the two kallikreins.

E. Glandular Kallikreins of the Rat

I. Rat Pancreatic Kallikrein

Table 9 shows the isolation and properties of the kallikrein from rat pancreas. By preparative disc electrophoresis, one sharp peak of kallikrein activity and some trailing material were obtained, that gave only a single sharp band each on analytical disc electrophoresis in pH 8.9 buffer (HOJIMA et al., 1975b). Kallikrein isolated by preparative isoelectric focusing also was homogenous in disc electrophoresis (HOJIMA et al., 1977). Whereas in carrier-free electrofocusing one rather broad peak of enzymic activity indicating the presence of several components was obtained, gel isoelectric focusing resolved four to five (HOJIMA et al., 1975b) or two (HOJIMA et al., 1977) protein bands.

At 280 nm, pH 8, $A_{1\,cm}^{1\%}$ was 20.3 (HOJIMA et al., 1975b). The amino acid composition, yielding a molecular weight of 31,585, is given in Table 10.

More than 90% of the enzyme activity was retained after 24 h incubation at 25 °C in the pH 4–10 range (HOJIMA et al., 1975b). At pH 4.5, the enzyme lost 50% of its activity in 1 h even at 45 °C, while at pH 8.0, 25 and 50% were lost at 60 and 80 °C, respectively (HOJIMA et al., 1977).

In the dog, rat pancreatic kallikrein proved to be a potent vasodilator. BAEe (pH optimum, 9.2; $K_m = 0.065$ mM) was hydrolyzed very fast and at a seven to 10-fold higher rate than TAMe ($K_m = 0.058$ mM) at 1 mM concentrations. At concentrations of 1 or 2 mM, respectively, a slight substrate inhibition has been observed (HOJIMA et al., 1977). Bz-Tyr-OEt was hydrolyzed only slowly at 0.06 µmol/min/A_{280} (HOJIMA et al., 1975b), while the rate of hydrolysis of BANA by this kallikrein (Table 9) was comparable to that of bovine trypsin, 0.74 µmol/min/mg (HOJIMA et al., 1975a). Hydrolysis of casein was also detected (HOJIMA et al., 1975b, 1977).

Table 9. Isolation and properties of pancreatic and submandibular kallikreins of the rat

	Pancreatic kallikrein		Submandibular kallikrein	
	HOJIMA et al. (1975b)	(MORIYA et al., 1975; HOJIMA et al., 1977)	EKFORS et al. (1967b)	BRANDTZAEG et al. (1976)
Assay method used in purification:	Dog vasodilation; BAEe	Dog vasodilation; BAEe	BANA	BAEe
Purification steps: 1.	Homogenate, 2 h at 25 °C (pH 6.2)	Water homogenate 10 h at room temp.	Freezing and thawing	Na-deoxycholate solubilization
2.	Acetone fractionation	Acetone fractionation	Ammonium sulfate fractionation	DEAE-Sephadex
3.	Acetone fractionation	Acetone fractionation	Sephadex G-100	Hydroxyapatite
4.	Disc electrophoresis	DEAE-Sephadex	DEAE-cellulose	Bio-Gel P-150
5.	Sephadex G-100	Sephadex G-100	DEAE-cellulose	Electrofocusing
6.		Electrofocusing	DEAE-Sephadex	
7.		Sephadex G-50		
Purification factor:	2500–2700	2700–4700		
Yield:	22–24%	27% (dog); 15% (BAEe)		
Components:			A B C D	C_1 C_2 C_3 C_4
Specific activity:				
Biologic (dog, KU):	$301/A_{280}$	810–870/mg		
Kinin release (µg BK/min):				(Rat kininogen II) 42 55 36 42/mg
BAEe (µmol/min):	(1 m*M*, pH 8; 25 °C) $124/A_{280}$	(1 m*M*; pH 8;25 °C) 300–390/mg	(5 m*M*; pH 8; 37 °C) 600 230 250 120/mg protein	(20 m*M*; pH 8.5; 37 °C) 603 700 610 636/mg protein
TAMe (µmol/min):	(1 m*M*; pH 8; 25 °C) $18.9/A_{280}$	(1 m*M*; pH 8; 25 °C) 33–43/mg	(5 m*M*; pH 8; 37 °C) 175 68 63 68/mg protein	
BANA (µmol/min):	(0.77 m*M*; pH 8; 25 °C) $0.061/A_{280}$	(0.77 m*M*; pH 8; 25 °C) 0.35–0.68/mg	(0.5 m*M*; pH 8; 37 °C) 6.7 3.6 3.1 3.1/mg protein	
Molecular weight:				
Gel filtration:	30,000		24,800 24,800 28,000 24,800	
SDS electrophoresis:				34,000 (C_1–C_4)
Isoelectric point:	around 4.1 (3.84–4.18) (broad peak with some structure)	around 4.1		3.87 3.96 4.07 4.16

Table 10. Amino acid compositions of pancreatic and urinary kallikreins of the rat (residues per molecule)

	Pancreatic kallikrein HOJIMA et al. (1977)	Urinary kallikrein PORCELLI et al. (1975)
Asp	35	28
Thr	14	15
Ser	17	16
Glu	28	24
Pro	24	19
Gly	25	25
Ala	10	21
Cys/2	8	12
Val	17	10
Met	6	5
Ile	13	11
Leu	32	23
Tyr	9	10
Phe	6	8
Lys	13	15
His	6	7
Arg	2	10
Trp	12	
Glucosamine (or galactosamine)		5

Sulfhydryl compounds or chelating agents stimulated the activity of this kallikrein by only 20% at most. Up to 1 m*M* Mg^{2+} or Ca^{2+} had no influence on BAEe hydrolysis, and Mn^{2+} or Cu^{2+} were only weak inhibitors, while Ni^{2+}, Co^{2+}, Hg^{2+}, Cd^{2+}, and Zn^{2+} inhibited the reaction with increasing potency (HOJIMA et al., 1977).

II. Rat Submandibular Kallikrein

Kallikreins from rat submandibular glands were purified by EKFORS et al. (1967b) and recently by BRANDTZAEG et al. (1976) (Table 9). The latter authors isolated by preparative electrofocusing four kallikrein fractions C_1–C_4 with isoelectric points at acid pH similar to that of rat pancreatic kallikrein. Some displayed additional components on gel electrofocusing. In gel electrophoresis at pH 8.9, C_1–C_3 showed essentially one protein band, whereas C_4 split to two components of somewhat higher anodic mobility. Specific activities of all four enzyme fractions measured with BAEe, that was hydrolyzed very fast, were nearly identical, as were those obtained from kinin release (Table 9). Caseinolytic activity was only 0.09% of that of trypsin. The fall of rat blood pressure after i.v. injection demonstrated the kallikrein nature of all four enzyme fractions. Each also contracted the isolated rat uterus. All four forms of this kallikrein produced reactions of identity to rat urinary kallikrein with antiserum to rat urinary kallikrein.

In addition, in step 2 of the isolation procedure of BRANDTZAEG et al. (1976), two further BAEe esterases A and B (MW of B, 37,500) were separated from kallikrein.

These had only a very low caseinolytic activity, could not release kinin from rat kininogen, and caused a very small or no fall in blood pressure of rats. They shared, however, some antigenic determinants with rat urinary kallikrein.

EKFORS et al. (1967b) separated by repeated chromatography on DEAE ion exchangers four components A–D hydrolyzing BANA from rat submandibular glands. These four enzymes showed different anodic mobilities in starch gel electrophoresis at pH 8.6. When injected i.v. into a rabbit, preparations A–C (D has evidently not been tested) produced a pronounced fall in blood pressure (EKFORS et al., 1967a). The main hypotensive activity was, however, found in an enzyme preparation called salivain, a potent caseinolytic enzyme previously isolated from rat submandibular glands (RIEKKINEN et al., 1966). Rabbit antiserum to salivain showed reactions of identity with salivain and all four kallikrein fractions (EKFORS et al., 1967b). BRANDTZAEG et al. (1976) quote evidence that salivain is indeed a mixture of a caseinolytic enzyme and of kallikrein.

Hydrolysis of BAEe by the kallikrein preparation A of highest specific activity is comparable to that of the preparations of BRANDTZAEG et al. (Table 9). EKFORS et al. (1967b) believe that the four components were not obtained in equal purity. TAMe is hydrolyzed several times more slowly. The data with BANA (Table 9; pH-optima, 8.2–8.3) or Bz-DL-Arg-β-naphthylamide (0.18–0.40 µmol/min/mg at 0.25 mM) are comparable to those obtained with trypsin as determined by these authors (3.2 or 0.75 µmol/min/mg at 1 mM substrate; RIEKKINEN et al., 1966). ArgMe and LysMe were only slowly attacked, and Arg- or Lys-β-naphthylamide not at all. The rates of hydrolysis of casein or hemoglobin were very low. All four enzyme fractions behaved similarly (EKFORS et al., 1967b). 10 mM tetra-N-methyl ammonium iodide had in some cases a marginally activating effect. The corresponding tetrabutyl compound, as well as 0.2 mM iodoacetamide, diethyl-p-nitrophenyl phosphate, or DFP were void of any action. A lack of inhibition by the latter serine proteinase inhibitor would be a remarkable property, but a slow inhibition could have been overlooked.

The data reported support the conclusion that both groups of investigators have isolated multiple forms of the same rat submandibular kallikrein. The four kallikrein components C_1–C_4 described by BRANDTZAEG et al. (1976) differing only in their isoelectric points might well be identical with the four kallikrein isozymes A–D isolated by EKFORS et al. (1967b).

III. Rat Urinary Kallikrein

1. Isolation and Molecular Aspects

NUSTAD and PIERCE (1974) found that about 50% of the TAMe esterase activity of the urine from female Sprague-Dawley rats was not due to kallikrein, but to another enzyme called esterase A which was not absorbed to DEAE-Sephadex. This enzyme did not lower the blood pressure of the rat or contract the rat uterus, though it formed a smooth muscle-contracting substance with heated dog plasma. Esterase A did not hydrolyze casein and was only weakly inhibited by BPTI, but strongly by SBTI. In the Ouchterlony assay, it did not react with antibodies against rat urinary kallikrein. OZA et al. (1976) found 66% of the BAEe esterase of rat urine to be bound to DEAE-cellulose. PORCELLI et al. (1975) reported that 30% of the BAEe activity absorbed to DEAE-cellulose is eluted in a broad peak preceding the sharp main activity peak that was purified further.

Purification methods applied in the isolation of this kallikrein are compiled in Table 11. Besides affinity chromatography (SILVA et al., 1974; PORCELLI et al., 1975; OZA et al., 1976), binding to Sepharose-coupled antibody (NUSTAD et al., 1975) or immune precipitation (NUSTAD and PIERCE, 1974) were successfully used. SILVA et al. (1974) observed a large increase in kininogenase, but not esterase or amidase, activity only after the Sephadex G-150 steps. This finding was interpreted as removal of a ligand that affected binding of only large protein substrates.

When preparations of rat urinary kallikrein were subjected to electrofocusing, several more or less well resolved components were observed with isoelectric points in the acid range of pH similar to those of other glandular kallikreins of the rat (Tables 11 and 9). NUSTAD and PIERCE (1974) isolated this way four kallikrein fractions called B_1–B_4 with specific BAEe esterase activities of 14.5–22.8 U/A_{280}. Component B_3 (pI, 3.73) was by far the most prominent one. On disc gel electrophoresis at pH 8.9, the mobilities differed little. As with porcine pancreatic kallikrein, treatment with neuraminidase did not change the mobilities under these conditions. Small differences in mobility which led to somewhat different MWs of fractions B_1 and B_4 were also observed in SDS electrophoresis (Table 11). Kallikrein components B_1–B_4 proved immunologically identical.

The traces of BANA hydrolyzing activity observed in electrofocusing by SILVA et al. (1974) with isoelectric points of 4.5 and higher are reminiscent of the fraction with pI 4.83 obtained from rat pancreas that was tentatively identified as an anionic trypsin (HOJIMA et al., 1975b). On gel electrophoresis at pH 8.2, the preparation of SILVA et al. (1974) showed a single component but on cellogel electrophoresis at pH 9.5 microheterogeneity also became evident. PAS staining demonstrated the glycoprotein nature of the enzyme. Using a MW of 33,100, the preparation has been found to be 97.4% pure by active site titration.

OZA et al. (1976) observed a minor second protein component in their kallikrein preparation after disc gel electrophoresis which also exhibited esterase and kininogenase activity, while PORCELLI and CROXATTO (1971) and PORCELLI et al. (1975) obtained only a single protein band. The latter preparation also gave a single protein band in SDS electrophoresis.

The amino acid composition of a preparation of rat urinary kallikrein is given in Table 10. PORCELLI et al. (1975) stated that it contained only galactosamine, but in a table of their paper the amino sugar is designated glucosamine. $A_{280\,nm}^{1\,cm}$ has been determined as 1.51 for a solution containing 1 mg protein/ml (OZA et al., 1976).

Solutions of this kallikrein in distilled water slowly lost activity even when kept frozen (PORCELLI and CROXATTO, 1971). Samples frozen and thawed four times gave, on gel filtration, one peak of esterase activity eluted earlier than native enzyme, and additional enzymically inert material (PORCELLI et al., 1975). Lability and a tendency to adhere to glass and plastic surfaces, were overcome by use of siliconized glassware (OZA et al., 1976). The TAMe esterase of the enzyme survived isolation in 8 *M* urea (NUSTAD and PIERCE, 1974).

2. Catalytic Properties

All four groups of investigators found a lowering of the blood pressure of rats, confirming the kallikrein nature of the various preparations. Direct contraction of the rat uterus by the enzyme has also been observed (Table 11). The various preparations also readily released kinin, though the specific activities reported differ widely

Table 11. Isolation and properties of urinary kallikrein of the rat

	PORCELLI and CROXATTO (1971)	NUSTAD and PIERCE (1974)	
Assay method used in purification:	Kinin release, BAEe	TAMe	
Purification steps: 1.	Acetone precipitation	Pressure dialysis	Pressure dialysis
2.	Sephadex G-100	DEAE-Sephadex	Immune precipitate
3.	CM-cellulose	Hydroxyapatite	Sephadex G-100 (8 *M* urea)
4.	DEAE-cellulose	Electrofocusing	
5.	DEAE-cellulose	(Bio-Gel P-200)	
6.			
Purification factor:	390	50–86	72
Yield:	19%	36%	72%
Rat uterus contraction (amount necessary to elicit an equal response as 1 part BK):	10–12×	5–7×	
Specific activity:			
Kinin release (μg BK/min):	(dog serum) 450/mg	(heated dog plasma) 20–32/mg	
BAEe (μmol/min):		(20 m*M*; pH 8; 25 °C) 193/A_{280}	
TAMe (μmol/min):		(20 m*M*; pH 8; 25 °C) 25/A_{280}	
BANA (μmol/min):		(L, 2.4 m*M*; pH 8.5; 37 °C) 0.5/A_{280}	
Molecular weight:			
Gel filtration:		38,500 (B_3)	
SDS electrophoresis:		35,500; 33,600; 33,100; 32,300	
Isoelectric point:		3.50; 3.68; 3.73; 3.80	

(Table 11). The especially high value of OZA et al. (1976) was obtained by determining kinin in the dog using kallidin as a standard and not as usual on an isolated organ using bradykinin as a standard.

Widely different values have also been given for the specific activities of rat urinary kallikrein with BAEe or TAMe (Table 11). In part, this might be due to the different reaction conditions. PORCELLI et al. (1975) mention a lag period often observed in the determination of activity with BAEe. Under comparable conditions, BAEe is hydrolyzed about eight times faster than TAMe (NUSTAD and PIERCE, 1974). The pH optimum for TAMe hydrolysis was 8.5, the K_m 0.130 m*M* and k_{cat} was 4.0 s^{-1} (0.1 *M* KCl, pH 8, 25 °C) at TAMe concentrations lower than 1 m*M* (SILVA et al., 1974). At higher concentrations, substrate activation has been observed, as observed with several trypsin-type enzymes. Substituted guanidines (p-tolyl and p-ethyl-phenylguanidine, ethyl p-guanidinobenzoate) also proved to be activators of this kallikrein.

Introduction of the carbobenzoxy group, largely isosteric to a phenylalanine residue, into position P_2 of a substrate also favours hydrolysis by rat urinary kallikrein. The rate of hydrolysis of Z-ArgOMe was as high as 346 μmol/min/A_{280} (20 m*M*, pH 8, 25 °C) (NUSTAD and PIERCE, 1974). Bz-DL-methionine methyl ester was not attacked. BANA is hydrolyzed at an appreciable rate (Table 11), but no hydrolysis of casein has been observed (NUSTAD and PIERCE, 1974).

Competitive inhibitors of rat urinary kallikrein were β-naphthamidine (K_i = 0.046 m*M*), benzamidine (0.24 m*M*), p-amino-benzamidine (0.036 m*M*), and a

SILVA et al. (1974)	PORCELLI et al. (1975)	OZA et al. (1976)
BANA, TAMe, kinin release	BAEe	BAEe
Pervaporation Acetone fractionation Sephadex G-100 ArgOMe-Sepharose Sephadex G-150 Sephadex G-150	DEAE-cellulose BPTI-Bio-Gel P-200 Sephadex G-100 Sephadex G-100	Ammonium sulfate precipitation DEAE-cellulose DEAE-cellulose BPTI-Sepharose Sephadex G-100
87	330	694
19%	17%	17%
75×		
(partially purified dog plasma) 100/mg (V_{max})		(partially purified dog kininogen) 1795/mg protein
	(1 mM; pH 8; 25 °C) 51.5/mg protein	(1 mM; pH 8.5; 25 °C?) 124.3/mg protein
(pH 8; 25 °C) 7.42/mg protein		(20 mM; pH 8.5; 37 °C?) 123/mg
(DL, 0.83 mM; pH 8.15; 25 °C) 0.348/mg protein		
33,100		(< 45,000)
	32,000	
3.97; 4.18; (4.50; 4.87; 5.30)		

number of other substituted benzamidines (0.079–0.422 mM), phenylguanidine (1.0 mM), and p-aminophenylguanidine (0.251 mM). p-Tolyl-guanidine had a slight inhibitory action that changed to activation at higher concentrations (SILVA et al., 1974).

Several active site reagents of trypsin were tested against rat urinary kallikrein. p-Nitrophenyl p′-guanidinobenzoate was useful for active site titration. The initial burst of nitrophenol was followed by a slow hydrolysis. The corresponding ethyl ester, however, did not inhibit but slightly activated. Tos-Lys-CH_2Cl caused only a weak reversible inhibition. p-Amidinophenacyl bromide did not inactivate the enzyme, but p-guanidinophenacyl bromide did so with a second-order rate constant of 3.0 M^{-1} min^{-1} (pH 8.1) (SILVA et al., 1974). DFP has previously been shown to inhibit rat urinary kallikrein (BERALDO et al., 1966).

IV. Comparison of Rat Glandular Kallikreins

Values reported for the specific activities of pancreatic, submandibular, and urinary kallikreins of the rat differ widely. In part, this is due to differing reaction conditions, but different states of purity of the various preparations are certainly also involved. Nevertheless, there is agreement as to the very high rate of BAEe hydrolysis (this being several times faster than the hydrolysis of TAMe), and as to a significant hydrolysis of BANA by all three rat kallikreins. All three enzymes are inhibited by BPTI (VOGEL, this volume). Rat submandibular and urinary kallikrein are also directly oxytocic on the rat uterus. Immunologically, the latter two enzymes are identical. All these observations indicate that the three glandular kallikreins of the rat have identical protein portions. Minor differences in the electrofocusing pattern might be due to some differences in the carbohydrate parts of the enzymes.

The differences of the amino acid compositions reported for pancreatic and urinary kallikrein of the rat (Table 10) might appear to definitely argue against identity of the two proteins. The specific activity of the preparation of urinary kallikrein of PORCELLI et al. (1975) was, however, less than half of that stated by other authors and much lower than that of the pancreatic kallikrein of HOJIMA et al. (1977). From the data reported it is impossible to judge the reliability of either amino acid determination. The question of possible identity must still be regarded as an open one.

F. Glandular Kallikreins of Other Species

I. Mouse Submaxillary Kallikrein

As in the case of rat, a number of BAEe esterases have been found in submaxillary glands of the mouse. PORCELLI et al. (1976) described the isolation of an enzyme under the name of kallikrein from a DEAE-cellulose fraction comprising only 28% of the eluted BAEe esterase, but 74% of the kininogenase activity. Regarding the different assay conditions, the specific activity measured with BAEe as substrate appears comparable to that of other enzyme preparations from mouse submaxillary glands (Table 12) or to that of rat submandibular kallikrein (Table 9). BPTI, in concentrations up to 30 μg/ml, inhibited the esterase activity to only about 70%. In spite of its kininogenase activity, the enzyme was reported to have renin-like activity, evidently attributed to contaminating isorenin. The kallikrein nature of this enzyme preparation is thus not well documented.

ANGELETTI et al. (1967) isolated an enzyme, called R-esteroprotease, from the main peak (60%) of BAEe esterase from submaxillary glands of male mice eluted from DEAE-cellulose (Table 12). The enzyme hydrolyzed casein at only 3% the rate of trypsin, but the rates of BANA hydrolysis were comparable. In these respects, it resembles rat submandibular kallikrein. The mouse enzyme, however, had only 6% of the activity of trypsin with Bz-DL-Arg-β-naphthylamide. It was inhibited by DFP and by mercaptoethanol, but not by EDTA, ovomucoid, or SBTI. It may be noteworthy that with BPTI, 80% inhibition of the esterase activity was observed. Antiserum raised with this enzyme preparation demonstrated immunologic homogeneity. It cross-reacted with two other BAEe hydrolyzing enzymes from mouse submaxillary glands to 15% and 70%, respectively.

An esteroprotease comprising 62% of the BAEe esterase activity of the submaxillary glands of male mice was purified 100-fold by ANGELETTI et al. (1973). These authors evidently assumed the latter enzyme was identical with the above mentioned R-esteroprotease. Though the specific activity measured with BAEe was lower than that of other enzyme preparations from this source (Table 12), the preparation was homogeneous in disc electrophoresis. Ultracentrifugation in a sucrose gradient re-

Table 12. Isolation and properties of BAEe esterases from submaxillary glands of the mouse

	Angeletti et al. (1967)	Angeletti et al. (1973)	(Ekfors et al., 1972a; Ekfors and Hopsu-Havu, 1972)		Porcelli et al. (1976)
Assay method used in purification:	BAEe	BAEe	BANA		BAEe, kinin release
Purification steps: 1.	DEAE-cellulose	Ethanol fractionation	pH and ammonium sulfate precipitation		Streptomycin supernatant
2.	DEAE-cellulose	DEAE-cellulose	Sephadex G-100		Sephadex G-100
3.	Sephadex G-100	CM-cellulose (pH 4.2)	DEAE-cellulose		DEAE-cellulose
4.	CM-cellulose	Bio-Gel P-100	CM-cellulose (pH 5.7)		Gel electrophoresis
5.	Sephadex G-100		DEAE-cellulose		Sephadex G-25
6.	DEAE-cellulose				
7.	DEAE-cellulose				
Specific activity:			Main component C	Other components	
Kinin release (μg BK/min):		(rabbit serum) 4×10^8/mg (?)			(dog serum; rat kininogen II?) 20/mg protein
BAEe (μmol/min):	(pH 9) 1,500/mg	133/mg protein (1.86×10^6/mg(?) after ultracentrifugation)	(6.7 m*M*; pH 8.2; 37 °C) 930/mg protein	290...2500/mg protein	(1 m*M*; pH 8; 25 °C) 350/mg protein
TAMe (μmol/min):			(6.7 m*M*; pH 8.2; 37 °C) 310/mg protein	100...1400/mg protein	
BANA (μmol/min):	(pH 9) 4.2/mg		(0.25 m*M*; pH 8.2; 37 °C) 0.67/mg protein	0.22...0.50/mg protein	
Bz-DL-Arg-β-naphthylamide (μmol/min):	(pH 9) 0.05/mg		(0.25 m*M*; pH 8.2; 37 °C) 0.070/mg protein	0.016...0.110/mg protein	
Molecular weight:					
Gel filtration:	32,000	31,000			
SDS electrophoresis:					32,000
Sucrose gradient centrifugation:	32,000				

sulted in a single protein peak (sedimentation coefficient, about 2.5) coinciding with the esterase activity. The reported enormous increase in specific activity in this procedure may involve some error. The stated rate of kinin release from rabbit serum is also incredibly high. Injected into a rabbit, the enzyme preparation (3 ng/kg) produced a fall in arterial blood pressure of about 40 mm Hg, lasting for about 4 min. In these respects, criteria for kallikrein activity were fulfilled. The enzyme preparation had a low proteolytic activity. Its esterase activity was not inhibited by ovomucoid or SBTI, but inhibited about 80% by BPTI.

EKFORS et al. (1972a) isolated six esteropeptidases A–F from mouse submandibular glands (Table 12). All the enzymes had low caseinolytic and high arginine esterase activities (EKFORS and HOPSU-HAVU, 1972). BAEe was a distinctly better substrate than TAMe and was hydrolyzed three times faster by component C, as is the case with rat submandibular kallikrein. AMe was much better substrate than LysOMe. Ac-TyrOEt was hydrolyzed only slowly. The rate of hydrolysis of BANA was of the same order of magnitude as found with rat urinary kallikrein. Component C was slowly inhibited by DFP and by diethyl p-nitrophenylphosphate. EDTA or cysteine increased the activity of components A–C by 24–45%, while mercaptoethanol or iodoacetamide were without influence. These three components were also sensitive to inhibition by Co^{2+} and especially by Hg^{2+}. SBTI or LBTI and ovomucoid trypsin inhibitors did not inhibit but BPTI did to a variable extent. All six enzymes were antigenetically related. Some had plasminogen activating activities, and four increased the vascular permeability of rabbit skin (EKFORS et al., 1972b).

EKFORS and HOPSU-HAVU (1972) summarize evidence that the principal component C (representing 69% of the gland's activity in hydrolyzing BANA, EKFORS et al., 1972a) is identical with the esteroprotease R of ANGELETTI et al. (1967), the latter preparation possibly contains still other enzyme components. If this is true, component C might be mouse kallikrein, though besides increasing vascular permeability it also had the highest plasminogen activator action.

Two esteroproteolytic enzymes from mouse submaxillary glands, called A and D, were isolated by LEVY et al. (1970). These have many properties in common with the enzymes mentioned above. Both enzymes are antigenetically related and have similar amino acid compositions (BOESMAN et al., 1976). The latter authors quote evidence for an identity of enzyme D with the epithelial growth factor binding protein described by TAYLOR et al. (1974). This arginine esterase is devoid of proteolytic activity and contains 12 half-cystine residues, but no free sulfhydryl groups, structural features resembling those of the family of pancreatic serine proteinases. Epidermal growth factor binding protein is a glycoprotein and is antigenetically related to nerve growth factor binding protein. It was reported to have no physiologically significant effect on the blood pressure of rats (TAYLOR et al., 1974). As, in contrast to rat kallikrein, mouse submaxillary kallikrein has no oxytocic effect on the isolated rat uterus (CHIANG et al., 1968) it is also possible that mouse kallikrein does not affect the blood pressure of the rat.

The relationships of all of these evidently closely related arginine esterases of the mouse submaxillary gland are far from clear. The question which of these enzymes is really kallikrein and whether it has been obtained in a high state of purity has not been settled conclusively. Studies on blood pressure of mice would help here.

II. Cat Submaxillary Kallikrein

Kallikrein from cat submaxillary glands was highly purified by MORIWAKI et al. (1976a) (Table 13). The enzyme obtained in high yield gave a single broad band in disc electrophoresis. The broadness of this band, the lower electrophoretic mobility in comparison to other glandular kallikreins and the relatively high MW determined by gel filtration were tentatively attributed to a high carbohydrate content. On isoelectric focusing, the enzyme was resolved into six enzymically active components with isoelectric points in the acid range (Table 13).

Cat submaxillary kallikrein was a potent vasodilator in the dog. BAEe was hydrolyzed twice as fast as TAMe, whereas a tyrosine ester was only very slowly cleaved (Table 13). No hydrolysis of BANA has been detected.

III. Dog Pancreatic Kallikrein

The two purification procedures developed for dog pancreatic kallikrein are summarized in Table 13. Chromatography on DEAE-Sephadex separated the enzyme from the more tightly bound anionic trypsin (HOJIMA et al., 1975c). By preparative isoelectric focusing, three components (from up to five observed) have been isolated (HOJIMA et al., 1977). These were homogeneous in disc gel electrophoresis. $A^{1\%}_{280\ \mathrm{nm}}$ has been determined as 14.8, 14.8, and 13.9 for the three fractions. Their catalytic activities and behaviour against inhibitors were very similar. The small differences in MW observed after gel filtration were attributed to differences in carbohydrate content. The amino acid composition of one of the fractions is shown in Table 14.

Dog pancreatic kallikrein lost less than 10% of activity during lyophilization. Incubated at pH 4–10 for 24 h at 25 °C, it remained more than 95% active. When kept at 80 °C for 1 h, the enzyme lost 50–80% of its activity at pH 4.5 or 8, but only 10% at 45 °C (HOJIMA et al., 1977).

In the dog, dog pancreatic kallikrein was a strong vasodilator in relation to its esterolytic potency (Table 13). BAEe (K_m, 0.27–0.33 mM) is hydrolyzed several times faster than TAMe (K_m, 0.14–0.26 mM). Casein or BANA were not attacked (HOJIMA et al., 1977). The pH optimum for TAMe hydrolysis was 8.0 (MORIWAKI et al., 1976b), and pH 9.0–9.2 for BAEe (HOJIMA et al., 1977).

After a 30 min incubation at pH 8 and 37 °C, with up to 1 mM L-cysteine, thioglycol, BAL, EDTA, or 8-hydroxyquinoline-5-sulfonate, the activity of dog pancreatic kallikrein was in the range of 83–120% of the controls. Among several heavy metal ions tested, Cd^{2+}, Hg^{2+}, and Zn^{2+} were especially effective inhibitors. 10 mM DFP inhibited 63–89% after 30 min at pH 8, 37 °C, but 1 mM Tos-LysCH_2Cl and Tos-PheCH_2Cl were inactive.

IV. Horse Urinary Kallikrein

1. Isolation and Molecular Aspects

The isolation procedure for horse urinary kallikrein has been vastly improved with regards to yield and specific activity by the introduction of an affinity chromatography step (Table 15). The material thus obtained was homogeneous by the criteria of a single symmetric peak with constant specific activity in gel filtration and of single

Table 13. Isolation and properties of cat submaxillary and dog pancreatic kallikreins

	Cat submaxillary kallikrein	Dog pancreatic kallikrein	
	MORIWAKI et al. (1976a)	HOJIMA et al. (1975b)	(MORIYA et al., 1975; HOJIMA et al., 1977)
Assay method used in purification:	Vasodilation, BAEe	Vasodilation, BAEe	Vasodilation, BAEe
Purification steps: 1.	Water extraction	Water extract, activated 8 h at 20 °C	Water homogenate, activated 6 h at pH 7.5, room temperature
2.	Acetone fractionation	Acetone fractionation	Acetone fractionation
3.	DEAE-Sephadex	Gel electrophoresis	Acetone fractionation
4.	Sephadex G-75	Sephadex G-75	DEAE-Sephadex
5.	Electrofocusing		Sephadex G-100
6.	Sephadex G-50		Electrofocusing
7.			Sephadex G-50
Purification factor:	80	1,500–2,000	3,300
Yield:	45%	28–36%	32–39%
Specific activity:			
Biologic (dog, KU):	1,260/mg	867/mg	606–1,350/mg
BAEe (μmol/min):	(1 mM; pH 8; 25 °C) 24.5/mg	(1 mM; pH 8; 25 °C) 18.3/mg	(1 mM; pH 8; 25 °C) 14.3–23.4/mg
TAMe (μmol/min):	11.6/mg	(1 mM; pH 8; 25 °C) 10.0/mg	(1 mM; pH 8; 25 °C) 2.4–4.8/mg
Bz-TyrOEt (μmol/min):	0.06/mg	(1 mM; pH 8; 25 °C) 0.05/mg	(1 mM; pH 8; 25 °C) <0.1/mg
Molecular weight:			
Gel filtration:	50,000		30,000; 28,000; 27,000
Composition:			27,026 (protein only)
Isoelectric point:	4.27; 4.41; 4.55; 4.70; 4.89; 4.94	4.22; 4.30; 4.40; 4.53	4.09; 4.16; 4.36

Table 14. Amino acid composition (residues per molecule) of various glandular kallikreins

	Dog pancreatic kallikrein III HOJIMA et al. (1977)	Rabbit urinary kallikrein PORCELLI et al. (1974b)	Kallikrein from guinea pig coagulating gland MORIWAKI et al. (1974b)
Asp	25	22	32
Thr	15	27	13
Ser	14	28	12–13
Glu	26	29	25
Pro	15	14	31
Gly	20	26	20–21
Ala	15	20	15
Cys/2	8	1	8–9
Val	17	19	20
Met	4	0	7
Ile	12	9	9
Leu	23	13	24–25
Tyr	8	11	6
Phe	8	14	4
Lys	8	12	4
His	13	5	10
Arg	5	6	7
Trp	4		7

bands in gel electrophoresis at pH 8.7 and 4.8 and also in the presence of SDS (GIUSTI et al., 1976). On gel electrofocusing with Ampholine pH 3.5–5, the material was resolved into five enzymically active protein bands. MWs obtained by gel filtration under different conditions varied considerably (Table 15).

The highly purified enzyme loses considerable activity on storage in water or pH 8 buffer even in the frozen state. Following exhaustive dialysis, the kallikrein is no longer able to release kinin, Na^+, K^+, Li^+, Rb^+, or Ca^{2+} being required for reactivation (WEBSTER and PRADO, 1970). Incubation at pH 3.0 (4 h at 37 °C) did not inactivate this kallikrein, but inactivation was observed at lower pH values (SAMPAIO and PRADO, 1975). Heating for 15 min at 70 ° or 98 °C led to activity losses of 30 and 49%; 30 min treatment with 8 *M* urea reduced the activity by 50%.

At 37 °C, the activity of horse urinary kallikrein was stable against the attack of trypsin, chymotrypsin, papain, subtilisin BPN′, pepsin, or carboxypeptidase B, but pronase inactivated it (SAMPAIO and PRADO, 1975). Trypsin, chymotrypsin, or subtilisin inactivated only after pretreatment of the kallikrein at 55 ° to 60 °C and incubation at this temperature.

2. Catalytic Properties

Horse urinary kallikrein was hypotensive in the dog, but not in the rat (PRADO et al., 1962). The kinin released from horse plasma has been identified as kallidin. Met-kallidin (Met-Lys-bradykinin) is not an intermediate of this reaction (PRADO et al., 1971). The rate of kinin formation at 37 °C, expressed in bradykinin equivalent, under condition of zero-order kinetics was calculated as 0.8 μmol/min/mg from heated horse plasma and as 0.14 μmol/min/mg from partially purified bovine kininogen (WEBSTER and PRADO, 1970).

Table 15. Isolation and properties of horse and rabbit urinary kallikreins and the kallikrein from the coagulating gland of the guinea pig

	Horse urinary kallikrein	
	WEBSTER and PRADO (1970)	GIUSTI et al. (1976)
Assay method used in purification:	Kinin release (TAMe)	
Purification steps: 1.	Ammonium sulfate fractionation	Ultrafiltration
2.	Acetone fractionation	Aluminium sulfate treatment
3.	DEAE-cellulose	Acetone fractionation
4.	Acetone fractionation	p-(ε-Aminocaprylamido)-benzamidine-Sepharose
5.	Sephadex G-75	Sephadex G-150
6.		
Purification factor:	2200	
Yield:	5%	46%
Specific activity:		
Biologic (dog, KU):		
Kinin release (μgBK/min):	(heated dog plasma) 800/mg	
BAEe (μmol/min):		
TAMe (μmol/min):	(6 mM; pH 8.5; 30 °C) 65/mg protein	112/mg protein
Molecular weight:		
Gel filtration:		57,000 (Sephadex G-150) 34,000 (Biogel A-0.5M)
SDS electrophoresis:		
Ultracentrifugation:		
Isoelectric point:		5 peaks (Ampholine pH 3.5–5)

Bradykinyl-Ser is readily hydrolyzed at the Arg-Ser bond (BABEL et al., 1968). Bradykinyl-Ser-Val-Gln-Val-Ser, a peptide with an amino acid sequence as occurs in bovine kininogen (see the section on porcine pancreatic kallikrein), is also very rapidly hydrolyzed at this bond. Though the K_m is less favourable, k_{cat} is comparable to that observed for the hydrolysis of the ester bond in bradykinylOMe, and amounts to 5–10% of k_{cat} of trypsin (Table 16). The rate observed is enough to account for the rate of kinin liberation from kininogen as by cleavage at the C-terminus.

A slow hydrolysis of Met-Lys-bradykinin, as well as of Lys-Lys-bradykinin, has been reported to occur at the Lys-Arg bond (BABEL et al., 1968), though the first-mentioned substrate was not attacked by highly purified horse urinary kallikrein (GIUSTI et al., 1976). Besides traces of bradykinin, the main product of the hydrolysis of Gly-Leu-Met-Lys-bradykinyl-Ser-Val-Gln-Val-Ser was kallidin (PRADO et al., 1977). From the corresponding Gly-Lys-Met-Lys-peptide, only about 10% each of kallidin and bradykinin and 4% Met-Lys-bradykinin were obtained on prolonged hydrolysis. These results show the hydrolysis of methionyl bonds and of some lysyl bonds by horse urinary kallikrein. The corresponding Gly-Arg-Val-Lys-peptide was cleaved mainly at this arginyl bond and to some extent at the lysyl bond, while in Asp-Arg-Met-Lys-bradykinin the lysyl, methionyl, and arginyl bonds seem to have been cleaved in decreasing order. The reaction-rates in all these experiments, however, were exceedingly low. 1 μmol of substrate has been incubated at pH 8.5, 37 °C,

Rabbit urinary kallikrein	Guinea pig coagulating gland kallikrein	
Porcelli et al. (1974b)	Moriwaki et al. (1974b)	Moriwaki et al. (1974a)
BAEe	Vasodilation, kinin release, TAMe	
Benzoic acid precipitation Acetone extraction DEAE-cellulose CM-cellulose Sephadex G-100 (3 times) Sephadex G-100	Extraction, ultrafiltration DEAE-cellulose DEAE-cellulose Sephadex G-200	
	34–48	
4 mg/30 l urine	38%	
	$420/A_{280}$ (crude bovine kininogen)	$333/A_{280}$ (crude bovine kininogen)
	$5.38/A_{280}$	$4.4/A_{280}$
(1 mM; pH 8; 25 °C) 3.4/mg protein		(1 mM; pH 8; 30 °C) $2.40/A_{280}$
	(33 mM; pH 8; 30 °C) $38.0/A_{280}$	(20 mM; pH 8.5; 30 °C) $9.7/A_{280}$
		(33 mM; pH 8.5; 30 °C) $8.30/A_{280}$
	40,000	
31,000		
	31,000	
	3.4	

with as much as 1.3 mg of horse urinary kallikrein for several hours. Though interestingly the highest yield of kallidin was obtained from the peptide with leucine in position P_2 to the bond cleaved, as it is reported to occur in bovine kininogen (Han et al., 1976), the low yields of identifiable products on prolonged hydrolysis suggest the possible presence of contaminating peptidases. Fragments other than those comprising the kinin part have in no case been identified. At any rate, the observed cleavage of methionyl bonds is orders of magnitude slower than that of kininogen.

Horse urinary kallikrein does not hydrolyze casein or hemoglobin (Prado et al., 1962; Brandi et al., 1965; Sampaio et al., 1977). Polyarginine and tetraarginine were hydrolyzed, but not triarginine, polylysine, a number of arginyl or lysyl dipeptides, or LysOEt (Prado et al., 1966). Salmine and histones are also hydrolyzed (Brandi et al., 1965; Sampaio et al., 1977).

Kinetic constants for the hydrolysis of several synthetic substrates by horse urinary kallikrein and by trypsin are compiled in Table 16. The K_m for TAMe is in accordance with a previous result of 1.0–1.5 mM (Kramer et al., 1966). BAEe is hardly a better substrate than TAMe. The extended ester substrate with kinin structure, bradykinylOMe, has a drastically lowered K_m. It is remarkable that k_{cat} is less favourable and is as high as with the bradykinyl peptide. With pig pancreatic kallikrein, the related peptide bradykinyl-Ser-Val-Gln has quite similar kinetic constants, and the shorter peptide Ac-Phe-Arg-Ser-Val-Gln has a comparable k_{cat} value, but k_{cat} for Ac-Phe-ArgOMe is 130-fold higher (Tables 3 and 4). When trypsin is used,

Table 16. Kinetic constants for the hydrolysis of ester and peptide substrates by horse urinary kallikrein and by trypsin (pH 8.0 or 8.1, 30 °C) (SAMPAIO et al., 1976)

	Horse urinary kallikrein			Trypsin		
	K_m (mM)	k_{cat} (s^{-1})	k_{cat}/K_m (mM^{-1} s^{-1})	K_m (mM)	k_{cat} (s^{-1})	k_{cat}/K_m (mM^{-1} s^{-1})
BAEe	2.02	87	43			
TAMe	1.30	51	39	0.041	160	3,900
BradykinylOMe	0.013	16	1,200	0.025	115	4,600
				0.052	225	4,300
Bradykinyl-Ser-Val-Gln-Val-Ser	0.19	9	47	1.70	250	150
	0.44	14	32	0.91	148	160

k_{cat} for the bradykinin ester is also similar to that of the bradykinyl peptide, but these values are much higher than found with kallikrein and are as high as described for the very good trypsin substrate TAMe (Table 16).

Nevertheless, a comparison of the specificity constants k_{cat}/K_m shows that the small ester substrate TAMe is hydrolyzed 100 times less efficiently by horse urinary kallikrein than by trypsin. In contrast, this constant for the bradykinin ester is only four times lower with the kallikrein than with trypsin. The specificity constants in tryptic hydrolysis are similar for TAMe and bradykinylOMe, while the smaller ester is a 30 times worse substrate of kallikrein than the peptide ester is. An extended peptide sequence to the left of the bond cleaved has thus a large favourable effect on the hydrolysis of substrates by horse urinary kallikrein, but not by trypsin. This result suggests that additional subsites, not essential in trypsin catalyzed hydrolysis, are of importance for the recognition of substrates by this kallikrein (SAMPAIO et al., 1976).

3. Low Molecular Weight Inhibitors

The importance of alkali metal or Ca^{2+} ions for the catalytic activity of horse urinary kallikrein has been mentioned above. 0.1–0.5 M Ca^{2+} or Mg^{2+} had some inhibitory effect but heavy metal ions were inhibitors at concentrations of 1 mM or lower, Cu^{2+}, Co^{2+}, Ni^{2+}, and above all, Hg^{2+}, being especially effective (KRAMER et al., 1966). Benzamidine inhibits the action of the enzyme on BAEe, kininogen (DINIZ et al., 1965), and peptides (BABEL et al., 1968), and protects from inhibition by a chloromethyl ketone (SAMPAIO and PRADO, 1976).

Incubation for 2 h with 10 mM DFP completely (and 5 mM partially) inhibited horse urinary kallikrein (PRADO et al., 1962). Tos-LysCH_2Cl did not inhibit the enzyme (DINIZ et al., 1965), but a more extended chloromethyl ketone in which a phenylalanine residue in P_2 as found in kininogen precedes the basic residue, Ala-Phe-LysCH_2Cl, proved inhibitory with a low K_i of 0.084 mM and $k_2 = 1.02 \times 10^{-3}\,s^{-1}$ (pH 7.4; 30 °C) (SAMPAIO and PRADO, 1976). p-Nitrophenyl p′-guanidinobenzoate was useful as an active site titrant of this kallikrein (SAMPAIO and PRADO, 1976). These observations indicate that horse urinary kallikrein is also a serine proteinase.

V. Rabbit Urinary Kallikrein

A BAEe esterase was purified from rabbit urine and called kallikrein by PORCELLI et al. (1974b) (Table 15). This enzyme behaved as a less acidic protein than human or rat urinary kallikrein. Specific activity measured with BAEe was low, but comparable to that of several other glandular kallikreins. No evidence for characterising this enzyme as a kallikrein was given. The enzyme contained four glucosamine and 13 hexose residues per molecule. Especially striking is the low content of cysteine (Table 14). In control experiments with BSA, correct cysteine and methionine values were obtained by these authors.

Upon Sephadex G-200 gel filtration and isoelectric focusing, a kininogenase from rabbit urine associated with albumin was observed in the pH 4.85 region by HAMBERG and YOUTSIMO (1974). This partially purified preparation had a specific activity of 0.48 nmol/min/mg measured with 0.7 μ*M* tritiated TAMe and had no plasminogen activator activity.

VI. Guinea Pig Coagulating Gland Kallikrein

A kininogenase has been highly purified from the coagulating gland of male guinea pigs (Table 15). The preparation behaved as a homogeneous enzyme during gel filtration and in the ultracentrifuge. On disc electrophoresis, a single protein band staining also with a BAEe-formazane system was observed, while more bands had been obtained with a less pure preparation (FUJIMOTO et al., 1972). On electrofocusing, the enzyme formed a single rather narrow peak with a pI of 3.4 (MORIWAKI et al., 1974b). The amino acid composition is given in Table 14. The preparation contained 6–7% of amino sugars, 6.0% hexoses, and 2.4% sialic acid. The MW determined by gel filtration (Table 15) was much higher than that found in ultracentrifugation ($s_{20,w}=2.7$), even though a partial specific volume of 0.749 (a value seemingly too high for a glycoprotein) had been assumed in the latter calculations. Similar observations have been made with other glandular kallikreins and are probably due to anomalous behaviour of glycoproteins in gel filtration. The enzyme was rather stable on heat treatment; 60% of the TAMe esterase activity survived 60 min incubation at 75 °C, pH 8.0.

The enzyme showed significant vasodilator activity in dog (Table 15), indicating that it was a kallikrein. The kinin released from crude dog kininogen was mainly kallidin with traces of bradykinin (MORIWAKI et al., 1975). The previous report on the liberation of bradykinin (MORIWAKI and SCHACHTER, 1971) was traced to a conversion of kallidin to bradykinin by the dog kininogen preparation used.

The kallikrein preparation from guinea pig coagulating gland showed no kininase or caseinolytic activity (MORIWAKI et al., 1974b). The pH optimum of TAMe hydrolysis was 9. K_m values for BAEe or TAMe were 0.213 and 0.780 m*M*. The ratio of the rate of hydrolysis of the two esters was 0.75. However, there are some inconsistencies with the results of MORIWAKI et al. (1974a) who used a preparation with the specific activity of 80% of the former in biologic or kininogenase assays, but of only 22% in the TAMe esterase assay (Table 15).

In each case, the kininogenase from guinea pig coagulating gland behaved as a glandular kallikrein. Nevertheless, it is not known whether the physiologic function of this enzyme is due to its ability to release kinin (MORIWAKI and SCHACHTER, 1971) but such questions arise with any kallikrein. A comparison with other glandular kallikreins of the guinea pig would be required before it can be finally decided whether this kininogenase is a glandular kallikrein.

Purification and properties of a kallikrein recently isolated from guinea pig submandibular gland are outlined in the chapter on Kallikrein in Exocerine Glands by BHOOLA et al.

G. Glandular Kallikreins as a Distinct Group of Related Enzymes[1]

I. Glandular Kallikreins as Acid Glycoproteins Belonging to the Serine Proteinases of Pancreatic Type

In the group of glandular kallikreins, similarities among the enzymes derived from different organs and body fluids of a single mammalian species have been noted early, but usually the apparent differences have been stressed. Recent immunologic and other work on the glandular kallikreins of man, rat, and especially pig have demonstrated, however, a rather high degree of similarity, if not identity, of the kallikreins from different organs and body fluids in each of these species. In the case of the pig, convincing evidence for the identity of the protein parts – apart from some secondary degradation – of the glandular kallikreins from pancreas, submandibular glands, and urine has accumulated. Differences have been found, however, in the carbohydrate parts of porcine pancreatic and submandibular kallikreins. The three porcine enzymes have definitely been shown to be of the serine proteinase family of the pancreatic type, indicating that all the glandular kallikreins may belong to this class of enzymes.

Among the serine proteinases of pancreatic type, the glycoprotein nature of glandular kallikreins, demonstrated regrettably in only a number of examples, is quite unique. It is not known, however, whether this possibly highly characteristic property is indeed essential for the physiologic function of a glandular kallikrein. The same holds true for the low isoelectric point observed with each glandular kallikrein investigated. The glycoprotein nature of these enzymes is probably responsible for the existence of multiple forms demonstrated for quite a number of glandular kallikreins. Heterogeneity of the carbohydrate part of glycoproteins is a well-known phenomenon.

The class of mammalian serine proteinases of the pancreatic type is characterized by an identical catalytic apparatus and, in addition, by further extensive structural homology, shown also by the similar number of constituent amino acid residues of the order of 200–240. Consequently, the MW of the protein part of a possible glandular kallikrein may be important for its classification. Regrettably, hardly any data on this are available. Reliable data are even lacking on MWs of the whole glycoproteins from which the MW of the protein part could be derived if the complete amino acid and carbohydrate composition is known. MWs of glandular kallikreins determined by different authors and techniques usually differ widely. To obtain reliable values for the MW of a glycoprotein is indeed not an easy task. Gel filtration tends to give falsely high values for glycoproteins (ANDREWS, 1970). During SDS gel electrophoresis the glycoprotein nature, low isoelectric point, and other individual features are known to influence the results since the introduction of the method (SHAPIRO et al., 1967; DUNKER and RUECKERT, 1969; BRETSCHER, 1971;

[1] For references see the sections on the individual glandular kallikreins.

SEGREST et al., 1971; WILLIAM and GRATHER, 1971; TUNG and KNIGHT, 1972; CAMACHO et al., 1975). The most reliable MWs appear to be expected from ultracentrifugation studies. These require, however, knowledge of the partial specific volume of the respective glycoprotein which is highly dependent on content and composition of carbohydrate and is generally much lower than that for proteins.

Conceivably, alternative methods for the direct determination of the MW of the protein part of a glandular kallikrein are active site titration in combination with quantitative amino acid analysis or quantitative end group determinations. The latter method is likely to involve errors of a magnitude defeating this approach and both would require enzyme preparations of very high purity, difficult to ascertain for a glycoprotein with inherent carbohydrate heterogeneity. Reported values for the total number of amino acids in glandular kallikreins are usually either based on doubtful MWs, do not take into consideration the possible glycoprotein nature of the preparations, or are derived by statistical analysis based on the occurrence of the amino acids in proteins in integral numbers. To produce meaningful results in the case of relatively large molecules, however, calculations of the latter type would require extreme purity of the material under study and knowledge of the precision of the amino acid analyses (HOY et al., 1974).

The known mammalian serine proteinases of pancreas have 8–12 half cystine residues that apparently occur always in even numbers and are all involved in the formation of disulfide bridges. Significantly lower figures for the cystine content of glandular kallikreins have been reported by one group of workers for rabbit and human urinary kallikreins. Both of these preparations were characterized only as arginine esterases and neither by kininogenase nor by depressor effects. The yield of the human kallikrein was only 0.8%. Other investigators found a much higher cysteine value for the latter enzyme. A low cystine content is also reported for human salivary kallikrein. All the low values were not obtained by the application of special techniques as performic acid oxidation or carboxymethylation. The occurrence of sulfhydryl groups in a particular preparation of human urinary kallikrein has been commented on there.

II. Glandular Kallikreins as Serine Proteinases

Data on the demonstration of the serine proteinase nature of glandular kallikreins are also scarce. One characteristic of the serine proteinases is their inhibition by DFP which reacts with the single catalytically active serine residue that has given its name to this class of enzymes. Besides the porcine glandular kallikreins, DFP inhibits horse, human, and rat urinary kallikreins, dog pancreatic kallikrein, and mouse submaxillary kininogenase (see also CHIANG et al., 1968). (The negative result reported for rat submandibular kallikrein is discussed elsewhere.) It would be interesting to learn from quantitative studies – in comparison with other serine proteinases from the respective species – whether the relatively low rate of inhibition by this compound is a common feature of glandular kallikreins. This could be a useful characteristic and indicator of some unique conformation of the active site of these enzymes.

A further indication of a common mechanism of catalysis in serine proteinases is their irreversible inhibition by chloromethyl ketone derivatives of amino acids which react with the catalytically active histidine residue. The trypsin inhibitor Tos-

$LysCH_2Cl$, in all cases investigated, does not inhibit glandular kallikreins. However, extended peptide chloromethyl ketones more closely resembling the structure of the natural kallikrein substrate, kininogen, inhibited horse urinary and all porcine glandular kallikreins.

Reactions of serine proteinases are generally accepted to follow an acyl enzyme mechanism. Demonstration of acyl enzyme formation was also possible for porcine pancreatic kallikrein by its reaction with cinnamoyl imidazole causing formation of cinnamoyl kallikrein with the characteristic difference spectrum of this class of acyl enzymes. A biphasic course of nitrophenol release (an initial stoichiometric burst followed by a slower steady state reaction phase) was observed in the reactions with p-nitrophenyl p′-guanidinobenzoate of pig pancreatic as well as rat and horse urinary kallikreins. This phenomenon is also indicative of the formation of an acyl enzyme intermediate in glandular kallikreins and allows active site titration in favourable cases. The remarkable lack of reactivity of this compound with a preparation of human urinary kallikrein showing very low activity with BAEe or TAMe may be a peculiarity of that particular preparation.

III. Glandular Kallikreins as Kininogenases Which Release Kallidin

Since their discovery, kallikreins just as other enzymes are defined by their function, i.e., the ability to liberate a kinin from kininogen. A definite proof that this is the only physiologic role of these enzymes is lacking. Nevertheless, this criterion still appears to be an essential – though by far not enough to define a kallikrein.

As to the identity of the kinin released by glandular kallikreins, release of kallidin from autologous serum has been demonstrated only with human (PIERCE and WEBSTER, 1961) and horse urinary kallikreins. Kallidin is also the principal kinin liberated from dog serum by guinea pig coagulating gland kallikrein or from bovine kininogen by porcine submandibular (WERLE et al., 1961) or pancreatic kallikrein or human urinary kallikrein. In nearly all of these experiments formation of some bradykinin has also been observed. The kinin liberated by trypsin – as well as by serum kallikrein – is generally bradykinin. It should not be ignored, however, that (bovine) trypsin also releases a small amount of kallidin (PRADO, 1970). From citraconylated bovine HMW kininogen, where the cleavage at lysine leading to bradykinin release is blocked, trypsin liberated Met-kallidin as well as kallidin, suggesting the cleavage of X-Met and also Met-Lys(ε-citraconyl) bonds by this enzyme (IWANAGA et al., 1977). All experiments of this kind, however, are very sensitive to contamination by aminopeptidase or possibly by chymotrypsin type enzymes or could be interpreted by the existence of minor fractions of kininogen with somewhat different sequence. Though kallidin liberation might turn out to be one of the most stringent criteria for the definition of a glandular kallikrein, the various kininogenases mentioned may differ only in the degree of preferential formation of bradykinin or kallidin.

IV. Glandular Kallikreins as Enzymes Highly Specific in Interactions With Proteins

As far as is known, glandular kallikreins possess only a very limited general proteolytic activity with proteins such as casein or hemoglobin. The reason for this is unknown, and so the question of whether this lack of proteolytic activity is essential for a glandular kallikrein must remain open. There are notable differences in their interaction with HMW proteinase inhibitors though quantitative data in the form of inhibition constants are regretably scarce. BPTI, once regarded as a universal inhibitor of glandular kallikreins, evidently reacts only with some of the enzymes.

The varying sensitivity of glandular kallikreins to heterologous protein inhibitors appears to be of no special significance. For the function of glandular kallikreins as kininogenases, reactions with inhibitors of the same species certainly will be of much higher importance. Differences in this inhibition pattern are probably responsible for differences in the ability of kallikreins and trypsins to liberate kinins, e.g., when injected into the circulation. This point is also in need of further exploration. Incidentally, reactions with HMW substrates and inhibitors are presumably the ones where differences in the carbohydrate content of various forms of a kallikrein may have an effect.

V. Glandular Kallikreins as Arginine-Specific Hydrolases With Pronounced Secondary Specificity

Amino acid specificity in the hydrolysis of smaller model substrates might also help to identify a glandular kallikrein. The specificity for arginyl bonds places glandular kallikreins closer to the serine proteinase trypsin, and it might be a general property of these enzymes. The few experiments with a typical chymotryptic substrate such as a tyrosine ester, point in this direction. It would be especially interesting to elucidate whether the big difference in hydrolysis of arginine- and lysine-containing substrates by the porcine enzymes is indeed a general property of the glandular kallikreins, distinguishing them from trypsins of the same species.

In these studies, however, the big influence of the α-N-acyl substituent in ester substrates should be borne in mind. Ratios of the rates of BAEe versus TAMe hydrolysis by glandular kallikreins of different species vary widely. Such ratios are useful in comparing kallikreins from different organs with each other or with other esterases of the same species. Substrate activation during TAMe hydrolysis might be a general property of enzymes related to trypsin. Nevertheless, such substrates evidently are of limited value for characterizing a glandular kallikrein. Acyl substituents such as benzoyl or tosyl residues are artificial; these enzymes have not been selected against them during evolution. Their interaction with an enzyme might differ considerably from that of a natural kallikrein substrate. In this respect, acyl substituents such as Ac-Phe, or perhaps the benzyloxycarbonyl group, that resemble kininogen more closely would be preferable for a comparison of relative amino acid specificities of kallikreins. Arginine esters of this type are much better substrates of porcine glandular kallikreins than are benzoylated or tosylated compounds. This also applies to rat and horse urinary kallikreins. These are better substrates because of the pronounced secondary specificity of these kallikreins to amino acid residues adjacent in N-terminal direction to the amino acid at the cleavage site (which is recognized on the basis of primary specificity). Such a high secondary specificity in ester or peptide hydrolysis or in inhibition reactions – not found in bovine trypsin – might be a very stringent criterion for characterizing a glandular kallikrein. Arginine esters of the aforementioned type might also yield more meaningful values for the ratios of esterase versus kininogenase activities than ratios obtained when the esterolytic activity is determined with benzoylated or tosylated esters.

The same is true for the hydrolysis of small amide substrates. The rate of BANA hydrolysis reported for different glandular kallikreins varies widely between practically zero and a rate comparable to that of tryptic hydrolysis. Use of compounds with less artificial acyl substituents might lead to more uniform and realistic values for the ability of these enzymes to hydrolyze nitroanilides or other amides.

In all of these studies, the degraded forms of an enzyme show different catalytic activities. Probably degraded forms occur in preparations of kallikreins that have been subjected to drastic procedures, e.g., for activation of proenzymes.

This attempt to give the general picture of glandular kallikreins regrettably reads more like a listing of information gaps and desirable experiments. Nevertheless, no known facts contradict the impression that glandular kallikreins form a closely related group of enzymes belonging to the family of serine proteinases of pancreatic type. More work is needed, however, before this view can be either definitely confirmed or disproved.

References

Amundsen, E., Svendsen, L., Vennerød, A.M., Laake, K.: Determination of plasma kallikrein with a new chromogenic tripeptide derivative. In: Chemistry and biology of the kallikrein-kinin system in health and disease. Pisano, J.J., Austen, K.F. (eds.), pp. 215–220. Washington: U.S. Gov. Printing Office 1976

Andrews, P.: Estimation of molecular size and molecular weights of biological compounds by gel filtration. Methods Biochem. Anal. *18*, 1–53 (1970)

Angeletti, R.A., Angeletti, P.U., Calissano, P.: Testosterone induction of estero-proteolytic activity in the mouse submaxillary gland. Biochim. Biophys. Acta *139*, 372–381 (1967)

Angeletti, M., Sbaraglia, G., De Campora, E., Frati, L.: Biological properties of esteroprotease isolated from the submaxillary gland of mice. Life Sci. II *12*, 297–305 (1973)

Arens, A., Haberland, G.L.: Determination of kallikrein activity in animal tissue using biochemical methods. In: Kininogenases – kallikrein. Haberland, G.L., Rohen, J.W. (eds.), pp. 43–53. Stuttgart, New York: Schattauer 1973

Babel, I., Stella, R.C.R., Prado, E.S.: Action of horse urinary kallikrein on synthetic derivatives of bradykinin. Biochem. Pharmacol. *17*, 2232–2234 (1968)

Beaven, V.H., Pierce, J.V., Pisano, J.J.: A sensitive isotopic procedure for the assay of esterase activity: measurement of human urinary kallikrein. Clin. Chim. Acta *32*, 67–73 (1971)

Béchet, J.-J., Dupaix, A., Roucous, C., Bonamy, A.-M.: Inactivation of proteases and esterases by halomethylated derivatives of dihydrocoumarins. Biochimie *59*, 241–246 (1977)

Bender, M.L., Kézdy, F.J.: Mechanism of action of proteolytic enzymes. Annu. Rev. Biochem. *34*, 49–76 (1965)

Beraldo, W.T., Araujo, R.L., Mares-Guia, M.: Oxytocic esterase in rat urine. Am. J. Physiol. *211*, 975–980 (1966)

Berrens, L.: Digestion of atopic allergens with trypsin α-chymotrypsin and pancreatic kallikrein, and influence of the allergens upon the proteolytic and esterolytic activity of these enzymes. Immunochemistry *5*, 585–605 (1968)

Bodanszky, M., Klausner, Y.S., Lin, C.Y., Mutt, V., Said, S.I.: Synthesis of the vasoactive intestinal peptide (VIP). J. Am. Chem. Soc. *96*, 4973–4978 (1974)

Boesman, M., Levy, M., Schenkein, I.: Esteroproteolytic enzymes from the submaxillary gland. Kinetics and other physicochemical properties. Arch. Biochem. Biophys. *175*, 463–476 (1976)

Brandi, C.M.W., Mendes, J., Paiva, A.C.M., Prado, E.S.: Proteolysis of salmine by horse urinary kallikrein. Biochem. Pharmacol. *14*, 1665–1671 (1965)
Brandtzaeg, P., Gautvik, K.M., Nustad, K., Pierce, J.V.: Rat submandibular gland kallikreins: Purification and cellular localization. Br. J. Pharmacol. *56*, 155–167 (1976)
Bretscher, M.S.: Major human erythrocyte glycoprotein spans the cell membrane. Nature (New Biol.) *231*, 229–232 (1971)
Bretzel, G., Hochstrasser, K.: Liberation of an acid stable proteinase inhibitor from the human inter-α-trypsin inhibitor by the action of kallikrein. Hoppe Seylers Z. Physiol. Chem. *357*, 487–489 (1976)
Camacho, A., Carrascosa, J.L., Vinuela, E., Salas, M.: Discrepancy in the mobility of a protein of phage *Φ* 29 in two different SDS polyacrylamide-gel systems. Anal. Biochem. *69*, 395–400 (1975)
Chambers, D.A., Bosser, C., Greep, J.M., Nardi, G.L.: Enzymatic investigations of partially purified hog kallikrein. Nature Lond. *197*, 1300–1301 (1963)
Chiang, T.S., Erdös, E.G., Miwa, I., Tague, L.L., Coalson, J.J.: Isolation from a salivary gland of granules containing renin and kallikrein. Circulation Res. *23*, 507–517 (1968)
Cohen, I., Zur, M., Kaminsky, E., De Vries, A.: Isolation and characterization of kinin-releasing enzyme of Echis coloratus venom. Biochem. Pharmacol. *19*, 785–793 (1970)
Diniz, C.R., Pereira, A.A., Barroso, J., Mares-Guia, M.: On the specificity of urinary kallikreins. Biochem. Biophys. Res. Commun. *21*, 448–453 (1965)
Dunker, A.K., Rueckert, R.R.: Observations on molecular weight determinations on polyacrylamide gel. J. Biol. Chem. *244*, 5074–5080 (1969)
Eeckhout, Y., Vaes, G.: Activation of the inactive precursor of collagenase by kallikrein and plasmin. Arch. Int. Physiol. Biochim. *82*, 786 (1974)
Eeckhout, Y., Vaes, G.: Further studies on the activation of procollagenase, the latent precursor of bone collagenase. Biochem. J. *166*, 21–31 (1977)
Eichner, H., Eichner, V., Fiedler, F., Hochstrasser, K.: Zum Sekretionsverhalten der BAEE-Esterase (Kallikrein) im gesunden menschlichen Parotissekret unter fraktionierter Abnahme bei Ruhe und Reiz. Laryng. Rhinol. *55*, 239–244 (1976)
Ekfors, T.O., Hopsu-Havu, V.K.: Properties of the esteropeptidases purified from the mouse submandibular gland. Enzymologia *43*, 177–189 (1972)
Ekfors, T.O., Malmiharju, T., Hopsu-Havu, V.K.: Isolation of six trypsin-like esteropeptidases from the mouse submandibular gland. Enzymologia *43*, 151–165 (1972a)
Ekfors, T.O., Malmiharju, T., Riekkinen, P.J., Hopsu-Havu, V.K.: The depressor activity of trypsin-like enzymes purified from rat submandibular gland. Biochem. Pharmacol. *16*, 1634–1636 (1967a)
Ekfors, T.O., Riekkinen, P.J., Malmiharju, T., Hopsu-Havu, V.K.: Four isozymic forms of a peptidase resembling kallikrein purified from the rat submandibular gland. Hoppe Seylers Z. Physiol. Chem. *348*, 111–118 (1967b)
Ekfors, T.O., Suominen, J., Hopsu-Havu, V.K.: Increased vascular permeability and activation of plasminogen by the trypsin-like esterases from the mouse submandibular gland. Biochem. Pharmacol. *21*, 1370–1373 (1972b)
Feinstein, G., Hofstein, R., Koifmann, J., Sokolovsky, M.: Human pancreatic proteolytic enzymes and protein inhibitors. Isolation and molecular properties. Eur. J. Biochem. *43*, 569–581 (1974)
Fiedler, F.: Heterogenität und enzymatische Eigenschaften von Pankreaskallikrein. Hoppe Seylers Z. Physiol. Chem. *349*, 926 (1968)
Fiedler, F.: Pig pancreatic kallikreins A and B. Methods Enzymol. *45*, 289–303 (1976)
Fiedler, F.: Pig pancreatic kallikrein: structure and catalytic properties. In: Chemistry and biology of the kallikrein-kinin system in health and disease. Pisano, J.J., Austen, K.F. (eds.), pp. 93–95. Washington: U.S. Gov. Printing Office 1977
Fiedler, F., Ehret, W., Godec, G., Hirschauer, C., Kutzbach, C., Schmidt-Kastner, G., Tschesche, H.: The primary structure of pig pancreatic kallikrein B. In: Kininogenases – kallikrein. Vol. 4. Haberland, G.L., Rohen, J.W., Suzuki, T. (eds.), pp. 7–14. Stuttgart, New York: Schattauer 1977b
Fiedler, F., Hirschauer, C., Werle, E.: Characterization of pig pancreatic kallikreins A and B. Hoppe Seylers Z. Physiol. Chem. *356*, 1879–1891 (1975)

Fiedler, F., Hirschauer, C., Fritz, H.: Inhibition of three porcine glandular kallikreins by chloromethyl ketones. Hoppe Seylers Z. Physiol. Chem. *358*, 447–451 (1977a)

Fiedler, F., Hirschauer, C., Werle, E.: Anreicherung von Präkallikrein B aus Schweinepankreas und Eigenschaften verschiedener Formen des Pankreaskallikreins. Hoppe Seylers Z. Physiol. Chem. *351*, 225–238 (1970a)

Fiedler, F., Leysath, G., Werle, E.: Hydrolysis of aminoacid esters by pig-pancreatic kallikrein. Eur. J. Biochem. *36*, 152–159 (1973)

Fiedler, F., Müller, B., Werle, E.: The inhibition of porcine pancreas kallikrein by di-isopropylfluorosphosphate. Kinetics, stoichiometry, and nature of the group phosphorylated. Eur. J. Biochem. *10*, 419–425 (1969)

Fiedler, F., Müller, B., Werle, E.: Charakterisierung verschiedener Schweinekallikreine mittels Diisopropylfluorophosphat. Hoppe Seylers Z. Physiol. Chem. *351*, 1002–1006 (1970b)

Fiedler, F., Müller, B., Werle, E.: Die Aminosäuresequenz im Bereich des Serins im aktiven Zentrum des Kallikreins aus Schweinepankreas. Hoppe Seylers Z. Physiol. Chem. *352*, 1463–1464 (1971)

Fiedler, F., Müller, B., Werle, E.: The reaction of pig pancreatic kallikrein with cinnamoyl and indoleacryloyl imidazoles. FEBS Lett. *22*, 1–4 (1972a)

Fiedler, F., Müller, B., Werle, E.: Active site titration of pig pancreatic kallikrein with p-nitrophenyl p′-guanidinobenzoate. FEBS Lett. *24*, 41–44 (1972b)

Fiedler, F., Werle, E.: Vorkommen zweier Kallikreinogene im Schweinepankreas und Automation der Kallikrein- und Kallikreinogenbestimmung. Hoppe Seylers Z. Physiol. Chem. *348*, 1087–1089 (1967)

Fiedler, F., Werle, E.: Activation, inhibition, and pH-dependence of the hydrolysis of α-N-benzoyl-L-arginine ethyl ester catalyzed by kallikrein from porcine pancreas. Eur. J. Biochem. *7*, 27–33 (1968)

Figarella, C., Negri, G.A., Guy, O.: The two human trypsinogens. Inhibition spectra of the two human trypsins derived from their purified zymogens. Eur. J. Biochem. *53*, 457–463 (1975)

Foucault, G., Seydoux, F., Yon, J.: Comparative kinetic properties of α, β, and ψ forms of trypsin. Eur. J. Biochem. *47*, 295–302 (1974)

Fräki, J.E., Jansén, C.T., Hopsu-Havu, V.K.: Human sweat kallikrein. Acta Derm. Venereol. (Stockh.) *50*, 321–326 (1970)

Fritz, H., Brey, B., Schmal, A., Werle, E.: Verwendung wasserunlöslicher Derivate des Trypsin-Kallikrein-Inhibitors zur Isolierung von Kallikreinen und Plasmin. Hoppe Seylers Z. Physiol. Chem. *350*, 617–625 (1969)

Fritz, H., Eckert, I., Werle, E.: Isolierung und Charakterisierung von sialinsäurehaltigem und sialinsäurefreiem Kallikrein aus Schweinepankreas. Hoppe Seylers Z. Physiol. Chem. *348*, 1120–1132 (1967)

Fritz, H., Fiedler, F., Dietl, T., Warwas, M., Truscheit, E., Kolb, H.J., Mair, G., Tschesche, H.: On the relationships between porcine pancreatic, submandibular, and urinary kallikreins. In: Kininogenases – kallikrein. Vol. 4. Haberland, G.L., Rohen, J.W., Suzuki, T. (eds.), pp. 15–28. Stuttgart, New York: Schattauer 1977

Fritz, H., Förg-Brey, B.: Zur Isolierung von Organ- und Harnkallikreinen durch Affinitätschromatographie. Spezifische Bindung an wasserlösliche Inhibitorderivate und Dissoziation der Komplexe mit kompetitiven Hemmstoffen (Benzamidin). Hoppe Seylers Z. Physiol. Chem. *353*, 901–905 (1972)

Fujimoto, Y., Moriwaki, C., Moriya, H.: Studies on human salivary kallikrein. II. Properties of purified salivary kallikrein. J. Biochem. (Tokyo) *74*, 247–252 (1973a)

Fujimoto, Y., Moriya, H., Yamaguchi, K., Moriwaki, C.: Detection of arginine esterase of various kallikrein preparations on gellified electrophoretic media. J. Biochem. (Tokyo) *71*, 751–754 (1972)

Fujimoto, Y., Moriya, H., Moriwaki, C.: Studies on human salivary kallikrein. I. Isolation of human salivary kallikrein. J. Biochem. (Tokyo) *74*, 239–246 (1973b)

Geratz, J.D.: Synthetic inhibitors and ester substrates of pancreatic kallikrein. Experientia *25*, 483–484 (1969)

Geratz, J.D.: Kinetic aspects of the irreversible inhibition of trypsin and related enzymes by p-[m(m-fluorosulfonyl-phenylureido) phenoxyethoxy]benzamidine. FEBS Lett. *20*, 294–296 (1972)

Geratz, J.D., Cheng, M.C.-F., Tidwell, R.R.: Novel bis(benzamidino) compounds with an aromatic central link. Inhibitors of thrombin, pancreatic kallikrein, trypsin, and complement. J. Med. Chem. *19*, 634–639 (1976)
Geratz, J.D., Fox, L.L.B.: On the irreversible inhibition of α-chymotrypsin, trypsin, pancreatic kallikrein, thrombin, and elastase by N-(β-pyridylmethyl)-3,4-dichlorophenoxyacetamide-p-fluorosulfonylacetanilide bromide. Biochim. Biophys. Acta *321*, 296–302 (1973)
Geratz, J.D., Whitmore, A.C., Cheng, M.C.-F., Piantadosi, C.: Diamidino-α, ω-diphenoxyalkanes. Structure-activity relationships for the inhibition of thrombin, pancreatic kallikrein, and trypsin. J. Med. Chem. *16*, 970–975 (1973)
Giusti, E.P., Sampaio, C.A.M., Prado, E.S.: Purification of horse urinary kallikrein by affinity chromatography. Abstr. No. 43. Kinin 76, International Symposium, Rio de Janeiro, Brazil 1976
Greene, L.J., Di Carlo, J.J., Sussman, A.J., Bartelt, D.C., Roark, D.E.: Two trypsin inhibitors from porcine pancreatic juice. J. Biol. Chem. *243*, 1804–1815 (1968)
Habermann, E.: Trennung und Reinigung von Pankreaskallikreinen. Hoppe Seylers Z. Physiol. Chem. *328*, 15–23 (1962)
Habermann, E.: Strukturaufklärung kininliefernder Peptide aus Rinderserum-Kininogen. Naunyn Schmiedebergs Arch. Pharmakol. *253*, 474–483 (1966)
Habermann, E., Blennemann, G.: Über Substrate und Reaktionsprodukte der kininbildenden Enzyme Trypsin, Serum- und Pankreaskallikrein sowie von Crotalusgift. Naunyn Schmiedebergs Arch. Pharmakol. *249*, 357–373 (1964)
Habermann, E., Helbig, J.: Untersuchungen zur Struktur des Rinderserum-Kininogens unter Verwendung von Bromcyan und Carboxypeptidase B. Naunyn Schmiedebergs Arch. Pharmakol. *258*, 160–180 (1967)
Habermann, E., Müller, B.: Zur enzymatischen Spaltung peptischer kininliefernder Fragmente (PKF) sowie von Rinderserum-Kininogen. Naunyn Schmiedebergs Arch. Pharmakol. *253*, 464–473 (1966)
Halabi, M., Back, N.: Kinetic studies with serine proteases and protease inhibitors utilizing a synthetic nitro-anilide chromogenic substrate. In: Kininogenases-kallikrein. Vol. 4. Haberland, G.L., Rohen, J.W., Suzuki, T. (eds.), pp. 35–46. Stuttgart, New York: Schattauer 1977
Hamberg, U., Joutsimo, L.: Heterogeneity of urokinase and urinary albumin. Biochem. Soc. Transact. *2*, 564–566 (1974)
Han, Y.N., Kato, H., Iwanaga, S.: Identification of Ser-Leu-Met-Lys-bradykinin isolated from chemically modified high-molecular-weight bovine kininogen. FEBS Lett. *71*, 45–48 (1976)
Hartley, B.S.: Amino-acid sequence of bovine chymotrypsinogen-A. Nature (Lond.) *201*, 1284–1287 (1964)
Hermodson, M.A., Ericsson, L.H., Neurath, H., Walsh, K.A.: Determination of the amino acid sequence of porcine trypsin by sequenator analysis. Biochemistry *12*, 3146–3153 (1973)
Hial, V., Diniz, C.R., Mares-Guia, M.: Purification and properties of a human urinary kallikrein (kininogenase). Biochemistry *13*, 4311–4318 (1974)
Hochstrasser, K., Werle, E.: Über kininliefernde Peptide aus pepsinverdauten Rinderplasmaproteinen. Hoppe Seylers Z. Physiol. Chem. *348*, 177–182 (1967)
Hojima, Y., Matsuda, Y., Moriwaki, C., Moriya, H.: Homogeneity and multiplicity forms of glandular kallikreins. Chem. Pharm. Bull. (Tokyo) *23*, 1120–1127 (1975a)
Hojima, Y., Moriwaki, C., Moriya, H.: Isolation of dog, rat, and hog pancreatic kallikreins by preparative disc electrophoresis and their properties. Chem. Pharm. Bull. (Tokyo) *23*, 1128–1136 (1975b)
Hojima, Y., Yamashita, M., Moriya, H.: Dog pancreatic arginine esterases spontaneously activated on DEAE-Sephadex. Chem. Pharm. Bull. (Tokyo) *23*, 225–228 (1975c)
Hojima, Y., Yamashita, M., Ochi, N., Moriwaki, C., Moriya, H.: Isolation and some properties of dog and rat pancreatic kallikreins. J. Biochem. (Tokyo) *81*, 599–610 (1977)
Hoy, T.G., Ferdinand, W., Harrison, P.M.: A computer-assisted method for determining the nearest integer ratios of amino acid residues in purified proteins. Int. J. Peptide Protein Res. *6*, 121–140 (1974)
Imanari, T., Kaizu, T., Yoshida, H., Yates, K., Pierce, J.V., Pisano, J.J.: Radiochemical assays for human urinary, salivary, and plasma kallikreins. In: Chemistry and biology of the kallikrein-kinin system in health and disease. Pisano, J.J., Austen, K.F. (eds.), pp. 205–213. Washington: U.S. Gov. Printing Office 1977

International Commission on Pharmaceutical Enzymes: Kallikrein. Farmaceutische Tijdschrift voor Belgie *51*, 1–9 (1974)

Iwanaga, S., Han, Y.N., Kato, H., Suzuki, T.: Actions of various kallikreins on HMW kininogen and its derivatives. In: Kininogenases – kallikrein. Vol. 4. Haberland, G.L., Rohen, J.W., Suzuki, T. (eds.), pp. 79–90. Stuttgart, New York: Schattauer 1977

Jollès, P., Alais, C., Jollès, J.: Action de la callicréine sur la caséine κ de vache. C.R. Acad. Sci. [D] (Paris) *256*, 4308–4310 (1963)

Kato, H., Han, Y.N., Iwanaga, S., Suzuki, T., Komiya, M.: Bovine plasma HMW and LMW kininogens: isolation and characterization of the polypeptide fragments produced by plasma and tissue kallikreins. In: Kinins – pharmacodynamics and biological roles. Sicuteri, F., Back, N., Haberland, G.L. (eds.), pp. 135–150. New York, London: Plenum Press 1976

Kato, H., Han, Y.N., Iwanaga, S., Hashimoto, N., Sugo, T., Fujii, S., Suzuki, T.: Mammalian plasma kininogens: their structures and functions. In: Kininogenases – kallikrein. Vol. 4. Haberland, G.L., Rohen, J.W., Suzuki, T. (eds.), pp. 63–72. Stuttgart, New York: Schattauer 1977

Kato, H., Suzuki, T.: Substrate specificities of kinin releasing enzymes: hog pancreatic kallikrein and snake venom kininogenase. J. Biochem. (Tokyo) *68*, 9–17 (1970)

Knights, R.J., Light, A.: Disulfide bond-modified trypsinogen. J. Biol. Chem. *251*, 222–228 (1976)

Kramer, C., Prado, E.S., Prado, J.L.: Inhibition by ions of the esterolytic activity of horse urinary kallikrein. Med. Pharmacol. Exp. *15*, 389–398 (1966)

Kutzbach, C., Schmidt-Kastner, G.: Kallikrein from pig pancreas: purification, separation of components A and B, and crystallization. Hoppe Seylers Z. Physiol. Chem. *353*, 1099–1106 (1972)

Kutzbach, C., Schmidt-Kastner, G.: Properties of highly purified hog pancreatic kallikrein. In: Kininogenases – kallikrein. Haberland, G.L., Rohen, J.W. (eds.), pp. 23–35. Stuttgart, New York: Schattauer 1973

Lemon, M., Förg-Brey, B., Fritz, H.: Isolation of porcine submaxillary kallikrein. In: Kinins – pharmacodynamics and biological roles. Sicuteri, F., Back, N., Haberland, G.L. (eds.), pp. 209–216. New York, London: Plenum Press 1976

Levy, M., Fishman, L., Schenkein, I.: Mouse submaxillary gland proteases. Methods Enzymol. *19*, 672–681 (1970)

Manivet, M., Figarella, C.: Purification of a kallikrein in human pancreatic juice. Irish J. Med. Sci. *146*, Suppl. 1, 11 (1977)

Mann, K., Geiger, R.: Radioimmunoassay of human urinary kallikrein. In: Kininogenases – kallikrein. Vol. 4. Haberland, G.L., Rohen, J.W., Suzuki, T. (eds.), pp. 55–61. Stuttgart, New York: Schattauer 1977

Mares-Guia, M., Diniz, C.R.: Studies on the mechanism of rat urinary kallikrein catalysis, and its relation to catalysis by trypsin. Arch. Biochem. Biophys. *121*, 750–756 (1967)

Markwardt, F., Walsmann, P., Richter, M., Klöcking, H.-P., Drawert, J., Landmann, H.: Aminoalkylbenzolsulfofluoride als Fermentinhibitoren. Pharmazie *26*, 401–404 (1971)

Martin, C.J., Golubow, J., Axelrod, A.E.: The hydrolysis of carbobenzoxy-L-tyrosine p-nitrophenyl ester by various enzymes. J. Biol. Chem. *234*, 1718–1725 (1959)

Matsuda, Y., Miyazaki, K., Moriya, H., Fujimoto, Y., Hojima, Y., Moriwaki, C.: Studies on urinary kallikreins. I. Purification and characterization of human urinary kallikreins. J. Biochem. (Tokyo) *80*, 671–679 (1976a)

Matsuda, Y., Moriya, H., Moriwaki, C., Fujimoto, Y., Matsuda, M.: Fluorometric method for the assay of kallikrein-like arginine esterases. J. Biochem. (Tokyo) *79*, 1197–1200 (1976b)

Mebs, D.: Isolierung und Eigenschaften eines Kallikreins aus dem Gift der Krustenechse Heloderma suspectum. Hoppe Seylers Z. Physiol. Chem. *350*, 821–826 (1969a)

Mebs, D.: Über Schlangengift-Kallikreine: Reinigung und Eigenschaften eines Kinin-freisetzenden Enzyms aus dem Gift der Viper Bitis gabonica. Hoppe Seylers Z. Physiol. Chem. *350*, 1563–1569 (1969b)

Modéer, T.: Human saliva kallikrein. Biological properties of saliva kallikrein isolated by use of affinity chromatography. Acta Odontol. Scand. *35*, 23–29 (1977a)

Modéer, T.: Characterization of kallikrein from human saliva isolated by use of affinity chromatography. Acta Odontol. Scand. *35*, 31–39 (1977b)

Montgomery, R.: Heterogeneity of the carbohydrate groups of glycoproteins. In: Glycoproteins. Their composition, structure, and function, 2nd ed. Part A. Gottschalk, A. (ed.), pp. 518–528. Amsterdam, London, New York: Elsevier 1972

Moriwaki, C., Hojima, Y., Moriya, H.: A proposal – use of combined assays of kallikrein activity measurement. Chem. Pharm. Bull. (Tokyo) *22*, 975–983 (1974a)
Moriwaki, C., Hojima, Y., Schachter, M.: Purification of kallikrein from cat submaxillary gland. In: Kinins – pharmacodynamics and biological roles. Sicuteri, F., Back, N., Haberland, G.L. (eds.), pp. 151–156. New York, London: Plenum Press 1976a
Moriwaki, C., Inoue, N., Hojima, Y., Moriya, H.: A new assay method for the esterolytic activity of kallikreins with chromotropic acid. Yakugaku Zasshi *91*, 413–416 (1971)
Moriwaki, C., Kizuki, K., Moriya, H.: Kininogenase from the coagulating gland. In: Kininogenases – kallikrein. Haberland, G.L., Rohen, J.W., Schirren, C., Huber, P. (eds.), Vol. 2, pp. 23–31. Stuttgart, New York: Schattauer 1975
Moriwaki, C., Miyazaki, K., Matsuda, Y., Moriya, H., Fujimoto, Y., Ueki, H.: Dog renal kallikrein: Purification and some properties. J. Biochem. (Tokyo) *80*, 1277–1285 (1976b)
Moriwaki, C., Schachter, M.: Kininogenase of the guinea-pig's coagulating gland and the release of bradykinin. J. Physiol. (Lond.) *219*, 341–353 (1971)
Moriwaki, C., Watanuki, N., Fujimoto, Y., Moriya, H.: Further purification and properties of kininogenase from the guinea pig's coagulating gland. Chem. Pharm. Bull. (Tokyo) *22*, 628–633 (1974b)
Moriya, H., Hojima, Y., Yamashita, Y., Moriwaki, C.: Some studies on dog and rat pancreatic kallikreins. In: Kininogenases – kallikrein. Haberland, G.L., Rohen, J.W., Blümel, G., Huber, P. (eds.), Vol. 3, pp. 19–26. Stuttgart, New York: Schattauer 1975
Moriya, H., Kato, A., Fukushima, H.: Further study on purification of hog pancreatic kallikrein. Biochem. Pharmacol. *18*, 549–552 (1969)
Moriya, H., Matsuda, Y., Fujimoto, Y., Hojima, Y., Moriwaki, C.: Some aspects of multiple components on the kallikrein. Human urinary kallikrein (HUK). In: Kininogenases – kallikrein. Haberland, G.L., Rohen, J.W. (eds.), pp. 37–42. Stuttgart, New York: Schattauer 1973
Moriya, H., Pierce, J.V., Webster, M.E.: Purification and some properties of three kallikreins. Ann. N.Y. Acad. Sci. *104*, 172–185 (1963)
Moriya, H., Todoki, N., Moriwaki, C., Hojima, Y.: A new sensitive assay method of kallikrein-like arginine-esterases. J. Biochem. (Tokyo) *69*, 815–817 (1971)
Moriya, H., Yamazaki, K., Fukushima, H., Moriwaki, C.: Biochemical studies on kallikreins and their related substances. II. An improved method of purification of hog pancreatic kallikrein and its some biological properties. J. Biochem. (Tokyo) *58*, 208–213 (1965)
Mutt, V., Said, S.I.: Structure of the porcine vasoactive intestinal octacosapeptide. The amino-acid sequence. Use of kallikrein in its determination. Eur. J. Biochem. *42*, 581–589 (1974)
Nustad, K., Gautvik, K.M., Pierce, J.V.: Glandular kallikreins: Purification, characterization, and biosynthesis. In: Chemistry and biology of the kallikrein-kinin system in health and disease. Pisano, J.J., Austen, K.F. (eds.), pp. 77–92. Washington: U.S. Gov. Printing Office 1977
Nustad, K., Pierce, J.V.: Purification of rat urinary kallikreins and their specific antibody. Biochemistry *13*, 2312–2319 (1974)
Nustad, K., Vaaje, K., Pierce, J.V.: Synthesis of kallikreins by rat kidney slices. Br. J. Pharmac. *53*, 229–234 (1975)
Olemoiyoi, O., Spragg, J., Halbert, S.P., Austen, K.F.: Immunologic reactivity of purified human urinary kallikrein (urokallikrein) with antiserum directed against human pancreas. J. Immunol. *118*, 667–672 (1977)
Oza, N.B., Amin, V.M., Mc Gregor, R.K., Scicli, A.G., Carretero, O.A.: Isolation of rat urinary kallikrein and properties of its antibodies. Biochem. Pharmacol. *25*, 1607–1612 (1976)
Palm, S., Fritz, H.: Components of the kallikrein-kinin-system in human midcycle cervical mucus and seminal plasma. In: Kininogenases – kallikrein. Haberland, G.L., Rohen, J.W., Schirren, C., Huber, P. (eds.), Vol. 2, pp. 17–21. Stuttgart, New York: Schattauer 1975
Paskhina, T.S., Zukova, V.P., Egorova, T.P., Narticova, V.F., Karpova, A.V., Guseva, M.V.: Reaction of N-α-tosyl-L-lysyl-chloromethane with kallicrein from blood plasm of rabbit and with kallicreins from urine and saliva of man. Biokhimiia *33*, 745–752 (1968)
Pierce, J.V.: Purification of mammalian kallikreins, kininogens, and kinins. In: Handbook of experimental pharmacology. Vol. XXV: Bradykinin, kallidin, and kallikrein. Erdös, E.G. (ed.), pp. 21–51. Berlin, Heidelberg, New York: Springer 1970
Pierce, J.V., Nustad, K.: Purification of human and rat urinary kallikreins. Fed. Proc. *31*, 623 (1972)

Pierce, J.V., Webster, M.E.: Human plasma kallidins: Isolation and chemical studies. Biochem. Biophys. Res. Commun. *5*, 353–357 (1961)
Porcelli, G., Cozzari, C., Di Iorio, M., Croxatto, R.H., Angeletti, P.: Isolation and partial characterization of a kallikrein from mouse submaxillary glands. Ital. J. Biochem. *25*, 337–348 (1976)
Porcelli, G., Croxatto, H.: Purification on kininogenase from rat urine. Ital. J. Biochem. *20*, 66–88 (1971)
Porcelli, G., Marini-Bettòlo, G.B., Croxatto, H.R., Di Iorio, M.: Purification and chemical studies on human urinary kallikrein. Ital. J. Biochem. *23*, 44–55 (1974a)
Porcelli, G., Marini-Bettòlo, G.B., Croxatto, H.R., Di Iorio, M.: Purification and chemical studies on rabbit urinary kallikrein. Ital. J. Biqchem. *23*, 154–164 (1974b)
Porcelli, G., Marini-Bettòlo, G.B., Croxatto, H.R., Di Iorio, M.: Purification and chemical studies on rat urinary kallikrein. Ital. J. Biochem. *24*, 175–187 (1975)
Prado, J.L.: Proteolytic enzymes as kininogenases. In: Handbook of experimental pharmacology. Vol. XXV: Bradykinin, kallidin, and kallikrein. Erdös, E.G. (ed.), pp. 156–192. Berlin, Heidelberg, New York: Springer 1970
Prado, J.L., Prado, E.S., Brandi, C.M.W., Katchburian, A.V.: Some properties of highly purified horse urinary kallikrein. Ann. N.Y. Acad. Sci. *104*, 186–189 (1963)
Prado, E.S., Aráujo-Viel, M.S., Sampaio, M.U., Prado, J.L., Paiva, A.C.M.: Enzymatic specificity of horse urinary kallikrein. In: Chemistry and biology of the kallikrein-kinin system in health and disease. Pisano, J.J., Austen, K.F. (eds.), pp. 103–105. Washington: U.S. Gov. Printing Office 1977
Prado, E.S., Prado, J.L., Brandi, C.M.W.: Further purification and some properties of horse urinary kallikrein. Arch. Int. Pharmacodyn. Ther. *87*, 358–374 (1962)
Prado, E.S., Stella, R.C.R., Roncada, M.J., Prado, J.L.: Action of horse urinary kallikrein on arginine and lysine-peptides. In: International symposium on vaso-active polypeptides: bradykinin and related kinins. Rocha e Silva, M., Rothschild, H.A. (eds.), pp. 141–147. Sao Paulo: Edart 1966
Prado, E.S., Webster, M.E., Prado, J.L.: Kallidin (lysylbradykinin), the kinin formed from horse plasma by horse urinary kallikrein. Biochem. Pharmacol. *20*, 2009–2015 (1971)
Riekkinen, P.J., Ekfors, T.O., Hopsu, V.K.: Purification and characteristics of an alkaline protease from rat-submandibular gland. Biochim. Biophys. Acta *118*, 604–620 (1966)
Roberts, D.V., Elmore, D.T.: Kinetics and mechanism of catalysis by proteolytic enzymes. A comparison of the kinetics of hydrolysis of synthetic substrates by bovine α- and β-trypsin. Biochem. J. *141*, 545–554 (1974)
Sach, E., Maillard, M., Toubiana, R., Choay, J.: Fractionnement par focalisation isoélectrique d'une estérase anionique pancréatique de porc et activité protéolytique de l'enzyme. C.R. Acad. Sci. [D] (Paris) *272*, 647–650 (1971)
Sampaio, C.A.M., Prado, E.S.: Action of proteolytic enzymes upon horse urinary kallikrein. Biochem. Pharmacol. *24*, 1438–1439 (1975)
Sampaio, C.A.M., Prado, E.S.: Active-site labelling of kallikreins by chloromethylketone derivatives. Gen. Pharmacol. *7*, 163–166 (1976)
Sampaio, C.A.M., Saad, A.D., Grisolia, D.: Hydrolysis of histones by horse urinary kallikreins. Experientia *33*, 292–294 (1977)
Sampaio, M.U., Galembeck, F., Paiva, A.C.M., Prado, E.S.: Kinetics of the hydrolysis of synthetic substrates by horse urinary kallikrein and trypsin. Gen. Pharmacol. *7*, 167–171 (1976)
Schröder, E., Lehmann, M.: Über Peptidsynthesen. XLVI. Synthese kininliefernder Kininogensequenzen. Experientia *25*, 1126–1127 (1969)
Schwert, G.W., Takenaka, Y.: A spectrophotometric determination of trypsin and chymotrypsin. Biochim. Biophys. Acta *16*, 570–575 (1955)
Segrest, J.P., Jackson, R.L., Andrews, E.P., Marchesi, V.T.: Human erythrocyte membrane glycoprotein: a re-evaluation of the molecular weight as determined by SDS polyacrylamide gel electrophoresis. Biochem. Biophys. Res. Commun. *44*, 390–395 (1971)
Shapiro, A.L., Viñueala, E., Maizel, J.V., Jr.: Molecular weight estimation of polypeptide chains by electrophoresis in SDS-polyacrylamide gels. Biochem. Biophys. Res. Commun. *28*, 815–820 (1967)
Silva, E., Diniz, C.R., Mares-Guia, M.: Rat urinary kallikrein: Purification and properties. Biochemistry *13*, 4304–4310 (1974)

Spragg, J., Austen, K.F.: Preparation of human kininogen. III. Enzymatic digestion and modification. Biochem. Pharmacol. *23*, 781–791 (1974)
Suzuki, T., Iwanaga, S.: Snake venoms. In: Handbook of experimental pharmacology. Vol. XXV: Bradykinin, kallidin, and kallikrein. Erdös, E.G. (ed.), pp. 193–212. Berlin, Heidelberg, New York: Springer 1970
Takami, T.: Action of hog pancreatic kallikrein on synthetic substrates and its some other enzymatic properties. J. Biochem. (Tokyo) *66*, 651–658 (1969a)
Takami, T.: Purification of hog pancreatic kallikreins and their proteolytic activities. Seikagaku (J. Jap. Biochem. Soc.) *41*, 777–785 (1969b)
Taylor, J.M., Mitchell, W.M., Cohen, S.: Characterization of the binding protein for epidermal growth factor. J. Biol. Chem. *249*, 2188–2194 (1974)
Trautschold, I.: Assay methods in the kinin system. In: Handbook of experimental pharmacology. Vol. XXV: Bradykinin, kallidin, and kallikrein. Erdös, E.G. (ed.), pp. 52–81. Berlin, Heidelberg, New York: Springer 1970
Trautschold, I., Werle, E.: Spektrophotometrische Bestimmung des Kallikreins und seiner Inaktivatoren. Hoppe Seylers Z. Physiol. Chem. *325*, 48–59 (1961)
Trowbridge, C.G., Krehbiel, A., Laskowski, M., Jr.: Substrate activation of trypsin. Biochemistry *2*, 843–850 (1963)
Tschesche, H., Ehret, W., Godec, G., Hirschauer, C., Kutzbach, C., Schmidt-Kastner, G., Fiedler, F.: The primary structure of pig pancreatic kallikrein B. In: Kinins – pharmacodynamics and biological roles. Sicuteri, F., Back, N., Haberland, G.L. (eds.), pp. 123–133. New York, London: Plenum Press 1976a
Tschesche, H., Mair, G., Förg-Brey, B., Fritz, H.: Isolation of porcine urinary kallikrein. In: Kinins – pharmacodynamics and biological roles. Sicuteri, F., Back, N., Haberland, G.L. (eds.), pp. 119–122. New York, London: Plenum Press 1976b
Tung, J.-S., Knight, C.A.: Relative importance of some factors affecting the electrophoretic migration of proteins in sodium dodecyl sulfate-polyacrylamide gels. Anal. Biochem. *48*, 153–163 (1972)
Webster, M.E.: Kallikreins in glandular tissues. In: Handbook of experimental pharmacology. Vol. XXV: Bradykinin, kallidin, and kallikrein. Erdös, E.G. (ed.), pp. 131–155. Berlin, Heidelberg, New York: Springer 1970
Webster, M.E., Pierce, J.V.: Action of kallikreins on synthetic ester substrates. Proc. Soc. Exp. Biol. Med. *107*, 186–191 (1961)
Webster, M.E., Prado, E.S.: Glandular kallikreins from horse and human urine and from hog pancreas. Methods Enzymol. *19*, 681–699 (1970)
Werle, E., Fiedler, F., Fritz, H.: Recent studies on kallikreins and kallikrein inhibitors. In: Pharmacology and the future of man, Vol. 5, pp. 284–295. Basel: Karger 1973
Werle, E., Trautschold, I., Leysath, G.: Isolierung und Struktur des Kallidins. Hoppe Seylers Z. Physiol. Chem. *326*, 174–176 (1961)
Williams, J.G., Gratzer, W.B.: Limitations of the detergent-polyacrylamide gel electrophoresis method for molecular weight determinations of proteins. J. Chromatogr. *57*, 121–125 (1971)
Worthington, K.J., Cuschieri, A.: A study on the kinetics of pancreatic kallikrein with the substrate benzoyl arginine ethyl ester using a spectrophotometric assay. Clin. Chim. Acta *52*, 129–136 (1974)
Yano, M., Magasawa, S., Suzuki, T.: Partial purification and some properties of high molecular weight kininogen, bovine kininogen-I. J. Biochem. (Tokyo) *69*, 471–481 (1971)
Zuber, M., Sache, E.: Isolation and characterization of porcine pancreatic kallikrein. Biochemistry *13*, 3098–3110 (1974)

Kallikrein Inhibitors

R. VOGEL

A. Introduction

During the last 10 years, a great number of naturally occuring enzyme inhibitors, besides proteinase inhibitors, have been detected. Their existence has often been indicated by yields of more than 100% during the first isolation steps of the enzyme. Thus, the mechanism of inhibition of proteinases in biologic systems is not unique as formerly thought.

The development of analytic instruments resulted in great progress in the understanding of proteinase inhibitors, especially of the polyvalent proteinase inhibitor of bovine organs (BPTI). Soybean inhibitor (SBTI), by 1968, had become commonly used for kinetic studies and was followed by BPTI. The three-dimensional structure of BPTI was among the first published of all protein molecules. Therefore, the emphasis of this review is on physicochemical information. The low MW of BPTI gave rise to exceptional theoretical and practical interest in the field of enzymic reaction mechanisms, especially kinetic studies of molecules with complicated conformations. BPTI is fundamentally a kallikrein-specific inhibitor and was used as a reference substance throughout this review.

According to X-ray analysis, the substrate binding site of proteinases is a deep pocket in the molecule with some residues representing the active center, connected with an S-S bond at the sides of the pocket (for review concerning trypsin and chymotrypsin see BLOW, 1974). The mechanism of inhibitor binding of this structure is the same for natural and synthetic inhibitors. Similar behavior is assumed for kallikreins with the restriction that the polysaccharide chain causes steric hindrance when bound to HMW proteins. The contact positions of kallikrein are not identical with those known for trypsin (see FIEDLER this Vol., p. 103).

In the sixties, LASKOWSKI, JR. initiated work on the kinetics of complex-formation, supporting the hypotheses founded on experimental work (review LASKOWSKI, JR. and SEALOCK, 1971). As a result of striking conclusions for protein-protein interactions in the complex form and the similarities found in flora and fauna, LASKOWSKI, JR.'s idea for the evolution of these substances is based on the genetic aspects of the subject (review LASKOWSKI, JR. et al., 1974). These papers cannot be reviewed. Anyone working in this field has to read them to gain an impression of the enthusiasm.

Because of the great interest in this field, besides symposia proceedings (FRITZ and TSCHESCHE, 1971; FRITZ et al., 1974a), a series of reviews were published: LIENER and KAKADE (1969): especially plant inhibitors; KASSELL (1970): especially isolation methods and assays; LASKOWSKI, JR. and SEALOCK (1971): general, estimation methods, constants, reactive site, kinetics; WERLE and ZICKGRAF-RÜDEL (1972): especially inhibition spectrum of all inhibitors so far known; RYAN (1973): especially plant inhibitors; TSCHESCHE (1974): general; FRITZ et al. (1974b, c): especially units and estimation methods; UHLIG and KLEINE (1974): general in tables; BIRK (1976): plants, especially isolation methods; CREIGHTON (1975a): mini-review, conformation; LORAND (1976): general.

A great number of the natural proteinase inhibitors are commercially available, although not all in pure state. For biochemical studies most of the preparations have to be tested and rechromatographed. Producers are Bayer, Sigma, Worthington, Boehringer and Behringwerke. For pharmaceutic purposes, other names are also used for BPTI: Trasylol, Aprotinin (GFR), Contrycal (DDR), Iniprol (France).

B. Methods and Definitions

I. Methods of Isolation

Affinity chromatography, one of the tools in analytic biochemistry, has been developed during the last 10 years and applied for purification of the natural inhibitors. The method is based on the complex binding capacity of proteins, i.e., enzymes coupled to insoluble resins. Enzymes linked to inhibitor-resins are of great interest in experimental work because they have some altered properties, e.g., stability or ease of handling in biologic tests (see review SEKI et al., 1970).

Coupling of enzymes to an insoluble carrier, initiated by KATCHALSKI (LEVIN et al., 1964; SILMAN and KATCHALSKI, 1966) was first applied to the purification of natural inhibitors by FRITZ (FRITZ et al., 1967, 1969a, b, c, 1971). After some years of experiments with various insoluble carriers alone, a great deal of separation of enzymes or natural inhibitors is now done via the coupled complex. This may yield the substance in question in nearly pure state from untreated biologic material. Isolation of inhibitors on carrier-bound enzymes is described below. The binding of enzymes to inhibitor-resins is summarized in Table 1. With this method, differentiation of enzymes is facilitated. Thus, the references include work done with different proteinase inhibitors, not just with kallikrein-specific ones.

II. Methods of Determination

The common method of inhibitor assay using the spectrophotometric measurement of synthetic enzyme substrates is described in detail by FRITZ et al. (1970b, 1974b, c) with regard to substrates, reaction conditions, units, and normal values. Besides spectrophotometric determination for kallikrein inhibitors bioassay remains an unavoidable method with the natural substrate kininogen (e.g., PEETERS et al., 1976, for SBTI, ovomucoid, BPTI; GEIGER and MANN, 1976, inhibitor in kidney tubules). In the tables, biologic assay on animal blood pressure is referred to as "in vivo" and assays on isolated organs as "in vitro".

Table 1. Affinity chromatography on inhibitor-containing resins

Inhibitor	Carrier	Enzyme bound	Author
SBTI	CM-cellulose	Serum kallikrein (human, pig)	FRITZ et al. (1972d)
SBTI	Sepharose 4B	Plasma kallikrein (human)	SAMPAIO et al. (1974)
SBTI	Sepharose	Pancreatic proteinases (mouse)	KASCHE et al. (1977)
SBTI	Sepharose 4B	Trypsin	SEKI et al. (1970)
SBTI	Woodward's reagent K	Trypsin	BARTLING and BARKER (1976)
SBTI dinitrophenylated	Dinitrophenyl-antibody column	Trypsin	WILCHEK and GORECKI (1973)
SBTI	Sepharose 4B	Trypsin	KNIGHTS and LIGHT (1976)
SBTI	Sepharose 4B	Trypsin (mouse) Chymotrypsin (mouse)	AMNÉUS et al. (1976)
SBTI Ovomucoid	Sepharose	Trypsin (starfish)	GILLIAM and KITTO (1976)
Ovomucoid	Sepharose	Trypsin	BURKHEAD et al. (1973)
Ovomucoid	Sepharose 2B	Trypsin chymotrypsin	FEINSTEIN (1970a, b)
BPTI	Copolymer of maleic acid and ethylene	Kallikrein submax., pancreas, urine (pig)	FRITZ et al. (1969a)
BPTI	Sepharose 4B	Kallikrein submax. (rat)	SEKI et al. (1970)
BPTI	CM-cellulose azide method	Kallikrein submax., pancreas, urine (pig)	FRITZ and FÖRG-BREY (1972)
BPTI	CM- and aminoalkyl cellulose	Serum kallikrein	FRITZ et al. (1972d)
BPTI	Guanylated derivative on CM-cellulose	Kallikrein submax., urine (pig)	WERLE et al. (1973)
BPTI	Cyanobromide-activated Sepharose 4B	Kallikrein saliva (human)	MODÉER (1977a, b)
BPTI	Cyanobromide-activated Sepharose 4B	Kallikrein urine (rat)	OZA et al. (1976)
BPTI	Sepharose	Kallikrein submax. (pig)	LEMON et al. (1976)
BPTI	Cyanobromide-activated Sepharose 4B	Kallikrein urine (pig)	MAIR et al. (1976)
BPTI	Sepharose 4B	α,β,ψ-trypsin DFP-trypsin chymotrypsin	CHAUVET and ACHER (1974)
BPTI	Sepharose 4B	Trypsin (rabbit)	JOHNSON (1976)
BPTI	Sepharose 4B	Trypsin (human) chymotrypsin (human)	JOHNSON and TRAVIS (1976)
BPTI	Sepharose 4B	Trypsin	CHAUVET and ACHER (1973)
BPTI	Sepharose 4B	Microbial trypsin-like enzyme	CHAUVET et al. (1976)
BPTI	Sepharose 4B	Trypsinogen chymotrypsinogen	CHAUVET and ACHER (1974)
BPTI	6-aminohexanoic-Sepharose	Trypsinogen	VINCENT and LAZDUNSKI (1976)

Table 2. Essential positions of inhibitor molecules for kallikrein inhibition (Taken from WUNDERER et al., 1975; FRITZ, 1976; KOIDE and IKENAKA, 1973)

Inhibitor	P_4	P_3	P_2	P_1	P'_1	P'_2	P'_{23}	P'_{24}	Kallikrein inhibited	
									Glandular	Serum
BPTI	Gly	Pro	Cys	Lys	Ala	Arg	Cys	Arg	++	+
Sea anemones	Gly	Pro	Cys	Arg	Ala	Arg	Cys	Arg	++	+
Snail isoinhibitor *K*	Gly	Pro	Cys	Lys	Ala	Ser	Cys	Arg	+	+
Cow colostrum (CTI)	Gly	Pro	Cys	Lys	Ala	Ala	Cys	Gln	(+)	−
Russell viper inhibitor II	Gly	Arg	Cys	Arg	Gly	His	Cys	Gly	+	++
SBTI (KUNITZ)	Pro	Ser	Tyr	Arg	Ile	Arg	Cys	Val	−	++

In the "biochemical assay", the spectrophotometric determination of a specific component of a system is made (ARENS and HABERLAND, 1973). Assay with the use of electrophoresis was described by URIEL and BERGES (1968). According to FINK and GREENE (1974) radioimmunoassay can be performed with BPTI. ^{125}I-labeled BPTI, separated with gel filtration and gel electrophoresis, can be assayed with rabbit antiserum at levels of 100–5000 pg with ±10% precision. Analysis may be done in automatic analyzers (STEWART, 1973) and kinetic measurement of complex formation is done with stopped-flow spectrophotometry. The complex formation of BPTI with chymotrypsin is determined by proflavin displacement from the enzyme (ENGEL et al., 1974) or by difference spectra of the complex and single proteins (LUTHY et al., 1973).

III. Labeling

Radioactive and fluorescent labeling is used in in vitro and in vivo studies. For example, the following labels have been used for BPTI: ^{14}C (VINCENT and LAZDUNSKI, 1972; LAZDUNSKI et al., 1974), ^{125}I (JUST and HABERMANN, 1973; FINK and GREENE, 1974), ^{131}I (ARNDTS et al., 1970), and fluorescent components (BÖSTERLING and ENGEL, 1976).

IV. Immunologic Methods

Antibodies have been prepared to differentiate inhibitors from serum (see TALAMO and GOODFRIEND, this Vol.). With FREUND'S adjuvant, antibodies against BPTI have been obtained by AUNGST et al. (1966) and FINK and GREENE (1974).

V. Estimation of Inhibitor Capacity

The complex binding capacity with different proteinases is determined by titration, i.e., addition of increasing amounts of inhibitor to constant levels of the enzyme. The titration curves give the percentage of remaining active enzyme (FRITZ et al., 1970b, 1974b, c).

VI. Determination of Reactive Site

The differentiation of the amino acid residues in the reactive site is of great importance. Modifying either the lysine residues or the arginine residues of the inhibitor molecule has been the method of approach (HAYNES and FEENEY, 1968a, b; FRITZ et al., 1969b). Identification of arginine via modification with butane-2,3-dione was used by YANKEELOW et al. (1966), GROSSBERG and PRESSMAN (1968), DIETL and TSCHESCHE (1976d). 1,2 Cyclohexanedione was used by DIETL and TSCHESCHE (1976d), the compound being complexed by borate. Such treatment results in reversible inactivation of Arg-type inhibitors, while the Lys-type inhibitors retain full activity.

The nomenclature introduced by SCHECHTER and BERGER (1967) is used to compare inhibitors independent of the amino acid sequence. According to this nomenclature, P_1–P'_1 indicates the specific cleavable bond of a protein, i.e., standing for positions 15–16 of BPTI. According to a theory of FRITZ and co-workers, based on comparison of different kallikrein inhibitors, a second configuration in the inhibitor molecule is essential for kallikrein inhibition (P_{23}–P_{24}, i.e., position 38–39 of BPTI). This postulated doublet may lie in the particular configuration of the natural kallikrein substrate, kininogen.

In comparing kallikrein inhibitors and specific inhibitors for other proteinases, a striking fact is noticed. In positions P'_2 and P'_{24} basic residues are essential for complex binding with kallikrein (WUNDERER et al., 1975; FRITZ, 1976) (Table 2). From this requirement, a number of inhibitors are excluded theoretically from kallikrein inhibitors, i.e., pancreatic secretory inhibitor, seminal plasma inhibitors, or lima bean inhibitor. In differentiation of other serine proteinases from the kallikreins, the use of these inhibitors in experimental work is of great importance.

VII. Kinetics of Complex Binding Reaction

Review of the estimation method of the inhibitor constant, i.e., dissociation constant of the complex formed, is given by BERGMEYER (1977).

The sensitivity of an inhibitor to enzymatic degradation and inactivation as a substrate of the initially inhibited enzyme has to be proved. Methods for studies on differentiation of "permanent inhibition" and the so-called "temporary inhibition" were reviewed by LASKOWSKI, JR. and SEALOCK (1971) and TSCHESCHE et al. (1971), based on publications of the two working groups (NIEKAMP et al., 1969; KOWALSKI and LASKOWSKI, JR., 1972; TSCHESCHE, 1967; TSCHESCHE and KLEIN, 1968). Theoretical studies which prompted kinetic experiments on the inhibition reaction are reviewed by LASKOWSKI, JR. and SEALOCK (1971), and FINKENSTADT et al. (1974).

C. Protein Inhibitors of Kallikrein

I. Polyvalent Bovine Proteinase Inhibitor (BPTI)

1. Isolation

Some isolation procedures have been undertaken to determine the similarity of inhibitors (e.g., of bovine liver and bovine pancreas inhibitor: CHAUVET and ACHER, 1970) or to improve isolation methods (FURUSAWA and KUROSAWA, 1974). Besides the well-known sources for preparation, additional sources in bovine organs were described: ovary (CHAUVET and ACHER, 1972), heart, thyroid gland, pituitary posterior lobe, and rumen mucosa (WILUSZ et al., 1973). A carbohydrate-free intracellular inhibitor has not yet been found in other animal species (TSCHESCHE et al., 1975).

2. Three-Dimensional Structure of BPTI

X-ray studies of conformation in single crystals showed that the crystals of BPTI were orthorhombic with a size of 0.5 × 0.5 × 0.8 mm. In 1970 the first stereo models of BPTI with a resolution of 2.5 Å were published (HUBER et al., 1970, 1971b). The length is estimated as 29 Å, with a thickness of 19 Å (HUBER et al., 1970, 1971a). With refinement of the methods according to DEISENHOFER and STEIGEMANN (1974), the amino acid sequence was resolved first to 1.9 Å (HUBER et al., 1974) and now to 1.5 Å (DEISENHOFER and STEIGEMANN, 1975). Data are obtained by Fourier analysis. The dihedral angles are 102° for Cys_{14}–Cys_{38}, 85° for Cys_{30}–Cys_{51}, and 87° for Cys_5–Cys_{55} (±5°). Those of the reactive site are registered in Table 16 (see also Fig. 3). An important residue is Asp_{43}, causing the distortion of the N-terminal helical segment by its internal location (HUBER et al., 1971b). For sequence and structure see Fig. 1 and Table 8.

3. Structure-Dependent Properties

BPTI exhibits an unusual stability within a wide pH range against heat and against denaturing agents (VINCENT et al., 1971). These authors published infrared and optical rotatory dispersion (ORD) spectra. The latter spectra of native inhibitor, partially reduced BPTI (Cys_{14}–Cys_{38}) and its different alkylated derivatives are identical. Cleavage of the Cys_{14}–Cys_{38} bond and subsequent alkylation does not change the conformation. The importance of the α-amino group of Arg_1 is discussed.

The strongest lines in Raman spectra of BPTI solutions, lyophilized powder, and of a single crystal were for vibration of the aromatic side chains, Phe and Tyr, and of S-S and C-S groups of the three disulfide bridges (BRUNNER and HOLZ, 1975). Of the four Tyr residues, Raman spectroscopy gave values only for exposed Tyr, whereas X-ray analysis, nitration, and UV spectrometry suggested that Tyr_{23} and Tyr_{25} are buried within the molecule (BRUNNER and HOLZ, 1975). In solid state, protein-solvent contacts are replaced by protein-protein contacts. Changes in the frequencies of the S-S and S-C stretching characterize such conformation in the lyophilized and crystallized states. Although BPTI is a compact protein, dissimilarities in the main chain between the different states are observed (BRUNNER and HOLZ, 1975).

Raman analyses of native inhibitor with respect to pH stability and heat stability are in good agreement with NMR-studies (BRUNNER et al., 1974; BRUNNER and HOLZ, 1974). Above 75 °C at pH 4.7 or at pH 1.7 and 65 °C, the line due to the β-structure decreases in intensity, whereas the α-helix seems to be unchanged. The modifications observed are reversible.

Reduced BPTI shows intense spectral changes when the temperature is increased. While with native inhibitor 50% of the intensity is lost at 90 °C, this amount of

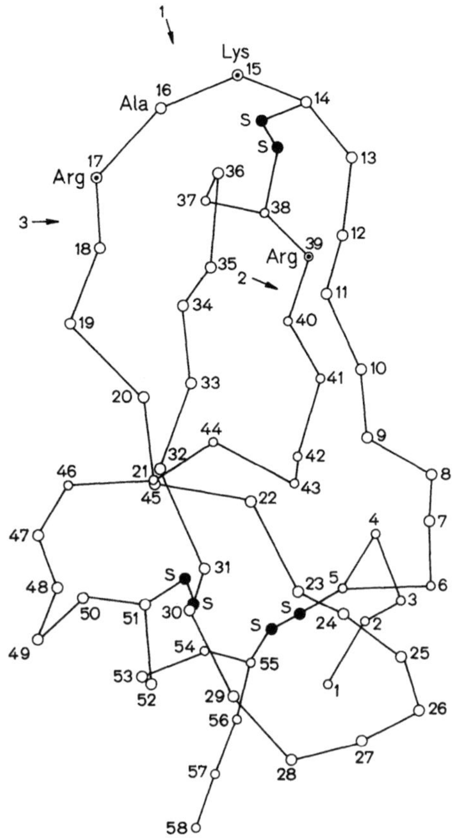

Fig. 1. Projection of the atomic structural model of the α-carbon atoms of BPTI. The arrows indicate the pepide bonds to be cleaved by trypsin after selective reduction of the Cys_{14}–Cys_{38} disulfide bond. ● = sulfur atoms. (Taken from TSCHESCHE et al., 1974b)

thermal denaturation occurs at 60 °C with an evident unfolding of the chain of the reduced inhibitor. Similar behavior is observed with reduced carboxamidomethyl inhibitor. This compound shows no inhibitory activity and the Raman spectrum of the unstable substance shows great differences from that of the native inhibitor obviously as a result of conformational changes near the reactive site (BRUNNER et al., 1974). In 1968 MELOUN et al. reported nitration of BPTI in positions Tyr_{10} and Tyr_{21} with maintenance of full activity (mononitro Tyr_{10} or dinitro Tyr_{10} Tyr_{21}-BPTI) and unchanged secondary structure (ORD-spectrum). The remaining two Tyr residues react very slowly or not at all.

The ring proton resonances of BPTI and the nitrated derivative have been located by SNYDER et al. (1975) and attributed to specific positions of specific rings. Because of the small size of the molecule, relatively narrow NMR lines resulted. Nine areas of resonances were found with individual buried backbone NH protons (KARPLUS et al., 1973; MASSON and WÜTHRICH, 1973; WAGNER et al., 1975). Position 22 is deeply buried; the assigned NH resonance is the most resistant to exchange with solvent D_2O (MASSON and WÜTHRICH, 1973; KARPLUS et al., 1973). The exchange rate of the amide protons with deuterium is reported with the first high resolution proton NMR spectra of BPTI (MASSON and WÜTHRICH, 1973), the values being in agreement with those reported by KARPLUS et al. (1973). Thermal denaturation is reversible as shown in the NMR experiments in accordance with Raman studies. The β-sheet and the α-helix were intact up to 87 °C; random coil conformation is found from 70 °C upwards. With the aide of nitrotyrosine-chelated lanthanides, MARINETTI et al. (1976) showed that the nitrotyrosyl side chain of BPTI binds lanthanides. Variation of pH allowed determination of the stability constant for bindings on nitro-Tyr_{10} and nitro-Tyr_{21} as 50 and 159 M^{-1} with Pr (III) and Eu (III). With the exception of one NH and a resolved α-CH, all nonexchangeable NH's are in a spherical shell of < 12 Å from position 21. Position 10 is the most exposed and nitro-Tyr motions at both sides may be possible. In contrast, nitro-Tyr_{21} has less of movement freedom (MARINETTI et al., 1976). These lanthanide studies were continued with nitro-Tyr_{21} of the dinitro-BPTI (MARINETTI et al., 1977) to obtain the distances of resolved backbone protons from this metal binding site. Shift and distance calculations for positions 19–22 and 31–33 are based on the data of X-ray structure analyses. Identical conformation in crystal and solvated states are compared with rigidity between 4 °C and 87 °C (WAGNER et al., 1976). The angles of the side chains at the surface are different in solvent and in solid state (GELIN and KARPLUS, 1975). Between 1 °C and < 40 °C the solvated state is stable between pH 0.5–12.0 (WAGNER et al., 1976). Using a combination of double resonance techniques, the dynamics of the aromatic rings were investigated. Tyr and Phe, fixed in the interior and hindered in rotation by the surrounding amino acids, partly show rapid rotation at high, and slow rotation at low temperatures (GELIN and KARPLUS, 1975; HETZEL et al., 1976).

With model calculations in 0.03 Å squares, HETZEL et al. (1976) got parameters for possible motions, taking account of the steric hindrance. Rotation of individual aromatic rings can only take place in a flexible structure and there is no model calculation permitting ring rotation of two or more aromatic residues simultaneously. This is an observation valid also for BPTI with reduced Tyr residues (ROCCHI et al., 1976). Reduction does not strongly influence the inhibitory capacity, but refolding of the molecule is evidently hindered.

Concerning the lysyl residues of BPTI, NMR-studies on single crystals and in solution gave the following results: Three of the four Lys residues freely extend into the hydration water. Lys_{41} reaching a position near Tyr_{10} interacts with this residue in solution. In solid crystal structure, Tyr_{10} is in proximity to Arg_{42} of the neighboring inhibitor molecule. The existence of a hydrogen bond in the soluble state is suggested. Thus, differences in the conformation of solution and crystal states can be inferred (BROWN et al., 1976).

The three disulfide bridges of the molecule with the capability of reduction and reoxydation are difficult to handle in reoxidizing experiments because of the accompanying folding of the protein. Earlier experiments with exposure to air have been replaced in effect by treatment with hydroxyethyl disulfide or dithiothreitol (in oxidized cyclic disulphide form) under anaerobic conditions (CREIGHTON, 1974a). After treatment with these reagents, the reactivated inhibitor shows the physicochemical and kinetic constants of the natural compound. Also it is stable against proteolytic cleavage. Quenching of the reactivation, by acidification or alkylation of the thiol groups followed by electrophoretic studies, allows isolation of intermediate states in the reactivation sequence (CREIGHTON, 1974b). Fractionation of these compounds yielded molecules with one disulfide bridge, 25% reoxidized in position Cys_{30}–Cys_{51}, ~25% in Cys_5–Cys_{30} and with a lower yield of Cys_{30}–Cys_{55} and Cys_5–Cys_{51}, only the first fraction being part of the natural conformation.

The three intermediates are formed with three different reoxidizing methods and can be attributed to steps in the folding mechanism (CREIGHTON, 1974c). From the statement that "the conformation of the protein determines the disulfide bonds, not vice versa" CREIGHTON concludes that bonding in position 30–51 is as facile as after the intramolecular interactions. In two disulfide intermediates, Cys_{30}–Cys_{51} is the preferred bond followed by 5–55 > 5–14 > 5–38 > 14–18 (CREIGHTON, 1975b). From these steps, an obligatory pathway of folding is derived. The latter bond represents the last step in folding the molecule (CREIGHTON, 1975c), the other three being intermediates (CREIGHTON, 1975b). Kinetic studies of the formation rate of the bond in this position support the conclusions of the conformational proximity of these residues (CREIGHTON, 1975c, d). The other S-S bridges are more stable intermediates of primary structure for starting points of folding to correct secondary structure. It is remarkable that the positions Cys_{14} and Cys_{38} near the reactive site are obviously not involved in the first folding; this bond being known as the point of fastening the rigid structure (CREIGHTON, 1974c). If this bond is reduced selectively, BPTI is inactive (e.g., against α-chymotrypsin) and becomes a substrate (CHAUVET and ACHER, 1975b). The proteolytic degradation results in a splitting at Lys_{15}, Tyr_{21}, Tyr_{35}, and Phe_{45} yielding two minor peptides and a major molecule. It could be that the bond Cys_{14}–Cys_{38} producing the configuration around the reactive site is the first site attacked during proteolysis.

Without denaturation, BPTI is resistant to 20 different enzymes (KASSELL, 1970). Only thermolysin is able to degrade native BPTI. This enzymic inactivation is temperature dependent because of the conformational changes at higher temperatures (WANG and KASSELL, 1970; KASSELL and WANG, 1971). Binding in a trypsin complex does not protect against degradation.

The UV absorption at 293 nm may be altered at pH 8 (up from pH 6) as an effect of Tyr_{23} and Tyr_{35} in the structure. At pH 5 the change in absorption starts at lower temperatures. This effect must be attributed to Tyr_{10} when compared with inhibitors of related structure (e.g., snail inhibitor) (DIETL and TSCHESCHE, 1976). Slight temperature and pH-dependent changes in fluorescence spectra are ascribed to aggregation effects at higher protein concentrations leading to limitation of conformational freedom in the regions of Tyr_{10} and Tyr_{21} (SIEMION and KANIA, 1975).

4. The Reactive Site

Since 1967/1968 the residue Lys_{15} has been considered responsible for the reactive site of BPTI in the complex with trypsin (CHAUVET and ACHER, 1967; KRESS and LASKOWSKI, 1968). With the aid of the anthraniloyl derivate of maleylated BPTI (ELKANA, 1974a, b), the reactive site for chymotrypsin was studied, the Lys_{15} residue being masked by this reaction. Whereas the K_i of the trypsin complex increases 10^6-fold, the inhibition of chymotrypsin is practically unchanged. These findings suggest that the BPTI derivative binds to chymotrypsin via the anthraniloyl group. This is the only possible explanation which could be in agreement with the studies of HUBER's group (BLOW et al., 1972). They conclude from model studies that Lys_{15} enters the tosyl pocket of the enzyme. For the sequence around the reactive site see Tables 2, 16, and Fig. 3.

5. Modification of the Reactive Site

The common complex binding reaction according to LASKOWSKI, JR. (see SBTI and reviews LASKOWSKI, JR. and SEALOCK, 1971; LUTHY et al., 1973; FINKENSTADT et al., 1974) does not apply to BPTI as shown by experiments analogous to those done with SBTI. No modified inhibitor was found (TSCHESCHE and OBERMEIER, 1971). Therefore, TSCHESCHE and co-workers developed a method for preparing "modified" inhibitor in accordance with known intermediates of SBTI (TSCHESCHE et al., 1974; JERING and TSCHESCHE, 1974a). If the P_1–P'_1 bond is split, changes of physicochemical values are found with different spectroscopic methods indicating the rotational freedom for the peptide chain residues P'_1–P'_5 (QUAST et al., 1975b).

JERING and TSCHESCHE (1976a) described artificial modification of BPTI by selective disulfide reduction of Cys_{14}–Cys_{38} with sodium borohydride. The reduced BPTI can be split with trypsin, reoxidized and rechromatographed carefully to avoid changes of the molecule other than those known for modified SBTI (JERING and TSCHESCHE, 1976a). The "modified" BPTI has an unchanged amino acid composition (JERING and TSCHESCHE, 1976a). With carboxypeptidase B, complete inactivation is reached by cleavage of P_1. Selective reduction of the Cys_{14}–Cys_{38} bond also inactivates. Cleavage of P'_1 to P'_3 with aminopeptidase K_1 also results in an inactive compound (JERING and TSCHESCHE, 1976a).

During incubation with trypsin the P_1–P'_1 bond is reformed and native inhibitor is obtained (JERING and TSCHESCHE, 1976a). This reaction, which does not go to completion, can also be performed with porcine pancreatic kallikrein, bovine α-chymotrypsin, and porcine plasmin (TSCHESCHE and KUPFER, 1976). The experiments reported were performed in concentrations of 10^{-5} *M* for very long times (over one year). The negative results reported by others were attributed to shorter reaction times (TSCHESCHE and OBERMEIER, 1971). The existence of an equilibrium between native and modified BPTI was described with an equilibrium constant $K=0.33$ at pH 5.0 with plasmin (JERING and TSCHESCHE, 1974b; TSCHESCHE and KUPFER, 1976).

This effect, the partial restoration of the P_1–P'_1 bond, indicates that the reactive site of the three enzymes is the same and BPTI is therefore a "single-headed" inhibitor. This immediate complex reaction can be followed with double-beam spectrophotometry or when the reaction is started with modified BPTI and enzyme (chymotrypsin) (QUAST et al., 1975a, 1976). The equilibrium between native and modified (see SBTI) inhibitor is unattainable. The half-life of trypsin complex with modified BPTI is 1.5×10^4 years. For that reason QUAST et al. (1976) started the reaction with modified inhibitor and found the intermediates (see also review TSCHESCHE et al., 1974b).

For changes in activity as a result of replacements of residues of the reactive site, see Table 3 (review: TSCHESCHE et al., 1974b). Similarly to the artificially

Table 3. Changes in activity of BPTI following replacements of residues in the reactive center

$P_1 = Lys_{15}$	
Des-Lys	Inactive (JERING and TSCHESCHE, 1974c)
Arg	Full activity (JERING and TSCHESCHE, 1974c)
Phe } Trp }	Preferably inhibits chymotrysin (JERING and TSCHESCHE, 1974c)
$P_1' - P_2' = Ala_{16} - Arg_{17}$	
Des-Ala-Arg	Inactive (JERING and TSCHESCHE, 1974d)
Phe_{16}	Weaker for trypsin (TAN and KAISER, 1977)

changes Lys_{15} to Arg_{15}, natural isoinhibitors are found in the snail (see p. 185). A tetrasuccinyl derivative of BPTI (in position Arg_1, Lys_{26}, Lys_{41}, Lys_{46}) is fully active if Lys_{15} is protected during succinylation. If Lys_{15} is acetylated the activity is lost (JERING et al., 1974).

6. Conformational Studies of the BPTI Complex With Trypsin and Chymotrypsin

According to current concepts, proteinase inhibitors are specific macromolecular substrates of proteinases but complex formation prevails over the cleavage as substrate. Observations concerning the configuration of the partner of the proteinase when acting as substrate and/or inhibitor have been reviewed by WRIGHT (1977).

The crystallization and the crystallogram of the complex were reported by COLE and PARTHASARATHY (1972) and RÜHLMANN et al. (1973). HUBER and co-workers (RÜHLMANN et al., 1973; HUBER et al., 1974b) counted over 200 interatomic contacts between trypsin and BPTI in the complex molecule (Table 4). The most important of them have been investigated by several groups. The conformation of the complex was determined by HUBER and co-workers, first by theoretical studies following X-ray analyses of BPTI and chymotrypsin (BLOW et al., 1972), of chymotrypsin and trypsin (RÜHLMANN et al., 1973), and finally with X-ray studies at 1.9 Å resolution (HUBER et al., 1974a; review: HUBER et al., 1974b).

For contact positions in the complex with trypsin and pancreas kallikrein see Table 4. The complex is tetrahedral; inhibitor and trypsin are connected by Lys_{15} (BPTI) and Ser_{195} (enzyme) (RÜHLMANN et al., 1973). The binding part of the molecule induces a conformational change in the main chain of BPTI, thus adapting its configuration to the enzyme's form (HUBER et al., 1975). Complex formation in general is assumed to be associated with dehydration (QUAST et al., 1974) and proceeds in different steps. This assumption has stimulated studies since 1968 (HAYNES and FEENEY, 1968).

Water is excluded from the contact area by means of the sequence Tyr_{35}–Cys_{38} and the bond Cys_{14}–Cys_{38} of the inhibitor molecule (RÜHLMANN et al., 1973). With enzymatically inactive anhydrotrypsin as reaction partner (Ser_{195} being converted to dehydroalanine), HUBER et al. (1975) got a crystallized complex with BPTI. They observed no significant changes in conformation of the complex formed, especially in view of angular changes of P_1. Ser_{183}-anhydrotrypsin also binds with similar constants to BPTI (VINCENT et al., 1974a). The first intermediate complex formed has a life time of $2 \times 10^{-4} - 2 \times 10^{-5}$ sec (ENGEL et al., 1974). The second

Table 4. Contact positions of BPTI complex with trypsin (RÜHLMANN et al., 1973) in comparison with the sequence of pancreatic kallikrein (modified taken from EHRET, 1976)

Kallikrein	Trypsin	Thr_{11}-	Gly_{12}-	P_3 Pro_{13}-	P_2 Cys_{14}-	P_1 Lys_{15}	P'_1 Ala_{16}-	P'_2 Arg_{17}-	P'_3 Ile_{18}	Val_{34}-	Tyr_{35}-	Gly_{36}-	P'_{22} Gly_{37}-	P'_{23} Cys_{38}-	P'_{24} Arg_{39}
?	Tyr_{39}							V							
?	His_{40}							H							
?	Phe_{41}						V	H, V	V						
Cys_{42}	Cys_{42}						V								
His_{57}	His_{57}				V	V	V					V	V	V	
Cys_{58}	Cys_{58}						V								
Lys_{59}	Tyr_{59}														
Asn_{60}	Lys_{60}								V						
Gly_{96}	Ser_{96}														
Lys_{97}	Asn_{97}														H, V
Asp_{98}	Thr_{98}														V
Tyr_{99}	Leu_{99}				V									V	V
X	Tyr_{151}							V, CT		V					
Lys_{175}	Gln_{175}														H
Asp_{189}	Asp_{189}					S									
Thr_{190}	Ser_{190}					H, V									
Cys_{191}	Cys_{191}					V									
Met_{192}	Gln_{192}	H?, H?, V			H	V	V								
Gly_{193}	Gly_{193}					H, V	V	V							
Asp_{194}	Asp_{194}														
Ser_{195}	Ser_{195}				V	C?, V, H	V								
Ser_{214}	Ser_{214}					H									
Trp_{215}	Tyr_{215}			V	V	V								V	
Gly_{216}	Gly_{216}			H, V											

C = Covalent bond; H = Hydrogen bond; V = Van der Waal interaction; CT = Charge transfer; S = Salt bridge.

reaction step is relatively slow because intermediate complex formation is necessary. Kinetic studies yielded a value of 350 sec^{-1} (at pH 7 for α-chymotrypsin) for the second complex conformation step, a minimal reaction mechanism proposed (QUAST et al., 1976):

$$I + E \rightleftharpoons L \rightleftharpoons C \rightleftharpoons X \rightleftharpoons L^* \rightleftharpoons I^* + E$$

I = native inhibitor $I^* = I$ with cleaved $P_1 \pm P_1'$ bond
L and L^* = labile precomplexes
C = final complex according to X-ray studies
X = intermediate found starting with $I^* + E$

The extreme stability of the complex with trypsin has been studied for years. The half-life was determined as 17 weeks (VINCENT and LAZDUNSKI, 1972). According to LAZDUNSKI et al. (1974) the dissociation constant at pH 8.0 is 6.0×10^{-14} M, the lowest so far known of interprotein reaction with an association energy higher than 19 Kcal/mol (VINCENT and LAZDUNSKI, 1972, 1973). Enthalpy calculations for the BPTI-trypsin complex were described by SWEET et al. (1974).

The dissociation of the ionic bridge, Lys_{15} (BPTI)-Asp_{177} (trypsin), is first order; pseudotrypsin (disconnected between positions 176 and 177) is only bound with a dissociation constant of 9.0×10^{-9} M and a half-life of 18 min (LAZDUNSKI et al., 1974). A change with similar consequences is P_1 transformation from Lys to homoarginine (LAZDUNSKI et al., 1974; VINCENT et al., 1974b). Stability of the complex also depends on the intact bridges Cys_{14}–Cys_{38} (BPTI) and Cys_{179}–Cys_{203} (trypsin), as established by various reduction experiments of both components (LAZDUNSKI et al., 1974). Shifting of binding capacity by the selective reduction of one component of the complex (BPTI reduced in position 14 and 38) was first observed by LASKOWSKI SR. (KRESS and LASKOWSKI SR., 1967; KRESS et al., 1968). From these drastic and easily obtained effects, VINCENT and LAZDUNSKI (1972) concluded that these disulfide bridges are the reactive sites of the complex binding reaction.

^1H–^2H exchange experiments with BPTI-trypsin complex in D_2O solution yield a slower exchange than the sum of the two proteins separately tested (PERSHINA and HVIDT, 1974). Obviously, as known from HUBER's studies, contact or entrance of hydrogen ions in the molecule and exchange within the peptide groups is impeded. BPTI itself in solution is relatively stable against proton exchange (KANIA et al., 1974; HVIDT and PEDERSEN, 1974). If the trypsin-BPTI complex is crosslinked with [^{14}C]-dimethyl adipimate, inter- and intramolecular cross-linking occur (WANG and KASSELL, 1974) with 10 modified Lys residues in the treated complex; at least one cross-link being formed between inhibitor and trypsin.

In experiments concerning the possible importance of arginine in BPTI (KEIL, 1971), phenylglyoxal treatment resulted in the disappearance of all Arg but Arg_{53}. The positions of Arg, therefore, are not essential for enzyme binding.

7. Synthesis of Models of the Reactive Site

The first work was done by WIEJAK in the field of the synthesis of fragments enclosing and surrounding the reactive site of BPTI. The compound

Ala_{16}-Lys_{15}-Cys_{14}
| |
Gly_{36}-Gly_{37}-Cys_{38}

and a partially protected amide derivative were inactive against proteinases, including kallikrein (WIEJAK and RZESZOTARSKA, 1974; RZESZOTARSKA and WIEJAK, 1976). WEBER and SCHMID (1975) described properties of

Gly-Gly-Cys-Cys-Lys-Ala ,

Gly-Gly-Cys
        |
Gly-Pro-Cys-Lys-Ala and

Cys-Lys-Ala-Gly-Gly-Cys – methyl ester. [the two Cys residues are joined by a drawn line]

The K_is of trypsin inhibition were $2.3 \times 10^{-2} - 5 \times 10^{-3}$ M. Widening of the ring formation resulted in

Gly-Pro-Cys-Lys-Ala-Arg-Phe-Gly-Gly-Cys [the two Cys residues are joined by a drawn line]

corresponding to positions 12–17 and 35–38 of BPTI (Tyr_{35} exchanged by Phe). With a K_i of 4.7×10^{-4} M, this model was no more effective (WEBER and SCHMID, 1976). The best model compound (TAN and KAISER, 1977) is a cyclic heptadecapeptide composed with respect to the known VAN DER WAAL contact points and hydrogen bonds (see Table 4) of the BPTI molecule:

Gly_{12}-Pro_{13}-Cys_{14}-Lys_{15}-Ala_{16}-Arg_{17}-Ile_{18}-Ile_{19}-Arg_{20}
| |
Ala_{40}-Arg_{39}-Cys_{38}-Gly_{37}-Gly_{36}-Tyr_{35}-Val_{34}-Phe_{33}

The complex formation of this compound with trypsin is of the temporary type and relatively strong with a $K_i = 1.8 \times 10^{-6}$ M. A "modified" molecule can be found after trypsin binding as is known for SBTI and for BPTI. Thus, it seems that the whole conformation of the protein is necessary for the high stability of the structure (TAN and KAISER, 1977).

8. Synthesis of BPTI

Using the Merrifield solid-phase method, NODA et al. (1971) obtained a preparation with around 35% of the activity of native BPTI against esterolytic activity of trypsin and an appreciable activity against kallikrein. YAJIMA and co-workers (YAJIMA and KISO, 1974; YAJIMA et al., 1974) described synthesis of a substance by fragment condensation which showed 82% of the trypsin-inhibiting capacity of BPTI. The possible experimental errors by these two groups are discussed by TAN and KAISER (1976). The first stable complete analog of native BPTI was synthetized by TAN and KAISER (1976). They used Merrifield solid-phase synthesis in an anaerobic system working with the reduced inhibitor. With the active substance high dilutions were used to ascertain correct pairing of the disulphide bridges. The substance prepared was purified by affinity chromatography and chromatography on CM-Sephadex C-25. The properties and constants, as compared with natural BPTI, were all identical within experimental error. Thus, amino acid composition, stability, competitive inhibition of β-trypsin with dissociation constant, circular dichroism spectra, and gel electrophoresis together indicate a molecule of synthetic BPTI with the same configuration as natural BPTI.

In further experiments, TAN and KAISER (1977) synthetized Phe_{16}-BPTI. The circular dichroism of the purified compound is identical with the Arg-inhibitor, thus demonstrating that the conformation was not perturbed. Inhibitory properties after the change in position 16 resemble those of a BPTI derivative.

9. Inhibition Spectrum

a) Trypsin

All data concerning the inhibition of trypsin were mentioned in the discussion of the complex binding reaction. The mechanism and kinetics of the trypsin inhibition were reviewed by FINKENSTADT et al. (1974), LAZDUNSKI et al. (1974) and LEVILLIERS et al. (1974). The inhibition against β- and ψ-trypsin, like α-trypsin, is confirmed by affinity chromatography (CHAUVET and ACHER, 1974) (see also Table 7).

b) Trypsinogen

Affinity chromatography experiments on BPTI-Sepharose 4B suggested complex binding forces with trypsinogen (CHAUVET and ACHER, 1974). With great excess of BPTI and the preenzyme in solution a similar observation was made (DLOUHÁ and KEIL, 1969; KEIL-DLOUHÁ and KEIL, 1972). In 1969 Ser_{197} was discussed as complex binding position of the preenzyme; later Trp_{199} (sequence numbers given are of free trypsin). Chromatography on Sephadex G-75 of the mixture of trypsinogen and BPTI yielded the complex molecule (VINCENT and LAZDUNSKI, 1976). With competition experiments (including chymotrypsin in the reaction) the dissociation constant was determined to be $1.8 \times 10^{-6} \pm 0.3 \times 10^{-6}$ M at pH 8.0 and 25 °C. Conformational changes connected with the activation of the enzyme therefore increase the stability of the complex by a factor of 3.3×10^{7}, especially with the connection by Asp_{189} (VINCENT and LAZDUNSKI, 1976).

c) Chymotrypsin

Reviews of the mechanism and kinetics of chymotrypsin inhibition are given by ENGEL et al. (1974) and LAZDUNSKI et al. (1974) and referred to here within "conformational studies of the BPTI complex." Nitration of chymotrypsin in complex form shows the same results as with free chymotrypsin (HOLT et al., 1972). It can be concluded that tyrosine of the enzyme is not involved in complex formation. Oxidizing experiments may support the notion that Trp_{215} of the enzyme is involved. Kinetic data of complex binding are given by VINCENT and LAZDUNSKI (1973)

Table 5. Inhibition spectra of BPTI with glandular kallikreins

Species	Gland	
Bird	pancreas	+C [1]
Rat	kidney	+B [2]
	urine	(+) [3]/−C [4]
	pancreas	+AC [5]/−□ [6]/+AC [7]/−C [4]
	submand.	+ABC [8]/±□ [6]/+B [9]/−C [4]
Mouse	urine	−□ [6]
	pancreas	−□ [6]
	submand.	−□ [6]/+A [9]/−B [22]/+A [23]
Guinea-pig	urine	−□ [6]
	pancreas	−□ [6]
	submand.	−□ [6]/−AB [10]
Hamster	submand.	−AB [10]
Rabbit	submand.	(+)AB [10]
Horse	urine	+□ [6]
Cattle	urine	+C [4]/+□ [6]
	pancreas	+C [4]/+□ [6]
	submand.	+C [4]/+□ [6]
Pig	udder	+B [11]
	urine	(+)A [12]/+C [4]/+□ [6]
	pancreas	+A [12]/+AB [13]/+C [4]/+□ [6]
	submand.	+A [12]/+C [4]/+□ [6]
Cat	urine	−C [4]/−□ [6]
	pancreas	
	submand.	−C [4]/±A [14]/−BC [10]/−□ [6]
Dog	colon	(+)AB [15]
	kidney	−C [16]
	urine	−C [4]/(+)C [16]/−□ [6]
	pancreas	−AC [5]/−C [4]/(+)C [16]/(+)AC [17]/−AC [7]/−□ [6]
	submand.	−C [4]/−AB [10]/−□ [6]
Monkey	colon	+AB [15]
Human	colon	+AB [15]
	urine	+C [4]/(+)C [16]/(+)A [18]/+AC [19]/+AB [20]/+□ [6]
	pancreas	+C [4]/+AC [19]/+□ [6]
	submand./saliva	+C [4]/+AB [13]/+AC [19]/+□ [21]/+□ [6]

A = Assay with synthetic substrate; B = Bioassay in vitro; C = Bioassay in vivo; □ = Different methods.

1. VOGEL and WERLE (1970); 2. CROXATTO et al. (1971); 3. NUSTAD (1969); 4. VOGEL (1968); 5. HOJIMA et al. (1975a); 6. VOGEL and WERLE (1970); 7. HOJIMA et al. (1975b); 8. ERDÖS et al. (1968a, b); 9. PORCELLI et al. (1976); 10. BHOOLA and DOREY (1971); 11. PEETERS et al. (1976); 12. WERLE et al. (1973); 13. MORIWAKI and SCHACHTER (1971); 14. MORIWAKI et al. (1976a); 15. SEKI et al. (1972); 16. MORIWAKI et al. (1976b); 17. HOJIMA et al. (1977); 18. MATSUDA et al. (1976); 19. ARENS and HABERLAND (1973); 20. MORIYA et al. (1972); 21. MODÉER (1977a); 22. SIQUEIRA and BERALDO (1973); 23. EKFORS and HOPSU-HAVU (1972).

Table 6. Inhibition of serum kallikrein of different species by BPTI

Animal	Test method	Inhibition	Author
Turtle	B	+	SEKI et al. (1973)
Alligator	B	+	SEKI et al. (1973)
Rat	A, C	±	MORIYA and HOJIMA (1972)
	□	(+)	VOGEL and WERLE (1970)
Mouse	□	(+)	VOGEL and WERLE (1970)
	B	−	BACK (1973)
Guinea-pig	□	(+)	VOGEL and WERLE (1970)
Horse	□	+	VOGEL and WERLE (1970)
Pig	A	(−)	WUNDERER et al. (1972)
	□	+	VOGEL and WERLE (1970)
Dog	□	(+)	VOGEL and WERLE (1970)
Man	C	+	MORIYA and HOJIMA (1972)
	□	+	VOGEL and WERLE (1970)
	A	+	ASGHAR et al. (1976)
	A	+	WUNDERER et al. (1972)
	A	+	VEREMIENKO et al. (1964)

A = Synthetic substrate; B = Bioassay in vitro; C = Bioassay in vivo; □ = Different methods.

and later by ENGEL et al. (1974) using displacement of proflavin from the enzyme by the inhibitor in measurements using fast stopped-flow spectrophotometry (see "reaction mechanism of complex formation"). With the same method, values for the dissociation constant are given (BÖSTERLING and ENGEL, 1976) as $6 \times 10^{-9}\,M$ at pH 7.2 and $1.7 \times 10^{-7}\,M$ at pH 5.0. The dissociation equilibrium is nearly constant from pH 7–10 and complex formation is observed around pH 12 with a velocity only three times slower. The complex is completely dissociated at pH 4.0 (CHAUVET and ACHER, 1975a). Trypsin competes with chymotrypsin in the complex binding reaction, e.g., on affinity chromatography of the chymotrypsin-BPTI complex on trypsin resin.

d) Kallikrein

Comparing the dissociation constants of the complexes with trypsin [$6 \times 10^{-14}\,M$ (VINCENT and LAZDUNSKI, 1972)], chymotrypsin [$9 \times 10^{-9}\,M$ (VINCENT and LAZDUNSKI, 1973)], and glandular kallikrein [$8 \times 10^{-9}\,M$ (FRITZ et al., 1969d)], the inhibition of the latter enzyme is not very strong. Kallikreins of different sources have been tested (Tables 5 and 6). It seems obvious that kallikrein inhibition has increased with the increasing purity of the kallikrein preparations. HOJIMA et al. (1975b) refer to such observations with crude and purified enzyme in testing rat pancreatic kallikrein.

The complex of inhibitor with porcine serum kallikrein has been reported as having the low dissociation constant of $1 \times 10^{-7}\,M$ (WUNDERER et al., 1972). In the test system, the complex is dissociated so that no titration curves were obtained. An equimolar complex formation cannot be observed. Elucidation of the structural differences of the kallikreins may explain the mechanism of complex formation. When the sequences of kallikrein and trypsin are compared, some residues in question

Table 7. Enzymes inhibited by BPTI

Trypsin human	+	FEENEY et al. (1969) MALLORY and TRAVIS (1973)
bovine	+	CHAUVET and ACHER (1974)
Trypsinogen bovine	+	CHAUVET and ACHER (1974)
Plasmin human	+	FEENEY et al. (1969)
Leukocyte proteinase	+	BRETZ et al. (1976)
(Kininogenase)	±	KOPITAR and LEBEZ (1975)
	+	KRUZE et al. (1969)
Kininogenase macrophages	−	GREENBAUM et al. (1969)
Kininogenase polymorphonuclear cells	−	GREENBAUM and KIM (1967)
Acrosin	(+)	FRITZ et al. (1972b)
Kininogenase snake venom	+	GEIGER and KORTMANN (1977)
Esteroprotease submaxillaris mouse, rat	+	ANGELETTI et al. (1973)
Human skin proteinase	(+)	FRÄKI and HOPSU-HAVU (1975)
Human pancreatic proteinase	+	MALLORY and TRAVIS (1974)
Kininase macrophages, polymorphonuclear cells	+	GREENBAUM et al. (1969)
Renin	−	KOKUBU et al. (1974)
Trypsin-like enzyme microbial	+	CHAUVET et al. (1976)

are quite different, e.g., Thr_{98} (neutral) of trypsin and Asp_{98} (with γ-carboxyl group) opposite to P'_{24} of BPTI (see Table 4).

Studies on kallikrein similar to those performed with trypsin are rare.

Circular dichroism spectra are changed when kallikrein and BPTI are assayed separately and in complex form (ROSENKRANZ, 1974a, b). Kallikrein CD-bands are different at different pH values, whereas the BPTI spectrum is pH-independent (ROSENKRANZ and SCHOLTAN, 1971). With the complex, changes are observed in the spectral regions concerning Tyr, Trp, and Cys; the importance of these residues indicated by comparison with trypsin (see Table 4).

e) Additional Inhibition Spectra (see Table 7)

The inhibition of acrosin is very weak (ČECHOVÁ and FRITZ, 1976). BAEe-cleaving esterases of human gastrointestinal tract are not inhibited (ARENS and HABERLAND, 1973). One µg human pancreatic proteinase E is inhibited 60% by 1 µg of BPTI (MALLORY and TRAVIS, 1974). An indirect kinin-releasing enzyme, clostridiopeptidase B (EC 3.4.22.8), is inhibited when assayed biologically (VARGAFTIG and GIROUX, 1976a, b). Cleavage of a synthetic substrate (i.e., direct activity) is not inhibited (SIFFERT et al., 1976). These findings are good examples of the use of inhibitors for differentiation of proteases.

BPTI inhibits the prostaglandin release induced by kininogen in a kidney preparation (COLINA-CHOURIO et al., 1976). This effect is explained by an indirect mechanism, i.e., inhibition of the kinin release by kallikrein.

It is suggested that BPTI is able to bind glycoproteins and mucopolysaccharides. This effect, produced via free uronyl and sialosyl groups, must be completely different from the enzyme-binding mechanism (STODDART and KIERNAN, 1973). It is also reported that BPTI binds in a complex to the stabilized double helix of DNA, whereas association with acetylated BPTI may result in destabilization of the DNA conformation (SZOPA, 1974).

10. Physiology

During development of the animal, BPTI content of the organs increases markedly: in lung, from 1% (fetal) to 5–30% (calf); in pancreas, from 0% (fetus) to 5–25% (calf), to normal adult (100%) values (WILUSZ et al., 1976).

a) Distribution and Elimination of BPTI

After i.v. application of BPTI in the rat, TRAUTSCHOLD et al. (1966) observed accumulation in the liver followed by fixation in the kidneys. With ^{3}H-labeled BPTI they found that the inhibitor was excreted in an inactive form after a few days. The same distribution is observed in the dog and (for blood and urine) in humans (FRITZ et al., 1969d). With ^{131}I-labeled BPTI in mice, autoradiography was used for localization of the inhibitor (ARNDTS et al., 1970). The experiments were done in parallel with radioimmunoassay studies of organ extracts of treated rats. Body autoradiography (ARNDTS et al., 1970) and immunofluorescence studies (TÖRÖK, 1972) suggest almost complete storage of BPTI in the renal cortex, the brush border having a special affinity for BPTI (JUST and HABERMANN, 1973; JUST et al., 1973; JUST, 1975). When compared with the distribution and elimination of other inhibitors, the retarded elimination in inactive form is a unique finding, obviously based on the basicity of BPTI (FRITZ et al., 1969d; JERING et al., 1974). The P_1-acetylated tetrasuccinyl derivative of BPTI is eliminated without storage in the kindey. 30% of the compound is deacetylated in vivo by acyl-lysine deacylase from the kidneys (JERING et al., 1974); these experiments were done in rats after proving the activity of the deacylase in vitro (see also TSCHESCHE et al., 1974b).

b) Relationship of Cow Colostrum Inhibitor and Bull Seminal Plasma Inhibitor to BPTI

By 1968, the inhibition of kallikrein in bioassay by unfractionated colostrum was known. The electrophoretically homogeneous inhibitor compound was resolved (for review see ČECHOVÁ, 1976) into three fractions, two being of high MW and one with MW 11,500.

Disregarding the carbohydrate component (ČECHOVÁ et al., 1969a), the sequence resembles that of BPTI especially around the reactive site (ČECHOVÁ and MUSZYNSKA, 1970) (see Table 2) and in the positions of the three disulfide bonds (ČECHOVÁ and BER, 1974). Together with the research group in Munich, these investigations succeded in the complete isolation and characterization (TSCHESCHE et al., 1975). DIETL and TSCHESCHE (1976d) definitely determined CTI to be a Lys-type inhibitor. JONÁKOVÁ and ČECHOVÁ (1976) reported the separation of nine fractions representing two isoinhibitors and confirmed the similarity to BPTI. There was up to 40% homology of the amino acid sequence to BPTI (see Table 8). In comparing the amino acid sequence, the positions 17–18 of BPTI are replaced in CTI by Ala-Ala, a position of importance in kallikrein inhibition (DIETL and TSCHESCHE, 1974; TSCHESCHE and DIETL, 1975).

A related compound occurs in colostrum of swine and humans indicating that it is a common principle. However, one must consider whether during metabolism of the bovine BPTI, it is conformationally changed in excretion because of its connection to the heterosaccharide chain. This conformation is the basis of the change in inhibitory activity as compared with BPTI.

c) Inhibition Spectrum of CTI

There is little known about kallikrein inhibition. Untreated cow colostrum was shown to inhibit the biologic activity of kallikrein (see Table 9). Investigations with one of the isolated fractions (or isoinhibitors) showed only weak or no inhibition. With regard to the different inhibition spectra of fractions isolated from different animal colostra (as mentioned above) it is possible to identify a specific kallikrein inhibitor within the fractions.

Concerning the special conditions in ruminants and the relation to structure, ČECHOVÁ et al. (1969b) assume two genes responsible for inhibitor synthesis. They postulate the differentiation from one original gene during evolution.

According to experiments done in ruminants by WERLE et al. (see FREY et al., 1968) and by HOUVENAGHEL (HOUVENAGHEL and PEETERS, 1968; HOUVENAGHEL et al., 1968a, b; REYNAERT et al., 1968; PEETERS et al., 1976) and in humans by YAMAZAKI and MORIYA (1969), the components of the kallikrein-kinin system play a role in colostrum and milk production. Therefore, there may be a physiological role of the proteinase (kininogenase) inhibitor(s) in colostrum in this regulation mechanism. In this respect the carbohydrate component of the inhibitor(s) may be important. TSCHESCHE et al. (1975) discussed facilitation of the inhibitor secretion by the cabohydrate side chain.

d) Bovine Seminal Plasma Inhibitor

A striking observation was made with seminal plasma inhibitors: one of the fractions isolated (II) from human semen was inactive against pancreatic kallikrein (SCHIESSLER et al., 1974). The same was true for boar and guinea-pig specimens (FINK et al., 1971b). On the other hand, bull seminal plasma has three fractions one containing a polyvalent inhibitor (ČECHOVÁ and FRITZ, 1976).

This fraction is the main inhibitor compound in sperm extracts. The MW of the pure fraction in question is 6800. This compound inhibits kallikreins (see Table 9). If the inhibitor fraction is a derivative of BPTI, structurally changed for secretion, this may be the subject of further studies. Nevertheless the derivatization is so extensive that cross reaction with BPTI-antiserum does not take place (ČECHOVÁ and FRITZ, 1976).

Table 8. Sequences of different proteinase inhibitors

Inhibitor	Sequence
	1 10 20
BPTI [1]	Arg Pro Asp Phe Cys Leu Glu Pro Pro Tyr Thr Gly Pro Cys Lys Ala Arg Ile Ile Arg Tyr Phe
Snail inhibitor K [2]	Glu Gly Arg Pro Ser Phe Cys Asn Leu Pro Ala Glu Thr Gly Pro Cys Lys Ala Ser Phe Arg Gln Tyr Tyr
Russell's viper inhibitor [3]	His Asp Arg Pro Thr Phe Cys Asn Leu Ala Pro Glu Ser Gly Arg Cys Arg Gly His Leu Arg Arg Ile Tyr
Bovine colostrum inhibitor [4]	Phe Gln Thr Pro Pro Asp Leu Cys Gln Leu Pro Gln Ala Arg Gly Pro Cys Lys Ala Ala Leu Leu Arg Tyr Phe
	30 40
BPTI [1]	Tyr Asn Ala Lys Ala Gly Leu Cys Gln Thr Phe Val Tyr Gly Gly Cys Arg Ala Lys Arg Asn Asn Phe Lys Ser
Snail inhibitor K [2]	Tyr Asn Ser Lys Ser Gly Gly Cys Gln Gln Phe Ile Tyr Gly Gly Cys Arg Gly Asn Gln Asn Arg Phe Asp Thr
Russell's viper inhibitor [3]	Tyr Asn Leu Glu Ser Asn Lys Cys Lys Val Phe Phe Tyr Gly Gly Cys Gly Gly Asn Ala Asn Asn Phe Glu Thr
Bovine colostrum inhibitor [4]	Tyr Asx Ser Thr Ser Asn Ala Cys Glu Pro Phe Thr Tyr Gly Gly Cys Gln Gly Asn Asn Asx Asn Phe Glu Thr
	50
BPTI [1]	Ala Glu Asp Cys Met Arg Thr Cys Gly Gly Ala
Snail inhibitor K [2]	Thr Gln Gln Cys Gln Gly Val Cys Val
Russell's viper inhibitor [3]	Arg Asp Glu Cys Arg Gln Thr Cys Gly Gly Lys
Bovine colostrum inhibitor [4]	Thr Glu Met Cys Leu Arg Ile Cys Glu Pro Pro Gln Gln Thr Asp Lys Ser

1. KASSELL and LASKOWSKI SR. (1965); 2. DIETL and TSCHESCHE (1974); 3. TAKAHASHI (1974c); 4. ČECHOVÁ et al. (1969b).

Table 9. Inhibition of different kallikreins by inhibitors from colostrum and semen

Kallikrein inhibitors	Porcine pancreas	urine	submand.	serum	Human urine	submand.	serum
Seminal inhibitors							
guinea-pig	− [1]/−AB [5]					−AB [5]	
human	± [2]/− [3]						
Bull fraction II	+A [6]	+A [6]					
Porcine colostrum				−A [10]			−A [10]
Cow colostrum							
whole			+C [7]		+C [7]		
isol. fraction	(+)A [8]	− [4]	− [4]				− [9]

A = Assay with synthetic substrate; B = Bioassay in vitro; C = Bioassay in vivo.
1. FRITZ et al. (1970); 2. SUOMINEN et al. (1971); SUOMINEN and NIEMI (1972); 3. FINK et al. (1971a); SCHIESSLER et al. (1974); 4. ČECHOVÁ (1976); 5. MORIWAKI and SCHACHTER (1971); 6. ČECHOVÁ and FRITZ (1976); 7. FREY et al. (1968); 8. DIETL and TSCHESCHE (1974); 9. FRITZ and WUNDERER (1972); 10. WUNDERER et al. (1972).

II. BPTI-Related Kallikrein Inhibitors in Various Animal Phyla

1. CNIDARIA: Trypsin-Kallikrein Inhibitor in Sea Anemones

In the phylum CNIDARIA, one species was successfully investigated: The sea anemone ANEMONIA SULCATA contains a proteinase-inhibiting compound (BÉRESS and BÉRESS, 1971). The substance in question was found during isolation of neurotoxins of this species. Together with FRITZ and co-workers the properties of the substance were established, and from ACTINARIA diverse species were analyzed (some of them containing inhibitor compounds although to a lesser degree) (BÉRESS et al., 1972). The highest concentrations were found in the tentacles (KORTMANN and FRITZ, cf. WUNDERER et al., 1974).

Isolation: The isolation process (BÉRESS et al., 1975a, b) is reviewed by WUNDERER et al. (1976b). Starting with extraction in hot 50% ethanol (FRITZ et al., 1972a), the acetone-ether preparation is chromatographed followed by affinity chromatography (WUNDERER et al., 1974). The five fractions with MW 6100–6620 (FRITZ et al., 1972a; WUNDERER et al., 1972) were analyzed and 54–59 amino acid residues found, two of the fractions being nearly identical (FRITZ et al., 1972a; WUNDERER et al., 1975). The 10 isoinhibitors are homogeneous in gel filtration, ion exchange chromatography, and gel electrophoresis (WUNDERER et al., 1975, 1976), purity 3.3–3.5 IU/mg (WUNDERER et al., 1976). A preliminary sequence study of one isoinhibitor showed a striking similarity to BPTI, especially around the reactive site. The similarity was a weak point when considering their importance for the inhibition of kallikrein, i.e., tissue or plasma kallikrein (WUNDERER et al., 1975) (see Table 2). Arg is the reactive site residue (WUNDERER et al., 1974), in isoinhibitors, isoleucine is located N-terminally (WUNDERER et al., 1975).

Properties: The inhibitor is highly stable against acid and high temperature (FRITZ et al., 1972a; WUNDERER et al., 1976). One of the three disulfide bonds is extraordinarily stable (WUNDERER et al., 1974).

Inhibition spectrum: (Table 10) Inhibition of trypsin: In 20 min equilibrium of the trypsin inhibition is reached (FRITZ et al., 1972a), the inhibition being of temporary type (FRITZ et al., 1972a; WUNDERER et al., 1974).

Inhibition of kallikrein: The equilibrium of the reaction is reached after 10 min incubation (FRITZ et al., 1972a). The inhibition of serum kallikrein is very interesting. Besides the similar inhibitory spectrum, BPTI and sea anemone inhibitor also inhibit serum kallikrein to the same extent as porcine pancreatic kallikrein (FRITZ et al., 1972a; WUNDERER et al., 1972). 90 mU pig serum kallikrein are inhibited totally by 100 µg inhibitor. In view of these parallel findings it is remarkable that Arg is in positions P'_2 and P'_{24} in both inhibitor molecules. (For kallikreins tested see Tables 11 and 12.) In comparing the inhibitor activity against organ and serum kallikrein, a certain relationship is to be seen: of the trypsin binding positions 13–17 and 38–39 the relevant P'_2 and P'_{24} positions are occupied by Arg (see also "Introduction").

Physiological function: The physiological function of this inhibitor compound may be for protection against proteinases of the gastrointestinal tract of the animal (FRITZ et al., 1972a).

Table 10. Inhibition of enzymes by inhibitors from sea anemones, snail, cuttle fish, and viper venom

Enzymes	Sea anemone inhibitor	Snail isoinhibitor	Cuttle fish inhibitor	Viper venom inhibitor
Trypsin	+ [1]	+ [2]	+ [6]	+ [3]
Chymotrypsin	+ [1]	+ [5]	+ [6]	+ [3]
Plasmin	+ [1]	+ [5]	+ [6]	+ [3]
Subtilisin	− [1]	− [2]		
Pepsin	− [2]			
Elastase	− [2]			
Acrosin	(+) [2; 4]			

1. FRITZ et al. (1972a); 2. DIETL and TSCHESCHE (1975); 3. TAKAHASHI et al. (1972, 1974c); 4. FRITZ et al. (1972c); 5. TSCHESCHE et al. (1972); 6. TSCHESCHE and v. RÜCKER (1973a).

2. GASTROPODA: Kallikrein Inhibitor of HELIX POMATIA

Occurence: The detection of a proteinase inhibitor in ANNELIDAE induced the search for inhibitors in hermaphrodite animals (MOLLUSCA).

Strong trypsin inhibiting activity is found in homogenates of the total body of the gastropod HELIX POMATIA with 1.1 mIU/mg fresh weight (TSCHESCHE and DIETL, 1972b). The kallikrein inhibitor in snail hemolymph was (WERLE et al., 1958) a thermolabile and acid labile component with HMW and different from the factors which inhibit trypsin. According to current definition this inhibition is of progressive type. One trypsin inhibitor was described as HMW and the other as thermostable, dialyzable and of LMW. The kallikrein inhibiting capacity of hemolymph is also reported for ACHATINA FULICA (family: PUPILLIDAE) by KAREEM (1973).

If the body of the edible snail is separated into foot, mantle, and mucus, and the inner organs, no proteinase inhibitor can be found in the inner organs; 55% of the other parts of the body is inactivated with perchloric acid and therefore is of HMW (TSCHESCHE and DIETL, 1972a).

Isolation: TSCHESCHE separated an inhibitor of trypsin and plasmin (soluble in 63% ammonium sulfate medium) and an inhibitor of kallikrein, trypsin, chymotrypsin, and plasmin (precipitated with 63% ammonium sulfate) (TSCHESCHE et al., 1972). The kallikrein inhibiting component, rechromatographed on Sephadex G-50 is heat stable. It is also resistant to 3% perchloric acid or TCA at 75 °C (TSCHESCHE and DIETL, 1976b).

From the fractions separated after rechromatography, five main components were characterized (TSCHESCHE and DIETL, 1972a). They were chromatographed repeatedly until homogeneous, i.e., with 3.3 IU/mg (see also review TSCHESCHE and DIETL, 1973, 1976b). The mixture with fractions of MW 6500 was resolved into one fraction with at least 17 isoinhibitors (low ionic strength fraction) and one additional fraction (high ionic strength) with one basic isoinhibitor, representing the majority of activity (DIETL and TSCHESCHE, 1975). This inhibitor, named fraction K, was stated to be homogeneous. The existence of large number of isoinhibitors may be due to biologic variation and/or species dependence. But it may also be the result of allelomorphism (TSCHESCHE and DIETL, 1972b).

Structure and reactive site: For amino acid composition see TSCHESCHE and DIETL (1972b) and Table 8. From the striking similarity to the sequence of BPTI, a similar three dimensional structure is postulated (TSCHESCHE and DIETL, 1972b). For details see DIETL and TSCHESCHE, 1974; TSCHESCHE and DIETL, 1975, 1976; DIETL and TSCHESCHE, 1976b, c).

Maleation only slightly affected inhibition. Modification of arginine of the maleated inhibitor with butane-2,3-dione (see Methods) resulted in inactivity against the proteinases (TSCHESCHE and DIETL, 1972b, 1973). Therefore, it was concluded that the reactive site is not lysine but arginine (TSCHESCHE and DIETL, 1972b). However, Lys is the reactive site residue of isoinhibitor K, whereas in the 17 isoinhibitors Arg-reactive site inhibitors are also found (DIETL and TSCHESCHE, 1975, 1976d).

The sequence, corresponding in a great part to BPTI, differs in position 19–20 of snail inhibitor from the corresponding position 17–18 of BPTI. Arg-Ile of BPTI is replaced by Ser-Phe (DIETL and TSCHESCHE, 1974). Because the trypsin inhibiting capacity of the two inhibitors is practically identical, one has to conclude that these positions are not essential in the complex formation with trypsin, but highly effective in kallikrein inhibition, especially serum kallikrein (DIETL and TSCHESCHE, 1974, 1976a). The authors discuss this specificity to be attributed to position 17 (BPTI) or 19 (snail), respectively.

Properties: Broad stability against proteolytic breakdown was reviewed by TSCHESCHE and DIETL (1976a). The inhibitor is only digested by thermolysin at higher temperatures just as BPTI is. However, in contrast to BPTI, the snail inhibitor is relatively heat labile. At pH 8.0, the molecule is irreversibly denatured at 60 °C resulting in precipitation of the substance (DIETL and TSCHESCHE, 1976b). At this pH and temperature, conformational changes around the positions Tyr_{25} and Tyr_{37} are recorded by an increase in tyrosine absorption at 293 nm (DIETL and TSCHESCHE, 1976b). In contrast to BPTI, the snail inhibitors are not cleavable in vivo by acyl-lysine deacylase (described in BPTI), because of their much lower basicity. In rats, i.v. application of snail inhibitors results in 30% excretion within 8 h and in 100% excretion within 48 h (JERING et al., 1974).

Inhibitory capacity: The reaction with trypsin takes place in a 1:1 ratio. In contrast to BPTI, which takes 20 min to reach equilibrium with the trypsin-BPTI complex, the inhibitor fraction I of snail reaches equilibrium within 1 min (TSCHESCHE and DIETL, 1972a, b). Fraction I also needs 1 min to obtain equilibrium with pancreatic kallikrein (TSCHESCHE and DIETL, 1972b). Extended preincubation of inhibitor and enzyme without substrate does not change the hydrolysis rate indicating the reaction to be of a non-temporary type (TSCHESCHE and DIETL, 1972b).

Kallikrein inhibition: See Tables 11 and 12. The mixture of isoinhibitors (TSCHESCHE et al., 1972) inhibits porcine pancreatic kallikrein more strongly than the isolated isoinhibitors do (TSCHESCHE and DIETL, 1972b). The authors expected a specific kallikrein inhibitor fraction to be present in the mixture because the mixture inhibited both porcine pancreatic and porcine serum kallikrein (75 μg inhibitor: 33 KU) but the latter is not inhibited by isolated isoinhibitors (TSCHESCHE and DIETL, 1972a, b). Obviously the sequence of snail inhibitor BPTI corresponding

Table 11. Inhibition of glandular kallikreins by inhibitors from sea anemones, snail, cuttle fish and viper venom

Kallikrein	Sea anemone	Snail	Cuttle fish	Viper venom
Porcine pancreas	+A [2] +A [4]	+ [5] gland −A [6] gland +A [8]	+A [9]	+ [1] +A [3]
Urine		+A [7]		

1. SUZUKI (1974); 2. FRITZ et al. (1972a); 3. TAKAHASHI et al. (1972); 4. WUNDERER et al. (1974); 5. UHLENBRUCK et al. (1971a); 6. TSCHESCHE and DIETL (1972a); 7. DIETL and TSCHESCHE (1975); 8. DIETL and TSCHESCHE (1974); 9. TSCHESCHE and v. RÜCKER (1973a).

Table 12. Inhibition of serum kallikrein by inhibitors from sea anemones, snail, cuttle fish, and viper venom

Kallikrein	Sea anemone	Snail isoinhib.	Cuttle fish	Viper venom
Bovine				+A [1]
Porcine	+A [2] +A [6]	+A [2] (+)A [3] +A [5, 7]	−A [4]	
Human	+A [6] +A [2]	+A [2] Snail tissue: porcine −A [5, 7]		

A = Assay with synthetic substrate.
1. TAKAHASHI et al. (1972, 1974c); 2. WUNDERER et al. (1972); 3. DIETL and TSCHESCHE (1976a); 4. TSCHESCHE (1976); 5. TSCHESCHE et al. (1972); 6. FRITZ et al. (1972a); 7. TSCHESCHE and DIETL (1972b).

to P'_1–P'_3 is of importance in complex formation with the kallikreins (TSCHESCHE and DIETL, 1975).

Among the isoinhibitors both Lys and Arg type compounds were detected; the main fraction K being of Lys-type (DIETL and TSCHESCHE, 1974). For a further inhibition spectrum see DIETL and TSCHESCHE (1976c) and Table 10. In general, the inhibitory spectrum changes markedly with the fractionation and separation of the isoinhibitors more or less for each enzyme. Substitution of just one or two residues may change the inhibitor constants (DIETL and TSCHESCHE, 1975).

Differentiation of the kallikrein inhibitor and other proteinase inhibitors in snails: In extracts of prepared albumin glands of some snail species and in their eggs, UHLENBRUCK and co-workers found four isoinhibitors and isolated these substances in fibrin-agar (immuno) electrophoresis (UHLENBRUCK et al., 1971a, b; SPRENGER et al., 1972). Two of these fractions are described as inhibitors of bovine pancreatic kallikrein, as tested in fibrin-agar electrophoresis (UHLENBRUCK et al., 1971a; SPRENGER et al., 1972). Besides these findings (discussed later), the inhibitory spectra of these compounds is very different from the LMW kallikrein isoinhibitors, including papain, ficin, bromelain, and microbial proteinases. Furthermore, according to gel filtration experiments, the albumin gland inhibitor is of HMW. So far, similarities with the inhibitor isolated by WERLE et al. (1958) have not been found.

TSCHESCHE and DIETL (1972a) found the compound in question during preparation of the LMW kallikrein inhibitor (review DIETL and TSCHESCHE, 1976a) and were unable to state a kallikrein-inhibiting capacity. These findings were confirmed independently by HERRMANN (1972). TSCHESCHE and DIETL (1973) differentiated organs with regard to trypsin and kallikrein inhibition and stated that the HMW compound occurs only in the albumin gland. According to TSCHESCHE and DIETL (1972b) the LMW kallikrein inhibitor and the inhibitor of UHLENBRUCK differ in the following properties: heat lability, irreversible inactivation with 3% perchloric acid, lack of binding to trypsin resin, solubility in 63% ammonium sulfate. No immunologic cross-reactions of the isoinhibitor preparation I with antibodies against BPTI or the albumin gland inhibitor were found by TRUSCHEIT or UHLENBRUCK (cf., TSCHESCHE and DIETL, 1976).

TSCHESCHE and DIETL (1976) reported that during isolation of the isoinhibitors, the inhibitor described by WERLE could not be found. The authors concluded that these former findings were the effects of cross contamination of the LMW inhibitor with the HMW inhibitor together with salt effects.

Biology and Physiology: In artificial hibernation the whole trypsin-inhibiting activity of the body of the snail is as high as in active life. In contrast, the kallikrein-inhibiting activity increases 100% (TSCHESCHE and DIETL, 1972a). In consequence, the existence of another LMW kallikrein inhibitor was suggested, with high concentration during hibernation and separable from the others described on SE-Sephadex C 25 (TSCHESCHE and DIETL, 1972a).

If the kallikrein-inhibiting compounds have a protective function this may be part of further investigations in view of the fact that they do not inhibit microbial proteinases (TSCHESCHE and DIETL, 1972a). However, the broad inhibitory spectrum is obviously a protective need of an animal exposed to a great number of microbial organisms and their enzymes (DIETL and TSCHESCHE, 1976c). Therefore, they are secreted as proteins, after biosynthesis in the subepithelial glands of the skin, and eliminated in the mucus (TSCHESCHE and DIETL, 1973). When injected intravenously into rats, the kallikrein inhibitor is almost completely excreted in the urine within 48 h, in contrast to BPTI (JERING et al., 1974).

3. MOLLUSCA: Kallikrein Inhibitor From Cuttle-Fish

Study of the phylum MOLLUSCA resulted in the detection of a polyvalent proteinase inhibitor in the cephalopod LOLIGO VULGARIS.

Occurrence: The inhibitor concentrations differ significantly in the different organs of the animal (TSCHESCHE and v. RÜCKER, 1973b). Most was found in the regions of the gastrointestinal tract and lower concentrations in the mantle, skin, and tentacles. In sexual organs an additional specific trypsin-inhibitor group was found, characterized by lack of stability against acid and heat. In female organs it occurs alone and in male organs it occurs together with the stable polyvalent inhibitor (TSCHESCHE and v. RÜCKER, 1973b). In contrast to the stable inhibitor of snail, the kallikrein inhibitor of squid is not secreted by the skin (TSCHESCHE and V. RÜCKER, 1973a).

Isolation: For special information on the isolation steps, see TSCHESCHE (1976). With rechromatography, four isoinhibitors were separated in pure state (90%) with specific activities of 3.8 IU/mg; one with 4.4 IU/mg (not homogeneous) with a MW of 6800–7200 (TSCHESCHE and V. RÜCKER, 1973a).

Amino acid composition and reactive site: Each inhibitor consists of 62 amino acid residues with four disulfide bridges. Slight differences are found in the content of histidine and proline. The authors conclude the existence of isoinhibitors from these findings (TSCHESCHE and V. RÜCKER, 1973a). The differences are discussed with respect to variations of the amino acid composition in the reactive site. An interesting rare fact is the variation in the reactive site of these isoinhibitors, occuring perhaps as results of mutants in *one* animal species (TSCHESCHE and V. RÜCKER, 1973a). Maleation and treatment with butane-2,3-dione (see "Methods") indicate that Lys is the reactive site residue for one isoinhibitor and Arg is the reactive site residue for another; two of the inhibitor fractions being underivatized (TSCHESCHE and V. RÜCKER, 1973a, 1974).

Properties: The outstanding stability against heat and acid denaturation tested in the first studies resulted in precleaning steps of the isolation method (TSCHESCHE and V. RÜCKER, 1973a).

Inhibition Spectrum (see Tables 10–12): The kallikrein inhibiting capacity of extracts increases with acid and heat treatment, perhaps by the dissociation of a naturally existing kallikrein-inhibitor complex (TSCHESCHE and V. RÜCKER, 1973b). An interesting fact is that the isoinhibitors A and B, which inhibit pancreatic kallikrein, are neither Lys- nor Arg-type inhibitors (TSCHESCHE and V. RÜCKER, 1974).

Association constants of the complexes of pancreatic kallikrein with the fractions differ over a wide range (TSCHESCHE and V. RÜCKER, 1973a).

Although having almost the same composition, the four isoinhibitors differ slightly in their specificity (dependent on the reactive site residue), especially against plasmin, and differ in the time needed to reach equilibrium (3–8 min, according to inhibitor or proteinase). In general, the inhibition ratio for trypsin is 1:1. Two of the isoinhibitors, ineffective against plasmin, inhibit chymotrypsin in a ratio 1:2 as known for "double-headed" inhibitors. This inhibition is permanent inhibition (TSCHESCHE and V. RÜCKER, 1973a).

4. Kallikrein Inhibitors in REPTILIA (PROTEROGLYPHA)

During studies on snake venom factors connected with the kallikrein-kinin system, SUZUKI and co-workers detected a specific kallikrein inhibitor.

The first isolation procedures from venom of VIPERA RUSSELLI (TAKAHASHI et al., 1972) included rechromatography and yielded 6 mg pure inhibitor substance from 100 mg venom; the highest concentration so far found in all snake species investigated (TAKAHASHI et al., 1974d, c). Three species from VIPERIDAE and six from ELAPIDAE were found to contain inhibitors in the venom (TAKAHASHI et al., 1974d). However, this is not a common principle because the inhibition spectra are different (e.g., for kallikrein) and no inhibitor was found in around 30 species.

Isolation and properties: For isolation steps see reviews (TAKAHASHI et al., 1974c; IWANAGA et al., 1976). From the two main fractions, the one representing the larger part was extensively examined. RUSSELL's viper venom inhibitor fraction II is characterized as follows: basic protein, MW ~ 7000 (TAKAHASHI et al., 1972). Fraction I has a lower MW. The amino acid composition for inhibitors I and II is given (TAKAHASHI et al., 1974c); inhibitor II was sequenced (TAKAHASHI et al., 1974b, c). The sequence is more than 50% identical with BPTI (TAKAHASHI et al., 1974a) with three disulfide bridges in identical positions. The authors conclude from the parallel sequence a similar conformation (see Tables 8 and 2). Data of the two inhibitors resemble those compounds later found in cobra venoms (HOKAMA et al., 1976) (review IWANAGA et al., 1976), but differ by content of Trp; the number of disulfide bridges is also different.

Inhibition spectrum (see Tables 10–12): From the common specification, snake venom inhibitors are of polyvalent character. Trypsin, chymotrypsin, and plasmin are inhibited; $K_i = 7.6 \times 10^{-10}\,M$ (trypsin), $1.4 \times 10^{-10}\,M$ (chymotrypsin), and $1.0 \times 10^{-9}\,M$ (plasmin) have been reported (TAKAHASHI et al., 1974c). The resemblance, but not identity, of the sequence with BPTI explains the strong inhibition of serum kallikrein by all RUSSELL's viper venom inhibitor fractions examined (TAKAHASHI et al., 1974c; HOKAMA et al., 1976), K_i for bovine plasma kallikrein-fraction II complex is estimated to be $2.9 \times 10^{-10}\,M$.

Biology: Variations in the structure of the snake inhibitors may contribute to theories on the phylogenesis of the widespread BPTI analogs. From the studies of STRYDOM (for references see STRYDOM, 1977) one can conclude that substances with similar structure are found in other species. The sequence of the venom compound of DENDROASPIS is homologous to BPTI, including the reactive site, Lys_{26}, responsible for a weak trypsin inhibiting activity. A sequence change in Lys–Arg results in marginal inhibitory properties.

III. Kallikrein Inhibitors of Animal Origin of HMW and/or Not Fully Characterized

1. Kallikrein Inhibitors in ANNELIDA

Till 1974, only the trypsin and chymotrypsin inhibitors of ASCARIS were known in ASCHELMINTHES. Now, in ANNELIDA two species were found with kallikrein inhibiting compounds in the tissue (see Table 13).

From POLYCHAETAE, SABELLASTARTE INDICA was investigated by GAUWERKY et al. (1975). The extract from tentacles, only utilized for raw preparation, was fractionated in disc electrophoresis and yielded five active compounds. The inhibitory capacity of the crude preparation was 4–5 IU/g dry weight (i.e., 9.6 IU/mg protein) determined with trypsin or 5.7 IU/mg protein determined with pig pancreatic kallikrein. Chymotrypsin, plasmin, and thrombin are also inhibited.

Properties: The substance is stable against 0.08 M perchloric acid at normal temperature. During electrophoresis the inhibitor migrates towards the anode. The MW was estimated by gel filtration and disc electrophoresis as 25,100. The molecule is a glycoprotein.

Table 13. Kallikrein inhibition by inhibitors of *Annelida*, submandibular gland and kidney tubules

Species	Kallikreins		Authors
Polychaetae spec.	Porcine pancreas	+A	GAUWERKY et al. (1975)
Oligochaetae spec.	Porcine pancreas	+A	ILLCHMANN and WERLE (1974)
Rat submand.	Rat submand.	+B	BERALDO et al. (1974)
Dog submand.	Porcine serum	−A	WUNDERER et al. (1972)
	Human serum	−A	WUNDERER et al. (1972)
Kidney tubules rat	Rat kidney	−A	GEIGER and MANN (1976)
		+B	GEIGER and MANN (1976)
	Rat urinary	−A	GEIGER and MANN (1976)
		+B	GEIGER and MANN (1976)
	Porcine pancreas	−A	GEIGER and MANN (1976)
		+B	GEIGER and MANN (1976)
	Porcine submand.	−A	GEIGER and MANN (1976)
		+B	GEIGER and MANN (1976)
	Human urine	−A	GEIGER and MANN (1976)
		+B	GEIGER and MANN (1976)

A = Assay with synthetic substrate; B = Bioassay in vitro.

From OLIGOCHAETA, the tissue of LUMBRICUS TERRESTRIS has a trypsin-inhibiting capacity of 150 ± 30 mIU/g wet weight (ILLCHMANN and WERLE, 1974). The substance, partially purified by affinity chromatography, had a specific activity of 3.7 IU/mg protein. Preliminary studies resulted in 62 amino acid residues in the molecule of MW 6100 (as determined by gel chromatography). Electrophoretically, the preparation could be separated into several components. Besides porcine pancreatic kallikrein, trypsin, and plasmin are also inhibited. The inhibition of trypsin was determined to be of temporary type.

Physiological function: Studies of the function of the inhibitor of earth worm gave indication for the occurence of the substance in the gastrointestinal tract in a masked form, i.e., as a proteinase complex (ILLCHMANN and WERLE, 1974). The function may be protection against self-digestion and/or microbial action.

2. Kallikrein Inhibition by Egg White

Kallikreins are inhibited by an extremely labile fraction of egg white (FREY et al., 1968). The components ovomucoid and ovoinhibitor differ strongly from each other (for differentiation see FEENEY, 1971; LIU et al., 1971). So far, no experiments have been published concerning the specificity of "ovoinhibitor" (see review VOGEL et al., 1968) against kallikreins. This is also true for the "ficin and papain inhibitor" (for characterization see SEN and WHITAKER, 1973) and the rennin inhibitor "ovomucin" (KATO et al., 1974).

All results reported were based on experiments using commercial egg white trypsin inhibitor "EWTI". Preparations from whole egg white obviously contain mixtures of all inhibitor fractions (e.g., Sigma preparation II-O; a mixture of ovomucoid and ovoinhibitor). ZANEVELD et al. (1971) report inhibition of plasma kallikrein by chicken ovomucoid, the only ovomucoid species of Arg-type; all other avian

Table 14. Inhibition of kallikreins by egg white fractions

Kallikreins	Ovomucoid	EWTI
Serum, rat		±AC [2] ±C [4]
Serum, porcine	−A [1]	
Serum, human	−A [1] +A [3] ±C [4] −A [5]	 −AC [2]
Rat submand.	±ABC [6, 8]	
pancreas		−AC [7]
Guinea-pig submand.	−AB [8]	
Hamster submand.	−AB [8]	
Rabbit submand.	−AB [8]	
Bovine pancreas	−B [9]	
Porcine pancreas	−AB [10]	±C [4]
udder	−C [11]	
Cat submand.	−AB [8]	
Dog pancreas		−AC [7]
submand.	−AB [8]	
colon	(−)AB [12]	
Monkey colon	−AB [12]	
Human submand.	−AB [10], −A [14]	±C [4]
urine	−A [13]	±C [4]

A = Assay with synthetic substrate; B = Bioassay in vitro; C = Bioassay in vivo.
1. WUNDERER et al. (1972); 2. MORIYA and HOJIMA (1972); 3. FRITZ and WUNDERER (1972); 4. HOJIMA et al. (1973b); 5. VEREMIENKO et al. (1974); 6. ERDÖS et al. (1968a); 7. HOJIMA et al. (1975b); 8. BHOOLA and DOREY (1971); 9. BACK (1973); 10. MORIWAKI and SCHACHTER (1971); 11. PEETERS et al. (1976);12. SEKI et al. (1972); 13. MATSUDA et al. (1976); 14. MODÉER (1977b).

species have Lys-type ovomucoids, (LIU et al., 1971). HOJIMA et al. (1973b) state that the egg white trypsin inhibitor, Sigma II-O, "hardly showed inhibitory activities" against various kallikreins (see Table 14). All other experiments were negative with exception of some doubtful positive bioassays.

In conclusion, the egg white factors so far studied are not inhibitors of kallikreins.

3. Kallikrein Inhibitor in Rat Submaxillary Gland

A compound was separated with inhibitory activity from acetone precipitate of submandibular glands after gel filtration on Sephadex G-100 (SIQUEIRA and BERALDO, 1973; RODRIGUES and BERALDO, 1973; BERALDO et al., 1974). This substance was tested against rat submaxillary kallikrein in bioassay (uterus-contracting activity) (see Table 14). The substance in question is of lower MW than kallikrein. In bioassay, trypsin was not inhibited. The inhibitor content of submaxillary glands increases during development of the rats; a period when the kallikrein content is still low (see FREY et al., 1968).

4. Rat Kidney Tubule Kallikrein-Specific Inhibitor

In 1976, studies on the synthesis of urinary kallikrein resulted in the detection of an inhibitor in rat kidney (GEIGER and MANN, 1976).

Isolation: Kidney tubules were prepared by decomposing the tissue with collagenase. From the supernatant of the mixture, obtained without harsh treatment, kallikrein, kininase, and inhibitor were separated on Sephadex G-100 in one step.

Properties: In gel electrophoresis the inhibitor was homogeneous and consisted of one acid stable fraction with a LMW of 4700.

Specific kallikrein inhibition: All kallikreins are inhibited: 30 μg pure inhibitor binds 93% of 200 mU rat urinary kallikrein or 75% of the same amount of human urinary kallikrein. 400 mU of other kallikreins (see Table 13) were 62–75% inhibited. Only the kininogenase activity of the kallikreins is influenced. Inhibition of the cleavage of synthetic substrates (BAEe) was not observed (GEIGER and MANN, 1976).

The rat kidney kallikrein inhibitor is the only inhibitor reported which binds all kallikreins, but *not* trypsin. GEIGER and MANN (1976) discuss several reasons: The inhibitor may be attached to the enzyme in a position different from the active center of the enzyme; the inhibition may be a result of allosteric effects; the synthetic substrate competes with the inhibitor and the complex dissociates. In any case, the authors observed BAEe cleavage by the kallikrein-inhibitor complex. Therefore, the inhibition is not due to breakdown of the enzyme as discussed by MILLS et al. (1975) in preliminary studies with rabbit kidney and bovine pancreatic kallikrein in vitro and in vivo.

Biology: Inhibition of the kinin system may affect components of other regulatory systems, e.g., prostaglandins (GEIGER and MANN, 1976). Previous reports concerning the presence of kallikrein inhibitor in rat urine after experimental injuries of the renal tubules (VOGEL et al., 1968) point to pathophysiological imbalance.

IV. Protein Proteinase Inhibitors in Plants

1. Soybean Inhibitor (Kunitz)

From the soybean inhibitors isolated (see review BIRK, 1976) only "Kunitz soybean trypsin inhibitor" (SBTI) has a configuration essential for kallikrein, especially serum kallikrein, inhibition.

a) Isolation and Purification of Commercial Preparations

In comparing the gel electrophoretically separated fractions of different seed specimens, CLARK and HYMOWITZ (1972) found statistically significant variants of SBTI with regard to trypsin-inhibiting activity. Most of the experiments were done with commercial SBTI preparations (i.e., Merck, Serva, Sigma, Worthington). For studies on kallikrein inhibition it is recommended that critical tests should be made of uncharacterized SBTI preparations. The inhibitor compound "Bowman-Birk soybean trypsin inhibitor" lacks kallikrein inhibiting capacity and can be separated quantitatively from SBTI by gel filtration (WUNDERER et al., 1972; FRITZ and WUNDERER, 1972; FRITZ et al., 1972c). Gel chromatography on Sephadex G-100

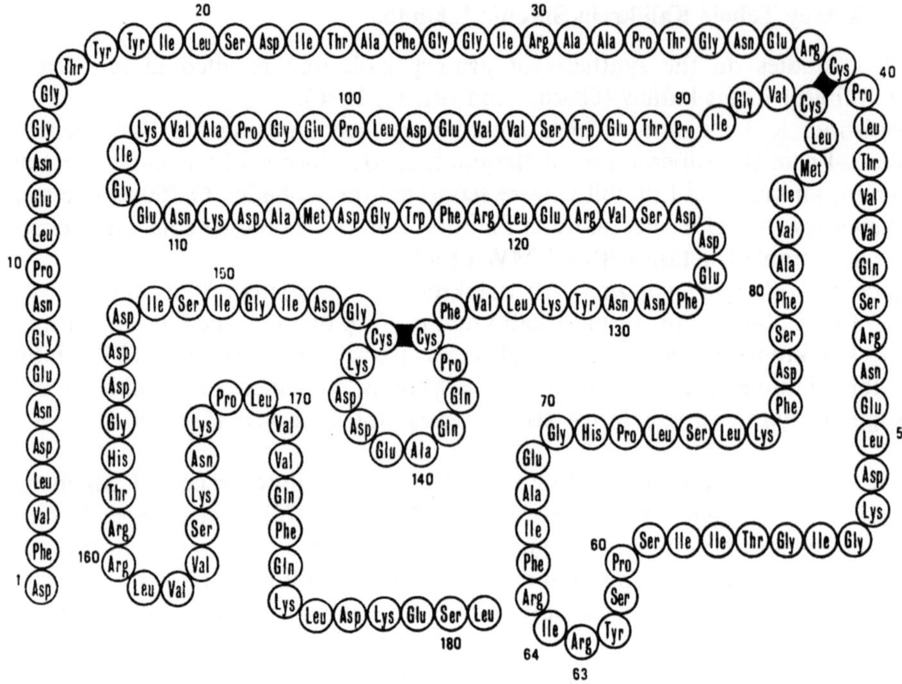

Fig. 2. Complete amino acid sequence of SBTI (KOIDE and IKENAKA, 1973b)

resulted in a preparation with two bands of impurities (<5% of the amount tested) (QUAST and STEFFEN, 1975). Gel electrophoretic separation (CLARK and HYMOWITZ, 1972; BIETH and FRECHIN, 1974) suggested that the impurities were elastase inhibitors (BIETH and FRECHIN, 1974). The amount by which small methodic errors can change the structure of SBTI are reported by ODANI et al. (1971).

b) Structure

From fragment studies, the amino acid composition must be revised from 202 to 181 residues and the MW to 20,100 (KOIDE and IKENAKA, 1973a). Initial work for characterization was done with sequence studies of four fragments (KOIDE and IKENAKA, 1973a). Further proteolytic breakdown and Edman degradation isolated the amino-terminal part of the molecule with 84 residues including the reactive site P_1–P'_1 as Arg_{63}–Ile_{64}[1] (KOIDE et al., 1973) (see Table 2). In finishing these experiments, the group published the amino acid sequence of SBTI (KOIDE and IKENAKA, 1973b) (Fig. 2).

Circular dichroism and optical rotatory dispersion studies showed no α-helix conformation (IKEDA et al., 1968). This conclusion has been confirmed in recent studies. Although experiments suggest partial helical structure (NAKANISHI and TSUBOI, 1974), KOIDE and IKENAKA (1973b) assumed a similar conformation as

[1] The full sequence resulted in change of the residue numbers: Arg_{63} is referred to in former papers as Arg_{64}.

BPTI with an equal exposed reactive site on the surface of the molecule. X-ray studies of SWEET et al. (1974) confirm that no α-helix structure exists.

From X-ray studies of the trypsin complex in comparison with the known data for trypsin, SWEET et al. (1974) calculated the radius of the molecule as 18 Å. In 6 *M* guanidine a slight unfolding was observed by viscosity measurements. At 25 °C in 2 weeks or at 70 °C in 15 min there was a remarkable change in hydrodynamic radius from 24 Å to 38 Å without loss of activity (FISH and LEACH, 1973).

The partial sequences 1–135 and 136–197 are both inactive, but KATO and TOMINAGA (1970) regained a compound with 80% of the native activity by recombining fractions obtained after gel filtration of the fragments. They observed up to 30% association of the fragments. These fragments have no regular tertiary structure as shown by circular dichroism spectra (KOIDE et al., 1974). In association, the configuration is similar to the native configuration. The time for this conformational reconstitution is 1 h with 70% yield. If this compound is concentrated by lyophilization, a "temporary inhibition" is observed (KOIDE et al., 1974). Selectively oxidizing Trp_{93} obviously accounts for the incomplete inhibitory capacity of the reconstituted compound, either in the inhibitor activity or in the formation of the essential tertiary structure.

From the 170 peptide NH groups known from the X-ray studies (see complex), 83 are involved in peptide-peptide hydrogen bonds of SBTI, as determined by the deuterium exchange reaction (NAKANISHI and TSUBOI, 1974). The resulting number does not correspond with the results of ELLIS et al. (1975). They state that only eight protons are not exchangeable. It was indicated that in complex reaction the solvent accessibility is reduced (WOODWARD and ELLIS, 1975). The proton exchange rate is markedly reduced as compared with the rates of the two single proteins. A reduction by hydrogen bonding alone can be excluded (WOODWARD and ELLIS, 1975). Reduced SBTI, reoxidized even under special conditions, e.g., in the presence of protein disulfide isomerase, cannot recover the original structure. Although enzymatically supported, the disulfide bridges do not reorganize in precise conformational order (HAWKINS and FREEDMAN, 1975).

c) Reactive Site

The sequence around the reactive site Arg_{63}–Ile_{64}(LIU et al., 1968; for chymotrypsin BIDLINGMEYER et al., 1972) including P_4–P'_4 is unique in the molecule, although other partial sequences are repeated (KOIDE and IKENAKA, 1973b). For chymotrypsin, besides P_1–P'_1, a second reactive site exists, SBTI being a "double-headed" inhibitor of this proteinase (LASKOWSKI JR. et al., 1974; QUAST and STEFFEN, 1975), but not through duplication or elongation of the molecule as reported for other inhibitors (QUAST and STEFFEN, 1975).

The reactive site is reshaped during complex formation (for review see LASKOWSKI JR. and SEALOCK, 1971) changing from "native" to "modified" inhibitor (see complex with trypsin). NMR-studies of histidine residues in native and modified SBTI make it obvious that His_{71}, although not involved in the reactive site, is altered during reactive site-modifying reactions (MARKLEY, 1973a, b; MARKLEY and KATO, 1975). X-ray analysis shows a position close to the reactive site (JANIN et al., 1974). The abnormal pK value of native SBTI is normalized in modified SBTI perhaps with structural loosening (MATTIS and LASKOWSKI JR., 1973). The Arg_{63} carboxyl terminal in modified SBTI cleaved by trypsin has a pK value of 3.56; the Ile_{64} amino terminal has a pK of 7.89 (MATTIS and LASKOWSKI JR., 1973).

Treatment of SBTI with N-acetylimidazole resulted in acetylation of two Tyr, and to a smaller degree, of a third Tyr residue. Low percentage acetylation does not affect inhibitor activity but a 50% reduction is obtained by acetylation of an average of two Tyr residues per mole SBTI. The only reason seems to be a neighboring Tyr residue in P_2 of the reactive site (GORBUNOFF, 1968, 1970). This theory was supported by findings of PAPAIOANNOU and LIENER (1970). If the trypsin-SBTI complex is acetylated and the proteins cleaved, four free Tyr are found, two belonging to trypsin and two to SBTI. Tyr-acetylated SBTI itself is fully active.

LASKOWSKI JR. and co-workers gained insight into the role of the amino acid residues around the reactive site. Their experiments were performed partly by chemical treatment and partly enzymatically (see Table 15). In position P'_1 smaller residues than Ile are tolerated. If the chain is elongated, e.g., Arg_{63}-endo amino acid-Ile_{64} (with Ile, Ala, or Glu as for the endo amino acid), the incubation with trypsin does not result in inhibition of the enzyme but in partial restitution of the P_1–P'_1 bond (KOWALSKI and LASKOWSKI JR., 1976b). Insertion of an amino acid between P_1 and P'_1 changes the inhibitor to a substrate for trypsin.

d) Complex Formation with Trypsin

Calorimetric measurement of the complex formation with trypsin at pH 5 gave $\Delta H = 8.6$ Kcal/mol at 25 °C. This changed to an apparent positive enthalpy at pH 6.5, and to 4 Kcal/mol at pH 8 (BAUGH et al., 1973). Measurements of BARNHILL and TROWBRIDGE (1975) gave values of 4 Kcal/mol less at pH 5 but other values agreed. This effect is discussed by SWEET et al. (1974) in relation to the tight binding of SBTI and BPTI. The exothermic effect obviously is attributable to one of the His residues (His_{71}) of SBTI (BARNHILL and TROWBRIDGE, 1975); this residue being perturbed by the modification of SBTI.

e) X-ray Studies on the Three-Dimensional Structure

Based on studies of BPTI, parallel experiments were made on crystallized SBTI-trypsin complex. After innoculation, crystallization settles in 3–12 weeks to orthorhombic crystals (SWEET et al., 1974). At a resolution of 2.6 Å, it could be seen that only a small part of the molecule is integrated in the complex formation (BLOW et al., 1974), the total molecule structure not being determined. For the SBTI-trypsin complex a tetrahedral intermediate was assumed similar to that of BPTI. In the crystals of the complex of porcine trypsin with SBTI, at least 300 interatomic contacts were counted (SWEET et al., 1974). From the X-ray studies, the contact sequences of SBTI are referred to as residues 1–2, 13, 61–66, 68, 71–72, and 116 (JANIN et al., 1974).

SWEET et al. (1974), studied the dimeric molecular aggregate of the complex and found that the positions around 63 and 64 had high electron density and filled the trypsin pocket. The structure around these positions is a sphere of 35 Å in diameter. A second contact site is located 15 Å distant from the reactive site and is interesting in view of the selective inhibition of serum kallikreins. In comparing

Table 15. Effect of Arg_{63} or Ile_{64} replacement in the reactive site of SBTI

$P_1 = Arg_{63}$ changed to:	
Lys	Complex dissociates more slowly (Kowalski et al., 1974[a])
Trp	Specific and strong chymotrypsin inhibitor (Kowalski et al., 1974) (Leary and Laskowski Jr., 1973)
Phe	Faster rate of dissociation (Kowalski et al., 1974)
Des-Arg	Inactive (Sealock and Laskowski Jr., 1969)
$P_1' = Ile_{64}$ changed to:	
Gly	As native (Kowalski et al., 1974) (Kowalski and Laskowski Jr., 1976a)
Ala	As native (Kowalski et al., 1974) (Kowalski and Laskowski Jr., 1976a)
Leu	As native (Kowalski et al., 1974) (Kowalski and Laskowski Jr., 1976a)
Des-Ile	Inactive (Kowalski et al., 1974) (Kowalski and Laskowski Jr., 1976a)
Carbamyl-Ile	Inactive (Kowalski et al., 1974)
Acetamido-Ile	Inactive (Kowalski et al., 1974)
$P_1 - X - P_1'$	Change from inhibitor to substrate (Kowalski and Laskowski Jr., 1976b)

[a] Kowalski et al. (1974) = Review.

Table 16. Conformation of the main chain at the reactive site of BPTI nd SBTI complexes (Taken from Sweet et al. (1975)

	BPTI[a]	Site	SBTI	
Pro_{13}	$\phi = -86$ $\psi = -28$	P_3	$\phi = -46$ $\psi = -21$	Ser_{61}
Cys_{14}	$\phi = -64$ $\psi = 152$	P_2	$\phi = -77$ $\psi = 136$	Tyr_{62}
Lys_{15}	$\phi = -116$ $\psi = 87$	P_1	$\phi = -89$ $\psi = 85$	Arg_{63}
Ala_{16}	$\phi = -135$ $\psi = 166$	P_1'	$\phi = -135$ $\psi = -115$	Ile_{64}
Arg_{17}	$\phi = -116$ $\psi = -87$	P_2'	$\phi = -175$ $\psi = -179$	Arg_{65}

[a] Huber and coworkers, personal communication to Sweet.

the dihedral angles of BPTI and SBTI (see Table 16) in the reactive site and corresponding configuration (see Fig. 3), there is a striking similarity; the differences are partly due to experimental errors (Sweet et al., 1974; Janin et al., 1974).

The formation of SBTI-trypsin complex is also indirect as described for BPTI, a series of several reaction steps (see review Laskowski Jr. and Sealock, 1971; Finkenstadt et al., 1974), at least:

$$E + I \underset{k-1}{\overset{k1}{\rightleftharpoons}} L \underset{k-2}{\overset{k2}{\rightleftharpoons}} C \underset{k-3}{\overset{k3}{\rightleftharpoons}} L^* \underset{k-4}{\overset{k4}{\rightleftharpoons}} E + I^*$$

E = free enzyme
I = native inhibitor I^* = modified (P_1–P_1' hydrolyzed) inhibitor
C = stable comlex
L = loose complex E–I L^* = loose complex E–I^*

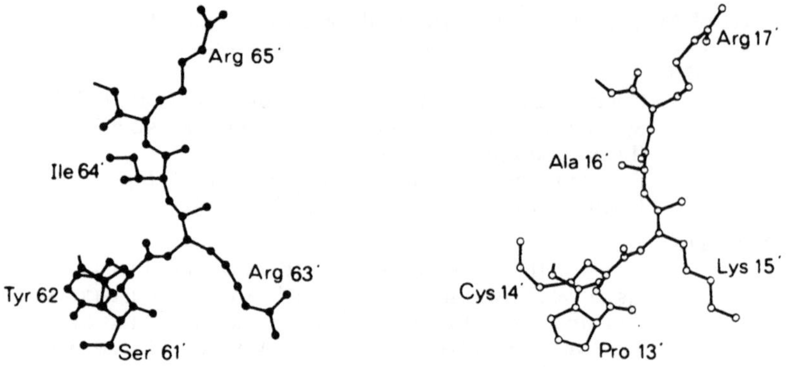

a b

Fig. 3a and b. Comparison of the reactive site of SBTI, **a** (SWEET et al., 1974) and BPTI, **b** (RÜHLMANN et al., 1973)

The first step results in a relatively loose Michaelis-Menten complex, L ($K_i \sim 10^{-4}$–10^{-6} M for trypsin). The following reaction step is the rate-determining one ($K_i < 10^{-8}$ M). This reaction mechanism, theoretically postulated by LASKOWSKI JR. was established by stopped-flow analysis of the system (LUTHY et al., 1973). The first order rate of the reaction was shown by HIXON JR. and LASKOWSKI JR. (1970). It follows that other considerations based on the form of a second order reaction are unimportant. In the reaction steps an acyl-enzyme intermediate in equilibrium with the tetrahedral compound seems to be involved (HUANG and LIENER, 1977). The abnormal rigid region of the inhibitor molecule results in low K_{hyd} values because only relatively little relaxation follows the hydrolysis of $P_1 - P_1'$ (MATTIS and LASKOWSKI JR., 1973; FINKENSTADT et al., 1974).

f) Inhibition of Kallikrein (see Tables 17 and 18)

SBTI is an example of a serum kallikrein inhibitor. The inhibitor constant is low $K_i = 5 \times 10^{-9}$ M (pig serum kallikrein) when compared with BPTI ($K_i = 1 \times 10^{-7}$ M for serum kallikrein and $K_i = 1 \times 10^{-8}$ M for glandular kallikrein) (WUNDERER et al., 1972). However, in the test medium of porcine serum kallikrein and SBTI a remarkable dissociation can be observed so that the estimation of K_i only gives an approximate value (WUNDERER et al., 1972). The lack of inhibition of glandular kallikreins may be explained by comparing the configuration of trypsin and pancreatic kallikrein. With X-ray studies (SWEET et al., 1974), a close relationship is found between Leu_{99} of trypsin and P_2 of SBTI. In pig pancreatic kallikrein, the corresponding residue is Tyr (TSCHESCHE et al., 1976). For discussion of substrate/inhibitor affinity see FIEDLER (this Vol., p. 103). For additional inhibition spectra see Table 19.

2. LEGUMINOSAE: Inhibitors of Other Species

In addition to known plasmin inhibitors in peanuts (see VOGEL et al., 1968), the search for kallikrein inhibitors was successful. Extracts from peanuts (ARACHIS HYPOGAEA) were separated by affinity chromatography (HOCHSTRASSER et al., 1969a) and after rechromatography yielded two inhibitor fractions with a MW

Table 17. Inhibition of glandular kallikreins by inhibitors from soybean, peanut, and potato

Kallikrein	SBTI	Peanut	Potato: PKI	Potato: Hochstrasser	Potato: Ryan I
Rat					
pancreas	(+)ABC [1]/(+)AC [2]		(+)AC [2]		
submand.	+AB [3]				
Mouse					
submand.	−A [4]				
Guinea-pig					
submand.	−AB [3]			−C [5]	
Hamster					
submand.	−AB [3]				
Rabbit					
submand.	+AB [3]				
Pig					
udder	−B [10]				
urine		−C [5]	−C [11]	−C [5]	
pancreas	−AC [9]	−C [5]	+AB [7]/+AC [6, 8, 11, 12]	−C [5]	−AC [6]
submand.		−C [5]		−C [5]	
Cat					
submand.	+AB [3]				
Dog					
colon	+AB [13]				
urine	−C [11]				
pancreas	−AC [2, 12]/−C [11]		+AC [2]		
submand.	−AB [3]				
Monkey					
colon	+AB [13]				
Human					
colon	+AB [13]				
urine	−ABC [17]/−C [11]/−AC [9]/−A [15]		(+)AC [6]/−AC [9]		+AC [6]
pancreas			−C [11]		
submand., saliva	−AC [9]/(+)A [16]	±A [14]	+AB [7]/(+)AC [6]/−AC [9]		+AC [6]

A = Assay with synthetic substrate; B = Bioassay in vitro; C = Bioassay in vivo.
1. Erdös et al. (1968a, b); 2. Hojima et al. (1975b); 3. Bhoola and Dorey (1971); 4. Ekfors and Hopsu-Havu (1972); 5. Hochstrasser et al. (1969a); 6. Hojima et al. (1971); 7. Moriwaki and Schachter (1971); 8. Hojima et al. (1973a, 1975a); 9. Hojima et al. (1973b); 10. Peeters et al. (1976); 11. Moriwaki et al. (1976b); 12. Hojima et al. (1977); 13. Seki et al. (1972); 14. Fujimoto et al. (1973); 15. Matsuda et al. (1976); 16. Modéer (1977b); 17. Moriya et al. (1973).

Table 18. Inhibition of serum kallikrein of different species by soybean, peanut, and potato inhibitors

Kallikrein species	SBTI	Peanut	Potato			
			PKI	Commercial Preparation (Behring)	Ryan I	Ryan II
Turtle	+C [1]					
Alligator	(+)B [1]					
Rat	+C [2]		+C [2]			
	±AC [3]		±AC [3]		−AC [3]	
Porcine	+A [4]	+A [4]			−A [4]	+A [4]
Human					−A [4]	+A [4]
	±AC [2, 3]		+AC [3]		−AC [5]	−A [3]
	+A [4]	+A [4]				
	+A [6]		+A [6]			
				−A [6]		
			+C [2]		−AC [5]	
	+A [7]	+A [4]	+AC [5]		−A [4]	+A [4]
	+A [4]					
	+A [8]					
	Bowman-Birk fraction					
	human − A [4]					
	porcine − A [4]					

A = Assay with synthetic substrate; B = Bioassay in vitro; C = Bioassay in vivo.
1. SEKI et al. (1973); 2. HOJIMA et al. (1973b); 3. MORIYA and HOJIMA (1972); 4. WUNDERER et al. (1972); 5. HOJIMA et al. (1971); 6. FRITZ and WUNDERER (1972); 7. ASGHAR et al. (1976); 8. VEREMIENKO et al. (1974).
Footnote: A trypsin inhibitor which inhibits serum kallikrein was used by MASON and SPARROW (1965). Correction of Table 7 in VOGEL and WERLE (1970).

of 17,000. The mixture of the partly characterized (HOCHSTRASSER et al., 1969a) isoinhibitors had an inhibitory capacity of 4.8 IU/mg protein (FRITZ et al., 1972c). The potent chymotrypsin inhibitors inhibit only serum kallikrein of the kallikreins tested (see Tables 17–19) (HOCHSTRASSER et al., 1969a). This inhibitor belongs to the Arg-type (Table 20).

3. Kallikrein Inhibitors in SOLANACEAE

a) Inhibitors of Potatoes

Different working groups found several inhibitors in potatoes with different inhibition spectra (for review see BIRK, 1976; RYAN and SANTARIUS, 1976). In the last years only one group described a specific kallikrein inhibitor in detail, this being different from the inhibitor described by WERLE's group (see review VOGEL et al., 1968). From the observations on animal material (e.g., snails) the differences observed may be attributed to species variation. However, there are certainly at least two groups of different MW.

Table 19. Inhibition spectrum of SBTI, peanut and potato inhibitors

Enzyme	SBTI	Peanut	Potato		
			PKI	Ryan I	Ryan II
Trypsin, human	(+) [1, 4]			– [1]	
animal			(+) [2]		
Chymotrypsin			(+) [2]		
Plasmin, human	+ [1]			– [1]	
Acrosin	+ [3, 13]	+ [3]			
Leukocyte	(+) [5]				
proteinase (kininogenase)	+ [6, 9]				
Kininogenase microbial	+ [7]				
Human pancreas proteinase	+ [8]				
Kininogenase snake venom	+ [10]				
Esteroprotease submand. mouse, rat	– [11]				
Skin human proteinase	+ [12]				
Kininogenase macrophages	+ [14]				

1. Feeney et al. (1969); 2. Hojima et al. (1973b); 3. Fritz et al. (1972c); 4. Mallory and Travis (1973); 5. Movat et al. (1976); 6. Bretz et al. (1976); 7. Vargaftig and Giroux (1976a, b); 8. Mallory and Travis (1974); 9. Kruze et al. (1976); 10. Geiger and Kortmann (1977); 11. Angeletti et al. (1973); 12. Fräki and Hopsu-Havu (1975); 13. Stambaugh et al. (1969); 14. Greenbaum et al. (1969).

Table 20. Reactive site amino acids of plant inhibitors

	P_1	P'_1	
Peanut	Arg	Ser	Hochstrasser et al. (1970)
Potato, Ryan I	Leu	Asp	Kiyohara et al. (1973); Richardson and Cossins (1974)
Potato, Ryan II	Lys	Ser	Iwasaki et al. (1973)

The HMW potato fraction "(chymotrypsin) inhibitor I" (Ryan, 1966) with a MW of 32,000 has an activity in the pure state of 0.8 IU/mg (Ryan cf. Wunderer et al., 1972). It is also an inhibitor of human salivary and urinary kallikreins, but not of hog pancreatic or human plasma kallikrein (Hojima et al., 1971; Melville and Ryan, 1972). Ryan and co-workers, separating RUSSET BURBANK potato tuber inhibitors, obtained fraction II which preferentially inhibited trypsin and chymotrypsin, but also inhibited kallikrein. Isolation (Bryant et al., 1976) on Sephadex G-75 and rechromatography on phosphocellulose in the presence of 8 *M* urea yielded four isoinhibitor fractions. Amino acid composition suggested a MW of 10,000 ± 1000 for the monomer. A dimeric form was also found. The compound is stable between pH 2.2 and 10.6. With this "fraction II," WUNDERER et al. (1972) observed weak inhibition of pig and human serum kallikrein. At this time this fraction was only partially separated and characterized from fraction I (RYAN and SHUMWAY, 1971; MELVILLE and RYAN, 1972), which has no serum kallikrein inhibiting capacity (WUNDERER et al., 1972). For the reactive site of fraction I and II (RYAN) see Table 20.

The nine different inhibitor fractions of BELITZ and co-workers from various German species of potato (KAISER and BELITZ, 1973; KAISER et al., 1974) were not extensively tested for kallikrein inhibition. Unfractionated extracts do not inhibit pancreatic kallikrein (KAISER and BELITZ, 1973). HOCHSTRASSER et al. (1969 b) described three main trypsin-chymotrypsin inhibiting fractions isolated by affinity chromatography. These Arg-type inhibitors with a mean MW of 24,000 inhibit serum kallikrein (HOCHSTRASSER et al., 1969 b). Inhibitors in Japanese potato species (for references see IWASAKI et al., 1976) mostly have not been tested for kallikrein inhibition. Only SAWADA et al. (1974) reported separation of a pure inhibitor fraction of MW 5500 into six isoinhibitors during rechromatography. Two of them were weak kallikrein inhibitors, one of which obviously inhibits kallikrein preferentially (kallikrein source not indicated). Properties of this compound: isoelectric point > 10, stable for 30 min at 75 °C in acid medium (SAWADA et al., 1974).

MORIYA and co-workers described two potato kallikrein inhibitors in detail (MORIYA et al., 1970; HOJIMA et al., 1971). The two main fractions with the unusual isoelectric points at pH 5.6 and pH 6.4 were named PKI-56 and PKI-64 (MORIYA et al., 1970; HOJIMA et al., 1973 a). The isolated inhibitors were homogeneous in disc electrophoresis. The sedimentation coefficients were $S_{20,w} = 2.20$ and 2.27 for the two inhibitors. From amino acid composition and gel filtration on Sephadex, the MWs were calculated as 22,000–24,000 (HOJIMA et al., 1973 a). No carbohydrate component was found in the molecule. Comparison of the amino acid composition showed no relationship to the trypsin inhibitors of HOCHSTRASSER et al. (1969 b). For reactive site see Table 20. From the MW of the complex, a binding of kallikrein in a 1:1 ratio was concluded (HOJIMA et al., 1973 a). The inhibition of both esterolytic and vasodilator activity of pig pancreatic kallikrein was described (HOJIMA et al., 1973 a). Using highly purified pig pancreatic kallikrein, the inhibitory activity of the preparation was reported as 395 IU/mg for PKI-56 and 611 IU/mg for PKI-64.

After further experiments it was stated that the inhibitory capacity is dependent on the purity of the kallikrein preparations. Partially purified kallikrein preparations are inhibited only with an activity of around 210 IU/mg (HOJIMA et al., 1975 b).

Pure dog pancreatic kallikrein preparations are inhibited by PKI-56 and PKI-64 with an activity of 350 and 800 IU/mg, respectively (HOJIMA et al., 1977). The inhibition by PKI-64 is stoichiometric up to 70% inhibition. Thus, 2 KU are inhibited 95% by 10 µg PKI-56 and 85% by 10 µg PKI-64 (MORIWAKI et al., 1976 b).

For complex formation with porcine pancreatic kallikrein there are two pH optima, pH 8.0, and pH 6.0, the latter being unusual (HOJIMA et al., 1973 b). The dissociation constant using porcine pancreatic kallikrein was $K_i = 4.0 \times 10^{-6}\,M$ for PKI-56 and $2.2 \times 10^{-6}\,M$ for PKI 64 with BAEe as substrate (HOJIMA et al., 1973 b). Stronger inhibition was observed against plasma kallikrein and weaker inhibition against salivary and urine kallikrein (HOJIMA et al., 1973 b). Trypsin and chymotrypsin are inhibited very weakly (Hojima et al., 1973a, b). Thus, these inhibitors are not related to the typical trypsin or chymotrypsin inhibitors. For inhibition spectra of the different compounds see Tables 17–19.

b) Inhibitors of Other Species

From SCOPOLIA JAPONICA, five inhibitors were isolated by affinity chromatography and rechromatography (Sakato et al., 1975), and the amino acid composition given. The relatively stable inhibitors are of LMW (3700–6000). Together with high activity against trypsin, chymotrypsin, and plasmin, pancreatic kallikrein is inhibited in the same order of magnitude when tested with synthetic substrate. Inhibition of the first two enzymes is noncompetitive.

V. Peptide Inhibitors of Kallikrein From Microorganisms

Proteinase inhibitors from ACTINOMYCETES: Among all microbial inhibitors (see review Wingender, 1974; Iwanaga et al., 1976) two are of special interest because of their activity against kallikrein.

In 1969 the occurence of proteinase inhibitors in culture media of microorganisms (different species of ACTINOMYCETES) was reported (Aoyagi et al., 1969a, b). The substance, named leupeptin, was isolated and characterized as two peptide aldehydes (Kondo et al., 1969; Maeda et al., 1971) and was synthetized in the same year (Kawamura et al., 1969). For isolation methods see review Umezawa (1976).

Experiments were made with the mixture of the two compounds Acetyl–Leu–Leu-argininal and Propionyl–Leu–Leu-argininal. Another substance, named antipain,

┌─Phe

with the structure OC–Arg–Val-argininal was found by Umezawa et al. (1972). For isolation steps see Umezawa (1976). Physicochemical data of this peptide were reported by Suda et al. (1972) and reviewed by Umezawa (1972, 1976).

The broad spectrum of competitive inhibition – plasmin, trypsin, papain, thrombokinase, and kallikrein – of leupeptin was reported in the first publications (Aoyagi et al., 1969a; Suda et al., 1972; Ikezawa et al., 1972). Together with the Munich group, the kallikrein inhibition was investigated. The dissociation constants for porcine pancreatic, submandibulary and urinary kallikrein (9.6 mU, substrate BAEe) were with leupeptin $4.1 \times 10^{-6}\,M$, $1.0 \times 10^{-5}\,M$, and $1.3 \times 10^{-5}\,M$, respectively and with antipain $1.6 \times 10^{-5}\,M$, $3.2 \times 10^{-5}\,M$ and $9.5 \times 10^{-5}\,M$ (Fritz et al., 1973). Complex formation is of competitive character and reversible. Dialysis results in complete reactivation of kallikrein (Fritz et al., 1973).

From experiments with other serine proteinases and synthetized derivatives of leupeptin, conclusions may be drawn about the complex binding reaction with kallikrein: The aldehyde group is important for inhibition, that is in the form of L-argininal; D-argininal derivatives are ineffective (Aoyagi et al., 1969a). In naturally occuring proteinase inhibitors, the conformation of an inhibitor must have 30–50 amino acid residues stabilizing the reactive conformation; with the exception of compounds with unusual configuration such as the peptide aldehydes of microorganisms.

VI. Synthetic Model Inhibitors of Kallikreins

A variety of compounds, mostly cyclic, have been studied as competitive inhibitors first for replacing natural inhibitors (especially in vivo) and second for simulating complex formation for conformational studies.

As shown by X-ray studies, the conformation of proteolytic enzymes contains a substrate-binding pocket. Distances between residues and the angles of side chains give space for natural or synthetic substrates/inhibitors (for review see BLOW, 1974). Theoretical studies concerning the interaction of these "organic chemical models for proteinase inhibitors" are given by KAISER (1974) and SHAW (1974).

Studies with other proteinases and synthetic inhibitors may help explain the mechanism of the reaction between the substances described here as inhibitors for kallikrein (KAISER, 1974; SHAW, 1974). All synthetic inhibitors inhibit the enzyme by formation of covalent bonds in the active center of the enzyme (see Introduction).

With respect to the pathophysiologic role of kininogenases, the search for synthetic inhibitors of kinin-releasing enzymes is important. Besides the known inhibitors of all serine proteinases, the synthesis of substances with low-grade toxicity and their analogs was pursued to find inhibitors acting in vivo. However, in vivo inhibition is usually tested in model experiments on isolated organs. Less is known about blocking of the effects of kinin release in pathologic conditions than about the kinins themselves.

1. Di-Isopropyl-Fluorophosphate (DFP), (Serine Proteinase Specific)

Enzymatic studies of the similarities and differences in trypsin, chymotrypsin, and the kallikreins led to detailed experiments with DFP (FIEDLER et al., 1968, 1969; FIEDLER, 1971); Using porcine pancreatic kallikrein and ^{32}-P-labeled DFP, the same binding mechanism was reported as for trypsin and chymotrypsin. One serine residue, located in the active center of kallikrein, is phosphorylated and the enzyme is rendered inactive.

2. Chloromethyl Ketones: Selective His-Alkylating Agents

Because kallikreins are serine proteinases, other inhibitors of trypsin and chymotrypsin were tested as inhibitors of kallikreins. The substances in question were substrate analogs which inhibit irreversibly by covalent bond formation with histidine in the active center, e.g., Tos–LysCH$_2$Cl(TLCK).

Studies during the last 10 years confirmed TLCK – in contrast to other serine proteinases – to be ineffective on the following kallikreins:
Human saliva (PASKHINA et al., 1968; MODÉER, 1977b)
Human urine (PASKHINA et al., 1968; HIAL et al., 1974)
Human serum (WUNDERER et al., 1972)
Porcine submandibulary gland (FIEDLER et al., 1977)
Porcine urine (FIEDLER et al., 1977)
Porcine pancreas (MARES-GUIA and DINIZ, 1967; FIEDLER, 1968)
Porcine serum (WUNDERER et al., 1972)
Rat submandibulary gland (BERALDO et al., 1974)

Rat urine (DINIZ et al., 1965; MARES-GUIA and DINIZ, 1967; SILVA et al., 1974)
Horse urine (DINIZ et al., 1965; SAMPAIO and PRADO, 1976)
Horse plasma (SAMPAIO and PRADO, 1976).

Concerning TLCK, peptides of arginine chloromethyl ketone should be synthetized according to the structure of natural substrates, but there are technical difficulties (SHAW, 1974). One of the synthetic structures similar to kininogen has Ala-Phe-Lys (COGGINS et al., 1974; SHAW, 1974), with a K_i for plasma kallikrein of 3×10^{-6} M. SAMPAIO and PRADO (1976) described the inhibition of horse urinary kallikrein by the same compound with a $K_i = 0.084$ mM and for horse plasma kallikrein $K_i = 0.018$ mM.

FIEDLER et al. (1977) tested Phe–Ala–LysCH_2Cl, Ala–Val–LysCH_2Cl, Ala–Leu–LysCH_2Cl, and Gly–Val–ArgCH_2Cl – the first of them was ineffective in a concentration of 5 mM. The rates of inhibition increase with increasing size of the residue in position P_2, although Gly–Val–ArgCH_2Cl was proved to be the most potent inhibitor; this being in accordance with the substrate specificity of the kallikreins.

For Ala–Leu–LysCH_2Cl (0.5–5 mM) the values of K_i are 1.04, 1.95, and 1.97 mM with pig pancreatic, submandibulary and urinary kallikrein; for Gly–Val–ArgCH_2Cl (0.1–2 mM) 0.37, 0.74, and 0.63 mM, respectively. The inhibition became constant within 10 min, demonstrating the irreversibility of the reaction (FIEDLER et al., 1977).

3. Compounds Resembling the Aromatic Residues of the Synthetic Kallikrein Substrates (Arg)

Derivatives of benzamidine and benzylamine and aromatic diamidines have been synthesized with various ring structures.

Benzamidine – long known for kallikrein inhibition – and benzylamine derivatives were described by MARKWARDT and co-workers to be inhibitors of serum kallikrein. Porcine serum kallikrein but not porcine pancreatic kallikrein was inhibited in esterolytic (MARKWARDT et al., 1971 a) and kinin-liberating (rabbit blood pressure) (MARKWARDT et al., 1971 b) activity by benzamidine. The in vivo effect was demonstrated for 4-amidinophenylpyruvic acid by GERATZ (1969) and MARKWARDT et al. (1971 b, c) as well as for other inhibitors.

As a result of these experiments MARKWARDT et al. (1974), using porcine serum kallikrein, tested around 60 derivatives of benzylamine, benzamidine, and phenylpyruvic acid (aminophenylcarboxyl acid, esters of amidino- and guanidinobenzoic acid, 4-amidino-phenylbenzoate, and benzenesulfonyl fluorides are inhibitors). Among them they found competitive, temporary, and irreversible inhibitors. Tests were performed by active site titration of the enzyme or by bioassay in vitro.

Inhibitory benzylamine derivatives were obtained by halogenation or by aromatic substitution. Benzamidine itself is much more active than benzylamine. Of the derivatives, 4-aminomethylbenzamidine ($I_{50} = 30 \times 10^{-6}$ M) and 4-amidinophenylpyruvic acid ($I_{50} = 6 \times 10^{-6}$ M) are the most potent inhibitors for serum kallikrein of this group (MARKWARDT et al., 1974).

Derivatives of phenylpyruvic acid esterification were without effect but esterification of 3-amidinophenylpyruvic acid ($I_{50} = 5 \times 10^{-6}$ M) was effective. Substituted phenyl-amidinobenzoates, -guanidinobenzoates, and amidinophenylbenzoates inhibit temporarily ($I_{50} > 0.4 \times 10^{-6}$ *M*). As specific irreversible inhibitors, amino-alkyl benzenesulfonyl fluorides surpassed the effect of DFP (MARKWARDT et al., 1974).

Mono- and diamidino-compounds inhibit guinea-pig plasma kallikrein (DAVIES and LOWE, 1970). Porcine pancreatic kallikrein is inhibited by aromatic diamidines (GERATZ, 1969). The strongest reversible inhibitor of the group of 19 diamidines tested is 2,2′-dibromopropamidine with $K_i = 1.3 \times 10^{-6}$ *M* (GERATZ and WEBSTER, 1971). For p[m(m-fluorosulfonylphenylureido)phenoxyethoxy]benzamidine $K_i = 4.3 \times 10^{-6}$ *M* with porcine pancreatic kallikrein (GERATZ, 1972). Kinetically, all substances behaved as competitive inhibitors (GERATZ and WEBSTER, 1971).

Human plasma kallikrein is competitively and strongly inhibited ($K_i \simeq 10^{-5}$ *M*) by propamidine, stilbamidine, pentamidine, 2-hydroxybamidine, and dibromopropamidine in esterolytic and biologic activity (ASGHAR et al., 1976).

Of about 45 compounds of diamidino-α, ω-diphenoxyalkanes synthetized 2′,2″-diiodo-4′-4″diamidino-1,8-diphenoxypentane inhibited porcine pancreatic kallikrein with $K_i = 4.5 \times 10^{-7}$ *M*. Elongation of the bridge was most effective with n = 12 ($K_i = 1.7$ μ*M*) (GERATZ et al., 1973). From α,ω-bis-4-amidino-2,6-dibromophenoxyalkanes elongation to n = 5 showed $K_i = 0.8$ μ*M* (GERATZ et al., 1973).

The in vitro inhibition by aromatic diamines was not of practical importance because diamines themselves lower blood pressure to shock level (GERATZ and WEBSTER, 1971; GERATZ et al., 1973). The results are of interest for in vitro experiments. The studies of GERATZ and co-workers included derivatives of p-amidinophenylpyruvic acid. They synthesized esters or halogen-substituted compounds. In comparison to the potent bisamidino derivatives, ethyl 4-amidino-2-iodophenoxyacetate is markedly less toxic, inhibiting porcine pancreatic kallikrein with $K_i = 1.4 \times 10^{-4}$ *M* (LOEFFLER et al., 1975).

4. Inactivation by Conversion to Acyl-Enzyme. Inhibition With Aliphatic and Aromatic Acid Esters

MURAMATU and FUJII (1968) reported inhibition of human plasma kallikrein by various saturated aliphatic esters of ω-guanidino acids in addition to effects of esters of ε-aminocaproic acid, a known inhibitor (BACK and STEGER, 1968). They also described the effect of trans-4-aminomethylcyclohexanecarboxylic acid on human plasma kallikrein (MURAMATU and FUJII, 1971). Aromatic esters were more effective than saturated aliphatic esters.

MURAMATU and FUJII (1971b) further tested ω-guanidino acid esters for inhibition of BAEe-hydrolysis activity of human plasma kallikrein. Whereas hexyl δ-guanidinovalerate and hexyl γ-guanidinobutyrate were without effect, benzyl ε-guanidinocaproate inhibited with $K_i = 3.2 \times 10^{-5}$ *M*. With TAMe as substrate for human plasma kallikrein, this substance inhibited 50% at a concentration of 0.19 m*M*. Phenyl ε-guanidinocaproate p-toluenesulfonate inhibited 50% at 7.5×10^{-6} *M* and p-carbethoxy-phenyl ε-guanidinocaproate at 7.4×10^{-6} *M*. K_i-values were not given. Phenyl trans-4-aminomethylcyclohexane carboxylate had little effect (50% inhibition at 0.13 mM). Some of these substances are reversible inhibitors, i.e., the inhibition could be reversed by dialysis (MURAMATU and FUJII, 1972).

Porcine pancreatic kallikrein was tested for inhibition by halomethylated derivatives of dicoumarins (BECHET et al., 1977); possibly they inhibit by conversion of active-center His into an acyl-derivate.

5. Other Compounds

According to MAKI and SASAKI (1972), 4-(2-carboxyethyl)phenyl-trans-4-aminomethyl cyclohexane is a kallikrein inhibitor in vivo (skin test with trypan blue). The esterolytic activity of pig pancreatic kallikrein is irreversibly inhibited by N-(β-pyridylmethyl)-3,4-dichlorophenoxyacetamide-p-fluorosulfonylacetanilide bromide, one of the strongest chymotrypsin inhibitors, with a $K_i = 3.1 \times 10^{-5}\,M$ (GERATZ and FOX, 1973).

Human plasma kallikrein is competitively inhibited by p- and m-nitrophenylamidino phenyl methanesulfate (SHAW, 1974), a reagent which sulfonates other proteinases (e.g., thrombin).

VII. Influence of Metal Ions on Kallikrein

FIEDLER (1968) reported that pig pancreatic kallikrein is inhibited by Cu^{2+}, Zn^{2+}, and Fe^{2+} in a concentration of $10^{-5}\,M$. Cd^{2+}, Mn^{2+}, Ni^{2+}, and Co^{2+} inhibit this kallikrein at $10^{-3}\,M$ concentrations.

Metal ions at a concentration of $10^{-4}\,M$ were tested on the esterolytic activity of human salivary kallikrein (MODÉER, 1977b): Co^{2+} is strongest inhibitor (55% inhibited), followed by Fe^{2+}, Zn^{2+}, Cu^{2+}, and Hg^{2+}. At a concentration of $10^{-3}\,M$ Fe^{2+} inhibits 57%, followed by Zn^{2+} (29%), Hg^{2+} (19%). Ca^{2+}, Mn^{2+}, Mg^{2+}, and Ni^{2+} were ineffective (MODÉER, 1977b). Fe^{2+}, Co^{2+}, Zn^{2+}, Hg^{2+}, and Cu^{2+} also inhibit kallikrein from porcine pancreas (ZUBER and SACHE, 1974). Zn^{2+}, Hg^{2+}, and Cd^{2+} inhibit pancreatic kallikrein from dog and rat (HOJIMA et al., 1977).

References

Amnéus, H., Gabel, D., Kasche, V.: Resolution in affinity chromatography. The effect of the heterogeneity of immobilized soybean trypsin inhibitor on the separation of pancreatic proteases. J. Chromatogr. *120*, 391–397 (1976)

Angeletti, M., Sbaraglia, G., de Campora, E., Fratti, L.: Biological properties of esteroprotease isolated from the submaxillary gland of mice. Life Sci. II *12*, 297–305 (1973)

Aoyagi, T., Miyata, S., Nanbo, M., Kojima, F., Matsuzaki, M., Ishizuka, M., Takeuchi, T., Umezawa, H.: Biological activities of leupeptins. J. Antibiot. (Tokyo) *22*, 558–568 (1969a)

Aoyagi, T., Takeuchi, T., Matsuzaki, M., Kawamura, K., Kondo, S., Hamada, M., Maeda, K., Umezawa, H.: Leupeptins, new protease inhibitors from actinomycetes. J. Antibiot. (Tokyo) *22*, 283–286 (1969b)

Arens, A., Haberland, G.L.: Determination of kallikrein activity in animal tissue using biochemical methods. In: Kininogenases. Haberland, G.L., Rohen, J.W. (eds.), pp. 43–53. Stuttgart, New York: Schattauer 1973

Arndts, D., Räker, K.-O., Török, P., Habermann, E.: Studien zur Verteilung und Elimination eines Proteinasen-Inhibitors mit Isotopentechniken. Arzneim. Forsch. *20*, 667–674 (1970)

Ashgar, S.S., Meijlink, F.C.P.W., Pondman, K.W., Cormane, R.H.: Human plasma kallikreins and their inhibition by amidino compounds. Biochim. Biophys. Acta *438*, 250–264 (1976)

Aungst, C.W., Back, N., Barlow, B., Tsukada, G.A.: Immunologic studies of components of the kallikrein-kinin system. In: Hypotensive peptides. Erdös, E.G., Back, N., Sicuteri, F. (eds.), pp. 211–230. Berlin, Heidelberg, New York: Springer 1966

Back, N.: Protease studies with cecal contents from germ-free and conventional mice. In: Kininogenases. Haberland, G.L., Rohen, J.W. (eds.), pp. 159–160. Stuttgart, New York: Schattauer 1973

Back, N., Steger, R.: Effect of inhibitors on kinin-releasing activity of proteases. Fed. Proc. *27*, 96–99 (1968)

Barnhill, M.T., Jr., Trowbridge, C.G.: Reaction heat variation with pH in formation of the trypsin-soybean inhibitor complex. J. Biol. Chem. *250*, 5501–5507 (1975)

Bartling, G.J., Barker, C.W.: Separation of trypsin and peroxidase by ultrafiltration using cross-linked soybean trypsin inhibitor. Biotechnol. Bioeng. *18*, 1023–1027 (1976)

Baugh, R.J., Barnhill, M.T., Jr., Trowbridge, C.G.: pH dependence of the trypsin-soybean trypsin inhibitor heat of reaction. Fed. Proc. *32*, 571 (Abstract) (1973)

Béchet, J.-J., Dupaix, A., Roucous, C., Bonamy, A.-M.: Inactivation of proteases and esterases by halomethylated derivatives of dihydrocoumarins. Biochimie *59*, 241–246 (1977)

Beraldo, W.T., Siqueira, G., Heneine, I.F.: Kallikrein and kallikrein inhibitor in rats. Acta Physiol. Lat. Am. *24*, 460–463 (1974)

Béress, L., Béress, R.: Reinigung zweier krabbenlähmender Toxine aus der Seeanemone Anemonia sulcata. Kieler Meeresforsch. *27*, 117–127 (1971)

Béress, L., Béress, R., Wunderer, G.: Isolation and characterization of three polypeptides with neurotoxic activity from Anemonia sulcata. FEBS Letters *50*, 311–314 (1975a)

Béress, L., Béress, R., Wunderer, G.: Purification of three polypeptides with neuro- and cardiotoxic activity from the sea anemone Anemonia sulcata. Toxicon *13*, 359–367 (1975b)

Béress, L., Kortmann, H., Fritz, H.: Über das Vorkommen polyvalenter Proteaseinhibitoren in Seeanemonen *(Actinaria)* mit einem dem Trypsin-Kallikrein-Inhibitor aus Rinderorganen analogen Hemmspektrum. Hoppe Seylers Z. Physiol. Chem. *353*, 111–112 (1972)

Bergmeyer, H.U.: Grundlagen der enzymatischen Analyse. Weinheim, New York: Verlag Chemie 1977

Bhoola, K.D., Dorey, G.: Kallikrein, trypsin-like proteases and amylase in mammalian submaxillary glands. Br. J. Pharmacol. *43*, 784–793 (1971)

Bidlingmeyer, U.D.V., Leary, T.R., Laskowski, M., Jr.: Identity of the tryptic and α-chymotryptic reactive site on soybean trypsin inhibitor (Kunitz). Biochemistry *11*, 3303–3310 (1972)

Bieth, J., Frechin, J.-C.: Elastase inhibitors as impurities in commercial preparations of soybean trypsin inhibitor (Kunitz). In: Proteinase inhibitors. Fritz, H., Tschesche, H., Greene, L.J., Truscheit, E. (eds.), pp. 291–304. Berlin, Heidelberg, New York: Springer 1974

Birk, Y.: Proteinase inhibitors from plant sources. In: Methods of enzymology. Lorand, L. (ed.), Vol. XLV/B, pp. 695–697. London, New York: Academic Press 1976

Blow, D.M.: Stereochemistry of substrate binding and hydrolysis in the trypsin family of enzymes. In: Proteinase inhibitors. Fritz, H., Tschesche, H., Greene, L.J., Truscheit, E. (eds.), pp. 473–483. Berlin, Heidelberg, New York: Springer 1974

Blow, D.M., Janin, J., Sweet, R.M.: Mode of action of soybean trypsin inhibitor (Kunitz) as a model for specific protein-protein interactions. Nature (Lond.) *249*, 54–57 (1974)

Blow, D.M., Wright, C.S., Kukla, D., Rühlmann, A., Steigemann, W., Huber, R.: A model for the association of bovine pancreatic trypsin inhibitor with chymotrypsin and trypsin. J. Mol. Biol. *69*, 137–144 (1972)

Bösterling, B., Engel, J.: Influence of various fluorescent and non-fluorescent labels on the kinetics of the complex formation of α-chymotrypsin with basic pancreatic trypsin inhibitor. Hoppe Seylers Z. Physiol. Chem. *357*, 1297–1307 (1976)

Bretz, U., Dewald, B., Baggiolini, M., Vischer, T.L.: In vitro stimulation of lymphocytes by neutral proteinases from human polymorphonuclear leukocyte granules. Schweiz. Med. Wochenschr. *106*, 1373–1374 (1976)

Brown, L.R., De Marco, A., Wagner, G., Wüthrich, K.: A study of the lysyl residues in the basic pancreatic trypsin inhibitor using ^{1}H nuclear magnetic resonance at 360 MHz. Eur. J. Biochem. *62*, 103–107 (1976)

Brunner, H., Holz, M.: Raman studies of native and partially (Cys 14–Cys 38) reduced basic pancreatic trypsin inhibitor. In: Proteinase inhibitors. Fritz, H., Tschesche, H., Greene, L.J., Truscheit, E. (eds.), pp. 455–457. Berlin, Heidelberg, New York: Springer 1974
Brunner, H., Holz, M.: Raman studies of the conformation of the basic pancreatic trypsin inhibitor. Biochim. Biophys. Acta *379*, 408–417 (1975)
Brunner, H., Holz, M., Jering, H.: Raman studies on native, reduced, and modified basic pancreatic trypsin inhibitor. Eur. J. Biochem. *50*, 129–133 (1974)
Bryant, J., Green, T.R., Gurusaddaiah, T., Ryan, C.A.: Proteinase inhibitor II from potatoes: Isolation and characterization of its protomer components. Biochemistry *15*, 3418–3423 (1976)
Burkhead, R.J., Shaffer, A.G., Jr., Hamrin, C.E., Jr.: Equilibrium studies in a Sepharose CVB ovomucoid-trypsin system. Biotechnol. Bioeng. *15*, 811–815 (1973)
Čechová, D.: Trypsin inhibitor from cow colostrum. In: Methods in enzymology. Lorand, L. (ed.), Vol. XLV/B, pp. 806–813. London, New York: Academic Press 1976
Čechová, D., Ber, E.: Disulfide bonds of trypsin inhibitor from cow colostrum. Collect. Czech. Chem. Commun. *39*, 680–688 (1974)
Čechová, D., Fritz, H.: Unpublished results, cit. in: Werle, E., Fiedler, F., Fritz, H.: Recent studies on kallikreins and kallikrein inhibitors. Pharmacology and the future of man. Proc. Vth. Int. Congr. Pharmacol. San Francisco 1972, Vol. V, pp. 284–295. Basel: Karger 1973
Čechová, D., Fritz, H.: Characterization of the proteinase inhibitors from bull seminal plasma and spermatozoa. Hoppe Seylers Z. Physiol. Chem. *357*, 401–408 (1976)
Čechová, D., Muszyńská, G.: Role of lysine 18 in active center of cow colostrum trypsin inhibitor. FEBS Letters *8*, 84–86 (1970)
Čechová-Pošpísilová, D., Švestková, V., Šorm, F.: Trypsin inhibitors from cow colostrum. VIth FEBS Meeting, Abstr. No. 225, Madrid 1969a
Čechová, D., Švestková, V., Keil, B., Šorm, F.: Similarities in primary structures of cow colostrum trypsin inhibitor and bovine basic pancreatic trypsin inhibitor. FEBS Letters *4*, 155–156 (1969b)
Chauvet, J., Acher, R.: The reactive site of the basic trypsin inhibitor of pancreas. J. Biol. Chem. *242*, 4274–4275 (1967)
Chauvet, J., Acher, R.: Identity of trypsin inhibitors isolated from bovine liver and pancreas. Int. J. Protein Res. *2*, 165–167 (1970)
Chauvet, J., Acher, R.: Isolation of a trypsin inhibitor (Kunitz inhibitor) from bovine ovary by affinity chromatography through trypsin-Sepharose. FEBS Letters *23*, 317–320 (1972)
Chauvet, J., Acher, R.: Chromatographie d'affinité des trypsines sur l'inhibiteur de Kunitz lié au Sépharose. Biochimie *55*, 1323–1324 (1973)
Chauvet, J., Acher, R.: A study of the active center of trypsinogen by comparative affinity chromatography of trypsinogen, α-, β-,ψ-trypsins, DIP-trypsin, chymotrypsinogen, α-chymotrypsin, and elastase. Int. J. Protein Res. *6*, 37–41 (1974)
Chauvet, J., Acher, R.: The reactive sites of Kunitz bovine-trypsin inhibitor. Role of lysine-15 in the interaction with chymotrypsin. Eur. J. Biochem. *54*, 31–38 (1975a)
Chauvet, J., Acher, R.: Conformation-directed proteolysis of Kunitz bovine trypsin inhibitor. In: Peptides: chemistry, structure, and biology. Walter, R., Meienhofer, J. (eds.), pp. 915–920. Ann Arbor: Ann Arbor Science 1975b
Chauvet, J., Dostal, J.-P., Acher, R.: Isolation of a trypsin-like enzyme from *Streptomyces paromomycinus* (Paromotrypsin) by affinity adsorption through Kunitz inhibitor-Sepharose. Int. J. Protein Res. *8*, 45–55 (1976)
Clark, R.W., Hymowitz, T.: Activity variation between and within two soybean trypsin inhibitor electrophoretic forms. Biochem. Genet. *6*, 169–182 (1972)
Coggins, J.R., Kray, W., Shaw, E.: Affinity labelling of proteinases with tryptic specificity by peptides with C-terminal lysine chloromethylketone. Biochem. J. *138*, 579–585 (1974)
Cole, F.E., Parthasarathy, R.: The trypsin-trypsin inhibitor complex: Crystallization, unit cells and space groups. J. Mol. Biol. *71*, 105–106 (1972)
Colina-Chourio, J., McGiff, J.C., Miller, M.P., Nasjletti, A.: Possible influence of intrarenal generation of kinins on prostaglandin release from the rabbit perfused kidney. Br. J. Pharmacol. *58*, 165–172 (1976)

Counitchansky, Y., Berthillier, G., Got, R.: Mise en évidence, dans le colostrum humain, de protéines formant des complexes avec la trypsine et la chymotrypsine. Clin. Chim. Acta *26*, 223–229 (1969)
Creighton, T.E.: Renaturation of the reduced bovine pancreatic trypsin inhibitor. J. Mol. Biol. *87*, 563–577 (1974a)
Creighton, T.E.: Intermediates in the refolding of reduced pancreatic trypsin inhibitor. J. Mol. Biol. *87*, 579–602 (1974b)
Creighton, T.E.: The single-disulphide intermediates in the refolding of reduced pancreatic trypsin inhibitor. J. Mol. Biol. *87*, 603–624 (1974c)
Creighton, T.E.: Homology of protein structures: Proteinase inhibitors. Nature (Lond.) *255*, 743–744 (1975a)
Creighton, T.E.: The two-disulphide intermediates and the folding pathway of reduced pancreatic trypsin inhibitor. J. Mol. Biol. *95*, 167–199 (1975b)
Creighton, T.E.: Interactions between cysteine residues as probes of protein conformation: The disulphide bond between Cys-14 and Cys-38 of the pancreatic trypsin inhibitor. J. Mol. Biol. *96*, 767–776 (1975c)
Creighton, T.E.: Reactivities of the cysteine residues of the reduced pancreatic trypsin inhibitor. J. Mol. Biol. *96*, 777–782 (1975d)
Croxatto, H.R., Porcelli, G., Noé, G., Roblero, J., Cruzat, H.: Kininogenasa urinaria, caracterización y propiedades. Acta Cient. Venez. *22*, 154–157 (1971)
Davies, G.E., Lowe, J.S.: The inhibition of guinea-pig plasma kallikrein by amidines. Adv. Exp. Med. Biol. *8*, 453–460 (1970)
Deisenhofer, J., Steigemann, W.: The model of the basic pancreatic trypsin inhibitor refined at 1.5 Å resolution. In: Proteinase inhibitors. Fritz, H., Tschesche, H., Greene, L.J., Truscheit, E. (eds.), pp. 484–496. Berlin, Heidelberg, New York: Springer 1974
Deisenhofer, J., Steigemann, W.: Crystallographic refinement of the structure of bovine pancreatic trypsin inhibitor at 1.5 Å resolution. Acta Cryst. *B31*, 238–250 (1975)
Dietl, T., Tschesche, H.: Amino acid sequence of snail inhibitor K and correlation of structure and specificity. In: Proteinase inhibitors. Fritz, H., Tschesche, H., Greene, L.J., Truscheit, E. (eds.), pp. 254–264. Berlin, Heidelberg, New York: Springer 1974
Dietl, T., Tschesche, H.: Trypsin-kallikrein isoinhibitor K (type Kunitz) from snails *(Helix pomatia)*. Purification and characterization. Eur. J. Biochem. *58*, 453–460 (1975)
Dietl, T., Tschesche, H.: Albumin gland inhibitor from snails *(Helix pomatia)*. In: Methods in enzymology. Lorand, L. (ed.), Vol. XLV/B, pp. 785–792. London, New York: Academic Press 1976a
Dietl, T., Tschesche, H.: Die Disulfidbrücken des Trypsin-Kallikrein-Inhibitors K aus Weinbergschnecken *(Helix pomatia)*. Thermische Denaturierung und thermolysinolytische Inaktivierung. Hoppe Seylers Z. Physiol. Chem. *357*, 139–145 (1976b)
Dietl, T., Tschesche, H.: Characterization and inhibitory properties of snail secretory proteinase inhibitors. In: Protides of the biological fluids. 23rd Colloquium. Peeters, H. (ed.), pp. 271–278. Oxford, New York: Pergamon Press 1976c
Dietl, T., Tschesche, H.: Determination of arginine in the reactive site of proteinase inhibitors by selective and reversible derivatization of the arginine side chain. Hoppe Seylers Z. Physiol. Chem. *357*, 657–665 (1976d)
Diniz, C.R., Pereira, A.A., Barroso, J., Mares-Guia, M.: On the specificity of urinary kallicreins. Biochem. Biophys. Res. Commun. *21*, 448–453 (1965)
Dlouhá, V., Keil, B.: Interaction of basic pancreatic trypsin inhibitor with trypsinogen. FEBS Letters *3*, 137–140 (1969)
Ehret, W.: Die Primärstruktur des Kallikreins aus Schweinepankreas. Inaug.-Diss. München 1976
Ekfors, T.O., Hopsu-Havu, V.K.: Properties of the esteropeptidases purified from the mouse submandibular gland. Enzymologia *43*, 177–189 (1972)
Elkana, Y.: Interaction between the basic inhibitor of bovine pancreas and chymotrypsin and trypsin. Selective anthraniloylation of the maleylated inhibitor. J. Mol. Biol. *84*, 523–538 (1974a)
Elkana, Y.: The use of fluorescence techniques in the study of the interaction of the basic trypsin inhibitor of bovine pancreas, selectively labelled at lysine 15, with chymotrypsin and trypsin.

In: Proteinase inhibitors. Fritz, H., Tschesche, H., Greene, L.J., Truscheit, E. (eds.), pp. 445–453. Berlin, Heidelberg, New York: Springer 1974b
Ellis, L.M., Bloomfield, V.A., Woodward, C.K.: Hydrogen-tritium exchange kinetics of soybean trypsin inhibitor (Kunitz). Solvent accessibility of the folded conformation. Biochemistry *14*, 3413–3419 (1975)
Engel, J., Quast, U., Heumann, H., Krause, G., Steffen, E.: Kinetic studies of the binding of bovine basic pancreatic trypsin inhibitor to α-chymotrypsin. In: Proteinase inhibitors. Fritz, H., Tschesche, H., Greene, L.J., Truscheit, E. (eds.), pp. 412–419. Berlin, Heidelberg, New York: Springer 1974
Erdös, E.G., Tague, L.L., Miwa, I.: Kallikrein in granules of the submaxillary gland. Biochem. Pharmacol. *17*, 667–674 (1968a)
Erdös, E.G., Tague, L.L., Miwa, I.: Kallikrein in granules of a salivary gland. Proc. West. Pharmacol. Soc. *11*, 26–28 (1968b)
Feeney, R.E.: Comparative biochemistry of avian egg white ovomucoids and ovoinhibitors. In: Proc. int. res. conf. on proteinase inhibitors. Fritz, H., Tschesche, H. (eds.), pp. 189–195. Berlin, New York: de Gruyter 1971
Feeney, R.E., Means, G.E., Bigler, J.C.: Inhibition of human trypsin, plasmin, and thrombin by naturally occurring inhibitors of proteolytic enzymes. J. Biol. Chem. *244*, 1957–1960 (1969)
Feinstein, G.: Purification of trypsin by affinity chromatography on ovomucoid-sepharose resin. FEBS Letters 7, 353–355 (1970a)
Feinstein, G.: Interaction of insoluble protein inhibitors with proteases. Biochim. Biophys. Acta *214*, 224–227 (1970b)
Fiedler, F.: Heterogenität und enzymatische Eigenschaften von Pankreaskallikrein. Hoppe Seylers Z. Physiol. Chem. *349*, 926 (1968)
Fiedler, F., Hirschauer, C., Fritz, H.: Inhibition of three porcine glandular kallikreins by chloromethyl ketones. Hoppe Seylers Z. Physiol. Chem. *358*, 447–451 (1977)
Fiedler, F., Müller, B., Werle, E.: Hemmung von Schweinepankreaskallikrein durch Diisopropylfluorophosphat. Hoppe Seylers Z. Physiol. Chem. *349*, 942 (1968)
Fiedler, F., Müller, B., Werle, E.: The inhibition of porcine kallikrein by Di-isopropyl-fluorophosphate. Eur. J. Biochem. *10*, 419–425 (1969)
Fiedler, F., Müller, B., Werle, E.: Die Aminosäuresequenz im Bereich des Serins im aktiven Zentrum des Kallikreins aus Schweinepankreas. Hoppe Seylers Z. Physiol. Chem. *352*, 1463–1464 (1971)
Fink, E., Greene, L.J.: Measurement of the bovine pancreatic trypsin inhibitors by radioimmunoassay. In: Proteinase inhibitors. Fritz, H., Tschesche, H., Greene, L.J., Truscheit, E. (eds.), pp. 243–249. Berlin, Heidelberg, New York: Springer 1974
Fink, E., Jaumann, E., Fritz, H., Ingrisch, H., Werle, E.: Protease-Inhibitoren im menschlichen Spermaplasma. Isolierung durch Affinitätschromatographie und Hemmverhalten. Hoppe Seylers Z. Physiol. Chem. *352*, 1591–1594 (1971a)
Fink, E., Klein, G., Hammer, F., Müller-Bardorff, G., Fritz, H.: Protein proteinase inhibitors in male sex glands. In: Proc. int. res. conf. on proteinase inhibitors. Fritz, H., Tschesche, H. (eds.), pp. 225–235. Berlin, New York: de Gruyter 1971b
Finkenstadt, W.R., Hamid, M.A., Mattis, J.A., Schrode, J., Sealock, R.W., Wang, D., Laskowski, M., Jr.: Kinetics and thermodynamics of the interaction of proteinases with protein inhibitors. In: Proteinase inhibitors. Fritz, H., Tschesche, H., Greene, L.J., Truscheit, E. (eds.), pp. 389–411. Berlin, Heidelberg, New York: Springer 1974
Fish, W.W., Leach, B.S.: Soybean trypsin inhibitor in 6 M guanidinium chloride: To unfold or not to unfold? Fed. Proc. *32*, 496 (Abstract) (1973)
Fräki, J.E., Hopsu-Havu, V.K.: Human skin proteases. Separation and characterization of two alkaline proteases, one splitting trypsin and the other chymotrypsin substrates. Arch. Dermatol. Res. *253*, 261–276 (1975)
Frey, E.K., Kraut, H., Werle, E., Vogel, R., Zickgraf-Rüdel, G., Trautschold, I.: Das Kallikrein-Kinin-System und seine Inhibitoren. Stuttgart: Enke 1968
Fritz, H.: Inhibition specificity. In: Chemistry and biology of the kallikrein-kinin system in health and disease. Pisano, J.J., Austen, K.F. (eds.), pp. 181–193. Washington: U.S. Gov. Printing Office 1976
Fritz, H., Brey, B., Béress, L.: Polyvalente Isoinhibitoren für Trypsin, Chymotrypsin, Plasmin und Kallikreine aus Seeanemonen *(Anemonia sulcata)*, Isolierung, Hemmverhalten und Aminosäurezusammensetzung. Hoppe Seylers Z. Physiol. Chem. *353*, 19–30 (1972a)

Fritz, H., Brey, B., Müller, M., Gebhardt, M.: Specific isolation and modification methods for proteinase inhibitors and proteinases. In: Proc. int. res. conf. on proteinase inhibitors. Fritz, H., Tschesche, H. (eds.), pp. 28–37. Berlin, New York: de Gruyter 1971
Fritz, H., Brey, B., Schmal, A., Werle, E.: Verwendung wasserunlöslicher Derivate des Trypsin-Kallikrein-Inhibitors zur Isolierung von Kallikreinen und von Plasmin. Hoppe Seylers Z. Physiol. Chem. *350*, 617–625 (1969a)
Fritz, H., Fink, E., Gebhardt, M., Hochstrasser, K., Werle, E.: Identifizierung von Lysin- und Argininresten als Hemmzentren von Proteinaseninhibitoren mit Hilfe von Maleinsäureanhydrid und Butandion-(2.3). Hoppe Seylers Z. Physiol. Chem. *350*, 933–944 (1969b)
Fritz, H., Fink, E., Meister, R., Klein, G.: Isolierung von Trypsininhibitoren und Trypsin-Plasmin-Inhibitoren aus den Samenblasen von Meerschweinchen. Hoppe Seylers Z. Physiol. Chem. *351*, 1344–1352 (1970a)
Fritz, H., Förg-Brey, B.: Zur Isolierung von Organ- und Harnkallikreinen durch Affinitätschromatographie. Hoppe Seylers Z. Physiol. Chem. *353*, 901–905 (1972)
Fritz, H., Förg-Brey, B., Fink, E., Schiessler, H., Jaumann, E., Arnhold, M.: Charakterisierung einer Trypsin-ähnlichen Proteinase (Akrosin) aus Eberspermien durch ihre Hemmbarkeit mit verschiedenen Protein-Proteinase-Inhibitoren, I. Seminale Trypsin-Inhibitoren und Trypsin-Kallikrein-Inhibitoren aus Rinderorganen. Hoppe Seylers Z. Physiol. Chem. *353*, 1007–1009 (1972b)
Fritz, H., Förg-Brey, B., Schiessler, H., Arnhold, M., Fink, E.: Charakterisierung einer Trypsin-ähnlichen Proteinase (Akrosin) aus Eberspermien durch ihre Hemmbarkeit mit verschiedenen Protein-Proteinase-Inhibitoren, II. Inhibitoren aus Blutegeln, Sojabohnen, Erdnüssen, Rindercolostrum und Seeanemonen. Hoppe Seylers Z. Physiol. Chem. *353*, 1010–1012 (1972c)
Fritz, H., Förg-Brey, B., Umezawa, H.: Leupeptin and antipain. Hoppe Seylers Z. Physiol. Chem. *354*, 1304–1306 (1973)
Fritz, H., Gebhardt, M., Fink, E., Schramm, W., Werle, E.: Verwendung wasserunlöslicher Enzymharze mit polyanionischer und polyamphoterer Harzmatrix zur Isolierung von Proteaseinhibitoren. Hoppe Seylers Z. Physiol. Chem. *350*, 129–138 (1969c)
Fritz, H., Oppitz, K.-H., Meckl, D., Kemkes, B., Haendle, H., Schult, H., Werle, E.: Verteilung und Ausscheidung von natürlich vorkommenden und chemisch modifizierten Proteaseinhibitoren nach intravenöser Injektion bei Ratte, Hund (und Mensch). Hoppe Seylers Z. Physiol. Chem. *350*, 1541–1550 (1969d)
Fritz, H., Schult, H., Hutzel, M., Wiedemann, M., Werle, E.: Über Proteaseinhibitoren. IV. Isolierung von Protease-Inhibitoren mit Hilfe wasserunlöslicher Enzym-Harze. Hoppe Seylers Z. Physiol. Chem. *348*, 308–312 (1967)
Fritz, H., Schult, H., Meister, R., Werle, E.: Herstellung und Eigenschaften von aktiven Derivaten des Trypsin-Kallikrein-Inhibitors aus Rinderorganen. Hoppe Seylers Z. Physiol. Chem. *350*, 1531–1540 (1969e)
Fritz, H., Trautschold, I., Werle, E.: Protease-Inhibitoren. In: Methoden der enzymatischen Analyse, 1st. ed. Bergmeyer, H.U. (ed.), pp. 1021–1038. Weinheim: Verlag Chemie 1970b
Fritz, H., Trautschold, I., Werle, E.: Protease-Inhibitoren. In: Methoden der enzymatischen Analyse. 3rd ed. Bergmeyer, H.U. (ed.), pp. 1105–1122. Weinheim: Verlag Chemie 1974b
Fritz, H., Trautschold, I., Werle, E.: Protease inhibitors. In: Methods of enzymatic analysis. 2nd ed. Bergmeyer, H.U. (ed.), pp. 1064–1080. Weinheim, New York, London: Verlag Chemie, Academic Press 1974c
Fritz, H., Tschesche, H.: Proceedings of the international research conference on proteinase inhibitors. Berlin, New York: de Gruyter 1971
Fritz, H., Tschesche, H., Greene, L.J., Truscheit, E.: Proteinase inhibitors. Berlin, Heidelberg, New York: Springer 1974a
Fritz, H., Wunderer, G.: Unpublished, cit. in: Serumkallikreine von Schwein und Mensch: Isolierung durch Affinitätschromatographie und Charakterisierung durch die Hemmbarkeit mit synthetisch und natürlich vorkommenden Inhibitoren. Dipl.-Arbeit. Techn. Univ. München 1972
Fritz, H., Wunderer, G., Dittmann, B.: Zur Isolierung von Schweine- und Human- Serumkallikrein durch Affinitätschromatographie. Hoppe Seylers Z. Physiol. Chem. *353*, 893–900 (1972d)

Fujimoto, Y., Moriwaki, C., Moriya, H.: Studies of human salivary kallikrein. II. Properties of purified salivary kallikrein. J. Biochem. (Tokyo) *74*, 247–252 (1973)
Furusawa, Y., Kurosawa, Y.: Studies on preparation and purification of kallikrein inhibitor from lungs. Agr. Biol. Chem. *38*, 1087–1089 (1974)
Gauwerky, C., Corman, G., Uhlenbruck, G.: Über neue Proteaseinhibitoren mit breiter Wirkungsspezifität bei dem Polychaeten *Sabellastarte indica* (Savingny). I. Mitteilung. Z. Klin. Chem. Klin. Biochem. *13*, 429–435 (1975)
Geiger, R., Kortmann, H.: Esterolytic and proteolytic activities of snake venoms and their inhibition by proteinase inhibitors. Toxicon *15*, 257–259 (1977)
Geiger, R., Mann, K.: A kallikrein-specific inhibitor in rat kidney tubules. Hoppe Seylers Z. Physiol. Chem. *357*, 553–558 (1976)
Gelin, B.R., Karplus, M.: Sidechain torsional potentials and motion of amino acids in proteins: bovine pancreatic trypsin inhibitor. Proc. Natl. Acad. Sci. USA *72*, 2002–2006 (1975)
Geratz, J.D.: Synthetic inhibitors and ester substrates of pancreatic kallikrein. Experientia *25*, 483–484 (1969)
Geratz, J.D.: Kinetic aspects of the irreversible inhibition of trypsin and related enzymes by *p*-[*m*(*m*-fluorosulfonylphenylureido)phenoxyethoxy]benzamidine. FEBS Letters *20*, 294–296 (1972)
Geratz, J.D., Cheng, M.C.-F., Tidwell, R.R.: New aromatic diamidines with central α-oxyalkane or α,ω-dioxyalkane chains. Structure-activity relationships for the inhibition of trypsin, pancreatic kallikrein, and thrombin and for the inhibition of the overall coagulation process. J. Med. Chem. *18*, 477–481 (1975)
Geratz, J.D., Cheng, M.C.-F., Tidwell, R.R.: Novel bis(benzamidino) compounds with an aromatic central link. Inhibitors of thrombin, pancreatic kallikrein, trypsin, and complement. J. Med. Chem. *19*, 634–639 (1976)
Geratz, J.D., Fox, L.L.B.: On the irreversible inhibition of α-chymotrypsin, trypsin, pancreatic kallikrein, thrombin and elastase by *N*-(β-pyridylmethyl)-3,4-dichlorophenoxyacetamide-*p*-fluorosulfonylacetatanilide bromide. Biochim. Biophys. Acta *321*, 296–302 (1973)
Geratz, J.D., Webster, W.P.: Inhibition of the amidase and kininogenase activities of pancreatic kallikrein by aromatic diamidines and an evaluation of diamidines for their in vivo use. Arch. Int. Pharmacodyn. Ther. *194*, 359–370 (1971)
Geratz, J.D., Whitmore, A.C., Cheng, M.C.-F., Piantadosi, C.: Diamidino-α, ω-diphenoxyalkanes. Structure-activity relationships for the inhibition of thrombin, pancreatic kallikrein, and trypsin. J. Med. Chem. *16*, 970–975 (1973)
Gilliam, E.B., Kitto, G.B.: Isolation of a starfish trypsin by affinity chromatography. Comp. Biochem. Physiol. [B] *54*, 21–26 (1976)
Gorbunoff, M.J.: Exposure of tyrosine residues in proteins. II. The reactions of cyanuric fluoride and *N*-acetylimidazole with pepsinogen, soybean trypsin inhibitor, and ovomucoid. Biochemistry 7, 2547–2554 (1968)
Gorbunoff, M.J.: On the role of hydroxyl-containing amino acids in trypsin inhibitors. Biochim. Biophys. Acta *221*, 314–325 (1970)
Greenbaum, L.M., Freer, R., Chang, J., Semente, G., Yamafuji, K.: PMN-kinin and kinin metabolizing enzymes in normal and malignant leucocytes. Br. J. Pharmacol. *36*, 623–634 (1969)
Greenbaum, L.M., Kim, K.S.: The kinin forming and kininase activities of rabbit polymorphonuclear leucocytes. Br. J. Pharmacol. Chemother. *29*, 238–247 (1967)
Grossberg, A.L., Pressman, D.: Modification of arginine in the active sites of antibodies. Biochemistry 7, 272–279 (1968)
Havsteen, B.H.: Kinetic studies of elementary steps in interaction of chymotrypsin with inhibitors. Stud. Biophys. *57*, 117–122 (1976)
Hawkins, H.C., Freedman, R.B.: Randomly reoxidised soybean trypsin inhibitor and the possibility of conformational barriers to disulphide isomerization in proteins. FEBS Letters *58*, 7–11 (1975)
Haynes, R., Feeney, R.E.: Transformation of active-site lysine in naturally occurring trypsin inhibitors. A basis for a general mechanism for inhibition of proteolytic enzymes. Biochemistry 7, 2879–2885 (1968a)
Haynes, R., Feeney, R.E.: Properties of enzymatically cleaved inhibitors of trypsin. Biochim. Biophys. Acta. *159*, 209–211 (1968b)

Hermann, G.: Personal communication, cit. in: Tschesche, H., Dietl, T., 1972a
Hetzel, R., Wüthrich, K., Deisenhofer, J., Huber, R.: Dynamics of the aromatic amino acid residues in the globular conformation of the basic pancreatic trypsin inhibitor (BPTI). II. Semi-empirical energy calculations. Biophys. Struct. Mech. *2*, 159–180 (1976)
Hial, V., Diniz, C.R., Mares-Guia, M.: Purification and properties of a human urinary kallikrein (kininogenase). Biochemistry *13*, 4311–4318 (1974)
Hixson, H.F., Jr., Laskowski, M., Jr.: Formation from trypsin and modified soybean trypsin inhibitor of a complex which upon kinetic control dissociation yields trypsin and virgin inhibitor. J. Biol. Chem. *245*, 2027–2035 (1970)
Hochstrasser, K., Illchmann, K., Werle, E.: Über pflanzliche Proteaseninhibitoren. VI. Reindarstellung der polyvalenten Proteaseninhibitoren aus *Arachis hypogaea*. Hoppe Seylers Z. Physiol. Chem. *350*, 929–932 (1969a)
Hochstrasser, K., Illchmann, K., Werle, E., Hössl, R., Schwarz, S.: Die Aminosäuresequenz des Trypsininhibitors aus Samen von *Arachis hypogaea*. Hoppe Seylers Z. Physiol. Chem. *351*, 1503–1512 (1970)
Hochstrasser, K., Werle, E., Siegelmann, R., Schwarz, S.: Über pflanzliche Proteaseninhibitoren. V. Isolierung und Charakterisierung einiger polyvalenter Proteaseninhibitoren aus *Solanum tuberosum*. Hoppe Seylers Z. Physiol. Chem. *350*, 897–902 (1969b)
Hojima, Y., Matsuda, Y., Moriwaki, C., Moriya, H.: Homogeneity and multiplicity forms of glandular kallikreins. Chem. Pharm. Bull. (Tokyo) *23*, 1120–1127 (1975a)
Hojima, Y., Moriwaki, C., Moriya, H.: Studies on kallikrein inhibitors from potatoes. IV. Isolation of two inhibitors and determination of molecular weights and amino acid composition. J. Biochem. (Tokyo) *73*, 923–932 (1973a)
Hojima, Y., Moriwaki, C., Moriya, H.: Studies on kallikrein inhibitors from potatoes. V. Characterization of two isolated inhibitors. J. Biochem. (Tokyo) *73*, 933–943 (1973b)
Hojima, Y., Moriwaki, C., Moriya, H.: Isolation of dog, rat, and hog pancreatic kallikreins by preparative disc electrophoresis and their properties. Chem. Pharm. Bull. (Tokyo) *23*, 1128–1136 (1975b)
Hojima, Y., Moriya, H., Moriwaki, C.: Studies of kallikrein in potatoes. II. Effect of potato kallikrein inhibitors on various kallikreins and other proteases. J. Biochem. (Tokyo) *69*, 1027–1032 (1971)
Hojima, Y., Yamashita, M., Ochi, N., Moriwaki, C., Moriya, H.: Isolation and some properties of dog and rat pancreatic kallikrein. J. Biochem. (Tokyo) *81*, 599–610 (1977)
Hokama, Y., Iwanaga, S., Tatsuki, T., Suzuki, T.: Snake venom proteinase inhibitors. III. Isolation of five polypeptide inhibitors from the venoms of *Hemachatus haemachatus* (Ringhal's Cobra) and *Naja nivea* (Cape Cobra), and the complete amino acid sequences of two of them. J. Biochem. (Tokyo) *79*, 559–578 (1976)
Holt, J.C., Meloun, B., Šorm, F.: Nitration by tetranitromethane of the complex of chymotrypsin with the basic pancreatic trypsin inhibitor. Collect. Czech. Chem. Commun. *37*, 1401–1407 (1972)
Houvenaghel, A., Peeters, G.: Influence de la bradykinine sur l'éjection du lait chez la brebis et la chèvre. Arch. Int. Physiol. Biochim. *76*, 647–657 (1968)
Houvenaghel, A., Peeters, G., Djordjeviç, N.: Influence des kinines du plasma et des kallikréines sur l'éjection du lait chez la brebis. Arch. Int. Pharmacodyn. *171*, 231–232 (1968a)
Houvenaghel, A., Peeters, G., Vandaele, G., Djordjeviç, N.: Influence des kinines du plasma et des kallikréines sur l'éjection du lait chez les ruminants. Arch. Int. Physiol. Biochim. *76*, 658–679 (1968b)
Huang, J.-S., Liener, I.E.: Interaction of the Kunitz soybean trypsin inhibitor with bovine trypsin. Evidence for an acylenzyme intermediate during complexation. Biochemistry *16*, 2474–2478 (1977)
Huber, R., Bode, W., Kukla, D., Kohl, U., Ryan, C.A.: The structure of the complex formed by bovine trypsin and bovine pancreatic trypsin inhibitor. III. Structure of the anhydro-trypsin-inhibitor complex. Biophys. Struct. Mech. *1*, 189–201 (1975)
Huber, R., Kukla, D., Bode, W., Schwager, P., Bartels, K., Deisenhofer, J., Steigemann, W.: Structure of the complex formed by bovine trypsin and bovine pancreatic trypsin inhibitor. II. Crystallographic refinement at 1.9 Å resolution. J. Mol. Biol. *89*, 73–101 (1974a)
Huber, R., Kukla, D., Rühlmann, A., Epp, O., Formanek, H.: The basic trypsin inhibitor of bovine pancreas. I. Structure analysis and conformation of the polypeptide chain. Naturwissenschaften *57*, 389–392 (1970)

Huber, R., Kukla, D., Rühlmann, A., Steigemann, W.: Pancreatic trypsin inhibitor (Kunitz). Cold Spring Harbour Symp. Quant. Biol. *36*, 141–150 (1971 a)

Huber, R., Kukla, D., Rühlmann, A., Steigemann, W.: The atomic structure of the basic trypsin inhibitor of bovine organs (kallikrein inactivator). In: Proc. int. res. conf. on proteinase inhibitors. Fritz, H., Tschesche, H. (eds.), pp. 56–63. Berlin, New York: de Gruyter 1971 b

Huber, R., Kukla, D., Steigemann, W., Deisenhofer, J., Jones, A.: Structure of the complex formed by bovine trypsin and bovine pancreatic trypsin inhibitor refinement of the crystal structure analysis. In: Proteinase inhibitors. Fritz, H., Tschesche, H., Greene, L.J., Truscheit, E. (eds.), pp. 497–512. Berlin, Heidelberg, New York: Springer 1974 b

Hvidt, A., Pedersen, E.J.: A comparative study on the basic pancreatic trypsin inhibitor and insulin by the hydrogen-exchange method. Eur. J. Biochem. *48*, 333–338 (1974)

Ikeda, K., Hamaguchi, K., Yamamoto, M., Ikenara, T.: Circular dichroism and optical rotatory dispersion of trypsin inhibitors. J. Biochem. (Tokyo) *63*, 521–531 (1968)

Ikezawa, H., Yamada, K., Aoyagi, T., Takeuchi, T., Umezawa, H.: Effect of antipain on lysosomal peptide-hydrolases from swine liver. J. Antibiot. (Tokyo) *25*, 738–740 (1972)

Illchmann, K., Werle, E.: A polyvalent proteinase inhibitor in the earthworm *(Lumbricus terrestris)*. In: Proteinase inhibitors. Fritz, H., Tschesche, H., Greene, L.J., Truscheit, E. (eds.), pp. 282–283. Berlin, Heidelberg, New York: Springer 1974

Iwanaga, S., Takahashi, H., Suzuki, T.: Proteinase inhibitors from the venom of Russell's viper. In: Methods in enzymology. Lorand, L. (ed.), Vol. XLV/B, pp. 874–881. London, New York: Academic Press 1976

Iwasaki, T., Kiyohara, T., Yoshikawa, M.: Identification of the reactive site of potato proteinase inhibitor II-b for bovine chymotrypsin and a bacterial proteinase. J. Biochem. (Tokyo) *74*, 335–340 (1973)

Iwasaki, T., Kiyohara, T., Yoshikawa, M.: Amino acid sequence of an active fragment of potato proteinase inhibitor II a. J. Biochem. (Tokyo) *79*, 381–391 (1976)

Janin, J., Sweet, R.M., Blow, D.M.: The mode of action of soybean trypsin inhibitor as revealed by crystal structure analysis of the complex with porcine trypsin. In: Proteinase inhibitors. Fritz, H., Tschesche, H., Greene, L.J., Truscheit, E. (eds.), pp. 513–520. Berlin, Heidelberg, New York: Springer 1974

Jering, H., Schorp, G., Tschesche, H.: Enzymatic cleavage of the N^{ε}-acetyl protecting group from lysine in proteins (Kunitz trypsin-kallikrein inhibitor) in vivo and in vitro. Hoppe Seylers Z. Physiol. Chem. *355*, 1129–1134 (1974)

Jering, H., Tschesche, H.: Darstellung des aktiven Derivates von Rinder-Trypsin-Kallikrein-Inhibitor (Kunitz) mit im reaktiven Zentrum geöffneter Peptidbindung. Angew. Chem. *86*, 702–703 (1974 a); Angew. Chem. (Engl.) *13*, 660 (1974a)

Jering, H., Tschesche, H.: Proteinase-katalysierte Resynthese der Peptidbindung Lys 15-Ala 16 im Derivat des Trypsin-Kallikrein Inhibitors (Kunitz) mit geöffneter Peptidbindung. Angew. Chem. *86*, 703 (1974 b); Angew. Chem. (Engl.) *13*, 661 (1974 b)

Jering, H., Tschesche, H.: Austausch von Lysin gegen Arginin, Phenylalanin und Tryptophan im reaktiven Zentrum des Trypsin-Kallikrein-Inhibitors (Kunitz). Angew. Chem. *86*, 704–705 (1974 c)

Jering, H., Tschesche, H.: Inaktivierung des Trypsin-Kallikrein-Inhibitors (Kunitz) durch Abspaltung des Dipeptides Ala 16-Arg 17 im reaktiven Zentrum. Angew. Chem. *86*, 705 (1974 d)

Jering, H., Tschesche, H.: Preparation and characterization of the active derivative of bovine trypsin-kallikrein inhibitor (Kunitz) with the reactive site lysine-15–alanine-16 hydrolyzed. Eur. J. Biochem. *61*, 443–452 (1976 a)

Jering, H., Tschesche, H.: Replacement of lysine by arginine, phenylalanine, and tryptophan in the reactive site of the bovine trypsin-kallikrein inhibitor (Kunitz) and change of the inhibitory properties. Eur. J. Biochem. *61*, 453–463 (1976 b)

Johnson, D.A.: Purification and properties of rabbit trypsin. Biochim. Biophys. Acta *452*, 482–487 (1976)

Johnson, D.A., Travis, J.: Rapid purification of human trypsin and chymotrypsin I. Anal. Biochem. *72*, 573–576 (1976)

Jonáková, V., Čechová, D.: Two trypsin inhibitors from cow colostrum differing in primary structure. Collect. Czech. Chem. Commun. *42*, 759–769 (1977)

Just, M.: In vivo interaction of the Kunitz protease inhibitor and of insulin with subcellular structures from rat renal cortex. Naunyn Schmiedebergs Arch. Pharmakol. *287*, 85–95 (1975)

Just, M., Habermann, E.: The bovine protease inhibitor as a tool for studying the renal reabsorption of peptides. Naunyn Schmiedebergs Arch. Pharmakol. *282*, R 43 (1974)
Just, M., Török, P., Habermann, E.: Interaction of trasylol with subcellular structures of the kidney. In: Kininogenases. Haberland, G. L., Rohen, J. W. (eds.), pp. 123–127. Stuttgart, New York: Schattauer 1973
Kaiser, E. T.: Organic chemical models for proteinase inhibitors. In: Proteinase inhibitors. Fritz, H., Tschesche, H., Greene, L. J., Truscheit, E. (eds.), pp. 523–530. Berlin, Heidelberg, New York: Springer 1974
Kaiser, K.-P., Belitz, H.-D.: Specifity of potato isoinhibitors towards various proteolytic enzymes. Z. Lebensmittel-Untersuch. Forsch. *151*, 18–22 (1973)
Kaiser, K.-P., Bruhn, L. C., Belitz, H.-D.: Proteaseinhibitors in potatoes. Protein-, trypsin-, and chymotrypsininhibitor patterns by isoelectric focusing in polyacrylamidgel. A rapid method for identification of potato varieties. Z. Lebensmittel-Untersuch. Forsch. *154*, 339–347 (1974)
Kaminogawa, S., Mizobuchi, H., Yamauchi, K.: Comparison of bovine milk protease with plasmin. Agr. Biol. Chem. *36*, 2163–2167 (1972)
Kania, L., Siemion, I. Z., Zabża, A.: Studies on hydrogen-deuterium exchange in basic trypsin inhibitor. Acta Biochim. Pol. *21*, 23–31 (1974)
Kareem, A.: Personal communication (1973), cit. in: Gauwerky, C., Corman, G., Uhlenbruck, G.: Über neue Proteaseinhibitoren mit breiter Wirkungsspezifität bei dem Polychaeten *Sabellastarte indica* (Sauvingny). I. Mitteilung. Z. Klin. Chem. Klin. Biochem. *13*, 429–435 (1975)
Karplus, S., Snyder, G. H., Sykes, B. D.: A nuclear magnetic resonance study of bovine pancreatic trypsin inhibitor. Tyrosine titrations and backbone NH groups. Biochemistry *12*, 1323–1329 (1973)
Kasche, V., Amnéus, H., Gabel, D., Näslund, L.: Rapid zymogen activation and isolation of serine proteases from an individual mouse pancreas by affinity chromatography. Genetical heterogeneity of chymotrypsins of *Mus musculus*. Biochim. Biophys. Acta *490*, 1–18 (1977)
Kassell, B.: Naturally occurring inhibitors of proteolytic enzymes. In: Methods in enzymology. Colowick, S. P., Kaplan, N. O. (eds.), Vol. XIX, pp. 839–883, 890–906. New York, London: Academic Press 1970
Kassell, B., Laskowski, M., Sr.: The basic trypsin inhibitor of bovine pancreas. V. The disulfide linkages. Biochem. Biophys. Res. Commun. *20*, 463–468 (1965)
Kassell, B., Wang, T.-W.: The action of thermolysin on the basic trypsin inhibitor of bovine organs. In: Proc. int. res. conf. on proteinase inhibitors. Fritz, H., Tschesche, H. (eds.), pp. 89–94. Berlin, New York: de Gruyter 1971
Kato, A., Hayashi, H., Yagishita, K.: The inhibitory properties of chicken egg white ovomucin against aggregation of *k*-casein by rennin. Agr. Biol. Chem. *38*, 1137–1140 (1974)
Kato, I., Tominaga, N.: Soybean trypsin inhibitor-C: An active derivative of soybean trypsin inhibitor composed of two noncovalently bonded peptide fragments. FEBS Letters *10*, 313–316 (1970)
Kawamura, K., Kondo, S., Meada, K., Umezawa, H.: Structures and synthesis of leupeptins Pr-LL and Ac-LL. Chem. Pharm. Bull. (Tokyo) *17*, 1902–1909 (1969)
Keil, B.: Reaction of arginine residues in basic pancreatic trypsin inhibitor with phenylglyoxal. FEBS Letters *14*, 181–184 (1971)
Keil-Dlouha, V., Keil, B.: A tryptophan residue in bovine trypsinogen essential for its potential enzymic activity and for its interaction with basic pancreatic trypsin inhibitor. J. Mol. Biol. *67*, 495–505 (1972)
Kiyohara, T., Fujii, M., Iwasaki, T., Yoshikawa, M.: Identification of the reactive site of potato proteinase inhibitor I of various proteinases. J. Biochem. (Tokyo) *74*, 675–682 (1973)
Knights, R. J., Light, A.: Disulfide bond-modified trypsinogen. J. Biol. Chem. *251*, 222–228 (1976)
Koide, T., Ikenaka, T.: Studies on soybean trypsin inhibitors. 1. Fragmentation of soybean trypsin inhibitor (Kunitz) by limited proteolysis and by chemical cleavage. Eur. J. Biochem. *32*, 401–407 (1973a)
Koide, T., Ikenaka, T.: Studies on soybean trypsin inhibitors. 3. Amino-acid-sequence of the carboxyl-terminal region and the complete amino-acid sequence of soybean trypsin inhibitor (Kunitz). Eur. J. Biochem. *32*, 417–431 (1973b)
Koide, T., Ikenaka, T., Ikeda, K., Hamaguchi, K.: Studies on soybean trypsin inhibitors. IX. Reconstitution of an active derivative from two inactive fragments and the contribution of tryptophan-93. J. Biochem. (Tokyo) *75*, 805–823 (1974)

Koide, T., Tsunasawa, S., Ikenaka, T.: Studies on soybean trypsin inhibitors. 2. Amino-acid sequence around the reactive site of soybean trypsin inhibitor (Kunitz). Eur. J. Biochem. *32*, 408–416 (1973)

Kokubu, T., Hiwada, K., Nagasaka, Y., Yamamura, Y.: Effect of several proteinase inhibitors on renin reaction. Jap. Circ. J. *38*, 955–958 (1974)

Kondo, S., Kawamura, K., Iwanaga, J., Hamada, M., Aoyagi, T., Maeda, K., Takeuchi, T., Umezawa, H.: Isolation and characterization of leupeptins produced by actinomycetes. Chem. Pharm. Bull. (Tokyo) *17*, 1896–1901 (1969)

Kopitar, M., Lebez, D.: Intracellular distribution of neutral proteinases and inhibitors in pig leucocytes. Eur. J. Biochem. *56*, 571–581 (1975)

Kowalski, D., Laskowski, M., Jr.: Inactivation of enzymatically modified trypsin inhibitors upon chemical modification of the α-amino group in the reactive site. Biochemistry *11*, 3451–3459 (1972)

Kowalski, D., Laskowski, M., Jr.: Chemical-enzymatic replacement of Ile^{64} in the reactive site of soybean trypsin inhibitor (Kunitz). Biochemistry *15*, 1300–1308 (1976a)

Kowalski, D., Laskowski, M., Jr.: Chemical-enzymatic insertion of an amino acid residue in the reactive site of soybean trypsin inhibitor (Kunitz). Biochemistry *15*, 1309–1315 (1976b)

Kowalski, D., Leary, T.R., McKee, R.E., Sealock, R.W., Wang, D., Laskowski, M., Jr.: Replacements, insertions, and modifications of amino acid residues in the reactive site of soybean trypsin inhibitor (Kunitz). In: Proteinase inhibitors. Fritz, H., Tschesche, H., Greene, L.J., Truscheit, E. (eds.), pp. 311–324. Berlin, Heidelberg, New York: Springer 1974

Kress, L.F., Laskowski, M., Sr.: The basic trypsin inhibitor of bovine pancreas. VII. Reduction with borohydride of disulfide bond linking half-cystine residues 14 and 38. J. Biol. Chem. *242*, 4925–4929 (1967)

Kress, L.F., Laskowski, M., Sr.: The basic trypsin inhibitor of bovine pancreas. IX. Location of the reactive site in the carboxamidomethyl derivative. J. Biol. Chem. *243*, 3548–3550 (1968)

Kress, L.F., Wilson, K.A., Laskowski, M., Sr.: The basic trypsin inhibitor of bovine pancreas. VIII. Changes in activity following substitution of reduced half-cystine residues 14 and 38 with sulfhydryl reagents. J. Biol. Chem. *243*, 1758–1762 (1968)

Kruze, D., Menninger, H., Fehr, K., Böni, A.: Purification and some properties of a neutral protease from human leukocyte granules and its comparison with pancreatic elastase. Biochim. Biophys. Acta *438*, 503–513 (1976)

Laskowski, M., Jr., Kato, I., Leary, T.R., Schrode, J., Sealock, R.W.: Evolution of specificity of protein proteinase inhibitors. In: Proteinase inhibitors. Fritz, H., Tschesche, H., Greene, L.J., Truscheit, E. (eds.), pp. 597–611. Berlin, Heidelberg, New York: Springer 1974

Laskowski, M., Jr., Sealock, R.W.: Protein proteinase inhibitors – molecular aspects. In: The enzymes, 3rd ed. Boyer, P.D. (ed.), Vol. III, pp. 375–473. London, New York: Academic Press 1971

Laskowski, M., Sr., Schneider, S.L., Wilson, K.A., Kress, L.F., Mozejko, J.H., Martin, S.R., Kucich, U., Andrews, M.: Naturally occurring trypsin inhibitors: Further studies on purification and temporary inhibition. In: Proc. int. res. conf. on proteinase inhibitors. Fritz, H., Tschesche, H. (eds.), pp. 66–73. Berlin, New York: de Gruyter 1971

Lazdunski, M., Vincent, J.-P., Schweitz, H., Péron-Renner, M., Pudles, J.: The mechanism of association of trypsin (or chymotrypsin) with the pancreatic trypsin inhibitors (Kunitz and Kazal). Kinetics and thermodynamics of the interaction. In: Proteinase inhibitors. Fritz, H., Tschesche, H., Greene, L.J., Truscheit, E. (eds.), pp. 420–431. Berlin, Heidelberg, New York: Springer 1974

Leary, T.R., Laskowski, M., Jr.: Enzymatic replacement of Arg^{63} by Trp^{63} in the reactive site of soybean trypsin inhibitor (Kunitz) – an intentional change from tryptic to chymotryptic specificity. Fed. Proc. *32*, 465 (Abstract) (1973)

Lemon, M., Förg-Brey, B., Fritz, H.: Isolation of porcine submandibular kallikrein. Agents Actions *6*, 431 (1976)

Levilliers, N., Péron-Renner, M., Pudles, J.: Kinetic studies on the interactions between native, acetylated and succinylated trypsin and natural proteinase inhibitors. In: Proteinase inhibitors. Fritz, H., Tschesche, H., Greene, L.J., Truscheit, E. (eds.), pp. 432–444. Berlin, Heidelberg, New York: Springer 1974

Levin, Y., Pecht, M., Goldstein, L., Katchalski, E.: A water-insoluble polyanionic derivative of trypsin. I. Preparation and properties. Biochemistry *3*, 1905–1919 (1964)

Liener, I.E., Kakade, M.: Protease inhibitors. In: Toxic constituents of plant foodstuffs. Liener, I.E. (ed.), pp. 7–68. London, New York: Academic Press 1969
Liu, W.-H., Feinstein, G., Osuga, D.T., Haynes, R., Feeney, R.E.: Modification of arginines in trypsin inhibitors by 1,2-cyclohexanedione. Biochemistry 7, 2886–2892 (1968)
Liu, W.-H., Means, G.E., Feeney, R.E.: The inhibitory properties of avian ovoinhibitors against proteolytic enzymes. Biochim. Biophys. Acta *229*, 176–185 (1971)
Loeffler, L.J., Mar, E.-C., Geratz, J.D., Fox, L.B.: Synthesis of isosteres of *p*-amidinophenylpyruvic acid. Inhibitors of trypsin, thrombin, and pancreatic kallikrein. J. Med. Chem. *18*, 287–292 (1975)
Lorand, L.: Methods in enzymology, Vol. XLV/B. London, New York: Academic Press 1976
Luthy, J.A., Praissman, M., Finkenstadt, W.R., Laskowski, M., Jr.: Detailed mechanism of interaction of bovine β-trypsin with soybean trypsin inhibitor (Kunitz). I. Stopped flow measurements. J. Biol. Chem. *248*, 1760–1771 (1973)
Maeda, K., Kawamura, K., Kondo, S., Aoyagi, T., Takeuchi, T., Umezawa, H.: The structure and activity of leupeptins and related analogs. J. Antibiot. (Tokyo) *24*, 402–404 (1971)
Mair, G., Tschesche, H., Förg-Brey, B., Fritz, H.: Isolation of porcine urinary kallikrein. Agents Actions *6*, 433 (1976)
Maki, M., Sasaki, K.: A new broad spectrum inhibitor of esteroproteases, 4-(2-carboxyethyl) phenyl-trans-aminomethyl cyclohexane carboxylate hydrochloride (DV 1006). Tohoku J. Exp. Med. *106*, 233–248 (1972)
Mallory, P.A., Travis, J.: Human pancreatic enzymes. Characterization of anionic human trypsin. Biochemistry *12*, 2847–2851 (1973)
Mallory, P.A., Travis, J.: Properties and inhibition spectrum of a new human pancreatic protease. In: Proteinase inhibitors. Fritz, H., Tschesche, H., Greene, L.J., Truscheit, E. (eds.), pp. 250–251. Berlin, Heidelberg, New York: Springer 1974
Mares-Guia, M., Diniz, C.R.: Studies on the mechanism of rat urinary kallikrein catalysis, and its relation to catalysis by trypsin. Arch. Biochem. Biophys. *121*, 750–756 (1967)
Marinetti, T.D., Snyder, G.H., Sykes, B.D.: Nuclear magnetic resonance determination of intramolecular distances in bovine pancreatic trypsin inhibitor using nitrotyrosine chelation of lanthanides. Biochemistry *15*, 4600–4608 (1976)
Marinetti, T.D., Snyder, G.H., Sykes, B.D.: Nitrotyrosine chelation of nuclear magnetic resonance shift probes in proteins: Application to bovine pancreatic trypsin inhibitor. Biochemistry *16*, 647–653 (1977)
Markley, J.L.: High-resolution proton magnetic resonance studies of two trypsin inhibitors: Soybean trypsin inhibitor (Kunitz) and ovomucoid (hen egg white). Ann. N.Y. Acad. Sci. *222*, 347–373 (1973a)
Markley, J.L.: Nuclear magnetic resonance studies of trypsin inhibitors. Histidines of virgin and modified soybean trypsin inhibitor (Kunitz). Biochemistry *12*, 2245–2250 (1973b)
Markley, J.L., Kati, I.: Assignment of the histidine proton magnetic resonance peaks of soybean trypsin inhibitor (Kunitz) by a differential deuterium exchange technique. Biochemistry *14*, 3234–3237 (1975)
Markwardt, F., Drawert, J., Walsmann, P.: Einfluß von Benzamidinderivaten auf die Aktivität von Serum- und Pankreaskallikrein. Acta Biol. Med. Ger. *26*, 123–128 (1971a)
Markwardt, F., Drawert, J., Walsmann, P.: Synthetic low molecular weight inhibitors of serum kallikrein. Biochem. Pharmacol. *23*, 2247–2256 (1974)
Markwardt, F., Klöcking, H.-P., Nowak, G.: Hemmung der Kininbildung im Blut durch *p*-Amidinophenylbrenztraubensäure. Experientia *27*, 812 (1971b)
Markwardt, F., Walsmann, P., Drawert, J.: Suppression of kinin formation with benzamidine derivatives. Farmakol. Toksikol. *34*, 195–198 (1971c)
Mason, B., Sparrow, E.M.: The relationship between the permeability-increasing and the hypotensive proteases of plasma. Br. J. Pharmacol. Chemother. *25*, 257–269 (1965)
Masson, A., Wüthrich, K.: Protein magnetic resonance investigation of the conformational properties of the basic pancreatic trypsin inhibitor. FEBS Letters *31*, 114–118 (1973)
Matsuda, Y., Miyazaki, K., Moriya, H., Fujimoto, Y., Hojima, Y., Moriwaki, C.: Studies on urinary kallikrein. I. Purification and characterization of human urinary kallikreins. J. Biochem. (Tokyo) *80*, 671–679 (1976)
Mattis, J.A., Laskowski, M., Jr.: pH dependence of the equilibrium constant for the hydrolysis of the Arg^{63}-Ile reactive-site peptide bond in soybean trypsin inhibitor (Kunitz). Bichemistry *12*, 2239–2244 (1973)

Meloun, B., Frič, I., Šorm, F.: Nitration of tyrosine residues in the pancreatic trypsin inhibitor with tetranitromethane. Eur. J. Biochem. *4*, 112–117 (1968)

Melville, J.C., Ryan, C.A.: Chymotrypsin inhibitor I from potatoes. J. Biol. Chem. *247*, 3445–3453 (1972)

Mills, I.H., Paterson, C.L., Ward, P.E.: The role of the kidney in the inactivation of injected [^{125}I]kallikrein. J. Physiol. (Lond.) *251*, 281–286 (1975)

Modéer, T.: Human saliva kallikrein. Acta Odontol. Scand. *35*, 23–29 (1977a)

Modéer, T.: Characterization of kallikrein from human saliva isolated by use of affinity chromatography. Acta Odontol. Scand. *35*, 31–39 (1977b)

Moriwaki, C., Hojima, Y., Schachter, M.: Purification of kallikrein from cat submaxillary gland. Agents Actions *6*, 436 (1976a)

Moriwaki, C., Miyazaki, K., Matsuda, Y., Moriya, H., Fujimoto, Y., Ueki, H.: Dog renal kallikrein: Purification and some properties. J. Biochem. (Tokyo) *80*, 1277–1285 (1976b)

Moriwaki, C., Schachter, M.: Kininogenase of the guinea-pig's coagulating gland and the release of bradykinin. J. Physiol. (Lond.) *219*, 341–353 (1971)

Moriya, H., Hojima, Y.: Studies on kinin-forming enzymes in human plasma and their heterogeneity. In: Vasopeptides. Back, N., Sicuteri, F. (eds.), pp. 167–184. New York: Plenum Press 1972

Moriya, H., Hojima, Y., Moriwaki, C., Tajima, T.: Specificity of potato kallikrein inhibitors for kallikreins. Experientia *26*, 720–721 (1970)

Moriya, H., Matsuda, Y., Fujimoto, Y., Hojima, Y., Moriwaki, C.: Some aspects of multiple components on the kallikrein human urinary kallikrein (HUK). In: Kininogenases. Haberland, G.L., Rohen, J.W. (eds.), pp. 37–42. Stuttgart, New York: Schattauer 1973

Movat, H.Z., Habal, F.M., MacMorine, D.R.L.: Neutral proteases of human PMN leukocytes with kininogenase activity. Int. Arch. Allergy Appl. Immunol. *50*, 257–281 (1976)

Muramatu, M., Fujii, S.: Inhibitory effects of ω-guanidino acid esters on trypsin, plasmin, thrombin, and plasma kallikrein. J. Biochem. (Tokyo) *64*, 807–814 (1968)

Muramatu, M., Fujii, S.: Inhibitory effects of ω-amino acid esters on trypsin, plasmin, plasma kallikrein, and thrombin. Biochim. Biophys. Acta *242*, 203–208 (1971)

Muramatu, M., Fujii, S.: Inhibitory effects of ω-guanidino acid esters on trypsin, plasmin, plasma kallikrein and thrombin. Biochim. Biophys. Acta *268*, 221–224 (1972)

Muszyńska, G., Čechová, D.: Effect of modification of lysine residues of cow colostrum trypsin inhibitor on its antitryptic and antichymotryptic activity. FEBS Letters *8*, 274–276 (1970)

Nakanishi, M., Tsuboi, M.: A slow fluctuation in the molecular conformation of a soya bean trypsin inhibitor. J. Mol. Biol. *83*, 379–391 (1974)

Niekamp, C.W., Hixon, M., Jr., Laskowski, M., Jr.: Peptide-bond hydrolysis equilibria in native proteins. Conversion of virgin into modified soybean trypsin inhibitor. Biochemistry *8*, 16–22 (1969)

Nustad, K.: Observations on the kininogenase activity of rat kidney and urine. Scand. J. Clin. Lab. Invest. *24*, Suppl. 107, 97–99 (1969)

Odani, S., Koide, T., Ikenaka, T.: Studies on soybean trypsin inhibitors. II. Accidentally modified Kunitz soybean trypsin inhibitor. J. Biochem. (Tokyo) *70*, 925–936 (1971)

Oza, N.B., Amin, V.M., McGregor, R.K., Scicli, A.G., Carretero, O.A.: Isolation of rat urinary kallikrein and properties of its antibodies. Biochem. Pharmacol. *25*, 1607–1612 (1976)

Papaioannou, S.E., Liener, I.E.: The involvement of tyrosyl and amino groups in the interaction of trypsin and a soybean trypsin inhibitor. J. Biol. Chem. *245*, 4931–4938 (1970)

Paskhina, T.S., Zukova, V.P., Egorova, T.P., Narticova, V.F., Karpova, A.V., Guseva, M.V.: Reaction of N-α-tosyl-L-lysyl-chloromethane with kallicrein from blood plasma of rabbit and with kallicreins from urine and saliva of man. Biokhimiya *33*, 745–752 (1968)

Peeters, G., Verbeke, R., Houvenaghel, A., Reynaert, R.: Isolation of kallikrein from mammary gland of cows. Q. J. Exp. Physiol. *61*, 1–14 (1976)

Pershina, L., Hvidt, A.: A study by the hydrogen-exchange method of the complex formed between the basic pancreatic trypsin inhibitor and trypsin. Eur. J. Biochem. *48*, 339–344 (1974)

Porcelli, G., Cozzari, C., Di Iorio, M., Croxatto, R.H., Angeletti, P.: Isolation and partial characterization of a kallikrein from mouse submaxillary glands. Ital. J. Biochem. *25*, 337–348 (1976)

Quast, U., Engel, J., Heumann, H., Krause, G., Steffen, E.: Kinetics of interaction of bovine pancreatic trypsin inhibitor (Kunitz) with α-chymotrypsin. Biochemistry *13*, 2512–2520 (1974)

Quast, U., Engel, J., Steffen, E., Mair, G., Tschesche, H., Jering, H.: Kinetics of binding of bovine trypsin-kallikrein inhibitor (Kunitz) in which the reactive-site peptide bond Lys-15–Ala-16 is cleaved, to α-chymotrypsin and β-trypsin. Eur. J. Biochem. *52*, 505–510 (1975a)

Quast, U., Engel, J., Steffen, E., Tschesche, H., Jering, H., Kupfer, S.: The effect of cleaving the reactive-site peptide bond Lys-15–Ala-16 on the conformation of bovine trypsin-kallikrein inhibitor (Kunitz) as revealed by solvent-perturbation spectra, circular dichroism and fluorescence. Eur. J. Biochem. *52*, 511–514 (1975b)

Quast, U., Engel, J., Tschesche, H.: Interaction of α-chymotrypsin or β-trypsin with basic pancreatic trypsin inhibitor. Experientia *32*, 807 (1976)

Quast, U., Steffen, E.: The soybean trypsin inhibitor (Kunitz) is a doubleheaded inhibitor. Hoppe Seylers Z. Physiol. Chem. *356*, 617–620 (1975)

Reynaert, H., Peeters, G., Verbeke, R., Houvenaghel, A.: Further studies of the physiology of plasma kinins and kallikreins in the udder of ruminants. Arch. Int. Pharmacodyn. Ther. *176*, 473–475 (1968)

Richardson, M., Cossins, L.: Chymotryptic inhibitor I from potatoes: The amino acid sequences of subunits B, C, and D. FEBS Letters *45*, 11–13 (1974)

Rocchi, R., Benassi, C.A., Tomatis, R., Ferroni, R., Menegatti, E.: On the reaction of acetamidomethanol with native and reduced bovine pancreatic trypsin inhibitor (Kunitz inhibitor). Int. J. Peptide Protein Res. *8*, 167–175 (1976)

Rodrigues, J.A.A., Beraldo, W.T.: Studies on the vascular reaction produced by proteolytic enzymes in the rat. Agents Actions *3*, 384 (1973)

Rosenkranz, H.: A study on the interaction of Trasylol with trypsin and kallikrein by circular dichroism. In: Proteinase inhibitors. Fritz, H., Tschesche, H., Greene, L.J., Truscheit, E. (eds.), pp. 458–462. Berlin, Heidelberg, New York: Springer 1974a

Rosenkranz, H.: Circular dichroism of globular proteins – a review of the limits of the CD methods for the calculation of secondary structure. Z. Klin. Chem. Klin. Biochem. *12*, 415–422 (1974b)

Rosenkranz, H., Scholtan, W.: Eine verbesserte Methode zur Konformationsbestimmung von helicalen Proteinen aus Messungen des Circulardichroismus. Hoppe Seylers Z. Physiol. Chem. *352*, 896–904 (1971)

Rühlmann, A., Kukla, D., Schwager, P., Bartels, K., Huber, R.: Structure of the complex formed by bovine trypsin and bovine pancreatic trypsin inhibitor. J. Mol. Biol. *77*, 417–436 (1973)

Ryan, C.A.: Chymotrypsin inhibitor I from potatoes: Reactivity with mammalian, plant, bacterial, and fungal proteinases. Biochemistry *5*, 1592–1596 (1966)

Ryan, C.A.: Proteolytic enzymes and their inhibitors in plants. Annu. Rev. Plant. Physiol. *24*, 173–196 (1973)

Ryan, C.A., Santarius, K.: Immunological similarities of proteinase inhibitors from potatoes. Plant. Physiol. *58*, 683–685 (1976)

Ryan, C.A., Shumway, L.K.: Studies on the structure and function of chymotrypsin inhibitor I in the Solanaceae family. In: Proc. int. res. conf. on proteinase inhibitors. Fritz, H., Tschesche, H. (eds.), pp. 175–188. Berlin, New York: de Gruyter 1971

Rzeszotarska, B., Wiejak, S.: Struktura i funkcja zasadowego inhibitora trypsyny. Postepy. Biochem. *22*, 123–142 (1976)

Sakato, K., Tanaka, H., Misawa, M.: Broad-specificity proteinase inhibitors in *Scopolia japonica* (Solanaceae) cultured cells. Eur. J. Biochem. *55*, 211–219 (1975)

Sampaio, C.A.M., Prado, E.S.: Active-site labelling of kallikreins by chloromethylketone derivatives. Gen. Pharmacol. *7*, 163–166 (1976)

Sampaio, C., Wong, S.-C., Shaw, E.: Human plasma kallikrein. Purification and preliminary characterization. Arch. Biochem. Biophys. *165*, 133–139 (1974)

Sawada, J., Yasui, H., Amamoto, T., Yamada, M., Okazaki, T., Tanaka, I.: Isolation and some properties of anti-proteolytic polypeptides from potato. Agr. Biol. Chem. *38*, 2559–2561 (1974)

Schechter, I., Berger, A.: On the size of the active site in proteases. I. Papain. Biochem. Biophys. Res. Commun. *27*, 157–162 (1967)

Schiessler, H., Arnhold, M., Fritz, H.: Characterization of two proteinase inhibitors from human seminal plasma and spermatozoa. In: Proteinase inhibitors. Fritz, H., Tschesche, H., Greene, L.J., Truscheit, E. (eds.), pp. 147–155. Berlin, Heidelberg, New York: Springer 1974
Schiessler, H., Arnhold, M., Ohlsson, K., Fritz, H.: Inhibitors of acrosin and granulocyte proteinases from human genital tract secretions. Hoppe Seylers Z. Physiol. Chem. *357*, 1251–1260 (1976)
Sealock, R.W., Laskowski, M., Jr.: Enzymatic replacement of the arginyl by a lysyl residue in the reactive site of soybean trypsin inhibitor. Biochemistry *8*, 3703–3710 (1969)
Seki, T., Miwa, I., Nakajima, T., Erdös, E.G.: Plasma kallikrein-kinin system in nonmammalian blood: Evolutionary aspects. Am. J. Physiol. *224*, 1425–1430 (1973)
Seki, T., Nakajima, T., Erdös, E.G.: Colon kallikrein, its relation to the plasma enzyme. Biochem. Pharmacol. *21*, 1227–1235 (1972)
Seki, T., Yang, H.Y.T., Levin, Y., Jenssen, T.A., Erdös, E.G.: Application of water-insoluble complexes of kininogenases, inhibitors, and kininases to kinin research. Adv. Exp. Med. Biol. *8*, 23–30 (1970)
Sen, L.C., Whitaker, J.R.: Some properties of a ficin-papain inhibitor from avian egg white. Arch. Biochem. Biophys. *158*, 623–632 (1973)
Shaw, E.: Progress in designing small inhibitors which discriminate among trypsin-like enzymes. In: Proteinase inhibitors. Fritz, H., Tschesche, H., Greene, L.J., Truscheit, E. (eds.), pp. 531–540. Berlin, Heidelberg, New York: Springer 1974
Siemion, I.Z., Kania, L.: Fluorescence of tyrosine residues in the basic trypsin inhibitor from bovine lungs. Acta Biochim. Pol. *22*, 195–200 (1975)
Siffert, O., Emöd, I., Keil, B.: Interaction of clostripain with natural trypsin inhibitors and its affinity labeling by N^{α}-*p*-nitrobenzyloxycarbonyl arginine chlormethyl ketone. FEBS Letters *66*, 114–119 (1976)
Silman, I.H., Katchalski, E.: Water-insoluble derivatives of enzymes, antigens, and antibodies. Annu. Rev. Biochem. *35*, 873–904 (1966)
Silva, E., Diniz, C.R., Mares-Guia, M.: Rat urinary kallikrein: Purification and properties. Biochemistry *13*, 4304–4310 (1974)
Siqueira, G., Beraldo, W.T.: Attempts to isolate a kallikrein inhibitor from rat salivary gland. Agents Actions *3*, 323–325 (1973)
Snyder, G.H., Rowan III, R., Karplus, S., Sykes, B.D.: Complete tyrosine assignments in the high field ^{1}H nuclear magnetic resonance spectrum of the bovine pancreatic trypsin inhibitor. Biochemistry *14*, 3765–3777 (1975)
Sprenger, I., Uhlenbruck, G., Hermann, G.: Snail albumin gland: A new source of proteinase inhibitors. Enzymologia *43*, 83–88 (1972)
Stambaugh, R., Brackett, B.G., Mastroianni, L.: Inhibition of in vitro fertilization of rabbit ova by trypsin inhibitors. Biol. Reprod. *1*, 223–227 (1969)
Stewart, K.K.: A method for automated analyses of the activities of trypsin, chymotrypsin, and their inhibitors. Anal. Biochem. *51*, 11–18 (1973)
Stoddart, R.W., Kiernan, J.A.: Aprotinin: A carbohydrate-binding protein. Histochemie *34*, 275–280 (1973)
Strydom, D.J.: Snake venom toxins. The amino acid sequence of toxin Vi2, a homologue of pancreatic trypsin inhibitor, from *Dendroaspis polylepis polylepis* (black mamba) venom. Biochim. Biophys. Acta *491*, 361–369 (1977)
Suda, H., Aoyagi, T., Hamada, M., Takeuchi, T., Umezawa, H.: Antipain, a new protease inhibitor isolated from actinomycetes. J. Antibiot. (Tokyo) *25*, 263–265 (1972)
Suominen, J., Multamäki, S., Niemi, M.: Trypsin inhibitors in human semen. Scand. J. Clin. Lab. Invest. *27*, Suppl. 116, 8 (1971)
Suominen, J.J.O., Niemi, M.: Human seminal trypsin inhibitors. J. Reprod. Fertil. *29*, 163–172 (1972)
Suzuki, T.: Personal communication (1974), cit. in: Fritz, H., 1976
Sweet, R.M., Wright, H.T., Janin, J., Chothia, C.H., Blow, D.M.: Crystal structure of the complex of porcine trypsin with soybean trypsin inhibitor (Kunitz) at 2.6-Å resolution. Biochemistry *13*, 4212–4228 (1974)
Szopa, J.: Interaction with DNA of the acetylated and nonacetylated polyvalent basic trypsin inhibitor of the Kunitz type. Acta Biochim. Pol. *21*, 151–157 (1974)

Takahashi, H., Iwanaga, S., Kitagawa, T., Hokama, Y., Suzuki, T.: Snake venom proteinase inhibitors II. Chemical structure of inhibitor II isolated from the venom of Russell's viper *(Vipera russelli)*. J. Biochem. (Tokyo) *76*, 721–733 (1974b)
Takahashi, H., Iwanaga, S., Kitagawa, T., Hokama, Y., Suzuki, T.: Novel proteinase inhibitors in snake venoms: Distribution, isolation, and amino acid sequence. In: Proteinase inhibitors. Fritz, H., Tschesche, H., Greene, L.J., Truscheit, E. (eds.), pp. 265–276. Berlin, Heidelberg, New York: Springer 1974c
Takahashi, H., Iwanaga, S., Hokama, Y., Suzuki, T., Kitagawa, T.: Primary structure of proteinase inhibitor II isolated from the venom of Russell's viper *(Vipera russelli)*. FEBS Letters *38*, 217–221 (1974a)
Takahashi, H., Iwanaga, S., Suzuki, T.: Isolation of a novel inhibitor of kallikrein, plasmin, and trypsin from the venom of Russell's viper *(Vipera russelli)*. FEBS Letters *27*, 207–210 (1972)
Takahashi, H., Iwanaga, S., Suzuki, T.: Distribution of proteinase inhibitors in snake venoms. Toxicon *12*, 193–197 (1974d)
Tan, N.H., Kaiser, E.T.: Studies on the solid-phase synthesis of bovine pancreatic trypsin inhibitor (Kunitz) and the characterization of the synthetic material. J. Org. Chem. *41*, 2787–2793 (1976)
Tan, N.H., Kaiser, E.T.: Synthesis and characterization of a pancreatic trypsin inhibitor homologue and a model inhibitor. Biochemistry *16*, 1531–1541 (1977)
Török, P.: Die Lokalisation eines Proteinasen-Inhibitors in der Niere der Maus durch Immunfluoreszenz. Arzneim. Forsch. *22*, 1534–1538 (1972)
Trautschold, I., Werle, E., Fritz, H., Eckert, I.: Zur Biochemie des Trasylol. In: Neue Aspekte der Trasylol-Therapie. Gross, R., Kroneberg, G. (eds.), pp. 3–19. Stuttgart; Schattauer 1966
Tschesche, H.: Über die Modifizierung des spezifischen Trypsin-Inhibitors aus Schweinepankreas bei der Hemmung von Trypsin. Hoppe Seylers Z. Physiol. Chem. *348*, 1216–1218 (1967)
Tschesche, H.: Biochemie natürlicher Proteinase-Inhibitoren. Angew. Chem. *86*, 21–40 (1974); Biochemistry of natural proteinase inhibitors. Angew. Chem. (Engl.) *13*, 10–28 (1974)
Tschesche, H.: Trypsin-kallikrein inhibitors from cuttlefish *(Loligo vulgaris)*. In: Methods of enzymology. Lorand, L. (ed.), Vol. XLV/B, pp. 792–797. London, New York: Academic Press 1976
Tschesche, H., Dietl, T.: Identifizierung der Proteaseinhibitoren synthetisierenden Organe der Weinbergschnecke *(Helix pomatia)*. Hoppe Seylers Z. Physiol. Chem. *353*, 1189–1193 (1972a)
Tschesche, H., Dietl, T.: Broad-specificity protease-isoinhibitors for trypsin, chymotrypsin, plasmin, and kallikrein from snails *(Helix pomatia)*. Eur. J. Biochem. *30*, 560–570 (1972b)
Tschesche, H., Dietl, T.: Low-molecular-weight proteinase isoinhibitors of broad specificity from the skin of snails. In: Protides of the biological fluids. Peeters, H. (ed.), Vol. XX, pp. 437–445. London: Pergamon Press 1973
Tschesche, H., Dietl, T.: The amino-acid sequence of isoinhibitor K from snails *(Helix pomatia)*. Eur. J. Biochem. *58*, 439–451 (1975)
Tschesche, H., Dietl, T.: Trypsin-kallikrein inhibitors from snails *(Helix pomatia)*. In: Methods in enzymology. Lorand, L. (ed.), Vol. XLV/B, pp. 772–785. London, New York: Academic Press 1976
Tschesche, H., Dietl, T., Kolb, H.J., Standl, E.: An insulin degrading proteinase from human erythrocytes and its inhibition by proteinase inhibitors. In: Proteinase inhibitors. Fritz, H., Tschesche, H., Greene, L.J., Truscheit, E. (eds.), pp. 586–593. Berlin, Heidelberg, New York: Springer 1974a
Tschesche, H., Dietl, T., Marx, R., Fritz, H.: Neue polyvalente Proteasen-Inhibitoren für Trypsin, Chymotrypsin, Plasmin und Kallikreine aus der Weinbergschnecke *(Helix pomatia)*. Hoppe Seylers Z. Physiol. Chem. *353*, 483–486 (1972)
Tschesche, H., Ehret, W., Godec, G., Hirschauer, C., Kutzbach, C., Schmidt-Kastner, G., Fiedler, F.: The primary structure of pig pancreatic kallikrein B. In: Kinins: pharmacodynamics and biological roles. Sicuteri, F., Back, N., Haberland, G.L. (eds.), pp. 123–133. New York, London: Plenum Press 1976
Tschesche, H., Jering, H., Schorp, G., Dietl, T.: Reactive site cleavage, thermodynamic control resynthesis, and properties of chemically derivatized trypsin-kallikrein-inhibitors. In: Proteinase inhibitors. Fritz, H., Tschesche, H., Greene, L.J., Truscheit, E. (eds.), pp. 362–377. Berlin, Heidelberg, New York: Springer 1974b

Tschesche, H., Klauser, R., Čechová, D., Jonáková, V.: On the carbohydrate composition of bovine colostrum trypsin inhibitor. Hoppe Seylers Z. Physiol. Chem. *356*, 1759–1764 (1975)
Tschesche, H., Klein, H.: Modifizierung und Hemmverhalten des spezifischen Trypsininhibitors aus Schweinepankreas – eine im Sauren katalysierbare tryptische Hydrolyse. Hoppe Seylers Z. Physiol. Chem. *349*, 1645–1656 (1968)
Tschesche, H., Klein, H., Reidel, G.: On the mechanism of temporary inhibition. In: Proc. int. res. conf. on proteinase inhibitors. Fritz, H., Tschesche, H. (eds.), pp. 299–304. Berlin, New York: de Gruyter 1971
Tschesche, H., Kupfer, S.: Hydrolysis-resynthesis equilibrium of the lysine-15–alanine-16 peptide bond in bovine trypsin inhibitor (Kunitz). Hoppe Seylers Z. Physiol. Chem. *357*, 769–776 (1976)
Tschesche, H., Obermeier, R.: Mass spectral determination of peptide bond hydrolysis equilibrium in protein proteinase-inhibitors. In: Proc. int. res. conf. on proteinase inhibitors. Fritz, H., Tschesche, H. (eds.), pp. 135–141. Berlin, New York: de Gruyter 1971
Tschesche, H., Rücker, A. v.: Proteinase-Isoinhibitoren mit breiter Spezifität für Trypsin, Chymotrypsin, Plasmin und Kallikrein aus Tintenfischen *(Loligo vulgaris)*. Hoppe Seylers Z. Physiol. Chem. *354*, 1447–1461 (1973a)
Tschesche, H., Rücker, A. v.: Über die Organverteilung der Proteinase-Inhibitoren breiter Spezifität aus Tintenfischen *(Loligo vulgaris)*. Hoppe Seylers Z. Physiol. Chem. *354*, 1510–1512 (1973b)
Tschesche, H., Rücker, A. v.: Proteinase inhibitors from cuttle fish *(Loligo vulgaris)*. In: Proteinase inhibitors. Fritz, H., Tschesche, H., Greene, L. J., Truscheit, E. (eds.), pp. 284–285. Berlin, Heidelberg, New York: Springer 1974
Uhlenbruck, G., Sprenger, I., Hermann, G.: Heterogeneity of polyvalent proteinase-inhibitors from certain snails demonstrated by fibrin-agar-electrophoresis. Z. Klin. Chem. Klin. Biochem. *9*, 494–496 (1971a)
Uhlenbruck, G., Sprenger, I., Ishiyama, I.: A new polyvalent proteinase-inhibitor occurring in the albumin gland of *Helix pomatia*. Z. Klin. Chem. Klin. Biochem. *9*, 361–362 (1971b)
Uhlig, H., Kleine, R.: Natürlich vorkommende Protein-Proteinase-Inhibitoren aus tierischen und pflanzlichen Organismen. Pharmazie *29*, 81–89 (1974)
Umezawa, H.: Enzyme inhibitors of microbial origin. Baltimore, London, Tokyo: Univ. Park Press 1972
Umezawa, H.: Structures and activities of protease inhibitors of microbial origin. In: Methods in enzymology. Lorand, L. (ed.), Vol. XLV/B, pp. 678–695. London, New York: Academic Press 1976
Umezawa, S., Tatsuta, K., Fujimoto, K., Tsuchiya, T., Umezawa, H., Naganawa, H.: Structure of antipain, a new sakaguchi-positive product of streptomycetes. J. Antibiot. (Tokyo) *25*, 267–270 (1972)
Uriel, J., Berges, J.: Characterization of natural inhibitors of trypsin and chymotrypsin by electrophoresis in acrylamide-agarose gels. Nature (Lond.) *218*, 578–580 (1968)
Vargaftig, B.B., Giroux, E.L.: Indirect release of kinin-like activity by clostripain. Agents Actions *6*, 285 (1976a)
Vargaftig, B.B., Giroux, E.L.: Mechanism of clostropain-induced kinin release from human, rat, and canine plasma. Agents Actions *6*, 446 (1976b)
Veremienko, K.M., Volokhonska, L.I., Kyzym, O.J., Mehed, N.F.: Study of kallikreinogens and inhibitors of kallikrein in blood plasma. Ukr. Biokhim. Zh. *46*, 246–251 (1974)
Vincent, J.-P., Chicheportiche, R., Lazdunski, M.: The conformational properties of the basic pancreatic trypsin-inhibitor. Eur. J. Biochem. *23*, 401–411 (1971)
Vincent, J.-P., Lazdunski, M.: Trypsin-pancreatic trypsin inhibitor association. Dynamics of the interaction and role of disulfide bridges. Biochemistry *11*, 2967–2977 (1972)
Vincent, J.-P., Lazdunski, M.: The interaction between α-chymotrypsin and pancreatic trypsin inhibitor (Kunitz inhibitor). Eur. J. Biochem. *38*, 365–372 (1973)
Vincent, J.-P., Lazdunski, M.: Pre-existence of the active site in zymogens, the interaction of trypsinogen with the basic pancreatic trypsin inhibitor (Kunitz). FEBS Letters *63*, 240–244 (1976)
Vincent, J.-P., Peron-Renner, M., Pudles, J., Lazdunski, M.: The association of anhydrotrypsin with the pancreatic trypsin inhibitors. Biochemistry *13*, 4205–4211 (1974a)

Vincent, J.-P., Schweitz, H., Lazdunski, M.: Guanidination of lysine-15 in the active site of the basic pancreatic trypsin inhibitor. Eur. J. Biochem. *42*, 505–510 (1974b)
Vogel, R.: Differenzierung der Kallikreine untereinander und Abgrenzung gegen andere vasoaktive Substanzen. Hoppe Seylers Z. Physiol. Chem. *349*, 926–927 (1968)
Vogel, R., Trautschold, I., Werle, E.: Natural proteinase inhibitors. London, New York: Academic Press 1968
Vogel, R., Werle, E.: Kallikrein inhibitors. In: Handbook of experimental pharmacology. Vol. XXV: Bradykinin, kallidin, and kallikrein. Erdös, E.G. (ed.), pp. 213–249. Berlin, Heidelberg, New York: Springer 1970
Wagner, G., De Marco, A., Wüthrich, K.: Convolution difference ^{1}H NMR Spectra at 360 MHz of the basic pancreatic trypsin inhibitor. J. Magn. Reşon. *20*, 565–569 (1975)
Wagner, G., De Marco, A., Wüthrich, K.: Dynamics of the aromatic amino acid residues in the globular conformation of the basic pancreatic trypsin inhibitor (BPTI). I. ^{1}H NMR studies. Biophys. Struct. Mech. *2*, 139–158 (1976)
Wagner, G., Wüthrich, K.: Proton NMR studies of the aromatic residues in the basic pancreatic trypsin inhibitor (BPTI). J. Magn. Reson. *20*, 435–445 (1975)
Wang, T.-W., Kassell, B.: Digestion of the basic trypsin inhibitor of bovine pancreas by thermolysin. Biochem. Biophys. Res. Commun. *40*, 1039–1045 (1970)
Wang, T.-W., Kassell, B.: The preparation of a chemically cross-linked complex of the basic pancreatic trypsin inhibitor with trypsin. Biochemistry *13*, 698–702 (1974)
Weber, U., Schmid, H.: Synthese und biologische Aktivität von Cystinpeptiden aus dem aktiven Zentrum des basischen Trypsininhibitors aus Rinderorganen (Kunitz-Inhibitor). Hoppe Seylers Z. Physiol. Chem. *356*, 1505–1515 (1975)
Weber, U., Schmid, H.: Synthese und biologische Aktivität des Dekapeptids Gly-Pro-Cys-Lys-Ala-Arg-Phe-Gly-Cys als Modell für das aktive Zentrum des basischen Trypsininhibitors aus Rinderorganen (Kunitz-Inhibitor). Hoppe Seylers Z. Physiol. Chem. *357*, 1359–1363 (1976)
Werle, E., Appel, W., Happ, E.: Über Hemmkörper für Trypsin und Kallikrein im Blut der Weinbergschnecke *(Helix pomatia)* und über eine Kreislauf-Schockwirkung des Schneckenblutes. Naunyn Schmiedebergs Arch. Pharmakol. *234*, 364–372 (1958)
Werle, E., Fiedler, F., Fritz, H.: Recent studies on kallikreins and kallikrein inhibitors. In: Proc. Vth Int. Congr. Pharmacol. San Francisco 1972, Vol. V, pp. 284–295. Basel: Karger 1973
Werle, E., Zickgraf-Rüdel, G.: Natural proteinase inhibitors. Distribution, specificity, mode of action, and physiological significance. Z. Klin. Chem. Klin. Biochem. *10*, 139–150 (1972)
Wiejak, S., Rzeszotarska, B.: Synthesis of peptides from the region essential for biological reactivity of basic pancreatic trypsin inhibitor. Part III. Synthesis of oxidized-L-cysteinyl-L-lysyl-L-alanylglycylglycyl-L-cysteine and its N^{α}-acetyl amide. Rocz. Chemii Ann. Soc. Chim. Pol. *48*, 2207–2215 (1974)
Wilchek, M., Gorecki, M.: A new approach for the isolation of biologically active compounds by affinity chromatography: Isolation of trypsin. FEBS Letters *31*, 149–152 (1973)
Wilusz, T., Łomako, J., Mejbaum-Katzenellenbogen, W.: An improved method of isolation of crystalline basic trypsin inhibitor from bovine tissues. Acta Biochim. Pol. *20*, 25–31 (1973)
Wilusz, T., Wilimowska-Pelc, A., Mejbaum-Katzenellenbogen, W.: Trypsin inhibitors in bovine lung and pancreas during development. Acta Biochim. Pol. *23*, 269–275 (1976)
Wingender, W.: Proteinase inhibitors of microbial origin. A review. In: Proteinase inhibitors. Fritz, H., Tschesche, H., Greene, L.J., Truscheit, E. (eds.), pp. 548–559. Berlin, Heidelberg, New York: Springer 1974
Woodward, C.K., Ellis, L.M.: Hydrogen exchange kinetics changes upon formation of the soybean trypsin inhibitor-trypsin complex. Biochemistry *14*, 3419–3423 (1975)
Wright, H.T.: Secondary and conformational specificities of trypsin and chymotrypsin. Eur. J. Biochem. *73*, 567–578 (1977)
Wunderer, G., Béress, L., Machleidt, W., Fritz, H.: Broad specificity proteinase inhibitors from sea anemones. In: Protides of the biological fluids. Peeters, H. (ed.), pp. 285–288. London: Pergamon Press 1973
Wunderer, G., Béress, L., Machleidt, W., Fritz, H.: Broad-specificity inhibitors from sea anemones. In: Methods in enzymology. Lorand, L. (ed.), Vol. XLV/B, pp. 881–888. London, New York: Academic Press 1976
Wunderer, G., Fritz, H., Brümmer, W., Hennrich, N., Orth, H.-D.: Isolation of proteinase and proteinase inhibitor by affinity chromatography on cellulose matrices. Biochem. Soc. Trans. *2*, 1324–1327 (1974a)

Wunderer, G., Kummer, K., Fritz, H.: Charakterisierung des Schweine- und Human-Serumkallikreins durch die Hemmbarkeit mit Protein-Proteinase-Inhibitoren. Hoppe Seylers Z. Physiol. Chem. *353*, 1646–1650 (1972)
Wunderer, G., Kummer, K., Fritz, H.: Broad specificity inhibitors from sea anemones. In: Proteinase inhibitors. Fritz, H., Tschesche, H., Greene, L.J., Truscheit, E. (eds.), pp. 277–281. Berlin, Heidelberg, New York: Springer 1974b
Wüthrich, K., Wagner, G.: NMR investigations of the dynamics of the aromatic amino acid residues in the basic pancreatic trypsin inhibitor. FEBS Letters *50*, 265–268 (1975)
Yajima, H., Kiso, Y.: Studies on peptides. 44. Synthesis of basic trypsin-inhibitor from bovine pancreas (Kunitz and Northrop) by the fragment condensation procedure on polymer support. Chem. Pharm. Bull. (Tokyo) *22*, 1087–1094 (1974)
Yajima, H., Kiso, Y., Okada, Y., Watanabe, H.: Synthesis of the basic trypsin inhibitor from bovine pancreas (Kunitz and Northrop) by fragment condensation on a polymer support. J.C.S. Chem. Commun. 106–107 (1974)
Yamazaki, K., Moriya, H.: Isolation and purification of colostrokinin from bovine colostrum. Biochem. Pharmacol. *18*, 2303–2311 (1969)
Yankeelov, J., Jr., Kochert, M., Page, J., Westphal, A.: A reagent for the modification of arginine residues under mild conditions. Fed. Proc. *25*, 590 (1966)
Zanefeld, L.J.D., Polakoski, K.L., Robertson, R.T., Williams, W.L.: Trypsin inhibitor and fertilization. In: Proc. int. res. conf. on proteinase inhibitors. Fritz, H., Tschesche, H. (eds.), pp. 236–244. Berlin, New York: de Gruyter 1971
Zuber, M., Sache, E.: Isolation and characterization of porcine pancreatic kallikrein. Biochemistry *13*, 3098–3110 (1974)

Chemistry and Biologic Activity of Peptides Related to Bradykinin

J. M. STEWART

A. Introduction

The great physiologic importance of the kinin system has prompted much investigation, during the last decade, of the chemistry, pharmacology and physiology of the peptides which constitute and affect this system. Since the earlier tabulation of bradykinin analogs in this work (SCHRÖDER, 1970), nearly 150 peptides related in structure to bradykinin have been synthesized and described. These new kinin analogs are tabulated in this chapter and the information gained from the study of these peptides is discussed. The attempts to make good peptide inhibitors of bradykinin will also be discussed.

Several new fields related to the kinins have appeared since the earlier work and have received much attention. The chemical nature of the bradykinin potentiating peptides in the venom of *Bothrops jararaca* has been established and the identification of these peptides has triggered a large program of synthetic investigation. This has been directed not only toward the potentiation of the kinin response, but even more toward inhibition of angiotensin I converting enzyme.

Since bradykinin and related peptides must presumably assume the proper shape to fit the cellular receptors which mediate the physiologic action of these peptides, several groups have investigated the conformation of bradykinin and related peptides in solution. The techniques of circular dichroism, proton and carbon nuclear magnetic resonance, and electron paramagnetic resonance have been applied to this problem and a nearly complete understanding of the shape of the bradykinin molecule in solution has been reached.

In all this work, chemical synthesis of the peptides in question is of paramount importance. While the major methods used in such synthetic work were described in an earlier volume (STEWART, 1970), recent significant work in this area will be described. The literature is surveyed to the middle of 1977.

Note added in proof: The last year has seen much activity in this field. For that reason the supplementary tables 1A (for bradykinin analogs) and 4A (for bradykinin potentiating peptides) have been added to bring the chapter to date on the important new compounds.

Shortly before his death, RUDINGER (1971) completed a major work on the design of peptide hormone analogs. That work contains many interesting and provocative observations, and should be consulted by anyone seriously interested in the field.

Table 1. Synthetic analogs of bradykinin (BK)
(see footnote for explanation of abbreviations)

Peptide No.	Variation in position	Name	Amino acid sequences	Biological activities (BK = 100): Isolated rat uterus	Isolated guinea pig ileum	Rat blood pressure (i. V.)	Rabbit blood pressure (i. V.)	Other	References
		Bradykinin	H-Arg-Pro-Pro-Gly-Phe-Ser-Pro-Phe-Arg-OH (1 2 3 4 5 6 7 8 9)						
(1)	Bradykinin analogs obtained by replacement of one amino acid								
1	1	Desamino-BK	GUV-Pro-Pro-Gly-Phe-Ser-Pro-Phe-Arg	23	—	—	—	—	LAW et al. (1971)
2	1	α-Guanido-BK	GAR-Pro-Pro-Gly-Phe-Ser-Pro-Phe-Arg	200	100	—	—	—	PINKER et al. (1976)
3	1	δ-AcetimidoylOrn^{1}-BK	DAO-Pro-Pro-Gly-Phe-Ser-Pro-Phe-Arg	—	—	—	—	—	PINKER et al. (1976)
4	1	ε-aminocaproic^{1}-BK	EAC-Pro-Pro-Gly-Phe-Ser-Pro-Phe-Arg	—	0	0	—	—	STEWART (unpublished)
5	1	HomoArg^{1}-BK	HAR-Pro-Pro-Gly-Phe-Ser-Pro-Phe-Arg	24	23	—	—	—	REISSMANN et al. (1974)
				—	—	—	—	6[b]	SAFDY and LYONS (1974)
				100	100	—	—	—	FLETCHER and YOUNG (1972)
6	1	ω-MethylArg^{1}-BK	OMA-Pro-Pro-Gly-Phe-Ser-Pro-Phe-Arg	23	—	—	—	—	PINKER et al. (1976)
7	1	NorArg^{1}-BK	NAR-Pro-Pro-Gly-Phe-Ser-Pro-Phe-Arg	0.8	0.4	—	0.1	+[a]	REISSMANN et al. (1974)
8	1	Val^{1}-BK	Val-Pro-Pro-Gly-Phe-Ser-Pro-Phe-Arg	< 0.2	< 10	—	—	—	FLETCHER and YOUNG (1972)
9	2	HydroxyPro^{2}-BK	Arg-Hyp-Pro-Gly-Phe-Ser-Pro-Phe-Arg	200	100	500[c]	—	1600[d]	STEWART et al. (1974)
10	2	Pipecolic^{2}-BK	Arg-Pip-Pro-Gly-Phe-Ser-Pro-Phe-Arg	—	5	—	—	—	NEUBERT et al. (1972)
11	3	Azetidinecarbox.^{3}-BK	Arg-Pro-AZC-Gly-Phe-Ser-Pro-Phe-Arg	46	68	26	—	—	FELIX et al. (1973)
12	3	DehydroPro^{3}-BK	Arg-Pro-DHP-Gly-Phe-Ser-Pro-Phe-Arg	97	82	71	—	[e]	FELIX et al. (1973)
13	3	HydroxyPro^{3}-BK	Arg-Pro-Hyp-Gly-Phe-Ser-Pro-Phe-Arg	100	35	300[c]	—	80[d]	STEWART et al. (1974)
				114	61	63	—	[e]	FELIX et al. (1973)
14	3	Lys^{3}-BK	Arg-Pro-Lys-Gly-Phe-Ser-Pro-Phe-Arg	0.4	0.1	1	—	—	FELIX et al. (1973)
15	3	MethylPro^{3}-BK	Arg-Pro-MPr-Gly-Phe-Ser-Pro-Phe-Arg	32	45	55	—	—	FELIX et al. (1973)
16	3	Pipecolic^{3}-BK	Arg-Pro-Pip-Gly-Phe-Ser-Pro-Phe-Arg	—	0	—	—	—	NEUBERT et al. (1972)
17	3	Thiazolidinecarboxylyl^{3}-BK	Arg-Pro-TZC-Gly-Phe-Ser-Pro-Phe-Arg	41	51	15	—	[e]	FELIX et al. (1973)
18	3–4	AminoethylGly^{3}-BK	Arg-Pro-AEG ——-Phe-Ser-Pro-Phe-Arg	—	0	—	—	—	ATHERTON et al. (1971)
19	4	D-Ala^{4}-BK	Arg-Pro-Pro-*ala*-Phe-Ser-Pro-Phe-Arg	0.01	—	—	—	—	MATSUEDA and STEWART (unpublished)
				0	—	0	—	—	TURK et al. (1975b)
20	4	Glycolic^{4}-BK	Arg-Pro-Pro-Glc-Phe-Ser-Pro-Phe-Arg	0.1	—	0.1	—	0.1[d]	SHEMYAKIN et al. (1966)
21	4	Leu^{4}-BK	Arg-Pro-Pro-Leu-Phe-Ser-Pro-Phe-Arg	—	—	"low"	—	0[f]	KAMEYAMA and SASAKI (1970)
22	4	Thr^{4}-BK	Arg-Pro-Pro-Thr-Phe-Ser-Pro-Phe-Arg	—	0	0	—	—	PEÑA and STEWART (unpublished)
23	5	*p*-AminoPhe^{5}-BK	Arg-Pro-Pro-Gly-PAP-Ser-Pro-Phe-Arg	0.7	—	2	—	—	TURK et al. (1975a)
24	5	β-MethylPhe^{5}-BK	Arg-Pro-Pro-Gly-BMP-Ser-Pro-Phe-Arg	3	3	—	1	+[a]	REISSMANN et al. (1974)
25	5	CyclohexylAla^{5}-BK	Arg-Pro-Pro-Gly-Cha-Ser-Pro-Phe-Arg	—	100	—	—	—	FLETCHER and YOUNG (1972)
				—	"less than BK"	—	—	—	FILATOVA et al. (1975)
26	5	Leu^{5}-BK	Arg-Pro-Pro-Gly-Leu-Ser-Pro-Phe-Arg	5	—	—	—	—	STEWART (unpublished)

27	5	α-MethylPhe^{5}-BK	Arg-Pro-Pro-Gly-AMP-Ser-Pro-Phe-Arg	3.5	—	1	—	—	TURK et al. (1975b)
28	5	N-MethylPhe^{5}-BK	Arg-Pro-Pro-Gly-NMP-Ser-Pro-Phe-Arg	0.3	1	0.1	—	—	PENA and STEWART (unpublished)
29	5	O-MethylTyr^{5}-BK	Arg-Pro-Pro-Gly-OMT-Ser-Pro-Phe-Arg	1	—	50	—	—	KEELING, BALL, and STEWART (unpublished)
30	5	e-β-PhenylSer^{5}-BK	Arg-Pro-Pro-Gly-ePS-Ser-Pro-Phe-Arg	8	2	—	3	+[a]	REISSMANN et al. (1974)
31	5	t-β-PhenylSer^{5}-BK	Arg-Pro-Pro-Gly-tPS-Ser-Pro-Phe-Arg	52	33	—	18	+[a]	REISSMANN et al. (1974)
32	5	ThienylAla^{5}-BK	Arg-Pro-Pro-Gly-Thi-Ser-Pro-Phe-Arg	200	40	150	—	—	DUNN and STEWART (1971)
			Ac						
33	6	AcetylSer^{6}-BK	Arg-Pro-Pro-Gly-Phe-Ser-Pro-Phe-Arg	—	—	"strong"	—	20[f]	KAMEYAMA and SASAKI (1970)
			Ac						
34	6	AcetylThr^{6}-BK	Arg-Pro-Pro-Gly-Phe-Thr-Pro-Phe-Arg	—	—	"strong"	—	45[f]	KAMEYAMA and SASAKI (1970)
35	6	Gly^{6}-BK	Arg-Pro-Pro-Gly-Phe-Gly-Pro-Phe-Arg	38	19	—	—	+[a]	REISSMANN et al. (1974)
36	6	Glycolyl^{6}-BK	Arg-Pro-Pro-Gly-Phe-Glc-Pro-Phe-Arg	150	—	10	—	50[d]	FILATOVA et al. (1975)
37	6	Leucine^{6}-BK	Arg-Pro-Pro-Gly-Phe-Leu-Pro-Phe-Arg	—	—	—	—	0.1[f]	SUZUKI et al. (1966)
38	6	Ornithine^{6}-BK	Arg-Pro-Pro-Gly-Phe-Orn-Pro-Phe-Arg						PINKER et al. (1976)
39	6	SuccinylOrn^{6}-BK	Arg-Pro-Pro-Gly-Phe-SuO-Pro-Phe-Arg						PINKER et al. (1976)
40	7	β-HomoPro^{7}-BK	Arg-Pro-Pro-Gly-Phe-Ser-HPR-Phe-Arg	—	—	100	—	100[g]	BALASPIRI et al. (1975) ONDETTI and ENGEL (1975)
41	7	HydroxyPro^{7}-BK	Arg-Pro-Pro-Gly-Phe-Ser-Hyp-Phe-Arg	2	3	2	—	20[d]	STEWART et al. (1974)
42	8	p-Amino-Phe^{8}-BK	Arg-Pro-Pro-Gly-Phe-Ser-Pro-PAP-Arg	53	—	18	—	—	TURK et al. (1975a)
43	8	β-MethylPhe^{8}-BK	Arg-Pro-Pro-Gly-Phe-Ser-Pro-BMP-Arg	52	21	—	14	+[a]	REISSMANN et al. (1974)
44	8	α-Aminophenylbutyric^{8}-BK	Arg-Pro-Pro-Gly-Phe-Ser-Pro-APB-Arg	0.1	0.05	—	0.1	+[a]	REISSMANN et al. (1974)
45	8	CyclohexylAla^{8}-BK	Arg-Pro-Pro-Gly-Phe-Ser-Pro-Cha-Arg	—	100	—	—	—	FLETCHER and YOUNG (1972)
				10	10	—	—	2[d]	POPKOVA et al. (1976)
				14	11	—	—	—	REISSMANN et al. (1975a)
46	8	β-HomoPhe^{8}-BK	Arg-Pro-Pro-Gly-Phe-Ser-Pro-HPH-Arg	—	—	3	—	—	ONDETTI and ENGEL (1975)
47	8	Leu^{8}-BK	Arg-Pro-Pro-Gly-Phe-Ser-Pro-Leu-Arg	0.3	—	2	—	3[d]	STEWART (1971)
48	8	α-MethylPhe^{8}-BK	Arg-Pro-Pro-Gly-Phe-Ser-Pro-AMP-Arg	31	—	1	—	—	TURK et al. (1975)
49	8	N-MethylPhe^{8}-BK	Arg-Pro-Pro-Gly-Phe-Ser-Pro-NMP-Arg	0.1	0	0.2	—	—	PEÑA and STEWART (unpublished)
				10	10	—	—	—	POPKOVA et al. (1976)
50	8	PhenylGly^{8}-BK	Arg-Pro-Pro-Gly-Phe-Ser-Pro-PhG-Arg	0.09	0.02	—	—	+[a]	REISSMANN et al. (1974)
51	8	e-PhenylSer^{8}-BK	Arg-Pro-Pro-Gly-Phe-Ser-Pro-ePS-Arg	13	6	—	8	+[a]	REISSMANN et al. (1974)
52	8	t-PhenylSer^{8}-BK	Arg-Pro-Pro-Gly-Phe-Ser-Pro-tPS-Arg	8	3	—	7	+[a]	REISSMANN et al. (1974)
53	8	Pro^{8}-BK	Arg-Pro-Pro-Gly-Phe-Ser-Pro-Pro-Arg	0	—	—	—	—	MATSUEDA and STEWART (unpublished)
54	8	ThienylAla^{8}-BK	Arg-Pro-Pro-Gly-Phe-Ser-Pro-Thi-Arg	400	40	150	—	—	DUNN and STEWART (1971)
55	9	δ-AcetimidoylOrn^{9}-BK	Arg-Pro-Pro-Gly-Phe-Ser-Pro-Phe-AIO	1	—	—	—	—	PINKER et al. (1976)
56	9	Agmatine^{9}-BK (des-Carboxy-BK)	Arg-Pro-Pro-Gly-Phe-Ser-Pro-Phe-Agm	0.3	—	—	—	—	LAW et al. (1971)
57	9	HomoArg^{9}-BK	Arg-Pro-Pro-Gly-Phe-Ser-Pro-Phe-HAR	10	24	—	59	+[a] 5[b]	REISSMANN et al. (1974) SAFDY and LYONS (1974)
58	9	ω-MethylArg^{9}-BK	Arg-Pro-Pro-Gly-Phe-Ser-Pro-Phe-OMA	63	—	—	—	—	PINKER et al. (1976)
59	9	NorArg^{9}-BK	Arg-Pro-Pro-Gly-Phe-Ser-Pro-Phe-NAR	2	1	—	3	+[a]	REISSMANN et al. (1974)
60	9	Phe^{9}-BK	Arg-Pro-Pro-Gly-Phe-Ser-Pro-Phe-Phe	< 0.01	—	0.02	—	3[d]	STEWART (1971)

Table 1 (continued

Peptide No.	Variation in position	Name	Amino acid sequences	Biological activities (BK = 100)					
				Isolated rat uterus	Isolated guinea pig ileum	Rat blood pressure (i. V.)	Rabbit blood pressure (i. V.)	Other	References
(2)	Bradykinin Analogs obtained by replacement of more than one amino acid								
61	1+5	HAR^{1}, Cha^{5}-BK	HAR-Pro-Pro-Gly-Cha-Ser-Pro-Phe-Arg	—	"full potency"	—	—	—	FLETCHER and YOUNG (1972)
62	1+6	Leu^{1}, Thr^{6}-BK	Leu-Pro-Pro-Gly-Phe-Thr-Pro-Phe-Arg	—	0	—	—	—	FLETCHER and YOUNG (1972)
63	1+6	Val^{1}, Gly^{6}-BK	Val-Pro-Pro-Gly-Phe-Gly-Pro-Phe-Arg	0.01	0.04	—	—	+[a]	REISSMANN et al. (1974)
64	1+6	Val^{1}, Thr^{6}-BK	Val-Pro-Pro-Gly-Phe-Thr-Pro-Phe-Arg	0.03	0.1	—	0.02	+[a]	REISSMANN et al. (1974)
				0	10	—	—	—	FLETCHER and YOUNG (1972)
65	1+9	GUV^{1}, Agm^{9}-BK (des-Amino, des-Carboxy-BK)	GUV-Pro-Pro-Gly-Phe-Ser-Pro-Phe-Agm	0.01	—	—	—	—	LAW et al. (1971)
66	1+9	Homoarg^{1,9}-BK	HAR-Pro-Pro-Gly-Phe-Ser-Pro-Phe-HAR	6	3	—	3	+[a]	REISSMANN et al. (1974)
				—	—	—	—	2[b]	SAFDY and LYONS (1974)
67	1+9	NorArg^{1,9}-BK	NAR-Pro-Pro-Gly-Phe-Ser-Pro-Phe-NAR	0.02	0.02	—	0.05	+[a]	REISSMANN et al. (1974)
68	1+9	Orn^{1,9}-BK	Orn-Pro-Pro-Gly-Phe-Ser-Pro-Phe-Orn	0	—	—	—	—	PINKER et al. (1976)
69	1+6+8	Lys^{1}, Gly^{6}, PhL^{8}-BK	Lys-Pro-Pro-Gly-Phe-Gly-Pro-PhL-Arg						KRIT et al. (1976)
70	2+3+7	FluoroPro^{2,3,7}-BK	Arg-FPr-FPr-Gly-Phe-Ser-FPr-Phe-Arg	—	—	—	—	—	EL-MAGHRABY (1976)
71	2+5+8	Hyp^{2}, Thi^{5,8}-BK	Arg-Hyp-Pro-Gly-Thi-Ser-Pro-Thi-Arg	100	50	—	—	—	STEWART (unpublished)
72	4+6	Phe^{4,6}-BK	Arg-Pro-Pro-Phe-Phe-Phe-Pro-Phe-Arg	0.01	—	0.05	—	0.001[d]	STEWART (unpublished)
73	5+6	Tyr^{5}, Gly^{6}-BK	Arg-Pro-Pro-Gly-Tyr-Gly-Pro-Phe-Arg						REISSMANN et al. (1976)
74	5+8	CyclohexylAla^{5,8}-BK	Arg-Pro-Pro-Gly-Cha-Ser-Pro-Cha-Arg	—	100	—	—	—	FLETCHER and YOUNG (1972)
				"less than BK"		—	—	—	FILATOVA et al. (1975)
75	5+8	e-β-MethylPhe^{5,8}-BK	Arg-Pro-Pro-Gly-BMP-Ser-Pro-BMP-Arg	5	4	—	4	+[a]	REISSMANN et al. (1974)
76	5+8	OMT^{5}, PNP^{8}-BK	Arg-Pro-Pro-Gly-OMT-Ser-Pro-PNP-Arg	—	5	—	—	—	ABIKO (1974)
77	5+8	PNP^{5},OMT^{8}-BK	Arg-Pro-Pro-Gly-PNP-Ser-Pro-OMT-Arg	—	10	—	—	—	ABIKO (1974)
78	5+8	e-PhenylSer^{5,8}-BK	Arg-Pro-Pro-Gly-ePS-Ser-Pro-ePS-Arg	2	0.05	—	0.1	+[a]	REISSMANN et al. (1974)
79	5+8	t-PhenylSer^{5,8}-BK	Arg-Pro-Pro-Gly-tPS-Ser-Pro-tPS-Arg	0.4	0.1	—	0.5	+[a]	REISSMANN et al. (1974)
80	5+8	ThienylAla^{5,8}-BK	Arg-Pro-Pro-Gly-Thi-Ser-Pro-Thi-Arg	1000	200	100	—	—	DUNN and STEWART (1971)
81	5+6+8	Gly^{5,6,8}-BK	Arg-Pro-Pro-Gly-Gly-Gly-Pro-Gly-Arg	0.01	—	0	—	—	STEWART (unpublished)
82	5+6+8	Tyr^{5,8},Gly^{6}-BK	Arg-Pro-Pro-Gly-Tyr-Gly-Pro-Tyr-Arg						REISSMANN et al. (1976)
83	6+8	Gly^{6},Cyclohexyl Ala^{8}-BK	Arg-Pro-Pro-Gly-Phe-Gly-Pro-Cha-Arg						KRIT et al. (1976)
84	6+8	Gly^{6},N-Methyl Phe^{8}-BK	Arg-Pro-Pro-Gly-Phe-Gly-Pro-NMP-Arg						KRIT et al. (1976)
85	6+8	Gly^{6}, Tyr^{8}-BK	Arg-Pro-Pro-Gly-Phe-Gly-Pro-Tyr-Arg	0.4	0.6	—	—	—	REISSMANN et al. (1975a)
86	8+9	Amino-γ-PheBu^{8}, HomoArg^{9}-BK	Arg-Pro-Pro-Gly-Phe-Ser-Pro-APB-HAR	0.1	0.04	—	0.05	+[a]	REISSMANN et al. (1974)
87	8+9	APB^{8},NorArg^{9}-BK	Arg-Pro-Pro-Gly-Phe-Ser-Pro-APB-NAR	0.1	< 0.01	—	< 0.05	+[a]	REISSMANN et al. (1974)
88	8+9	PhenylGly^{8},HomoArg^{9}-BK	Arg-Pro-Pro-Gly-Phe-Ser-Pro-PhG-HAR	0.06	0.14	—	—	+[a]	REISSMANN et al (1974)
89	8+9	PhenylGly^{8},NorArg^{9}-BK	Arg-Pro-Pro-Gly-Phe-Ser-Pro-PhG-NAR	0.07	0.004	—	—	+[a]	REISSMANN et al. (1974)

(3)	Bradykinin fragments and analogs having shorter peptide chains								
90	—	All possible fragments of BK		No significant activity except compound #91					Suzuki et al. (1969)
91	1–4	BK C-terminal pentapeptide	Phe-Ser-Pro-Phe-Arg	0.005	0.02	—	—	+[a]	Reissmann et al. (1974)
				—	2.9	0.007	—	—	Suzuki et al. (1969)
92	1–4+6	Gly^6-C-terminal pentapeptide	Phe-Gly-Pro-Phe-Arg	0.001	0.002	—	—	h	Reissmann et al. (1974)
93	1–4+6	Thr^6-C-terminal pentapeptide	Phe-Thr-Pro-Phe-Arg	0.1	1.7	—	—	+[a]	Reissmann et al. (1974)
94	1–4+5	β-MethylPhe^5-C-terminal pentapeptide	BMP-Ser-Pro-Phe-Arg	0.01	0.005	—	—	+[a]	Reissmann et al. (1974)
95	1–4+8+9	PhenylGly^8,Homoarg^9-C-terminal pentapeptide	Phe-Ser-Pro-PhG-HAR	0.03	0.07	—	—	+[a]	Reissmann et al. (1974)
96	1+5	des-(Arg^1)-O-MeTyr^5-BK	Pro-Pro-Gly-OMT-Ser-Pro-Phe-Arg	0.1	—	10	—	—	Keeling, Ball, and Stewart (unpublished)
97	1+6	des-(Arg^1)-Gly^6-BK	Pro-Pro-Gly-Phe-Gly-Pro-Phe-Arg	0.34	0.02	—	—	+[a]	Reissmann et al. (1974)
(4)	Bradykinin analogs having longer peptide chains (peptides are numbered as corresponding bradykinin positions)								
98	1	Glu^1-Kallidin	Glu-Arg-Pro-Pro-Gly-Phe-Ser-Pro-Phe-Arg	41	8	32	—	—	Felix et al. (1973)
99	1	Tyr^1-Kallidin	Tyr-Arg-Pro-Pro-Gly-Phe-Ser-Pro-Phe-Arg	40	33	74	—	—	Felix et al. (1973)
				95	40	—	—	—	Peña and Stewart (unpublished)
100	1	Aminocaproic^1-Kallidin	EAC-Arg-Pro-Pro-Gly-Phe-Ser-Pro-Phe-Arg		100	200	—	—	Stewart (unpublished)
101	1+3	Glu^1,DehydroPro^3-Kallidin	Glu-Arg-Pro-DHP-Gly-Phe-Ser-Pro-Phe-Arg	39	44	32	—	—	Felix et al. (1973)
102	1+3	Glu^1,HydroxyPro^3-Kallidin	Glu-Arg-Pro-Hyp-Gly-Phe-Ser-Pro-Phe-Arg					e	McGee et al. (1973)
103	1	Arg-Gly-BK	Arg-Gly-Arg-Pro-Pro-Gly-Phe-Ser-Pro-Phe-Arg	10	—	80	—	35[d]	Stewart (1971)
104	1+6	Polistes Kinin-R (Ala-Arg-Thr^6-BK)	Ala-Arg-Arg-Pro-Pro-Gly-Phe-Thr-Pro-Phe-Arg						Watanabe et al. (1976)
105	1+6	Gly-Gly-Lys-Ser(Ac)^6-BK	Ac (on Ser) Gly-Gly-Lys-Arg-Pro-Pro-Gly-Phe-Ser-Pro-Phe-Arg	—	0	—	—	—	Kameyama et al. (1971)
106	1	Gly-Arg-Met-Lys-BK	Gly-Arg-Met-Lys- -Arg-Pro-Pro-Gly-Phe-Ser-Pro-Phe-Arg	150	—	1500	—	—	Stewart (1971)
				—	7	—	—	1500[d]	Ribeiro and Rocha e Silva (1973)
107	1	Ser-Leu-Met-Lys-BK (Kininogen sequence)	Ser-Leu-Met-Lys- -Arg-Pro-Pro-Gly-Phe-Ser-Pro-Phe-Arg	35	—	—	—	—	Han et al. (1976)
108	1	Vespulakinin-2	CHO CHO (on Thr, Thr) Thr - Thr-Arg-Arg-Arg-Gly- -Arg-Pro-Pro-Gly-Phe-Ser-Pro-Phe-Arg	active	active	200	—	—	Yoshida et al. (1976)
109	1	Vespulakinin-1	CHO CHO (on Thr, Thr) Thr-Ala- Thr - Thr-Arg-Arg-Arg-Gly- -Arg-Pro-Pro-Gly-Phe-Ser-Pro-Phe-Arg	active	active	active	—	—	Yoshida et al. (1976)
110	1	Angiotensinyl-BK	Asp-Arg-Val-Tyr-Ile-His-Pro-Phe- -Arg-Pro-Pro-Gly-Phe-Ser-Pro-Phe-Arg	10	—	—	—	—	Merrifield (1967)
				—	—	25	—	2[d]	Stewart and Roblero (unpublished)
111	1	Bradykininyl-BK	Arg-Pro-Pro-Gly-Phe-Ser-Pro-Phe-Arg- -Arg-Pro-Pro-Gly-Phe-Ser-Pro-Phe-Arg	10	—	—	—	—	Najjar and Merrifield (1966)
				—	—	35	—	5[d]	Stewart and Roblero (unpublished)

Table 1 (continued

Peptide No.	Variation in position	Name	Amino acid sequences	Biological activities (BK = 100): Isolated rat uterus	Isolated guinea pig ileum	Rat blood pressure (i. V.)	Rabbit blood pressure (i. V.)	Other	References
112	1	Polisteskinin	<Glu-Thr-Asn-Lys-Lys-Lys-Leu-Arg-Gly- -Arg-Pro-Pro-Gly-Phe-Ser-Pro-Phe-Arg	100	—	1000	—	250[d]	STEWART (1968b)
113	9	Bradykininyl-Glu	Arg-Pro-Pro-Gly-Phe-Ser-Pro-Phe-Arg-Glu	—	0.2	—	—	—	MATSUEDA and STEWART (unpublished)
114	9	Bradykininyl-Ile-Tyr (des-SO_4-Phyllokinin)	Arg-Pro-Pro-Gly-Phe-Ser-Pro-Phe-Arg-Ile-Tyr	40	45	—	70	300[j]	ANASTASI et al. (1966)
				35	—	125	—	10[d]	ROBLERO and STEWART (unpublished)
115	9	Phyllokinin	Arg-Pro-Pro-Gly-Phe-Ser-Pro-Phe-Arg-Ile-Tyr(SO_4)	25	20	—	25	70[j]	ANASTASI et al. (1966)
116	9	BK-Ser-Val-Gln	Arg-Pro-Pro-Gly-Phe-Ser-Pro-Phe-Arg-Ser-Val-Gln	—	0.1	—	—	—	SCHRÖDER (1969)
117	6+9	Ser(Ac)[6]-BK-Ser-Val-Gln	Ac Arg-Pro-Pro-Gly-Phe-Ser-Pro-Phe-Arg-Ser-Val-Gln	—	0	—	—	—	KAMEYAMA et al. (1971)
118	9	BK-Ser-Val-Gln-Val	Arg-Pro-Pro-Gly-Phe-Ser-Pro-Phe-Arg-Ser-Val-Gln-Val	—	0.1	—	—	—	SCHRÖDER (1969)
119	9	Bombinakinin-O (BK-Gly-Lys-Phe-His)	Arg-Pro-Pro-Gly-Phe-Ser-Pro-Phe-Arg-Gly-Lys-Phe-His					33[k]	YASUHARA et al. (1973)
120	9	Ranakinin-N (BK-Val-Ala-Pro-Ala-Ser)	Arg-Pro-Pro-Gly-Phe-Ser-Pro-Phe-Arg- -Val-Ala-Pro-Ala-Ser	7	6			29[k]	YANAIHARA et al. (1973)
121	6+9	Ranakinin-R (Thr[6]-BK-Ile-Ala-Pro-Glu-Ile-Val)	Arg-Pro-Pro-Gly-Phe-Thr-Pro-Phe-Arg- -Ile-Ala-Pro-Glu-Ile-Val	10				22[k]	ISHIKAWA et al. (1974)
122	1+9	Vespakinin-X (Ala-BK-Ile-Val)	Ala-Arg-Pro-Pro-Gly-Phe-Ser-Pro-Phe-Arg- -Ile-Val	12				96[k]	YASUHARA and NAKAJIMA (1977)
123	1+9	Kininogen sequence (PKFL)	Met-Lys-Arg-Pro-Pro-Gly-Phe-Ser-Pro-Phe-Arg- -Ser-Val-Gln	—	0.3	—	—	—	SCHRÖDER (1969)
124	1+9	Kininogen sequence (PKFS)	Met-Lys-Arg-Pro-Pro-Gly-Phe-Ser-Pro-Phe-Arg- -Ser-Val-Gln-Val	—	0.3	—	—	—	SCHRÖDER (1969)
125	1+3+9	Vespakinin-M	Gly-Arg-Pro-Hyp-Gly-Phe-Ser-Pro-Phe-Arg- -Ile-Asp					29[k]	KISHIMURA et al. (1976)
(5)	Derivatives of bradykinin, analogs, and fragments								
126	1	t-Butyloxycarbonyl-BK	Boc-Arg-Pro-Pro-Gly-Phe-Ser-Pro-Phe-Arg	0	0	—	—	—	FLETCHER and YOUNG (1972)
127	1	Bromoacetyl-BK	BrAc-Arg-Pro-Pro-Gly-Phe-Ser-Pro-Phe-Arg	100	—	20	—	100[d]	FREER and STEWART (unpublished)
				62	—	80	—	—	TURK et al. (1975a)
128	1	Chlorambucilyl-BK	Chl-Arg-Pro-Pro-Gly-Phe-Ser-Pro-Phe-Arg	100	10	—	—	—	FREER and STEWART (1972)
129	1	1-Chlorambucil-BK	Chl-Pro-Pro-Gly-Phe-Ser-Pro-Phe-Arg	0.1	0.3	—	—	—	FREER and STEWART (1972)
130	1	Lys(ε-Chl)[1]-BK	Chl Lys-Pro-Pro-Gly-Phe-Ser-Pro-Phe-Arg	25	2	—	—	—	FREER and STEWART (1972)
131	Various Chl derivatives of all C-terminal BK fragments			negligible BK-like activity in any system					FREER and STEWART (1972)

Table 1 (continued

Peptide No.	Variation in position	Name	Amino acid sequences	Biological activities (BK = 100)					
				Isolated rat uterus	Isolated guinea pig ileum	Rat blood pressure (i. V.)	Rabbit blood pressure (i. V.)	Other	References
132	1	Chloroacetyl-BK	ClAc-Arg-Pro-Pro-Gly-Phe-Ser-Pro-Phe-Arg	1000	—	25	—	100[d]	FREER and STEWART (unpublished)
133	1	Dextran(CNBr)-BK	Dex-Arg-Pro-Pro-Gly-Phe-Ser-Pro-Phe-Arg	6	—	—	—	—	ODYA et al. (1978)
134	1	Dextran(IO_4)-BK	Dex-Arg-Pro-Pro-Gly-Phe-Ser-Pro-Phe-Arg	29	—	—	—	—	ODYA et al. (1978)
135	1	Palmitoyl-BK	Palm-Arg-Pro-Pro-Gly-Phe-Ser-Pro-Phe-Arg	0.3	—	—	—	3[d]	FREER and STEWART (unpublished)
136	1	Spin-labeled BK	TMP-Arg-Pro-Pro-Gly-Phe-Ser-Pro-Phe-Arg	0.5	0.15	—	—	—	REISSMANN et al. (1975a)
137	1+5	N-Bromoacetyl, (BrAcNH-Phe)^5-BK	BrAc-Arg-Pro-Pro-Gly-BAP-Ser-Pro-Phe-Arg	0	—	0	—	—	TURK et al. (1975a)
138	1+8	N-Bromoacetyl, (BrAcNH-Phe)^8-BK	BrAc-Arg-Pro-Pro-Gly-Phe-Ser-Pro-BAP-Arg	1	—	0.4	—	—	TURK et al. (1975a)

[a] BK-like on rat duodenum (relaxes); [b] Rat fundus, colon, and duodenum; [c] Due to decreased pulmonary inactivation. See Table 2. [d] Vascular permeability increase in guinea pig skin assay; [e] Inhibits collagen proline hydroxylase; [f] Mouse ileum; [g] Rat ileum; [h] Contracts rat duodenum, in contrast to BK; [j] Dog blood pressure; [k] Guinea pig colon.

Abbreviations: 1. AEG – N-aminoethylglycine; 2. Agm – Agmatine-(5-guanido pentylamine); 3. AIO – δ-Acetimidoylornithine; 4. AMP – α-Methylphenylalanine; 5. APB – α-Amino-γ-phenylbutyric acid; 6. AZC – Azetidine-2-carboxylic acid; 7. BAP – 4-Bromoacetylaminophenylalanine; 8. BK – Bradykinin; 9. BMP – *erythro*-β-Methylphenylalanine; 10. Boc – *tert*-Butyloxycarbonyl; 11. Cha – β-cyclohexylalanine; 12. Chl – Chlorambucil (phenybutyric acid nitrogen mustard); 13. DAO – δ-Acetimidoylornithine; 14. Dex – Dextran (MW 500,000) activated by cyanogen bromide or periodate; 15. DHP – 3,4-Dehydroproline; 16. EAC – ε-aminocaproic acid; 17. *e*PS – *erythro*-β-Phenylserine; 18. FPr – 4-Fluoroproline; 19. GAR – α-guanidoarginine; 20. Glc – Glycolic acid; 21. <Glu – Pyroglutamic acid; 22. GUV – 4-Guanidovaleric acid; 23. HAR – Homoarginine; 24. HPH – β-Homophenylalanine; 25. HPR – β-Homoproline; 26. Hyp – *trans*-4-Hydroxyproline; 27. MPr – *cis, trans*-4-Methyl-D,L-Proline 28. NAR – Norarginine; 29. NMP – N-Methylphenylalanine; 30. OMA – O-Methylarginine; 31. OMT – O-Methyltyrosine; 32. Palm – Palmitic acid; 33. PAP – *p*-aminophenylalanine; 34. PhG – α-Phenylglycine; 35. PhL – Phenyllactic acid; 36. Pip – Pipecolic acid; 37. PNP – *p*-Nitrophenylalanine; 38. SuO – N-Succinylornithine; 39. Thi – β-(2-Thienyl) alanine; 40. TMP – 2,6-Tetramethylpiperidine(N→O)-4-acetic acid; 41. *t*PS – *threo*-β-Phenylserine; 42. TZC – Thiazolidine-4-carboxylic acid. D-Amino acid residues are uncapitalized in italics.

Table 1A. Recently published analogs of bradykinin
(see Footnote and footnote to table 1 for explanation of abbreviations)

Peptide No.	Variation in position	Name	Amino acid sequences	Biological activities (BK = 100)				References
				Isolated rat uterus	Isolated guinea pig ileum	Isolated cat ileum	Rat blood pressure (i. v.)	
139	1	*p*GuanidoPhe^{1}-BK	GUP-Pro-Pro-Gly-Phe-Ser-Pro-Phe-Arg	2	2	—	—	Moore et al. (1977)
140	2	DehydroPro^{2}-BK	Arg-DHP-Pro-Gly-Phe-Ser-Pro-Phe-Arg	120	93	—	90	Fisher et al. (1977)
141	3	DehydroPro^{3}-BK	Arg-Pro-DHP-Gly-Phe-Ser-Pro-Phe-Arg	97	82	—	71	Fisher et al. (1977)
142	5	*p*-NitroPhe^{5}-BK	Arg-Pro-Pro-Gly-PNP-Ser-Pro-Phe-Arg	3.5	4	—	11	Fisher et al. (1977)
143	5	*p*-FluoroPhe^{5}-BK	Arg-Pro-Pro-Gly-FPh-Ser-Pro-Phe-Arg	180	127	—	143	Fisher et al. (1978)
144	5	*p*-ChloroPhe^{5}-BK	Arg-Pro-Pro-Gly-CPh-Ser-Pro-Phe-Arg	5	3	—	4	Fisher et al. (1977)
145	5	*p*-BromoPhe^{5}-BK	Arg-Pro-Pro-Gly-BPh-Ser-Pro-Phe-Arg	18	56	—	22	Fisher et al. (1977)
146	5	*p*-IodoPhe^{5}-BK	Arg-Pro-Pro-Gly-IPh-Ser-Pro-Phe-Arg	3	4	—	7	Fisher et al. (1977)
147	6	γ-Aminobutyric^{6}-BK	Arg-Pro-Pro-Gly-Phe-ABU-Pro-Phe-Arg	—	—	52	2	Park et al. (1978)
148	6	D-Ala^{6}-BK	Arg-Pro-Pro-Gly-Phe-*ala*-Pro-Phe-Arg	—	—	0.7	1	Park et al. (1978)
149	7	Aminocyclopentanecarboxylic^{7}-BK	Arg-Pro-Pro-Gly-Phe-Ser-ACC-Phe-Arg	—	—	5	25	Park et al. (1978)
150	7	DehydroPro^{7}-BK	Arg-Pro-Pro-Gly-Phe-Ser-DHP-Phe-Arg	25	12	—	23	Fisher et al. (1977)
151	8	*p*-NitroPhe^{8}-BK	Arg-Pro-Pro-Gly-Phe-Ser-Pro-PNP-Arg	52	26	—	30	Fisher et al. (1977)
152	8	*p*-FluoroPhe^{8}-BK	Arg-Pro-Pro-Gly-Phe-Ser-Pro-FPh-Arg	150	140	—	171	Fisher et al. (1978)
153	8	*p*-ChloroPhe^{8}-BK	Arg-Pro-Pro-Gly-Phe-Ser-Pro-CPh-Arg	68	92	—	134	Fisher et al. (1977)
154	8	*p*-BromoPhe^{8}-BK	Arg-Pro-Pro-Gly-Phe-Ser-Pro-BPh-Arg	143	153	—	360	Fisher et al (1977)
155	8	*p*-IodoPhe^{8}-BK	Arg-Pro-Pro-Gly-Phe-Ser-Pro-IPh-Arg	67	78	—	150	Fisher et al. (1977)
156	8	O-MethylTyr^{8}-BK	Arg-Pro-Pro-Gly-Phe-Ser-Pro-OMT-Arg	—	—	285	240	Park et al (1978)
157	8	NorLeu^{8}-BK	Arg-Pro-Pro-Gly-Phe-Ser-Pro-Nle-Arg	—	—	0.3	0.7	Park et al. (1978)
158	8	Trp^{8}-BK	Arg-Pro-Pro-Gly-Phe-Ser-Pro-Trp-Arg	—	—	180	150	Park et al. (1978)
159	9	Glu^{9}-BK	Arg-Pro-Pro-Gly-Phe-Ser-Pro-Phe-Glu	—	—	0.04	0	Park et al. (1977)
160	9	*p*-GuanidoPhe^{9}-BK	Arg-Pro-Pro-Gly-Phe-Ser-Pro-Phe-GUP	0.1	2	—	—	Moore et al. (1977)
161	9	Ile^{9}-BK	Arg-Pro-Pro-Gly-Phe-Ser-Pro-Phe-Ile	—	—	0.3	0.001	Park et al. (1978)
162	9	NorLeu^{9}-BK	Arg-Pro-Pro-Gly-Phe-Ser-Pro-Phe-Nle	—	—	0.001	0.01	Park et al. (1978)
163	9	Ser^{9}-BK	Arg-Pro-Pro-Gly-Phe-Ser-Pro-Phe-Ser	—	—	0.1	0.01	Park et al. (1978)
164	1+9	Glu^{1,9}-BK	Glu-Pro-Pro-Gly-Phe-Ser-Pro-Phe-Glu	—	—	0	0	Park et al. (1978)
165	1+9	*p*-GuanidoPhe^{1,9}-BK	GUP-Pro-Pro-Gly-Phe-Ser-Pro-Phe-GUP	0.001	2	—	—	Moore et al. (1977)
166	5+8	Ala^{5,8}-BK	Arg-Pro-Pro-Gly-Ala-Ser-Pro-Ala-Arg	—	—	0	0.05	Park et al. (1978)
167	5+8	Leu^{5,8}-BK	Arg-Pro-Pro-Gly-Leu-Ser-Pro-Leu-Arg	—	—	0	0.2	Park et al. (1978)
168	5+8	*p*-NitroPhe^{5,8}-BK	Arg-Pro-Pro-Gly-PNP-Ser-Pro-PNP-Arg	9	6	—	29	Fisher et al. (1977)
169	5+8	*p*-Fluoro^{5,8}-BK	Arg-Pro-Pro-Gly-FPh-Ser-Pro-FPh-Arg	33	31	—	25	Fisher et al. (1978)
170	5+8	*p*-ChloroPhe^{5,8}-BK	Arg-Pro-Pro-Gly-CPh-Ser-Pro-CPh-Arg	16	12	—	50	Fisher et al. (1977)
171	5+8	*p*-Bromo^{5,8}-BK	Arg-Pro-Pro-Gly-BPh-Ser-Pro-BPh-Arg	22	36	—	113	Fisher et al. (1977)
172	5+8	*p*-IodoPhe^{5,8}-BK	Arg-Pro-Pro-Gly-IPh-Ser-Pro-IPh-Arg	10	19	—	45	Fisher et al. (1977)
173	8+9	Ala^{8,9}-BK	Arg-Pro-Pro-Gly-Phe-Ser-Pro-Ala-Ala	—	—	0	0	Park et al. (1978)
174	8+9	Arg^{8}, Phe^{9}-BK	Arg-Pro-Pro-Gly-Phe-Ser-Pro-Arg-Phe	—	—	0.06	0.16	Park et al. (1978)
175	5+9	Leu^{5}-BK Octapeptide (1-8)	Arg-Pro-Pro-Gly-Leu-Ser-Pro-Phe	—	—	0.001	0	Park et al. (1978)
176	5+9	Tyr^{5}-BK Octapeptide (1-8)	Arg-Pro-Pro-Gly-Tyr-Ser-Pro-Phe	—	—	0.02	0.001	Park et al. (1978)

177[a]	8+9	Ala^8-BK Octapeptide (1-8)	Arg-Pro-Pro-Gly-Phe-Ser-Pro-Ala	—	—	0.001	0[a]	PARK et al. (1978)
178[a]	8+9	Leu^8-BK Octapeptide (1-8)	Arg-Pro-Pro-Gly-Phe-Ser-Pro-Leu	—	—	0.001	0[a]	PARK et al. (1978)
179[a]	8+9	$NorLeu^8$-BK Octapeptide (1-8)	Arg-Pro-Pro-Gly-Phe-Ser-Pro-Nle	—	—	0.001	0.001[a]	PARK et al. (1978)
180[a]	8+9	Leu^8-BK Octapeptide (1-8) methyl ester	Arg-Pro-Pro-Gly-Phe-Ser-Pro-Leu-OMe	—	—	0.05	0.001[a]	PARK et al. (1978)
181	7+	*endo*-Ala^7-BK	Arg-Pro-Pro-Gly-Phe-Ser-Ala-Pro-Phe-Arg	—	—	3.4	0.2	PARK et al. (1978)
182	8+	*endo*-Ala^9-BK	Arg-Pro-Pro-Gly-Phe-Ser-Pro-Phe-Ala-Arg	—	—	0.8	0.1	PARK et al. (1978)
183	0	D-Ala^1-Kallidin	*ala*-Arg-Pro-Pro-Gly-Phe-Ser-Pro-Phe-Arg	—	—	71	200	PARK et al. (1978)
184	0	Sar^1-Kallidin	Sar-Arg-Pro-Pro-Gly-Phe-Ser-Pro-Phe-Arg	—	—	260	180	PARK et al. (1978)
185	10	BK-Ala	Arg-Pro-Pro-Gly-Phe-Ser-Pro-Phe-Arg-Ala	—	—	2	0.1	PARK et al. (1978)
186	10+11	BK-Ala-Ala	Arg-Pro-Pro-Gly-Phe-Ser-Pro-Phe-Arg-Ala-Ala	—	—	2.9	4	PARK et al. (1978)
187	9	BK Methyl ester	Arg-Pro-Pro-Gly-Phe-Ser-Pro-Phe-Arg-OMe	—	—	62	9	PARK et al. (1978)

[a] Competitively inhibited the action of BK on rabbit aorta, but not other tissues.

New Abbreviations: 43. ABU-γ-Aminobutyric acid; 44. ACC- Aminocyclopentanecarboxylic acid; 45. BPh- *p*-Bromophenylalanine; 46. CPh- *p*-Chlorophenylalanine; 47. FPh- *p*-Fluorophenylalanine; 48. GUP- *p*-Guanidophenylalanine; 49. IPh- *p*-Iodophenylalanine; 50. Nle- Norleucine.

B. Structure-Activity Relationships of Bradykinin Analogs

The analogs, homologs, and fragments of bradykinin and related kinins which have been described in the literature since the publication of the prior volume are listed in Table 1. These and the previously described analogs have been synthesized by many investigators with several goals in mind. In order to understand the mechanism of interaction of bradykinin with its receptors, one must know which groups in the molecule are responsible for receptor binding (affinity) and which are responsible for activation of the receptor (intrinsic activity) after binding has occurred. A closely related question is that of the nature of the amino acid residues responsible for determining and maintaining the shape of the peptide molecule in solution and during combination with receptors. Introduction of amino acid residues which restrict or alter the shape of the molecule can provide significant information on this point. Identification of the amino acid residue or residues responsible for the intrinsic activity of the peptide hormone is an essential prerequisite for the design of inhibitors of the action of that hormone. Unfortunately, this information is not yet available for bradykinin, although it has been deduced for certain other peptide hormones.

An understanding of the metabolism of the peptide hormone is essential to the design and synthesis of analogs with enhanced or prolonged activity. Although the nature of the in vivo degradation of bradykinin is quite well understood, and some analogs have been synthesized which show significantly enhanced potency, there have not as yet been described any analogs which show a significantly prolonged duration of action.

The wide range of biologic activities displayed by the bradykinin molecule has made the study of analogs in several different bioassay systems imperative. Unfortunately, most of the work has been done in laboratories in which only one or two assays are in routine use and very little work has been done where a given analog has been studied in all the different assays in one laboratory. The great differences which exist in biologic test systems and in test procedures in different laboratories mean that the data presented here, as well as previously, can only be interpreted as generalizations and not as exact comparisons. This problem has caused the reassay and even the resynthesis of previously described analogs in order that the characteristics governing their behavior may be more completely understood. This problem of assay technique is particularly important with respect to the in vivo depressor action of bradykinin and its analogs. The realization of the very extensive pulmonary destruction of bradykinin came only after years of work on synthesis and assay of analogs had taken place. All of those earlier analogs, and unfortunately many even today, are studied only by intravenous injection. The results of these assays then do not represent the true biologic potency of the bradykinin analog itself, but rather a composite of the potency of the analog and its resistance to pulmonary degradation, since the peptide must pass through the pulmonary circulation following intravenous injection before it can exert its biologic effect.

I. Effects of Bradykinin Analogs on Isolated Rat Uterus

In studying general structure-activity relationships in the bradykinin molecule, it is most helpful to examine first the activities on isolated rat uterus. This tissue is very sensitive and very selective for bradykinin and is essentially devoid of kininases. The bradykinin receptors of guinea pig ileum appear to have approximately the same characteristics as those of rat uterus, although some differences in specificity are obvious. The clarity of the structure-activity analysis on ileum may be confused by tachyphylaxis and the presence of kininases.

In the bradykinin molecule an intact peptide chain of nine amino acids having an arginine or other large basic residue at each end and possessing a free carboxyl group are essential requirements for high potency in the rat uterus. Removal of either arginine yields an octapeptide with little activity, although this deletion is more harmful at the amino end (peptide #210)[1] than at the carboxyl end (#235). While two arginine residues separated by a peptide chain of proper length may be necessary for biologic activity, this is not a sufficient criterion, as shown by ABRAMSON et al. (1970) who found that Arg-Gly_7-Arg was without activity. Introduction of either one or both phenylalanine residues at the appropriate places in this glycine chain still did not confer activity on the peptide. Reasoning that the conformation of the peptide chain, which can to a great extent be expected to be a function of the proline residues, is important, we investigated the molecule containing only prolines and glycines between the two arginine residues (#81); this was also inactive. It is clear that both phenylalanine and at least two of the proline residues are important for high potency, in addition to the two arginine residues. Investigations of the importance of the spacing of the basic guanidine group in the side-chain of the residues in position 1 and 9 have yielded interesting results. At position 1, the guanidine can be moved further from the peptide backbone by one additional methylene group without serious loss of potency (#5), while bringing it one methylene group closer to the backbone causes almost total loss of activity (#7). Somewhat similar results are seen at position 9 (#57 and #59), although here the homoarginine analog is not quite as active, nor is the norarginine analog as inactive as in the case of similar substitutions at position 1.

In sharp contrast to the importance of the basic group in the side-chain at position 1, the α-amino group is of little importance. It can be eliminated (#1) or acylated (see examples in SCHRÖDER, 1970, and peptides #202–209 in this chapter) with retention of high or even increased activity. Replacement of the amino group by the highly basic guanido group (#2) yields one of the most potent analogs known. Gly-Arg-Met-Lys-bradykinin has received much attention because these added amino acids were found in the bovine kininogen sequence by HOCHSTRASSER and WERLE (1967). HAN et al. (1976) in recent work have questioned this result and proposed a different sequence (peptide #107). In some assays, particularly in vivo, it appears that the high potency of these N-extended homologs of bradykinin is due to marked resistance to enzymatic degradation. However, in the case of the rat uterus, where kininase activity is not readily demonstrable, we should probably consider that these homologs have enhanced ability to bind to and activate the receptors.

The crucial importance of an unmodified free carboxyl group at the C-terminus of the bradykinin chain stands in sharp contrast to the lack of importance of the α-amino group (STEWART and WOOLLEY, 1965a). Elimination of the carboxyl group

1 In this chapter, peptides cited in the tables are numbered consecutively. All peptides having serial numbers less than 200 appear in Table 1, those in the 200 series in Table 2, etc.

(#56) or modification to the amide (SCHRÖDER, 1970; peptide #3) caused essentially total loss of activity. Addition of amino acid residues to the carboxyl end of bradykinin generally causes nearly total loss of activity (#116–118, 236, 237). It was suggested (STEWART, 1968a) that the reason for this extreme importance of the C-terminus of the bradykinin molecule may indicate that this is the initial point of attachment of the peptide to its receptors on smooth muscles. This attachment probably involves ionic bonds between the free carboxyl and arginine^9 guanidinium group of the peptide with oppositely charged groups on the receptor. The remainder of the peptide chain may then "zipper up" into contact with the remainder of the receptor. If the converse were true and the initial attachment of the peptide to the receptor took place at the amino end of the chain, we would expect modifications at that end to interfere seriously with the activity. This great importance of the carboxyl part of the peptide molecule is shared by several other small peptide hormones, although it is by no means an absolute rule. Further support for this hypothesis comes from the extreme importance of the optical configuration of the Arg^9 residue in bradykinin. Inversion of this residue (#234) leads to a very inactive analog. Of all the bradykinin analogs studied so far having inversion of one amino acid, only D-Pro^3-bradykinin (#216) is less potent. If the original receptor binding involves the carboxyl and guanidinium groups of the arginine residue, it can be appreciated that when these points of attachment have been established in the D-Arg^9 analog, all the remainder of the peptide chain would project into space in the wrong direction for effective alignment with the receptor to take place.

Phyllokinin (#115) is a remarkable exception to this general principle concerning extension of the chain in the C-direction. It has been suggested (STEWART, 1971) that the acidic sulfate residue on the C-terminal tyrosine of phyllokinin may be able to provide for the initial correct attachment of this molecule to the bradykinin receptors. The high in vivo potency of this peptide is clearly due to its resistance to inactivation by pulmonary kininases (see #238). Highest depressor potency is seen in the dog, a species which has a much less active pulmonary kininase system than the rat (SCHOLTZ and BIRON, 1969).

Proline residues, because of their cyclic structure, impose significant restrictions on the shape that peptides may adopt. For example, proline residues, as well as glycine, do not occur in α-helical sequences in peptides and proteins. Furthermore, acyl-proline bonds in peptides and proteins are the only ones known to be able to adopt freely the *cis* conformation about the peptide bond. The normal, and usually most stable, conformation is the *trans* arrangement. The presence in bradykinin of a glycine and three prolines eliminates the possibility of any helical structure of the peptide and restricts significantly the conformations available when the peptide combines with receptors. For these reasons it might be expected that the proline residues in bradykinin would play an important role in determining the biologic potency of this hormone.

Studies with alanine analogs (#211, 214, 226) suggested that Pro^2, Pro^7, and Pro^3 were most important, in that order, for the biologic activity. Surprisingly, Ala^3-bradykinin showed full potency on rat uterus, suggesting that the ring of the proline at this position did not play any significant role in receptor combination and that flexibility at this point in the molecule was not a disadvantage. While the ring of this proline is apparently not important for receptor binding, there seems to be limited space available on the receptor at this point since substitution here of amino acids having bulky side-chains yields inactive analogs. There is room to accommodate an added hydroxyl group (#215) since hydroxyproline^3-bradykinin is fully active. A methyl group added to the proline ring can also be accommodated (#15) but enlarging the ring to six members destroys activity (#16). It is interesting that hydroxyproline^2-bradykinin (#212) is one of the most potent analogs known. Its high potency is particularly impressive in the vascular permeability assay (see Table 2). The stringent structural specificity requirements about position 7 are further exemplified by the lack of potency of other analogs with substitutions in this position, even those containing hydroxyproline (#227). It is conceivable that the low potency of analogs substituted at position 7 may be related to the kinetics of hormone-receptor interaction, as discussed above.

The incorporation of D-proline residues into the bradykinin molecule has yielded puzzling results. In the case of positions 2 and 7, substitution of D-proline has approximately the same effect on potency as does substitution of L-alanine. In sharp contrast is position 3, where D-proline (#216) causes nearly complete loss of activity, while alanine or hydroxyproline yield fully potent analogs. Incorporation of all three prolines in the D-configuration (#240) yields an analog with extremely low potency; inversion of all the remaining optically active centers of the molecule causes no further loss of potency (#239, all-D-bradykinin). The interpretation of the effects of incorporation of D-amino acid residues into the bradykinin molecule is by no means clear at the present time. Although the work done so far with over 300 bradykinin analogs allows one to hazard some guesses about the chemical and topologic characteristics of the bradykinin receptor on smooth muscles, we do not have a sufficiently comprehensive picture of the receptor to allow us to explain these puzzling results.

Until very recently it had been stated categorically that the aromatic rings of the two phenylalanine residues were both crucially important for biologic activity of the bradykinin molecule, since all aliphatic substitutions (for example #219, 229, and other analogs see SCHRÖDER) yielded analogs with very low potency even when the residues substituted possessed large aliphatic hydrophobic side-chains (for example see SCHRÖDER, #89). The announcement by FLETCHER and YOUNG (1972) that cyclohexylalanine analogs of bradykinin possessed essentially full potency (#25, 45, 74) created much surprise and forced a reassessment of this conclusion. Just how the cyclohexyl residue substitutes for the phenyl ring and how it interacts with receptors is uncertain at the moment. If the aromatic side-chains do not play an essential role, it is not clear why the introduction of the "superaromatic" thiophene ring at these positions (#32, 54, 80) leads to superactive analogs. Indeed, the analog containing two thienylalanine residues in place of phenylalanine is the most potent bradykinin analog yet studied on rat uterus. Resistance to kininases cannot be the explanation, even if uterus should contain some as yet unstudied enzyme, since the high in vivo potency of these thienylalanine analogs is clearly not due to resistance to kininases (#221, 231). Chloroacetyl bradykinin (#132) also shows a very high potency on rat uterus, but its high potency is not sustained in other assay systems. Replacement of phenylalanine by N-methylphanylalanine in angiotensin II (PEÑA et al., 1974) yielded an excellent inhibitor. The conformational restriction imposed upon the molecule by this methylation apparently prevented the aromatic ring (which is the trigger for intrinsic activity) from interacting properly with the receptor. Similar replacement of

Table 2. Permeability and pulmonary results with selected bradykinin in analogs

Peptide number	Structure	Rat uterus (in %)	G.P. permeability[a] (in %)	Rat B. P. (i.a. adm)[b] (in %)	Pulmonary inactivation[c] (in %)
201	Bradykinin	100	100	100	98
202	Lys-BK	50	100	200	95
203	Met-Lys-BK	100	500	35	82
204	Gly-Arg-Met-Lys-BK	150	1500	50	0
205	Polistes Kinin	100	250	25	0
206	Lys-Lys-BK	35	120	750	0
207	Gly-BK	150	100	75	96
208	Arg-Gly-BK	10	35	8	75
209	Acetyl-BK	50	20	40	95
210	des-Arg^1-BK	10^{-5}	0.3	10^{-4}	65
211	Ala^2-BK	0.3	0.2	—	—
212	Hyp^2-BK	200	1600	90	90
213	D-Pro^2-BK	0.2	0.3	0.15	80
214	Ala^3-BK	100	100	120	97
215	Hyp^3-BK	100	70	85	94
216	D-Pro^3-BK	0.01	0.1	2×10^{-5}	30
217	des-Gly^4-BK	10^{-5}	0.5	$< 10^{-5}$	—
218	Ala^4-BK	0.03	0.2	—	—
219	Ala^5-BK	0.01	0.2	—	—
220	D-Phe^5-BK	1	3	2	80
221	Thi^5-BK	200	—	10	95
222	des-Ser^6-BK	0.03	1	0.1	93
223	Ala^6-BK	10	25	—	—
224	Phe^6-BK	0.1	1	0.3	94
225	Lys(Tos)^6-BK	0.05	1	0.05	80
226	Ala^7-BK	1.5	2.5	—	—
227	Hyp^7-BK	2	20	5	97
228	D-Pro^7-BK	1.5	0.3	0.5	0
229	Ala^8-BK	0.05	0.2	—	—
230	D-Phe^8-BK	15	15	5	80
231	Thi^8-BK	4	—	10	95
232	Leu^8-BK	0.3	3	0.05	0
233	Ala^9-BK	0.2	0.2	—	—
234	D-Arg^9-BK	0.1	1	0.2	70
235	des-Arg^9-BK	1	0.1	0.5	0
236	BK-Gly	0.7	1	1	90
237	BK-Arg	4	1	20	85
238	Phyllokinin	25	10	14	85
239	all-D-BK	5×10^{-6}	0.5	10^{-5}	—
240	tri-D-Pro^{2,3,7}-BK	5×10^{-6}	0.3	—	—
241	di-D-Phe^{5,8}-BK	0.3	0.2	0.1	45

Abbreviations are those of Table 1 with the addition of: Tos – *p*-Toluenesulfonyl.

[a] By intradermal injection into a guinea pig previously injected intravenously with Evan's blue dye. Data form MELROSE et al. (1970), RIBEIRAO and ROCHA E SILVA (1973), STEWART (1967, 1968, 1971 and unpublished results), and DONALDSON and RATNOFF (1967).

[b] Injected into the aortic arch of the rat via a carotid artery cannula. Data from ROBLERO et al. (1973), STEWART (1971) and ROBLERO and STEWART (unpublished results).

[c] In the rat, by comparison of the amount needed to cause a 25 mm Hg depressor response by i.a. and i.v. injection. The i.v. injections were into the right atrium via a jugular vein cannula. References as in Footnote b.

phenylalanine in bradykinin (#28, 49) served only to destroy all activity. Addition of an α-methyl group to the phenylalanine (#27, 48), which also severely restricts the conformational flexibility of the molecule, had a much less deleterious effect on activity and did not produce an inhibitor.

Glycine and serine residues in bradykinin appear to function principally as spacers to hold the essential amino acid residues in the proper arrangement for interaction with the receptor. These residues can be replaced by other small amino acids without significant loss of activity, although replacement by large residues leads to loss of activity (#223–225, and SCHRÖDER). These results imply the existence of a very limited amount of space at the receptor in these loci and that large side-chains probably interfere with the close approximation of the hormone to the receptor. The presence of these spacer residues is quite important, however, since omission of either the glycine (#217) or the serine (#222) leads to analogs with essentially no activity. In this context, it is very surprising that omission of one of the prolines near the amino end of the molecule yields an analog with significant potency (5%, SCHRÖDER, #177). It is also surprising that substitution of N-aminoethylglycine for the Pro^3-Gly^4 pair of amino acids in the bradykinin molecule led to an analog completely devoid of activity (#18). At first one might assume that this result implies an essential interaction of the peptide bond between positions 3 and 4 with the receptor. However, it may be better interpreted as demonstrating a deleterious effect of a basic group at this position since the aminoethyl glycine residue possesses a positive charge at physiologic pH. This basic group may form a strong ionic bond with the receptor and force the peptide into a conformation which prevents the proper receptor binding and activation from taking place. Perhaps insertion of a δ-aminovaleric acid residue at this position would lead to an analog with significant potency.

A closer examination of the possible role of the glycine residue in bradykinin was carried out by MATSUEDA and STEWART (unpublished), who compared the effects of D- and L-alanine substitutions at this position on the biologic activity of bradykinin. In the peptide hormones, luteinizing hormone-releasing hormone (LRH) and enkephalin, it has been found that replacement of a glycine residue by D-alanine leads to peptides with greatly enhanced biologic potency. In these cases, the major reason for the increased potency appears to be resistance to the action of degrading enzymes. High potency of D-alanine analogs implies also that the peptide hormone in its combination with receptors must be acceptable in this D-conformation. Since all amino acids other than glycine appear normally only in the L configuration, glycine is the only natural amino acid which can be used to give a peptide hormone the conformation imposed upon it by a D-amino acid. Glycine has no side-chain and can be effectively either (or both) D or L. Investigation of the types of cleavage in the bradykinin molecule observed upon passage through the pulmonary circulation (RYAN et al., 1968, 1970) had shown that the bradykinin molecule is cleaved on both sides of the glycine residue. If the bradykinin receptor, like those for LRH and enkephalin, should be designed to need the D conformation at this position, insertion of a D-alanine residue at this point might be expected to lead to superpotent bradykinin analogs. With respect to activity on rat uterus, however, this was found not to be the case. Both D- and L-$alanine^4$ analogs of bradykinin had very low activity, but the D-alanine analog (#19) had only about 30% of the activity of the L-alanine analog

(#218). As was pointed out above, there appears to be very little space available on the bradykinin receptor to accommodate an amino acid side-chain at this position. This may also be an important factor in the low biologic activity of these analogs. The case of LRH stands in sharp contrast, since very large groups may be substituted in the LRH molecule in place of the glycine residue with retention of very high potency.

Experiments with all-D-bradykinin, retro-bradykinin and all-D-retro-bradykinin (see SCHRÖDER) have not cast much additional light on the fine details of hormone-receptor interactions. All of these analogs possessed extremely low potency on smooth muscles. All-D-retro-bradykinin did appear to be somewhat more potent on uterus than all-D-bradykinin, suggesting that the direction of projection of the side-chains might be better in this case. A serious problem with this analog and retro-bradykinin is the lack of a carboxyl group in the essential position to combine with the receptor. However, the potencies of all these analogs were so low that one questions the significance of these data. Recent experiments with similar analogs of other peptide hormones where the investigator has attempted to make the necessary provision for a carboxyl and/or amino group suggest that the receptor may be able to sense the direction of the peptide bond.

Investigation of kinins from nonmammalian sources has continued to yield interesting new compounds (#104, 108, 109, 112, 119–122, 125). The defense secretions of insect venoms and amphibian skin glands have been the richest sources for bradykinin-related peptides. These peptides usually contain the intact bradykinin sequence with residues added to one or both ends of the molecule, although substitutions in the bradykinin portion are beginning to appear (e.g., Val^1 and Thr^6). Of particular interest are the vespulakinins (#108, 109), the first bradykinin analogs found which contain carbohydrate chains in the molecule. These carbohydrate residues are not within the bradykinin portion, but in the portion added to the amino end of the molecule. Nothing is known at this time about the possible importance of these carbohydrates for biologic activity of the peptides. Little comparative information is available on these new nonmammalian kinins since many of them have not been synthesized and tested extensively. The available information suggests that the same general rules previously determined will also hold here and that peptides having intact carboxyl ends but with added residues at the amino end will have high potency, while those with residues added to the carboxyl end of the bradykinin moiety will have very low potency in the usual bradykinin assays. Since these peptides occur in defense secretions, one should probably examine them in pain assays. As is discussed below, N-extended homologs of bradykinin seem generally to have very high potencies for permeability increase, which probably bears a relationship to pain production, at least in the compounds investigated to date.

II. Effects of Bradykinin Analogs on Intestinal Smooth Muscle

The response of the smooth muscles of small intestine to bradykinin depends on the position in the gut from which the test muscle is taken. Ileum responds to bradykinin with a characteristic slow contraction, while bradykinin relaxes the tonus of duodenum. Guinea pig ileum has been the classical assay tissue for kinins, and in general it responds to variations in the bradykinin structure in much the same way as does rat uterus. The ileum assay is, however, complicated by two characteristics which do not appear to be important in the rat uterus assay; tachyphylaxis and kininase action. If an ED_{50} dose (the amount needed to produce a half-maximal contraction) of bradykinin is applied to rat uterus and left in contact with the tissue without washing, the initial contraction is followed by a series of rhythmic relaxations and contractions, the contractions increasing in amplitude until a plateau is reached. This behavior will continue for many minutes. In contrast, application of an ED_{50} of bradykinin to guinea pig ileum induces a single contraction, followed by relaxation to the baseline. Although kininase action may play a role in this behavior, rapid desensitization appears to be more important. Examination of Table 1 for bradykinin analogs which have been compared in the same laboratory on rat uterus and guinea pig ileum shows that while many analogs have the same potency in both assay systems, as compared to bradykinin itself, many analogs are less potent on ileum than on uterus. In most cases it is not clear whether this decreased potency on ileum is due to more stringent requirements for peptide-receptor interaction, rapid onset of tachyphylaxis, or greater susceptibility to kininases. In one case, however, kininase action was shown to play a significant role (see Section D below).

Several bradykinin analogs having added residues at the amino end of the molecule are much less potent in the ileum assay. Gly-Arg-Met-Lys-bradykinin (#106) and Met-Lys-bradykinin (25% as potent as bradykinin on ileum) are examples of this. ROCHA E SILVA has called these larger kinins "pachykinins" (RIBEIRO and ROCHA E SILVA, 1973) and suggested that they may be formed in the body with the purpose of differentiating the various functions of kinins. Compared to bradykinin, these large kinins are much more potent for permeability increase than for ileum contraction. A striking exception to this rule about large kinins and ileum is the case of polisteskinin (#112). It is equipotent with bradykinin on ileum on a weight basis and twice as potent on a molar basis (since the molecular weight is twice that of bradykinin).

Several analogs of bradykinin have been tested for their ability to cause relaxation of rat duodenum. Rather surprisingly, the results in this assay roughly paralleled those found in rat uterus. The relaxation induced in duodenum by bradykinin has been the subject of much speculation. It has been proposed (MONTGOMERY and KROEGER, 1967) that this action was mediated by catecholamine β-receptors responding to catecholamines released in the tissue by bradykinin. Extensive experiments with catecholamine blockers have failed to substantiate this claim (STEWART, unpublished). Furthermore, bradykinin analogs which were found to be particularly effective in promoting catecholamine release in other assays were no more active on duodenum than on uterus. More recently it has been suggested that the different response of duodenum and ileum to bradykinin is due to the release of different prostaglandins in these tissues (see TERRAGNO and TERRAGNO, this volume, for a review). Preliminary efforts to inhibit the response of intestine to bradykinin by pretreatment with indomethacin (T. PAIVA, personal communication; STEWART, unpublished) have not supported this postulate. Final delineation of the mechanism of action of bradykinin and related kinins on gut awaits further investigation.

III. Effects of Bradykinin Analogs on Vascular Permeability

Except for eledoisin and substance P, bradykinin is the most potent substance known for increasing vascular permeability (BISSET and LEWIS, 1962). This effect is not due to any change in the permeability of vascular endothelial cell membranes, but rather to a weakening of the cell junctions so that the blood vessels become "leaky" and allow macromolecules and leucocytes to pass out into the extravascular space (GABBIANI et al., 1970). In general, structural requirements for permeability-increasing activity were found to be much less stringent than for uterotonic activity. Analogs modified in one or more of the groups found to be essential for uterotonic activity usually also had impaired potency in the permeability assay, but the loss was not so great. In the rat uterus several analogs were found to have less than 10^{-5} times the potency of bradykinin, while in the guinea pig vascular permeability assay none was found to have an activity lower than 10^{-4} times that of bradykinin. It is believed, however, that such low activities do represent activation of bradykinin receptors regulating permeability, and not nonspecific irritation, since other arginine-containing peptides having structures unlike bradykinin were found to be much less active. Rather surprisingly, an intact carboxyl end was found to be even more important in the permeability assay than in the uterus; the only analogs found to be less active in the permeability assay than in uterus were those with carboxyl end changes (#235, 237). Extension of the peptide chain at the amino end produced analogs more active in increasing permeability than on the uterus. Met-Lys-bradykinin and polisteskinin are notable in this respect, both being five times as active as bradykinin on a molar basis (the data in Table 2 are on a weight basis). Most potent of all is Gly-Arg-Met-Lys-bradykinin (#204), which is 20 times as potent as bradykinin. Hydroxyproline^2-bradykinin (#212) is nearly as potent (16 × bradykinin), and is the most potent simple bradykinin analog in this assay. Some N-extended analogs are thus strikingly different in their effects on permeability and on ileum contraction. In contrast, hydroxyproline^2-bradykinin (#9) shows very high potency in all bradykinin assays.

As mentioned above, the occurrence of these N-extended bradykinin homologs ("pachykinins") in venoms may be related to their preferential potency for permeability increase. Although only very limited studies have been done so far on the relationship of structure to pain production in bradykinin analogs, the evidence already obtained (ARMSTRONG, 1970) suggests that the N-extended homologs will also show very high potency for pain production. The resistance of these N-extended homologs to degradation by kininases is also very impressive and may be important in their function as chemical defense substances. Several of these [Gly-Arg-Met-Lys-bradykinin, Lys-Lys-bradykinin, and polisteskinin, (#204–206)] were found to be totally resistant to the action of normal pulmonary kininases in the rat, and recent work with purified angiotensin-converting enzyme (DORER et al., 1974) showed a similar resistance to in vitro degradation by kininase II.

IV. Effects of Bradykinin Analogs on Blood Pressure

The action of bradykinin on the vascular system is complex. Arterioles dilate, venules constrict, and small vessels leak. The net result of these actions in all species is the production of a sharp fall in arterial blood pressure. This hypotensive effect is minimized by the action of efficient kininases and by the pressor effect of the catecholamines released by the bradykinin. Kininases are present in plasma (half-life of bradykinin in blood is 15–20 s in most species) and in all capillary beds. Most efficient of these latter is the lung, which in the rat destroys 98–99% of the plasma

Lung: Arg↓Pro-Pro↓Gly↓Phe-Ser↓Pro↓Phe↓Arg

Arg-Pro-Pro-Gly-Phe-Ser-Pro-Phe-Arg

Plasma: Arg-Pro-Pro-Gly-Phe-Ser-Pro↑Phe↑Arg

Fig. 1. Observed points of cleavage of the bradykinin molecule by kininases in lung and plasma

bradykinin on a single passage. This very efficient pulmonary destruction is caused by several enzymes apparently attached to the capillary walls and freely exposed to the passing blood. As indicated in Fig. 1, these enzymes cleave the peptide chain in several places (RYAN et al., 1968, 1970) throughout the molecule, in contrast to the plasma enzymes which cause two cleavages at the carboxyl end (see ERDÖS, this volume).

Previously published data on the effects of bradykinin analogs on blood pressure (SCHRÖDER, 1970) were all obtained by intravenous injection. When administered in this way, the peptides must first pass through the lung and be subjected to its kininases before they can reach the arterial side of the circulation and produce a hypotensive effect. Data thus obtained represent only the net result of the combined inherent hypotensive potency of the peptide and its susceptibility or resistance to the pulmonary and plasma kininases and do not provide accurate data for structure-activity studies.

In this laboratory (ROBLERO et al., 1973), we have compared the hypotensive effects of bradykinin analogs in the rat by both intravenous (into the right atrium) and intra-arterial (into the ascending aorta) routes of administration. The result of the intra-arterial injection represents the true hypotensive potency of the peptide, and comparison of this effect with that produced by intravenous injection gives a measure of the pulmonary destruction. It is realized, of course, that intra-aortic injection does not provide a result totally free of the effects of kininase action since the peptides are exposed to the plasma kininases for a few seconds before they reach their sites of action. Pretreatment of rats with 2-mercaptoethanol, which inhibits plasma kininases, approximately doubles the intra-aortic potency of bradykinin. In this way, the effect of plasma kininases on the bradykinin analogs can be estimated. Catecholamine release was assessed in animals pretreated with phenoxybenzamine which blocks the pressor effect of these amines (FREER and STEWART, 1975; STEWART, 1976a).

In general, the hypotensive effect of bradykinin analogs, as judged by intra-arterial injection, paralleled the rat uterus activity (see Table 2). Differences between the two assays of as much as an order of magnitude either way were sometimes seen, but there was no reason to believe that the vascular receptors had significantly different structural specificities than did those of uterus. The N-extended homologs (#202–208) were generally somewhat less potent on blood pressure but kallidin was a notable exception. Thienylalanine^5-bradykinin (#221) was much less potent than on uterus. On the other hand, potencies of the analogs observed by intravenous injection varied very widely because of their differing susceptibility to the pulmonary kininases. For example, Met-Lys-bradykinin, Gly-Arg-Met-Lys-bradykinin, polisteskinin, and phyllokinin are all inherently less active than bradykinin but appear to be more active when administered intravenously because they are not extensively degraded by the pulmonary kininases. The most active analog found by intravenous injection is Lys-Lys-bradykinin (#206), which is not only highly active inherently but is totally resistant to the pulmonary kininases during pulmonary passage. It is up to 1000 times as active as bradykinin given intravenously to the rat. Of all the analogs examined so far, only Gly-Arg-Met-Lys-bradykinin, polisteskinin, Lys-Lys-bradykinin, D-Phe^{5}-bradykinin, D-Pro^{7}-bradykinin, D-Phe^{5,8}-bradykinin, Leu^{8}-bradykinin, des-Arg^{9}-bradykinin, and Phe^{9}-bradykinin are totally resistant to pulmonary kininases in the rat. Three of these (des-Arg^{9}-, D-Phe^{5}-, and D-Phe^{5,8}-) appeared to be inactivated in normal animals, but pretreatment with phenoxybenzamine showed that this was due to efficient catecholamine release, apparently from stores in the lung. In fact, infusions of des-Arg^{9}-bradykinin are pressor because the weak depressor potency of the peptide is overwhelmed by the pressor effect of the released catecholamine. It is interesting that des-Arg^{9}-bradykinin, having lost the C-terminal arginine, is now quite similar to angiotensin II at this end of the molecule. Like angiotensin II, it is stable to pulmonary kininases and is a very effective releaser of catecholamines. Potent release of adrenal catecholamines by des-Arg^{9}-bradykinin was also observed by DAMAS and CESSION-FOSSION (1973).

It is clear from examination of these analogs that there is no correlation between bradykinin potency of analogs and their susceptibility to pulmonary kininases. Some of the totally resistant analogs have very high potency (#204–206), while others have very low inherent potency (#228, 235). Substrate specificity requirements for the kininases thus are totally different from receptor binding requirements.

A knowledge of the mechanism of action and substrate specificity of all significant kininases is essential to the design of bradykinin derivatives or analogs able to accomplish specific purposes in vivo. An illustration of this point is D-Arg^{9}-bradykinin. After ERDÖS had discovered plasma kininase I, which removes the C-terminal arginine from bradykinin, NICOLAIDES et al. (1965) synthesized D-Arg^{9}-bradykinin in the expectation that it would not be degraded and would thus have a prolonged action in vivo. Much to their surprise, this analog had very low potency and no more prolonged action on blood pressure than did bradykinin itself. At that time, the existence of the pulmonary kininases was not even suspected, and we now know that this analog is destroyed by the lung to the extent of 70% on a single passage (see Table 2). Future work should be significantly aided by the rudimentary knowledge we now possess concerning peptides which are resistant to these enzymes.

The pulmonary kininases, like those in plasma, are inhibited by 2-mercaptoethanol, 2,3-dimercaptopropanol (BAL), and other metal chelating agents. The pulmonary kininases differ greatly in their susceptibility to these agents. While infusion of mercaptoethanol at extremely high rates will completely block all pulmonary destruction of bradykinin in the rat, more moderate doses (75 mg/kg, intramuscularly) show a great deal of selectivity in protection of the different homologs and analogs of bradykinin. Among the analogs which are extensively inactivated in normal rats, pretreatment with mercaptoethanol may show no effect, significant but partial protection, or complete protection. For example, mercaptoethanol at this level has no effect on the pulmonary inactivation of D-Pro^{2}-, D-Phe^{8}-, and D-Arg^{9}-bradykinins, while Met-Lys-bradykinin, bradykininyl-arginine, and D-Pro^{3}-bradykinin are completely protected. Most analogs, like bradykinin itself, are partially protected by this level of mercaptoethanol (ROBLERO et al., 1973).

As discussed by FREER and STEWART (1975), several lines of evidence suggested that angiotensin I converting enzyme is not the rate-determining pulmonary kininase in the rat, although removal of the C-terminal dipeptide from bradykinin was observed when radioactive bradykinin was perfused through rat lung. The recent discovery (DORER et al., 1974) that the resistance to rat pulmonary kininases of several N-extended bradykinin homologs is mirrored by the action of pure hog lung angiotensin I converting enzyme in vitro further confuses this point. The physiologic significance of this finding is not completely clear, since the most dramatic resistance to hydrolysis was obtained in solution free of chloride. At chloride concentrations nearing physiologic, a trend was still visible, but the absolute failure to hydrolyze Gly-Arg-Met-Lys-bradykinin and polisteskinin was not seen. Another analog, D-Pro^7-bradykinin (# 228), was not hydrolyzed by converting enzyme under any conditions. In my opinion these results cast angiotensin I converting enzyme (peptidyl dipeptidase; kininase II) in quite a different light from that of the nonspecific carboxydipeptidase in which it has usually been portrayed. It is very interesting that modification at the amino terminus of the peptide can block the action of an enzyme which acts upon the carboxyl end. Examination of the circular dichroism spectra of certain of these resistant analogs did not provide evidence that resistance to hydrolysis might be due to a solution conformation unlike that of bradykinin (BRADY et al., 1971). There appear to be significant differences in the activity of pulmonary kininases in different species; human and dog lungs seem to be much less active than those of the rat. Pulmonary inactivation of bradykinin has not been studied in the hog in vivo, although the enzyme has been purified from this tissue: It is not clear how many of the apparent contradictions in this field may be due to species differences. Further work is needed to clarify many of these points. Some other characteristics of kininases are discussed in the section on bradykinin-potentiating peptides, below.

V. Structure-Activity Relationships in Other Assays

A few bradykinin analogs have been examined by ARMSTRONG (1970) for their ability to produce pain on the exposed human blister base. Although this assay is extremely difficult to quantitate, a few generalizations can be made. Here again is seen the importance of an intact carboxyl end of the kinin molecule. Amino acid residues can be added to the amino end of the molecule with retention of high activity (RIBEIRO and ROCHA E SILVA, 1973).

The ability of bradykinin to cause bronchoconstriction has implicated it in asthma and anaphylaxis. It was of considerable interest, therefore, to study the effects of structural alteration on this phenomenon. Several analogs have been examined in the guinea pig for both hypotensive and bronchoconstrictor action, and generally show roughly parallel activities by these two indices (SCHRÖDER, 1970). Since these assays were done in vivo with intravenous administration of the peptides, much of the effect seen may be a reflection of the resistance of the peptides to guinea pig pulmonary kininases. A further complication arose with the discovery, by PIPER and VANE (1969), that the observed bronchoconstriction is not caused by direct action of bradykinin but that bradykinin causes the lungs to secrete into the circulation a hitherto undiscovered substance, called RCS, which is a potent bronchoconstrictor and the mediator of the observed effect. RCS is now known to be a prostaglandin (prostacyclin, or PGI; see TERRAGNO and TERRAGNO, this volume).

As yet, no studies have appeared on the relationship of peptide structure to leucocyte chemotaxis.

C. Antagonists of Bradykinin Action

Extensive work on analogs of peptide hormones over more than two decades has demonstrated clearly that few generalizations can be made in this field. The different hormones are very individualistic, and their receptors demonstrate very different specificity requirements. As a consequence, principles operating in the design of inhibitors of the action of one peptide hormone are generally not applicable to other peptide systems. Synthesis of inhibitors has been particularly successful in the cases of angiotensin II and luteinizing hormone-releasing hormone, and much valuable information has been learned from use of these inhibitors. The search for competitive inhibitors of bradykinin among structural analogs of the hormone has been singularly unrewarding, although several analogs were found which did show some antibradykinin action in certain circumstances. In general, they showed only partial antagonism and also possessed agonist action at higher concentration (STEWART and WOOLLEY, 1966). The first structural modification of bradykinin by STEWART and WOOLLEY in 1962 (substitution of leucine for phenylalanine) (see STEWART and WOOLLEY, 1966) was much later found to yield effective inhibitors of angiotensin II. As discussed in Sect. B-I, the aliphatic replacements of phenylalanine yield merely inactive peptides, except in the case of the cyclohexyl derivatives which show good agonist potency. The failure of N-methylphenylalanine substitutions to yield inhibitors was discussed above.

Several bradykinin analogs containing D-amino acids and with or without acetylated amino termini appeared initially to be useful inhibitors of the action of bradykinin on vascular permeability increase in guinea pigs (STEWART, 1968a; STEWART and WOOLLEY, 1965b). These analogs also suffered from the same defect of partial antagonism, with agonist activity appearing at higher concentrations. It was later found that this antagonism was demonstrable only in a special strain of guinea pigs. This was a strain developed by Dr. M.W. Chase for extremely uniform response in delayed hypersensitivity, most likely a kinin-mediated phenomenon. Repetition of the tests with standard strains of albino guinea pigs showed no antagonism with these peptides. Moreover, the initial demonstration of antibradykinin activity (STEWART and WOOLLEY, 1966) could be done only on rat uterus from a special type of animal, in which the tissue was probably not normal.

FREER and STEWART (1972) synthesized a series of fragments and analogs of bradykinin containing the nitrogen mustard, chlorambucil, as a potential affinity label (see Table 1, # 127–132). If the bradykinin receptor contains a nucleophilic group that can be alkylated by the nitrogen mustard, the peptide should be permanently linked to the receptor by a covalent bond. This should inhibit the receptor permanently. Although none of these chlorambucil derivatives proved to be an effective bradykinin inhibitor, certain of them did have the ability to potentiate permanently the response to bradykinin; they are discussed in Sect. D, below. The use of chlorambucil as an affinity label was later applied with great success to inhibitors of angiotensin II (PAIVA et al., 1972). TURK et al. (1975a) also unsuccessfully sought bradykinin inhibitors among reactive derivatives.

Very recently, REGOLI and BARABÉ (1977) have disclosed that the leucine analog of the bradykinin 1–8 octapeptide is a competitive inhibitor of the action of bradykinin on isolated rabbit aortic strips. This is quite analogous to the effectiveness of leucine^8-angiotensin II as an angiotensin II inhibitor. They state that this peptide, Arg-Pro-Pro-Gly-Phe-Ser-Pro-Leu, is not a bradykinin inhibitor in any other standard bradykinin assay system. These investigators emphasize that the bradykinin receptors of rabbit aorta are very different from those of other tissues. They state that des-Arg^9-bradykinin, which normally possesses about 1% the potency of bradykinin, is 10 times as potent as bradykinin in this assay. As was discussed earlier, des-Arg^9-bradykinin has some characteristics in common with angiotensin II and one wonders if these investigators are not actually dealing with an angiotensin receptor in the aorta. Aortic angiotensin receptors are well known and have been much studied. REGOLI and BARABÉ state, however, that the response of aorta to bradykinin is not inhibited by Leu^8-angiotensin II, a well known angiotensin inhibitor and that the action of angiotensin on the tissue is not inhibited by the Leu^8-bradykinin octapeptide. Although this discovery reveals an interesting new type of bradykinin receptor which may have physiologic significance – for example, if there is a significant circulating level of des-Arg^9-bradykinin – it does not appear that the key to useful general bradykinin inhibitors has been found.

Several nonpeptide antagonists of the action of bradykinin on isolated smooth muscles have been described, but these are generally polycyclic aromatic amines that probably do not act upon bradykinin receptors directly, since no structural analogy exists between these inhibitors and bradykinin. Although such sweeping generalizations must be made with some caution these days since the discovery that morphine acts by occupying receptors for a peptide (enkephalin) (FREDRICKSON, 1977), these types of kinin inhibitors probably act by interfering with microtubule function in the smooth muscle cells. These inhibitors are not specific for kinins, generally affect the response of the tissue to other agonists, and usually show noncompetitive inhibition. This work has been reviewed by ROCHA E SILVA (1970). Recently, GECSE et al. (1976) showed that high concentrations of phenylglycine heptyl ester, phenylalanine heptyl ester, and arginine heptyl ester (10^4 times the concentration of bradykinin) would inhibit the action of bradykinin on isolated rat uterus. The same compounds given at 2.5 mg/kg would inhibit the vascular permeability increase in guinea pigs due to bradykinin, histamine, and serotonin. Another group of in vivo bradykinin inhibitors consists of compounds such as indomethacin and aspirin that block the bradykinin-mediated release of prostaglandin. (This subject is reviewed elsewhere in this volume by TARRAGNO and TARRAGNO.)

D. Potentiators of Responses to Kinins

Although no useful inhibitors of bradykinin action have yet been found, useful potentiators of the kinin response have been known for over a decade. In this section I will discuss the bradykinin-potentiating peptides found in snake venoms, the synthetic peptides related to these naturally occurring potentiators, derivatives of peptides containing alkylating agents, enzymes, and enzyme inhibitors.

I. Naturally Occurring Bradykinin-Potentiating Peptides

The most important peptide potentiators of kinins are found in the venoms of crotalid snakes. Shortly after bradykinin was first synthesized in 1960, ROCHA E SILVA (personal communication) obtained a sample of the synthetic material and compared it to bradykinin prepared in his laboratory by treatment of plasma with *Bothrops jararaca* venom. The venom-derived material was more potent and had a longer duration of action. FERREIRA (1965), investigating this difference, found that the snake venom contains, in addition to the enzyme which produces bradykinin, a low molecular weight alcohol-soluble substance that potentiates the action of bradykinin. This material appeared to be of peptide nature and was found in the venoms of a number of crotalid snakes (FERREIRA, 1966). Nine bradykinin-potentiating peptides were isolated from *B. jararaca* venom by FERREIRA et al. (1970) (Table 3); the amino acid sequence of the smallest, a pentapeptide called BPP5a, was determined, and it was synthesized (STEWART et al., 1971). KATO and SUZUKI (1971) later found other bradykinin-potentiating peptides in the venom of the Japanese snake, *Agkistrodon halys blomhoffii*. The discovery that bradykinin-potentiating factor inhibits angiotensin I converting enzyme (BAKHLE, 1968; NG and VANE, 1970) stimulated vigorous work on these peptides and the structures of the remaining *Bothrops* peptides were soon determined (ONDETTI et al., 1971). Table 3 gives the structures of all the venom bradykinin-potentiating peptides that have been determined. Although the complete structure of *Agkistrodon* potentiator D (#314) has not been published, it is most likely a close structural analog of potentiator C (#313), with arginine replacing the glycine residue in potentiator C. Most of the pharmacologic work has been done with the pentapeptide (#310, BPP5a, SQ-20,475) and the nonapeptide (#309, BPP9a, SQ-20,881). This nonapeptide has been given the generic name Teprotide.

Of several snake venoms examined, FERREIRA (1966) found that from *Crotalus viridi viridi* to be the most potent for bradykinin potentiation. (It has double the potency of *B. jararaca* venom.) More recently, SANDER et al. (1972) found *C. horridus horridus* venom to be 10 times as potent as that of *B. jararaca* for converting-enzyme inhibition. It is unknown at the present time whether these increased potencies are due to a greater concentration of bradykinin-potentiating peptides in the venom or if these species of venoms contain other, more potent, bradykinin-potentiating peptides.

Determination of the amino sequences of the bradykinin-potentiating peptides has not been an easy project. A pyroglutamic acid residue blocks the amino terminus of all of them and makes the peptides resistant to the action of the Edman degradation procedure which is normally used. The presence of multiple proline residues has added confusion to amino acid analysis and made specific enzymatic cleavage procedures poorly applicable, since X-Pro bonds are not cleaved by most proteolytic enzymes.

The standard assay for bradykinin-potentiating peptides uses the isolated guinea pig ileum (FERREIRA et al., 1970; STEWART et al., 1971). One unit of bradykinin-potentiating activity is defined as that amount of the potentiating peptide which when dissolved in 1 ml Tyrode solution causes a moderate dose of bradykinin to give a response equivalent to that normally produced by twice the amount of bradykinin. This is a mirror-image analogy of the agonist dose ratio (x) used in calculation of

Table 3. Bradykinin-potentiating peptides isolated from snake venoms

Peptide number	Ferreira and Greene[a]	Ondetti[b]	Kato and Suzuki[c]	Structure	Biologic activity[d]
301	IV-1-Bα	V–A		<Glu-Trp-Pro-Arg-Pro-Thr-Pro-Gln-Ile-Pro-Pro	34[k]
302	III-1-A	V–D		<Glu-Gly-Gly-Trp-Pro-Arg-Pro-Gly-Pro-Glu-Ile-Pro-Pro	200[k]
303	II-1-A[e]			<Glu-Gly-Gly-Leu-Pro-Arg-Pro-Gly-Pro-Glu-Ile-Pro-Pro	90
304	IV-1-A	V–B_2		<Glu-Ser-Trp-Pro-Gly-Pro-Asn-Ile-Pro-Pro	80[k]
305	V-3-B[e]			<Glu-Ser-Trp-Pro-Gly-Pro	9
306	IV-1-Bβ	V–B_1		<Glu-Asn-Trp-Pro-His-Pro-Gln-Ile-Pro-Pro	47[k]
307		V–C_2^e		<Glu-Asn-Trp-Pro-Arg-Pro-Gln-Ile-Pro-Pro	100[k]
308	V-1-A[e]			<Glu-Glx-Trp-Ala-Trp-Pro-Arg-Pro-Gln-Ile-Pro-Pro	380
309(BPP9a)[h]	IV-1-D	V–C_1^e		<Glu-Trp-Pro-Arg-Pro-Gln-Ile-Pro-Pro	410[j,k]
310(BPP5a)[i]	V-3-A			<Glu-Lys-Trp-Ala-Pro	100[k]
311			A	<Glu-Gly-Arg-Pro-Pro-Gly-Pro-Pro-Ile-Pro	0.2[f]
312			B	<Glu-Gly-Leu-Pro-Pro-Arg-Pro-Lys-Ile-Pro-Pro	280[g]
313			C	<Glu-Gly-Leu-Pro-Pro-Gly-Pro-Pro-Ile-Pro-Pro	20[g]
314			D	<Glu-Gly-(Arg, Ile, Leu, Pro_6)	5[f]
315			E	<Glu-Lys-Trp-Asp-Pro-Pro-Pro-Val-Ser-Pro-Pro	0.3[f]

[a] Ferreira et al. (1970)
[b] Ondetti et al. (1971)
[c] Kato and Suzuki (1971).
[d] Relative specific activity, on a molar basis, for the potentiation of the action of bradykinin on guinea pig ileum. The activity of BPP5a is arbitrarily taken as 100.
[e] Sequences of these peptides were not determined. The sequences shown were deduced from physical properties and by comparison with related peptides.
[f] As no direct comparison of these peptides with the others has been made, the activities given were estimated from the literature.
[g] Based on a new comparison of these peptides with BPP5a (Tominaga et al., 1975). See also Kato and Suzuki (1976).
[h] Also known as Teprotide and SQ 20,881.
[i] Also known as SQ 20,475.
[j] Also reported as 960 by Sabia et al. (1977).
[k] Rat in vivo ID_{80} (for 80% inhibition of the pressor response to angiotensin I): #301—1.5 mg/kg; 302—>8; 304—>32; 306—2; 307—1.5; 309—0.5; 310—6. Bradykinin potentiation was parallel, but at much lower doses. From Engel et al. (1972).

pA_2 of antagonists. The potencies found in this way for the venom peptides are given in Table 3. Activities are expressed relative to BPP5a (#310). The concentration of BPP5a needed to double the effect of bradykinin on the guinea pig ileum is seven times the concentration of bradykinin used, and is typically 10^{-8}-10^{-7} *M*. BPP5a is remarkable for having very high potency in a relatively small molecule. The most potent venom peptide isolated so far is BPP9a (#309), which has four times the potency of BPP5a. This nonapeptide, now called Teprotide, has been very extensively used in both in vitro and in vivo studies of bradykinin and angiotensin pharmacology. Its greatest emphasis has been as an inhibitor of angiotensin I converting enzyme.

These venom peptides potentiate the action of bradykinin both by inhibition of kininases and by a direct effect on tissue. Potentiation in vivo is clearly due principally to kininase inhibition, while potentiation in isolated tissues is apparently due to a mixed action. Potencies in vivo differ greatly from those given above from in vitro determinations (ENGEL et al., 1972). Part of this difference is due to the presence of enzymes which can cleave the potentiating peptides and thus destroy their activity. ONDETTI et al. (1972) showed that BPP5a is a substrate for angiotensin-converting enzyme, which cleaves a dipeptide from the carboxyl end of the potentiator. In contrast, the penultimate proline residue in BPP9a prevents it from serving as a substrate for this enzyme. While BPP5a does not block completely the pulmonary destruction of bradykinin in the rat, BPP9a is able to do this very effectively, and has a very persistent action. Some in vivo potencies are given in Table 3.

Potentiation of the kinin response in isolated smooth muscles by bradykinin-potentiating peptides occurs mainly in those tissues where significant kininase action can be demonstrated, suggesting that kininase inhibition is the mode of action. *Agkistrodon* potentiator E (#315) is an exception to this rule, since it is much more potent for potentiation of bradykinin on rat uterus than on guinea pig ileum. It has recently been shown (TOMINAGA et al., 1975) that other bradykinin-potentiating peptides can also act in rat uterus but at very high concentrations. Kininase inhibition is not the only mode of potentiation in ileum as is demonstrated by the fact that pre-addition of the potentiator before the challenge bradykinin dose, or addition of the potentiator when the contraction in response to the same dose of bradykinin has reached its peak, yields the same degree of potentiation (STEWART et al., 1971). Furthermore, bradykinin-potentiating peptides potentiate the ileum response to bradykinin analogs which are not degraded by kininases. GREENE et al. (1972) showed that D-Pro^7-bradykinin and des-Arg^9-bradykinin, which had been earlier found by ROBLERO et al. (1973) to be fully resistant to rat pulmonary kininases, were also completely resistant to the action of degrading enzymes in guinea pig ileum homogenates. However, the action of these two analogs on ileum was potentiated fully by the same dose of BPP5a that was needed to potentiate the response of the tissue to bradykinin. The nature of this non-kininase-related potentiation has yet to be elucidated.

TOMINAGA et al. (1975) and SABIA et al. (1977) have observed that some bradykinin-potentiating peptides have the ability to increase the response of ileum to bradykinin for several hours after application, even though the tissue is washed thoroughly. This so-called "sensitization" was greatest for *Agkistrodon* potentiator B

(# 312), which caused a 2.4-fold increase in the response to bradykinin after application of the potentiator 4×10^{-7} *M* and washing. The ability to sensitize was not related to the potentiating potency; all those peptides which sensitized had their maximum effect at 4×10^{-7} *M*. Significant sensitization was also seen with synthetic peptides # 477 (2.2-fold) and # 490 (1.5-fold). The ability to sensitize appeared to be correlated with the number of basic residues in the peptide; BPP9a, with one basic residue, was a very weak sensitizer (1.2-fold). The mechanism of this long-lasting effect was not elucidated; it may be due to slow dissociation of the peptide from the tissue, which is also seen with some angiotensin inhibitors.

The occurrence in insect and amphibian chemical defense secretions of braydkinin homologs resistant to the action of kininases in the victims was noted above. The crotalid snakes have also done a very beautiful job of designing a system to cause the victim maximum difficulty and discomfort. Injection of the snake venom causes massive hemolysis, thrombosis, and kinin liberation in the affected tissue area. The consequent great vasodilation and permeability increase contribute to hemostasis in the affected area, and produce extensive edema and pain. The accompanying bradykinin-potentiating peptides protect the liberated bradykinin from destruction, potentiate its action, and block the effective utilization by the victim of the renin-angiotensin system for increasing the blood pressure in an effort to re-establish the circulation through the affected area. This concatenation of events also contributes to systemic shock and prostration of the victim. Peptide chemists and pharmacologists can still learn lessons in drug design from lower species.

In addition to the venom peptides, other kinds of peptides also potentiate the action of bradykinin. GLADNER (1966) observed that fibrinopeptides (byproducts of the action of thrombin on fibrinogen) potentiated the action of bradykinin and several analogs on smooth muscles. These results were further investigated by FABER (1969). The structures of two fragments of fibrinopeptides found by GLADNER to be potent bradykinin potentiators are given in Table 4 (# 505, 506). The intact fibrinopeptides from which these were derived (human fibrinopeptide A and bovine fibrinopeptide B) were also found to be effective. It should be pointed out that the assay system used by GLADNER for bradykinin potentiation was very different from the standard ileum system described above. He showed that the fibrinopeptides, when incubated with isolated rat uterus for periods of 15–60 min, potentiated subsequent addition of bradykinin. It is possible that these fibrinopeptides may be acting on uterus in a manner similar to the *Agkistrodon* potentiator E. Several investigators have reported that peptides obtained by the action of trypsin on plasma proteins potentiate the action of bradykinin (AARSEN, 1968; HAMBERG et al., 1968; WEYERS et al., 1972; TEWKSBURY, 1972). The structures of synthetic peptides related to those isolated by WEYERS are given in Table 4 (# 496–499). It should be pointed out that the sequences of these tryptic peptides and the fibrinopeptides studied by GLADNER bear no relationship whatever to the sequences of the venom bradykinin-potentiating peptides. These peptides are generally much less potent than the best venom potentiators, but since they are materials that could be present in the circulatory system they may play a role in modulating the physiologic effects of kinins. HAMBERG et al. (1968) also have suggested that they may potentiate the action of bradykinin by serving as alternate substrates or inhibitors for plasma kininases and thus prolong the life of bradykinin in vivo.

Table 4. Synthetic analogs of bradykinin potentiating peptides

Peptide number	Structure	Biologic activity	
		BK[b]	ANG[c]
401	<Glu-Lys-Trp-Ala-Pro(BPP5a)	100	100
402	Glu-Lys-Trp-Ala-Pro	6.3	—
403	<Glu-Lys(Ac)-Trp-Ala-Pro	15	—
404	Pro-Lys-Trp-Ala-Pro	100	—
405	<Glu-Pro-Lys-Trp-Ala-Pro	100	—
406	PhB-Pro-Lys-Trp-Ala-Pro	17	—
407	<Glu-Lys-Trp-Ala-Pro-NH_2	< 0.5	—
408	<Glu-Lys-Trp(Ox)-Ala-Pro	0.5	—
409	<Glu-Lys-Trp — Pro	< 0.5	—
410	<Glu-Lys-Trp-Ala	< 0.1	—
411	<Glu-Lys-Phe-Ala	—	0.7
412	Lys-Trp-Ala-Pro	0.5	4
413	Trp-Ala-Pro	0.2	—
414	Phe-Ala-Pro	—	3.6
415	Ala-Pro	< 0.1	0.1
416	<Glu-Lys	0	—
417	<Glu-Lys-Phe	—	0.1
418	<Glu-Lys-Phe — Pro	—	< 0.02
419	<Glu — Phe-Ala-Pro	—	2
420	Boc — Phe-Ala-Pro	—	0.3
421	<Glu-Lys-Phe-Ala-Pro-Pro	—	1
422	<Glu-Lys-Phe-Ala-Pro	—	100
423	Cpc-Lys-Phe-Ala-Pro	—	83
424	Boc-Lys-Phe-Ala-Pro	—	1
425	<Glu-Nle-Phe-Ala-Pro	—	25
426	<Glu-Gln-Phe-Ala-Pro	—	12
427	<Glu-Glu-Phe-Ala-Pro	—	2
428	<Glu-Thr-Phe-Ala-Pro	—	1
429	<Glu-Lys-Pro-Ala-Pro	—	4.5
430	<Glu-Lys-Ser-Ala-Pro	—	3
431	<Glu-Lys-Ser-Ala-Pro	—	2
432	<Glu-Lys-*trp*-Ala-Pro	—	0.07
433	<Glu-Lys-Phe-Lac-Pro	—	83
434	<Glu-Lys-Phe-Gly-Pro	—	50
435	<Glu-Lys-Phe-Pro-Pro	—	1.5
436	<Glu-Lys-Phe-Ala-Ala	—	83
437	<Glu-Lys-Phe-Ala-Glu	—	2.5
438	<Glu-Lys-Phe-Ala-Pyn	—	< 0.02
439	<Glu-Lys-Trp-Ala-Pro-Ile-Pro-Pro	< 0.1	—
440	<Glu-Lys-Trp-Ala-Pro-Phe-Arg	20	—
441	Lys-Trp-Ala-Pro-Phe-Arg	2	—
442	<Glu-Lys-Trp-Pro-Arg-Pro	5	—
443	<Glu — Trp-Pro-Arg-Pro	< 0.1	0.4
444	<Glu-Pro-Pro-Gly-Trp-Ser	< 0.1	—
445	<Glu — Pro-Gly-Trp-Ser-Pro	1	—
446	<Glu-Ser-Trp-Pro-Gly-Pro	2	—
447	Chl-Pro-Lys-Trp-Ala-Pro	"potent"[d]	—
448	Chl-Lys-Trp-Ala-Pro	"potent"	—
449	Chl-Trp-Ala-Pro	"potent"[d]	—
450	Chl-Ala-Pro	0[d]	—
451	Chl-Lys-Trp-Ala-Pro-Phe	0	—

Table 4 (continued)

Peptide number	Structure	Biologic activity	
		BK[b]	ANG[c]
452	Chl-Trp-Ala-Pro-Phe	0	—
453	Chl-Ala-Pro-Phe	0[d]	—
454	Chl-Lys-Trp-Ala-Pro-Phe-Arg	"potent"	—
455	Chl-Trp-Ala-Pro-Phe-Arg	"potent"	—
456	Chl-Ala-Pro-Phe-Arg	"potent"[d]	—
457	<Glu-Trp-Pro-Arg-Pro-Gln-Ile-Pro-Pro(BPP9a)	410[j]	4.5
458	Cpc-Trp-Pro-Arg-Pro-Gln-Ile-Pro-Pro	—	25
459	<Glu-Tyr-Pro-Arg-Pro-Gln-Ile-Pro-Pro	—	2
460	<Glu-Phe-Pro-Arg-Pro-Gln-Ile-Pro-Pro	—	2
461	<Glu-Leu-Pro-Arg-Pro-Gln-Ile-Pro-Pro	—	0.8
462	<Glu-Gly-Pro-Arg-Pro-Gln-Ile-Pro-Pro	—	0.8
463	<Glu-*trp*-Pro-Arg-Pro-Gln-Ile-Pro-Pro	—	0.7
464	<Glu-Trp-Pro-Lys-Pro-Gln-Ile-Pro-Pro	—	3
465	<Glu-Trp-Pro-His-Pro-Gln-Ile-Pro-Pro	—	3
466	<Glu-Trp-Pro-Gly-Pro-Gln-Ile-Pro-Pro	—	3
467	<Glu-Trp-Pro-Orn-Pro-Gln-Ile-Pro-Pro	—	2
468	<Glu-Trp-Pro-*arg*-Pro-Gln-Ile-Pro-Pro	—	0.5
469	<Glu-Trp-Pro-Arg-Pro-Gln-Phe-Pro-Pro	—	20
470	<Glu-Trp-Pro-Arg-Pro-Gln-Ile-Ala-Pro	—	13
471	<Glu-Trp-Pro-Arg-Pro-Gln-Ile-Pro-Pyn	—	< 0.02
472	<Glu-Ile-Pro-Pro-Lys-Phe-Ala-Pro	—	20
473	<Glu-Lys-Phe-Ala-Pro-Gln-Ile-Pro-Pro	—	1.5
474	<Glu-Trp-Pro-Arg-Pro-Lys-Phe-Ala-Pro	—	100
475	<Glu-Trp-Pro-Arg-Pro-Lys-Trp-Ala-Pro	720	—
476	<Glu-Trp-Pro-Arg-Pro-Lys-Trp-Pro-Pro	110	—
477	<Glu-Trp-Pro-Arg-Pro-Lys-Ile-Pro-Pro	580	—
478	EAC-Trp-Pro-Arg-Pro-Gln-Ile-Pro-Pro	300	450[e]
479	<Glu-Glu-Trp-Pro-Arg-Pro-Gln-Ile-Pro-Pro	—	1
480	<Glu-Lys-Trp-Pro-Arg-Pro-Gln-Ile-Pro-Pro	—	1
481	Pro-Arg-Pro-Gln-Ile-Pro-Pro	—	0.5
482	Arg-Pro-Gln-Ile-Pro-Pro	—	0.2
483	Z-Pro-Gln-Ile-Pro-Pro	—	0
484	<Glu-Ile-Pro-Pro	—	0.06
485	Pro-Arg-Pro-Gln-Ile	—	0.07
486	<Glu-Arg-Pro-Gln-Ile-Pro	—	< 0.02
487	<Glu-Trp-Pro	—	< 0.02
488	<Glu-Trp	—	< 0.02
489	<Glu-Gly-Leu-Pro-Pro-Gly-Pro-Lys-Ile-Pro-Pro	60	—
490	<Glu-Gly-Leu-Pro-Pro-Lys-Pro-Gln-Ile-Pro-Pro	80	—
491	<Glu-Gly-Leu-Pro-Pro-Arg-Pro-Gln-Ile-Pro-Pro	320	—
492	Leu-Pro-Pro-Arg-Pro-Gln-Ile-Pro-Pro	200	—
493	<Glu-Gly-Leu-Pro-Pro-Gly-Pro-Gln-Ile-Pro-Pro	28	—
494	Leu-Pro-Pro-Gly-Pro-Gln-Ile-Pro-Pro	58	—
495	<Glu-Gly-Arg-Pro-Pro-Gly-Pro-Gln-Ile-Pro-Pro	200	—
496	Leu-Val-Glu-Ser-Ser-Lys	0.011[f]	—
497	Thr-Pro-Val-Ser-Glu-Lys	0.014	—
498	Ile-Glu-Thr-Met-Arg	0.007	—
499	Val-Glu-Ser-Ser-Lys	< 0.001	—
		Conc. to double BK response[g]	
500	Arg-Gly-Phe-Ser-Pro-Phe-Arg	8.2×10^{-10}	

Table 4 (continued)

Peptide number	Structure	Biologic activity	
		BK[b]	ANG[c]
501	Arg-Phe-Ser-Pro-Phe-Arg	2.7×10^{-3}	
502	Arg-Ser-Pro-Phe-Arg	6.0×10^{-9}	
503	Arg-Pro-Phe-Arg	6.7×10^{-9}	
504	Arg-Phe-Arg	4.2×10^{-8}	
505	Ala-Asp-Ser-Gly-Glu-Gly-Asp-Phe[h]		
506	<Glu-Phe-Pro-Thr-Asp-Tyr-Asp-Glu-Gly--Gln-Asp-Asp-Arg-Pro-Lys[i]		

[a] Abbreviations are those used in Table 1, with the following additions: Ac – Acetyl, Cpc – Cyclopentanecarboxylic acid, Lac – Lactic acid, Nle – Norleucine, Pyn – Pyrrolidine (des-carboxy proline), PhB – Phenylbutyric acid, Z – Benzyloxycarbonyl. D-Amino acids are uncapitalized and italicized.

[b] Expressed as a percentage of the molar activity of BPP5a (peptide #401) for potentiation of the action of bradykinin on guinea pig ileum. Data from FREER and STEWART (1971); FREER and STEWART (1972); KATO and SUZUKI (1971, 1976); KATO et al. (1973); SABIA et al. (1977); STEWART et al. (1971); TOMINAGA et al. (1975) and unpublished results in the author's laboratory, unless otherwise specified.

[c] Expressed as a percentage of the activity (weight basis) of BPP5a for half-maximal inhibition of the hydrolysis of benzoyl-Gly_3 by angiotensin I converting enzyme in vitro. Data from CUSHMAN et al. (1973). The ID_{50} for BPP5a was 8.2×10^{-8} *M*.

[d] Caused irreversible potentiation (see text).

[e] J. M. STEWART and I. B. WILSON, unpublished.

[f] Tryptic peptides from bovine and rabbit serum albumin (WEYERS et al., 1972).

[g] From SAKAKIBARA and NARUSE (1975). The assay was not specified.

[h] Human fibrinopeptide A fragment which potentiates the action of bradykinin on rat uterus (GLADNER, 1966). Larger natural peptides were also studied.

[i] Bovine fibrinopeptide B fragment (GLADNER, 1966).

[j] Also reported as 960 by SABIA et al. (1977).

II. Synthetic Bradykinin-Potentiating Peptides

The synthetic peptides which have been described as possessing the ability to potentiate the bradykinin response or inhibit angiotensin I converting enzyme are listed in Table 4. Unfortunately, very few analogs have been examined for both these activities. It is striking that BPP9a (#457), one of the most potent bradykinin potentiators known, is only 5% as potent as BPP5a as an inhibitor of angiotensin converting enzyme in vitro. However, it is much more potent in vivo than the pentapeptide because of its resistance to degradation by kininases. If the pyroglutamyl residue in BPP9a is replaced by an ε-amino caproyl residue (#478), the resulting analog is approximately equipotent for kinin potentiation and angiotensin conversion inhibition in vitro. Unfortunately, this peptide (#478) did not prove to be an effective inhibitor of the pressor response to angiotensin I in vivo in the rat (STEWART, unpublished observation).

Examination of the synthetic analogs of BPP5a (#402–446) shows that very few modifications can be made in the native molecule without serious loss of potency.

Table 4A. Recently published fragments and analogs of BPP9a

Peptide number	Structure[a]	Biologic activity[b]
457	<Glu-Trp-Pro-Arg-Pro-Gln-Ile-Pro-Pro (BPP9a)	100
507	<Glu-Trp-Pro-Arg-Pro-Gln-Ile-Pro	3.4
508	<Glu-Trp-Pro-Arg-Pro-Gln-Ile	52
509	<Glu-Trp-Pro-Arg-Pro-Gln	0.04
510	<Glu-Trp-Pro-Arg-Pro	1.2
511	<Glu-Trp-Pro-Arg	0.006
512	<Glu-Trp-Pro	0.07
513	Trp-Pro-Arg-Pro-Gln-Ile-Pro-Pro	56
514	Trp-Pro-Arg-Pro-Gln-Ile-Pro	5.1
515	Trp-Pro-Arg-Pro-Gln-Ile	82
516	Trp-Pro-Arg-Pro	0.5
517	Pro-Arg-Pro-Gln-Ile-Pro	16
519	Pro-Arg-Pro-Gln-Ile	0.4
520	Pro-Arg-Pro-Gln	0.04
521	Pro-Arg-Pro	0.3
522	Arg-Pro-Gln-Ile-Pro	0.2
523	Arg-Pro-Gln-Ile	0.4
524	Pro-Gln-Ile-Pro-Pro	1.9
525	Pro-Gln-Ile-Pro	0.05
526	Pro-Gln-Ile	0.03
527	Ile-Pro-Pro	9
528	<Glu-Trp-DHP-Arg-Pro-Gln-Ile-Pro-Pro	3100
529	<Glu-Trp-Pro-Arg-DHP-Gln-Ile-Pro-Pro	3100
530	<Glu-Trp-Pro-Arg-Pro-Gln-Ile-DHP-Pro	25
531	<Glu-Trp-Pro-Arg-Pro-Gln-Ile-Pro-DHP	9300

[a] Abbreviations are those used in Table 1.
[b] Activity relative to BPP9a for inhibition of hydrolysis of Benzoyl-Gly-His-Leu by purified kininase II. Data from FISHER et al. (1979).

Substitution of proline for pyroglutamic acid (#404) and addition of pyroglutamic acid to that pentapeptide (#405) yielded analogs with full potency for bradykinin potentiation; substitution of phenylalanine for the tryptophan gave an analog with full potency for converting-enzyme inhibition. Oxidation of the tryptophan residue, on the other hand, destroyed most of the bradykinin-potentiating activity (#408). This is somewhat reminiscent of the situation with calcitonin, where a methionine residue can be replaced by leucine with retention of full potency but oxidation of the methionine to the sulfoxide destroys all activity. In both these cases, the oxidation causes a marked increase in polarity of the amino acid residue in question and probably interferes with an essential hydrophobic receptor binding function of that residue in the native hormone. The chemical nature of the oxidized tryptophan in peptide 408 was not determined. As far as is known, the phenylalanine-containing analogs have not been tested for bradykinin potentiation. Peptide 405 served as a model for the synthesis of analogs having a reactive group (an alkylating agent) in the amino terminal position of BPP 5a (compounds 447–456). These peptides contain the nitrogen mustard alkylating agent chlorambucil at the N-terminus of the chain and were synthesized as potential irreversible inhibitors of bradykinin receptors or of bradykinin metabolizing enzymes (FREER and STEWART, 1972).

Several of these chlorambucil peptides had significant bradykinin-potentiating activity while they were in the ileum bath (see Table 4), although this potency was not determined accurately. After the ileum had been treated with the chlorambucil derivative for 60 min, the tissue was washed exhaustively and again tested for its response to bradykinin and angiotensin. None of the derivatives caused a significant permanent inhibition of the bradykinin response, but several did significantly potentiate the action of bradykinin on ileum. Most potent among these were Chl-Trp-Ala-Pro (#449) and Chl-Pro-Lys-Trp-Ala-Pro (#447). Two chlorambucil derivatives of bradykinin, Chl-Pro-Pro-Gly-Phe-Ser-Pro-Phe-Arg and Chl-Pro-Gly-Phe-Ser-Pro-Phe-Arg, also caused marked permanent potentiation of the ileum response to bradykinin. The mechanism of the potentiation evoked by these latter alkylating peptides was shown (STEWART et al., 1973) to be inhibition of kininase activity. It was mentioned above that two bradykinin analogs which were resistant to ileum kininases were still potentiated fully by treatment with BPP 5a. On the other hand, the response of ileum to these two peptides, D-Pro^7-bradykinin and des-Arg^9-bradykinin, was not changed by treatment with chlorambucil^1-bradykinin. The substance alkylated by the affinity label must then be the kininase and not the receptor. The mechanism of the permanent potentiation evoked by the chlorambucil derivatives of bradykinin-potentiating peptides has not been similarly examined. The response of isolated rat uterus to bradykinin was significantly and permanently potentiated by Chl-Trp-Ala-Pro-Phe (#452). Several chlorambucil peptides examined in this study also permanently inhibited the response of uterus and ileum to angiotensin II. The response of ileum to angiotensin I was not examined in this study. These chlorambucil derivatives were also studied for their ability to cause prolonged inhibition of angiotensin I conversion and pulmonary bradykinin inactivation in the rat in vivo. Chl-Pro-Lys-Trp-Ala-Pro (#447) significantly inhibited bradykinin inactivation during infusion of the peptide but none of the treatments showed any prolonged effectiveness in either assay.

The BPP 5a analogs containing the added phenylalanine and phenylalanine-arginine residues at the carboxy terminus were synthesized to cause the potentiator to resemble more closely the bradykinin structure. This did not prove to be a successful maneuver for increasing the potency of the peptides.

No synthetic analogs of BPP 9a have been found to possess greater potency for bradykinin-potentiation or angiotensin I conversion inhibition than does the native peptide itself. Several analogs have been synthesized to examine the effects of combining parts of BPP 5a and BPP 9a in the same molecule. For example, peptide 475 combines the amino part of BPP 9a with the carboxy part of BPP 5a while peptide 473 makes the reverse combination. Peptide 475 is the most potent of all known peptides for potentiation of the response of ileum to bradykinin.

The bradykinin fragments reported to potentiate the action of bradykinin (#500–504) were described in a Japanese patent and no further details were given on the assay used. These peptides probably function as alternate substrates for kininases, particularly kininase II (angiotensin-converting enzyme).

III. Potentiation of the Bradykinin Response by Enzymes

EDERY (1965) discovered that if isolated guinea pig ileum or rat uterus is treated for a time with chymotrypsin or other proteolytic enzyme, the response of these tissues to bradykinin and related kinins is permanently increased. This effect is specific for kinins, since no potentiation of the response of the tissues to other agonists (including other peptides) is observed. The mechanism of this action is unknown, although the enzyme may possibly modify the receptors to make them more accessible to bradykinin.

IV. Potentiation by Chelating Agents

Many substances that chelate divalent metals potentiate the actions of kinins both in vitro and in vivo. Those most widely used in kinin pharmacology include 2,3-dimercaptopropanol (BAL), cysteine, ethylenediaminetetraacetic acid (EDTA), 2-mercaptoethanol, and 1,10-phenanthroline. Since it is well established that these compounds inhibit kininases, both in vitro and in vivo, it is assumed that this inhibition is the mechanism of their potentiating action (ERDÖS and YANG, 1970, and this volume; ROBLERO et al., 1973; FREER and STEWART, 1975). Evidently, the kininases are metalloenzymes and require a divalent cation which the chelating agent removes. Angiotensin I converting enzyme, which hydrolyzes bradykinin very effectively and may be an important kininase in vivo, appears to be a zinc enzyme (DORER et al., 1970).

Chelating agents generally potentiate the actions of kinins only in those tissues that contain significant amounts of kininases, e.g., there is no significant potentiation of the action of bradykinin on rat uterus. That kininase inhibition cannot be the entire mechanism for potentiation of kinin action, however, is shown by experiments on guinea pig ileum using analogs of bradykinin that are resistant to the action of kininase (GREENE et al., 1972). For example, the action of D-Pro^7-bradykinin, which is not destroyed by guinea pig ileum kininases, is effectively potentiated on that tissue by BAL as well as by BPP 5a, as noted above.

After a long and exhaustive search for more potent analogs of the bradykinin-potentiating peptides (CUSHMAN et al., 1973), the investigators at Squibb turned to simpler compounds as converting-enzyme inhibitors with potential clinical usefulness. Several investigations had shown that BPP9a was an active inhibitor of converting enzyme in vivo but the quantities required for human use made the expense of treatment with this compound prohibitive. An analysis of the hypothetical active site of angiotensin-converting enzyme suggested that it must have (1) a cationic site to combine with peptide carboxyl groups (since it is a carboxypeptidase enzyme), (2) a region capable of forming hydrogen bonds with the peptide bond adjacent to the C-terminal residue of the substrate peptide (since it cleaves dipeptides and not compounds lacking this peptide bond in the middle of the cleaved moiety), and (3) a zinc atom which probably chelates with the carbonyl group of the peptide bond to be hydrolyzed (the second peptide bond from the carboxyl end of the substrate). Proline was found to be the best amino acid for incorporation at the C-terminus of inhibitors, as exemplified in all the naturally occurring bradykinin-potentiating peptides. Presence of a proline in this position also makes the substrate resistant to degradation by carboxypeptidases A and B. The Squibb investigators found that effective

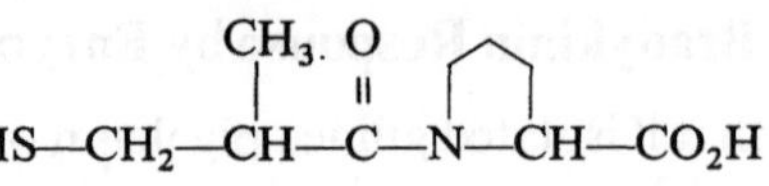

Fig. 2. The structure of SQ 14,225

converting-enzyme inhibitors could be synthesized by acylating proline with an acid which contained a thiol group in a position where it might bind strongly to the zinc residue in the enzyme active site. Examination of a series of such compounds led ultimately to the synthesis of 2-D-methyl-3-mercaptopropionyl-L-proline, designated SQ 14,225, or Captopril (Fig. 2) (ONDETTI et al., 1977; CUSHMAN et al., 1977).

This compound is 200 times as potent as BPP9a for inhibition of rabbit lung angiotensin-converting enzyme in vitro, 14 times as potent as BPP9a for inhibition of the response of isolated guinea pig ileum to angiotensin I, and 2.5 times as potent as BPP9a for potentiation of the response of ileum to bradykinin. The compound was also shown to be highly effective in vivo as an inhibitor of angiotensin-converting enzyme, even by oral administration, and may be useful in therapy of some forms of renal hypertension. The successful design of SQ 14,225 is a triumph of the rational design of an enzyme inhibitor.

E. Conformation of Bradykinin in Solution

Conformation of the bradykinin molecule in solution has been investigated by a wide variety of physical techniques, among them optical rotatory dispersion (ORD), circular dichroism (CD), proton and ^{13}C-nuclear magnetic resonance (NMR), electron spin resonance, and fluorescence energy transfer. Theoretical calculations of minimum energy conformations of bradykinin have also been made. Although elucidation of the conformation of bradykinin has not been easy, knowledge at the present time at least approaches a definition of the solution structure.

Initial observation of the ORD and CD spectra of bradykinin were made by BODANSZKY et al. (1970), followed shortly by a study of bradykinin and several analogs by BRADY et al. (1971) and work of TONIOLO (1972). The CD studies revealed a weak negative band at 234 nm, a relatively strong positive band at 221 nm, and a very strong negative band at about 195 nm. These investigators suggested that bradykinin had neither α-helix nor β-pleated sheet structure, but probably existed in an extended conformation, perhaps resembling a random coil (BRADY et al., 1971). In any case, helix formation would be ruled out by the presence of the three proline residues in the bradykinin structure. BRADY et al. (1971), in their study of bradykinin analogs, observed that all analogs possessing significant biologic activity had CD spectra similar to that of bradykinin, although several analogs with essentially no biologic activity also appeared to have solution conformations similar to bradykinin, as indicated by CD. In a careful study of the CD of bradykinin, its fragments and model compounds, CANN et al. (1973) concluded that at least two conformational characteristics of the molecule contribute to the CD spectrum. They assigned the 234 nm band to a hydrogen bond in the C-terminal part of the molecule (most likely across Pro^7) and the 221 nm band to independent contributions from two chromophores, the phenylalanine residues plus a structural contribution from the amino end of the molecule having to do with the Pro-Pro sequence there. Determination of the thermodynamic parameters of the H-bond around Pro^7 showed that the structure of water plays an important role in determining this conformation. It was suggested that under physiologic conditions of temperature and pH, approximately 30% of the bradykinin molecules exist in this bonded form, while elevation of the temperature or addition of nonpolar solvents increases the strength of this bond. Subsequent studies by this group (CANN et al., 1976; LONDON et al., 1978) have further refined these structural predictions and have shown (by means of ^{13}C-NMR) that approximately 15% of the bradykinin molecules exist with one or more X-Pro bonds in the *cis* configuration. Nearly complete assignments of proton and carbon resonances have been made and spin-lattice relaxation times of the various atoms in the molecule have been measured. These measurements are consistent with the involvement of the carbonyl of Ser^6 in a hydrogen bond and in general support the earlier conclusions. They show no evidence of involvement of any of the charged groups of the molecule in ionic bonds or any interaction between the two phenylalanine residues. CD studies of additional analogs by MARLBOROUGH et al. (1976) and MARLBOROUGH and RYAN (1977) have tended to support the general ideas presented above for the solution conformation of bradykinin.

A group of Russian investigators has studied the solution conformation of bradykinin by a variety of techniques over a period of years. Preliminary communications of this work have appeared in German (FILATOVA et al., 1973) and English (IVANOV et al., 1975a), and the details of the studies have just appeared in Russian (IVANOV et al., 1977; EFREMOV et al., 1977; FILATOVA et al., 1977; and GALAKTIONOV et al., 1977). Many of the observations on bradykinin they have reported agree with data cited above, although they have encountered some difficulty due to chemical problems with their peptides. The conclusions reached by IVANOV et al. (1975a and 1975b) must be revised for this reason. They have placed a great deal of reliance upon theoretical molecular orbital calculations of lowest energy conformation of bradykinin (GALAKTIONOV et al., 1977; IVANOV et al., 1975a). They predict, for example, a cyclic conformation for the bradykinin molecule stabilized by an ionic bond between the guanidinium group of Arg^1 and the carboxyl group of Arg^9. However, this prediction is not supported by careful analysis of the pKs of the functional groups by ^{13}C-NMR (LONDON et al., 1978). KIER and GEORGE (1970) had earlier calculated a minimum energy conformation for bradykinin and predicted a close phenylalanine-phenylalanine interaction, for which no evidence can be seen in any physical measurements. Theoretical calculations of bradykinin conformation have also been published by ARKHIPOVA et al. (1977).

Such studies of the solution conformation of a peptide hormone such as bradykinin provide interesting and valuable insights into the intramolecular forces which are acting upon molecules in solution. It is clear that the medium in which the peptide is placed plays an important role; the conformation in water is quite different from that in nonpolar solvents. The observed enhancement of conformational structure in nonpolar solvents suggests that bradykinin may be influenced by the postulated nonpolar environment around tissue receptors. It is very doubtful if the observed conformational features of bradykinin contribute to our knowledge of the conformation of bradykinin when it binds to tissue receptors. This is especially true in light of the fact that the observed interactions within the bradykinin molecule appear to be relatively weak, while peptide-receptor interactions are clearly very strong. Only when it is possible to make actual measurements of the conformation of the peptide on the receptor, or at least comparisons of the receptor-bound conformation with solution conformations, will we understand the nature of the peptide-receptor binding and the environment of the receptor.

BODANSZKY et al. (1971) reported the ORD spectra of seven bradykinin-potentiating peptides. They did not see evidence of solution structure in these peptides, and proposed that flexibility in solution was required for effective inhibition of angiotensin-converting enzyme.

F. Chemical Synthesis of Bradykinin, Bradykinin Analogs, and Bradykinin-Potentiating Peptides

Methods used for the chemical synthesis of bradykinin-related peptides were reviewed in Volume XXV of the Handbook (STEWART, 1970). Since that time there has been much general improvement in techniques of peptide synthesis, both in solution and by the solid-phase method. Excellent reviews of the state of the art of solution synthesis (FINN and HOFMANN, 1976) and of the solid-phase method (ERICKSON and MERRIFIELD, 1976) have appeared. Additional useful suggestions for improvements in solid-phase synthesis have been made in reviews by STEWART (1976b) and STEWART et al. (1976).

I. Solution Synthesis of Bradykinin and Related Peptides

Some new techniques of peptide synthesis in solution have been applied to bradykinin and related peptides. HIRSCHMANN and DENKEWALTER (1974) applied their rapid stepwise N-carboxyanhydride method of peptide synthesis to the synthesis of bradykinin. This is probably not a method for the novice to attempt to use as success apparently depends on precise control of reaction conditions. If the procedures are successful, great speed can be achieved in synthesis. YOUNG has applied his picolyl ester method to the synthesis of bradykinin (SCHAFER et al., 1971). In this method, the synthesis is begun with the C-terminal amino acid, which is introduced as a picolyl ester. This basic functional group facilitates purification of the product at every stage of the synthesis.

Widespread adoption of anhydrous hydrogen fluoride as a reagent for deprotection of blocking groups in peptide synthesis has eliminated some serious chemical problems and greatly facilitated the synthesis of bradykinin and related peptides. The use of nitroarginine in synthesis of bradykinin and related peptides has caused some difficulties, due to problems introduced by reductive cleavage of the nitro group from the finished peptide. HF removes the nitro group cleanly and eliminates these problems. Even better results are obtained with the use of *p*-toluenesulfonyl (tosyl) arginine in synthesis, both in solution and in the solid-phase method. The tosyl group is removed readily by HF and is now the preferred blocking group for arginine in peptide synthesis. Use of this system in the synthesis of bradykinin was described by MAZUR and PLUME (1968). Oximinopyrazoline active esters were applied to the synthesis of bradykinin by TOMATIS et al. (1973).

II. Solid-Phase Synthesis of Bradykinin and Related Peptides

Part of the initial appeal of solid-phase synthesis was the greatly increased speed with which peptides could be synthesized by this method. The original bradykinin synthesis described by MERRIFIELD (1967) showed that the entire peptide chain could be assembled on the polymeric support in 32 h, starting with arginine-resin. It has recently been shown that even greater savings in time are possible, especially with peptides such as bradykinin which are very easy to synthesize by the solid-phase method. For example, CORLEY et al. (1972) showed that by repetitive short-time treatment with deprotection and coupling reagents, the eight residues of bradykinin could be added to the polymer in less than 5 h. They used the manual method of solid-phase synthesis with 10-fold excesses of Boc-amino acids and dicyclohexylcarbodiimide (DCC), repeating the coupling a second time. This procedure was therefore very wasteful of reagents. TAKAHASHI and SHIMONISHI (1974) showed that a similar advance in speed of solid-phase synthesis of bradykinin could be achieved by using ultrasonic mixing of the resin with the reagents. They also claimed to be able to add all the eight amino acids to the polymer in 5 h. Reinvestigation of the coupling reactions in the synthesis of bradykinin (MATSUEDA and STEWART, unpublished) showed that even when the standard 2.5-fold excess of Boc-amino acid and DCC were used in the coupling reactions, all of the coupling reactions in the bradykinin synthesis were complete in 10 min. This finding made possible the completely automatic synthesis of bradykinin in much less time than before; total coupling reaction time could be reduced to 2 h, instead of 16, and the total elapsed time for automatic assembly of eight amino acids to the arginine-resin was 18 h, an easy overnight run of the automatic synthesizer. One should not assume from this result that all solid-phase coupling reactions are complete in this short a period of time. As mentioned above, bradykinin is a very easy peptide to synthesize by the solid-phase method. Some coupling reactions are not complete even in the standard 2 h coupling time normally used, particularly if sterically hindered amino acids are involved.

Anhydrous HF appears to be the reagent of choice for cleavage of peptides from the solid-phase resin after synthesis, although for ideal use of this reagent rather expensive equipment is needed. Other techniques that have been proposed for cleavage of solid-phase peptide-resins do not appear to give as good yields or as pure products as does HF. We routinely use tosyl arginine in all solid-phase syntheses.

When bradykinin is synthesized in this laboratory by our standard automatic solid-phase procedures, the crude product obtained is nearly homogeneous. It is clear that significant methodologic improvements are not badly needed for the satisfactory synthesis of bradykinin. However, bradykinin has been used as a demonstration peptide for testing some newer techniques of solid-phase peptide synthesis. SANDBERG and RAGNARSSON (1974) have used Ppoc amino acids in the synthesis of bradykinin by the solid-phase method. The Ppoc (phenylisopropyloxycarbonyl) blocking group is much more labile than the Boc group, and is removed from the peptide-resin by treatment with quite dilute (1–2%) solutions of trifluoroacetic acid in dichloromethane. While it is difficult to demonstrate a clear superiority of this procedure for the synthesis of bradykinin, such labile blocking groups are needed in the solid-phase synthesis of some types of peptides. RAGNARSSON et al. (1975) also applied fragment condensation techniques to the synthesis of bradykinin by the solid-phase method. They showed that it was possible to synthesize bradykinin in good yield and without racemization by coupling two tripeptide fragments followed by a dipeptide to a nitroarginine-polymer. This synthesis demonstrates the use of fragment condensation methods in solid-phase synthesis, but does not offer any significant advantage for the synthesis of bradykinin itself. Several kinds of radioactive bradykinin have been synthesized by the solid-phase method (RYAN et al., 1968, 1970) and one form has been made available for general scientific investigation (PISANO, 1969).

III. Synthesis of Bradykinin-Potentiating Peptides

Nearly all of the syntheses of the bradykinin-potentiating peptides and analogs described in Sect. D of this chapter were done by the solid-phase method. Some solution syntheses of bradykinin-potentiating peptides have been reported by VARDEL et al. (1975) and ALI et al. (1976). The occurrence in these peptides of multiple proline residues, tryptophan, glutamine, and arginine caused significant problems in solution synthesis. Using the best techniques of solid-phase synthesis currently available, these peptides can be synthesized readily without any significant problems. Certain pitfalls do exist, however, and those who attempt to synthesize peptides in this group by the solid-phase method should be forewarned. The methods currently used in this laboratory to avoid these problems will be described briefly.

Prolyl-proline sequences in peptides are particularly prone to diketopiperazine formation. When the Pro-Pro sequence occurs in the C-terminal position of peptides synthesized by the solid-phase method, this dipeptide can be lost from the resin as a diketopiperazine by intramolecular aminolysis of the peptide-resin ester link. This can be readily prevented by addition of DCC before the Boc-amino acid in coupling the third residue on the resin (isoleucine, in the case of BPP9a), as shown by GISIN and MERRIFIELD (1972). In this laboratory, this reversed-addition procedure is programmed automatically on the Beckman 990 Synthesizer; this program is used routinely for coupling the third residue of peptides where diketopiperazine formation might be expected. In addition to proline, other dipeptides which have been found to cyclize readily are those involving N-methyl amino acids and valine or isoleucine.

In the synthesis of BPP9a, glutamine must be coupled to isoleucine. Glutamine has traditionally been introduced in solid-phase synthesis by using the nitrophenyl ester for coupling in order to avoid nitrile formation in DCC-mediated coupling reactions. These active ester couplings are much slower, particularly when the coupling is to a hindered amino acid such as isoleucine. This one step was the weakest point in the solid-phase synthesis of BPP9a. When the side-chain amide of glutamine is blocked by conversion to the xanthydryl derivative (SOUTHARD, 1971), DCC can be used as the coupling agent with attendant greater speed and efficiency. Introduction of this single change into the synthesis of BPP9a improved the yield by 20%.

Tryptophan is used routinely in this laboratory without any protecting group on the indole ring. We avoid oxidation of tryptophan during the acidic deprotection step by incorporating into the deprotection reagent (trifluoroacetic acid in dichloromethane) indole (1 mg/ml) to serve as a scavenger for substances which might react with or otherwise degrade the tryptophan. The deprotection reagent is made by mixing the indole, trifluoroacetic acid, and dichloromethane and allowing them to stand overnight before use. In this way the indole scavenges harmful substances from the reagent. This indole-containing reagent is routinely used for all solid-phase synthesis in this laboratory. The oxidation of tryptophan that occurred in the first synthesis of BPP 5a (Table 4, peptide #408) occurred before indole was introduced for protection of this amino acid in solid-phase synthesis. Pyroglutamic acid is introduced into the peptide as such, rather than by using a carbobenzoxy or Boc-derivative. No problems have been encountered in this procedure.

IV. Purity of Synthetic Peptides

The purity of synthetic peptides used in various types of research is a subject that has caused much concern and discussion, but which still causes problems. Chemists who synthesize peptides should always be aware of the types of problems that can arise in synthesis and be sure that adequate methods of purification and analysis are applied to their products before they are used in research. The great improvements in peptide synthesis, particularly in the solid-phase method, have made synthesis appear so simple that everyone is tempted to try it. Fortunately, the synthesis of bradykinin and related peptides is very easy and if the novice adheres rigorously to published procedures serious problems should be avoided. The temptation often arises, however, to take short-cuts or to try to "improve" on established procedures, without the sound basis in knowledge and experience required for such changes. Unfortunately, serious embarrassments have arisen on more than one occasion in the bradykinin field when investigators were using peptides presumed to have a particular structure when the chemist had unwittingly provided them a different material.

Analytical techniques available today leave no excuse for this kind of problem, especially with peptides the size of those under discussion here. Accurate amino acid analysis of all synthetic products is an absolute essential and cannot be bypassed. Paper or thin-layer electrophoresis is particularly useful with charged peptides such as the kinins because direct correlations with the presence of the expected functional groups and molecular size can be made. We have found this technique to be much more useful as an indicator of purity and composition than thin-layer chromatography. The naturally occurring kinins can be readily separated by electrophoresis (LALKA and BACK, 1971). The recent application of high performance liquid chromatography (HPLC) to synthetic peptides has provided an incredibly sensitive and selective technique for the analysis and purification of these substances (BURGUS and RIVIER, 1976). Fluorimetric techniques provide even greater sensitivity (GRUBER et al., 1976). The kinins may be chromatographed quite readily on available systems of HPLC (MORRIS and STEWART, unpublished). Elemental analysis of synthetic peptides is frequently of very little use in establishment of purity. Adequate attention to these matters will greatly accelerate the progress of research in the kinin field.

References

Aarsen, P. N.: Sensitization of guinea pig ileum to the action of bradykinin by trypsin hydrolysate of ox and rabbit plasma. Br. J. Pharmacol. *32*, 453–465 (1968)

Abiko, T.: Syntheses of 4-nitrophenylalanine[5], O-methyltyrosine[8]-, and O-methyltyrosine[5], 4-nitrophenylalanine[8]-BK. Chem. Pharm. Bull. (Tokyo) *22*, 2191–2196 (1974)

Abramson, F.B., Elliott, D.F., Lindsay, D.G., Wade, R.: Synthesis of peptides related to bradykinin. J. Chem. Soc. (C), 1042–1048 (1970)

Ali, A., Guidicci, M.A., Stevenson, D.: Synthesis of bradykinin-potentiating peptide BPP5a. Experientia *32*, 1503–1504 (1976)

Anastasi, A., Bertaccini, G., Erspamer, V.: Pharmacological data on phyllokinin and bradykinin-isoleucine-tyrosine. Br. J. Pharmacol. *27*, 479–485 (1966)

Arkhipova, S.F., Sevastyanova, N.N., Lipkind, G.M., Popov, E.M.: Theoretical conformational analysis of BPP9a. Bioorganicheskaya Khimiya *3*, 335–347 (1977)

Armstrong, D.: Pain. In: Handbook experimental pharmacology. Vol. XXV: Bradykinin, kallidin, and kallikrein. Erdös, E.G. (ed.), p. 434. Berlin, Heidelberg, New York: Springer 1970

Atherton, E., Law, H.D., Moore, S., Elliott, D.F., Wade, R.: Synthesis of peptides containing N-2-aminoethyl glycine – Reduction analogues. J. Chem. Soc. (C) 3393–3396 (1971)

Bakhle, Y.S.: Conversion of angiotensin I to angiotensin II by cell-free extracts of dog lung. Nature *220*, 919–921 (1968)

Balaspiri, L., Penke, B., Papp, G., Dombi, G., Kovacs, K.: Rational synthesis of α-L-homoproline and its derivatives. Production of 7-α-L-homoproline bradykinin. Helv. Chim. Acta *58*, 969–973 (1975)

Bisset, G.W., Lewis, G.P.: A spectrum of pharmacological activity in some biologically active peptides. Br. J. Pharmacol. *19*, 168–182 (1962)

Bodanszky, A., Bodanszky, M., Jorpes, E.J., Mutt, V., Ondetti, M.A.: Molecular architecture of peptide hormones. Optical rotatory dispersion of cholecystokinin, bradykinin, and 6-glycine bradykinin. Experientia *26*, 948–950 (1970)

Bodanszky, A., Ondetti, M.A., Ralofsky, C.A., Bodanszky, M.: Optical rotatory dispersion of proline-rich peptides from the venom of *Bothrops jararaca*. Experientia *27*, 1269–1270 (1971)

Brady, A.H., Ryan, J.W., Stewart, J.M.: Circular dichroism of bradykinin and related peptides. Biochem. J. *121*, 179–184 (1971)

Burgus, R., Rivier, J.: Use of high pressure liquid chromatography in the purification of peptides. In: Peptides 1976. Loffet, A. (ed.), p. 85. Brussels: Editions de l'Université de Bruxelles 1976

Cann, J.R., Stewart, J.M., Matsueda, G.R.: A circular dichroism study of the secondary structure of bradykinin. Biochemistry *12*, 3780–3788 (1973)

Cann, J.R., Stewart, J.M., London, R.E., Matwiyoff, N.: On the solution conformation of bradykinin and certain fragments. Biochemistry *15*, 498–504 (1976)

Corley, L., Sachs, D.H., Anfinsen, C.B.: Rapid solid-phase synthesis of bradykinin. Biochem. Biophys. Res. Commun. *47*, 1353–1359 (1972)

Cushman, D.W., Pluscec, J., Williams, N.J., Weaver, E.R., Sabo, E.F., Kocy, O., Cheung, H.S., Ondetti, M.A.: Inhibition of angiotensin-converting enzyme by analogs of peptides from *Bothrops jararaca* venom. Experientia *29*, 1032–1035 (1973)

Cushman, D.W., Cheung, H.S., Sabo, E.F., Ondetti, M.A.: Design of potent competitive inhibitors of angiotensin-converting enzyme. Biochemistry *16*, 5484–5491 (1977)

Damas, J., Cession-Fossion, A.: Are the smooth muscle and adrenal medulla receptors for BK different? C. R. Soc. Biol. (Paris) *167*, 1478–1482 (1973)

Donaldson, V.H., Ratnoff, O.D.: Effect of some analogs of bradykinin on vascular permeability. Proc. Soc. Exp. Biol. Med. *125*, 145–148 (1967)

Dorer, F.E., Skeggs, L.T., Kahn, J.R., Lentz, K.E., Levine, M.: Angiotensin converting enzyme: method of assay and partial purification. Anal. Biochem. *33*, 102–113 (1970)

Dorer, F.E., Ryan, J.W., Stewart, J.M.: Hydrolysis of bradykinin and its higher homologues by angiotensin-converting enzyme. Biochem. J. *141*, 915–917 (1974)

Dunn, F.W., Stewart, J.M.: Analogs of bradykinin containing β-2-thienyl-L-alanine. J. Med. Chem. *14*, 779–781 (1971)

Edery, H.: Further studies of the sensitization of smooth muscle to the action of plasma kinins by proteolytic enzymes. Br. J. Pharmacol. *24*, 485–496 (1965)

Efremov, E.S., Filatova, M.P., Reutova, T.O., Stepanova, L.N., Reissmann, S., Ivanov, V.T.: Conformational states of bradykinin and its analogs in solution. II. Fluorescence spectra. Bioorganicheskaya Khimiya *3*, 1169–1180 (1977)

El-Maghraby, M.A.: New synthetic analogue of bradykinin. Journal of the Indian Chemical Society *53*, 65–67 (1976)

Engel, S.L., Schaeffer, T.R., Gold, B.I., Rubin, B.: Inhibition of pressor effects of angiotensin I and augmentation of depressor effects of bradykinin by synthetic peptides. Proc. Soc. Exp. Biol. Med. *140*, 240–244 (1972)

Erdös, E.G., Yang, H.Y.T.: Kininases. In: Handbook of experimental pharmacology. Vol. XXV: Bradykinin, kallidin, and kallikrein. Erdös, E.G. (ed.), p. 289. Berlin, Heidelberg, New York: Springer 1970

Erickson, B.W., Merrifield, R.B.: Solid phase peptide synthesis. In: The proteins, 3rd ed. Neurath, H., Hill, R.L. (eds.), Vol. II, p. 257. London, New York: Academic Press 1976

Faber, D.B.: Pharmacology of peptides which enhance the action of bradykinin. Acta Physiologica et Pharmacologica Neerlandica *15*, 101–102 (1969)

Felix, A.M., Jiminez, M.H., Vergona, R., Cohen, M.R.: Synthesis and biological studies of novel bradykinin analogues. Int. J. Pept. Protein Res. *5*, 201–206 (1973)

Ferreira, S.H.: Bradykinin potentiating factor (BPF) present in venom of *Bothrops jararaca*. Br. J. Pharmacol. *24*, 163–169 (1965)

Ferreira, S.H.: Bradykinin-potentiating factor. In: Hypotensive peptides. Erdös, E.G., Back, N., Sicuteri, F. (eds.), p. 356. Berlin, Heidelberg, New York: Springer 1966

Ferreira, S.H., Bartelt, D.C., Greene, L.J.: Isolation of bradykinin-potentiating peptides from *Bothrops jararaca* venom. Biochemistry *9*, 2583–2593 (1970)

Filatova, M.P., Reissmann, S., Ravdel, G.A., Ivanov, V.T., Grigoryan, G.L., Shapiro, A.B.: Konformationsuntersuchungen an Bradykinin und Bradykininanaloga mit Hilfe von CD-, NMR und ESR-Messungen. In: Peptides 1972. Hanson, H., Jakubke, H.-D. (eds.), p. 333. New York: American Elsevier 1973

Filatova, M.P., Krit, N.A., Suchkova, G.S., Ravdel, G.A., Ivanov, V.T.: New synthesis of bradykinin and its analogs. Bioorganicheskaya Khimiya *1*, 437–446 (1975)

Filatova, M.P., Reissmann, S., Reutova, T.O., Ivanov, V.T., Grigoryan, G.L., Shapiro, A.M., Rozantsev, E.G.: Conformational states of bradykinin and its analogs in solution. III. ESR spectra of spin-labeled analogs. Bioorganicheskaya Khimiya *3*, 1181–1189 (1977)

Finn, F.M., Hofmann, K.: The synthesis of peptides by solution methods. In: The proteins, 3rd ed. Neurath, H., Hill, R.L. (eds.), Vol. II, p. 106. London, New York: Academic Press 1976

Fisher, G.H., Chung, A., Ryan, J.W.: Para-Halogenated phenylaline analogs of bradykinin: Effects on blood pressure. Circulation *55* and *56* (Suppl III), 241 (1977)

Fisher, G.H., Marlborough, D.I., Ryan, J.W., Felix, A.M.: L-3,4-Dehydroproline analogs of bradykinin: synthesis, biological activity, and solution conformation. Arch. Biochem. Biophys. *189*, 81–85 (1978)

Fisher, G.H., Ryan, J.W., Martin, L.C., Pena, G.: Strucutre-activity relationships for kininase II inhibition by lower homologs of the bradykinin potentiating peptide BPP9a. In: Proceedings, International Symposium on Kinins (Kinin 78 Tokyo). Moriya, H. (ed.). New York, London: Plenum Press 1979 (in press)

Fletcher, G.A., Young, G.T.: Amino acids and peptides. The synthesis of analogues of bradykinin by the picolyl ester method. J. Chem. Soc. (Perkin I) 1867–1874 (1972)

Fredrickson, R.C.A.: Enkephalin pentapeptides – a review. Life Sci. *21*, 23–42 (1977)

Freer, R.J., Stewart, J.M.: Synthetic bradykinin potentiating peptides related to those isolated from snake venoms. Ciencia e Cultura *23*, 539–542 (1971)

Freer, R.J., Stewart, J.M.: Alkylating analogs of peptide hormones. Synthesis and properties of *p*-[N,N-Bis(2-chloroethyl)amino]phenylbutyryl derivatives of bradykinin and bradykinin potentiating factor. J. Med. Chem. *15*, 1–5 (1972)

Freer, R.J., Stewart, J.M.: In vivo pulmonary metabolism of bradykinin, angiotensin I, and 5-hydroxytryptamine in the rat. Arch. Int. Pharmacodyn. Ther. *217*, 97–109 (1975)

Gabbiani, G., Baddonel, M.C., Majno, G.: Vascular leakage induced by intra-arterial histamine, serotonin or bradykinin. Proc. Soc. Exp. Biol. Med. *135*, 447–452 (1970)

Galaktionov, S.G., Sherman, S.A., Shenderovich, M.D., Nikiforovich, G.V., Leonova, V.I.: Conformational states of bradykinin in solution. Calculation of stable conformations. Bioorganicheskaya Khimiya *3*, 1190–1197 (1977)

Gaponyuk, P.Y., Oivin, V.I.: Comparative study of the effect of BK, kallidin, methionyl-lysyl-BK, and eledoisin on the permeability of skin vessels and the mechanism of their action. In: Histo-hematic barriers. Rosin, Y.A. (ed.), p. 115. Moscow: Nauka 1971

Gecse, A., Zsilinszky, E., Szekeres, L.: Bradykinin antagonism. In: Advances in experimental medicine and biology. Vol. 70: Kinins. Sicuteri, F., Back, N., Haberland, G. (eds.), pp. 5–13. New York, London: Plenum Press 1976
Gisin, B.F., Merrifield, R.B.: Carboxyl-catalyzed intramolecular aminolysis. A side reaction in solid-phase peptide synthesis. J. Am. Chem. Soc. *94*, 3102–3106 (1972)
Gladner, J.A.: Potentiation of the effect of bradykinin. In: Hypotensive peptides. Erdös, E.G., Back, N., Sicuteri, F. (eds.), p. 344. Berlin, Heidelberg, New York: Springer 1966
Greene, L.J., Camargo, A.C.M., Krieger, E.M., Stewart, J.M., Ferreira, S.H.: Inhibition of the conversion of angiotensin I to II and potentiation of bradykinin by small peptides present in *Bothrops jararaca* venom. Circ. Res. *30* II, 62–71 (1972)
Gruber, K.A., Stein, S., Brink, L., Radhakrishnan, A., Udenfriend, S.: Fluorimetric assay of vasopressin and oxytocin: A general approach to the assay of peptides in tissues. Proc. Nat. Acad. Sci. USA *73*, 1314–1318 (1976)
Hamberg, U., Elg, P., Stellwagen, P.: On the mechanism of bradykinin potentiation. In: Pharmacology of hormonal polypeptides and proteins. Back, N., Martini, L., Paoletti, R. (eds.), pp. 626–631. New York, London: Plenum Press 1968
Han, Y.N., Kato, H., Iwanaga, S.: Identification of Ser-Leu-Met-Lys-bradykinin isolated from chemically modified high-molecular-weight bovine kininogen. FEBS Lett. *71*, 45–48 (1976)
Hirschmann, R.F., Denkewalter, R.G.: Controlled stepwise synthesis of polypeptides. US Pat. *3*, 846, 399 (1974)
Hochstrasser, K., Werle, E.: Kinin-yielding peptides from pepsin-treated bovine plasma proteins. Hoppe Seylers Z. Physiol. Chem. *348*, 177–182 (1967)
Ishikawa, O., Yasuhara, T., Nakajima, T., Tachibana, S.: Ranakinin N, a new bradykinin analog from *Rana nigromaculata*. 12th Peptide Symp., Tokyo 1974
Ivanov, V.T., Filatova, M.P., Reissmann, S., Reutova, T.O., Efremov, E.S., Pashkov, U.S., Galaktionov, S.G., Grigoryan, G.L., Ovchinnikov, Y.A.: The solution conformation of bradykinin. In: Peptides: Chemistry, structure, and biology. Walter, R., Meienhofer, J. (eds.), pp. 151–157. Ann Arbor: Ann Arbor Science Publishers 1975a
Ivanov, V.T., Filatova, M.P., Reissmann, S., Reutova, T.O., Kogan, G.A., Efremov, E.S., Pashkov, V.S., Galaktionov, S.G., Grigoryan, G.L., Bystrov, V.F.: Conformational state of bradykinin in solution. Bioorganicheskaya Khimiya *1*, 1241–1244 (1975b)
Ivanov, V.T., Filatova, M.P., Reissmann, S., Reutova, T.O., Chekhlyaeva, N.M.: Conformational states of bradykinin and its analogs in solution. I. Circular dichroism spectra. Bioorganicheskaya Khimiya *3*, 1157–1168 (1977)
Kameyama, T., Sasaki, K.: Comparison of hypotensive activities of synthetic bradykinin and bradykinin analogs in rats. Nippon Yakubutsugaku Zasshi *66*, 503–510 (1970)
Kameyama, T., Sasaki, K., Suzuki, K.: Interaction between contractile action of low-molecular kininogen-like peptides on guinea pig ileum and trypsin. Nippon Yakubutsugaku Zasshi *91*, 1–5 (1971); Chem. Abstr. *74*, 10754p (1971)
Kato, H., Suzuki, T.: Bradykinin potentiating peptides from the venom of *Agkistrodon halys blomhoffii*. Biochemistry *10*, 972–980 (1971)
Kato, H., Suzuki, T.: Bradykinin-potentiating peptides from the venom of *Agkistrodon halys blomhoffii*: Their amino acid sequence and the inhibitory activity on angiotensin I-converting enzyme from rabbit lung. In: Chemistry and biology of the kallikrein-kinin system in health and disease. Pisano, J.J., Austen, K.F. (eds.), pp. 299–303. Fogarty Internat. Center Proc. No. 27. Washington: U.S. Gov. Printing Office 1977
Kato, H., Suzuki, T., Okada, K., Kimura, T., Sakakibara, S.: Structure of potentiator A, one of the five bradykinin potentiating peptides from the venom of *Agkistrodon halys blomhoffii*. Experientia *29*, 574–575 (1973)
Kier, L.B., George, J.M.: Molecular orbital consideration of amino acid conformation. In: Molecular orbital studies in chemical pharmacology. Kier, L.B. (ed.), pp. 82–104. Berlin, Heidelberg, New York: Springer 1970
Kishimura, H., Yasuhara, T., Yoshida, H., Nakajima, T.: Vespakinin-M, a novel bradykinin analogue containing hydroxyproline, in the venom of *Vespa mandarinia* Smith. Chem. Pharm. Bull. (Tokyo) *24*, 2896–2897 (1976)
Krit, N.A., Ravdel, G.A., Ivanov, V.T.: Synthesis of bradykinin analogs modified in position 8. Bioorganicheskaya Khimiya *2*, 1455–1463 (1976)

Lalka, D., Back, N.: The high voltage paper electrophoresis of kinin peptides K9, K10, and K11. Biochim. Biophys. Acta *236*, 47–51 (1971)

Law, H.D., Johnson, W.H., Studer, R.D.: Synthesis and properties of bradykinin analogs: 1-deamino-, 9-decarboxy-, and 1-deamino-9-decarboxy-bradykinin. J. Chem. Soc. (C) 748–753 (1971)

London, R.E., Stewart, J.M., Cann, J.R., Matwiyoff, N.A.: ^{13}C and ^{1}H NMR studies of bradykinin and selected peptide fragments. Biochemistry *17*, 2270–2277 (1978)

Marlborough, D.I., Ryan, J.W.: Circular dichroism spectra of bradykinin analogs containing β-homoamino acids. Biochem. Biophys. Res. Commun. *75*, 757–765 (1977)

Marlborough, D.I., Ryan, J.W., Felix, A.M.: Conformative response of bradykinin and analogs to solvent variation. Arch. Biochem. Biophys. *176*, 582–590 (1976)

Mazur, R.H., Plume, G.: Improved synthesis of bradykinin. Experientia *24*, 661 (1968)

Mc Gee, J.O., Jimenez, M.H., Felix, A.M., Cardinale, G.J., Udenfriend, S.: Inhibition of prolyl hydroxylase activity by bradykinin analogs containing a prolyl-like residue. Arch. Biochem. Biophys. *154*, 483–487 (1973)

Melrose, G.J.H., Muller, H.K., Vagg, W.J.: Capillary permeability activity of alanine analogs of bradykinin. Nature *225*, 547–548 (1970)

Merrifield, R.B.: New approaches to the chemical synthesis of peptides. Recent Prog. Horm. Res. *23*, 451–482 (1967)

Montgomery, E.H., Kroeger, D.C.: Bradykinin relaxation of duodenum. Fed. Proc. *26*, 465 (1967)

Moore, S., Law, H.D., Brundish, D.E., Elliott, D.F., Wade, R.: Synthesis of analogs of bradykinin with replacement of arginine residues by 4-guanidinophenylalanine. J. Chem. Soc. (Perkin I) 2025–2030 (1977)

Najjar, V.A., Merrifield, R.B.: The use of the *o*-nitrophenylsulfenyl group in the synthesis of the octadecapeptide bradykinylbradykinin. Biochemistry *5*, 3765–3770 (1966)

Neubert, K., Balaspiri, L., Losse, G.: Solid phase synthesis of 2-L- and 2-D-pipecolic acid-bradykinin. Monatshefte für Chemie *103*, 1575–1584 (1972)

Ng, K.K.F., Vane, J.R.: Some properties of angiotensin converting enzyme in the lung in vivo. Nature *225*, 1142–1144 (1970)

Nicolaides, E.D., Mc Carthy, D.A., Potter, D.E.: Bradykinin: configuration of the arginine moieties and biological activity. Biochemistry *4*, 190–195 (1965)

Odya, C.E., Levin, Y., Erdös, E.G., Robinson, C.J.G.: Soluble dextran complexes of kallikrein, bradykinin, and enzyme inhibitors. Biochem. Pharmacol. *27*, 173–179 (1978)

Ondetti, M.A., Engel, S.L.: Bradykinin analogs containing β-homoamino acids. J. Med. Chem. *18*, 761–763 (1975)

Ondetti, M.A., Williams, N.J., Sabo, E.F., Pluscec, J., Weaver, E.R., Kocy, O.: Angiotensin-converting enzyme inhibitors from the venom of *Bothrops jararaca*. Biochemistry *10*, 4033–4039 (1971)

Ondetti, M.A., Pluscec, J., Weaver, E.R., Williams, N., Sabo, E.F., Kocy, O.: Mode of action of peptide inhibitors of angiotensin converting enzyme. In: Chemistry and biology of peptides. Meienhofer, J. (ed.), pp. 525–531. Ann Arbor: Ann Arbor Science Publishers 1972

Ondetti, M.A., Rubin, B., Cushman, D.W.: Design of specific inhibitors of angiotensin converting enzyme. Science *196*, 441–443 (1977)

Paiva, T.B., Paiva, A.C.M., Freer, R.J., Stewart, J.M.: Alkylating analogs of peptide hormones. 2. Synthesis and properties of *p*-[N,N-Bis(2-chloroethyl)amino]phenylbutyryl derivatives of angiotensin II. J. Med. Chem. *15*, 6–8 (1972)

Park, W.K., St-Pierre, S.A., Barabé, J., Regoli, D.: Synthesis of peptides by the solid phase method. III. Bradykinin: fragments and analogs. Canad. J. Biochem. *56*, 92–100 (1978)

Peña, C., Stewart, J.M., Goodfriend, T.C.: A new class of angiotensin inhibitors: N-Methylphenylalanine analogs. Life Sci. *14*, 1331–1336 (1974)

Pinker, T.G., Young, G.T., Elliott, D.F., Wade, R.: Synthesis of analogs of bradykinin with modifications in positions 1, 6, and 9. J. Chem. Soc. (Perkin I), 220–228 (1976)

Piper, P.J., Vane, J.R.: Release of additional factors in anaphylaxis and its antagonism by anti-inflammatory drugs. Nature *223*, 29–35 (1969)

Pisano, J.J.: Availability of labeled bradykinin. Science *163*, 494 (1969)

Popkova, G.A., Astapova, M.V., Lisunkin, Y.Y., Ravdel, G.A., Krit, N.A.: A comparative study of biological activity and resistance to tissue kininases of bradykinin analogs modified in position 8. Bioorganicheskaya Khimiya *2*, 1606–1612 (1976)
Ragnarsson, U., Karlsson, S.M., Hamberg, U.: Synthesis of peptides by fragment condensation on a solid support. Int. J. Pept. Protein Res. *7*, 307–312 (1975)
Regoli, D., Barabé, J.: Receptors for peptide hormones. In: Proc. 5th American Peptide Symposium. Goodman, M. (ed.), pp. 157–160. New York: Wiley & Sons 1977
Reissmann, S., Pagelow, I., Arold, H.: Relationship between structure and activity of new bradykinin analogs. Acta Biol. Med. Ger. *33*, 77–88 (1974)
Reissmann, S., Arold, H., Filatova, M.P., Reutova, T.O., Ivanov, V.T.: Activated esters of spin labels and their use for substituting functional groups on the nonapeptide bradykinin. Z. Chem. *15*, 399–400 (1975a)
Reissmann, S., Pagelow, I., Leisner, H., Arold, H.: Bradykinin-binding cell fractions. Stability of some bradykinin analogs against kininase II. Experientia *31*, 1395–1396 (1975b)
Reissmann, S., Filatova, M.P., Reutova, T.O., Arold, H., Ivanov, V.T.: Synthesis of bradykinin analogs and partial sequences with tyrosine for electron spin resonance and fluorescence studies. Journal für praktische Chemie *318*, 429–440 (1976)
Ribeiro, S.A., Rocha e Silva, M.: Antinociceptive action of bradykinin and related kinins of larger molecular weight by the intraventricular route. Br. J. Pharmacol. *47*, 517–528 (1973)
Roblero, J., Ryan, J.W., Stewart, J.M.: Assay of kinins by their effects on blood pressure. Res. Commun. Chem. Pathol. Pharmacol. *6*, 207–212 (1973)
Rocha e Silva, M.: Kinin hormones. Springfield: Thomas 1970
Rudinger, J.: The design of peptide hormone analogs. In: Drug design. Ariëns, E.J. (ed.), pp. 319–419. London, New York: Academic Press 1971
Ryan, J.W., Roblero, J., Stewart, J.M.: Inactivation of bradykinin in the pulmonary circulation. Biochem. J. *110*, 795–797 (1968)
Ryan, J.W., Roblero, J., Stewart, J.M.: Inactivation of bradykinin in rat lung. In: Bradykinin and related kinins. Sicuteri, F., Rocha e Silva, M., Back, N. (eds.), pp. 263–271. New York, London: Plenum Press 1970
Sabia, E.B., Tominaga, M., Paiva, A.C.M., Paiva, T.B.: Bradykinin potentiating and sensitizing activities of new synthetic analogues of snake venom peptides. J. Med. Chem. *20*, 1679–1681 (1977)
Safdy, M.E., Lyons, P.A.: Synthesis and pharmacology of homoarginine bradykinin analogs. J. Med. Chem. *17*, 1227–1228 (1974)
Sakakibara, S., Naruse, M.: Bradykinin-like peptides. Japan Pat 7,503,306 (1975); Chemical Abstracts *83*, 10889 (1975)
Sandberg, B.E.B., Ragnarsson, U.: Preparation of some 2-phenylisopropyloxycarbonyl amino acids. Evaluation of their properties with particular reference to application in solid phase peptide synthesis. Int. J. Pept. Protein Res. *6*, 111–119 (1974)
Sander, G.E., West, D.W., Huggins, C.G.: Inhibitors of the pulmonary angiotensin I-converting enzyme. Biochim. Biophys. Acta *289*, 392–400 (1972)
Schafer, D.J., Young, G.T., Elliott, D.F., Wade, R.: A simplified synthesis of bradykinin by use of the picolyl ester method. J. Chem. Soc. (C) 46–49 (1971)
Scholtz, H.W., Biron, P.: Non-identity between pulmonary bradykininase and converting enzyme activity. Rev. Can. Biol. *28*, 197–198 (1969)
Schröder, E.: Synthesis of kinin-liberating kininogens. Experientia *25*, 1126–1127 (1969)
Schröder, E.: Structure-activity relationships of kinins. In: Handbook of experimental pharmacology. Vol. XXV: Bradykinin, kallidin, and kallikrein. Erdös, E.G. (ed.), pp. 324–350. Berlin, Heidelberg, New York: Springer 1970
Shemyakin, M., Shchukina, L.A., Vinogradova, E.I., Ravdel, G.A., Ovchinnikov, Y.A.: Mutual replaceability of amide and ester groups in biologically active peptides and depsipeptides. Experientia *22*, 535–536 (1966)
Southard, G.L.: Comments. In: Peptides 1969. Scoffone, E. (ed.), pp. 168–170. Amsterdam: North-Holland 1971
Stewart, J.M.: Effects of bradykinin analogs on capillary permeability. Abstract I-66, 7th Intl. Cong. Biochem., Tokyo 1967
Stewart, J.M.: Structure-activity relationships in bradykinin analogs. Fed. Proc. *27*, 63–66 (1968a)

Stewart, J.M.: Synthesis and pharmacology of polisteskinin, a bradykinin homolog. Fed. Proc. *27*, 534 (1968b)
Stewart, J.M.: The kinins: Methods of chemical synthesis. In: Handbook of experimental pharmacology. Vol. XXV: Bradykinin, kallidin, and kallikrein. Erdös, E.G. (ed.), pp. 14–20. Berlin, Heidelberg, New York: Springer 1970
Stewart, J.M.: Structure-activity relationships among the kinins. In: Structure-activity relationships of protein and polypeptide hormones. Margoulies, M., Greenwood, F.C. (eds.), pp. 23–30. Amsterdam: Excerpta Medica 1971
Stewart, J.M.: Solid phase peptide synthesis. Journal of Macromolecular Science-Chemistry *A 10*, 259–288 (1976)
Stewart, J.M.: Modifiers of the response to kinins and their interactions with other systems. In: Chemistry and biology of the kallikrein-kinin system in health and disease. Pisano, J.J., Austen, K.F. (eds.), pp. 287–294. Fogarty Internat. Center Proc. No. 27. Washington: U.S. Gov. Printing Office 1977
Stewart, J.M., Woolley, D.W.: Importance of the carboxyl end of bradykinin and other peptides. Nature (Lond.) *207*, 1160–1161 (1965a)
Stewart, J.M., Woolley, D.W.: Effect of proline configuration on pro and anti activity of bradykinin peptides. In: Abstracts, p. 81c. 150th Meeting of the American Chemical Society, Atlantic City, N.J. 1965b
Stewart, J.M., Woolley, D.W.: The search for peptides with specific antibradykinin activity. In: Hypotensive peptides. Erdös, E.G., Back, N., Sicuteri, F. (eds.)., pp. 23–33. Berlin, Heidelberg, New York: Springer 1966
Stewart, J.M., Ferreira, S.H., Greene, L.J.: Bradykinin potentiating peptide PCA-Lys-Trp-Ala-Pro. Biochem. Pharmacol. *20*, 1557–1567 (1971)
Stewart, J.M., Freer, R.J., Ferreira, S.H.: Two mechanisms for potentiation of the response of smooth muscle to bradykinin. Fed. Proc. *32*, 846 (Abstract) (1973)
Stewart, J.M., Ryan, J.W., Brady, A.H.: Hydroxyproline analogs of bradykinin. J. Med. Chem. *17*, 537–539 (1974)
Stewart, J.M., Peña, C., Matsueda, G.R., Harris, K.: Some improvements in the solid phase synthesis of large peptides. In: Peptides 1976. Loffet, A. (ed.), pp. 285–290. Brussels: Editions de l'Université de Bruxelles 1976
Suzuki, K., Asaka, M., Abiko, T.: Synthesis of 6-leucine-, 6-O-acetyl threonine-, and 6-threonine-bradykinin. Chem. Pharm. Bull. (Tokyo) *14*, 211–216 (1966)
Suzuki, K., Abiko, T., Endo, N.: Synthesis of every kind of peptide fragments of bradykinin. Chem. Pharm. Bull. (Tokyo) *17*, 1671–1678 (1969)
Takahashi, S., Shimonishi, Y.: Solid phase peptide synthesis using ultrasonic waves. Chem. Lett. *1*, 51–56 (1974)
Tewksbury, D.A.: Studies on bradykinin-potentiating peptides. In: Chemistry and biology of peptides. Meienhofer, J. (ed.), pp. 461–463. Ann Arbor: Ann Arbor Science Publishers 1972
Tomatis, R., Ferroni, R., Guarneri, M., Benassi, C.A.: Synthesis of bradykinin via oximinopyrazoline active esters. J. Med. Chem. *16*, 1053–1054 (1973)
Tominaga, M., Stewart, J.M., Paiva, T.B., Paiva, A.C.M.: Synthesis and properties of new bradykinin potentiating peptides. J. Med. Chem. *18*, 130–133 (1975)
Toniolo, C.: Relations between primary structures, conformations, and biological activities of polypeptide hormones. Il Farmaco (Pavia), Edizione Scientifica *27*, 156–178 (1972)
Turk, J., Needleman, P., Marshall, G.R.: Alkylating analogs of bradykinin. J. Med. Chem. *18*, 1135–1139 (1975a)
Turk, J., Needleman, P., Marshall, G.R.: Analogs of bradykinin with restricted conformational freedom. J. Med. Chem. *18*, 1139–1142 (1975b)
Vardel, G.A., Monapova, N.N., Krit, N.A., Filatova, M.P., Lisunken, V.I., Ivanova, V.T.: Synthesis and biological properties of bradykinin-potentiating peptides from snake venom. Khimiya Prirodnych Soedinenii *11*, 47–56 (1975)
Watanabe, M., Yasuhara, T., Nakajima, T.: Occurrence of Thr^{6}-bradykinin and its analogous peptide in the venom of *Polistes rothneyi iwatai*. In: Proc. 4th Int. Symp. Toxins, Tokyo 1974. Ohsaka, A., Hayashi, K., Sawai, Y. (eds.), pp. 105–112. New York, London: Plenum Press 1976
Weyers, R., Hagel, D., Das, B.C., Van der Meer, C.: Tryptic peptides from rabbit albumin enhancing the effect of bradykinin. Biochim. Biophys. Acta *279*, 331–355 (1972)

Yanaihara, N., Yanaihara, C., Sakagami, M., Nakajima, T., Nakayama, T., Matsumoto, K.: Chem. Pharm. Bull. (Tokyo) *21*, 616–621 (1973)
Yasuhara, T., Hira, M., Nakajima, T., Yanaihara, N., Yanaihara, C., Hashimoto, T., Sakura, N., Tachibana, S., Abaki, K., Besho, M., Yamanaka, T.: Active peptides on smooth muscle in the skin of *Bombina orientalis* Boulenger and characterization of a new bradykinin analogue. Chem. Pharm. Bull. (Tokyo) *21*, 1388–1391 (1973)
Yasuhara, T., Nakajima, T.: The structure of granuliberin-R, a potent mastocytolytic peptide obtained from the skin of *Rana rugosa*. In: Peptide chemistry 1976. Nakajima, T. (ed.), p. 159. Osaka: Protein Research Foundation 1977; Chem. Pharm. Bull. *25*, 936–941 (1977)
Yasuhara, T., Yoshida, H., Nakajima, T.: The structure of a new bradykinin analogue "Vespakinin-X". Chem. Pharm. Bull. (Tokyo) *25*, 936–941 (1977)
Yoshida, H., Geller, R. G., Pisano, J. J.: Vespulakinins: New carbohydrate-containing bradykinin derivatives. Biochemistry *15*, 61–64 (1976)

Kinins in Nature

J. J. PISANO

A. Bradykinins

Kinins are usually defined as hypotensive polypeptides which contract most extravascular isolated smooth muscle preparations but relax the rat duodenum. Kinins also increase vascular permeability, produce pain, and cause bronchoconstriction in the guinea pig (WEBSTER, 1970). In addition, structurally related peptides are classified as kinins even though they may have little or no biological activity.

Since the discovery of bradykinin (ROCHA E SILVA et al., 1949) the structure of 14 additional naturally occuring kinins have been reported (Table 1), and it is likely that many more exist. Three kinins have been found in man and other mammals: bradykinin, Lys-bradykinin (kallidin) and Met-Lys-bradykinin. Bradykinin is produced by plasma kallikrein; Lys-bradykinin, by glandular kallikreins (PIERCE and WEBSTER, 1961; WERLE et al., 1961); Met-Lys-bradykinin, by pepsin (GUIMARÃES et al., 1976). Bradykinin is generated throughout the body from components in blood; normally, plasma contains 0–3 ng/ml. Bradykinin also has been detected in somewhat higher concentrations in damaged or inflamed tissue such as arthritic joints. In certain pathological conditions, such as dumping and carcinoid syndromes, and pancreatitis, glandular kallikrein may enter the blood and form Lys-bradykinin (see COLMAN and WONG, this volume). Met-Lys-bradykinin was discovered in acidified blood (ELLIOTT and LEWIS, 1965) and probably was generated by pepsin (see below).

Bradykinin, Lys-bradykinin, and Met-Lys-bradykinin all occur in urine (MIWA et al., 1969; HIAL et al., 1976) (Table 2) but their relative significance merits comment. Bradykinin injected into the renal artery does not appear in urine, suggesting that urinary kinins are formed in the kidney (YOSHINAGA et al., 1964). The major urinary kinin is Lys-bradykinin, which is probably formed in the nephron by renal kallikrein acting on local kininogen (HIAL et al., 1976; PISANO et al., 1978). Bradykinin is probably generated from Lys-bradykinin through the action of a renal aminopeptidase (GUIMARÃES et al., 1973; BRANDI et al., 1976; see also ERDÖS, this volume). Any bradykinin filtered from blood would be destroyed in transit through the proximal tubules (CARONE et al., 1976). Consistent with this observation is the earlier report of kininase II in the brush border of the proximal tubules (WARD et al., 1975) and observations of YOSHINAGA et al. (1964) cited above.

The third urinary kinin, Met-Lys-bradykinin, was found in urine collected in acid (MIWA et al., 1969; HIAL et al., 1976). Acid was added to protect kinins from enzymatic destruction but it is now known that acid also activates uropepsinogen (HIAL et al., 1976) and that pepsin forms Met-Lys-bradykinin (GUIMARÃES et al., 1976) from kininogen in urine (PISANO et al., 1978). Men have more uropepsin and produce more

Table 1. Naturally occurring kinins

Bradykinin	Arg-Pro-Pro-Gly-Phe-Ser-Pro-Phe-Arg
Lys-bradykinin (Kallidin)	Lys-Arg-Pro-Pro-Gly-Phe-Ser-Pro-Phe-Arg
Met-Lys-bradykinin	Met-Lys-Arg-Pro-Pro-Gly-Phe-Ser-Pro-Phe-Arg
Polisteskinin	<Glu-Thr-Asn-Lys-Lys-Lys-Leu-Arg-Gly-Arg-Pro-Pro-Gly-Phe-Ser-Pro-Phe-Arg
Vespulakinin 1	Carb. Carb. Thr-Ala-Thr-Thr-Arg-Arg-Arg-Gly-Arg-Pro-Pro-Gly-Phe-Ser-Pro-Phe-Arg
Vespulakinin 2	Carb. Carb. Thr-Thr-Arg-Arg-Arg-Gly-Arg-Pro-Pro-Gly-Phe-Ser-Pro-Phe-Arg
Polisteskinin R	Ala-Arg-Arg-Pro-Pro-Gly-Phe-Thr-Pro-Phe-Arg
Vespakinin X	Ala-Arg-Pro-Pro-Gly-Phe-Ser-Pro-Phe-Arg-Ile-Val
Vespakinin M	Gly-Arg-Pro-Hyp-Gly-Phe-Ser-Pro-Phe-Arg-Ile-Asp
Thr^6-bradykinin	Arg-Pro-Pro-Gly-Phe-Thr-Pro-Phe-Arg
Phyllokinin	Arg-Pro-Pro-Gly-Phe-Ser-Pro-Phe-Arg-Ile-Tyr(SO_3H)
Val^1, Thr^6-bradykinin	Val-Pro-Pro-Gly-Phe-Thr-Pro-Phe-Arg
Bombinakinin O	Arg-Pro-Pro-Gly-Phe-Ser-Pro-Phe-Arg-Gly-Lys-Phe-His
Ranakinin N	Arg-Pro-Pro-Gly-Phe-Ser-Pro-Phe-Arg-Val-Ala-Pro-Ala-Ser
Ranakinin R	Arg-Pro-Pro-Gly-Phe-Thr-Pro-Phe-Arg-Ile-Ala-Pro-Glu-Ile-Val

Met-Lys-bradykinin than women (HIAL et al., 1976). When the pepsin inhibitor, pepstatin, was added to the collection bottle with the acid, only one of four male urines tested contained detectable Met-Lys-bradykinin. A 24-h urine specimen contained 2 μg; before pepstatin it contained 22 μg, the highest level ever detected. In

Table 2. Human urinary kinins

Subject	Lys-bradykinin	Bradykinin	Met-Lys-bradykinin[a]
		μg/24 h	
Men (n = 10)			
mean ± SEM	7.6 ± 1.1	3.4 ± 0.6	9.5 ± 1.6
Women (n = 7)			
mean ± SEM	5.1 ± 1.0	2.5 ± 0.7	1.2 ± 0.4

[a] This kinin was largely generated in acidigied urine by uropepsin after volding.

conclusion, urine may contain Met-Lys-bradykinin but it is the least abundant of the kinins. It also is generated after voiding when urine is acidified. It is interesting to note that Met-Lys-bradykinin was only detected in plasma that had been acidified (ELLIOTT and LEWIS, 1965). This treatment probably activated plasma pepsinogen.

The pharmacologic actions of the three kinins are qualitatively similar, but in quantitative tests with isolated guinea pig ileum, bradykinin was three and 10 times more potent than Lys-bradykinin and Met-Lys-bradykinin, respectively. The order of potency was reversed when vascular permeability of guinea pig skin and the hypotensive effects in rats were observed (REIS et al., 1971). The study also included an analysis of Gly-Arg-Met-Lys-bradykinin which was supposedly isolated from pepsin digests of crude bovine kininogen (HOCHSTRASSER and WERLE, 1967). The structural significance of this peptide is in question because recent studies with highly purified bovine kininogen indicate that the correct sequence within the larger molecule is -Ser-Leu-Met-Lys-bradykinin (KATO et al., 1977). Nonetheless, the activity of the synthetic Gly-Arg-Met-Lys-bradykinin is quite interesting. Although it was the least active in in vitro tests, it was the most potent of the four kinins tested for increasing vascular permeability and lowering blood pressure, being 10–20 times more potent than bradykinin (REIS et al., 1971). It would be interesting to know if this greater potency is due to intrinsic properties or to the longer survival time of the kinin in blood. Lys-bradykinin, Met-Lys-bradykinin, and especially Gly-Arg-Met-Lys-bradykinin are not as actively hydrolyzed by purified pulmonary kininase II (angiotensin-converting enzyme) as is bradykinin. However, the difference between bradykinin, Lys-bradykinin, and Met-Lys-bradykinin is not significant when the chloride ion is raised to 0.1 *M* (DORER et al., 1974). The possible physiologic significance of the larger kinins has been discussed by ROCHA E SILVA (1974, 1976) who terms them "pachykinins."

The extramammalian occurrence of bradykinin-like substances was first reported by JAQUES and SCHACHTER (1954) who demonstrated that extracts of venom sacs of the common European wasp, *Vespa vulgaris*, contained a potent smooth muscle stimulant which, like bradykinin, produced a delayed, slow contraction of the guinea pig ileum. SCHACHTER and THAIN (1954) further characterized the substance and named it wasp kinin. Later studies (MATHIAS and SCHACHTER, 1958) revealed the presence of three peptides with characteristic kinin-like activities on guinea pig ileum and rat uterus. Extracts of the venom sacs of the hornet, *Vespa crabro*, contained a single kinin which resembled bradykinin in all tests except that it was about 10% as active on the guinea pig ileum (BHOOLA et al., 1961).

In studies initiated to chemically characterize the venom kinins, PRADO et al. (1966) showed that the combined extracts of venom sacs of the American wasps, *Polistes annularis* Linnaeus, *P. fuscatus* Lepeletier, and *P. exclamans* Viereck, also contained three kinins as had been observed earlier in *Vespa vulgaris* (MATHIAS and SCHACHTER, 1958). The total kinin activity per wasp produced a response equivalent to 1.5 μg bradykinin in the rat uterus assay. The structure of the major kinin (about 90% of the total activity) was determined by T. Nakajima in the author's laboratory (PISANO, 1968). Polisteskinin is a highly basic octadecapeptide which contains three lysine, three arginine, and no acidic amino acid residues. The potency of the synthetic peptide was compared to bradykinin; on a molar basis it was twice as potent on rat uterus and duodenum, five times more potent in increasing vascular permeability in guinea pig, and 10 times more potent in producing pain on human forearm (STEWART, 1968). Administered intravenously, polisteskinin was 20 times more potent in lowering rat blood pressure but only half as active when given intra-arterially. The explanation for this arteriovenous difference is that polisteskinin is not inactivated during passage through rat lung while more than 80% of bradykinin is (RYAN et al., 1970).

In a study of histamine release from rat mast cells by vasoactive peptides (JOHNSON and ERDÖS, 1973), it was shown that the potency of polisteskinin was surpassed only by the well known histamine releaser, compound 48/80. About 50% of the amine was released by 0.8, 3, 10, 20, and 45 μ*M* compound 48/80, polisteskinin, substance P, Met-Lys-bradykinin, and Lys-bradykinin, respectively. A peptide much more potent than compound 48/80 (but not a kinin), granuliberin R (Phe-Gly-Phe-Leu-Pro-Ile-Tyr-Arg-Arg-Pro-Ala-Ser-NH_2), was recently isolated from the skin of *Rana rugosa* (YASUHARA and NAKAJIMA, 1977). In a personal communication NAKAJIMA has revealed that his laboratory has discovered another unique mast cell degranulating peptide. Mastoparan was isolated from wasp venom and has the structur: Ile-Asn-Leu-Lys-Ala-Leu-Ala-Ala-Leu-Ala-Lys-Lys-Ile-Leu-NH_2.

Vespulakinins 1 and 2 were isolated from yellow jacket *(Vespula (Vespula) maculifrons)* venom sacs (YOSHIDA et al., 1976). Extracts of 1300 sacs contained activity equivalent to 1.1 mg bradykinin. Vespulakinins are similar to polisteskinin; bradykinin forms the carboxy end, both peptides are very basic and they are about the same size. The most distinguishing feature of vespulakinins is the prosthetic groups of carbohydrates. They consist of N-acetylgalactosamine and galactose. Vespulakinins are the first reported vasoactive glycopeptides. Vespulakinin 1 is at least twice as potent as bradykinin (on a weight basis) in lowering rat blood pressure after i.v. injection but the duration of the response is not significantly longer. Presumably, vespulakinin, similar to bradykinin, is rapidly inactivated by lung. The high basicity of vespulakinins and their unique carbohydrate content invite further pharmacologic testing. Especially interesting would be a determination of their potency in releasing histamine from mast cells and leucocytes and in producing pain, since polisteskinin is very active in these tests. It would be important to know the contribution of vespulakinins to the toxicity of yellow jacket venom because the yellow jacket sting probably causes more deaths every year in the United States than ony other venomous animal (BARR, 1974).

Polisteskinin R (WATANABE et al., 1974) contains 11 amino acid residues. The two additional residues to the bradykinin sequence (Ala-Arg) are located at the amino-terminal end of the molecule (Table 1). Also noteworthy is the replacement of serine with threonine. Vespakinins X (YASUHARA et al., 1978) and M (KISHIMURA et al., 1976) contain substituents at both the amino and the carboxyl end of a bradykinin moiety. Especially interesting is the replacement of one proline residue with hydroxyproline in vespakinin M. Thr^6-Bradykinin was first isolated from turtle *(Pseudemys scripta elegans)* plasma where it was generated by contact with glass beads (DUNN and PERKS, 1970). The free peptide was isolated from wasp *(Polistes rothneyi)* venom (WATANABE et al., 1974) and frog *(Rana rugosa)* skin (ISHIKAWA et al., 1974). Compared to bradykinin, Thr^6-bradykinin was equipotent in rat uterus and in rat blood pressure tests. However, it was only 40% as active on guinea pig ileum and 14% as active in reducing rabbit blood pressure (DUNN and PERKS, 1970).

Amphibian skin is an extraordinarily rich source of biologically active compounds, including peptides. This important observation comes from the pioneering research of Italian workers led by Dr. Vittorio Erspamer (see the reviews by ERSPAMER and MELCHIORRI, 1973; ERSPAMER et al., 1976, 1977; BERTACCINI, 1976). ANASTASI et al. (1965) were the first to demonstrate the extramammalian occurrence of bradykinin itself. They showed that the skin of the common European frog, *Rana temporaria*, contains a remarkable 200–250 μg bradykinin/g fresh tissue. The common American frog, *Rana pipiens*, contains similar quantities (NAKAJIMA and PISANO, unpublished).

The first potent bradykinin homolog with the additional amino acids at the carboxy-terminal end, phyllokinin, was isolated from the South American tree frog, *Phyllomedusa rohdei* (ANASTASI et al., 1966). Phyllokinin is pharmacologically very similar to bradykinin except that it is somewhat more potent on dog blood pressure and less on extravascular smooth muscles. Using dog blood pressure it was shown that the activity is due to the intact molecule and not to bradykinin which might be released from the molecule. Removal of the O-sulfate caused a considerable reduction in activity. The activity of phyllokinin, and the subsequently discovered bombinakinin O and ranakinins N and R, is especially interesting in light of the fact that organic chemists have never been able to prepare highly active homologs with substituents at the carboxyl end of bradykinin (SCHRÖDER, 1970).

Val^1, Thr^6-Bradykinin was the first reported nonapeptide analog of bradykinin. It was isolated from the skin of the Japanese frog, *Rana nigromaculata* (NAKAJIMA, 1968a). Thr^6-Bradykinin is the only other naturally occurring analog known.

Bombinakinin O was isolated from the skin of the Korean discoglosid frog *Bombina orientalis* (YASUHARA et al., 1973), ranakinin N from the skin of the Japanese frog *Rana nigromaulata* (NAKAJIMA, 1968b), and ranakinin R from the skin of the Japanese frog *Rana rugosa* (ISHIKAWA et al., 1974). The peptides contain, respectively, 4, 5, and 6 additional amino acid residues at the carboxyl end of bradykinin. The activity of ranakinin N on smooth muscle (and presumably ranakinin R and bombinakinin O) is increased about 20-fold when the additional amino acids are removed with trypsin (NAKAJIMA, 1968b).

Virtually all the reports cited above have been primarily concerned with announcing the discovery of a new kinin and have not included systematic studies of its biologic properties. Such studies are needed for a better understanding of the significance of naturally occurring kinins.

B. Tachykinins

The term kinin was coined in 1954 (SCHACHTER and THAIN, 1954) and further defined by a special committee in 1970 (WEBSTER, 1970). In the interim, ERSPAMER and his colleagues had isolated several peptides which caused the rapid (tachy) rather than slow (brady) contraction of the guinea pig ileum. Tachykinins are a group of hypotensive peptides, typified by physalaemin, which are structurally different from the bradykinins (Table 3) but which share many of their biologic properties (Table 4). A notable exception is the opposite effects of the two classes of kinins on rat duodenum, hen cecum, and rabbit uterus, which are all relaxed by the bradykinins and contracted by the tachykinins. In addition, the tachykinins are characteristically potent stimulants of salivary and lachrymal glands. In fact, it was the sialogogic action of substance P which ultimately led to its isolation and the determination of its structure (CHANG et al., 1971).

Physalaemin was isolated from methanol extracts of the skin of the South American frog, *Physalaemus bigilonigerus* (fuscumaculatus), which contains 370–700 μg physalaemin/g dried skin. Phyllomedusin was isolated from extracts of the skin of *Phyllomedusa bicolor*, an Amazonian hylid frog; dried skin contained 1100 μg peptide/g. Uperolein was isolated from the Australian leptodactylid frogs, *Uperoleia rugosa* and *Uperoleia marmorato*, which contained 500–1500 μg peptide/g dried skin. Kassinin was recently isolated from the African frog, *Kassina senegalensis* (ANASTASI et al., 1977). It most closely resembles substance P.

Tachykinins have an almost identical spectrum of biologic activities. A discussion of these properties is outside the scope of this review. The authoritative reviews by their discoverer ERSPAMER (ERSPAMER and MELCHIORRI, 1973; ERSPAMER et al., 1976, 1977) and the also excellent review by his colleague BERTACCINI (1976) should be consulted. A brief statement about the cardiovascular effects of tachykinins seems appropriate because they are much more potent than the bradykinins. Comparative studies have not been done in man but, in the dog, the hypotensive threshold dose of physalaemin is 0.25 ng/kg while eledoisin and bradykinin were 25 and 0.5% as potent, respectively (NAKANO, 1970). Substance P is as potent or slightly more potent than physalaemin (ERSPAMER et al., 1977). Substance P infused I.V. at the rate of 0.5–0.8 ng/kg/min caused a vasodilation in the skin, skeletal muscle, and small intestine of the dog. The peptide had no effect on vascular permeability and no direct action on the heart (BURCHER et al., 1977).

C. Putative Kinins

The skin of the lamprey, *Eudontomyzon danfordi vladykovi* (FISHER and ALBERT, 1971), contains two partially characterized peptides which appear to be pharmacologically similar to bradykinin. A kinin-like peptide also has been isolated from the urinary bladder of the toad, *Bufo marinus paracnemis* (Lutz). The peptide, which was hypotensive in dogs and cats, contracted isolated rat uterus, guinea pig ileum, rat stomach, cat jejunum, and rabbit duodenum but it relaxed rat duodenum as kinins do. The peptide appears to be five times more active than bradykinin as an inhibitor of the permeability-increasing effect of oxytocin or vasopression on the isolated toad bladder. The activity of the peptide increased when incubated with trypsin but

Table 3. Tachykinins

Physalaemin[a]	<Glu-Ala-Asp-Pro-Asn-Lys-Phe-Tyr-Gly-Leu-Met-NH_2
Uperolein[a]	<Glu-Pro-Asp-Pro-Asn-Ala-Phe-Tyr-Gly-Leu-Met-NH_2
Phyllomedusin[a]	< Glu-Asn-Pro-Asn-Arg-Phe-Ile-Gly-Leu-Met-NH_2
Eledoisin[b]	<Glu-Pro-Ser-Lys-Asp-Ala-Phe-Ile-Gly-Leu-Met-NH_2
Kassinin[a]	Asp-Val-Pro-Lys-Ser-Asp-Gln-Phe-Val-Gly-Leu-Met-NH_2
Substance P[c]	Arg-Pro-Lys-Pro-Gln-Gln-Phe-Phe-Gly-Leu-Met-NH_2

[a] Discovered in amphibian skin.
[b] Discovered in the posterior salivary glands of a Mediterranean octopod.
[c] Discovered in mammalian brain and intestine.

Table 4. Comparison of some properties of bradykinins and tachykinins

Test	Bradykinins	Tachykinins
Blood pressure	Hypotension	Hypotension
Pain	Stimulation	Stimulation
Vascular permeability	Increase	Increase
Guinea pig ileum, many other extravascular smooth muscles	Contraction	Contraction
Rat uterus	Contraction	Variable response
Rabbit uterus, rat duodenum, and hen cecum	Relaxation	Contraction
Salivary and lachrymal glands	No response	Powerful stimulation

chymotrypsin abolished activity completely. The peptide is acidic and its estimated MW is 1000 (FURTADO, 1972).

Colostrokinin is released from colostrokininogen by salivary, urinary, and pancreatic kallikrein, trypsin, and chymotrpysin (see the review by ERDÖS, 1970). The estimated MW of the peptide is 2000; the amino-terminal amino acid is phenylalanine and serine is at the carboxyl end (YAMAZAKI and MORIYA, 1969b). The peptide is qualitatively similar to bradykinin but appears to be relatively more active in increasing vascular permeability in the guinea pig than in contracting smooth muscle preparations (YAMAZAKI and MORIYA, 1969b). Bovine colostrokinin generated by hog pancreatic kallikrein has been partially purified by modifying (CASELLATO et al., 1977) the procedure of YAMAZAKI and MORIYA (1969a). The peptide, which is not inactivated by pepsin, is partially inactivated by trypsin and completely by papain (CASELLATO et al., 1977).

Ornithokinin is generated from avian plasma (chicken, goose, pigeon, duck) incubated with pancreatic ornithokallikrein. A kinin may also be generated spontaneously in avian plasma preincubated for a short time at pH 2 and then incubated at pH 7.5 (WERLE et al., 1966; WERLE and LEYSATH, 1967). The MW of both kinins is about 6000. Ornithokinin is hypotensive in birds but not in mammals. It also contracts the chicken ileum, a tissue insensitive to mammalian kinins. In a more recent study (SEKI et al., 1973), a kinin was generated from goose plasma (and presumably from the duck and pigeon as well) by the addition of mammalian plasma prekallikrein activator or by acid activation of the plasma. This kinin, unlike WERLE's kinin, was indistinguishable from bradykinin when compared on a CM-Sephadex column and in bioassay using rat uterus and guinea pig ileum. Two additional active substances were isolated from activated goose plasma: One was less basic than bradykinin and raised the blood pressure of the pithed rat; the other one was more basic but less active on rat uterus. The kinin produced in acidified pigeon plasma was relatively more active on guinea pig ileum than on rat uterus when compared with bradykinin. Apparently, two kinins were produced in acidified duck plasma. One peptide differed from bradykinin in that it eluted earlier on a CM-Sephadex column and was relatively more active on guinea pig ileum and in reducing blood flow in dog hind limbs. The other substance detected in acidified duck plasma lowered blood pressure in the goose. The authors (SEKI et al., 1973) stated that it could be the ornithokinin of WERLE and LEYSATH (1967). In mammals, acidification of plasma probably causes activation of pepsinogen and formation of Met-Lys-bradykinin (GUIMARÃES et al., 1976) whereas bradykinin is formed by plasma kallikrein and Lys-bradykinin by glandular kallikrein (PIERCE and WEBSTER, 1961; WERLE et al., 1961).

D. Comparative Studies of Plasma Kallikrein-Kinin Systems

In man and other mammals little or no kinin is found normally in blood or other tissues. Rather than being stored, kinins are generated locally from blood-born components and for this reason they are sometimes classified as local hormones to distinguish them from other hormones that are synthesized or stored in specific tissues or glands. Kinins are rapidly inactivated in blood and other tissues, especially lung. In all mammals so far studied, two types of kallikrein have been observed; plasma kallikrein and glandular kallikrein (which is found in exocrine glands and their secretions). Plasma and glandular kallikreins differ in their physiochemical properties, rates of reaction with kininogens (PIERCE and GUIMARÃES, 1976) and synthetic substrates, kinins produced, and in their response to synthetic and natural inhibitors (see also MOVAT and FRIEDLER, this volume). Kinins also may be generated by nonspecific proteases such as trypsin, plasmin, pepsin, ficin, and Nagarse (PRADO, 1970).

In contrast with the low concentration in mammalian tissue, high levels of free kinins have been detected in the venoms of wasps, yellow jackets, and hornets and especially in amphibian skin (which can contain hundreds of μg/g dried skin). It is not known whether these kinins are generated from precursor proteins, as in mammals, or if they are synthesized de novo. Their activity on isolated smooth muscle preparations may be enhanced by partial degradation to the bradykinin moiety. It is interesting that the higher MW kinins found in venom and skin contain the amino acid sequence of bradykinin but the remainder of the molecule bears no other structural resemblance to the regions surrounding the kinin in bovine kininogen (the only kininogen substantially sequenced to date).

In an attempt to gain a better understanding of its significance, comparative studies of components of the plasma kallikrein-kinin system have been undertaken. The components studied include: prekallikrein activator (coagulation factor XII, i.e., Hageman factor), prekallikrein, kininogens, kinins, and kininases. In general, plasmas from mammals and reptiles (alligator and turtle but not snake plasma) contain all the components. Birds lack the activator but snake, frog, and fish appear to lack prekallikrein and kininogen as well (SEKI et al., 1973). However, in another study, hog pancreatic kallikrein generated an oxytocic substance after addition to all of the above plasmas as well as in plasmas from the amphibians *Amphiuma tridactylum* and *Rana catesbeiana* and the teleost *Salmo gairdnerii* (DUNN and PERKS, 1975).

In a seemingly conflicting report (RABITO et al., 1972), kininogen was found in the pigeon and turtle as observed by others but not in the toad, chicken, or turkey. An explanation for this discrepancy may lie in the fact that trypsin was used to generate the kinin from kininogen and that the kinin was assayed only by estimating its vasodilator effect on perfused dog leg. This study points to the difficulty in interpreting the significance of negative findings. Factors which must be considered before any conclusions are drawn are the mode of kinin generation (contact activation, trypsin, kallikrein) and the bioassay employed. Specifically, trypsin could generate, destroy, or modify a kinin-like peptide, or trypsin may not generate kinin in all species. Kallikreins could be species specific, and finally, the kinin-like substance generated could be active in the animal from which it was generated or in certain bioassays but inactive in the screening test employed. LAVRAS et al. (1970) could not generate a kinin from plasma of the snake *Bothrops jararaca* by contact activation or by incubation with either trypsin or the snake venom, procedures which actively generate kinins in mammalian plasma. However, when they incubated the snake plasma with hog pancreatic kallikrein, Nagarse, or bacterial fibrinolysin, a peptide was generated which, unlike bradykinin, was more active on guinea pig ileum than on rat uterus, contracted rat duodenum, was hypertensive in rat, and did not increase vascular permeability.

The mode of biosynthesis of kinins in venoms and in amphibian skin is unknown. In an interesting report, DOCKRAY and HOPKINS (1975) showed that the decapeptide, caerulein, is contained in secretory granules of cutaneous granular (as opposed to mucous) glands of *Xenopus laevis*. The glands release the granules by a holocrine mechanism upon stimulation of cutaneous nerves or upon direct injection of epinephrine or norepinephrine into the dorsal lymph sac or into subepidermal tissue. Secreted granules may be harvested by centrifugation. Granules are replenished in about 2 weeks. As noted by the authors, *Xenopus* may be well suited for the study of peptide biosynthesis.

E. Concluding Remarks

Research in the last 20 years has clearly shown that nervous tissue and the gastrointestinal tract as well as amphibian skin are extraordinarily rich sources of peptide hormones, many of which are similar or identical from tissue to tissue. To explain this apparently strange distribution, PEARSE (1976, 1977) proposed that cells found in nervous tissue, intestine, pituitary gland, placenta, and skin are derived at different periods from the embryonic ectoblast and share a common neuroendocrine program. Environmental circumstances determine the final expression of their endocrine programs.

While peptides in nervous tissue and gastrointestinal tract can act to release or inhibit release of hormones, to contract or relax muscle, and possibly act as neurotransmitters, the role played by the enormous quantities of active peptide found in amphibian skin is unknown. They may to some extent be involved in the regulation of the local vasculature or in the control of water and salt movement, but their uneven distribution in amphibians, their location in glandular granules, and the release of granules by an adrenergic mechanism (DOCKRAY and HOPKINS, 1975) suggests that they have a defensive role. Such a role is easy to accept in the case of hymenoptera venom which also may contain histamine, acetylcholine, serotonin, phospholipase, hyaluronidase, and other biologically active agents. The number and concentration of these compounds in venom (GELLER et al., 1976; TU, 1977) as in amphibian skin is very different in different species.

Although they are not in the focus of this report, other active peptides have been discovered in amphibian skin and insect venom. ERSPAMER and his colleagues have, in addition to the bradykinins and tachykinins, discovered and classified other peptides including: 1. Caerulein and phyllocaerulein, which bear pharmacologic properties very similar to cholecystokinin and gastrin: 2. Bombesin-like peptides (bombesin, alytesin, ranatensin, and litorin) which possess an unusual spectrum of activities because they release or inhibit the release of other hormones and act directly on a number of smooth muscles; 3. New peptide families currently under investigation. Ranatensin was the first peptide in the bombesin family to be sequenced (NAKAJIMA et al., 1970). Xenopsin is an interesting octapeptide isolated from the skin of *Xenopus laevis* (ARAKI et al., 1973). It resembles neurotensin which was isolated from bovine hypothalami at about the same time (CARRAWAY and LEEMAN, 1973, 1975). Thyrotropin-releasing hormone (<Glu-His-Pro-NH_2), first isolated in mammalian brain, also occurs in the skin (40 μg/g wet weight) of the Korean frog, *Bombina orientalis* (YASUHARA and NAKAJIMA, 1975).

Bee venom does not contain kinin-like peptides. However, it does contain other pharmacologically active peptides including melittin (which causes cell lysis), apamin (a neurotoxin), mast cell degranulating peptide, secapin, and tertiapin (GAULDIE et al., 1976).

There is no doubt that continued study of the distribution of active peptides in nature can be interesting and important. Among the possible rewards are the discovery of uniquely active peptides and the likelihood that some of these will provide valuable clues to the presence and function of identical or related peptides in man.

References

Anastasi, A., Erspamer, V., Bertaccini, G.: Occurrence of bradykinin in the skin of *Rana temporaria.* Comp. Biochem. Physiol. *14*, 43 (1965)

Anastasi, A., Erspamer, V., Bertaccini, G., Cei, J.M.: Isolation, amino acid sequence, and biological activity of phyllokinin (bradykinyl-isoleucyl-tyrosine O-sulfate), a bradykinin-like endecapeptide of the skin of *Phyllomedusa rohdei.* In: Hypotensive peptides. Erdös, E.G., Back, N., Sicuteri, F. (eds.), p. 76. Berlin, Heidelberg, New York: Springer 1966

Anastasi, A., Montecucchi, P., Erspamer, V., Visser, J.: Amino acid composition and sequence of kassinin, a tachykinin dodecapeptide from the skin of the African frog *Kassina senegalensis.* Experientia *33*, 857 (1977)

Araki, K., Tachibana, S., Uchiyama, M., Nakajima, T., Yasuhara, T.: Isolation and structure of a new active peptide "Xenopsin" on the smooth muscle, especially on a strip of fundus from a rat stomach, from the skin of *Xenopus laevis.* Chem. Pharm. Bull. *21*, 2801 (1973)

Barr, S. E.: Allergy to hymenoptera stings. J. Am. Med. Assoc. *228*, 718 (1974)
Bertaccini, G.: Active polypeptides of nonmammalian origin. Pharmacol. Rev. *28*, 127 (1976)
Bhoola, K.D., Calle, J., Schachter, M.: Identification of acetylcholine, 5-hydroxy-tryptamine, histamine, and a new kinin in hornet venom *(Vespa crabro)*. J. Physiol. *159*, 167 (1961).
Brandi, C.M.W., Prado, E.S., Prado, M.J.B.A., Prado, J.L.: Kinin-converting aminopeptidase from human urine partial purification and properties. Int. J. Biochem. 7, 335 (1976)
Burcher, E., Atterhög, J.H., Pernow, B., Rosell, S.: Cardiovascular effects of substance P: effects on the heart and regional blood flow in the dog. In: Substance P. Euler, U.S., Pernow, B. (eds.), p. 261. New York: Raven 1977
Carone, F.A., Pullman, T.N., Oparil, S., Nakamura, S.: Micropuncture evidence of rapid hydrolysis of bradykinin by rat proximal tubule. Am. J. Physiol. *230*, 1420 (1976)
Carraway, R.E., Leeman, S.E.: The isolation of a new hypotensive peptide, Neurotensin, from bovine hypothalami. J. of Biol. Chem. *248*, 6854–6861 (1973)
Carraway, R.E., Leeman, S.E.: The amino acid sequence of a hypothalamic peptide, Neurotensin. J. Biol. Chem. *250*, 1907–1911 (1975)
Casellato, M.M., Lugaro, G., Pasta, P., Manera, E., Ormas, P., Beretta, C.: A new approach to preparation and purification of colostrokinin from bovine colostrum. Experientia *33*, 485 (1977)
Chang, M.M., Leeman, S.E., Niall, H.D.: Amino acid sequence of substance P. Nature New Biol. *232*, 86 (1971)
Dockray, G.J., Hopkins, C.R.: Caerulein secretion by dermal glands in *Xenopus laevis*. J. Cell. Biol. *64*, 724 (1975)
Dorer, F.E., Ryan, J.W., Stewart, J.M.: Hydroysis of bradykinin and its higher homologues by angiotensin-converting enzyme. Biochem. J. *141*, 915 (1974)
Dunn, R.S., Perks, A.M.: A new plasma kinin in the turtle, *Pseudemys scripta elegans*. Experientia *26*, 1220 (1970)
Dunn, R.S., Perks, A.M.: Comparative studies on plasma kinins: the kallikrein-kinin system in poikilotherm and other vertebrates. Gen. Comp. Endocrinol. *26*, 165 (1975)
Elliott, D.F., Lewis, G.P.: Methionyl-lysyl-bradykinin, a new kinin from oxblood. Biochem. J. *95*, 437 (1965)
Erdös, E.G.: Urinary kinins and colostrokinin. In: Handbook of experimental pharmacology. Vol. XXV: Bradykinin, kallidin, and kallikrein. Erdös, E.G. (ed.), p. 579. Berlin, Heidelberg, New York: Springer 1970
Erspamer, V., Erspamer, G.F., Linari, G.: Occurrence of tachykinins (physalemin- of substance P-like peptides) in the amphibian skin and their actions on smooth muscle preparations. In: Substance P. Euler, U.S., Pernow, B. (eds.), p. 67. New York: Raven 1977
Erspamer, V., Erspamer, G.F., Negri, L.: Naturally occurring kinins. In: Chemistry and biology of the kallikrein-kinin system in health and disease. Pisano, J.J., Austen, K.F. (eds.), p. 153. Fogarty Internat. Center Proc. No. 27. Washington: U.S. Gov. Printing Office 1976
Erspamer, V., Melchiorri, P.: Active polypeptides of the amphibian skin and their synthetic analogues. Pure Appl. Chem. *35*, 463 (1973)
Fischer, G., Albert, W.: A biological active peptide in the skin of lampreys *(Eudontomyzon danfordi vladykovi)*. Z. Naturforsch. *26b*, 1021 (1971)
Furtado, M.R.F.: Occurrence of a kinin-like peptide in the urinary bladder of the toad *Bufo marinus paracnemis* Lutz. Biochem. Pharmacol. *21*, 118 (1972)
Gauldie, J., Hanson, J.M., Runjanek, F.D., Shipolini, R.A., Vernon, C.A.: The peptide components of Bee Venom. Eur. J. Biochem. *61*, 369 (1976)
Geller, R.G., Yoshida, H., Beaven, M.A., Horakova, Z., Atkins, F.L., Yamabe, H., Pisano, J.J.: Pharmacologically active substances in venoms of the bald-faced hornet, *Vespula (Dolichovespula) maculata*, and the yellow jacket, *Vespula (Vespula) maculifrons*. Toxicon *14*, 27 (1976)
Guimarães, J.A., Borges, D.R., Prado, E.S., Prado, J.L.: Kinin-converting aminopeptidase from human serum. Biochem. Pharmacol. *22*, 3157 (1973)
Guimarães, J.A., Pierce, J.V., Hial, V., Pisano, J.J.: Methionyl-lysyl-bradykinin: the kinin released by pepsin from human kininogens. In: Advances in experimental medicine and biology. Kinins: pharmacodynamics and biological roles. Sicuteri, F., Back, N., Haberland, G.L. (eds.), Vol. 70, p. 265. New York, London: Plenum Press 1976

Hial, V., Keiser, H.R., Pisano, J.J.: Origin and content of methionyl-lysyl-bradykinin, lysyl-bradykinin, and bradykinin in human urine. Biochem. Pharmacol. *25*, 2499 (1976)

Hochstrasser, K., Werle, E.: Über kininliefernde Peptide aus Pepsin-verdauten Rinderplasma-proteinen. Hoppe Seylers Z. Physiol. Chem. *348*, 177 (1967)

Ishikawa, O., Yasuhara, T., Nakajima, T., Tachibana, S.: On the biological active peptides in the skin of *Rana rugosa*. Paper presented at the 12th Symposium on Peptide Chemistry (Kyoto, Japan) (1974)

Jaques, R., Schachter, M.: The presence of histamine, 5-hydroxytryptamine and a potent, slow-contracting substance in wasp venom. Br. J. Pharmacol. *9*, 53 (1954)

Johnson, A.R., Erdös, E.G.: Release of histamine from mast cells by vasoactive peptides. Proc. Soc. Exp. Biol. Med. *142*, 1252 (1973)

Kato, H., Han, Y.N., Iwanaga, S.: Primary structure of bovine plasma low-molecular-weight kininogen. J. Biochem. *82*, 377 (1977)

Kishimura, H., Yasuhara, T., Yoshida, H., Nakajima, T.: Vespakinin-M, a novel bradykinin analogue containing hydroxyproline, in the venom of *Vespa madarina* Smith. Chem. Pharm. Bull. *24*, 2896 (1976)

Lavras, A.A.C., Fichman, M., Hiraichi, E., Schmuziger, P., Picarelli, Z.P.: Active pharmacological principle released by different enzymatic preparations from *Bothrops jararaca* plasma. In: Advances in experimental medicine and biology. Bradykinin and related kinins, cardiovascular, biochemical, and neural actions. Sicuteri, F., Rocha e Silva, M., Back, N. (eds.), Vol. 8, p. 89. New York, London: Plenum Press 1970

Mathias, A.P., Schachter, M.: The chromatographic behaviour of wasp venom kinin, kallidin, and bradykinin. Br. J. Pharmacol. *13*, 326 (1958)

Miwa, I., Erdös, E.G., Seki, T.: Separation of peptide components of urinary kinin (substance Z). Proc. Soc. Exp. Biol. Med. *131*, 768 (1969)

Nakajima, T.: Occurrence of a new active peptides on smooth muscle and bradykinin in the skin of *Rana nigromaculata* Hallowell. Chem. Pharm. Bull. *16*, 769 (1968a)

Nakajima, T.: On the third active peptide on smooth muscle in the skin of *Rana nigromaculata* Hallowell. Chem. Pharm. Bull. *16*, 2088 (1968b)

Nakajima, T., Tanimura, T., Pisano, J.J.: Isolation and structure of a new vasoactive peptide. Fed. Proc. *29*, 282 (Abstract) (1970)

Nakajima, T., Yasuhara, T.: A new mast cell degranulating peptide, granuliberin-R, in the frog (*Rana rugosa*) skin. Chem. Pharm. Bull. *25*, 2464 (1977)

Nakano, J.: Effects of bradykinin, eledoisin, and physalaemin on cardiovascular dynamics. In: Advances in experimental medicine and biology. Bradykinin and related kinins, cardiovascular, biochemical, and neural actions. Sicuteri, F., Rocha e Silva, M., Back, N. (eds.), Vol. 8, p. 157. New York, London: Plenum Press 1970

Pearse, A.G.E.: Peptides in brain and intestine. Nature (London) *262*, 92 (1976)

Pearse, A.G.E.: The diffuse endocrine system and the APUD concept: related "endocrine" peptides in brain, intestine, pituitary, placenta and anuran cutaneous glands. Med. Biol. *55*, 115 (1977)

Pierce, J.V., Guimarães, J.A.: Further characterization of highly purified human plasma kininogens. In: Chemistry and biology of the kallikrein-kinin system in health and disease. Pisano, J.J., Austen, K.F. (eds.), p. 121. Fogarty Internat. Center Proc. No. 27. Washington: U.S. Gov. Printing Office 1976

Pierce, J.V., Webster, M.E.: Human plasma kallidins: Isolation and chemical studies. Biochem. Biophys. Res. Commun. *5*, 353 (1961)

Pisano, J.J.: Vasoactive peptides in venoms. Fed. Proc. *27*, 58 (1968)

Pisano, J.J., Corthorn, J., Yates, K., Pierce, J.V.: Kallikrein-kinin system in the kidney. In: Contributions to Nephrology. Eisenbach, G.M., Brod, J. (eds.), Vol. 12, p. 116. Basel: Karger, 1978

Prado, J.L.: Proteolytic enzymes as kininogenases. In: Handbook of experimental pharmacology. Vol. XXV: Bradykinin, kallidin, and kallikrein. Erdös, E.G. (ed.), p. 156. Berlin, Heidelberg, New York: Springer 1970

Prado, J.L., Tamura, Z., Furano, E., Pisano, J.J., Udenfriend, S.: Characterization of kinins in wasp venom. In: Hypotensive peptides. Erdös, E.G., Back, N., Sicuteri, F. (eds.), p. 93. Berlin, Heidelberg, New York: Springer 1966

Rabito, S.F., Binia, A., Segovia, R.: Plasma kininogen content of toads, fowl, and reptiles. Comp. Biochem. Physiol. *41 A*, 281 (1972)
Reis, M.L., Okino, L., Rocha e Silva, M.: Comparative pharmacological actions of bradykinin and related kinins of larger molecular weights. Biochem. Pharmacol. *20*, 2935 (1971)
Rocha e Silva, M.: Present trends in kinin research. Life Sci. *15*, 7 (1974)
Rocha e Silva, M.: Bradykinin and bradykininogen – introductory remarks. In: Chemistry and biology of the kallikrein-kinin system in health and disease. Pisano, J.J., Austen, K.F. (eds.), p. 7. Fogarty Internat. Center Proc. No. 27. Washington: U.S. Gov. Printing Office 1976
Rocha e Silva, M., Beraldo, W.T., Rosenfeld, G.: Bradykinin, a hypotensive and smooth muscle stimulating factor released from plasma by snake venoms and by trypsin. Am. J. Physiol. *156*, 261 (1949)
Ryan, J.W., Roblero, J., Stewart, J.M.: Inactivation of bradykinin in rat lung. In: Advances in experimental medicine and biology. Bradykinin and related kinins, cardiovascular, biochemical and neural actions. Sicuteri, F., Rocha e Silva, M., Back, N. (eds.), Vol. 8, p. 263. New York, London: Plenum Press 1970
Schachter, M., Thain, E.M.: Chemical and pharmacological properties of the potent, slow contracting substance (kinin) in wasp venom. Br. J. Pharmacol. *9*, 352 (1954)
Schröder, E.: Structure-activity relationships of kinins. In: Handbook of experimental pharmacology. Vol. XXV: Bradykinin, kallidin, and kallikrein. Erdös, E.G. (ed.), p. 324. Berlin, Heidelberg, New York: Springer 1970
Seki, T., Miwa, I., Nakajima, T., Erdös, E.G.: Plasma kallikrein-kinin system in nonmammalian blood: evolutionary aspects. Am. J. Physiol. *224*, 1425 (1973)
Stewart, J.M.: Synthesis and pharmacology of Polistes kinin, a bradykinin homolog. Fed. Proc. *27*, 534 (1968)
Tu, A.T.: Venoms of bees, hornets, and wasps. In: Venoms: chemistry and molecular biology, p. 501. New York: Wiley & Sons 1977
Ward, P.E., Gedney, C., Dowben, R.M., Erdös, E.G.: Isolation of membrane-bound renal kallikrein and kininase. Biochem. J. *151*, 755 (1975)
Watanabe, M., Yasuhara, T., Nakajima, T.: Paper presented at the 4th International symposium on animal, plant, and microbial toxins, Tokyo (1974)
Webster, M.E.: Recommendations for nomenclature and units. In: Handbook of experimental pharmacology. Vol. XXV: Bradykinin, kallidin, and kallikrein. Erdös, E.G. (ed.), p. 659. Berlin, Heidelberg, New York: Springer 1970
Werle, E., Hochstrasser, K., Trautschold, I.: Studies of bovine plasma kininogen, ornitho-kallikrein, and ornitho-kinin. In: Hypotensive peptides. Erdös, E.G., Back, N., Sicuteri, F. (eds.), p. 105. Berlin, Heidelberg, New York: Springer 1966
Werle, E., Leysath, G.: Über das Molekulargewicht des Plasmakinins von Vögeln. Hoppe Seylers Z. Physiol. Chem. *348*, 352 (1967)
Werle, E., Trautschold, I., Leysath, G.: Isolierung und Struktur des Kallidins. Hoppe Seylers Z. Physiol. Chem. *326*, 174 (1961)
Yamazaki, K., Moriya, H.: Isolation and purification of colostrokinin from bovine colostrum. Biochem. Pharm. *18*, 2303 (1969a)
Yamazaki, K., Moriya, H.: Properties of colostrokinin from bovine colostrum. Biochem. Pharm. *18*, 2313 (1969b)
Yasuhara, T., Hira, M., Nakajima, T., Yanaihara, N., Yanaihara, C., Hashimoto, T., Sakura, N., Tachibana, S., Araki, K., Bessho, M., Yamanaka, T.: Active peptides on smooth muscle in the skin of *Bombina orientalis* Boulenger and characterization of a new bradykinin analogue. Chem. Pharm. Bull. *21*, 1388 (1973)
Yasuhara, T., Nakajima, T.: Occurrence of Pyr-His-Pro-NH_2 in the frog skin. Chem. Pharm. Bull. *23*, 3301 (1975)
Yasuhara, T., Nakajima, T.: A new mast cell degranulating peptide, granuliberin-*R*, in the frog *(Rana rugosa)* skin. Chem. Pharm. Bull. *25*, 2464 (1977)
Yasuhara, T., Yoshida, H., Nakajima, T.: Vespakinin X. Submitted to Chem. Pharm. Bull. (1978)
Yoshida, H., Geller, R.G., Pisano, J.J.: Vespulakinins: new carbohydrate-containing bradykinin derivatives. Biochemistry *15*, 61 (1976)
Yoshinaga, K., Abe, K., Miwa, I., Furuyama, T., Suzuki, Ch.: Evidence for the Renal Origin of Urinary Kinin. Experientia *XX*/7, Vol. 20, 396 (1964)

Bradykinin Receptors

C. E. Odya and T. L. Goodfriend

A. Introduction

As discussed by Goldstein et al. (1974), the modern receptor concept was proposed in the first part of this century by Langley and Ehrlich. Observations of the effects of drugs on biologic systems led them to hypothesize that responsive cells contain specialized components which recognize the drugs. Although this idea was controversial at first, it is now commonly accepted that most drugs and hormones affect cells by interacting with specific receptors. Deductions from physiologic and pharmacologic experiments suggest that receptors have the properties listed in Table 1.

Conclusions about receptors have been drawn from a variety of indirect experimental approaches. Because of the complexity of biologic responses it is usually difficult to determine whether a given manipulation has affected receptors and not the agonist itself, the systems that degrade the agonist, receptor-effector coupling, or the effectors themselves. The experiments reviewed here were analyzed bearing these ambiguities in mind. Virtually every experimental manipulation that alters a tissue's response to bradykinin could be viewed as involving bradykinin receptors. Therefore, we have narrowed our citations from the literature to those that we believe reveal the most about receptors. The chapter is divided into sections according to experimental approach:

(1) Direct binding studies
(2) Modification of receptors and responses in vitro
(3) Modification of receptors and responses in vivo
(4) Receptor-effector coupling
(5) Structure-activity relationships and theoretical approaches.

B. Experimental Approaches

I. Direct Binding Studies

The study of binding reactions is the most direct experimental approach to receptors used today. Tissues known to respond to a given agonist are prepared in various ways and exposed to radioactive derivatives of that agonist. Binding of a labeled ligand that is avid, saturable, and specific is taken as an indication that receptor-ligand interaction has occurred.

Radioactive ligands used in binding studies of putative receptors must be of sufficiently high specific activity to be detected when bound by the small number of receptors on responsive tissues. This number is currently estimated to be thousands

Table 1. Properties of a receptor

1. Interaction with agonists enables other parts of the cell to change when hormone concentrations exceed the threshold.
2. Isolated receptors can restore a specific response to a cell that has had its receptors removed or destroyed.
3. Interacts with agonists by binding.
4. Binds all active analogs and competitive inhibitors.
5. Found in all target tissues.
6. Binds agonists at a rate adequate to account for the rates of response.
7. Binding is saturated by an agonist concentration equal to or higher than maximum effective physiologic concentration.
8. All inhibitors of binding also inhibit effects of hormone and destruction of a receptor eliminates the response to hormone (but not necessarily other responses of tissue).
9. Function exceeds that of a hormone-degrading system, but may include degradation.
10. Interaction with an agonist affects the shape and location of the dose-response curve.

or tens of thousands per cell. Radioactive ligands must also be of sufficient structural similarity to the native hormone or drug to be "recognized" by the receptor. The best test of this similarity is a biologic response to the radioactive ligand.

Biologically active ^{3}H- and ^{14}C-labeled bradykinins have been prepared (SPRAGG et al., 1966; RINDERKNECHT et al., 1967) but their specific activities were usually too low to allow detection of the amount of hormone specifically bound by target tissues. Higher specific activities are commonly obtained by the use of radioactive iodine, ^{125}I or ^{131}I. However, the introduction of this bulky atom can greatly alter a molecule's structure, which can result in drastic loss of biologic activity. The easiest residue to iodinate, tyrosine, is not present in bradykinin, which makes it necessary to use unnatural analogs that contain tyrosine, a change that also reduces the biologic activity of the ligands.

To test the usefulness of iodinated bradykinin analogs that contain tyrosine we prepared and bioassayed nonradioactive ^{127}iodo-derivatives of tyr 1-kallidin, tyr^{5}-bradykinin, and tyr^{8}-bradykinin (ODYA, 1975). The monoiodo derivative of tyr^{1}-kallidin exhibited 88% of the activity of native bradykinin on rat uterus and 69% of the activity of native bradykinin on bovine uterine strips. The iodinated derivative of tyr^{5}-bradykinin was essentially inert in these bioassays and the tyr^{8}-analog had about 20% of the activity of bradykinin.

The monoiodo derivative ^{125}I-tyr^{1}-kallidin was used as a probe for bradykinin receptors. ^{125}I-tyr^{5}-bradykinin was used as a control for other binding sites with different specificity. The specific activities of these ligands were 1–2 Ci/μmol. ^{125}I-tyr^{8}-bradykinin is a good substrate for the angiotensin I converting enzyme, kininase II (CHIU et al., 1975). In our early attempts to study bradykinin receptors using this radioactive derivative, we found that most of the binding to a subcellular fraction from pig kidney medulla was inhibited by the kininase II inhibitor, BPP_{9a} (SQ 20,881) (ODYA and GOODFRIEND, 1973). Most of the binding was probably to kininase II in subcellular particles, not to receptors. This illustrates a common pitfall in studies of receptors by the binding measurement method: enzymes that can attack ligands may mimic receptors in specificity, saturability, and affinity. Inhibition of binding by enzyme inhibitors suggests that binding has taken place to enzymes, not to receptors.

Most or all tissues that respond to bradykinin contain kininases as well as receptors. Kininases presumably have lower affinities for kinins but higher binding capacities than receptors. Their presence in receptor preparations could make it difficult, if not impossible, to study receptor binding. To minimize this problem, receptor preparations could be purified until they no longer exhibit kininase activity, or kininase inhibitors could be included in incubation mixtures. We used the second approach, and added BPP_{9a} (SQ 20,881) to our incubation buffer. Competitive kininase inhibitors are preferred because they block the binding of the substrate to the enzyme. Noncompetitive inhibitors, although they block hydrolysis, may still allow kinin to bind to kininases.

We found that subcellular particles isolated from uterine myometrium from pregnant cows bind monoiodo ^{125}I-tyr^{1}-kallidin in a way expected of a bradykinin receptor (ODYA, 1975; ODYA and GOODFRIEND, 1975). The apparent K_{assoc} for bradykinin was high ($10^9\ M^{-1}$). The binding was specific; angiotensins I and II and oxytocin, serotonin, BPP_{9a} (SQ 20,881) and biologically inactive elision analogs of bradykinin did not inhibit binding at concentrations of 5 µg/ml. Biologically active kinin analogs inhibited binding proportionately to their biologic activities.

REISSMANN et al. (1977) used tritium-labeled acetyl-bradykinin analogs with specific activities of about 2 Ci/mmol to study bradykinin binding to plasma membranes isolated from rat uterus. Their experiments showed that [^{3}H]-acetyl-(8-erythro-amino-β-phenylbutyric acid)-bradykinin was bound to these membranes at a site with an apparent K_{assoc} of $3.6 \times 10^9\ M^{-1}$. The comparable value for [^{3}H]-acetyl-(1,9-di-norarginine)-bradykinin was $2.2 \times 10^{10}\ M^{-1}$. Lower affinity sites were also found, ($3.6 \times 10^8\ M^{-1}$ and $4.8 \times 10^8\ M^{-1}$). The high affinity sites have apparent K_{assoc} constants similar to those we found with bovine uterine particles.

Proof that the binding studies described above pertained to receptors and not other sites requires knowledge of the cellular events the receptors modulate, or the use of specific inhibitors of their interaction with bradykinin. Lacking these tools we must interpret binding data with caution.

II. Modification of Receptors and Responses in Vitro

1. General

FLEISCH and EHRENPRIES (1968b) studied the effect of urea on the bradykinin response of the isolated rat fundal strip. Treatment of the strip with 2 *M* urea for 19 min had no effect on the response to KCl, but significantly shifted the bradykinin dose-response curve to the right and decreased its slope. The maximal response was elicited at a bradykinin concentration 19 times higher than control levels. It was presumed that the decrease in slope reflected partial inactivation of the entire bradykinin receptor population. The shift in the dose-response curve was presumed to be caused by a conformational change in the receptors which altered their affinity for bradykinin. Since proteins are more labile in urea than nonprotein macromolecules, these investigators suggested that the bradykinin receptor is composed primarily of protein.

The influence of the hydrogen ion concentration on the bradykinin response of the isolated guinea pig ileum was studied over a range of pH 5–10 by WALASZEK and

DYER (1966). They found that bradykinin was most active at pH 6.0 and least active at pH 10. To explain that finding they theorized that bradykinin, with an isoelectric point of 10–10.5, is positively charged at pH 6.0 and interacts with a receptor that contains anionic groups. At pH 10, bradykinin would be neutral and would not interact as well with its receptors. WIEGERSHAUSEN et al. (1972) confirmed the results of WALASZEK and DYER.

EDERY (1964, 1965) showed that treatment of isolated guinea pig ileum with chymotrypsin and trypsin specifically sensitized this preparation to kinins. The response to angiotensin, eledoisin, and substance P were either not affected or were reduced. Similar treatment of the isolated rat uterus had a less specific effect, sensitizing not only to kinins but also to oxytocin and eledoisin. Edery suggested recently that the potentiation by proteolytic enzymes involves prostaglandins, since it is abolished by indomethacin, (personal communication).

WOOLLEY and GOMMI (1964) treated the isolated rat uterus and stomach strip with neuraminidase in the presence of EDTA. The bradykinin responsiveness of the tissues was greatly reduced only when enzyme concentrations 10–100 times greater than those abolishing the response to serotonin were used. Under these conditions the response of the tissues to acetylcholine was also reduced while that to calcium ions remained constant. The possibility was not ruled out that the effects with higher enzyme concentrations were due to contamination of the enzyme preparation. If the decreased response to bradykinin was a specific effect of neuraminidase then the bradykinin receptor may have an essential ganglioside or a glycoprotein containing sialic acid.

The effects of thiol compounds on the action of bradykinin have been studied by a number of investigators. CÎRSTEA (1965) hypothesized that the potentiation of bradykinin-induced contractions of the isolated guinea pig ileum and rat uterus by thiol compounds was caused by an increased number of bradykinin receptors following the rupture of disulfide bridges and the subsequent unfolding of protein macromolecules. The results of MANN et al. (1975) are consistent with this hypothesis. They reported that *p*-chloromercuribenzoic acid, a specific SH-blocking agent, coupled to 10,000 MW dextran could reversibly increase the sensitivity of the isolated rat uterus to bradykinin. Since the size of the reagent probably restricted its sites of action to the cell membrane, they believed that the bradykinin response was enhanced by alteration of SH-groups near the exterior cell surface.

Other explanations proposed for the potentiation of bradykinin's actions by thiols include: kininase inhibition (PICARELLI et al., 1962); alteration of excitation-contraction coupling AUERSWALD and DOLESCHEL (1967); facilitation of acetylcholine release (POTTER and WALASZEK, 1972); and increased permeability to bradykinin (TEWKSBURY, 1968). Since thiol compounds are known to inhibit kininases, potentiation could not be interpreted as an effect on the bradykinin receptor unless it could be demonstrated that kininase activity was not limiting. This example illustrates a recurring difficulty in the interpretation of indirect experiments designed to study drug or hormone receptors.

AUERSWALD and DOLESCHEL (1967) observed a reversible inhibition of bradykinin's action on the guinea pig ileum by thiol compounds in concentrations higher than those resulting in potentiation. This probably was not caused by a direct action on the receptor, but rather by a nonspecific interference with the contractile mechanism, since responses to angiotensin and eledoisin were also inhibited. This too is typical of problems encountered in interpreting experiments on intact tissues with respect to receptors.

FLEISCH and EHRENPREIS (1968a) tested the effect of heat on the bradykinin responsiveness of the rat stomach fundal strip. Heating the strip at 47 °C for 20 min had no effect on the bradykinin response measured at 37.5 °C, although it did reduce the response to angiotensin and vasopressin. They offered three possible explanations for the relative heat-resistance of the bradykinin response: bradykinin receptors in rat stomach are nonprotein; the receptors are heat-stable proteins; or the receptors are proteins that undergo rapid renaturation. Available data do not permit a clear explanation of the observations.

2. Potentiators

All compounds that inhibit kininases can potentiate the actions of kinins if the assay system includes active kininases and if the compounds do not inhibit the response mechanism itself. A list of compounds that inhibit kininases has been compiled by ERDÖS (1970). We will discuss those believed to affect receptors directly, or the receptor-effector coupling.

The bradykinin potentiator peptides discovered in the venom of the Brazilian snake, Bothrops jararaca (FERREIRA, 1965; FERREIRA et al., 1970; STEWART et al., 1971) have been employed in many investigations. The most commonly used is designated BPP_{9a} or SQ 20,881. Although this peptide inhibits the destruction of bradykinin by angiotensin I converting enzyme (kininase II) (ERDÖS, 1975), this is probably not its sole mechanism for bradykinin potentiation (CARMARGO and FERREIRA, 1971; GREENE et al., 1972). REISSMANN et al. (1977) believe that BPP_{5a}, another of the peptides isolated from B. jararaca, and potentiator B (BPP_{11a}), a bradykinin potentiator peptide isolated from the Japanese snake Agkistrodon halys blomhoffii (KATO and SUZUKI, 1971), potentiate bradykinin's action on the isolated guinea pig ileum by increasing the intracellular calcium concentration. UFKES et al. (1977) believe this potentiation by BPP_{5a} is due to a sensitization of bradykinin receptors resulting from an increased affinity of the receptor for bradykinin. BPP_{5a} also potentiates the actions of bradykinin on guinea pig lung, rat duodenum, uterus and ileum, and rabbit ileum (UFKES et al., 1976).

Peptide derivatives of the bradykinin potentiators isolated from the venoms of B. jararaca and A. halys blomhoffii have been tested on guinea pig ileum and rat uterus preparations (TOMINAGA et al., 1975). A peptide with even greater bradykinin potentiating activities than the naturally occurring peptides was found. A feature common to all of the peptides, both naturally-occurring and synthetic, is that they only potentiate the actions of kinins. This distinguishes them from the other kininase inhibitors (e.g., sulfhydryl reagents) that potentiate the actions of other biologically active agents as well as kinins (CÎRSTEA, 1965; POTTER and WALASZEK, 1972). Whether any of these kininase inhibitors exerts a direct effect on the bradykinin receptor is unknown.

3. Inhibitors

Antibodies elicited in laboratory animals are specific inhibitors of bradykinin (DAVIS and GOODFRIEND, 1969; MARTIN et al., 1971; MARIN-GREZ et al., 1974;

Table 2. Nonspecific bradykinin antagonists

Compound	Test preparation	Reference
Khellin (a furochromone) Apiin and Hesperitin (flavonoids)	Guinea pig ileum	GARCIA-LEME and WALASZEK, 1973
Promethazine, antazoline, diphenhydramine, L-isoproterenol, cyproheptadine	Rat hindpaw inflammation	MALING et al., 1974
Gallic acid and some of its esters	Guinea pig ileum	POSTATI et al., 1970
Butylated hydroxyanisole	Guinea pig ileum	POSTATI and PALLAUSCH, 1970
Butylated hydroxyanisole, methylene blue, D- and L-ascorbic acid	Guinea pig ileum	DONALDSON, 1973
Dibenzazepine, thiaxanthene, cycloalkindole, dihydrodibenzocycloheptene, benzodiazepine, dihydrodibenzazepine, dibenzocycloheptene, phenothiazine and some of their derivatives	Guinea pig ileum	ROCHA e SILVA, 1970a
Dimethindenmaleate, p-bromtripelenamine, neclastinum, antazoline, alimemazine, phenindamine, diphenhydramine	Rat uterus	WERLE and LORENZE, 1970
Ouabain	Guinea pig ileum	GRIFFIN et al., 1972
Cryogenine, chloropromazine, flufenamic acid, indomethacin, and tetrabenazine	Rat uterus	MALONE and TROTTIER, 1973

MARIN GREZ, 1974). Presumably, the antibodies inhibit the actions of bradykinins by competing with the receptors for the available kinin. They do not block kinin receptors directly. Antibodies must be used cautiously because they can also compete with degradative systems and potentiate the agonist (GOODFRIEND et al., 1970).

Many bradykinin analogs have been synthesized and tested for bradykinin receptor blocking activity (STEWART, J.M. in this Volume). The most potent inhibitor of bradykinin's action on rat uterus is 5,8-di-(O-methyl-tyrosine) bradykinin (STEWART and WOOLLEY, 1966). Although this and some other bradykinin analogs could block part of bradykinin's actions on this preparation, inhibition was not complete. At high concentrations the "antagonists" displayed agonist activity.

REGOLI et al. (1977) reported that bradykinin analogs that lack the C-terminal arginine residue and that have aliphatic residues replacing phenylalanine in position 8 are specific inhibitors of bradykinin action on isolated rabbit aorta. The most potent antagonist was (des-Arg^9)-Leu^8-bradykinin. None of the inhibitors displayed agonist activity. The analogs that inhibit the action of bradykinin in rabbit aorta have no effect in rat uterus, guinea pig ileum, or cat ileum. Furthermore, the rabbit aorta is singularly responsive to agonists lacking C-terminal arginine. These observations provide strong evidence for the existence of more than one type of bradykinin receptor.

Many nonpeptide compounds have been screened for antikinin activity. Some active ones are listed in Table 2. Although their exact mechanisms of action are not known, their site of action is probably distal to the bradykinin-receptor interaction, because none of them antagonizes bradykinin alone. We know of no compound that specifically blocks kinin receptors.

III. Modification of Receptors and Responses in Vivo

Ileum of female guinea pig is more sensitive to bradykinin than that of male (WEINBERG et al., 1976). WEINBERG et al. reported that ilia from castrated male guinea pigs have bradykinin sensitivities closer to those of females than to intact males. Treating castrated males with testosterone reversed this effect. Similarly, treatment of castrated males with β-estradiol resulted in bradykinin sensitivities closely approaching those of females. Direct addition of the steroids into the media bathing isolated guinea pig ileum had no effect. The effects of hormone seemed to be specific for bradykinin since similar results were not obtained with acetylcholine and histamine. The authors suggested two possible explanations for their findings: modified receptors were synthesized as a result of steroid action; the conformation of bradykinin receptors can be changed by the action of some steroid hormones. Both explanations assumed that bradykinin sensitivity is a function of receptor affinity alone. Although this assumption has not been proved, it is favored by the specificity of the hormone-induced changes.

IV. Receptor-Effector Coupling

After the interaction of a hormone and its receptor, a sequence of cellular events occurs culminating in a response. In studies of kinin receptors, the response measured most often is the contraction or relaxation of smooth muscle. Cellular processes that might be part of a sequence triggered by the bradykinin-receptor interaction and that might lead to changes in muscle contraction include: movements of ions across the cell membrane; prostaglandin synthesis or catabolism; and synthesis or degradation of cyclic nucleotides.

1. Ions

Several investigators have studied simple systems in which the effects of bradykinin were linked to calcium. PERRIS and WHITFIELD (1969) showed that bradykinin in μM concentrations increased the mitotic activity of rat thymocytes in suspension. The response was calcium dependent. They suggested that bradykinin facilitated influx of calcium during mitosis. ZELCK et al. (1974) found that bradykinin, 1×10^{-6} M, reduced the ATP-dependent calcium uptake by microsomal fractions from pig coronary arteries and increased the release of membrane-incorporated calcium. Angiotensin II had no effect under similar conditions. In the same laboratory, intact isolated pig coronary arteries contracted in response to bradykinin but not to angiotensin II.

CLYMAN et al. (1975a) reported that bradykinin, 1.1×10^{-6} *M*, caused a calcium-dependent increase in cGMP in human umbilical artery segments. They were unable to determine whether the increase in cGMP was the result of increased synthesis, decreased degradation or both.

2. Prostaglandins

Bradykinin has been reported to affect the synthesis of prostaglandins by cells grown in tissue culture. HONG et al. (1976) showed that bradykinin at a concentration of 0.5 μg/ml increased the production of PGE_2 and $PGF_{2\alpha}$ in methylcholanthrene-transformed mouse fibroblasts. The increase was blocked by treatment of the cells with indomethacin, an inhibitor of prostaglandin synthetase. They also found that cells stimulated by one exposure to bradykinin were refractory to additional bradykinin stimulation, although other substances such as thrombin elicited a response. This indicated that the interaction of bradykinin was specific, suggesting mediation by receptors.

HONG and LEVINE (1976) reported that bradykinin at 1 μg/ml released primarily radioactive PGE_2 from mouse fibroblasts that had been exposed to [^{3}H]-arachidonic acid. They also found that 1 h after the removal of bradykinin, the response to bradykinin was fully restored. Hydrocortisone, an antiinflammatory steroid, and indomethacin blocked the release of prostaglandin into the medium. They proposed that bradykinin stimulates phospholipases followed by the conversion of arachidonic acid to prostaglandins. NEWCOMBE et al. (1977) had results consistent with that hypothesis in their study of the effects of bradykinin (8×10^{-6} *M*) on human synovial fibroblasts labeled with [^{3}H]-arachidonic acid. They also proposed that bradykinin activates a phospholipase.

Cultured human umbilical vein smooth muscle cells released prostaglandins in response to bradykinin (0.4 n*M*–4 μ*M*). This release was blocked by indomethacin (ALEXANDER and GIMBRONE, 1976). Angiotensin II and histamine produced an effect similar to that of bradykinin.

ZUSMAN and KEISER (1977a, b) reported that rabbit renomedullary interstitial cells in tissue culture released PGE_2 in response to bradykinin (2.5×10^{-8} *M*), angiotensin II (2×10^{-9} *M*) and arginine vasopressin (7.5×10^{-7} *M*). Indomethacin completely inhibited the synthesis of PGE_2 without affecting the release of arachidonic acid. Mepacrine, a phospholipase inhibitor, inhibited arachidonic acid release but not PGE_2 synthesis. These authors also suggested that the release of arachidonic acid by hormone-activated phospholipases and/or acylhydrolase is the mechanism by which bradykinin stimulated PGE_2 biosynthesis.

In addition to its effect on prostaglandin synthesis, bradykinin has been reported to increase the conversion of PGE_2 to $PGF_{2\alpha}$ by prostaglandin E 9-ketoreductase. LIMAS (1977) showed that bradykinin 50 μ*M*, more than doubled the conversion of PGE_2 to $PGF_{2\alpha}$ by prostaglandin E 9-ketoreductase that was purified about 600 times from canine mesenteric vein. The enzyme purified to the same degree from canine mesenteric artery was not affected even by bradykinin concentrations five times higher than those affecting reductase in the vein. WONG et al. (1977) found that bradykinin, 10 μ*M*, more than doubled the conversion of PGE_2 to $PGF_{2\alpha}$ by a crude PGE 9-ketoreductase preparation from bovine mesenteric vein and that under the same assay conditions the reductase from bovine mesenteric artery was not affected. However, with BPP_{9a} (SQ 20,881) in the incubation mixtures, bradykinin caused a similar increase in reductase activities from artery and vein. These results can be used to explain how bradykinin caused the differential release of PGE-like material from mesenteric artery and PGF-like material from vein (TERRAGNO et al., 1975). The activity of the reductase from vein is stimulated by bradykinin which leads to the production of PGF, while the enzyme in the artery is either not affected by bradykinin or the peptide never reaches levels high enough to stimulate the enzyme because of highly active kininases in this tissue.

3. Cyclic Nucleotides

It is likely that many hormones elicit their responses by means of changes in levels of cyclic nucleotides. One of the first publications that suggested that bradykinin acts through cyclic nucleotides was by WHITFIELD et al. (1970). They reported that bradykinin, (1 μM), increased the mitotic activity of rat thymocytes in vitro. They believed that this effect was mediated through cAMP because doses of bradykinin that normally were ineffective could elicit a response when caffeine, a phosphodiesterase inhibitor, was included in the incubation medium. In addition, bradykinin doses that normally increase mitotic activity were ineffective when imidazole was present. Imidazole is a compound that increases phosphodiesterase activity. Caffeine also blocked the inhibition by imidazole and exogenous cAMP mimicked the action of bradykinin.

The first report in which cAMP and cGMP level changes were measured in response to bradykinin was that of STONER et al. (1973), who studied guinea pig lung slices. They reported that levels of both cyclic nucleotides increased in response to bradykinin (1–100 μg/ml). Indomethacin blocked the rise in cAMP without affecting the increase in cGMP. The rise in cAMP was therefore thought to be mediated by prostaglandins, while the effect on cGMP was thought to be direct.

SCHÖNHÖFER et al. (1974) also measured a rise in cAMP when bradykinin, (0.1–1.0 μg/ml) was incubated with cultured mouse fibroblasts from embryonic vertebral columns. Whether this rise in cAMP was secondary to an increase in prostaglandins was not determined, as the experiments were not repeated with a prostaglandin synthetase inhibitor.

CLYMAN et al. (1975b) reported an increase in cGMP levels in segments of human umbilical artery incubated with bradykinin (1.1 μM). The levels of cAMP were not affected. They reported that the concentration of bradykinin required to produce a maximal rise in cGMP was similar to that reported to cause a maximal contraction of the artery in vitro. Other agents that constricted the artery also increased cGMP without affecting cAMP. PGE, which relaxes the umbilical artery, increased cAMP without affecting cGMP. These results are consistent with the hypothesis that agents that constrict the artery increase cGMP and those that relax it increase cAMP.

KAHN and BRACHET (1976) studied disks punched out of rat mesentery and found that bradykinin (10^{-7} M) doubled cAMP. The increase was not blocked by indomethacin. NEWCOMBE et al. (1977) detected an increase in cAMP in human synovial fibroblasts incubated with bradykinin (8×10^{-6} M). Hydrocortisone and indomethacin blocked this effect. Based on these and other results from the same laboratory

(FAHEY et al., 1977), the authors suggested that either a thromboxane, endoperoxide or some other product of the prostaglandin pathway mediates the changes in cAMP after bradykinin administration.

REISSMANN et al. (1977) measured increases in membrane-bound adenylate cyclase activity in response to bradykinin at concentrations from 10^{-12}–10^{-6} M using preparations from rat duodenum. Adenylate cyclase activity decreased in rat uterine membranes. These findings support the hypothesis that increases in cAMP in smooth muscle lead to relaxation, since bradykinin relaxes isolated rat duodenum and contracts the isolated rat uterus.

V. Structure-Activity Relationships, Physical Measurements, and Receptor Models

A common indirect approach to the study of receptors is to test the effects of systematic modifications of the agonist structure. It is assumed that the data relating structure to biologic activity can be used to deduce the complementary structure of the receptor. SCHRÖDER compiled a list of 173 bradykinin analogs reported by 1970 (1970). A more recent compilation appears elsewhere in this volume. STEWART (1971) discussed problems in studies of structure-activity relationships. Based on the available data, ROCHA E SILVA (1970b) proposed a topographic model for the bradykinin receptor. SMYTHIES (1971) also suggested a receptor model including polypeptides, prostaglandins, and phosphorylated nucleotides. The validity of these indirectly adduced models is questionable.

Several investigators have studied the conformation of bradykinin and its analogs in defined solvents (BODANSKY et al., 1970; BRADY et al., 1970, 1971; STEWART et al., 1972; CANN, 1972; CANN et al., 1973, 1976; IVANOV et al., 1975; FILATOVA et al., 1972; MARLBOROUGH et al., 1976a, b; MARLBOROUGH and RYAN, 1977). Insofar as the solvents mimic the receptor environment, the conformation of bradykinin in the solvent may reflect events at the receptor.

CANN et al. (1973) stated that bradykinin in aqueous solution has a partially ordered structure caused by a 3→1-type hydrogen bond across Pro^7. In organic solvents, additional hydrogen bonding was believed to occur across Pro^3 and Phe^8. MARBOROUGH et al. (1976a) postulated that the changes in bradykinin circular dichroism spectra obtained when changing from an aqueous to a hydrophobic solvent could be attributed partly to trans-to-cis isomerization around the prolyl bonds.

As in the case of models for the bradykinin receptor, the true test of a model proposed for bradykinin in solution is to make it possible to predict the effects that structural changes will have on biologic activity. This test has not been met by any model proposed.

References

Alexander, R.W., Gimbrone, M.A., Jr.: Stimulation of prostaglandin E synthesis in cultured human umbilical vein smooth muscle cells. Proc. Natl. Acad. Sci. USA *73*, 1617–1620 (1976)

Auerswald, W., Doleschel, W.: On the potentiation of kinins by sulfhydrylic compounds. Arch. Int. Pharmacodyn. Ther. *168*, 188–198 (1967)

Bodansky, A., Bodansky, M., Jorpes, E.J., Mutt, V., Ondetti, M.A.: Molecular architecture of peptide hormones. Optical rotatory dispersion of cholecystokinin-pancreozymin, bradykinin, and 6-glycine bradykinin. Experientia *26*, 948–950 (1970)
Brady, A.H., Stewart, J.M., Ryan, J.W.: Optical activity and conformation of bradykinin and related peptides. Adv. Exp. Med. Biol. *8*, 47–56 (1970)
Brady, A.H., Ryan, J.W., Stewart, J.M.: Circular dichroism of bradykinin and related peptides. Biochem. J. *121*, 179–184 (1971)
Camargo, A., Ferreira, S.H.: Action of bradykinin potentiating factor (BPF) and dimercaprol (BAL) on the responses to bradykinin of isolated preparations of rat intestines. Br. J. Pharmacol. *42*, 305–307 (1971)
Cann, J.R.: Circular dichroism of intramolecularly hydrogen-bonded acetylamino acid amides. Biochemistry *11*, 2654–2659 (1972)
Cann, J.R., Stewart, J.M., Matsueda, G.R.: A circular dichroism study of the secondary structure of bradykinin. Biochemistry *12*, 3780–3788 (1973)
Cann, J.R., Stewart, J.M., London, R.E., Matwiyoff, N.: On the solution conformation of bradykinin and certain fragments. Biochemistry *15*, 498–504 (1976)
Chiu, A.T., Ryan, J.W., Ryan, U.S., Dorer, F.E.: A sensitive radiochemical assay for angiotensin-converting enzyme (kininase II). Biochem. J. *149*, 297–300 (1975)
Cîrstea, M.: Potentiation of some bradykinin effects by thiol compounds. Br. J. Pharmacol. *25*, 405–410 (1965)
Clyman, R.I., Blacksin, A.S., Sandler, J.A., Manganiello, V.C., Vaughan, M.: The role of calcium in regulation of cyclic nucleotide content in human umbilical artery. J. Biol. Chem. *250*, 4718–4721 (1975a)
Clyman, R.I., Sandler, J.A., Manganiello, V.C., Vaughan, M.: Guanosine 3′, 5′-monophosphate and adenosine 3′, 5′-monophosphate content of human umbilical artery. Possible role in perinatal arterial patency and closure. J. Clin. Invest. *55*, 1020–1025 (1975b)
Davis, T.R.A., Goodfriend, T.L.: Neutralization of airway effects of bradykinin by antibodies. Am. J. Physiol. *217*, 73–77 (1969)
Donaldson, V.H.: Bradykinin inactivation by rabbit serum and butylated hydroxyanisole. J. Appl. Physiol. *35*, 880–883 (1973)
Edery, H.: Potentiation of the action of bradykinin on smooth muscle by chymotrypsin, chymotrypsinogen, and trypsin. Br. J. Pharmacol. *22*, 371–379 (1964)
Edery, H.: Further studies of the sensitization of smooth muscle to the action of plasma kinins by proteolytic enzymes. Br. J. Pharmacol. *24*, 485–496 (1965)
Erdös, E.G.: Kininases. In: Handbook exp. Pharmacol. Vol. XXV: Bradykinin, kallidin, and kallikrein. Erdös, E.G., Wilde, A.F. (eds.), pp. 289–323. Berlin, Heidelberg, New York: Springer 1970
Erdös, E.G.: Angiotensin I converting enzyme. Circ. Res. *36*, 247–255 (1975)
Fahey, J.V., Ciosek, C.P., Jr., Newcombe, D.S.: Human synovial fibroblasts: the relationships between cyclic AMP, bradykinin and prostaglandins. Agents Actions 7, 255–264 (1977)
Ferreira, S.H.: A bradykinin-potentiating factor (BPF) present in the venom of Bothrops jararaca. Br. J. Pharmacol. *24*, 163–169 (1965)
Ferreira, S.H., Bartelt, D.C., Greene, L.J.: Isolation of bradykinin-potentiating peptides from Bothrops jararaca venom. Biochemistry *9*, 2583–2593 (1970)
Filatova, M.P., Reissmann, S., Ravdel, G.A., Ivanov, V.T.: In: Peptides 1972. Hanson, H., Jakubka, H.D. (eds.), pp. 333–340. New York: American Elsevier 1973
Fleisch, J.H., Ehrenpreis, S.: Thermal alteration in receptor activity of the rat fundal strip. J. Pharmacol. Exp. Ther. *162*, 21–29 (1968a)
Fleisch, J.H., Ehrenpreis, S.: A study of the alteration in receptor activity of the rat fundal strip by urea. J. Pharmacol. Exp. Ther. *163*, 362–367 (1968b)
Garcia Leme, J., Walaszek, E.J.: Antagonists of pharmacologically active peptides. Effect on guinea pig ileum and inflammation. In: Pharmacology and the future of man. Maxwell, R.A., Acheson, G.H. (eds.), Vol. 5, pp. 328–335. Basel: Karger 1973
Goldstein, A., Aronow, L., Kalman, S.M.: Molecular mechanisms of drug action. In: Principles of drug action: the basis of pharmacology, 2nd ed., pp. 1–127. New York: Wiley & Sons 1974
Goodfriend, T., Webster, M., McGuire, J.: Complex effects of antibodies to polypeptide hormones. J. Clin. Endocrinol. Metab. *30*, 565–572 (1970)

Greene, L.J., Camargo, A.C.M., Krieger, E.M., Stewart, J.M., Ferreira, S.H.: Inhibition of the conversion of angiotensin I to II and potentiation of bradykinin by small peptides present in Bothrops jararaca venom. Circ. Res. [Suppl. II] 30 and 31, II-62-II-71 (1972)
Griffin, J.D., Szaro, R.P., Weltman, J.K.: Ouabain antagonism of smooth muscle contraction. J. Pharmacol. Exp. Ther. *182*, 378–387 (1972)
Hong, S.-C.L., Levine, L.: Stimulation of prostaglandin synthesis by bradykinin and thrombin and their mechanisms of action on MC5-5 fibroblasts. J. Biol. Chem. *251*, 5814–5816 (1976)
Hong, S.-C.L., Polsky-Cynkin, R., Levine, L.: Stimulation of prostaglandin biosynthesis by vasoactive substances in methylcholanthrene-transformed mouse BALB/3T3. J. Biol. Chem. *251*, 776–780 (1976)
Ivanov, V.T., Filatova, M.P., Reissmann, S., Reutova, T.O., Efremov, E.S., Pashkov, V.S., Galaktionov, S.G., Grigoryan, G.L., Ovchinnikov, Yu.A.: The solution conformation of bradykinin. In: Proceedings of the 4th American peptide symposium, pp. 151–157. Ann. Arbor: Ann Arbor Sciences 1975
Kahn, A., Brachet, E.: Effect of some mediators of inflammation on cyclic AMP concentrations in the incubated rat mesentery. Arch. Int. Physiol. Biochim. *84*, 553–555 (1976)
Kato, H., Suzuki, T.: Bradykinin-potentiating peptides from the venom of Agkistrodon halys blomhoffii. Isolation of five bradykinin potentiators and the amino acid sequences of two of them, potentiators B and C. Biochemistry *10*, 972–980 (1971)
Limas, C.J.: Selective stimulation of venous prostaglandin E 9-ketoreductase by bradykinin. Biochim. Biophys. Acta *498*, 306–315 (1977)
Maling, H.M., Webster, M.E., Williams, M.A., Saul, W., Anderson, W., Jr.: Inflammation induced by histamine, serotonin, bradykinin, and compound 48/80 in the rat: antagonists and mechanisms of action. J. Pharmacol. Exp. Ther. *191*, 300–310 (1974)
Malone, M.H., Trottier, R.W., Jr.: Evaluation of cryogenine on rat paw thermal oedema and rat isolated uterus. Br. J. Pharmacol. *48*, 255–262 (1973)
Mann, K., Bachhuber, F., Kather, H., Simon, B.: Amplification of the bradykinin response in rat uterus by pCMB-dextran T 10. Agents Actions *5*, 236–238 (1975)
Marin Grez, M.: The influence of antibodies against bradykinin on isotonic saline diuresis in the rat. Evidence for kinin involvement in renal function. Pflügers Arch. *350*, 231–239 (1974)
Marin Grez, M., Marin Grez, M.S., Peters, G.: Inhibition of oxytocic and hypotensive activities of bradykinin by bradykinin-binding antibodies. Eur. J. Pharmacol. *29*, 35–42 (1974)
Marlborough, D.I., Ryan, J.W.: Circular dichroism spectra of bradykinin analogs containing β-homoamino acids. Biochem. Biophys. Res. Commun. *75*, 757–765 (1977)
Marlborough, D.I., Ryan, J.W., Felix, A.M.: Conformative responses of bradykinin and bradykinin analogs to variations in solvents. Arch. Biochem. Biophys. *176*, 582–590 (1976a)
Marlborough, D.I., Ryan, J.W., Felix, A.M.: Conformation of bradykinin in relation to solvent environment. Adv. Exp. Med. Biol. *70*, 43–51 (1976b)
Martin, C.A., Mashford, M.L., Roberts, M.L.: Neutralization by an antibody of some vascular actions of bradykinin. Biochem. Pharmacol. *20*, 3179–3184 (1971)
Newcombe, D.S., Fahey, J.V., Ishikawa, Y.: Hydrocortisone inhibition of the bradykinin activation of human synovial fibroblasts. Prostaglandins *13*, 235–244 (1977)
Odya, C.E.: Iodobradykinins: Applications to bradykinin radioimmunoassay and to bradykinin receptor studies. Ph. D. thesis. University of Wisconsin, Madison, Wisconsin 1975
Odya, C.E., Goodfriend, T.L.: Bradykinin binding by tissues. Fed. Proc. *32*, 766 (Abstract) (1973)
Odya, C.E., Goodfriend, T.L.: Bradykinin receptors. Pharmacolog. *17*, 235 (Abstract) (1975)
Perris, A.D., Whitfield, J.F.: The mitogenic action of bradykinin on thymic lymphocytes and its dependence on calcium. Proc. Soc. Exp. Med. Biol. *130*, 1198–1201 (1969)
Picarelli, Z.P., Henriques, O.B., Oliveira, M.C.F.: Potentiation of bradykinin action on smooth muscle by cysteine. Experientia *18*, 77–79 (1962)
Posati, L.P., Fox, K.K., Pallansch, M.J.: Inhibition of bradykinin by gallates. J. Agric. Food Chem. *18*, 632–635 (1970)
Posati, L.P., Pallansch, M.J.: Bradykinin inhibition by butylated hydroxyanisole. Science *168*, 121–122 (1970)
Potter, D.E., Walaszek, E.J.: Potentiation of the bradykinin response by cysteine: mechanism of action. Arch. Int. Pharmacodyn. Ther. *197*, 338–349 (1972)

Regoli, D., Barabe, J., Park, W.K.: Receptors for bradykinin in rabbit aortae. Can. J. Physiol. Pharmacol. *55*, 855–867 (1977)
Reissmann, S., Paegelow, I., Liebmann, C., Steinmetzger, H., Jankova, T., Arold, H.: Investigations on the mechanism of bradykinin action on smooth muscles. In: Physiology and Pharmacology of Smooth Muscle. Papasova, M., Atanassova, E. (eds.), pp. 208–217. Sofia: Bulgarian Academy of Sciences 1977
Rinderknecht, H., Haverback, B.J., Aladjem, F.: Radioimmunoassay of bradykinin. Nature *213*, 1130–1131 (1967)
Rocha e Silva, M.: Antagonists of bradykinin. In: Kinin hormones. Kugelmann, I.N. (ed.), pp. 218–256. Springfield: Thomas 1970a
Rocha e Silva, M.: A hypothetical model for the bradykinin receptor. In: Kinin hormones. Kugelmann, I.N. (ed.), pp. 75–77. Springfield: Thomas 1970b
Schönhöfer, P.S., Peters, H.D., Karzel, K., Dinnendahl, V., Westhofen, P.: Influence of antiphlogistic drugs on prostaglandin E-stimulated cyclic 3′, 5′-AMP levels and glycosaminoglycan synthesis in fibroblast tissue culture. Pol. J. Pharmacol. Pharm. *26*, 51–60 (1974)
Schröder, E.: Structure-activity relationships of kinins. In: Handbook experimental pharmacology. Vol. XXV: Bradykinin, kallidin, and kallikrein. Erdös, E.G., Wilde, A.F. (eds.), pp. 324–350. Berlin, Heidelberg, New York: Springer 1970
Smythies, J.R.: The chemical anatomy of synaptic mechanisms: Receptors. Int. Rev. Neurobiol. *14*, 233–331 (1971)
Spragg, J., Austen, K.F., Haber, E.: Production of antibody against bradykinin: Demonstration of specificity by complement fixation and radioimmunoassay. J. Immunol. *96*, 865–871 (1966)
Stewart, J.M.: Structure-activity relationships among the kinins. In: Structure-activity relationships of protein and polypeptide hormones, Part I. Margoulies, M., Greenwood, F.E.C. (eds.), pp. 23–30. Amsterdam: Excerpta Medica 1971
Stewart, J.M., Woolley, D.W.: The search for peptides with specific antibradykinin activity. In: Hypotensive peptides. Erdös, E.G., Back, N., Sicuteri, F., Wilde, A.F. (eds.), pp. 23–31. Berlin, Heidelberg, New York: Springer 1966
Stewart, J.M., Ferreira, S.H., Greene, L.J.: Bradykinin potentiating peptide PCA-Lys-Trp-Ala-Pro. An inhibitor of the pulmonary inactivation of bradykinin and conversion of angiotensin I to II. Biochem. Pharmacol. *20*, 1557–1567 (1971)
Stewart, J.M., Brady, A.H., Ryan, J.W.: Hydroxyproline analogs of bradykinin: biological activities and solution structures. Adv. Exp. Med. Biol. *21*, 3–8 (1972)
Stoner, J., Manganiello, V.C., Vaughan, M.: Effect of bradykinin and indomethacin on cyclic GMP and cyclic AMP in lung slices. Proc. Natl. Acad. Sci. USA *70*, 3830–3833 (1973)
Terragno, D.A., Crowshaw, K., Terragno, N.A., McGiff, J.C.: Prostaglandin synthesis by bovine mesenteric arteries and veins. Circ. Res. [Suppl. I] *36* and *37*, I-76-I-80 (1975)
Tewksbury, D.A.: Studies on the mechanism of bradykinin potentiation. Arch. Int. Pharmacodyn. Ther. *173*, 426–432 (1968)
Tominaga, M., Stewart, J.M., Paiva, T.B., Paiva, A.C.M.: Synthesis and properties of new bradykinin potentiating peptides. J. Med. Chem. *18*, 130–133 (1975)
Ufkes, J.G.R., Aarsen, P.N., Van der Meer, C.: The bradykinin potentiating activity of two pentapeptides on various isolated smooth muscle preparations. Eur. J. Pharmacol. *40*, 137–144 (1976)
Ufkes, J.G.R., Aarsen, P.N., Van der Meer, C.: The mechanism of action of two bradykinin-potentiating peptides on isolated smooth muscle. Eur. J. Pharmacol. *44*, 89–97 (1977)
Walaszek, E.J., Dyer, D.C.: Polypeptide receptor mechanisms: Influence of pH. In: Hypotensive peptides. Erdös, E.G., Back, N., Sicuteri, F., Wilde, A.F. (eds.), pp. 329–338. Berlin, Heidelberg, New York: Springer 1966
Weinberg, J., Diniz, C.R., Mares-Guia, M.: Influence of sex and sexual hormones in the bradykinin-receptor interaction in the guinea pig ileum. Biochem. Pharmacol. *25*, 433–437 (1976)
Werle, E., Lorenz, W.: The antikinin action of some antihistaminic drugs on the isolated guinea pig ileum, rat uterus, and blood pressure of the anesthetized dog. Adv. Exp. Med. Biol. *8*, 447–452 (1970)
Whitfield, J.F., MacManus, J.P., Gillan, D.J.: Cyclic AMP mediation of bradykinin-induced stimulation of mitotic activity and DNA synthesis in thymocytes. Proc. Soc. Exp. Med. Biol. *133*, 1270–1274 (1970)

Wiegershausen, B., Paegelow, I., Arold, H., Reissmann, S.: The problem of latency at bradykinin and some analogues. In: Vasopeptides. Back, N., Sicuteri, F. (eds.), pp. 325–330. New York: Plenum Press 1972
Wong, P.Y.-K., Terragno, D.A., Terragno, N.A., McGiff, J.C.: Dual effects of bradykinin on prostaglandin metabolism: relationship to the dissimilar vascular actions of kinins. Prostaglandins *13*, 1113–1125 (1977)
Woolley, D.W., Gommi, B.W.: Serotonin receptors: V, Selective destruction by neuraminidase plus EDTA and reactivation with tissue lipids. Nature *202*, 1074–1075 (1964)
Zelck, U., Konya, L., Albrecht, E.: ATP-dependent calcium uptake by microsomal fractions of pig coronary artery and its dependence on bradykinin and angiotensin II. Acta Biol. Med. Ger. *32*, K1–K5 (1974)
Zusman, R.M., Keiser, H.R.: Prostaglandin biosynthesis by rabbit renomedullary interstitial cells in tissue culture. Stimulation by angiotensin II, bradykinin, and arginine vasopressin. J. Clin. Invest. *60*, 215–223 (1977a)
Zusman, R.M., Keiser, H.R.: Prostaglandin E_2 biosynthesis by rabbit renomedullary interstitial cells in tissue culture. J. Biol. Chem. *252*, 2069–2071 (1977b)

Bradykinin Radioimmunoassay

R. C. TALAMO* and T. L. GOODFRIEND

Introduction

Radioimmunoassay of kinins provides a useful tool for the investigation of clinical and basic research problems in kinin biology. While this method has the advantages of reproducibility, ease of multiple measurements, and relative immunologic specificity, there are several factors which make it less easy to perform and more difficult to interpret than similar methods employed to study a variety of other polypeptide hormones. As a small endogenous peptide, bradykinin is not very immunogenic. In addition, potent kinin-destroying enzymes are present in abundance in the circulation and in all body tissues (ERDÖS and YANG, 1970), probably decreasing the length of time the intact peptide might be available to stimulate an immune response. Finally, measurements in body fluids are complicated by the extremely rapid formation and degradation of kinin. For example, normal plasma has the capacity to generate amounts of bradykinin well over 1000 times its presumed normal baseline levels. Bradykinin has a half life of under 30 sec in plasma in vitro (ERDÖS and YANG, 1970). In spite of these drawbacks, it has been possible to develop and use kinin radioimmunoassay to great advantage. Antibodies to bradykinin were first successfully made by GOODFRIEND et al. (1964), and the first report of kinin radioimmunoassay was published by SPRAGG et al. (1966). Subsequent modifications published by TALAMO et al. (1969), GOODFRIEND and BALL (1969), MASHFORD and ROBERTS (1972), and SPRAGG et al. (1976) have allowed increased sensitivity and specificity of these methods.

A. Preparation of Subjects

When samples of body fluids are obtained for kinin radioimmunoassay, one must consider the animal species being used, the individual variation in levels among animals of the same species, the properties of the body fluid being studied, and in man, the clinical status of the individual subject.

The components of the plasma kinin system in man have been well characterized, including biochemical, functional and immunochemical data (PISANO and AUSTEN, 1977), as well as kinetic data on the rates of formation and destruction of kinin (GIREY et al., 1972). Other mammalian species in which the system is reasonably well known include the rabbit, cow, and dog. While the major kinin peptide produced in the plasma of all of these species appears to be the nonapeptide, bradykinin, the rate

* Supported in part by the Hospital for Consumptives of Maryland (Eudowood), Baltimore, Maryland

of formation of kinin may be quite different among them; e.g., in dog, kinin formation is dramatically slow in vitro (GREEN et al., 1974), in contrast to man.

There is considerable variation in baseline kinin levels among individuals of the same species. In man, several studies have agreed that normal levels are less than 3–5 ng/ml plasma and yet the range of values extends downward over 2 orders of magnitude below this. In one study, approximately 20% of normal healthy adult humans had plasma kinin levels less than 1.25 ng/ml (TALAMO et al., 1969).

Among the various body fluids studied, plasma appears to have the highest measured levels of kinin, and certainly the greatest potential for the production of kinin. The levels of kinin peptide in urine are considerably lower, and, in contrast to plasma, which contains bradykinin as the major kinin, human urine contains bradykinin, kallidin, and Met-Lys-bradykinin (MIWA et al., 1968).

The clinical factors which are of importance in determining plasma kinin levels are many. For example, in man the state of sodium balance in the body is of critical importance (WONG et al., 1975). Normal volunteers depleted of their body sodium by a low salt diet have significantly higher kinin levels than individuals with a normal sodium balance. In such sodium-depleted individuals, rapid infusion of a saline solution intravenously induces a rapid fall of plasma kinin levels within 15–20 min. Body position also has been shown to have an influence on kinin levels; human volunteers studied in the upright position have significantly higher kinin levels than those in the supine position. Both the changes induced by alterations in sodium balance and those related to posture appear to occur parallel to changes in the renin-angiotensin system.

Several genetic diseases in man, described in other sections of this volume, have an important influence on the detectability of kinin in plasma, as well as on the ability of plasma to produce kinin. Plasma from individuals with factor XII (Hageman factor) deficiency, lacking the central first step in kinin system activation, cannot be induced to form active kallikrein or bradykinin in vitro. Plasma from individuals with prekallikrein deficiency (Fletcher factor deficiency) (DONALDSON et al., 1977; WUEPPER, 1977) is also significantly deficient in kinin formation in vitro as well as in the active components of the pathways of coagulation and fibrinolysis. The same problems exist in plasma from individuals with a deficiency in HMW kininogen [Williams (COLMAN et al., 1967a), Fitzgerald (SAITO and RATNOFF, 1977), or Flaujeac trait]. Finally, individuals with a deficiency of C1 inhibitor and hereditary angioedema, lacking the major inhibitor of active kallikrein, may have elevated circulating plasma kinin levels (TALAMO et al., 1969).

Human or animal subjects with an inflammatory disease state, a systemic infection, shock or any tissue-damaging disease may show evidence of activation of the kinin system with free active kallikrein, decreased prekallikrein, decreased C1 inhibitor, and/or increased plasma kinin levels. These changes are documented well in other chapters.

Having considered the above features of the experimental subject, it is essential to measure bradykinin levels in plasma or other body fluids avoiding, as much as possible, both activation of the kinin-forming system and destruction of preformed kinin. Samples should be obtained through siliconized needles into plastic syringes, avoiding tissue trauma as much as possible since damaged tissues are readily able to activate the kinin-forming system. Several different detailed schemes of obtaining blood samples for kinin assay have been described in the literature and summarized previously (GOODFRIEND and ODYA, 1974). A simple procedure is to use a #18 siliconized "butterfly" needle, remove the tourniquet, allow 5–10 drops of blood to flow freely through the tubing attached to the needle, and then begin to draw the test sample (TALAMO et al., 1969).

B. Preparation and Preservation of Samples

Since kinin-forming and destroying enzymes are present in many body fluids, measurement of the true levels of free bradykinin requires the rapid handling of samples accompanied by the use of potent inhibitors of kinin formation and destruction. Hexadimethrine is an excellent inhibitor of the activation of factor XII, and has been demonstrated to prevent surface-induced kinin formation (ARMSTRONG and STEWART, 1962). Kinin release in blood, which contains potentially high levels of kinin-forming enzymes, as well as a variety of cell types which contribute to kinin formation, may be inhibited with hexadimethrine over a period of a few minutes while it is being centrifuged to remove cellular elements. Other anticoagulants, such as heparin and citrate do not provide effective inhibition of kinin formation.

Many different inhibitors have been used for the plasma kininases, and these are described in detail in another chapter. Several authors have found 1,10-phenanthroline to prevent kinin destruction (ERDÖS and YOUNG, 1970; MASHFORD and ROBERTS, 1972). Since the kininases are metalloenzymes and their activity is especially enhanced by cobalt, phenanthroline probably works by chelating cofactors. Disodium-EDTA is another chelating agent which may be effective for a few minutes while samples are processed. However, the latter agent is clearly not as potent as 1,10-phenanthroline. As an example of the use of these inhibitors, venous blood samples (drawn as noted above) may be added quickly with mixing to an ice-cold 12 ml polypropylene tube containing 3.6 mg hexadimethrine and 9 mg disodium-EDTA in 0.1 ml of 0.15 *M* saline. Instead of EDTA, 1,10-phenanthroline may be used in the blood sample in a final concentration of 3×10^{-3} *M*.

While the use of inhibitors may be suitable for a short period of time, more vigorous measures must be taken to counteract the effects of kinin-forming and -destroying enzymes during assay procedures. With hexadimethrine and 1,10-phenanthroline present in whole blood at 4 °C, no kinin formation appears to take place during the first 4–5 min but thereafter a progressive rise in kinin levels in the blood may be observed. To prevent this rise, following rapid centrifugation of the inhibited blood sample at $900 \times g$ for 5 min at 4 °C, plasma is removed with a siliconized glass transfer pipette, and the proteins in a measured amount are precipitated by addition of 0.05 ml of 20% TCA/ml plasma. After centrifugation, the precipitated plasma proteins may be washed with 0.9% TCA and centrifuged again. The combined supernatants may be stored at −70 °C for several months, or processed further for radioimmunoassay as noted below. Several alternative schemes for preparation of samples up to this point have been described in the literature. A particularly useful one is that of MASHFORD and ROBERTS (1971) involving the use of 1,10-phenanthroline in ethanol, which immediately precipitates enzymes, followed by lipid removal using acidification and ether extraction and the storage of samples for assay in the dried state. This latter method requires no further isolation procedure for kinin.

If the method described above (using hexadimethrine, 1,10-phenanthroline, centrifugation, and TCA-precipitation of plasma) is used, the kinin in the sample can be isolated on ion-exchange gels such as IRC-50 (CG-50), 100–200 mesh (Mallinckrodt) (TALAMO et al., 1969). Columns of this gel, 2×0.5 cm can be prepared in 0.1 N acetic acid in a 14.6 cm siliconized transfer pipette stoppered by glass wool. The column is washed with 7–8 ml of 0.1 N acetic acid, and the kinin remaining on the column is eluted with 5 ml of 50% acetic acid. This eluate is mixed with an equal volume of distilled water and flash evaporated in a siliconized glass flask. The dried sample is recovered from the flask with a small volume of barbiturate-buffered saline, pH 7.5, containing 1 mg muramidase per ml (Worthington Biochemical Corp.) or 1 mg gelatin per ml. Some authors, particularly SPRAGG et al. (1974), have added an additional step on a QAE-Sephadex column in order to remove possible traces of kininogen. Using intrinsically-labeled radioactive synthetic kinin tracers, these methods can be expected to yield 70–90% recovery of the kinin present initially in the biologic fluids.

Once the initial sample has been obtained with as much avoidance of kinin formation and destruction as possible, storage of samples maintaining stability of the kinin molecule can be accomplished at several steps. The supernatant of TCA-precipitated plasma, the 50% acetic acid eluate of ion-exchange gels or the final dried or buffered sample of kinin are all stable for several months. On the other hand, plasma in the presence of hexadimethrine and phenanthroline (or any other combination of inhibitors) cannot be expected to retain its original kinin level. Clearly, more potent inhibitors of these enzyme systems are desired.

C. Induction of Antibodies

Rabbits and sheep have been induced to make antibodies to bradykinin, despite the fact that it is a small polypeptide that occurs naturally in those animals. This has been accomplished by injecting the kinin in a macromolecular form in Freund's adjuvant. The macromolecular form has been either the endogenous substrate, kininogen, or a synthetic conjugate of bradykinin and a protein (GOODFRIEND et al., 1974; WEBSTER et al., 1970; SPRAGG et al., 1966). The success of this procedure depends on the individual animal immunized and the carrier protein. As an example of individual variability in animals, WEBSTER et al. (1970), reported successful induction of antibodies to bradykinin by injecting kininogen I into one sheep. When the same immunogen was injected into a sheep of another strain, the resulting antibodies to kininogen did not cross-react with bradykinin. We have observed variations among strains of rabbits injected with synthetic conjugates of bradykinin and protein.

The carrier protein to which bradykinin is coupled contributes to the success of immunization and determines in part the specificity of the resultant antibodies to bradykinin (TALAMO et al., 1969). No one has yet performed a single study that tests simultaneously the relative importance of species, strain, carrier, adjuvant, and schedule of immunization. The technique we now employ has been used successfully at two different times, with two groups of rabbits. We do not know which aspects of the method are essential or most conducive to this success, nor do we know whether it will work the third time that it is tried!

The immunogen we use is a mixture of bradykinin coupled to ovalbumin and bradykinin coupled to thyroglobulin. The former was suggested by TALAMO et al. (1969), and the latter by SKOWSKY and FISHER (1972). The coupling reagents used to make the bradykinin-thyroglobulin conjugate were a water-soluble carbodiimide and glutaraldehyde used in succession (GOODFRIEND et al., 1964; REICHLIN et al., 1968; ODYA et al., submitted). The rabbits were obtained from a variety of suppliers to make up a mixed population of strains such as Dutch Belted, Chinchilla, California, and the standard New Zealand albino. Useful antisera were obtained from 10–20% of the animals.

D. Labeled Antigens

All other things being equal, radioimmunoassays are more sensitive when the labeled antigen has a high specific activity. However, high specific activity is usually achieved in ways that alter the reactivity of a given antiserum to the labeled antigen. In most polypeptides, high specific activity can be achieved conveniently by incorporating radioactive iodine. Since bradykinin contains no tyrosine, it is difficult to label with iodine. While incorporation of ^{14}carbon or tritium results in a polypeptide very similar in structure to the native polypeptide, it has relatively low specific activity. We have chosen to use synthetic analogs that contain tyrosine in place of natural amino acids and to label these with ^{125}iodine (GOODFRIEND and BALL, 1969; ODYA et al., 1975). Although this enables production of polypeptides of very high specific activity, the products differ significantly in structure from the naturally occurring kinin and from the immunizing antigen. The derivatives have iodotyrosine in their structure in place of lysine (as in tyrosine^1-kallidin), or in place of phenylalanine (as in tyrosine^5- or tyrosine^8-bradykinin).

The availability of three labeled analogs of bradykinin has revealed heterogeneity among antisera produced in response to immunogenic complexes. Each antiserum displays a distinct but unpredictable preference for one of the three antigens, and use of the antigen bound most avidly results in the best reaction mixture for radioimmunoassay (ODYA et al., 1978). Iodotyrosine-5-bradykinin is generally bound more avidly by most antisera (GOODFRIEND and ODYA, 1974).

E. Reaction Conditions

All bradykinin radioimmunoassays reported to date have been performed with soluble reagents in aqueous media. Standard buffers and physiologic pH ranges have been employed. Customarily, the reaction is carried out at 4 °C for more than 12 h to permit equilibrium to be reached. The greatest variation has been in the choice of enzyme inhibitors added to the reaction mixture to preserve the kinins against the action of kininases present in the sample and in the antiserum. The most commonly employed inhibitors are 1,10-phenanthroline, EDTA, and the polypeptide inhibitor of kininase II originally found in *Bothrops jararaca* venom, also known as an inhibitor of converting enzyme, and known as SQ 20,881 (COLLIER et al., 1973).

Virtually all reagents that might logically be added to an incubation mixture containing kinins exert some effect on the net results of radioimmunoassay procedures. Some inhibit antigen-antibody binding by a direct effect on the antibody, some cause an apparent increase in binding by protecting the labeled antigen against degradation, and others probably prevent adsorption of the antigen to surfaces or precipitates. It is apparent that these effects of reagents and enzyme inhibitors depend on their concentration, the concentration of the antigen and antibody, the specific antibody and antigen used, and the contamination of the reaction mixture by enzymes and particles introduced with the antiserum itself or the sample to be measured. These effects must be measured for each set of assay reagents and each incubation condition employed.

Our current reagent mixture is: sodium phosphate, 0.01 *M*, pH 7.0; 1,10-phenanthroline, 3 m*M*, and autoclaved casein, 0.01%. The incubation is performed at 4 °C for 16 h. Using one antiserum, we found no deleterious effects of the following potentially useful reagents: EDTA, 9 m*M*; dithiothreitol, 4 m*M*; phenylmethylsulfonyl fluoride, 3 m*M*; and a kininase II inhibitor, (SQ 20,881), 0.005%. The casein is added to prevent adsorption of kinin to glass. It is autoclaved, (and antiserum is heat-treated at 60 °C for 30 min), in order to reduce the activity of contaminating proteolytic enzymes.

The incubation is terminated by one of a variety of techniques that separate antibody-bound peptide from free (unbound), peptide. The most commonly used procedures are precipitation of antibody by ammonium sulfate or anti-rabbit globulin, and adsorption of free peptide by charcoal. The choice and execution of this last step can be critical and should be individualized. Finally, the separated labeled peptide is counted and the results compared to a standard curve. The standard curve is plotted by measuring known amounts of unlabeled kinin in a medium identical to the vehicle of the unknown and carried through a simultaneous assay. It is difficult to find a medium identical to the vehicles containing samples, but essential because unknown components of plasma or tissue may accompany kinin through its assay and affect the antigen-antibody reaction in a way that can thoroughly confuse the interpretation of results.

F. Interpretation of Data

Care must be taken in interpretation of kinin levels obtained from biologic fluids. Single kinin values from an individual experimental subject are not particularly dependable because of the wide range of normal levels and the larger number of factors which may affect levels. Serial studies in animals or man are much more useful.

Because of the rapid kinetics of kinin formation and destruction (GIREY et al., 1972), the results of radioimmunoassay of kinin are not necessarily indicative of the in vivo state. Current radioimmunoassay methods, along with careful processing, have recorded levels as low as 25 pg/ml normal blood (MASHFORD and ROBERTS, 1972). In comparison with the known levels of other circulating peptide hormones, this is a reasonable normal value. Other reported values cover a range extending 10 or 100-fold above that value (TALAMO et al., 1969; GOODFRIEND and BALL, 1969). Without better enzyme inhibitors and/or more rapid processing techniques, one cannot approach the true normal values with any more certainty.

The radioimmunoassay designed to detect bradykinin is also capable of recognizing some other kinin peptides, such as kallidin and Met-Lys-bradykinin, but less well than bradykinin itself (CARRETERO et al., 1976). Thus, any results using these assays should allow for the possibility that one or all of these peptides might be present in the sample. In addition, plasma kininogen also reacts with the antibodies in most bradykinin radioimmunoassays. One should be careful to be certain that no intact kininogen is present in the final assay samples [1] (SPRAGG et al., 1974). The metabolic fragments of bradykinin react to a lesser extent in the kinin radioimmunoassay; for example, the octapeptide resulting from the action of kininase I is less than half as active as bradykinin in one radioimmunoassay (FISCHER et al., 1969).

G. Applications of the Radioimmunoassay

Kinin radioimmunoassay has been used in a wide variety of studies in vivo and in vitro in animals and man. The radioimmunoassay has been employed to detect kinin in plasma (SIPILA and LOUHIJA, 1976; TALAMO et al., 1969), synovial fluid (TALAMO et al., 1969), urine (CARRETERO et al., 1976), and lung lavage fluid (WEESE et al., 1976).

In vivo studies in animals and man utilizing the radioimmunoassay for kinins have included the study of endotoxin shock in the pig (WEISSER et al., 1973); patients with cirrhosis (WONG et al., 1972), sepsis (O'DONNELL et al., 1976), dengue hemorrhagic fever (EDELMAN et al., 1975), carcinoid syndrome (COLMAN et al., 1977), dumping syndrome (COLMAN et al., 1977b), hypertension (STREETEN et al., 1976), and the effects of sodium balance and body position on kinin levels (WONG et al., 1975).

In vitro studies of the kinin system by radioimmunoassay have explored the degradation of kinin by the isolated lung (LEVINE et al., 1973), the isolation and purification of kinin-forming enzymes (BAGDASARIAN et al., 1973, 1974), the mechanism of action of antithrombin III (LAHIRI et al., 1976), the presence of kinin-forming and destroying enzymes in hamster lung washes (WEESE et al., 1976), the kinetics of kinin formation and destruction in plasma (GIREY et al., 1972), and the measurement of kininogen (SIPILA and LOUHIJA, 1976).

References

Armstrong, D., Stewart, J.W.: Anti-heparin agents as inhibitors of plasma kinin formation. Nature (Lond.) *194*, 689 (1962)

Bagdasarian, A., Talamo, R.C., Colman, R.W.: Isolation of high molecular weight activators of human plasma prekallikrein. J. Biol. Chem. *248*, 3456–3463 (1973)

Bagdasarian, A., Lahiri, B., Talamo, R.C., Wong, P., Colman, R.W.: Immunochemical studies of plasma kallikrein. J. Clin. Invest. *54*, 1444–1454 (1974)

Carretero, O.A., Oza, N.B., Piwonska, A., Ocholik, T., Scicli, A.G.: Measurement of urinary kallikrein activity by kinin radioimmunoassay. Biochem. Pharmacol. *25*, 2265–2270 (1976)

Collier, J.G., Robinsin, B.F., Vane, J.R.: Reduction of pressor effects of angiotensin I in man by synthetic nonapeptide (B.P.P. or SQ 20,881) which inhibits converting enzyme. Lancet *1973/I*, 72–74

Colman, R.W., Wong, P.Y., Talamo, R.C.: Kallikrein-kinin system in carcinoid and postgastrectomy dumping syndromes. In: Chemistry and biology of the kallikrein-kinin system in health and disease. Pisano, J.J., Austen, K.F. (eds.), pp. 487–494. Washington: U.S. Gov. Printing Office 1977a

[1] This may be achieved by precipation with alcohol or the use of ion-exchange chromatography.

Colman, R.W., Bagdasarian, A., Talamo, R.C., Kaplan, A.P.: Williams trait: A new deficiency with abnormal levels of prekallikrein, plasminogen proactivator, and kininogen. In: Chemistry and biology of the kallikrein-kinin system in health and disease. Pisano, J.J., Austen, K.F. (eds.), pp. 65–72. Washington: U.S. Gov. Printing Office 1977b

Donaldson, V.H., Saito, H., Ratnoff, O.: Kallikrein-like activity in a fraction from Fletcher-trait plasma. In: Chemistry and biology of the kallikrein-kinin system in health and disease. Pisano, J.J., Austen, K.F. (eds.), pp. 53–54. Washington: U.S. Gov. Printing Office 1977

Edelman, R., Nimmannitya, S., Colman, R.W., Talamo, R.C., Top, F.H., Jr.: Evaluation of the plasma kinin system in dengue hemorrhagic fever. J. Lab. Clin. Med. *86*, 410–421 (1975)

Erdös, E.G., Yang, H.Y.T.: Kininases. In: Handbook of experimental pharmacology. Vol. XXV: Bradykinin, kallidin, and kallikrein. Erdös, E.G. (ed.), pp. 289–323. Berlin, Heidelberg, New York: Springer 1970

Fischer, J., Spragg, J., Talamo, R.C., Pierce, J.V., Suzuki, K., Austen, K.F., Haber, E.: Structural requirements for binding of bradykinin to antibody. III. The effect of carrier on antibody specificity. Biochem. J. *8*, 3750–3757 (1969)

Girey, G.J.D., Talamo, R.C., Colman, R.W.: The kinetics of the release of bradykinin by kallikrein in normal human plasma. J. Lab. Clin. Med. *80*, 496–505 (1972)

Goodfriend, T.L., Ball, D.L.: Radioimmunoassay of bradykinin: Chemical modification to enable use of radioactive iodine. J. Lab. Clin. Med. *73*, 501–511 (1969)

Goodfriend, T.L., Odya, C.E.: Bradykinin. In: Methods of hormone radioimmunoassay. Jaffee, B.M., Behrman, H.R. (eds.), pp. 439–454. London, New York: Academic Press 1974

Goodfriend, T.L., Levine, L., Fasman, G.D.: Antibodies to bradykinin and angiotensin: A use of carbodiimides in immunology. Science *144*, 1344–1346 (1964)

Goodfriend, T.L., Ball, D.L.: Radioimmunoassay of bradykinin: Chemical modification to enable use of radioactive iodine. J. Lab. Clin. Med. *73*, 501–511 (1969)

Green, J.G., Talamo, R.C., Colman, R.W.: Kinetics of kinin release in canine plasma. Am. J. Physiol. *226*, 784–790 (1974)

Lahiri, B., Bagdasarian, A., Mitchell, B., Talamo, R.C., Colman, R.W., Rosenberg, R.D.: Antithrombin-heparin cofactor: An inhibitor of plasma kallikrein. Arch. Biochem. Biophys. *175*, 737–747 (1976)

Levine, B.W., Talamo, R.C., Kazemi, H.: Action and metabolism of bradykinin in the dog lung. J. Appl. Physiol. *34*, 821–826 (1973)

Mashford, M.L., Roberts, M.L.: Determination of human urinary kinin levels by radioimmunoassay using a tyrosine analogue of bradykinin. Biochem. Pharmacol. *20*, 969–973 (1971)

Mashford, M.L., Roberts, M.L.: Determination of blood kinin levels by radioimmunoassay. Biochem. Pharmacol. *21*, 2727–2735 (1972)

Miwa, I., Erdös, E.G., Seki, T.: Presence of three peptides in urinary kinin (substance Z) preparations. Life Sci. II 7, 1339–1343 (1968)

Newball, H.H., Talamo, R.C., Lichtenstein, L.M.: Release of leukocyte kallikrein mediated by IgE. Nature (Lond.) *254*, 635–636 (1975)

O'Donnell, T.F., Jr., Clowes, G.H.A., Jr., Talamo, R.C., Colman, R.W.: Kinin activation in the blood of patients with sepsis. Surg. Gynecol. Obstet. *143*, 539–545 (1976)

Odya, C.E., Goodfriend, T.L., Stewart, J.M., Pena, C.: Aspects of bradykinin radioimmunoassay. J. Immunol. Methods *19*, 243–257 (1978)

Odya, C.E., Goodfriend, T.L., Pena, C., Stewart, J.M.: The use of tyr^1-kallidin, tyr^5-bradykinin, and try^8-bradykinin in the evaluation of bradykinin antisera for use in radioimmunoassay. Life Sci. II *16*, 800–801 (Abstract) (1975)

Pisano, J.J., Austen, K.F. (eds.): Chemistry and biology of the kallikrein-kinin system in health and disease. Washington: U.S. Gov. Printing Office 1977

Reichlin, M., Schnure, J.J., Vance, V.K.: Induction of antibodies to porcine ACTH in rabbits with nonsteroidogenic polymers of BSA and ACTH. Proc. Soc. Exp. Biol. Med. *128*, 347–350 (1968)

Rinderknecht, H., Haverback, B.J., Aladjem, F.: Radioimmunoassay of bradykinin. Nature (Lond.) *213*, 1130–1131 (1967)

Saito, H., Ratnoff, O.: Fitzgerald Trait: An asymptomatic disorder with impaired blood coagulation, fibrinolysis, kinin generation, and generation of permeability factor of dilution. In: Chemistry and biology of the kallikrein-kinin system in health and disease. Pisano, J.J., Austen, K.F. (eds.), pp. 73–74. Washington: U.S. Gov. Printing Office 1977

Sipila, R., Louhija, A.: The application of bradykinin radioimmunoassay to plasma kininogen determination. Biochem. Pharmacol. *25*, 543–545 (1976)
Skowsky, W.R., Fisher, D.A.: The use of the thyroglobulin to induce antigenicity to small molecules. J. Lab. Clin. Med. *80*, 134–144 (1972)
Spragg, J., Austen, K.F., Haber, E.: Production of antibody against bradykinin: Demonstration of specificity by complement fixation and radioimmunoassay. J. Immunol. *96*, 865–871 (1966)
Spragg, J., Talamo, R.C., Wintroub, B.U., Haber, E., Austen, K.F.: Immunoassay for bradykinin and kininogen. In: Methods in immunology and immunochemistry. Williams, C.A., Chase, M.W. (eds.), Vol. 5, pp. 149–157. London, New York: Academic Press 1976
Streeten, D.H.P., Kerr, L.P., Kerr, C.B., Prior, J.C., Dalakos, T.G.: Hyperbradykininism: A new orthostatic syndrome. Lancet *1972/II*, 1048–1053
Talamo, R.C.: Kinetics of kinin release and disappearance. In: Chemistry and biology of the kallikrein-kinin system in health and disease. Pisano, J.J., Austen, K.F. (eds.), pp. 307–312. Washington: U.S. Gov. Printing Office 1977
Talamo, R.C., Haber, E., Austen, K.F.: A radioimmunoassay for bradykinin in plasma and synovial fluid. J. Lab. Clin. Med. *74*, 816–827 (1969)
Webster, M.E., Pierce, J.V., Sampaio, M.U.: Studies on antibody to bradykinin. In: Bradykinin and related kinins: Cardiovascular, biochemical, and neural actions. Sicuteri, F., Rocha e Silva, M., Back, N. (eds.), pp. 57–64. New York, London: Plenum Press 1970
Weese, W.C., Talamo, R.C., Neyhard, N.L., Kazemi, H.: Presence of a bradykinin-like substance in pulmonary washings. Am. Rev. Resp. Dis. *113*, 181–187 (1976)
Weisser, A., Clowes, G.H.A., Colman, R.W., Talamo, R.C.: Sepsis and endotoxemia in pigs: A comparison of mortality and pathophysiology. In: New aspects of trasylol treatment – the lung in shock. Haberland, G.L., Lewis, D.H. (eds.), pp. 159–174. New York: Schappauer 1973
Wong, P. Y., Colman, R. W., Talamo, R. C.: Kallikrein-bradykinin system in chronic alcoholic liver disease. Ann. Int. Med. 77, 205–209 (1972)
Wong, P.Y., Talamo, R.C., Williams, G.H., Colman, R.W.: Response of the kallikrein-kinin and renin-angiotensin systems to saline infusion and upright posture. J. Clin. Invest. *55*, 691–698 (1975)
Wuepper, K.D.: Plasma prekallikrein: Its characterization, mechanism of activation, and inherited deficiency in man. In: Chemistry and biology of the kallikrein-kinin system in health and disease. Pisano, J.J., Austen, K.F. (eds.), pp. 37–51. Washington: U.S. Gov. Printing Office 1977

Kinins and the Peripheral and Central Nervous Systems

W. G. CLARK

A. Introduction

In the previous edition of this section of the Handbook, the primary focus on kinins, with regard to their relationships with the nervous system, was on their ability to stimulate chemoreceptors for pain in animals and especially in man (ARMSTRONG, 1970). Direct application of bradykinin to an exposed cantharidin blister area on the forearm of human subjects causes a slightly delayed, burning type of pain. This reaches maximum in about 1 min and gradually lessens if the kinin is not removed. An after-pain may occur when the kinin is washed from the area. Tachyphylaxis developes with repeated applications at short intervals to the blister area but not usually if pain is induced by administration of kinin by other routes such as by intra-arterial (i.a.) injection. Bradykinin, kallidin, and substance P were the most potent algesic agents evaluated with the cantharidin blister area technique. Burning pain is also evoked in man by intradermal and i.a. injections of bradykinin; i.p. administration causes pain most often described as cramping or colicky (LIM et al., 1967), although the pain was associated with sensations of pressure, distention, or burning in some subjects. The algesic effect of kinins, other peptides and agents such as histamine, acetylcholine, and 5-hydroxytryptamine is thought to be due primarily to stimulation of chemoreceptors on free nerve endings located in the paravascular connective tissue spaces around capillaries and venules (LIM, 1968; ARMSTRONG, 1970). Degeneration after dorsal root ganglionectomy of sensory nerves surrounding small blood vessels has been shown in animals to prevent elicitation of pain by i.a. injections of algesic agents to the denervated limb while sympathectomy, which did not alter the paravascular sensory nerves, had no effect on the response (GUZMAN et al., 1962; LIM, 1968). With few exceptions, when bradykinin is injected i.v., i.m., or s.c., it does not evoke pain (KANTOR et al., 1967; LIM, 1970), apparently because of rapid inactivation before it reaches the appropriate receptors.

KEELE (1969) discussed a number of pathologic states in which kinin formation might contribute to pain or other symptoms and signs. Since then, bradykinin-like material has been detected in fluid obtained from tooth sockets of patients with local inflammation of the bone marrow (BIRN, 1972), and local release has been evoked by electric and other types of stimulation of dentine or tooth pulp in the dog (INOKI et al., 1973; TÜRKER and TÜRKER, 1974; TÜRKER, 1975; KUDO et al., 1975). Other systems in which release of bradykinin-related materials has been suggested or reported include rat paws stimulated by heating (GARCIA LEME et al., 1970) or by pinching and sciatic nerve stimulation (INOKI et al., 1977), ischemic heart or skeletal muscle (BURCH and DEPASQUALE, 1963; SICUTERI et al., 1970; KIMURA et al., 1973; SICUTERI et al., 1974; VECCHIET et al., 1976), and rheumatoid joints (EISEN, 1970).

This chapter will cover primarily the literature reported since the extensive summary by ARMSTRONG (1970) of studies on peripheral aspects of kinin-induced pain. Since then, interest in the role of kinins in pain has focused on interactions between kinins, prostaglandins, and nonsteroidal anti-inflammatory agents and on determination of alterations in neuronal pathways as a result of i.a. administration of kinins. A small number of studies before 1968 dealt with the possibility that kinins exert direct actions within the central nervous system (WALASZEK, 1970). Interest in this area has greatly expanded and will also be discussed.

B. Use of Bradykinin in Conscious Animals for Inducing Pain and for Assessment of Analgesic Activity

As stated by ARMSTRONG (1970), "The verbal report of the subjective experience ... is the fundamental basis for all studies of pain ..." Man, therefore, is especially suitable for detecting and comparing algesic activities of chemical agents. However, various animal models have been useful for screening possible analgesic agents and for studies (1) of interactions of algesic agents with each other and with agents which enhance or antagonize their action, (2) of anatomic pathways involved in transmission of information about painful or other stimuli, (3) of reflexes evoked by these stimuli, etc. Administration of "algesic" agents is assumed to be painful to conscious animals because these same agents cause pain in man, because the responses elicited by these agents can usually be antagonized by drugs which are known to be analgesic in man and, to some extent, because responses of the animals may mimic responses of man to painful stimuli (COLLIER et al., 1968; ARMSTRONG, 1970). Bradykinin has been used as an algesic stimulus in many of these models. The earlier literature has been discussed by ARMSTRONG (1970) and, aspirin in particular, by COLLIER (1969). Conscious animals have been used primarily for screening new analgesic agents or for comparisons with known analgesics. The techniques have the general advantages of being relatively rapid and easy to perform. One problem with animal models has been that they are not entirely specific for analgesic agents. That is, drugs which are not considered to be analgesic in man may still reduce the activity of algesic agents in the model – a "false-positive" result.

Mice given i.p. injections of a variety of agents, including bradykinin, phenylquinone, and acetic acid, respond with "writhing" or "abdominal constriction." For example, mice given 2.5 μg bradykinin in 0.25 ml vehicle responded with "... abdominal torsion, drawing up of the hind legs to the body, marked contraction of the abdominal area and arching of the back ..." (EMELE and SHANAMAN, 1963). Writhing began in only a small percentage of animals within 10 min and in most by 20 min. When known analgesics and nonanalgesics were given orally 10 min prior to bradykinin or phenylquinone, fewer false-positive results were obtained after bradykinin. Examples of the use of this technique for evaluation of analgesic activity include those of EMELE et al. (1966), JULOU et al. (1966), EMELE and SHANAMAN (1967) and BHALLA et al. (1973).

COLLIER et al. (1968) indicated three general disadvantages of such antinociceptive tests involving i.p. injections: (1) multiple episodes of what they preferred to call "abdominal constriction" were excessively time consuming and harmful to the animals, (2) some of the so-called antinociceptive effect might be due to anti-inflammatory activity of some agents and (3) there are many false-positive results. They gave a wide variety of agents i.p. and recorded the percentages of mice which developed at least one abdominal constriction within 30 min. Sham injections and 0.9% saline solution both elicited responses in 23% of mice by 30 min but in only 0% and 2%, respectively, within 2 min of injection. Other vehicles caused even higher percentages of animals to respond progressively with time. On the other hand, a dose of 0.4 mg bradykinin/kg evoked contractions in 70–75% of mice within the first 2 min, after which the percentage responding in any given 2-min period, up to 10 min after injection, markedly declined. The explanation for this marked difference in pattern from that reported by EMELE and SHANAMAN (1963) is unknown. Acetylcholine, ATP, KCl, and tryptamine showed a similar ability to elicit responses within a few minutes of injection with a subsequent rapid reduction in responses. Since these algesic agents were most likely, and the vehicles were least likely, to cause writhing within 2 min of injection, this brief initial period was chosen for evaluation of analgesic activity. When mice were pretreated with known analgesics, the rank orders of analgesic potencies (ED 50) against these five rapidly acting algesic agents were virtually identical when the proportions of mice writhing within 2 min of algesic challenge were compared. Narcotic analgesics were uniformly more potent than anti-inflammatory analgesics. Thus, the primary modification from the technique as used by EMELE and SHANAMAN (1963) was that only responses elicited within the first 2 min of injection of the algesic agent were considered. This reduced the time required for the tests, but it is unlikely to have lessened the stress on the animals since bradykinin still evoked approximately 6 writhes per mouse – the same number reported by EMELE and SHANAMAN (1963). However, inflammation would be less likely to contribute to the algesic effect within 2 min, so that anti-inflammatory actions would probably not contribute significantly to reduction in the number of animals responding. Another advantage was that evocation of responses due to the injection process or to administration of vehicle seldom occurred within the 2-min period of observation. This would reduce the number of false-positive responses. Nevertheless, when acetylcholine was used as the algesic agent (COLLIER et al., 1968) many false-positives were still obtained when 81 agents were examined for their analgesic activity; so this particular problem still remains. Bradykinin was not evaluated against an extensive number of compounds so it is not known if it is a more specific discriminator than acetylcholine for analgesics.

Flexion of extremities following retrograde i.a. administration of bradykinin has also been used to compare analgesics (DEFFENU et al., 1966). Rats were given 0.125–0.5 μg bradykinin via a catheter implanted into the right carotid artery toward the heart. Responses were primarily a dextro-rotatory flexion of the neck and flexion of the right forelimb. These reactions appeared about 7–10 s after injection (BOTHA et al., 1969). The latter authors determined that acetic acid and acetylcholine also evoked flexion but were less potent than bradykinin. Suprathreshold doses of bradykinin could be given at 5-min intervals for 6–8 h without apparent changes in sensitivity, thereby allowing repeated evaluation of analgesic activity after administration of drugs. This technique has been employed in other studies (LUMACHI, 1972; THOMPKINS and LEE, 1975; PIERSON and ROSENBERG, 1976). Rabbits have also been used (DOI et al., 1976). The animal was restrained on its back, and the hindlimb ipsilateral to a femoral catheter was attached to a recording device to allow quantitation of the magnitude of the flexion.

In a brief report, JEZDINSKÝ and HÁLĚK (1974) noted that rats given a subplantar injection of bradykinin exhibited two responses – holding the limb above the surface (flexion), which was attributed to a nociceptive withdrawal reflex, and licking of the site of injection, which was considered an affective response. The recording technique apparently allowed separate quantitation of these responses. Aspirin and indomethacin primarily inhibited the flexion while narcotic analgesics, and also some phenothiazines, significantly decreased only the licking. Thus, this type of test may offer a means of differentiating effects of painful sensation from changes in the reaction to pain. One would expect, however, that a drug which decreased the sensation would secondarily reduce the reaction as well.

Another end point utilized to evaluate algesic and analgesic activity has been vocalization after i.a. injection of bradykinin (GUZMAN et al., 1964; LIM et al., 1964). One disadvantage was that about one-third of adult dogs did not vocalize appropriately (GUZMAN et al., 1964). Puppies responded more uniformly to injection of algesics into mesenteric or femoral arteries (TAIRA et al., 1968). Bradykinin and eledoisin were more potent than histamine, acetylcholine, or barium chloride while 5-hydroxytryptamine was ineffective. 5-Hydroxytryptamine potentiated somewhat the activity of acetylcholine and bradykinin (NAKANO and TAIRA, 1976). Synthetic fragments of the bradykinin molecule were also inactive (TAIRA and HASHIMOTO, 1973).

C. Cardiovascular Reflex Responses in Anesthetized Animals After Administration of Bradykinin

While rapid, easily performed tests with conscious animals have been useful in screening assays, determination of changes in systemic arterial blood pressure, usually in anesthetized animals, has been widely used for studies of physiologic and anatomic aspects of pain mechanisms. Administration of bradykinin and other algesic agents, i.a., to lightly anesthetized animals can evoke a number of reflex responses, including vocalization, hyperpnea, and usually hypertension (GUZMAN et al., 1962). These are not unlike some reactions of conscious animals (LIM et al., 1964) and constitute the reflex component of the response to pain according to LIM (1960). These reflexes can be elicited in decerebrate animals and have been termed "pseudaffective" (WOODWORTH and SHERRINGTON, 1904). It should be remembered that the kinins are also very potent vasodilators and cause hypotension when given i.v. The fall in blood pressure is sometimes followed by hypertension (HADDY et al., 1970). The only venous locations at which GUZMAN et al. (1962) were able to elicit pseudaffective responses were the splenic and portal veins.

When FERREIRA et al. (1973) injected bradykinin (0.05–10 μg) into a cannulated branch of the splenic artery in the dog, a dose-related increase in blood pressure occurred provided an optimal level of anesthesia was maintained. If anesthesia was excessive, no response to bradykinin developed. If anesthesia was too light, a dose-response relationship was not obtained. The pressor response began within 3–20 s after injection, and the latency was inversely related to the dose. RICCIOPPO NETO et al. (1974) also noted hypertension after intrasplenic injections of bradykinin.

Although GUZMAN et al. (1962) injected algesic agents via many different arterial routes, qualitatively similar responses, usually including hypertension, were obtained regardless of the specific route in their chloralose-anesthetized animals. However, there have been several reports of hypotensive or biphasic blood pressure changes after i.a. injection of bradykinin. These responses have been shown in many studies to be mediated by the autonomic nervous system and are not elicited by i.v. administration of the same amounts of bradykinin. RICCIOPPO NETO et al. (1974) produced only hypotension in dogs by intrafemoral injections of up to 40 μg bradykinin. Cats given 1–3 μg developed transient hypotension (DAMAS, 1974), sometimes followed by hypertension and agitation. Unanesthetized rabbits given very small doses of bradykinin (100–400 ng) intrafemorally developed a transient hypotension accompanied by bradycardia (TALLARIDA et al., 1974a, 1976). This was followed by hypertension and tachycardia. The latter phase could be selectively blocked by anesthesia which prolonged the duration of the hypotensive phase.

Bradykinin has also been injected into the carotid artery in many studies. There is no reason to believe that such injections would not stimulate paravascular pain receptors just as do injections into other arteries (GUZMAN et al., 1962). In addition, there is the possibility of a direct action on the central nervous system. However, a peptide such as bradykinin would not be expected to diffuse through the blood-brain barrier (DAMAS, 1971). BUMPUS et al. (1964) found some evidence of bradykinin in the brain of rats at the end of a 20-min infusion, but, unless bradykinin is actively transported, it is unlikely that there is significant penetration of the blood-brain barrier during the brief exposure to a high concentration after intracarotid injection. The blood pressure of cats given 10 μg doses of bradykinin or kallidin via this route primarily increased although initial hypotension was evoked in some tests (LANG and PEARSON, 1968; PEARSON et al., 1969). Eledoisin (0.1–10 μg) caused only hypotension (PEARSON et al., 1969). PEARSON and LANG (1969) were usually unable to block the pressor response to bradykinin in anesthetized cats and dogs, or in conscious dogs, with doses of aspirin or morphine which did antagonize bradykinin injected into the femoral artery (GUZMAN et al., 1964). PEARSON and LANG concluded, therefore, that the entire pressor response could not be pseudaffective and that part must be due to more direct stimulation of central control mechanisms. In the rat, to the contrary, indomethacin effectively antagonized both depressor and pressor responses to bradykinin (DAMAS, 1975). Just as after intrafemoral injection, DAMAS (1974) noted, in the cat, transient hypotension followed by hypertension and tachypnea, plus increased motor activity on the side of injection indicative of the pseudaffective response. TALLARIDA et al. (1974b) also obtained responses in conscious rabbits similar to those after intrafemoral administration; namely biphasic responses, the hypertensive phase of which was reduced by anesthesia. Bradykinin was more potent by the carotid than by the femoral route in both the cat (DAMAS, 1974) and rabbit (TALLARIDA et al., 1974a, b).

Anesthetized dogs given retrograde injections of 10–40 μg bradykinin into the carotid artery via the lingual artery exhibited bradycardia and systemic hypotension (RICCIOPPO NETO et al., 1974). The development of hypotension, rather than hypertension as obtained by GUZMAN et al. (1962), was attributed to a deeper level of anesthesia and possibly to some direct peripheral vasodilation after recirculation of the kinin. However, even dogs lightly anesthetized with thiopental became hypotensive after bradykinin (1 μg/kg) (CORRADO et al., 1974). Perhaps barbiturates more effectively inhibit the pressor activity than does chloralose. Responses to bradykinin were enhanced when the maxillary arteries were tied off to deliver a higher concentration into the occipital and internal carotid arteries. Furthermore, apnea occurred, and contractions of neck muscles caused flexion of the neck similar to that seen in unanesthetized rats (DEFFENU et al., 1966). Kallidin produced similar effects (RICCIOPPO NETO et al., 1970). Occlusion of the internal carotid artery in addition, which diverted bradykinin into the occipital artery and away from the central nervous system, did not diminish these responses so that they were not likely to be due to direct central nervous system stimulation. This idea was reinforced by observations that 5-hydroxytryptamine, which also does not penetrate the blood-brain barrier, potentiated bradykinin and that effects of bradykinin injection on one side of the brain could be selectively reduced by ipsilateral treatments with capsaicin which desensitizes pain receptors (KEELE and ARMSTRONG, 1964; SZOLCSÁNYI, 1977). Intravertebral arterial injection of bradykinin caused less intense effects than intracarotid injection. Pseudaffective responses could even be evoked in some animals by applying bradykinin to the dura mater.

JUAN and LEMBECK (1974) began an extensive series of studies on bradykinin with an isolated, perfused rabbit ear preparation. With the exception of the great auricular nerve which was left intact, the ear was separated from the anesthetized body. Carotid arterial pressure was recorded, and changes in vascular resistance within the ear were determined by measurement of venous outflow. Intra-arterial injections into the ear of substance P from bovine gut, bradykinin, synthetic substance P, acetylcholine, ATP, histamine, 5-hydroxytryptamine, and KCl, listed in order of decreasing potency, elicited reflex falls in systemic blood pressure. Responses to the peptides and 5-hydroxytryptamine began 4–10 s after injection and lasted longer than those after acetylcholine, ATP and KCl which had even shorter latencies. This preparation was stable for many hours, and tachyphylaxis did not occur with repeated injections. Brief bradycardia, changes in respiration and muscle contractions, especially in the neck, also occurred, particularly with higher doses. The level of anesthesia did not greatly affect the sensitivity of this preparation to these agents. The responses were attributed to stimulation of pain receptors since similar results could be elicited by heating or squeezing but not by merely touching or altering vasomotor tone in the ear (LEMBECK, 1957). All the agents listed above decreased venous outflow from the ear, indicative of local vasoconstriction, but this constriction did not evoke the systemic hypotension because it usually began later and showed no particular quantitative relationship to the change in systemic blood pressure.

Although depth of anesthesia cannot be the sole determinent of the type of cardiovascular response to bradykinin, the general pattern of response to i.a. administration which emerges in conscious or lightly anesthetized animals is the development of primarily pressor responses and tachycardia accompanied by vocalization, hyperpnea, and general struggling or flexion of muscles vascularized by the specific arterial tree. In some animals a transient hypotension precedes the hypertension. With increasing depth of anesthesia, pressor responses lessen as depressor responses and bradycardia become more prominent or become the only cardiovascular changes induced. Other factors which may contribute to the variability between results from different laboratories are the bradykinin dosage, the specific arterial route of administration, the specific anesthetic used, and species differences.

Injection of 0.5–10 μg bradykinin into knee joints of lightly anesthetized dogs evoked a dose-related increase in blood pressure within 7–40 s (MONCADA et al., 1975). The rate and depth of respiration increased as well. Evocation of reproducible responses required that Tris buffer or saline solution be infused into the joint cavity for 1–3 h before testing. As with the spleen (FERREIRA et al., 1973), excessive anesthesia abolished the pressor response. KCl, but not epinephrine or vehicle, also increased blood pressure.

The same group (STASZEWSKA-BARCZAK et al., 1976) has described a preparation in which topical application of bradykinin (0.02–1 μg) to the left ventricular epicardium of dogs elicited tachycardia and dose-related pressor responses. Both of these effects were due primarily to reflex sympathetic activity as evidenced by antagonism of the tachycardia by propranolol or spinal section at C 1, with or without vagotomy, and antagonism of the pressor response by phenoxybenzamine or spinal section (STASZEWSKA-BARCZAK and DUSTING, 1977).

D. Interactions Between Bradykinin and Prostaglandins

I. Algesic Effects of Prostaglandins

A totally new development since 1970 in the area of pain research has been the discovery that prostaglandins, primarily of the E series, can enhance a variety of painful stimuli (FERREIRA et al., 1974; FERREIRA and VANE, 1974; VANE, 1976). By themselves prostaglandins or related agents have been reported to cause writhing when given i.p. to mice (COLLIER et al., 1968; COLLIER and SCHNEIDER, 1972), to incapacitate dogs after injection into knee joints (ROSENTHALE et al., 1972), to increase the rate of discharge of single cutaneous C fibers from the heated hindpaw of the cat (HANDWERKER, 1976), to cause headache when infused i.v. in man (BERGSTRÖM et al., 1959) and to induce local pain in human subjects after i.v. (COLLIER et al., 1972; GILLESPIE, 1972), i.m. (KARIM, 1971), or intradermal administration or after application to the cantharidin blister area (FERREIRA, 1972).

On the other hand, when prostaglandins are given in small doses or concentrations likely to be present in vivo, they do not usually evoke responses indicative of pain (HORTON, 1963; CRUNKHORN and WILLIS, 1971; FERREIRA, 1972; FERREIRA et al., 1973; FERREIRA and VANE, 1974; JUAN and LEMBECK, 1974; SZOLCSÁNYI, 1977).

II. Enhancement of Bradykinin Potency by Co-Administration of Prostaglandins

The general topics of hyperalgesia and sensitization of tissues to kinins by other agents, such as 5-hydroxytryptamine, were discussed by ARMSTRONG (1970). Prostaglandins, in amounts too small to evoke pain or reflex responses alone, can also cause a state of hyperalgesia in which the potency of algesic stimuli is enhanced or in which usually non-noxious stimuli become painful. For instance, increased sensitivity to mechanical stimuli, associated with erythema or slight swelling, after local administration of prostaglandins has been reported in man (SOLOMON et al., 1968;

JUHLIN and MICHAËLSSON, 1969) and rats (WILLIS and CORNELSEN, 1973). FERREIRA (1972) found that 30-min subdermal infusions into the volar surface of the arm of certain concentrations of prostaglandin E_1 (PGE_1) or bradykinin did not consistently induce pain in man. However, infusions of the two agents in the same concentrations combined did cause moderate to strong pain which became continuous near the end of the infusion period. The possibility of an additive effect of subthreshold concentrations of both agents was not ruled out. Gradually increasing pain was also evoked if bradykinin was infused for 10 min into an area which had received a 30-min infusion of PGE_1 shortly before.

Several cardiovascular reflexes (Sect. C) have been used to study interactions between bradykinin and prostaglandins. In dogs, simultaneous injections or infusions of PGE_1 into the splenic artery enhanced and hastened the pressor response to bradykinin (FERREIRA et al., 1973). Prostaglandin alone either did not alter or slightly lowered blood pressure. Similar results were obtained with epicardial application of bradykinin and E-type prostaglandins (STASZEWSKA-BARCZAK et al., 1976). $PGF_{2\alpha}$ did not potentiate bradykinin. Reflex tachycardia was not altered by any of the prostaglandins.

Intra-arterial infusion of PGE_1 at concentrations up to 200 ng/ml into the rabbit ear preparation, isolated from the body except for the auricular nerve, did not lower systemic blood pressure (JUAN and LEMBECK, 1974). However, infusion of only 50 ng PGE_1/ml enhanced the ability of bradykinin and other agents to elicit a hypotensive response. The order of potentiation by prostaglandin was bradykinin (more than 10 fold) $\geqq$ substance P from bovine gut $>$ 5-hydroxytryptamine $>$ histamine $\geqq$ acetylcholine $>$ ATP $>$ KCl. The degree of enhancement increased with the duration of the infusion and reached maximum after 20–30 min with this concentration of PGE_1. Even 10 ng PGE_1/ml caused an equivalent potentiation if perfursion was continued for 2 or more hours. Again, reflex hypotension was not related to vasoconstriction in the ear since local vasoconstriction in response to the algesic agents was reduced or abolished during prostaglandin infusion while at the same time reflex hypotensive activity increased. In subsequent studies (see below), these authors have compared further the interactions of bradykinin and acetylcholine with prostaglandins. In their initial study, acetylcholine was potentiated about half as much as bradykinin by PGE_1. On the other hand, infusion of low doses of $PGF_{2\alpha}$ delayed the depressor response and reduced the potency of bradykinin but not of acetylcholine (JUAN and LEMBECK, 1977). Higher concentrations of 50 ng $PGF_{2\alpha}$/ml reversed the potentiation of both bradykinin and acetylcholine by 10 ng PGE_1/ml when these prostaglandins were infused simultaneously.

III. Release of Prostaglandins by Bradykinin

Potentiation by prostaglandins of the E series is likely to be of considerable importance in contributing to the algesic action of bradykinin because bradykinin causes the release of prostaglandins and related substances in many systems (TERRAGNO and TERRAGNO, this volume). Intra-arterial injection of 5–10 µg bradykinin into the dog spleen was followed by release of a PGE-like material assayed on a series of tissues bathed in the venous outflow from the spleen (FERREIRA et al., 1973).

JUAN and LEMBECK (1976a) obtained similar results with the isolated rabbit ear. The venous effluent, to which antagonists to acetylcholine, histamine, 5-hydroxytryptamine, and adrenergic agents had been added, was used to superfuse rat stomach strips (assay for prostaglandins of the E type) and rat colon (assay for prostaglandins of the F type). Effluent after i.a. injection of bradykinin contracted the stomach strip more than did direct application to the strip of the same amount of bradykinin, indicative of release of PGE-like material. The colon strip showed no response to the effluent so no F-type prostaglandin was detected. In contrast to bradykinin, little or no prostaglandin-like activity was found after acetylcholine administration. These experiments were later extended with the use of a radioimmunoassay for prostaglandin (LEMBECK et al., 1976). Injection of 0.3–10 μg bradykinin elicited dose-related release of PGE. A second dose 4 h later released much more PGE than did the first. Dose-related release of smaller amounts of PGF was also detected. Acetylcholine released half or less of the maximum amount of PGE liberated by an equipotent (hypotensive) dose of bradykinin, and synthetic substance P did not release any detectable prostaglandin. Release by bradykinin of PGE from chronically denervated ears was comparable to that from innervated ears. Release of prostaglandin-like materials by bradykinin has also been demonstrated in a wide variety of other preparations (TERRAGNO and TERRAGNO, this volume).

DAMAS and DEBY (1976) suggested that bradykinin may act early in the prostaglandin synthesis cascade (see TERRAGNO and TERRAGNO, Fig. 1, this volume) to increase the availability of fatty acid precursors, such as arachidonate. In their study with perfused rat lung, bradykinin released not only prostaglandins but also the precursors, and this release was inhibited by chloroquine, an agent previously reported to inhibit lipase activity (MARKUS and BALL, 1969). Studies with the isolated rabbit ear by JUAN (1977 a) showed that perfusion with another phospholipase inhibitor, quinacrine or mepacrine, almost completely prevented bradykinin-induced release of prostaglandin and reduced release after phospholipase A_2 administration to about half. It did not significantly decrease release of prostaglandin by arachidonic acid. JUAN concluded that bradykinin activates phospholipase A_2, thereby increasing the availability of precursors for conversion to prostaglandins, etc. If bradykinin acted further downstream to stimulate cyclo-oxygenase, prostaglandin synthetase, etc., it should not have been antagonized by quinacrine since arachidonic acid was not antagonized. Indomethacin, which reduces the synthesis from fatty acids of the cyclic endoperoxide precursors of prostaglandins (FLOWER, 1974), did prevent arachidonate-induced release of PGE as expected. Quinacine perfusion also markedly reduced the reflex hypotensive effects of bradykinin and acetylcholine (JUAN, 1977 b). Responses to bradykinin were restored by simultaneous infusion of PGE_1, while responses to acetylcholine were only partially restored.

It is, therefore, well established that bradykinin can release prostaglandins which in turn can potentiate the kinin. GUZMAN et al. (1962) noted that the latency for bradykinin-induced responses was quite long and suggested that this might partially be due to changes prior to excitation of the receptor.

IV. Inhibition of Bradykinin-Induced Effects by Nonsteroidal Anti-Inflammatory Agents and Prostaglandin Antagonists

It has long been known that aspirin and related agents can antagonize the algesic action of bradykinin (ARMSTRONG, 1970). Bradykinin was used in cross-perfusion studies by LIM et al. (1964) to show that aspirin can act peripherally to prevent vocalization while morphine and related agents did not exert a significant analgesic action peripherally. After the initial discoveries that aspirin and other nonsteroidal anti-inflammatory agents inhibited the synthesis of prostaglandins (FERREIRA et al., 1971; SMITH and WILLIS, 1971; VANE, 1971), VANE (1971) proposed that the anti-inflammatory, analgesic, and antipyretic actions of these drugs might all be the result of such inhibition.

1. Inhibition of Prostaglandin Release

Splenic venous blood from the anesthetized dog contained a small amount of prostaglandin-like material as indicated by the rat stomach strip (FERREIRA et al., 1973) whereas femoral arterial blood did not. Intravenous administration of 2–4 mg indomethacin/kg abolished the basal release of prostaglandin-like material and reduced or prevented release by bradykinin. Doses of indomethacin as low as 50–100 μg/kg partially blocked release by bradykinin. Likewise i.a. infusion of 1–5 μg indomethacin/ml virtually abolished bradykinin-induced release of PGE-like material from the isolated rabbit ear (JUAN and LEMBECK, 1976a; LEMBECK et al., 1976). Antagonism of bradykinin-induced prostaglandin release has also been reported in a number of other systems including guinea pig lung (PALMER et al., 1973) and rabbit heart (NEEDLEMAN et al., 1975; NEEDLEMAN, 1976). Inhibition by aspirin of release of bradykinin itself has been proposed by INOKI et al. (1973), KUDO et al. (1975) and INOKI et al. (1977). However, since the release of bradykinin was determined by bioassay, it is possible that the decrease in activity of the perfusates was due to reduced synthesis of prostaglandins (TÜRKER and TÜRKER, 1974) and, therefore, decreased sensitivity of the assay system to bradykinin.

2. Inhibition of Other Bradykinin-Induced Effects

Pretreatment with i.v. injections of 1–5 mg indomethacin/kg reduced pressor responses to injection of bradykinin into dog spleen (FERREIRA et al., 1973). The lower doses of bradykinin were inhibited by a greater percentage. The potency of bradykinin could be restored at least partially by infusion of exogenous PGE. Since responses to bradykinin were not abolished by doses of indomethacin which abolished release of prostaglandin-like material from the spleen, the authors concluded that release of prostaglandin did not *mediate* the algesic action of bradykinin but rather *sensitized* the receptors to bradykinin. Very similar results were obtained with the reflex rabbit ear preparation (LEMBECK and JUAN, 1974). Intra-arterial infusions of 1–25 μg indomethacin/ml produced dose-related reductions in the hypotensive potency of bradykinin injected into the ear. Substance P and acetylcholine were also antagonized but to lesser degrees. Thus bradykinin, which was potentiated more by exogenous PGE_1 (JUAN and LEMBECK, 1974) and was more potent in releasing prostaglandin (LEMBECK et al., 1976), was more effectively antagonized by indomethacin, as one would predict. It should, perhaps, be noted that bradykinin and acetylcholine are acting on different receptors (COLLIER et al., 1968; JUAN and LEMBECK, 1975; LEMBECK and JUAN, 1977). To continue, the magnitude of antagonism of the algesic agents by indomethacin increased with the duration of its infusion (LEMBECK and JUAN, 1974). After the infusion was stopped, the duration required for recovery of the response to bradykinin was directly related to the degree of antagonism (i.e., to both the concentration of indomethacin and the duration of infusion). As in dog spleen, conditions which abolished release of prostaglandin by bradykinin (1 μg indomethacin/ml for 20 min – LEMBECK et al., 1976) did not abolish the hypotensive response but simply reduced the potency of bradykinin, indicative of a desensitization. Infusion of exogenous PGE_1 along with indomethacin for a sufficient length of time not only restored the potency of bradykinin but even enhanced its activity, just as in an ear not treated with indomethacin. Thus the primary effect of indomethacin in these experiments was a reduction in release of prostaglandin and, therefore, a decrease in sensitivity to bradykinin. LEMBECK and JUAN (1974) also presented evidence of a more direct, but minor, action of indomethacin to antagonize either the prostaglandin or bradykinin.

JUAN and LEMBECK (1976b) produced a dose-related inhibition of the reflex hypotensive response to bradykinin, and a considerably less effective antagonism of acetylcholine, by infusion of a prostaglandin antagonist, polyphoretin phosphate. As with indomethacin, the degree of antagonism was related to the duration of the infusion. As expected of an agent that antagonizes prostaglandin, rather than inhibiting its synthesis, polyphoretin phosphate infusion also reversed potentiation of bradykinin by an infusion of PGE_1.

The inhibitory effect of low concentrations of $PGF_{1\alpha}$ on the activity of bradykinin (JUAN and LEMBECK, 1977) disappeared when endogenous release of PGE was inhibited by indomethacin. Therefore, these low concentrations apparently antagonized PGE sensitization to bradykinin and did not antagonize bradykinin per se. Thus the relative concentrations of F- and E-type prostaglandins released by various stimuli may be an important factor in determining the intensity of the response. Interestingly, a large dose of $PGF_{2\alpha}$ given during indomethacin infusion potentiated bradykinin action.

Infusion of indomethacin or aspirin into knee joints of dogs greatly reduced the potency of bradykinin, as indicated by reduction of the reflex pressor response (MONCADA et al., 1975). As usual, the sensitivity to bradykinin was restored by addition to the infusion of PGE_1 or E_2, but not $PGF_{2\alpha}$.

Transient myocardial ischemia produced in the dog by occlusion of a branch of coronary artery enhanced the pressor response to epicardial application of bradykinin (STASZEWSKA-BARCZAK et al., 1976). Indomethacin decreased such pressor responses to bradykinin and also abolished potentiation by ischemia.

Injection of bradykinin into the femoral artery of the rabbit increased the firing rate of cells in the dorsal horn (SATOH et al., 1976). This effect was inhibited by i.v. administration of indomethacin, aspirin, aminopyrine, and oxyphenbutazone in spinal as well as intact animals, indicative of a peripheral site of action.

Antagonism of miscellaneous bradykinin-induced responses by nonsteroidal anti-inflammatory agents has also been reported by VARGAFTIG (1966), BALDONI et al. (1974), DAMAS (1975), and NEEDLEMAN et al. (1975).

V. Conclusions

There is now considerable evidence that prostaglandins of the E series sensitize tissues to the action of algesic agents, especially bradykinin. Furthermore, bradykinin releases prostaglandins, thereby enhancing its algesic effect. The study by JUAN and LEMBECK (1977), however, suggests that the algesic potency of bradykinin is related to the relative release of prostaglandins with opposing actions. Much of the antagonism of bradykinin by nonsteroidal anti-inflammatory agents, of which primarily indomethacin and aspirin have been studied, can be attributed to inhibition of prostaglandin synthesis. When bradykinin is applied to the cantharidin blister area in man, it causes a somewhat delayed, slowly increasing pain (ARMSTRONG, 1970). This gradual increase in pain may reflect increasing synthesis of prostaglandin enhancing the sensitivity of the receptors. On the other hand, ARMSTRONG (1970) has observed that aspirin does not block bradykinin-induced pain in this preparation.

It should be mentioned here that the nonsteroidal anti-inflammatory agents which have also been called prostaglandin synthetase inhibitors do not specifically inhibit prostaglandin synthesis (FLOWER, 1974; VANE, 1978). Instead they inhibit the cyclo-oxygenase which is responsible for formation of cyclic endoperoxides from arachidonic and other fatty acids. Therefore, these drugs reduce synthesis not only of prostaglandins but also of more recently discovered derivatives such as thromboxanes and prostacyclin (PGI_2) (VANE, 1978; TERRAGNO and TERRAGNO, this volume). These other products, which are much less stable, are considerably more potent than prostaglandins in several systems. For instance, prostacyclin is 20–30 times more potent than PGE_1 in inhibiting human platelet aggregation. Thus, some of these other derivatives may turn out to be more important than prostaglandins in enhancing or antagonizing the algesic activity of bradykinin. In line with this idea is a recent report that prostacyclin can enhance the increases in capillary permeability produced by bradykinin in rabbit skin (PECK and WILLIAMS, 1978).

E. Neurophysiologic Studies in Which Bradykinin was Used as the Initial Stimulus

Since bradykinin is such a potent algesic agent, it should be especially useful for examination of pathways involved in transmission of information about painful chemical stimuli. All recording of neuronal activity in these studies was done extracellularly, and bradykinin was administered i.a. unless otherwise indicated.

I. Paravascular Pain Receptors

LIM (1968) and ARMSTRONG (1970) have discussed evidence that chemical agents which cause pain act on chemoreceptors associated with sensory neurons in the connective tissue spaces around capillaries and venules. LIM preferred the term chemoceptor to nociceptor because nociceptor, nociceptive, etc. imply injury which does not have to occur for chemical agents such as bradykinin to evoke pain, pseudaffective responses, etc. BOTHA et al. (1969) noted that when small doses of bradykinin were injected into the right carotid artery of rats, the typical flexion of the neck and ipsilateral forelimb could be evoked at 5-min intervals for several hours. The lack of tachyphylaxis or sensitization was interpreted as indicative of chemoreceptor stimulation. Actual injury would be expected to alter sensitivity to algesic agents. Consistent responses to repeated i.a. injections of bradykinin have been reported in many other studies, such as that of JUAN and LEMBECK (1974).

KHAYUTIN et al. (1976) perfused the vasculature of the small intestine of the cat, leaving the nerves intact. Perfusion of the gut with very low concentrations of many agents caused small increases in systemic blood pressure which they attributed to non-nociceptive stimulation of chemoreceptors on nerve endings. However, when the concentration of some agents was increased past a certain level, 0.5 μg/ml for bradykinin, much larger pressor responses occurred, and the log dose-response curve became much steeper. These larger responses were considered the result of nociceptive reflexes, probably due to direct stimulation of axons themselves rather than specific chemoreceptors.

About 7 s after injection of bradykinin (100–250 ng) into a femoral artery, the blood pressure of unanesthetized rabbits fell, and heart rate slowed (TALLARIDA et al., 1976). This response, which lasted less than 10 s, was immediately followed by hypertension, tachycardia and behavioral responses indicative of pain. Anesthesia reduced the second phase and enhanced the initial hypotension. Injection of acidic solutions or hypertonic solutions of NaCl or glucose, which are known to cause pain in man (KEELE and ARMSTRONG, 1964), caused responses similar to the second phase after bradykinin. TALLARIDA et al. (1976) proposed the existence of selective and sensitive K- (for kinin) receptors, stimulation of which caused the initial depressor phase, and P- (for pain) receptors, stimulation of which caused the pressor phase.

II. Primary Afferent Fibers

Primary afferents have been classified into several groups on the basis of their size, conduction velocity, myelination or lack of it, and whether they innervate receptors in skin, viscera or muscle (WILLIS and GROSSMAN, 1977). Afferents from muscle have been subdivided into groups I–IV and those from skin and viscera into Aβ, Aδ, and C. Group I fibers are the largest myelinated fibers with conduction velocities of 72–120 m/s. Group II and Aβ fibers have conduction velocities of 36–72 m/s, while Group III and Aδ fibers are the smallest myelinated fibers with conduction velocities of 6–36 m/s. Group IV and C fibers are unmyelinated with conduction velocities generally less than 2 m/s. The neurophysiology of nociceptors has recently been discussed by IGGO (1976), ZIMMERMAN (1976), and PRICE and DUBNER (1977). Neurons primarily concerned with nociception in the skin include high threshold Aδ mechanoreceptive and heat nociceptive afferents. These afferents have relatively small receptive fields and contribute to so-called fast (first) pain which is well localized. C polymodal nociceptive afferents, which make up a high proportion of the total C fibers, have high thresholds to mechanical and thermal stimuli and can also respond to topical application of irritant chemicals. These fibers mediate slow (second), burning pain which is not as well localized. Fibers of the same sizes also contribute to pain sensation from viscera and muscle. The observations that application of acetylcholine to the cantharidin blister base in man evokes an immediate "smarting pain" while bradykinin and 5-hydroxytryptamine elicit a slightly delayed, duller burning pain (ARMSTRONG, 1970) suggest that transmission of the response to acetylcholine may be via Aδ fibers while the response to the others is carried primarily by C fibers. However, as shown below, this is not necessarily the case.

All of the agents, including bradykinin, which caused reflex hypotension when injected into the isolated, perfused rabbit ear also elicited asynchronous action po-

Table 1. Excitation of primary afferent fibers in cats by close i.a. injection of algesic agents

Fiber type	Algesic agent	Total units tested	Percent excited	Reference
Aβ[a]	Bradykinin	30	30	BECK and HANDWERKER (1974)
	5-Hydroxytryptamine	30	37	
Aδ[a]	Bradykinin	17	53	
	5-Hydroxytryptamine	17	59	
C	Bradykinin	68	51	
	5-Hydroxytryptamine	54	44	
IV	Bradykinin	184	48	FRANZ and MENSE (1975)
IV	5-Hydroxytryptamine	131	44	FOCK and MENSE (1976)
	Histamine	37	51	
	KCl	98	42	
IV	One or more of the above		46	MENSE (1977a)
III	One or more of the above	63	71	
II	One or more of the above	33	0	
I	One or more of the above	51	4	

[a] From slowly adapting mechanoreceptors only.

tentials in the great auricular nerve (JUAN and LEMBECK, 1974). Physalaemin, eledoisin, and a variety of other agents including PGE_1, epinephrine, and vasopressin were inactive. Since the latter two agents greatly reduced venous outflow from the ear, the increase in neural discharge after bradykinin, etc. was clearly not secondary to vasoconstriction. In line with the biphasic change in blood pressure of unanesthetized rabbits after i.a. administration of bradykinin, TALLARIDA et al. (1976) noted that weak stimulation of the central end of somatic nerves usually causes the blood pressure to fall while stronger stimulation tends to raise the pressure. They cite the literature indicating that the former response may result from stimulation of small myelinated fibers and the latter response primarily from unmyelinated fibers.

Studies on excitation of single cutaneous and muscle afferents by bradykinin in anesthetized, immobilized cats are summarized in Table 1. Fiber types were determined by their conduction velocities. BECK and HANDWERKER (1974) compared the effects of 5–10 μg bradykinin with up to 30 μg 5-hydroxytryptamine on fibers from cutaneous nerves in the hind leg. Both bradykinin and 5-hydroxytryptamine, but not the vehicle, excited fibers of all types present in these nerves. However, a smaller proportion of Aβ fibers was activated, and Aβ and Aδ fibers innervating rapidly adapting receptors were not excited. When spike discharges of individual fibers to 10 μg doses of bradykinin and 5-hydroxytryptamine were compared in random order, about half of the myelinated fibers were more sensitive to bradykinin and the other half to 5-hydroxytryptamine. However, bradykinin was the more potent in over two-thirds of the unmyelinated fibers. Spike discharges began 10–20 s after the start of injection and peaked from 20–60 s. Tachyphylaxis, but not cross-tachyphylaxis, occurred with repeated injection, just as after repeated application of bradykinin or 5-hydroxytryptamine to a cantharidin blister area (ARMSTRONG, 1970). Bradykinin, but not 5-hydroxytryptamine, enhanced discharges of C fibers evoked by 10-s periods of heating the skin to 45 °C. HANDWERKER (1976) studied further the effect of bradykinin on the activity of C fibers which were stimulated by radiant heat. In one example, after tachyphylaxis had been produced, injection of bradykinin during an i.v. infusion of PGE_1 stimulated even more than the initial injection. Infusion or intracutaneous injection of PGE also enhanced the response of such fibers to stepwise heating.

MENSE and his co-workers have studied the effects of algesic agents on units from the gastrocnemius-soleus muscle. Potentials were recorded from fine strands of dorsal roots (L6-S1) or from the sciatic nerve in the upper thigh. At rest most group IV fibers fired irregularly at less than 3 impulses/s, and 64% were excited mechanically by vigorous squeezing of the tissues, not by stretching or simply touching (FRANZ and MENSE, 1975). Injections of bradykinin into the sural artery excited nearly half of the units examined whether they responded to vigorous or light squeezing or did not respond to either. When the usual dose of 26 µg bradykinin was given, the latency before increased discharge averaged 10 s, and the firing rate was elevated for 40 s. Infusions of the same concentration of bradykinin did not cause sustained increases in discharge activity. However, recovery of sensitivity to injection of bradykinin was fairly rapid after the infusion was stopped. Local application of bradykinin directly onto dissected fibers, onto intact muscle nerves or onto the muscle surface only rarely excited fibers which were sensitive to i.a. injections, seemingly ruling out the axons as the site of action. When bradykinin was injected i.m. in the vicinity of a unit stimulated by the injection needle, relatively long-lasting (40–1180 s) responses were obtained. However, in the only example shown, the maximum rate was only 2 impulses/s, much less than the maximum after i.a. injection of the same concentration. To determine if vasomotor changes could evoke responses similar to those after bradykinin, the vasodilator nylidrine and the vasoconstrictor norepinephrine were injected i.a. These had little or no effect on the rate of discharge. 5-Hydroxytryptamine, histamine, and KCl also excited group IV fibers (Table 1, FOCK and MENSE, 1976). KCl had the shortest mean latency (3 s) and duration (8 s). After 5-hydroxytryptamine and KCl a period of depression often followed excitation. Mean threshold doses of 2.6 µg for bradykinin, 30 µg for 5-hydroxytryptamine creatinine sulfate, 75 µg for histamine dihydrochloride, and 3.6 mg for KCl were in quite good agreement with those reported for hyperpnea after i.a. injection into the spleen of the dog (GUZMAN et al., 1962). The dose of KCl was so high that FOCK and MENSE postulated an unspecific depolarization by this agent. If this were the case, one would expect that a higher percentage or even all of the fibers would have been stimulated. Perhaps a still higher concentration of KCl would have done so. The chemoreceptive units did not respond uniformly to the different algesic agents. Responses to 5-hydroxytryptamine were evoked in only 20 of 42 units which responded to bradykinin, while histamine excited only 9 of 15 units sensitive to bradykinin. The authors note that of these agents, probably only bradykinin reaches concentrations in vivo comparable to those achieved by the i.a. injections. Tachyphylaxis occurred when 5-hydroxytryptamine, but not bradykinin, was injected at 1–2 min intervals (HISS and MENSE, 1976). Units rendered insensitive to 5-hydroxytryptamine still responded to bradykinin. MENSE (1977a) extended his studies to group I, II, and III muscle afferents. The patterns of the responses of group III fibers were similar in latency and duration to the patterns evoked by the specific agents in group IV afferents. Repeated injections of bradykinin at 4-min intervals did not cause tachyphylaxis.

Group III fibers were somewhat more sensitive to bradykinin in that the usual dose elicited 60% more impulses than in group IV afferents. Furthermore, a higher percentage of group III afferents responded to one or more of the algesic agents. Group I and group II fibers, which were excited by i.a. administration of succinylcholine and which were spontaneously active before injections, tended to be depressed, if anything, by the algesic agents. Thus, unlike slowly adapting Aβ fibers from cutaneous nerves (BECK and HANDWERKER, 1974), class II fibers from skeletal muscle are apparently not excited by algesic agents. A brief summary of these studies has recently been presented by MENSE (1977b).

Topical application of bradykinin to the heart has also been reported to excite mechanoreceptive afferents in cardiac sympathetic nerves (UCHIDA and MURAO, 1974; NISHI et al., 1977). In the latter study some of the units were identified as Aß fibers.

Thus, in agreement with current concepts of the neurophysiology of nociceptors, bradykinin and the other algesic agents tested in these studies excited primarily polymodal afferents which also responded to mechanical and/or thermal stimuli. There is recent evidence that some afferents respond solely to chemical stimuli (DASH and DESHPANDE, 1976; KNIFFKI et al., 1978). Contrary to the expectation that bradykinin would preferentially excite C fibers because of the burning quality of the response to its application, it excited essentially equal proportions of C and Aδ afferents and even a somewhat lesser proportion of Aβ mechanoreceptive afferents. Group III fibers actually tended to be somewhat more sensitive to the algesic agents than were the unmyelinated group IV afferents, but there was no appreciable excitation of the larger myelinated muscle afferents. Clearly the different algesic agents act on different receptive elements as indicated by lack of cross-tachyphylaxis, by differing sensitivities of specific units to these agents and by selective inhibition by pharmacologic antagonists (WATSON, 1970).

III. Dorsal Horn

The dorsal horn has been divided into a number of layers or laminae based on anatomic differences among the cells in each location (REXED, 1952). Lamina I, the outer layer, is also termed the marginal zone. Laminae II and III correspond to the substantia gelatinosa while laminae IV–VI correspond to the nucleus proprius (KERR, 1975). Cells which respond primarily to noxious stimuli via the high threshold Aδ mechanoreceptors and C polymodal afferents are highly concentrated in lamina I (BESSON and GUILBAUD, 1976) and in the monkey in laminae II and III as well (KUMAZAWA and PERL, 1976). Some of these cells are found in lamina V which also contains a high concentration of cells which respond to input from Aβ as well as from Aδ and C fibers (PRICE and DUBNER, 1977). Afferent fibers from muscle and viscera also converge upon cells in this layer. Lamina IV cells are more likely to be excited by large afferents from mechanoreceptors and less likely by small myelinated and unmyelinated fibers. Powerful inhibition of nociceptive inputs by the brainstem occurs primarily in laminae V and also I and II (FIELDS and BASBAUM, 1978). The functional demarcations between laminae are not exact, and units may be found in one lamina which have characteristics more in common with an adjacent lamina. There are also numerous quantitative and even qualitative differences between species with regard to innervation of specific laminae, spinal pathways, etc. Table 2 lists results of studies in which activity of dorsal horn cells in various laminae was recorded. Spinal section was done usually at C1, and recording was done at the appropriate level to correspond with the route of bradykinin administration.

BESSON et al. (1972) injected 5 μg bradykinin into the popliteal artery. Very few cells in lamina IV, which were excited by light touch or hair movement, responded to bradykinin. On the other hand, the firing rate of a majority of cells in lamina V (with perhaps some overlap into lamina VI) was enhanced an average of 700% with a 20-s latency. These cells were also excited by nociceptive pressure or pinching of the skin over a certain area or excitatory field. Repeated injections did not cause tachyphylaxis. Another 25% of cells in lamina V were inhibited to an average of 13% of their original activity with a 12-s latency. Although these cells could be excited by stimulation of an excitatory field, in contrast to cells which were excited by bradykinin they were also inhibited by light natural stimuli over a much larger inhibitory field. This was a general characteristic of units which were depressed by bradykinin in later studies also. It should perhaps be added here that in this and in studies to be discussed below, regardless of whether units were excited or depressed, there was marked quantitative variation among units. Depression after bradykinin was followed by excitation in 2% of lamina V cells (BESSON et al., 1974).

When 10 μg bradykinin was given to decerebrate, rather than spinal, cats only 5 of 21 lamina V cells were affected (BESSON et al., 1975). However, when the spinal cord was cooled above the recording level to produce a "reversible spinalization," the pattern of units responding to bradykinin became similar to the previous study. The spontaneous firing rate of nearly all these cells also increased during spinal cooling. These results demonstrate the strong inhibitory influence of the brainstem on spinal cord transmission.

GUILBAUD et al. (1976) indicate that dorsal horn cells receiving input from both A and C fibers in the sural nerve were always excited by intrafemoral injection of bradykinin. When the nerve was cooled to block input from A fibers, bradykinin still exerted about the same effect, suggesting that the primary effect of bradykinin on these dorsal horn cells was via C fibers. Since bradykinin can excite A afferents (BECK and HANDWERKER, 1974), one would expect that some dorsal horn cells innervated by slowly adapting mechanoreceptive afferents would also be affected by bradykinin. The question arises – are those dorsal horn cells which are depressed by bradykinin, therefore, receiving input only from A fibers? To the contrary, GUILBAUD et al. (1976) indicated that cells receiving input only from A fibers did not respond to bradykinin. This brings up another question – if dorsal horn cells receiving input from C fibers are always excited by bradykinin and cells receiving input only from A fibers don't show any response, how does bradykinin depress some cells?

When 5–20 μg bradykinin was injected into the inferior mesenteric artery (GUILBAUD et al., 1977a), no response was evoked in lamina IV units, which were excited by mild cutaneous stimulation. Nearly all units with the characteristics of lamina V cells (some of which were anatomically outside lamina V) were affected by bradykinin. Acetylcholine (5–10 μg), tested on 17 of these units, altered activity qualitatively the same as bradykinin, but with a shorter latency. Twelve of the 14 units inhibited by bradykinin were also inhibited by stimulation of a rather large cutaneous recep-

Table 2. Responses of dorsal horn neurons to i.a. injection of bradykinin in immobilized, ventilated, unanesthetized animals

Species	Condition	Laminae	Total units tested	Percent of units:				Reference
				Excited	Depressed	Biphasic	No change	
Cat	Spinal	IV	29	14	3	0	83	Besson et al. (1972)
		V (VI)	61	52	23	2	23	
	Decerebrate	V	21	20	5	0	75	Besson et al. (1975)
	Spinal[a]	V	21	43	20	14	23	
	Spinal	IV	20	0	0	0	100	Guilbaud et al. (1977a)
		V	27	30	52	11	8	
		IV–VI	65	37[b]	6	0[b]	57	Piercey and Hollister (1977)
		I, II	9	100	0	0	0	Randić and Yu (1976)
Rabbit	Spinal or intact	V	65	55	20	0	25	Satoh et al. (1971)

[a] Decerebrate, but with "reversible spinalization" produced by cooling the spinal cord.
[b] Unspecified number excited, then depressed.

tive field. These results indicate that visceral stimulation by bradykinin and acetylcholine projects primarily to lamina V rather than to lamina IV.

PIERCEY and HOLLISTER (1977), recording from laminae IV–VI at L 7, found that cells which responded most vigorously to 10–30 μg bradykinin were nearly always sensitive to electric stimulation of the hind paw, usually to both weak and strong stimulation.

When cats were given intrafemoral injections of 5–15 μg bradykinin, all units in laminae I and II were excited with latencies of 5–18 s depending on the dose (RANDIĆ and YU, 1976). These particular cells had been tested because they responded to electric stimulation of Aδ and C fibers in the dorsal root or to strong mechanical or thermal stimuli. Thus, a high proportion of cells which responded to noxious stimuli, like those in lamina V, were excited by peripheral administration of bradykinin. It is also of considerable interest that when bradykinin was applied microelectrophoretically directly onto 13 such cells, nine of them were excited. Direct application of 5-hydroxytryptamine, to the contrary, depressed 70% of cells in laminae I and II.

SATOH et al. (1971) studied lamina V cells which responded to squeezing of the ipsilateral hind limb. The overall pattern of responses to 1–2 μg bradykinin was similar to that reported by BESSON et al. (1972). Similar results were obtained in both spinal and intact rabbits.

The general pattern which has emerged so far is that i.a. injections of bradykinin excite afferent fibers which project largely to lamina V, where they are susceptible to presynaptic inhibition from higher centers, and also apparently to laminae I and II. The projection to lamina IV is minor.

Morphine and related analgesics are known to act centrally (LIM, 1968), and their ability to inhibit certain spinal reflexes in animals or in subjects with spinal cord transection indicates that a portion of the analgesia may be evoked at the spinal level (JAFFE and MARTIN, 1975). The presence of opiate receptors, or at least stereospecific binding sites, in the substantia gelatinosa has recently been established (SNYDER and SIMANTOV, 1977; SIMON and HILLER, 1978). There is evidence that morphine localized to the spinal cord can cause analgesia in the rat (YAKSH and RUDY, 1976) or applied microiontophoretically to dorsal horn neurons can depress their response to various stimuli (CALVILLO et al., 1974; ZIEGLGÄNSBERGER and BAYERL, 1976). More specifically with regard to bradykinin, LE BARS et al. (1976) reported that 2 mg/kg morphine i.v. reduced the response to 10 μg bradykinin of four lamina V units in decerebrate cats only when the response of the cells had been restored by cooling the spinal cord. In strictly decerebrate cats, the cells were not appreciably stimulated by bradykinin, and morphine-induced inhibition was not apparent. A similar dose of morphine in intact rabbits reduced the excitatory effect of 1–2 μg bradykinin in six of 10 units in lamina V, whereas none of six units in spinal animals was inhibited (TAKAGI et al., 1976b). A larger dose of morphine in spinal rabbits did antagonize bradykinin in three of four units. PIERCEY and HOLLISTER (1977) reduced the response to bradykinin in only one of six laminae IV–VI cells in spinal cats with 3 mg morphine sulfate/kg. Even 6 mg/kg was ineffective in two cells.

Although these few tests suggest that morphine can act at the spinal level to inhibit the response of dorsal horn cells to bradykinin, the overall poor antagonism in spinal animals indicates that actions at a higher level are of greater importance.

Direct injection of morphine into the medullary reticular formation of the rabbit has been reported to inhibit the effect of 2 μg bradykinin on a small number of cells in lamina V (TAKAGI et al., 1976a).

IV. Afferent Spinal Pathways

DENNIS and MELZACK (1977) divided ascending pain-signalling systems into two main groups. The lateral group consisting primarily of the neospinothalamic tract and the spinocervical tract, which is especially well developed in the cat, projects to somatosensory thalamic nuclei, such as the ventral posterior lateral (VPL) nucleus, and to several other regions. Nociceptive signals in the spinocervical tract appear to be particularly susceptible to descending inhibitory control. Fibers from the medial group, which includes the paleospinothalamic tract and the spinoreticular system, turn more medially to synapse in the reticular formation and midline-intralaminar thalamic nuclei.

In the lightly anesthetized, immobilized monkey, LEVANTE et al. (1975) studied the effect of bradykinin on cells, primarily in lamina V, which were identified as belonging to the neospinothalamic tract by their antidromic activation upon stimulation of the contralateral VPL nucleus. Intrafemoral injections of 5–10 μg bradykinin excited 11 of 21 such cells with latencies of 15–30 s and durations of 30–90 s. Two units were inhibited. Thus at least some of the lamina V cells activated by bradykinin project to the specific thalamic relay nuclei. In a preliminary report on a similar preparation, except that chemical stimulation was limited to muscle afferents (FOREMAN et al., 1977), 26 μg bradykinin increased discharge within 12 s after beginning injection whereas 135 μg 5-hydroxytryptamine increased activity after a latency of only 3 s in the examples given.

In the cat (KNIFFKI et al., 1977) stimulation of muscle afferents by bradykinin, as well as by 5-hydroxytryptamine and KCl, activated units in the spinocervical tract which projects ipsilaterally from the dorsal horn to the lateral cervical nucleus. Recordings were made at L3–L4 from axons which were excited by electric stimulation of the gastrocnemius-soleus nerves and also antidromically by stimulation of the ipsilateral dorsallateral funiculus at C3. In anesthetized, spinalized cats, eight of 28 spinocervical tract units were excited by 26 μg bradykinin, 12 of 17 by 135 μg 5-hydroxytryptamine, and 12 of 21 by 3.8 mg KCl. Evidence of descending inhibition from the brainstem was obtained for bradykinin, when only one of 24 units responded in unanesthetized, decerebrate cats. This inhibition was not general, however, since 20 of 26 units, which were mostly the same units which did not respond to bradykinin, did respond to 5-hydroxytryptamine and 18 of 19 cells responded to KCl.

V. Brainstem

Not only do afferent pathways project into and through the brainstem on their way to higher centers, but, as mentioned above, the brainstem exerts a considerable inhibitory influence, particularly on the dorsal horn, on pathways transmitting infor-

Table 3. Responses of brainstem and thalamic neurons to i.a. injection of bradykinin in immobilized, unanesthetized[a] but hyperventilated cats

Recording site	Total units tested	Percent of units:				Reference
		Excited	Depressed	Biphasic	No change	
Medulla (NRGC)	112	65	12	5	18	GUILBAUD et al. (1973)
Midbrain reticular formation	135	56	17	5	22	LOMBARD et al. (1975)
Thalamic nuclei:						
centromedian	64	48	14	3	35	CONSEILLER et al. (1972)
VPL	53	11	11	8	70	
dorsomedial	29	14	4	10	72	
lateral posterior	16	44	6	0	50	
posterior group	39	95	5	0	0	GUILBAUD et al. (1977b)
VPL	28	4	4	0	92	
VPL	69	39	13	0	48	KRAUTHAMER et al. (1977)

[a] With the exception of the last study; moderate hyperventilation was used in the other studies to obtain slow waves and spindles on the electrocorticogram.

mation about noxious stimuli (DENNIS and MELZACK, 1977; FIELDS and BASBAUM, 1978). Such inhibition was illustrated by reduction in responses to bradykinin after decerebration. Electric stimulation of the midbrain periaqueductal gray, the dorsal raphe, the nucleus raphe magnus and periventricular thalamic sites can inhibit transmission of impulses in the dorsal horn, and analgesia can be produced by injection of opiates into certain regions, such as the midbrain periaqueductal and diencephalic periventricular gray (FIELDS and BASBAUM, 1978). Very few studies have been reported on changes in the brainstem after peripheral injections of bradykinin (Table 3).

Injections of 5–10 μg bradykinin into axillary or femoral arteries of cats excited a majority of units in the medullary nucleus reticularis gigantocellularis (NRGC) with a mean latency of 14 s and duration of 17 s (GUILBAUD et al., 1973). Of these excited cells, 57% also responded to strong stimulation such as pinching of the appropriate limb, and the others were stimulated only by light stimuli. Cells in the NRGC which were inhibited by bradykinin showed variable responses to electric or mechanical stimulation with some being inhibited, some excited or both. Ninety percent of the cells which were unaffected by bradykinin were sensitive to gentle, but not strong, peripheral stimuli. Similar results were obtained when recording from the midbrain reticular formation (LOMBARD et al., 1975). Seventy-five percent of the cells excited by 5–10 μg bradykinin, which responded with a latency of 10–20 s and duration of 15–20 s and were designated as group B, required strong mechanical stimulation of the limb to evoke marked increases in discharge frequency. These units were considered to react specifically to nociceptive stimuli. Twenty-one percent of the units excited by bradykinin, which responded with a latency of at least 25 s and a duration of over

25 s, were also excited by touch or strong auditory stimuli. These "group A" units were considered to be associated with arousal reactions. Three units, designated group C, were variable in that they were activated by noxious stimuli but inhibited by touching or auditory stimuli. Cells which were inhibited by bradykinin were usually also inhibited by tactile or auditory stimuli.

VI. Thalamus

Administration of 20–50 µg bradykinin to immobilized, locally anesthetized cats excited medial thalamic regions, in particular the dorsomedial nucleus and the centromedian-parafascicular (intralaminar) complex, and laterally in the medial geniculate body, the posterior nuclei and the pulvinar (LIM et al., 1969). Some activation was recorded near the suprageniculate and ventral posterior medial (VPM) nuclei, but there was no response from the VPL nucleus. Control injections indicated that the responses were not secondary to bradykinin-induced vasomotor changes. Excitation was antagonized by morphine. Potentials evoked in the thalamus and brainstem by electrically shocking the foot pads were inhibited by bradykinin.

CONSEILLER et al. (1972) reported that 5–10 µg bradykinin excited about half of the units studied in the centromedian nucleus and a small number in the VPL nucleus. It was later noted that only one of the latter cells was actually in the VPL nucleus. Smaller numbers of cells were examined in other nuclei (see Table 3). Of 76 cells located, with one exception, in the posterior group nuclei, 41 were driven only by strong noxious stimuli such as pinching of the skin, usually on the contralateral side (87%), while 35 were excited by both weak and strong stimuli (GUILBAUD et al., 1977b). Bradykinin (5–10 µg) excited nearly all of 39 units tested in this group with latencies from 10–15 s and durations greater than 30 s. Another 59 cells were located with three exceptions, within the VPL or VPM nuclei. These were stimulated only by non-noxious stimulation, such as hair movement and light touch, applied contralaterally. Only one of 28 such cells located in the VPL nucleus was excited by bradykinin. The VPM nucleus was not tested since bradykinin was given into the limbs.

These results, as well as those in the previous section (E.V.), suggest that responses to bradykinin in the cat project primarily via the more medial pathways from the spinal cord to medial thalamic nuclei. Yet there was evidence in Sect. E.IV. for some transmission via the spinocervical tract in the cat and via the neospinothalamic tract in the monkey. Support for transmission to the VPL nucleus was obtained in lightly to moderately anesthetized cats (KRAUTHAMER et al., 1977). All of the cells studied in this nucleus were excited by low intensity mechanical stimuli, and none responded only to high intensity stimuli such as pinching or pin prick. About half of the units also responded to 2–50 µg bradykinin, three-fourths being excited and one-fourth inhibited. Latency was 5–25 s, and the responses lasted 40–60 s. Usually mechanical stimulation of a particular unit evoked greater excitation that did bradykinin injection. Although the peripheral field for mechanical stimulation of a particular cell was limited and contralateral (except for a few orofacial units studied), the same unit was affected by bradykinin given by a variety of routes – contralateral or ipsilateral, hindlimb or forelimb or even visceral. This convergence was not always complete. Bradykinin also blocked bursts of discharges in those units with rhythmic discharge patterns. A variety of control injections indicated that neither the injection procedure per se nor changes in blood pressure evoked by bradykinin were responsible for the changes in VPL nucleus activity.

VII. Cortex

Cortical activity in 11 of 16 lightly or moderately pentobarbitalized immobilized cats was altered by injection of 20–100 μg bradykinin into limbs or visceral organs (KRAUTHAMER et al., 1976). The amplitude of the discharge increased considerably, with a relatively regular frequency which ranged from about 4–11 cycles/s in different animals. Latency was from 5–20 s and duration 15–60 s. Barbiturate spindles were suppressed during this period. These responses were recorded most consistently from the primary somatosensory cortex. The response contralateral to the side of injection into a forelimb often had a slightly shorter latency and was more pronounced. The reverse did not occur. Deep anesthesia, sectioning afferent pathways within the appropriate limb or spinal section usually prevented the bradykinin-induced response. In chloralose-anesthetized cats, 20–50 μg bradykinin did not evoke field potentials but, as in the brainstem and thalamus, it did suppress responses to shocking the footpads (LIM et al., 1969).

F. Direct Application of Kinins to the Nervous System

I. Autonomic Ganglia and Postganglionic Nerves

Direct stimulation of the superior cervical ganglion by bradykinin and angiotensin was demonstrated in spinal cats by LEWIS and REIT (1965). Close retrograde arterial injections of 0.5–10 μg bradykinin and 0.1–0.3 μg angiotensin into the ganglion caused the nictitating membrane to contract. The contraction, which was not blocked by hexamethonium, was the result of direct stimulation of ganglion cells since it was not elicited by injections to the nictitating membrane, after cutting the postganglionic trunk or removal of the ganglion and was enhanced after denervation of the ganglion. In spinal or anesthetized cats, kallidin and Met-Lys-bradykinin were about half as potent as bradykinin; another analog, Arg-Pro-Pro-Gly-Ser-Phe-Phe-Arg, was much less potent (LEWIS and REIT, 1966). These relative potencies were similar to their relative activity as hypotensive agents and in releasing catecholamines from the adrenal medulla. Eledoisin (7–28 μg) and substance P (75 units) were inactive. Bradykinin was antagonized by a very low, systemic dose of morphine (10 μg/kg, i.v.) or by injection of morphine (0.1–1 μg, i.a.) into the ganglion. Angiotensin and 5-hydroxytryptamine were likewise antagonized. Bradykinin and angiotensin acted as non-nicotinic ganglionic stimulants in that their effects were inhibited during the initial depolarization phase of nicotine-induced block but were enhanced during the later competitive phase and were also enhanced by a period of preganglionic stimulation. In the dog and rabbit, unlike in the cat, only small contractions of the nictitating membrane were induced by 30–50 μg bradykinin. Potentiation of bradykinin and angiotensin by preganglionic stimulation and antagonism of these peptides during the depolarization block after nicotine or after morphine administration were also reported by TRENDELENBERG (1966), who, in addition, noted antagonism by cocaine. During the non-depolarization phase after nicotine, the response to angiotensin was enhanced, in agreement with LEWIS and REIT (1966), but the response to bradykinin had only partially recovered at best. Intravenous injections of hexamethonium during this repolarization phase tended to restore responses to both agents toward control levels; i.e., it prevented enhancement of the angiotensin effect and increased the response to bradykinin.

HAEFELY (1970), recording from the postganglionic nerve leaving the superior cervical ganglion of the cat, found that sensitive ganglia responded after about 10 s to intracarotid injections of about 1–10 μg bradykinin and angiotensin, but not to eledoisin or physalaemin, with asynchronous discharges which lasted 1–2 min. Little or no change in the ganglionic surface potential occurred. As usual, orthodromic tetanic stimulation potentiated bradykinin and angiotensin and even allowed detection of very transient, small postganglionic responses to eledoisin and physalaemin. Other potentiating factors were chronic denervation and isoproterenol administration. Subthreshold doses of the active peptides also facilitated ganglionic transmission.

In excised, isolated superfused superior cervical ganglia from the rabbit, a conditioning stimulus delivered to the preganglionic fibers ordinarily enhances the postganglionic response to a subsequent submaximal stimulus given within 1.5 s (WALLIS and WOODWARD, 1974). Addition of bradykinin (1–7.7 μ*M*) to the bathing solution abolished facilitation by a conditioning stimulus given 60 s before the test stimulus. At the same time, bradykinin enhanced the component of the postganglionic action potential produced by the conditioning stimulus. These effects could be due to a reduction of the subliminal fringe by bradykinin, if the first submaximal stimulus after bradykinin activated more postganglionic neurons so that fewer cells in a facilitated state (the subliminal fringe) were available for stimulation by the second stimulus.

The stellate ganglion of the cat contains adrenergic ganglionic cells innervating the sinoatrial node and cholinergic cells which innervate sweat glands in the forelimb footpads. Close i.a. injections of 10 μg/kg bradykinin toward the ganglion maximally increased the heart rate in three of four cats, but even 30 μg/kg did not initiate sweating (AIKEN and REIT, 1969). Angiotensin likewise stimulated only the adrenergic neurons.

Unlike the unresponsive cholinergic cells in the stellate ganglion of the cat, when bradykinin was perfused through isolated rabbit hearts (SCHUMACHER and STARKE, 1978) there was a dose-related decrease in heart rate indicative of stimulation of cholinergic postganglionic neurons in 30 of 45 hearts. Heart rate returned to normal even though the infusion was continued. However, only about 15 min between exposures to bradykinin was necessary for recovery of sensitivity. Hexamethonium did not antagonize the effect of bradykinin, but atropine, nicotine, and tetrodotoxin did. Antagonism by atropine suggests an action on muscarinic receptors in the ganglion. Antagonism of bradykinin by atropine was not seen in the superior cervical ganglion of the cat (TRENDELENBERG, 1966; LEWIS and REIT, 1965).

In general, bradykinin and angiotensin share many attributes of other non-nicotinic ganglionic stimulants such as histamine and 5-hydroxytryptamine. There are minor differences between these agents, and studies of cross tachyphylaxis or with specific antagonists indicate that they act on different receptors. Directly or indirectly, bradykinin can also cause the adrenal medulla to release catecholamines (TERRAGNO and TERRAGNO, this volume).

Strips of pulmonary artery and isolated hearts of rabbits, which lack sympathetic ganglia, were used to study the effects of bradykinin on sympathetic postganglionic transmission (STARKE et al., 1977). Bradykinin did not alter outflow of labeled material from superfused resting arterial strips which had been incubated with tritiated norepinephrine. However, when the strips were electrically stimulated, the usual contraction and release of radioactivity was reduced by bradykinin pretreatment. This inhibition by bradykinin was prevented by the prostaglandin-synthesis inhibitors indomethacin and 5,8,11,14-eicosatetraenoic acid. Bradykinin also increased the efflux of PGE from the tissue, and administration of PGE_2 mimicked the effects of bradykinin. Thus these effects of bradykinin apparently require and are mediated by prostaglandin. Similar results were obtained with the isolated hearts. Atropine had no effect on any of the effects of bradykinin so they were not the result of muscarinic or parasympathetic ganglionic stimulation.

II. Spinal Cord

KONISHI and OTSUKA (1974) have reported a direct effect of bradykinin on the spinal cord of the frog. An isolated cord was mounted in a cooled (15 °C) bath, and ventral and dorsal roots were drawn into separate compartments for recording and stimulating respectively. In one example, eledoisin (10^{-6} *M*), physalaemin (3×10^{-6} *M*), substance P (2×10^{-5} *M*), and glutamate (7×10^{-4} *M*) in the bath depolarized the ventral root about equally. These agents were effective even when synaptic transmission was blocked by tetrodotoxin or by reduced calcium concentration, indicative of a direct action on the ventral horn. Direct application of physalaemin to the isolated ventral root was without effect so that the site of action was apparently on the cell bodies or dendrites. Bradykinin was at least 10 times more potent than glutamate over the range of concentrations studied, but depolarization by bradykinin was delayed 10–20 s and was abolished by tetrodotoxin or low calcium concentration. Thus bradykinin apparently acted on interneurons which secondarily excited the motoneurons. Tachyphylaxis occurred with 10-min intervals between injections.

As mentioned above, microelectrophoretic application of bradykinin stimulated two-thirds of a small number of cells tested in laminae I and II of the dorsal horn (RANDIĆ and YU, 1976).

III. Brain

Since bradykinin and kallidin are released in blood during a variety of pathologic disorders (COLMAN and WONG, this volume), most studies of their biologic effects, pharmacokinetics, etc., have been limited to the periphery. However, kinins may also exert important physiologic or pathologic actions within the central nervous system (GRAEFF, 1971), possibly because they enter the brain after release in the periphery, but more likely because they are synthetized and released within the central nervous system where they mediate or modulate neuronal activity.

One technique for determining that a chemical agent can act within the central nervous system, rather than in the periphery, to cause a certain effect is to inject it

Table 4. Behavioral and cardiovascular responses to central administration of bradykinin

Species	Route	Dose (μg)	Volume (μl)	Vocalization	Level of activity	Change in blood pressure	Other responses; comments	Reference
Mouse	i.c.v.[a]	≦ 1	20		↓		↓ Exploration maximum at 5 min	Čapek et al. (1969)
	i.c.v.[a]	2–12.5	10–12.5		↓		Catatonia, tachypnea	Iwata et al. (1970)
		≧15			(1) ↑ (2) ↓		Jumping, rolling, struggling As with lower doses	
	i.c.v.[a]	0.5, 2.6 13	25		↓ ↑		↑ Pentobarbital sleeping time Jumping	Okada et al. (1977)
Rat	i.c.v.[ab]	0.1, 1	10			(1) ↓ (2) ↑	2–5 min; lessened with high dose 5–15 min; enhanced with high dose	Pearson et al. (1969)
	i.c.v.	1	?	+	(1) ↑ (2) ↓	↑	Piloerection, rapid movements	Lambert and Lang (1970)
	i.c.v.	1–4	5–10		(1) ↑ (2) ↓	↑	Restlessness, struggling	Corrêa and Graeff (1974)
	i.c.v.[a]	4	?		↓		↓ Walking, washing, standing	Moniuszko-Jakoniuk and Wiśniewski (1974a); Wiśniewski et al. (1974)
	i.c.v.	0.25–5	20		↓		Catatonia	Przesmycki and Kleinrok (1976)
	i.c.v.[b]	1	5			↑		Corrêa and Graeff (1975)
	septum[b]	0.5	1			↑	Ventral part of lateral septum	
	septum[b]	0.125–2	1			↑	Dose-related	Corrêa and Graeff (1976)
Rabbit	i.cist.	5–10	?	+			In each of 28 animals	Bertolini et al. (1969)
	i.c.v.	30		+			In three of five only	
	i.c.v.	~30	200	+	(1) ↑ (2) ↓		0–2 min; jumping, rotation 2–15 min; catatonia	Kaneko et al. (1969)
	i.c.v.	0.5–5	50	+	(1) ↑ (2) ↓	(1) ↓ (2) ↑	0–2 min; flight reaction, alertness ≧5–10 min; catatonia, ptosis, ear drop	Graeff et al. (1969)
	i.c.v.	2.5–5	50		↓		20–70 min; catatonia, ptosis	da Silva and Rocha e Silva (1971)
	i.cist.				↓↓		12–14 min; catatonia, death with 5 μg	

	i.c.v.	1–5.6	50		(1) ↑		Tachyphylaxis	MELO and GRAEFF (1975)
					(2) ↓		Impaired behavioral task	
	i.c.v.	0.5–2	50–100	+	(1) ↑		1–2 min; ↑ motor activity	RIBEIRO et al. (1971);
					(2) ↓		20–40 min; ↑ threshold for evoked activity	RIBEIRO and ROCHA E SILVA (1973)
	i.cist.	1			↑			
	aqueduct	2	100				↑ Threshold for evoked activity	CORRADO et al. (1974)
Cat	i.c.v.	0.5–10	200		↑		1–4 min; alertness, ↑ restlessness	GRAEFF et al. (1967)
		10–100			(1) ↑		As above	
				+	(2) ↓	↑	10–30 min; ptosis, ↓ mobility	
	i.c.v.[b]	5–10	50–200			↓	1–14 min	DAMAS (1974)
	i.cist.[b]	2–20			↑		0–5 min; agitation, polypnea	

[a] Acute puncture.
[b] Anesthetized.
(1) = First phase of a biphasic response; (2) = Second phase.
Times indicate periods after injection.

into the cerebral ventricular system (i.c.v.) in amounts too small to evoke the effect if given peripherally (FELDBERG, 1963). If a response occurs, one then knows it was not due to the agent leaving the brain to act at a peripheral site. There are modifications of this technique by which the spread of material can be limited somewhat to tissues near specific portions of the ventricular system, but to date none of these modifications has been used to study kinins. Probable sites of action may be narrowed further by prior knowledge of which structures in proximity to the ventricular system are involved in certain functions and by injecting chemicals directly into specific tissue sites. In the studies discussed below, unless otherwise indicated, injections were made into a lateral cerebral ventricle, usually in amounts sufficient to enter the third and fourth ventricles as well and often even the subarachnoid spaces surrounding the brainstem. Some injections were made directly into the cisterna magna (i.cist.). Injections were done through chronically implanted cannulas unless designated "acute," signifying a direct puncture into the cerebrospinal fluid system. Animals were unanesthetized unless otherwise indicated.

1. Behavioral Responses

The predominate change in behavior after i.c.v. administration of bradykinin has been depression in the level of activity (Table 4) often with a state of catatonia. In several studies, depression was preceded by a short period, usually no longer than 2–5 min, of excitation in which vocalization, jumping, struggling, etc., occurred. Certain fragments of bradykinin were more potent than bradykinin in enhancing pentobarbital-induced sleeping time in the mouse (OKADA et al., 1977).

In the rat, bradykinin, eledoisin, and kallidin caused excitation followed by depression (LAMBERT and LANG, 1970; CORRÊA and GRAEFF, 1974). Tachyphylaxis was noted in the latter study when injections were given at 20-min intervals. MONIUSZKO-JAKONIUK and WIŚNIEWSKI (1974a) and WIŚNIEWSKI et al. (1974), on the other hand, noted only decreased behavioral activity after bradykinin, although in the latter study, bradykinin did enhance the increase in walking produced by the monoamine oxidase inhibitor, nialamide. Doses of 1–2 μg bradykinin usually did not decrease activity in studies by these authors and their co-workers. Neither bradykinin (0.5–1 μg/μl) nor kallikrein (1–5 μg) injections, into diencephalic regions in which angiotensin elicited drinking, altered drinking activity (FITZSIMONS, 1971).

In rabbits, bradykinin injections into the cisterna magna always evoked vocalization while i.c.v. administration was only occasionally effective (BERTOLINI et al., 1969). Involvement of a beta-adrenergic link was implied by reduction of the percentage of animals vocalizing after pretreatment with propanolol and nifenolol (INPEA). Antagonism was also produced by the monoamine oxidase inhibitor pargyline but not by reserpine or phentolamine. A biphasic response to central administration of bradykinin was reported by KANEKO et al. (1969). Miosis, increased depth of respiration, bradycardia and EEG alerting were present in both phases. Procaine, i.c.v., antagonized all the effects of bradykinin. Aspirin given i.v. antagonized all but the EEG changes, while morphine and aminopyrine antagonized only the EEG alerting. A small dose of phenobarbital did not antagonize any of the effects. GRAEFF et al. (1969) also noted biphasic responses to bradykinin in rabbits as did GRAEFF et al. (1967) in cats. During the first phase, the electrocorticogram or EEG became desynchronized, while during the second phase it was synchronized with an increased number of spindles. Miosis was present during both phases in the rabbit, but with hourly injections miosis and the initial excitment phase became less apparent. Injection of 10 μg eledoisin i.c.v. in rabbits caused an immediate excitation and increased exploratory activity which persisted for more than 2 h. Catatonia, which was enhanced by morphine, was attributed by DA SILVA and ROCHA E SILVA (1971) to an action of bradykinin at some location accessible to the subarachnoid space since i.cist. injections caused more severe catatonia than i.c.v. administration and did not produce sedation. The animals given bradykinin i.cist. were in poor condition thereafter and usually died within 1 h of receiving the larger dose.

Bradykinin impaired the response of rabbits to a behavioral task; namely lifting of a lever to obtain sweetened water (MELO and GRAEFF, 1975). The response to the first bradykinin injection was excluded to avoid interpretation problems associated with the initial excitement. Thereafter, bradykinin evoked the usual sedative or catatonic phase during which responding was delayed and less consistent. It is unlikely that the change in behavior was in any way specific. Pretreatment with bradykinin potentiating peptides enhanced kinin activity about 20-fold. The order of potency in disrupting behavior was angiotensin > bradykinin = substance P > Gly-Arg-Met-Lys-bradykinin.

Threshold electric stimulation of tooth pulp in rabbits evoked chewing movements with or without licking (RIBEIRO et al., 1971; RIBEIRO and ROCHA E SILVA, 1973). Injection of bradykinin i.c.v., but not i.cist., caused a dose-related increase in the threshold. This increase was lessened by 4-h pretreatment with reserpine and was enhanced by bradykinin-potentiating factor (see STEWART, this volume) and aprotinin (kallikrein inhibitor) which by themselves induced moderate increases in threshold. Kallidin, Met-Lys-bradykinin, and Gly-Arg-Met-Lys-bradykinin were less potent than bradykinin in raising the threshold, and their relative potencies on guinea-pig ileum were similar. Injections of morphine (50–200 μg) i.c.v. also raised the threshold, and the authors noted a number of other similarities between morphine and bradykinin given centrally. They suggested the periaqueductal and periventricular gray regions of the brain as possible sites for an antinociceptive action of bradykinin. This idea is supported by elevation of the threshold when bradykinin was injected directly into the aqueduct (CORRADO et al., 1974). It at first appears strange that an agent which causes pain peripherally may have an analgesic effect when given centrally. However, similar paradoxes have been implicated in other systems. For instance, antihypertensive agents such as methyldopa and clonidine have been proposed to act by stimulating centrally located α-adrenergic receptors, an action which in the periphery would increase blood pressure (NICKERSON and RUEDY, 1975).

2. Cardiovascular Responses

Blood pressure usually increased after central bradykinin administration (Table 4). In two studies, hypertension was preceded by hypotension. Because of conflicting results with various antagonists, it is not possible to draw general conclusions regarding the neuroeffector systems responsible. In anesthetized rats, eledoisin as well as bradykinin caused an initial hypotension with hypertension ensuing after 2–5 min

(PEARSON et al., 1969). These effects were antagonized by hexamethonium but not significantly by atropine. Pretreatment with phentolamine antagonized the depressor response but not the hypertension. The depressor response was attributed to inhibition of sympathetic tone and could, therefore, not be evoked when tone was already minimal after the alpha-blocking agent. The pressor response was almost abolished by propranolol indicating that it was primarily due to cardiac stimulation. There was also probably some increased sympathetic tone to the vessels as well since phentolamine reduced the mean pressor response about 50% even though the difference from control was not statistically significant. Pretreatment with phentolamine and propranolol together prevented any marked change after bradykinin but only blocked the pressor response to eledoisin. The depressor response to eledoisin was enhanced as it also was after propranolol alone. In unanesthetized rats, bradykinin, eledoisin (1 μg) and kallidin (1 μg) produced only a pressor response (LAMBERT and LANG, 1970; CORRÊA and GRAEFF, 1974). The response to bradykinin began rapidly and ended within about 4 min while that to eledoisin developed more slowly and lasted for over 12 min. Kallidin caused a very transient response. Phentolamine i.p. or i.c.v. antagonized this response while propranolol did not. Diphenhydramine given i.a. or pyrilamine given i.c.v. shortened the duration of the response to bradykinin, suggestive of histaminergic as well as alpha-adrenergic mediation (CORRÊA and GRAEFF, 1974). Peripherally injected atropine or i.c.v. hexamethonium or methysergide were not effective antagonists. Morphine antagonized bradykinin, but not eledoisin, and the possibility that the effect of bradykinin was due to induction of pain was suggested (LAMBERT and LANG, 1970). Contrary to this, however, pretreatment with four closely-spaced i.c.v. injections of capsaicin, which can desensitize pain receptors to bradykinin (KEELE and ARMSTRONG, 1964; SZOLCSÁNYI, 1977), did not impair the pressor response to bradykinin (CORRÊA, and GRAEFF, 1974).

CORRÊA and GRAEFF (1975) injected bradykinin into several brain sites in rats. Injections into the pars ventralis of the lateral septum caused pressor responses but did not appreciably alter pulse pressure or heart rate. Bilateral lesions in the lateral septal region reduced or abolished the response. Bradykinin was ineffective at other sites in the septal region, hypothalamus, striatum, etc. Thus the lateral septum appears to be a relatively specific site for the pressor action of centrally injected bradykinin. The effect was not secondary to bradykinin-induced vasodilation, since substance P, which is also a powerful vasodilator, did not evoke a pressor response. DesArg^9-bradykinin was also inactive. The increase in pressure after intraseptal injection of bradykinin was dose-related and was antagonized by prior injection of phentolamine into the same sites (CORRÊA and GRAEFF, 1976). Although intraseptal histamine injections also caused pressor responses, bradykinin injected into the septum was not antagonized by doses of pyrilamine which antagonized histamine, contrary to results with i.c.v. administration.

About 30–60 s after rabbits were given bradykinin, blood pressure suddenly fell accompanied by bradycardia (GRAEFF et al., 1969). In the next 10–20 s hypotension was succeeded by hypertension, tachycardia, and tachypnea. When injections were repeated at 40-min intervals, tachyphylaxis occurred. Atropine pretreatment reduced the hypotension and enhanced the hypertension. Because of this antagonism by atropine and a decrease in brainstem norepinephrine concentration after bradykinin (see next section), both cholinergic and adrenergic systems were considered to be activated by bradykinin. Morphine (10 mg/kg, i.v.) pretreatment did not antagonize bradykinin in the four animals tested in this study. Hypotensive responses to i.c.v. administration of bradykinin in cats were antagonized by atropine and vagotomy and were attributed to parasympathetic activity (DAMAS, 1974). In contrast, when bradykinin was injected i.cist., blood pressure increased, associated with polypnea and agitation, and this response was attributed to stimulation of paravascular pain receptors.

Before the technique of evaluating central versus peripheral actions of drugs by i.c.v. injection was widely used, cross-perfusion studies were used to examine the same question. Bradykinin injected into the carotid artery of dogs' heads, cross-perfused with donors' blood, caused pressor responses in recipients with denervated carotid sinus baroreceptors (BENETATO et al., 1964). This response was blocked by adrenalectomy or pretreatment of the recipient's body with reserpine, chlorpromazine or ergotamine, but it was not inhibited when chlorpromazine was administered centrally via the carotid artery.

Unlike the reports above, neither i.c.v. nor suboccipital injections of bradykinin or eledoisin were found to cause any significant changes in blood pressure in anesthetized dogs (CUPARENCU et al., 1971).

3. Effects on Brain Amines

Injections of bradykinin i.c.v. can alter brain concentrations of amines and some of their metabolites. In most of these studies a dose of 1–5 μg bradykinin was injected directly into the lateral ventricle of rats, through a hole previously made in the skull, and amine concentrations were determined 30 min later. The volume injected, which was often not stated, was probably 20 μl in the rat, assuming that it was the same as the volume used in the original reference to the technique. One hour after injection of bradykinin or angiotensin, whole brain norepinephrine concentration in the mouse was about 40% of control levels (CAPEK et al., 1969). When tritiated norepinephrine was injected i.c.v. 30 min after these peptides and the brain was evaluated for radioactivity 1 h later, bradykinin had depressed the uptake of tritiated material somewhat more than had angiotensin. Injections of 1–2 μg bradykinin did not significantly alter norepinephrine concentration in any of seven regions of rat brain (MONIUSZKO-JAKONIUK et al., 1976), but 4 μg did decrease concentrations in the corpus striatum, midbrain and cerebellum. Small reductions in normetanephrine concentration were detected in the striatum, midbrain and hippocampus after bradykinin. Bradykinin (1 μg) partially prevented the increase in norepinephrine concentration in the hippocampus which occurred 24 h after oral administration of nialamide (MONIUSZKO-JAKONIUK and WIŚNIEWSKI, 1977). Bradykinin (2 μg) combined with 0.5 mg amphetamine/kg decreased norepinephrine concentration in the striatum (MONIUSZKO-JAKONIUK et al., 1978). Bradykinin (50 μg in 100 μl) decreased norepinephrine concentration in the brainstem of rabbits (GRAEFF et al., 1969) and, combined with bradykinin potentiating factor, of cats (GRAEFF et al., 1967). Intracarotid administration of bradykinin has been reported to rise the concentration of norepinephrine in blood leaving the brain of dogs (BENETATO et al., 1967). This observation and evidence that bradykinin can stimulate sympathetic ganglia (see Sect. F.I.) and the adrenal medulla (TERRAGNO and TERRAGNO, this volume) indicate that enhanced release of norepinephrine is likely to be the cause of the decreased concentration in several regions of the brain. Norepinephrine release has been suggested as the cause of the centrally-induced pressor activity of bradykinin (CORRÊA and GRAEFF, 1974).

PRZESMYCKI and KLEINROK (1976) reported increased turnover of dopamine in the striatum of rats given 5 µg bradykinin, as indicated by a decreased dopamine concentration when the rats were pretreated with alpha-methyltyrosine. Bradykinin alone did not change dopamine levels in their animals nor in the brainstem of rabbits (GRAEFF et al., 1969), but MONIUSZKO-JAKONIUK et al. (1976) observed a decrease in the striatum and increase in the cerebellum of rats after a dose of 4 µg. On the other hand, 1–2 µg bradykinin tended to enhance the increase in dopamine concentration induced in the striatum, cerebellum, hypothalamus, and elsewhere by nialamide or by a 2 mg/kg dose of amphetamine (MONIUSZKO-JAKONIUK and WIŚNIEWSKI, 1977; MONIUSZKO-JAKONIUK et al., 1978). PREZESMYCKI and KLEINROK (1976) reported a 68% increase in striatal levels of homovanillic acid, a metabolite of dopamine, after bradykinin injection while MONIUSZKO-JAKONIUK et al. (1976) reported a 46% decrease.

A dose of 1 µg bradykinin increased 5-hydroxytryptamine concentration in the cerebellum but decreased the level in the midbrain of the rat (BRASZKO and KOŚCIELAK, 1975; MONIUSZKO-JAKONIUK et al., 1976). Nialamide pretreatment also increased the cerebellar 5-hydroxytryptamine level, but when the two were combined the concentration increase was less than with either nialamide or bradykinin alone (MONIUSZKO-JAKONIUK and WIŚNIEWSKI, 1977). A 2 µg dose of bradykinin did not significantly alter 5-hydroxytryptamine level in any of the regions examined (MONIUSZKO-JAKONIUK et al., 1976), but it reduced an increase in cerebellar concentration induced by 0.5 mg/kg amphetamine (MONIUSZKO-JAKONIUK et al., 1978). A 4 µg dose of bradykinin increased 5-hydroxytryptamine concentration in the striatum and again lowered it in the midbrain (MONIUSZKO-JAKONIUK et al., 1976). Bradykinin did not significantly alter brainstem 5-hydroxytryptamine levels in the rabbit (GRAEFF et al., 1969).

Thus, i.c.v. administration of bradykinin, studied primarily in the rat, apparently releases norepinephrine or by some other mechanism tends to decrease its concentration in certain regions of the brain. No definate conclusions can be stated with regard to dopamine or 5-hydroxytryptamine. Dopamine was reported to be affected primarily in the striatum where there may be an increase in turnover and even a decreased concentration, but otherwise there has been little agreement between laboratories. Responses to 5-hydroxytryptamine in the rat do not appear to be dose-related in the range studied so far. It should be noted that many of the changes in amine concentrations after i.c.v. administration of bradykinin were also observed after i.p. injection of kallikrein 1 h prior to assay (MONIUSZKO-JAKONIUK et al., 1976). If i.p. injection of kallikrein increases endogenous kinin formation within the central nervous system (MONIUSZKO-JAKONIUK and WIŚNIEWSKI, 1974a), centrally injected bradykinin mimicks the actions of endogenously synthetized kinins reasonably well.

4. Miscellaneous Effects

Activation or desynchronization of the EEG or electrocorticogram after i.c.v. injection of bradykinin and eledoisin has been reported in the anesthetized rat (PEARSON et al., 1969) and after bradykinin in the conscious rabbit (GRAEFF et al., 1969) and cat

(GRAEFF et al., 1967). This effect was also produced by intracarotid injections of bradykinin, but not consistently by eledoisin, in anesthetized cats (PEARSON et al., 1969).

Microiontophoresis of bradykinin into the nucleus locus coeruleus of anesthetized rats evoked no change in activity of nine cells (GUYENET and AGHAJANIAN, 1977). Thyrotropin-releasing hormone and neurotensin likewise were inactive. Methionine-enkephalin, epinephrine, and norepinephrine inhibited activity while eledoisin-related peptide, physalaemin, substance P, and acetylcholine usually excited but occasionally caused no change in activity. Iontophoretic application of bradykinin to Betz cells and to other spontaneously active cortical neurons caused excitation in 91% of 42 units and 76% of 62 units, respectively (PHILLIS and LIMACHER, 1974). Similar results were obtained with substance P and physalaemin. Eledoisin excited most Betz cells but was inconsistent otherwise. Cells which were not spontaneously active, but were stimulated by glutamate, were not affected by any of the polypeptides studied.

Administration of equimolar concentrations of bradykinin, kallidin, and Met-Lys-bradykinin i.c.v. caused roughly equivalent hyperthermic responses in conscious rabbits (ALMEIDA E SILVA and PELÁ, 1978). These began within 15 min, with recovery after 3 h or more, and were antagonized by indomethacin and acetaminophen pretreatment, implicating a role of prostaglandins or related substances. Removal of the C-terminal arginine from bradykinin produced an inactive peptide.

In addition to effects which can be attributed to the usual stimulation of pain receptors, effects after intracarotid injection of bradykinin in the rat which may be due to direct central actions include release of ACTH (HAUGER-KLEVENE, 1970) and antidiuretic hormone (HARRIS, 1971; TERRAGNO and TERRAGNO, this volume).

5. Interactions With Drugs

Centrally injected bradykinin alters a variety of behavioral and motor responses to other agents. Rats were used in all the studies discussed below. Bradykinin delayed or prevented hypoglycemic convulsions after i.p. injection of insulin (WIŚNIEWSKI and MACKIEWICZ, 1974). Brain kinin formation after insulin alone was enhanced following seizures, and this increase appeared to protect against further seizures. Simultaneous administration of kallikrein i.p. with insulin also protected against seizures, without preventing hypoglycemia, while iniprol, which somewhat reduced brain kinin-forming activity after insulin, enhanced seizure intensity or recurrence.

Injection of 5-hydroxytryptamine and bradykinin separately i.c.v. increased the pain threshold for electric shock applied to the paws, but when given together the increase in threshold was less than with either alone (BRASZKO and KOŚCIELAK, 1975).

MONIUSZKO-JAKONIUK, WIŚNIEWSKI and their co-workers have used four behavioral states – walking (mobility), washing, standing-up and immobility (LÁT, 1965) – to examine interactions between bradykinin and a variety of drugs. Rats were used only if their number of standing-up reactions was relatively consistent during 10-min periods on three daily tests prior to drug testing. The number of times the animals stood and the amount of time spent in each of the other three activities were then determined for a control 10-min period before injection of bradykinin, vehicle, etc. The control result, whether number or duration for each activity, was considered

100%, and changes were determined from those baselines. At various times after injection, activities were again recorded. Although a given change is stated as being, for instance at 30 min, this must mean ±5 min. Unfortunately, an indication of the actual amounts of time spent in each of the four activities during the control periods is not given. This appears to be quite variable from study to study. For instance, 75 min after i.p. administration of kallikrein, walking had decreased about 60%, washing about 80%, and standing about 75%. Yet immobility had increased only about 25% (MONIUSZKO-JAKONIUK and WIŚNIEWSKI, 1974a). This sort of result would be obtained if the rats were immobile about 70–75% of the time. For other studies, quite different control activities would be calculated (WIŚNIEWSKI and BODZENTA, 1975). In most of the experiments, partly because of rather large variations between animals, 1–2 µg bradykinin did not statistically alter the four activities, usually evaluated 30 min after injection. Yet there was often a fairly large difference in mean values between the animals receiving vehicle and those receiving bradykinin. In testing for effects of bradykinin on the change in activity evoked by another agent, the statistical comparisons were usually made only between animals receiving the test drug alone versus test drug plus bradykinin. In many cases this difference is large enough that bradykinin clearly enhanced or antagonized the action of the drug, but in other cases it is likely that the effect of bradykinin was only additive with that of the other agent since bradykinin caused mean changes in the same direction even though they were not statistically significant. A better analysis would have been to compare the difference between bradykinin and vehicle versus the difference between test drug plus bradykinin and test drug alone.

Chlorpromazine (1 mg/kg, i.p.) caused depression as indicated by lessened walking, washing, and standing and, of course, concomitantly increased immobility (MONIUSZKO-JAKONIUK et al., 1974). Bradykinin (2 µg) most clearly enhanced the effect of chlorpromazine on standing and possibly on immobility as well. Injection of kallikrein i.p. also enhanced chlorpromazine-induced psychomotor depression. Thiopental (2.5 mg/kg, i.p.) caused depression, but the administration of bradykinin probably only produced an additive effect (MONIUSZKO-JAKONIUK and WIŚNIEWSKI, 1974b). Of the four parameters of Lát's test, definitive bradykinin-induced alterations of the activity of other agents appeared most consistently with walking. Walking was enhanced by 24-h prior administration of nialamide (WIŚNIEWSKI et al., 1974) or nialamide plus 90-min prior L-dopa (MONIUSZKO-JAKONIUK and WIŚNIEWSKI, 1976, 1977), by i.c.v. norepinephrine (MONIUSZKO-JAKONIUK and WIŚNIEWSKI, 1977), by norepinephrine after treatment with reserpine (WIŚNIEWSKI et al., 1974) and by amphetamine (MONIUSZKO-JAKONIUK et al., 1978). Bradykinin enhanced the effect of these treatments. Although when given alone dopamine (MONIUSZKO-JAKONIUK and WIŚNIEWSKI, 1977) and norepinephrine in one study (WIŚNIEWSKI et al., 1974) did not significantly affect walking, simultaneous treatment with bradykinin increased walking activity.

Bradykinin has been proposed both to increase dopaminergic transmission in the brain (MONIUSZKO-JAKONIUK, WIŚNIEWSKI and co-workers) and to inhibit dopamine receptors (PRZESMYCKI and KLEINROK, 1976). In Sect. F.III.3. it was noted that these two groups obtained different effects on striatal dopamine and homovanillic acid levels after bradykinin. PRZESMYCKI and KLEINROK found that 0.25–1 µg doses of bradykinin given i.c.v. 90 min after amphetamine (2.5 mg/kg, s.c.) or 2 µg bradykinin given 5–15 min prior to apomorphine (0.6–5 mg/kg, i.p.) inhibited stereotypic behavior for no more than 30 min. Bradykinin also enhanced flufenazine-induced catalepsy for a similar duration. These results are consistent with dopamine receptor blockade as they suggested. Animals given bradykinin (4 μg, i.c.v.) at the same time as amphetamine (10 mg/kg, i.p.) exhibited less stereotypy 10 min later, than when amphetamine was given alone (MONIUSZKO-JAKONIUK et al., 1978). Although this difference between groups was not statistically significant, the difference was in the same direction as reported by PRZESMYCKI and KLEINROK during the same time period. The group receiving bradykinin exhibited statistically greater stereotypy 90–180 min after injection. No direct correlation between striatal dopamine levels and stereotypy can be made from this study since striatal dopamine level was determined 30 min after administration of bradykinin (2 μg) plus amphetamine (2 mg/kg) and stereotypy was not enhanced until 90 min after bradykinin (4 μg) plus amphetamine (10 mg/kg). Thus, the difference in opinion regarding the effect of bradykinin on amphetamine-induced stereotypy may be partially dependent on the time period examined. Under conditions similar to those of PRZESMYCKI and KLEINROK, on the other hand, bradykinin enhanced apomorphine-induced stereotypy in the study by MONIUSZKO-JAKONIUK and WIŚNIEWSKI (1977). Because of enhancement by bradykinin of (1) stereotypy, (2) brain dopamine concentration, and (3) behavioral effects of nialamide plus L-dopa which were inhibited by the dopamine receptor blocker, spiroperidol (MONIUSZKO-JAKONIUK and WIŚNIEWSKI, 1977), these authors proposed an interaction of bradykinin with dopamine receptors. MONIUSZKO-JAKONIUK, WIŚNIEWSKI and co-workers used both i.c.v. injection of bradykinin and i.p. administration of kallikrein in many of their studies. Similar interactions with other agents were usually obtained in either case, and, perhaps surprisingly, in some instances kallikrein was the more effective.

As in the previous section, it appears most likely that bradykinin enhances activity in adrenergic systems, while there is disagreement with regard to dopaminergic systems and minimal information on agents such as acetylcholine (WIŚNIEWSKI and BODZENTA, 1975) and 5-hydroxytryptamine.

G. Kallikrein-Kinin System in the Brain

As discussed above, stimulation of peripheral chemoreceptors by bradykinin evokes a variety of motor responses, autonomic reflexes, etc. which involve the nervous system at all levels. Evidence has been provided by direct administration of bradykinin at various sites within the nervous system including ganglia, the cerebral ventricles, etc., that bradykinin can act pharmacologically at sites other than paravascular chemoreceptors. If kinins also act physiologically as transmitters or modulators of transmission within the nervous system, they must be synthetized, inactivated, and perhaps stored within brain tissue.

I. Kininases

Certainly the brain is capable of inactivating kinins. Overt effects of central administration of bradykinin were often short lived although changes in brain amine levels were frequently apparent 30 min after injection (Sect. F.III.3.). Kininase activity has been found in brain tissue of the mouse (IWATA et al., 1970), the rat (HORI et al., 1968,

1970; IWATA et al., 1969; SHIKIMI and IWATA, 1970; SHIKIMI et al., 1970; MARKS and PIROTTA, 1971; DAMAS, 1972; SHIKIMI et al., 1973), rabbit (HORI, 1968; HORI et al., 1968, 1970; KONDO, 1969; CAMARGO and GRAEFF, 1969; CAMARGO et al., 1972, 1973; OLIVEIRA et al., 1976a), cat (KRIVOY and KROEGER, 1964), guinea pig (HORI et al., 1968, 1970) and dog (HOOPER, 1962; KRIVOY and KROEGER, 1964). There is agreement that this activity is higher (about 60% of the total) in the supernatant or soluble fraction (HORI, 1968; HORI et al., 1970; CAMARGO and GRAEFF, 1969; IWATA et al., 1969) with considerably lesser amounts in the microsomal, nuclear, and mitochondrial fractions. HORI (1968) noted that the kininase activity associated with the microsomal fraction was tightly bound to the granules. Kininase activities were low and nearly equal in the microsomal, nuclear, and mitochondrial fractions from cortex or brainstem of the rat while in the cerebellum there were greater differences in activity among these subcellular fractions (IWATA et al., 1969). These same authors determined that lethal doses of pentylenetetrazol did not alter kininase activity in the cortex or brainstem but increased activity specifically in the nuclear fraction of the cerebellum. Picrotoxin likewise increased the cerebellar kininase activity, but strychnine did not. Neither ether nor amobarbital had any effect on total kininase activity in the three brain regions (SHIKIMI et al., 1973). Kininase activity was somewhat elevated in mouse brain after i.c.v. injection of 20–25 μg bradykinin (IWATA et al., 1970).

SHIKIMI and IWATA (1970) partially purified a kininase from the supernatant fraction of rat brain homogenates with an increase in potency of about 30-fold. Both arginine and phenylalanine were split from bradykinin by this enzyme. The enzyme was relatively specific for bradykinin, lacked trypsin- and chymotrypsin-like activity and, unlike kininase I, did not hydrolyze hippuryl-L-lysine (SHIKIMI et al., 1970; see ERDÖS, this volume).

CAMARGO et al. (1972) purified 50–75-fold two kininases from the soluble fraction of rabbit brain homogenates. One of these, "kinin converting enzyme" hydrolyzed Met-Lys-bradykinin to kallidin and kallidin to bradykinin. The other enzyme inactivated all three peptides by release of phenylalanine and arginine, similarly to the enzyme purified by SHIKIMI and IWATA (1970). CAMARGO et al. (1973) then isolated two endopeptidases, one of which hydrolyzed the Phe^5-Ser^6 bond of bradykinin (see also MARKS and PIROTTA, 1971) and was activated by dithiothreitol (OLIVEIRA et al., 1976b). The other enzyme was a peptidase which was initially thought to successively split Phe-Arg and then Ser-Pro dipeptides from the C-terminal end of bradykinin. These enzymes, designated kininases A and B, respectively, were further studied to determine substrate specificity (OLIVEIRA et al., 1976a). In contrast to the initial report, kininase B only split off the terminal Phe-Arg dipeptide and was unable to further hydrolyze the remaining heptapeptide. In this respect and in its inability to convert angiotensin I to angiotensin II, kininase B differs from kininase II from other tissues (ERDÖS, this volume).

II. Kininogenases

Kinin-forming activity has been reported in homogenates prepared from rabbit brains which were perfused with saline solution to avoid errors due to contamination by blood (HORI, 1968). The activity was found primarily in the microsomal fraction and was attributed to a kallikrein-like enzyme. In an examination of homogenates of several organs from the rabbit, HORI et al. (1969) found that the tissues in general contained very small amounts of kallikrein. However, treatment of the homogenates with acetone, which activates prekallikrein, increased the kallikrein-like activity. This activity was lower in brain homogenates than in homogenates from most of the other tissues with the exception of the spleen. Brain levels of kallikrein inhibitor, on the other hand, were comparable to other organs. DAMAS (1972) obtained evidence of kinin-forming activity in aqueous extracts of rat brain. To detect such activity, it was first necessary to inactivate kininase activity by acidification. Kininogenase activity was highest in cerebral cortex of rats, with less in brainstem and cerebellum (SHIKIMI et al., 1973) and was not affected by treatment with ether, amobarbital, or lethal amounts of pentylenetetrazol, strychnine or nitrogen gas. Administration of kallikrein to rats i.p. has been reported to increase brain kininogenase activity (MONIUSZKO-JAKONIUK and WIŚNIEWSKI, 1974a), but the mechanism has not been studied.

III. Kinin-Like Activity

Probably because of rapid destruction by kininases, reports of kinin-like activity in brain tissue have been few. As mentioned above, it was even necessary to inactivate kininase activity to demonstrate kinin-forming activity in aqueous extracts of rat brain (DAMAS, 1972). HORI (1968) reported partial purification of a peptide from bovine brain which was qualitatively similar to bradykinin in a variety of bioassay systems, in paper-electrophoretic mobility, and in sensitivity to several chemical treatments. An apparently similar material was also found in bullfrog brain. Kinin-like material has been extracted from regions of rabbit brain, in particular from the hypothalamus and lower brainstem (PELA et al., 1975). The activity was reduced during fevers induced by i.v. administration of a bacterial endotoxin. It was not decided if the decrease in activity was due to the fever per se or required the presence of endotoxin. SHIKIMI et al. (1973) determined that the cerebellum and brainstem of rats contained about three times more kininogen than did cerebral cortex. The guinea pig ileum was used to assay for bradykinin-like material in the subarachnoid spaces of the rat (DAMAS, 1971). Little or no kinin-like activity was found unless the perfusion fluid contained blood. This was also true when kininogenase-containing extract from the salivary gland was infused into the jugular vein, so that kinins do not pass readily through an intact blood-brain barrier.

Although it has been somewhat difficult to demonstrate the presence of kininogenases and kinin-like material in the brain, there is sufficient positive evidence to warrent further investigation into possible functions within the central nervous system of locally synthetized kinins.

References

Aiken, J.W., Reit, E.: A comparison of the sensitivity to chemical stimuli of adrenergic and cholinergic neurons in the cat stellate ganglion. J. Pharmacol. Exp. Ther. *169*, 211–223 (1969)
Almeida e Silva, T.C., Pelá, I.R.: Changes in rectal temperature of the rabbit by intracerebroventricular injection of bradykinin and related kinins. Agents Actions *8*, 102–107 (1978)
Armstrong, D.: Pain. In: Handbook of experimental pharmacology. Vol. XXV: Bradykinin, kallidin and kallikrein. Erdös, E.G. (ed.), pp. 434–481. Berlin, Heidelberg, New York: Springer 1970

Baldoni, F., Tallarida, G., Peruzzi, G., Semprini, A., Cesario, A., Cannata, D.: Effetti dell'acido acetilsalicilico sulle risposte cardiocircolatorie e respiratorie riflesse determinate dall'iniezione di bradichinina in arteria femorale. Boll. Soc. Ital. Biol. Sper. *50*, 1170–1175 (1974)

Beck, P.W., Handwerker, H.O.: Bradykinin and serotonin effects on various types of cutaneous nerve fibres. Pflügers Arch. *347*, 209–222 (1974)

Benetato, G., Hăulică, I., Muscalu, I., Bubuianu, E., Găleşanu, S.: On the central nervous action of bradykinin. Rev. roum. Physiol. *1*, 313–322 (1964)

Benetato, G., Bubuianu, E., Cîrmaciu, R., Găleşanu, S.: The action of bradykinin on the sympathico-adrenergic centers. Rev. roum. Physiol. *4*, 245–250 (1967)

Bergström, S., Duner, H., Euler, U.S., von, Pernow, B., Sjövall, J.: Observations on the effects of infusion of prostaglandin E in man. Acta Physiol. Scand. *45*, 145–151 (1959)

Bertolini, A., Mucci, P., Sternieri, E.: Behavioural effect of bradykinin injected into the cerebrospinal fluid. In: Prostaglandins, peptides and amines. Mantegazza, P., Horton, E.W. (eds.), pp. 129–134. London, New York: Academic Press 1969

Besson, J.-M., Guilbaud, G.: Modulation of the transmission of painful messages at the spinal level. In: Mechanisms in transmission of signals for conscious behavior. Desiraju, T. (ed.), pp. 137–162. Amsterdam: Elsevier 1976

Besson, J.M., Conseiller, C., Hamann, K.-F., Maillard, M.-C.: Modifications of dorsal horn cell activities in the spinal cord, after intra-arterial injection of bradykinin. J. Physiol. (Lond.) *221*, 189–205 (1972)

Besson, J.M., Guilbaud, G., Lombard, M.C.: Effects of bradykinin intra-arterial injection into the limbs upon bulbar and reticular unit activity. Adv. Neurol. *4*, 207–215 (1974)

Besson, J.M., Guilbaud, G., Le Bars, D.: Descending inhibitory influences exerted by the brain stem upon the activities of dorsal horn lamina V cells induced by intra-arterial injection of bradykinin into the limbs. J. Physiol. (Lond.) *248*, 725–739 (1975)

Bhalla, T.N., Sinha, J.N., Kohli, R.P., Bhargava, K.P.: A comparative study of the writhing response induced by phenylquinone, bradykinin and aconitine for the assessment of analgesic agents. Jpn. J. Pharmacol. *23*, 609–614 (1973)

Birn, H.: Kinines and pain in "dry socket." Int. J. Oral Surg. *1*, 34–42 (1972)

Botha, D., Müller, F.O., Krueger, F.G.M., Melnitzky, H., Vermaak, L., Louw, L.: Quantitative assessment of analgesia conferred by various analgesics, as determined by blocking the intra-arterial bradykinin-evoked pain-response in the rat. Eur. J. Pharmacol. *6*, 312–321 (1969)

Braszko, J., Kościelak, M.: Effect of kinins on the central action of serotonin. Pol. J. Pharmacol. Pharm. *27*, Suppl. 61–68 (1975)

Bumpus, F.M., Smeby, R.R., Page, I.H., Khairallah, P.A.: Distribution and metabolic fate of angiotensin II and various derivatives. Can. Med. Assoc. J. *90*, 190–193 (1964)

Burch, G.E., DePasquale, N.P.: Bradykinin. Am. Heart J. *65*, 116–123 (1963)

Calvillo, O., Henry, J.L., Neuman, R.S.: Effects of morphine and naloxone on dorsal horn neurones in the cat. Can. J. Physiol. Pharmacol. *52*, 1207–1211 (1974)

Camargo, A.C.M., Graeff, F.G.: Subcellular distribution and properties of the bradykinin inactivation system in rabbit brain homogenates. Biochem. Pharmacol. *18*, 548–549 (1969)

Camargo, A.C.M., Ramalho-Pinto, F.J., Greene, L.J.: Brain peptidases: conversion and inactivation of kinin hormones. J. Neurochem. *19*, 37–49 (1972)

Camargo, A.C.M., Shapanka, R., Greene, L.J.: Preparation, assay, and partial characterization of a neutral endopeptidase from rabbit brain. Biochemistry *12*, 1838–1844 (1973)

Čapek, R., Mašek, K., Šramka, M., Kršiak, M., Švec, P.: The similarities of the angiotensin and bradykinin action on the central nervous system. Pharmacology *2*, 161–170 (1969)

Collier, H.O.J.: A pharmacological analysis of aspirin. Adv. Pharmacol. *7*, 333–405 (1969)

Collier, H.O.J., Schneider, C.: Nociceptive response to prostaglandins and analgesic actions of aspirin and morphine. Nature New Biol. *236*, 141–143 (1972)

Collier, H.O.J., Dinneen, L.C., Johnson, C.A., Schneider, C.: The abdominal constriction response and its suppression by analgesic drugs in the mouse. Br. J. Pharmacol. *32*, 295–310 (1968)

Collier, J.G., Karim, S.M.M., Robinson, B., Somers, K.: Action of prostaglandins A_2, B_1, E_2, and $F_{2\alpha}$ on superficial hand veins of man. Br. J. Pharmacol. *44*, 374–375 P (1972)

Conseiller, C., Wyon-Maillard, M.-C., Hamann, K.-F., Besson, J.-M.: Effets de l'injection intra-artérielle de bradykinine au niveau des membres sur l'activité cellulaire de quelques structures thalamiques. C.R. Acad. Sci. (Paris) *274*, 3425–3427 (1972)

Corrado, A.P., Graeff, F.G., Ribeiro, S.A., Riccioppo Neto, F.: Comparison of effects of bradykinin administered intracarotideally and intraventricularly. Ciênc. Cult. (São Paulo) *26*, 589–596 (1974)
Corrêa, F.M.A., Graeff, F.G.: Central mechanisms of the hypertensive action of intraventricular bradykinin in the unanaesthetized rat. Neuropharmacology *13*, 65–75 (1974)
Corrêa, F.M.A., Graeff, F.G.: Central site of the hypertensive action of bradykinin. J. Pharmacol. Exp. Ther. *192*, 670–676 (1975)
Corrêa, F.M.A., Graeff, F.G.: On the mechanism of the hypertensive action of intraseptal bradykinin in the rat. Neuropharmacology *15*, 713–717 (1976)
Crunkhorn, P., Willis, A.L.: Cutaneous reactions to intradermal prostaglandins. Br. J. Pharmacol. *41*, 49–56 (1971)
Cuparencu, B., Tiçsa, I., Safta, L., Csutak, V., Mocan, R.: Der Einfluß von intraventrikulär verabreichten Angiotensin II, Bradykinin und Eledoisin auf den arteriellen Blutdruck, die Atmung und das Elektrokardiogramm. Acta Biol. Med. Ger. *27*, 435–441 (1971)
Damas, J.: Sur la présence de la bradykinine dans les espaces sous-arachnoïdiens du rat. C. R. Soc. Biol. (Paris) *165*, 2232–2234 (1971)
Damas, J.: La demi-vie de la bradykinine dans les espaces sous-arachnoïdiens du rat. C. R. Soc. Biol. (Paris) *166*, 740–744 (1972)
Damas, J.: Réactions cardiovasculaires déclenchées par l'introduction de la bradykinine dans les espaces sous-arachnoïdiens du chat anesthésié. Arch. Int. Physiol. Biochim. *82*, 669–677 (1974)
Damas, J.: Sur la stimulation des récepteurs paravasculaires carotidiens, par la bradykinine. Arch. Int. Physiol. Biochim. *83*, 111–121 (1975)
Damas, J., Deby, C.: Sur la libération des prostaglandines et de leurs précurseurs, par la bradykinine. Arch. Int. Physiol. Biochim. *84*, 293–304 (1976)
Dash, M.S., Deshpande, S.S.: Human skin nociceptors and their chemical response. In: Advances in pain research and therapy. Bonica, J.J., Albe-Fessard, D. (eds.), Vol. 1, pp. 47–51. New York: Raven 1976
Da Silva, G.R., Rocha e Silva, M.: Catatonia induced in the rabbit by intracerebral injection of bradykinin and morphine. Eur. J. Pharmacol. *15*, 180–186 (1971)
Deffenu, G., Pegrassi, L., Lumachi, B.: The use of bradykinin-induced effects in rats as an assay for analgesic drugs. J. Pharm. Pharmacol. *18*, 135 (1966)
Dennis, S.G., Melzack, R.: Pain-signalling systems in the dorsal and ventral spinal cord. Pain *4*, 97–132 (1977)
Doi, T., Akaike, A., Ohashi, M., Satoh, M., Takagi, H.: Bradykinin-induced flexor reflex of rabbit hindlimb for comparing analgesics. Jpn. J. Pharmacol. *26*, 634–637 (1976)
Eisen, V.: Plasma kinins in synovial exudates. Br. J. Exp. Path. *51*, 322–327 (1970)
Emele, J.F., Shanaman, J.: Bradykinin writhing: a method for measuring analgesia. Proc. Soc. Exp. Biol. Med. *114*, 680–682 (1963)
Emele, J.F., Shanaman, J.E.: Analgesic activity of namoxyrate (2-[4-biphenylyl] butyric acid 2-dimethylaminoethanol salt). Arch. Int. Pharmacodyn. Ther. *170*, 99–107 (1967)
Emele, J.F., Shanaman, J., Winbury, M.M.: The analgesic-antiinflammatory activity of papain. Arch. Int. Pharmacodyn. Ther. *159*, 126–134 (1966)
Feldberg, W.: A pharmacological approach to the brain from its inner and outer surface. Baltimore: Williams and Wilkins 1963
Ferreira, S.H.: Prostaglandins, aspirin-like drugs and analgesia. Nature New Biol. *240*, 200–203 (1972)
Ferreira, S.H., Vane, J.R.: New aspects of the mode of action of nonsteroid anti-inflammatory drugs. Annu. Rev. Pharmacol. *14*, 57–73 (1974)
Ferreira, S.H., Moncada, S., Vane, J.R.: Indomethacin and aspirin abolish prostaglandin release from the spleen. Nature New Biol. *231*, 237–239 (1971)
Ferreira, S.H., Moncada, S., Vane, J.R.: Prostaglandins and the mechanism of analgesia produced by aspirin-like drugs. Br. J. Pharmacol. *49*, 86–97 (1973)
Ferreira, S.H., Moncada, S., Vane, J.R.: Prostaglandins and signs and symptoms of inflammation. In: Prostaglandin synthetase inhibitors. Robinson, H.J., Vane, J.R. (eds.), pp. 175–187. New York: Raven 1974
Fields, H.L., Basbaum, A.I.: Brainstem control of spinal pain-transmission neurons. Annu. Rev. Physiol. *40*, 217–248 (1978)

Fitzsimons, J.T.: The effect on drinking of peptide precursors and of shorter chain peptide fragments of angiotensin II injected into the rat's diencephalon. J. Physiol. (Lond.) *214*, 295–303 (1971)
Flower, R.J.: Drugs which inhibit prostaglandin biosynthesis. Pharmacol. Rev. *26*, 33–67 (1974)
Fock, S., Mense, S.: Excitatory effects of 5-hydroxytryptamine, histamine and potassium ions on muscular group IV afferent units: a comparison with bradykinin. Brain Res. *105*, 459–469 (1976)
Foreman, R.D., Schmidt, R.F., Willis, W.D.: Convergence of muscle and cutaneous input onto primate spinothalamic tract neurons. Brain Res. *124*, 555–560 (1977)
Franz, M., Mense, S.: Muscle receptors with group IV afferent fibres responding to application of bradykinin. Brain Res. *92*, 369–383 (1975)
Garcia Leme, J., Hamamura, L., Rocha e Silva, M.: Effect of anti-proteases and hexadimethrine bromide on the release of a bradykinin-like substance during heating (46 °C) of rat paws. Br. J. Pharmacol. *40*, 294–309 (1970)
Gillespie, A.: Prostaglandin-oxytocin enhancement and potentiation and their clinical applications. Br. med. J. *1*, 150–152 (1972)
Graeff, F.G.: Kinins as possible neurotransmitters in the central nervous system. Ciênc. Cult. (São Paulo) *23*, 465–473 (1971)
Graeff, F.G., Corrado, A.P., Pelá, I.R., Capek, R.: Actions of bradykinin upon the central nervous system. In: International symposium on vaso-active polypeptides: bradykinin and related kinins. Rocha e Silva, M., Rothschild, H.A. (eds.), pp. 97–102. São Paulo: Edart 1967
Graeff, F.G., Pelá, I.R., Rocha e Silva, M.: Behavioural and somatic effects of bradykinin injected into the cerebral ventricles of unanaesthetized rabbits. Br. J. Pharmacol. *37*, 723–732 (1969)
Guilbaud, G., Besson, J.M., Oliveras, J.L., Wyon-Maillard, M.C.: Modifications of the firing rate of bulbar reticular units (nucleus gigantocellularis) after intra-arterial injection of bradykinin into the limbs. Brain Res. *63*, 131–140 (1973)
Guilbaud, G., Le Bars, D., Besson, J.M.: Bradykinin as a tool in neurophysiological studies of pain mechanisms. In: Advances in pain research and therapy. Bonica, J.J., Albe-Fessard, D. (eds.), Vol. 1, pp. 67–73. New York: Raven 1976
Guilbaud, G., Benelli, G., Besson, J.M.: Responses of thoracic dorsal horn interneurons to cutaneous stimulation and to the administration of algogenic substances into the mesenteric artery in the spinal cat. Brain Res. *124*, 437–448 (1977a)
Guilbaud, G., Caille, D., Besson, J.M., Benelli, G.: Single units activities in ventral posterior and posterior group thalamic nuclei during nociceptive and non nociceptive stimulations in the cat. Arch. Ital. Biol. *115*, 38–56 (1977b)
Guyenet, P.G., Aghajanian, G.K.: Excitation of neurons in the nucleus locus coeruleus by substance P and related peptides. Brain Res. *136*, 178–184 (1977)
Guzman, F., Braun, C., Lim, R.K.S.: Visceral pain and the pseudaffective response to intra-arterial injection of bradykinin and other algesic agents. Arch. Int. Pharmacodyn. Ther. *136*, 353–384 (1962)
Guzman, F., Braun, C., Lim, R.K.S., Potter, G.D., Rodgers, D.W.: Narcotic and non-narcotic analgesics which block visceral pain evoked by intra-arterial injection of bradykinin and other algesic agents. Arch. Int. Pharmacodyn. Ther. *149*, 571–588 (1964)
Haddy, F.J., Emerson, T.E., Jr., Scott, J.B., Daugherty, R.M.: The effect of the kinins on the cardiovascular system. In: Handbook of experimental pharmacology. Vol. XXV: Bradykinin, kallidin and kallikrein. Erdös, E. (ed.), pp. 362–384. Berlin, Heidelberg, New York: Springer 1970
Haefely, W.E.: Some actions of bradykinin and related peptides on autonomic ganglion cells. Adv. Exp. Med. Biol. *8*, 591–599 (1970)
Handwerker, H.O.: Influences of algogenic substances and prostaglandins on the discharges of unmyelinated cutaneous nerve fibers identified as nociceptors. In: Advances in pain research and therapy. Bonica, J.J., Albe-Fessard, D. (eds.), Vol. 1, pp. 41–45. New York: Raven 1976
Harris, M.C.: Release of an antidiuretic substance by bradykinin in the rat. J. Physiol. (Lond.) *219*, 403–419 (1971)
Hauger-Klevene, J.H.: Corticotrophin releasing activity of bradykinin in the rat. Acta Physiol. Lat.-Am. *20*, 238–241 (1970)
Hiss, E., Mense, S.: Evidence for the existence of different receptor sites for algesic agents at the endings of muscular group IV afferent units. Pflügers Arch. *362*, 141–146 (1976)

Hooper, K.C.: The catabolism of some physiologically active polypeptides by homogenate of dog hypothalamus. Biochem. J. *83*, 511–517 (1962)
Hori, S.: The presence of bradykinin-like polypeptides, kinin-releasing and destroying activity in brain. Jpn. J. Physiol. *18*, 772–787 (1968)
Hori, S., Hori, K., Masumura, S., Kondo, M.: Kinin-destroying activities of cell homogenates. Mie Med. J. *18*, 139–146 (1968)
Hori, S., Masumura, S., Mizuta, K., Kondo, M.: Kallikreins and their inhibitors in various tissues. Mie Med. J. *18*, 223–233 (1969)
Hori, S., Ota, S., Kondo, M.: Subcellular distribution of kininase activity in various tissues. Mie Med. J. *20*, 167–173 (1970)
Horton, E.W.: Action of prostaglandin E_1 on tissues which respond to bradykinin. Nature (Lond.) *200*, 892–893 (1963)
Iggo, A.: Peripheral and spinal "pain" mechanisms and their modulation. In: Advances in pain research and therapy. Bonica, J.J., Albe-Fessard, D. (eds.), Vol. 1, pp. 381–394. New York: Raven 1976
Inoki, R., Toyoda, T., Yamamoto, I.: Elaboration of a bradykinin-like substance in dog's canine pulp during electrical stimulation and its inhibition by narcotic and nonnarcotic analgesics. Naunyn Schmiedebergs Arch. Pharmacol. *279*, 387–398 (1973)
Inoki, R., Hayashi, T., Kudo, T., Matsumoto, K., Oka, M., Kotani, Y.: Effects of morphine and acetylsalicylic acid on kinin forming enzyme in rat paw. Arch. Int. Pharmacodyn. Ther. *228*, 126–135 (1977)
Iwata, H., Shikimi, T., Oka, T.: Pharmacological significances of peptidase and proteinase in the brain (report I)-enzymatic inactivation of bradykinin in rat brain. Biochem. Pharmacol. *18*, 119–128 (1969)
Iwata, H., Shikimi, T., Iida, M., Miichi, H.: Pharmacological significances of peptidase and proteinase in the brain. Report 4: Effect of bradykinin on the central nervous system and role of the enzyme inactivating bradykinin in mouse brain. Jpn. J. Pharmacol. *20*, 80–86 (1970)
Jaffe, J.H., Martin, W.R.: Narcotic analgesics and antagonists. In: The pharmacological basis of therapeutics, 5th ed. Goodman, L.S., Gilman, A. (eds.), pp. 245–283. New York: Macmillan 1975
Jezdinský, J., Hálek, J.: The effects of some analgesics and neuroleptics upon the reflexive and affective components of the formaldehyde- and bradykinin-induced nociceptive reactions in rats. Activ. Nerv. Sup. (Praha) *16*, 226–228 (1974)
Juan, H.: Mechanism of action of bradykinin-induced release of prostaglandin E. Naunyn Schmiedebergs Arch. Pharmacol. *300*, 77–85 (1977a)
Juan, H.: Inhibition of the algesic effect of bradykinin and acetylcholine by mepacrine. Naunyn Schmiedebergs Arch. Pharmacol. *301*, 23–27 (1977b)
Juan, H., Lembeck, F.: Action of peptides and other algesic agents on paravascular pain receptors of the isolated perfused rabbit ear. Naunyn Schmiedebergs Arch. Pharmacol. *283*, 151–164 (1974)
Juan, H., Lembeck, F.: Inhibition of the action of bradykinin and acetylcholine on paravascular pain receptors by tetrodotoxin and procaine. Naunyn Schmiedebergs Arch. Pharmacol. *290*, 389–395 (1975)
Juan, H., Lembeck, F.: Release of prostaglandins from the isolated perfused rabbit ear by bradykinin and acetylcholine. Agents Actions *6*, 642–645 (1976a)
Juan, H., Lembeck, F.: Polyphloretin phosphate reduces the algesic action of bradykinin by interfering with E-type prostaglandins. Agents Actions *6*, 646–650 (1976b)
Juan, H., Lembeck, F.: Prostaglandin $F_{2\alpha}$ reduces the algesic effect of bradykinin by antagonizing the pain enhancing action of endogenously released prostaglandin E. Br. J. Pharmacol. *59*, 385–391 (1977)
Juhlin, L., Michaëlsson, G.: Cutaneous vascular reactions to prostaglandins in healthy subjects and in patients with urticaria and atopic dermatitis. Acta Derm.-Venereol. (Stockh.) *49*, 251–261 (1969)
Julou, L., Ducrot, R., Bardone, M.C., Detaille, J.Y., Feo, C., Guyonnet, J.C., Loiseau, G., Pasquet, J.: Étude des propriétés pharmacologiques de la diméthyl sulfamido-3 (diméthylamino-2 propyl)-10 phénothiazine (8.599 R.P.). Arch. Int. Pharmacodyn. Ther. *159*, 70–86 (1966)
Kaneko, T., Satoh, M., Takagi, H.: Central actions of bradykinin in rabbit and their modification by analgesics. Folia Pharmacol. Jpn. *65*, 176–181 (1969)

Kantor, T.G., Jarvik, M.E., Wolff, B.B.: Bradykinin as a mediator of human pain. Proc. Soc. Exp. Biol. Med. *126*, 505–507 (1967)
Karim, S.: Action of prostaglandin in the pregnant woman. Ann. N.Y. Acad. Sci. *180*, 483–498 (1971)
Keele, C.A.: Clinical and pathological aspects of kinins in man. Proc. R. Soc. Lond. [Biol.] *173*, 361–369 (1969)
Keele, C.A., Armstrong, D.: Substances producing pain and itch. London: Arnold 1964
Kerr, F.W.L.: Neuroanatomical substrates of nociception in the spinal cord. Pain *1*, 325–356 (1975)
Khayutin, V.M., Baraz, L.A., Lukoshkova, E.V., Sonina, R.S., Chernilovskaya, P.E.: Chemosensitive spinal afferents: thresholds of specific and nociceptive reflexes as compared with thresholds of excitation for receptors and axons. Prog. Brain Res. *43*, 293–306 (1976)
Kimura, E., Hashimoto, K., Furukawa, S., Hayakawa, H.: Changes in bradykinin level in coronary sinus blood after the experimental occlusion of a coronary artery. Am. Heart J. *85*, 635–647 (1973)
Kniffki, K.-D., Mense, S., Schmidt, R.-F.: The spinocervical tract as a possible pathway for muscular nociception. J. Physiol. (Paris) *73*, 359–366 (1977)
Kniffki, K.-D., Mense, S., Schmidt, R.F.: Responses of group IV afferent units from skeletal muscle to stretch, contraction and chemical stimulation. Exp. Brain Res. *31*, 511–522 (1978)
Kondo, M.: Studies on the kallikrein-like substances, kininases and kallikrein inhibitors in the rabbit's organs. Mie Med. J. *18*, 235–241 (1969)
Konishi, S., Otsuka, M.: The effects of substance P and other peptides on spinal neurons of the frog. Brain Res. *65*, 397–410 (1974)
Krauthamer, G., Gottesman, L., McGuinness, C.: Synchronization of the electrocorticogram by visceral and somatic bradykinin stimulation in anesthetized cats. Electroencephalogr. Clin. Neurophysiol. *41*, 153–167 (1976)
Krauthamer, G., McGuinness, C., Gottesman, L.: Unit responses in the ventrobasal thalamus (VPL) of the cat to bradykinin injected into somatic and visceral arteries. Brain Res. Bull. *2*, 299–306 (1977)
Krivoy, W., Kroeger, D.: The preservation of bradykinin by phenothiazines in vitro. Br. J. Pharmacol. *22*, 329–341 (1964)
Kudo, T., Kawagoe, M., Hayashi, T., Takezawa, J., Inoki, R.: Inhibitory effect of Apernyl on production of bradykininlike substance in pulp. J. Dent. Res. *54*, 1082–1086 (1975)
Kumazawa, T., Perl, E.R.: Differential excitation of dorsal horn and substantia gelatinosa marginal neurons by primary afferent units with fine (Aδ and C) fibers. In: Sensory functions of the skin in primates. Zotterman, Y. (ed.), pp. 67–87. Oxford: Pergamon 1976
Lambert, G.A., Lang, W.J.: The effects of bradykinin and eledoisin injected into the cerebral ventricles of conscious cats. Eur. J. Pharmacol. *9*, 383–386 (1970)
Lang, W.J., Pearson, L.: Studies on the pressor responses produced by bradykinin and kallidin. Br. J. Pharmacol. *32*, 330–338 (1968)
Lát, J.: The spontaneous exploratory reactions as a tool for psychopharmacological studies. A contribution towards a theory of contradictory results in psychopharmacology. In: Proc. II Int. Pharmacol. Meet., Vol. 1: Pharmacology of conditioning, learning and retention. Mikhel'son, M.Ya., Longo, V.G., Votava, Z. (eds.), pp. 47–63. Oxford: Pergamon 1965
Le Bars, D., Menetrey, D., Besson, J.M.: Effects of morphine upon the lamina V type cells activities in the dorsal horn of the decerebrate cat. Brain Res. *113*, 293–310 (1976)
Lembeck, F.: Untersuchungen über die Auslösung afferenter Impulse. Naunyn Schmiedebergs Arch. exp. Path. Pharmak. *230*, 1–9 (1957)
Lembeck, F., Juan, H.: Interaction of prostaglandins and indomethacin with algesic substances. Naunyn Schmiedebergs Arch. Pharmacol. *285*, 301–313 (1974)
Lembeck, F., Juan, H.: Influence of changed calcium and potassium concentration on the algesic effect of bradykinin and acetylcholine. Naunyn Schmiedebergs Arch. Pharmacol. *299*, 289–294 (1977)
Lembeck, F., Popper, H., Juan, H.: Release of prostaglandins by bradykinin as an intrinsic mechanism of its algesic effect. Naunyn Schmiedebergs Arch. Pharmacol. *294*, 69–73 (1976)
Levante, A., Lamour, Y., Guilbaud, G., Besson, J.M.: Spinothalamic cell activity in the monkey during intense nociceptive stimulation: Intra-arterial injection of bradykinin into the limbs. Brain Res. *88*, 560–564 (1975)

Lewis, G.P., Reit, E.: The action of angiotensin and bradykinin on the superior cervical ganglion of the cat. J. Physiol. (Lond.) *179*, 538–553 (1965)
Lewis, G.P., Reit, E.: Further studies on the actions of peptides on the superior cervical ganglion and suprarenal medulla. Br. J. Pharmacol. *26*, 444–460 (1966)
Lim, R.K.S.: Visceral receptors and visceral pain. Ann. N.Y. Acad. Sci. *86*, 73–89 (1960)
Lim, R.K.S.: Neuropharmacology of pain and analgesia. In: Proc. III Int. Pharmacol. Meet., Vol. 9: Pharmacology of pain. Lim, R.K.S., Armstrong, D., Pardo, E.G. (eds.), pp. 169–217. Oxford: Pergamon 1968
Lim, R.K.S.: Pain. Annu. Rev. Physiol. *32*, 269–288 (1970)
Lim, R.K.S., Guzman, F., Rodgers, D.W., Goto, K., Braun, C., Dickerson, C.D., Engle, R.J.: Site of action of narcotic and non-narcotic analgesics determined by blocking bradykinin-evoked visceral pain. Arch. Int. Pharmacodyn. Ther. *152*, 25–58 (1964)
Lim, R.K.S., Miller, D.G., Guzman, F., Rodgers, D.W., Rogers, R.W., Wang, S.K., Chao, P.Y., Shih, T.Y.: Pain and analgesia evaluated by the intraperitoneal bradykinin-evoked pain method in man. Clin. Pharmacol. Ther. *8*, 521–542 (1967)
Lim, R.K.S., Krauthamer, G., Guzman, F., Fulp, R.R.: Central nervous system activity associated with the pain evoked by bradykinin and its alteration by morphine and aspirin. Proc. Natl. Acad. Sci. USA *63*, 705–712 (1969)
Lombard, M.-C., Guilbaud, G., Besson, J.-M.: Effects of the intra-arterial injection of bradykinin into the limbs, upon the activity of mesencephalic reticular units. Eur. J. Pharmacol. *30*, 298–308 (1975)
Lumachi, B.: Pharmacological investigations of 4-prenyl-1,2-diphenyl-3,5-pyrazolidinedione (DA 2370). Part 4: Analgesic activity on bradykinin evoked pain in rats. Arzneim.-Forsch. *22*, 201–202 (1972)
Marks, N., Pirotta, M.: Breakdown of bradykinin and its analogs by rat brain neutral proteinase. Brain Res. *33*, 565–567 (1971)
Markus, H.B., Ball, E.G.: Inhibition of lipolytic processes in rat adipose tissue by antimalarial drugs. Biochim. Biophys. Acta *187*, 486–491 (1969)
Melo, J.C., Graeff, F.G.: Effect of intracerebroventricular bradykinin and related peptides on rabbit operant behavior. J. Pharmacol. Exp. Ther. *193*, 1–10 (1975)
Mense, S.: Nervous outflow from skeletal muscle following chemical noxious stimulation. J. Physiol. (Lond.) *267*, 75–88 (1977a)
Mense, S.: Muscular nociceptors. J. Physiol. (Paris) *73*, 233–240 (1977b)
Moncada, S., Ferreira, S.H., Vane, J.R.: Inhibition of prostaglandin biosynthesis as the mechanism of analgesia of aspirin-like drugs in the dog knee joint. Eur. J. Pharmacol. *31*, 250–260 (1975)
Moniuszko-Jakoniuk, J., Kościelak, M., Wiśniewski, K.: Investigations into the mechanism of the influence of kinins on the action of amphetamine. Pharmacology *16*, 89–97 (1978)
Moniuszko-Jakoniuk, J., Wiśniewski, K.: The effects of kinins on the psychomotor activity of rats as evaluated by Lát's test. Acta Neurobiol. Exp. (Warsz.) *34*, 621–628 (1974a)
Moniuszko-Jakoniuk, J., Wiśniewski, K.: The activation of the kinin-forming system and the effects of thiopental. Psychopharmacology *40*, 269–277 (1974b)
Moniuszko-Jakoniuk, J., Wiśniewski, K.: The influence of bradykinin and drugs blocking alpha and beta-adrenergic receptor on the stimulating effect of nialamide and L-dopa. Acta Physiol. Pol. *27*, 395–399 (1976)
Moniuszko-Jakoniuk, J., Wiśniewski, K.: Interaction of bradykinin with dopaminergic receptors in the CNS. Pol. J. Pharmacol. Pharm. *29*, 301–311 (1977)
Moniuszko-Jakoniuk, J., Wiśniewski, K., Bodzenta, A.: Effect of the activation of the kinin-forming system on the potency of chlorpromazine. Pharmacology *12*, 216–223 (1974)
Moniuszko-Jakoniuk, J., Wiśniewski, K., Kościelak, M.: Investigations of the mechanism of central action of kinins. Psychopharmacology *50*, 181–186 (1976)
Nakano, T., Taira, N.: 5-Hydroxytryptamine as a sensitizer of somatic nociceptors for pain-producing substances. Eur. J. Pharmacol. *38*, 23–29 (1976)
Needleman, P.: The synthesis and function of prostaglandins in the heart. Fed. Proc. *35*, 2376–2381 (1976)
Needleman, P., Key, S.L., Denny, S.E., Isakson, P.C., Marshall, G.R.: Mechanism and modification of bradykinin-induced coronary vasodilation. Proc. Natl. Acad. Sci. USA *72*, 2060–2063 (1975)

Nickerson, M., Ruedy, J.: Antihypertensive agents and the drug therapy of hypertension. In: The pharmacological basis of therapeutics, 5th ed. Goodman, L.S., Gilman, A. (eds.), pp. 705–726. New York: Macmillan 1975
Nishi, K., Sakanashi, M., Takenaka, F.: Activation of afferent cardiac sympathetic nerve fibers of the cat by pain producing substances and by noxious heat. Pflügers Arch. *372*, 53–61 (1977)
Okada, Y., Tuchiya, Y., Yagyu, M., Kozawa, S., Kariya, K.: Synthesis of bradykinin fragments and their effect on pentobarbital sleeping time in mouse. Neuropharmacology *16*, 381–383 (1977)
Oliveira, E.B., Martins, A.R., Camargo, A.C.M.: Isolation of brain endopeptidases: influence of size and sequence of substrates structurally related to bradykinin. Biochemistry *15*, 1967–1974 (1976a)
Oliveira, E.B., Martins, A.R., De Camargo, A.C.M.: Rabbit brain thiol-activated endopeptidase. Hydrolysis of bradykinin and kininogen. Gen. Pharmacol. *7*, 159–161 (1976b)
Palmer, M.A., Piper, P.J., Vane, J.R.: Release of rabbit aorta contracting substance (RCS) and prostaglandins induced by chemical or mechanical stimulation of guinea-pig lungs. Br. J. Pharmacol. *49*, 226–242 (1973)
Pearson, L., Lambert, G.A., Lang, W.J.: Centrally mediated cardiovascular and EEG responses to bradykinin and eledoisin. Eur. J. Pharmacol. *8*, 153–158 (1969)
Pearson, L., Lang, W.J.: Effect of acetylsalicylic acid and morphine on pressor responses produced by bradykinin. Eur. J. Pharmacol. *6*, 17–23 (1969)
Peck, M.J., Williams, T.J.: Prostacyclin (PGI_2) potentiates bradykinin-induced plasma exudation in rabbit skin. Br. J. Pharmacol. *62*, 464P–465P (1978)
Pela, I.R., Gardey-Levassort, C., Lechat, P., Rocha e Silva, M.: Brain kinins and fever induced by bacterial pyrogens in rabbits. J. Pharm. Pharmacol. *27*, 793–794 (1975)
Phillis, J.W., Limacher, J.J.: Excitation of cerebral cortical neurons by various polypeptides. Exp. Neurol. *43*, 414–423 (1974)
Piercey, M.F., Hollister, R.P.: Morphine fails to block the discharges evoked by intra-arterial bradykinin in dorsal horn neurones of spinal cats. Neuropharmacology *16*, 425–429 (1977)
Pierson, A.K., Rosenberg, F.J.: WIN 35197-2: another benzomorphan with a unique analgesic profile. In: Proceedings of the thirty-eighth scientific meeting, committee on problems of drug dependence, pp. 949–965. Washington: National Academy of Sciences 1976
Price, D.D., Dubner, R.: Neurons that subserve the sensory-discriminative aspects of pain. Pain *3*, 307–338 (1977)
Przesmycki, K., Kleinrok, Z.: The effect of bradykinin on central dopamine receptors. Pol. J. Pharmacol. Pharm. *28*, 673–678 (1976)
Randić, M., Yu, H.H.: Effects of 5-hydroxytryptamine and bradykinin in cat dorsal horn neurones activated by noxious stimuli. Brain Res. *111*, 197–203 (1976)
Rexed, B.: The cytoarchitectonic organization of the spinal cord in the cat. J. Comp. Neurol. *96*, 415–495 (1952)
Riccioppo Neto, F., Reis, D.S., Corrado, A.P.: Stimulation of paravascular intracranial receptors by bradykinin and kallidin. Adv. Exp. Med. Biol. *8*, 547–554 (1970)
Riccioppo Neto, F., Corrado, A.P., Rocha e Silva, M.: Apnea, bradycardia, hypotension and muscular contraction induced by intracarotid injection of bradykinin. J. Pharmacol. Exp. Ther. *190*, 316–326 (1974)
Ribeiro, S.A., Corrado, A.P., Graeff, F.G.: Antinociceptive action of intraventricular bradykinin. Neuropharmacology *10*, 725–731 (1971)
Ribeiro, S.A., Rocha e Silva, M.: Antinociceptive action of bradykinin and related kinins of larger molecular weights by the intraventricular route. Br. J. Pharmacol. *47*, 517–528 (1973)
Rosenthale, M.E., Dervinis, A., Kassarich, J., Singer, S.: Prostaglandins and anti-inflammatory drugs in the dog knee joint. J. Pharm. Pharmacol. *24*, 149–150 (1972)
Satoh, M., Nakamura, N., Takagi, H.: Effect of morphine on bradykinin-induced unitary discharges in the spinal cord of the rabbit. Eur. J. Pharmacol. *16*, 245–247 (1971)
Satoh, M., Doi, T., Kawasaki, K., Akaike, A., Takagi, H.: Effects of indomethacin and the other anti-inflammatory agents on activation of dorsal horn cell in the spinal cord induced by intra-arterial injection of bradykinin. Jpn. J. Pharmacol. *26*, 309–314 (1976)
Schumacher, K.A., Starke, K.: Bradykinin-induced stimulation of cardiac parasympathetic ganglia. Experientia (Basel) *34*, 223–224 (1978)

Shikimi, T., Iwata, H.: Pharmacological significances of peptidase and proteinase in the brain – II. Purification and properties of a bradykinin inactivating enzyme from rat brain. Biochem. Pharmacol. *19*, 1399–1407 (1970)
Shikimi, T., Houki, S., Iwata, H.: Pharmacological significances of peptidase and proteinase in the brain. Report 3: Substrate specificity and amino acid composition of partially purified enzyme inactivating bradykinin in rat brain. Jpn. J. Pharmacol. *20*, 169–170 (1970)
Shikimi, T., Kema, R., Matsumoto, M., Yamahata, Y., Miyata, S.: Studies on kinin-like substances in brain. Biochem. Pharmacol. *22*, 567–573 (1973)
Sicuteri, F., Del Bianco, P.L., Fanciullacci, M.: Kinins in the pathogenesis of cardiogenic shock and pain. Adv. Exp. Med. Biol. *9*, 315–322 (1970)
Sicuteri, F., Franchi, G., Michelacci, S.: Biochemical mechanism of ischemic pain. Adv. Neurol. *4*, 39–44 (1974)
Simon, E.J., Hiller, J.M.: The opiate receptors. Annu. Rev. Pharmacol. Toxicol. *18*, 371–394 (1978)
Smith, J.B., Willis, A.L.: Aspirin selectively inhibits prostaglandin production in human platelets. Nature New Biol. *231*, 235–237 (1971)
Snyder, S.H., Simantov, R.: The opiate receptor and opioid peptides. J. Neurochem. *28*, 13–20 (1977)
Solomon, L.M., Juhlin, L., Kirschenbaum, M.B.: Prostaglandin on cutaneous vasculature. J. Invest. Dermatol. *51*, 280–282 (1968)
Starke, K., Peskar, B.A., Schumacher, K.A., Taube, H.D.: Bradykinin and postganglionic sympathetic transmission. Naunyn Schmiedebergs Arch. Pharmacol. *299*, 23–32 (1977)
Staszewska-Barczak, J., Dusting, G.J.: Sympathetic cardiovascular reflex initiated by bradykinin-induced stimulation of cardiac pain receptors in the dog. Clin. Exp. Pharmacol. Physiol. *4*, 443–452 (1977)
Staszewska-Barczak, J., Ferreira, S.H., Vane, J.R.: An excitatory nociceptive cardiac reflex elicited by bradykinin and potentiated by prostaglandins and myocardial ischaemia. Cardiovasc. Res. *10*, 314–327 (1976)
Szolcsányi, J.: A pharmacological approach to elucidation of the role of different nerve fibres and receptor endings in mediation of pain. J. Physiol. (Paris) *73*, 251–259 (1977)
Taira, N., Hashimoto, K.: Absence of the pain-producing activity of otherwise biologically active synthetic fragments of bradykinin. Tohoku J. Exp. Med. *110*, 191–194 (1973)
Taira, N., Nakayama, K., Hashimoto, K.: Vocalization response of puppies to intra-arterial administration of bradykinin and other algesic agents, and mode of action of blocking agents. Tohoku J. Exp. Med. *96*, 365–377 (1968)
Takagi, H., Doi, T., Akaike, A.: Microinjection of morphine into the medial part of the bulbar reticular formation in rabbit and rat: inhibitory effects on lamina V cells of spinal dorsal horn and behavioral analgesia. In: Opiates and endogenous opioid peptides. Kosterlitz, H.W. (ed.), pp. 191–198. Amsterdam: North-Holland 1976a
Takagi, H., Satoh, M., Doi, T., Kawasaki, K., Akaike, A.: Indirect and direct depressive effects of morphine on activation of lamina V cell of the spinal dorsal horn induced by intra-arterial injection of bradykinin. Arch. Int. Pharmacodyn. Ther. *221*, 96–104 (1976b)
Tallarida, G., Baldoni, F., Peruzzi, G.: Ricerche sulla regolazione neuro-umorale della circolazione. Studio delle risposte riflesse cardiovascolari e respiratorie determinate dalla stimolazione di chemocettori sensibili alla bradichinina nel distretto circolatorio femorale. Boll. Soc. Ital. Cardiol. *19*, 61–83 (1974a)
Tallarida, G., Baldoni, F., Peruzzi, G.: Ricerche sulla regolazione neuro-umorale della circolazione. Analisi delle risposte riflesse cardiovascolari e respiratorie indotte dall'iniezione intracarotidea di bradichinina. Boll. Soc. Ital. Cardiol. *19*, 85–106 (1974b)
Tallarida, G., Baldoni, F., Peruzzi, G., Semprini, A., Sangiorgi, M.: Cardiovascular and respiratory reflexes elicited by bradykinin acting on receptor sites (K&P) in the muscular circulatory area. Adv. Exp. Med. Biol. *70*, 301–314 (1976)
Thompkins, L., Lee, K.H.: Comparison of analgesic effects of isosteric variations of salicyclic acid and aspirin (acetylsalicyclic acid). J. Pharm. Sci. *64*, 760–763 (1975)
Trendelenberg, U.: Observations on the ganglion-stimulating action of angiotensin and bradykinin. J. Pharmacol. Exp. Ther. *154*, 418–425 (1966)
Türker, M.N.: A method for studying the peripheral mediators of the dental pain induced by electrical stimulation. Arch. Int. Physiol. Biochim. *83*, 553–561 (1975)

Türker, M.N., Türker, R.K.: A study on the peripheral mediators of dental pain. Experientia (Basel) *30*, 932–933 (1974)
Uchida, Y., Murao, S.: Bradykinin-induced excitation of afferent cardiac sympathetic nerve fibers. Jpn. Heart J. *15*, 84–91 (1974)
Vane, J.R.: Inhibition of prostaglandin synthesis as a mechanism of action for aspirin-like drugs. Nature New Biol. *231*, 232–235 (1971)
Vane, J.R.: Prostaglandins as mediators of inflammation. In: Advances in prostaglandin and thromboxane research. Samuelsson, B., Paoletti, R. (eds.), Vol. 2, pp. 791–801. New York: Raven 1976
Vane, J.R.: Inhibitors of prostaglandin, prostacyclin, and thromboxane synthesis. In: Advances in prostaglandin and thromboxane research. Coceani, F., Olley, P.M. (eds.), Vol. 4, pp. 27–44. New York: Raven 1978
Vargaftig, B.: Effet des analgésiques non narcotiques sur l'hypotension due à la bradykinine. Experientia (Basel) *22*, 182–183 (1966)
Vecchiet, L., Dolce, V., Galleti, R.: Algogenic activity of human plasma following muscular work. Adv. Exp. Med. Biol. *70*, 177–182 (1976)
Walaszek, E.J.: Effect of bradykinin on the central nervous system. In: Handbook of experimental pharmacology. Vol. XXV: Bradykinin, kallidin and kallikrein. Erdös, E.G. (ed.), pp. 430–433. Berlin, Heidelberg, New York: Springer 1970
Wallis, D.I., Woodward, B.: The facilitatory actions of 5-hydroxytryptamine and bradykinin in the superior cervical ganglion of the rabbit. Br. J. Pharmacol. *51*, 521–531 (1974)
Watson, P.J.: Drug receptor sites in the rabbit saphenous nerve. Br. J. Pharmacol. *40*, 102–112 (1970)
Willis, A.L., Cornelsen, M.: Repeated injection of prostaglandin E_2 in rat paws induces chronic swelling and a marked decrease in pain threshold. Prostaglandins *3*, 353–357 (1973)
Willis, W.D., Jr., Grossman, R.G.: Medical neurobiology, 2nd ed. St. Louis: Mosby 1977
Wiśniewski, K., Bodzenta, A.: Kinins and central effects of the acetylcholine. Acta Neurobiol. Exp. (Warcz.) *35*, 85–92 (1975)
Wiśniewski, K., Mackiewicz, W.: Kinins and hypoglycemic convulsions. Pol. J. Pharmacol. Pharm. *26*, 611–615 (1974)
Wiśniewski, K., Moniuszko-Jakoniuk, J., Sosnowska, Z.: The effects of kinins and their interactions with adrenergic mechanisms on the behavioural activity of rats. Clin. Exp. Pharmacol. Physiol. *1*, 519–526 (1974)
Woodworth, R.S., Sherrington, C.S.: A pseudaffective reflex and its spinal path. J. Physiol. (Lond.) *31*, 234–243 (1904)
Yaksh, T.L., Rudy, T.A.: Analgesia mediated by a direct spinal action of narcotics. Science *192*, 1357–1358 (1976)
Zieglgänsberger, W., Bayerl, H.: The mechanism of inhibition of neuronal activity by opiates in the spinal cord of cat. Brain Res. *115*, 111–128 (1976)
Zimmermann, M.: Neurophysiology of nociception. In: International review of physiology. Vol. 10: Neurophysiology II. Porter, R. (ed.), pp. 179–221. Baltimore: University Park 1976

Effects of Kinins on Organ Systems

A. R. Johnson

A. Introduction

Kinins have an impressive array of effects on various physiological functions. They can affect organ systems directly or indirectly through their interactions with neural pathways and with other mediators. The recently recognized effects of kinins on prostaglandin synthesis and metabolism (see next Chapter) emphasize the potentially broad-range effects these potent peptides may have. However, kinins presently have no generally accepted role in normal physiology. While many cellular and metabolic actions of kinins are reviewed elsewhere in this volume (see Terragno and Terragno; Odya and Goodfriend), this chapter will address some of the prominent actions of kinins of cardiovascular, pulmonary, gastrointestinal and reproductive functions.

B. Effects on the Cardiovascular System

Kinins exert their major effects on the cardiovascular system by acting directly on vascular smooth muscle. The resulting hemodynamic changes can influence cardiac functions via reflexes. Bradykinin causes either constriction or dilation of blood vessels, depending on the type of vessel and the animal species. The response of a particular vessel may be influenced by local metabolic conditions in the blood and surrounding tissues, e.g., as in hypoxia or during muscle work. In man and most other mammals, kinins act on peripheral arterioles to cause vasodilation and hypotension. They constrict venules and usually increase flow in capillary beds. In addition, kinins cause leakage of fluid from the microvascular system at the level of the postcapillary venules. These actions were reviewed comprehensively in an earlier volume of this series (Haddy et al., 1970).

I. Cardiac Effects

Both direct and indirect effects of kinins on hearts of experimental animals have been described, but the effects on cardiac muscle are insignificant compared with effects on coronary or peripheral vessels (Harrison et al., 1968; Nakano, 1970). Bradykinin dilates coronary arteries in isolated perfused hearts (Rocha e Silva et al., 1976; Needleman et al., 1975; Needleman, 1976; Regoli et al., 1977a) and in intact animals (Bassenge et al., 1970; 1972; Nakano, 1970). The fact that indomethacin blocks this effect of bradykinin suggests that prostaglandin synthesis or release may mediate the coronary vasodilation. There is not universal agreement on this mechanism, however. Regoli and associates (1977a) found that indomethacin only partially inhibits the

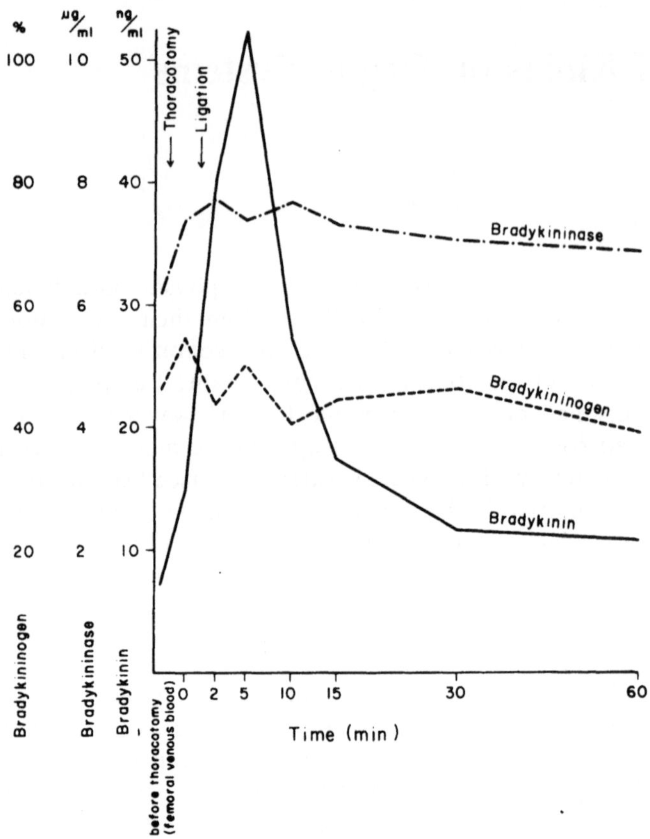

Fig. 1. Changes in mean values of kininogen, bradykinin and kininase in dog coronary sinus blood before and after ligation of coronary artery. (From KIMURA et al., 1973). Reproduced with permission from the authors

vasodilation by bradykinin in isolated rabbit hearts and that it does not influence other potent coronary vasodilators such as substance P or nitroglycerin.

BASSENGE and co-workers (1972) considered the possibility that kinins could regulate coronary resistance during reactive or functional hyperemia. However, their studies in conscious dogs indicated that kinins do not contribute to coronary regulation under physiological conditions. Others suggested that bradykinin stimulates a chemoreflex response similar to that provoked by veratrine (NETO et al., 1974).

While kinins probably do not affect cardiac dynamics under normal conditions, they may contribute to anginal pain (FURUKAWA et al., 1969; KIMURA et al., 1973) or cardiogenic shock (SICUTERRI et al., 1972; WILKENS et al., 1975). Changes in components of the kinin system during experimental myocardial ischemia suggest that kinin generation is involved. KIMURA and associates (1973) found that bradykinin increased threefold in coronary sinus blood within 5 min of ligation of the anterior descending artery in dogs (Fig. 1). Kininogen levels in the coronary sinus blood decreased slightly after ligation. Although dilation of the coronary vessels by bradykinin may be a compensatory response to ischemia of the heart, retention of the peptide within the area of the occluded vessel could cause pain by stimulation of afferent cardiac nerve fibers (UCHIDA and MURAO, 1974).

In experiments with acute coronary occlusion in dogs, WILKINS and associates (1975) found that treatment with aprotinin diminished the incidence of arrhythmias and prolonged survival times. Changes in plasma kininogen, fibrinogen and plasminogen occurred concomittantly with the hemodynamic events, but these authors were unable to detect kinin in coronary venous blood either before or after occlusion of the coronary artery. Any changes in components of the kinin system as indicative of kinin involvement in hypoxia or shock must be interpreted with caution, however, since kinins can be generated by plasmin and other kininogenases (see MOVAT, p. 1). Even a slight lowering of blood pH can activate both the kinin and fibrinolytic systems (WILKENS et al., 1970), and hypoxia alters the surface characteristics of vascular endothelium (FONKALSRUD et al., 1976), which in turn, may cause contact activation of blood.

Kinins probably do not affect energy metabolism in the heart, but may modify the actions of other hormones and mediators. MONIUSZKO-JAKONUIK and associates (1976) found that neither bradykinin nor kallikrein affected phosphorylase *a* activity in heart muscle of anesthetized rats, but that bradykinin diminished the stimulating effect of norepinephrine on this enzyme. Both bradykinin and kallikrein opposed the metabolic actions of catecholamines on phosphorylase *a*, fatty acids, and lactate, possibly through an effect on adenyl cyclase.

Studies of kinin system components in patients with acute myocardial infarction suggest that kinins are generated during myocardial ischemia in man as well as in experimental animals (DZIZINSKII and KUIMOV, 1972; KEDRA et al., 1973; HASHIMOTO et al., 1976, 1978). KEDRA et al. (1973) found that the kininogen levels decreased between the first and third days, and then returned toward normal by the eighth day after infarction. Patients who experienced tachycardia, hypotension, and decreased central venous pressure had lower kininogen levels than those without hemodynamic disturbances. HASHIMOTO and associates (1976) found that both prekallikrein and kininogen levels in blood were substantially decreased in patients with acute myocardial infarction, compared to normal subjects, during a three-day observation period. Survivors of the infarction had less pronounced changes than did nonsurvivors.

A possible beneficial effect of kinins was suggested by the finding of HASHIMOTO and associates (1976, 1978), viz., that survivors of acute myocardial infarction had lower kininase activity than nonsurvivors. This led the authors to speculate that kinins may reduce the work load of an injured heart by decreasing peripheral resistance. However, there is still no direct evidence to establish whether kinin generation is a cause or a result of hemodynamic changes following infarction.

II. Cardiac Nerves

The cardiovascular response to injected kinins depends on both the animal species and the route of administration. The situation is complicated by the frequent involvement of cardiovascular reflexes and direct stimulation of nerves. For example, intraarterial injection of bradykinin (0.3–1 μg/kg) into rats or cats causes a biphasic response: hypotension followed by elevation of blood pressure and polypnea (DAMAS, 1974, 1975). These latter effects may result from stimulation of the carotid sinus or of paravascular nociceptive receptors. In addition, bradykinin can alter blood pressure by stimulation of coronary receptors. Injection of 1 μg of bradykinin into coronary arteries of anesthetized dogs causes a simultaneous decrease in systemic blood pressure and heart rate, accompanied by a decrease in respiratory rate and amplitude. The bradycardia, but not the hypotension, was potentiated by neostigmine and abolished by atropine. Bilateral vagotomy abolished the bradycardia and decreased the hypotension caused by intracoronary injection of bradykinin (NETO et al., 1974).

Bradykinin generation within ischemic hearts may affect cardiac and hemodynamic functions by stimulation of nerves within the heart. STASZEWSKA-BARCZAK and DUSTING (1977) found that application of bradykinin to the epicardium of open-chest anesthetized dogs caused dose-related pressor effects and acceleration of the heart rate. The tachycardia was inhibited by the beta adrenergic blocking drug, propranolol, and the pressor response was inhibited by the alpha adrenergic antagonist, phenoxybenzamine. Neither vagotomy nor atropine affected the response to bradykinin, but spinal section at C-1 reduced it. Thus, bradykinin appears to stimulate both heart and blood vessels reflexly through sympathetic efferent nerves.

Bradykinin has a negative chronotropic effect on isolated rabbit hearts, probably via parasympathetic innervation of the heart. Pretreatment of the hearts with atropine or tetrodotoxin block this effect, but hexamethonium does not (SCHUMACHER and STARKE, 1978).

In addition, bradykinin may affect blood flow by an action on peripheral nerves. TALLARIDA et al. (1976) found that low doses of kinin (250 ng) injected into the femoral artery of rabbits caused a reflex vasodilation in the contralateral hindlimb. This effect was not blocked by atropine but was abolished by sectioning of femoral and sciatic nerves.

III. Vascular Effects

In general, small arterial vessels are relaxed by bradykinin and veins are constricted, but there may be regional variations. In isolated structures such as rabbit ear (SEKIYA et al., 1971) and rat mesentery (NORTHOVER and NORTHOVER, 1970), arterioles are dilated and venules are constricted, with a resultant increase in venular pressure. Infusion of bradykinin at a rate of 20–25 ng/min into the brachial artery of human subjects results in vasodilation and increased flow in the forearm without effect on either heart rate or systemic arterial pressure (LUDBROOK et al., 1973). These actions presumably result from direct stimulation of kinin receptors on vascular smooth muscle, but this can not be firmly established until specific receptor antagonists for kinins are available.

Injection of bradykinin into the marginal ear vein of rabbits causes venoconstriction at doses that do not affect the systemic circulation (BOBBIN and GUTH, 1968). Since venoconstriction is not affected by denervation of the ear or by antihistaminic and antiadrenergic drugs, it probably results from stimulation of kinin receptors associated with the vessels. Bradykinin does not have a uniform effect on all veins; helical strips of umbilical veins from sheep or monkeys are relaxed by application of bradykinin in vitro (DYER, 1970; DYER et al., 1972). Human saphenous vein strips are unresponsive to bradykinin in concentrations ranging from 50–2000 ng/ml (LEVY, 1972), but dog saphenous veins contract in response to as little as 1 ng/ml of the peptide (GOLDBERG et al., 1977).

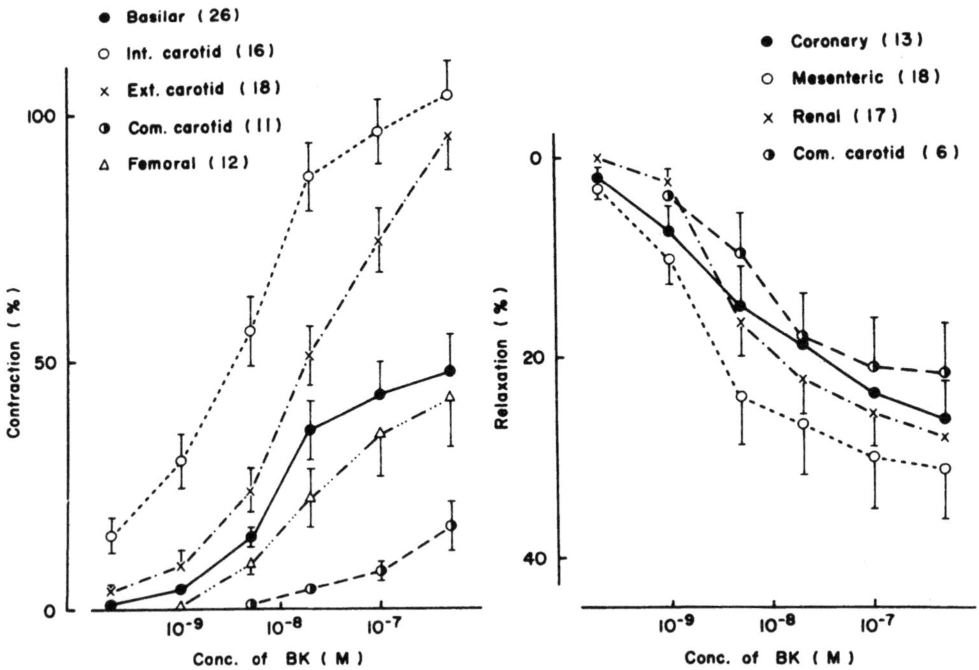

Fig. 2. Dose-response curves to bradykinin in arteries from dogs. The figures in parenthesis indicate the number of experiments. The left panel shows contractions relative to those induced by 30 mM K^+. The right panel shows relaxation of arterial preparations that were contracted with K^+. The relaxation is expressed relative to that caused by papaverine ($10^{-5}M$). (From TODA, 1977). Reproduced with permission from the author

TSURU et al. (1974; 1976) found that veins from various sites in the dog could be classified into two groups with respect to their response to bradykinin. One group, which included vessels from the visceral area, was highly sensitive to bradykinin. The other group, which included vessels from the extremities, was much less sensitive.

In studies of canine arterial strips in vitro, TODA (1977) found that bradykinin had opposite effects on similar-sized arteries from different sites. The kinin caused a dose-related contraction of helical strips of cerebral, carotid, and femoral arteries, but it relaxed coronary, renal and mesenteric arteries that had been contracted by K^+ or $PGF_{2\alpha}$ (see TERRAGNO and TERRAGNO, this volume). This pattern is illustrated in Fig. 2.

Taking these findings together with those of TSURU et al. (1974), an intriguing pattern emerges. In the neck and extremities (carotid and femoral vessels), bradykinin contracts arteries but has only a slight effect on veins. In the thoracic and abdominal cavities (coronary, mesentery, and renal vessels), bradykinin relaxes arteries but contracts veins (pulmonary, hepatic, and splenic vessels).

Bradykinin appears to promote flow through microcirculatory beds by increasing the number of functioning capillaries. This has been observed in tissues as diverse as the vasa vasorum of the dog aorta (SHIONOYA et al., 1971) and in the microcirculation of experimental tumors in rats (ACKERMAN and HECHMER, 1977).

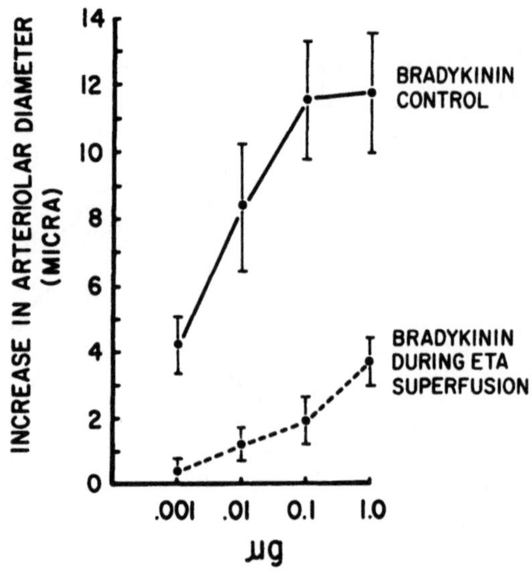

Fig. 3. Inhibition by 5,8,11,14-eicosatetraynoic acid (ETA) of bradykinin-induced vasodilation in rat cremaster muscle arterioles. Values are mean increases in diameter from control. Vertical lines are SEM. (From MESSINA et al., Circ. Res. *37*, 430–437, 1975). Reproduced with permission from the authors

Considerable evidence has accumulated to suggest that the actions of bradykinin on vessels in the heart, kidney, and mesentery involves release of prostaglandins (see TERRAGNO and TERRAGNO, next chapter). Experiments with indomethacin and other agents that block prostaglandin synthesis support this idea. For example, indomethacin decreases the duration of hypotension caused by injection of bradykinin in experimental animals (DAMAS and MOUSTY, 1976). MESSINA et al. (1975) found that local application of indomethacin or 5,8,11,14-eicosatetraynoic acid (ETA) to single arterioles in the rat cremaster muscle reduced the dilation caused by bradykinin (see Fig. 3). In addition, it has been shown that bradykinin releases prostaglandin-like materials from a variety of experimental preparations. These include: isolated perfused rabbit hearts (NEEDLEMAN et al., 1975; NEEDLEMAN, 1976; HSUEH et al., 1977), perfused rabbit ears (JUAN and LEMBECK, 1976), dog kidney (MCGIFF et al., 1972), vessels of mesentery (TERRAGNO et al., 1975; BLUMBERG et al., 1977), and cultured vascular smooth muscle cells (ALEXANDER and GIMBRONE, 1976; PITLICK et al., 1977).

The studies of TERRAGNO et al. (1975) and WONG et al. (1977b) offer an explanation for the differential effects of bradykinin on arteries and veins. It was initially observed that bradykinin increased prostaglandin synthesis by both bovine mesenteric arteries and veins in vitro, with a PGE-like material produced specifically by the arteries and PGF-like material produced by veins (TERRAGNO et al., 1975). The generation of $PGF_{2\alpha}$ in veins appears to depend on the conversion of $PGE_{2\alpha}$ by 9-ketoreductase, and this enzyme is stimulated by bradykinin (WONG et al., 1977b; LIMAS, 1977). In addition, release of prostaglandin by bradykinin may depend on phospholipase activation (DAMAS and DEBY, 1976; LIMAS, 1977; HSUEH et al., 1977).

Not all authors agree that prostaglandins mediate the response of vessels to bradykinin. CHAPNICK and co-workers (1977) found that, in the anesthetized cat, indomethacin did not block the response of renal vessels to bradykinin. In fact, the vasodilator response to bradykinin was enhanced by indomethacin. They concluded that, in contrast to vascular responses in the dog (MCGIFF et al., 1972), endogenous prostaglandins do not mediate the response to bradykinin in the cat, and they suggested that drugs such as indomethacin and meclofenamate have actions unrelated to prostaglandin synthesis. A similar conclusion was reached by TODA (1977) who used isolated canine arteries. The contractile response to bradykinin in various isolated canine vessels was not affected by specific receptor blocking agents such as phentolamine, diphenhydramine, or methysergide. While the response was attenuated by aspirin or indomethacin, polyphloretin phosphate (a prostaglandin antagonist) did not reduce it (TODA, 1977). This indicates that prostaglandins may not be directly responsible for the contractile effect.

Alternatively, postanglandins may modulate the effects of kinins on vessels. GOLDBERG and associates (1976) found that bradykinin caused contraction of helical strips of canine saphenous veins. The responsiveness of the tissue increased with time after isolation. Initially, when the tissue was least sensitive to bradykinin, either indomethacin or ETA enhanced the response, shifting the concentration-effect curve to the left. Later, when the tissue had become more sensitive to kinin stimulation, these inhibitors of prostaglandin synthesis did not affect the response. The authors speculated that prostaglandins attenuate the response of vein strips to bradykinin, and that in vitro prostaglandin synthesis declines with time. However, they did not measure prostaglandins in these experiments.

Bradykinin appears to have only a direct action on smooth muscle receptors in rabbit aorta in vitro (GARRETT and BROWN, 1972; REGOLI et al., 1977b). Kinin receptors in the aorta were studied with bradykinin and with des-Arg^1-bradykinin by REGOLI et al. (1977b). Since the kinin effects were not blocked by phentolamine, methysergide, mepyramine, 8-Leu-angiotensin II or indomethacin, REGOLI and associates concluded that kinins affected receptors distinct from those for catecholamines, histamine, or angiotensin. The kinin effects on aorta were competitively inhibited by octapeptide analogs with an aliphatic substitution at the 8-Phe position. However, the receptors for kinins in other tissues may be different since these substituted analogs did not block the actions of bradykinin on other smooth muscle preparations (BARABÉ et al., 1977).

Factors such as oxygen tension can also influence blood vessel reactivity and flow. SVENSJÖ and associates (1977b) found that the flow through the microvasculature of the hamster cheek pouch decreased under conditions where the pO_2 of the superfusing solution was elevated to 115 mm Hg. These experiments point out the need for rigid control of conditions in microcirculation experiments before conclusions can be made about drug effects.

The role of kinins in functional hyperemia has been explored by many investigators. While either bradykinin or kallidin causes hyperemia in the salivary gland that coincides with enzyme secretion from the gland, this may not be a general role for kinins. FASTH and associates (FASTH and MARTINSON, 1973; FASTH and HULTEN, 1973) concluded that kinins did not mediate functional hypermia in the cat stomach, since the pattern of vascular effects caused by vagal nerve stimulation was not reproduced by injected bradykinin.

The generation of kinins in proximity to vessels within specific vascular beds may cause functional changes either by a direct effect on vascular smooth muscle or by release of other mediators. ITO et al. (1973) found that bradykinin first increased and then decreased blood flow in the gingival circulation in dogs. Chlorpromazine reduced the initial phase of the response and completely blocked the secondary decrease in flow, but atropine did not affect the response.

Experiments on intact fetal animals indicate that kinins might play a role in the conversion of fetal circulation to that of the adult (MELMON et al., 1968). Bradykinin causes pulmonary arterial dilation in the fetal lamb and closure of the ductus arteriosus (CAMPBELL et al., 1968; ASSALI et al., 1971), and the levels of bradykinin in umbilical cord blood are higher than those in maternal circulation. Kininogen is present in arterial blood of fetal lambs as early as 61 days of gestation and increases toward term. Following birth the kininogen levels in left atrial blood decrease after ventilation with O_2, and bradykinin can be detected in left atrial blood (HEYMANN et al., 1969).

Since prostaglandins are thought to maintain the patency of the ductus in utero, this may be another tissue in which kinins and prostaglandins interact. Although PGs of the A and E series relax the isolated ductus from lambs (and would thus oppose the closing action of bradykinin), ($PGF_{2\alpha}$ and its 15-keto metabolites do not have this action (CLYMAN et al., 1978). It remains to be seen whether bradykinin selectively stimulates formation of a specific prostaglandin which mediates closure of the ductus at birth.

It was suggested that bradykinin mediates the decrease in pulmonary vascular resistance when fetal lungs are ventilated with air after birth (HEYMANN et al., 1969). GILBERT and co-workers (1973) studied the response of the pulmonary circulation in fetal goats and found that either air breathing or infusion of bradykinin into the pulmonary artery decreased pulmonary vascular resistance. The effect of air breathing depends on the oxygen concentration, since ventilation of the lung at the same oxygen tension as fetal arterial blood did not decrease vascular resistance. When the right lung was separately ventilated with gas of the same composition as in fetal blood (4% O_2 and 6% CO_2 in N_2) there was no change in resistance in the left lung. However, when the right lung was ventilated with air, resistance in the left lung decreased. GILBERT et al. suggested that bradykinin release may have caused the decrease in resistance in the left lung, but since they did not measure kinins in the blood and did not evaluate the influence of drugs that inhibit kallikrein or kininase, their conclusions are only speculative.

ALTURA (1972) found that not only bradykinin but also kallidin and Met-Lys-bradykinin contracted arteries and veins of human umbilical cord and suggested that these peptides could influence blood flow in the human umbilical cord in vivo. Similarly, kinins might influence blood flow and lactation following delivery. All three kinins (2–400 ng/kg) caused vasodilation and increased blood flow in the mammary glands when injected intravenously into lactating goats (HOUVENAGHEL and PEETERS, 1971). Intravenous kallikrein produced a similar but longer-lasting effect (HOUVENAGEL and PEETERS, 1972; PEETERS et al., 1972).

IV. Vascular Permeability

Among the most prominent effects of kinins are an increase in vascular permeability within the microcirculation and a net movement of water from blood into tissues. This has supported the idea that kinins are mediators of acute inflammation. However, how much kinins contribute to inflammation can not be assessed convincingly until appropriate specific antagonists are available. The major alteration of vessel permeability as determined by electron microscopy and tracer materials occurs at the level of postcapillary venules (GABBIANI et al., 1970, 1972), possibly as a result of endothelial cell contraction and widening of intracellular junctions (MAJNO et al., 1969; MAJNO et al., 1972; GABBIANI et al., 1975). This is presumably an active, energy-requiring process since the increase in permeability produced by bradykinin and other mediators in microcirculation can be prevented by application of sodium cyanide to the vessels (OYVIN et al., 1970, 1972).

HULTSTRÖM and SVENSJÖ (1977) combined vital staining with electron microscopy to study vessels in the hamster cheek pouch. They found that 1 μg bradykinin applied topically to the vessels caused formation of intracellular gaps as large as 0.4 microns between endothelial cells (Fig. 4). The passage of a fluorescent dextran tracer permitted the immediate identification of affected vessels by fluorescent microscopy. Other studies of microcirculation suggest that the increase in vascular permeability might be mediated by prostaglandins. NORTHOVER and NORTHOVER (1969) observed that indomethacin inhibited the effect of bradykinin on the rat mesentery, but the possibility of prostaglandin involvement was suggested only later by studies in various permeability models (see below).

The mechanism of edema formation by bradykinin is complex. The venular gaps caused by histamine or bradykinin are generally transient and last only 20–30 min (PIETRA et al., 1971), but edema formation continues beyond this time. JOYNER and associates (JOYNER et al., 1974; CARTER et al., 1974) found that bradykinin or histamine produced a sustained increase in lymph flow in the dog paw and increased the concentration of protein in lymph relative to plasma. They interpreted the increase in blood–lymph transport as a manifestation of increased flux of water and protein across a barrier of unchanged porosity rather than the result of a generalized increase in capillary permeability. They used a series of markers of different molecular weights (dextrans and plasma proteins) to measure efflux in the dog-paw preparation and found that subcutaneous injection of 5–100 μg bradykinin increased the efflux of a number of plasma proteins and dextrans regardless of molecular size. They suggested that bradykinin increased vesicular transport by the endothelium rather than causing gap (or large pore) formation.

The issue of whether bradykinin affects the formation of gaps between endothelial junctions or enhances formation of vesicles is still not resolved. Regional variation in vessels or differences in the types of receptors can also influence transport functions and edema formation. For example, SCHWARTZ and COTRAN (1972) found that the microvasculature of the kidney was impermeable to a carbon tracer even when bradykinin caused leakage of the marker in peripelvic, periureteral, and pericystic vessels. They attributed the insensitivity of the renal parenchymal vessels to the pecularities of their endothelial structure.

BAUMGARTEN and co-workers (1970) studied vascular permeability changes caused by histamine and bradykinin in cutaneous vessels of the guinea pig. By continuously monitoring the leakage of a circulating radioactive tracer, they determined the response to intracutaneous injections of histamine and bradykinin. They suggested that there were two types of receptors for these mediators on the vessels: one was responsive to both histamine and bradykinin and one to only bradykinin. The former sites became refractory to permeability mediators, but the latter sites (responsive only to bradykinin) did not.

Longer kinin peptides, such as Gly-Arg-Met-Lys-bradykinin and Met-Lys-bradykinin are more potent than the native nonapeptide in increasing vascular

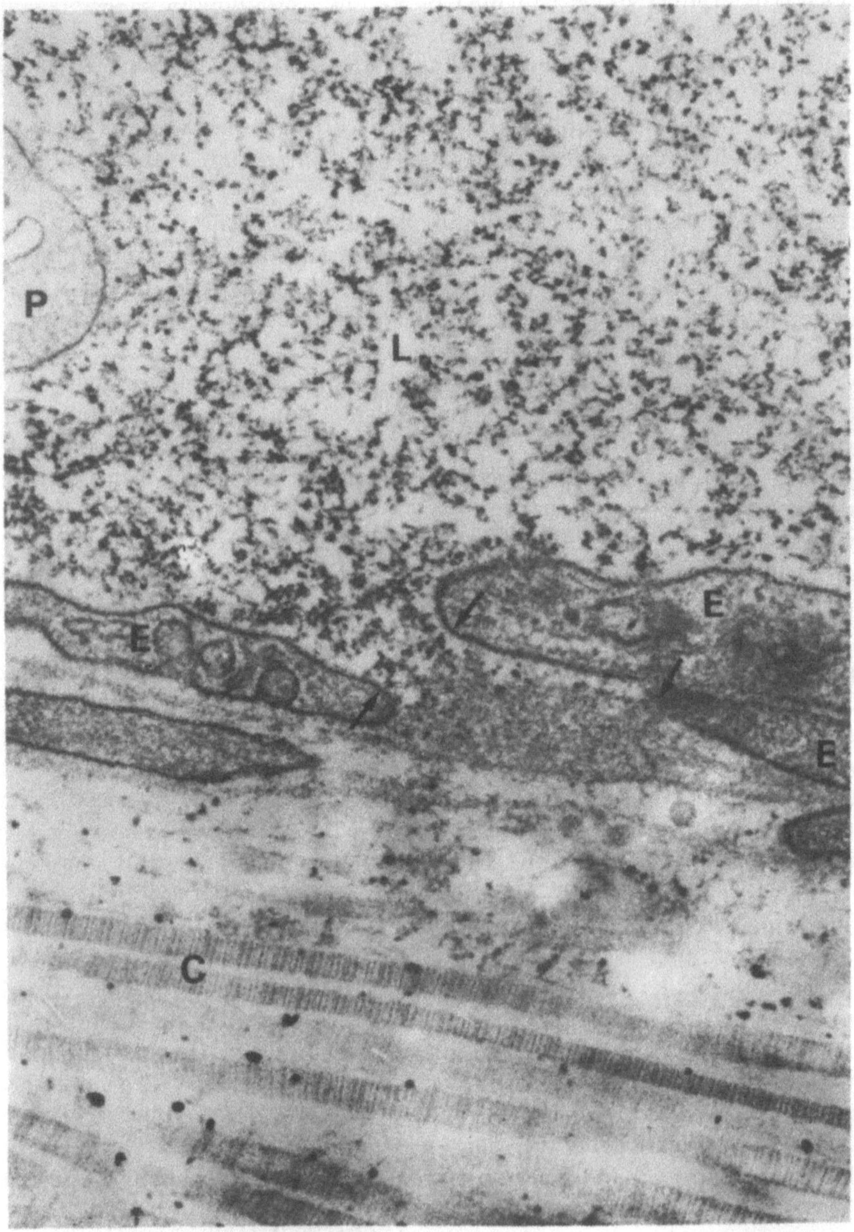

Fig. 4. Endothelial gap in vessel from hamster cheek pouch after treatment with bradykinin. The electron micrograph shows a gap between endothelial cells (E) as indicated by arrows. Dark precipitates are seen in the vessel lumen (L), in the gap, and between the collagen fibers (C). Platelet (P). Magnification, × 100,000. (From HULTSTRÖM and SVENSJÖ, 1977). Reproduced with permission from the authors

permeability, but are less potent in stimulation of smooth muscle (REIS et al., 1971; 1973). Since longer kinin derivatives may also be more resistant than bradykinin to inactivation by kininase II (DORER et al., 1974; JOHNSON and ERDÖS, 1977) they could be important mediators of inflammatory reactions.

Various endogenous mediators and added drugs can influence the development of vascular permeability in response to kinins. A fraction from human plasma inhibits carrageenin-induced edema in the rat paw (BOLAM et al., 1974) which may depend in part on kinin formation (DI ROSA and SORRENTINO, 1970). However, since this particular experimental model involves a number of phlogistic substances, the inhibitory effects of this plasma fraction can not be attributed to a specific blockade of kinins.

MACIEJKO and associates (1978) studied the effects of bradykinin on transvascular fluid and protein transfer in the forelimb of dogs and found that both norepinephrine and isoproterenol antagonized the protein efflux caused by an infusion of bradykinin (0.8 μg/min). The antagonism could be prevented by prior treatment with propranolol. Since there were only minimal effluxes of protein after systemic administration of bradykinin compared to the efflux that occurred after infusion directly into the brachial artery, the authors concluded that released catecholamines inhibited the effects of bradykinin. They suggested that when the levels of bradykinin increased enough to cause a fall in blood pressure, a reflex sympathoadrenal discharge would offset the increase in vessel permeability. Although these investigators attempted to circumvent the inactivation of bradykinin in the lungs by infusing it into the left ventricle, they did not block the metabolism by kininase in blood and peripheral vessels. Thus, it is not certain that released catecholamines, and not differences in kinin metabolism, can account for their observations.

SVENSJÖ and colleagues (1977a) found that the beta adrenergic agonist, terbutaline, inhibited bradykinin-induced permeability changes in the microcirculation of the hamster cheek pouch. Since there is evidence that endothelial cell contraction may cause formation of gaps between the cells (MAJNO et al., 1972; GABBIANI et al., 1975; HULTSTRÖM and SVENSJÖ, 1977) they suggested that terbutaline might prevent endothelial contraction.

Other investigators suggest that cyclic AMP is an important mediator in the permeability response to bradykinin. KAHN and BRACHET (1976) used sheets of isolated rat mesenteries as a model in which to study transfer properties of endothelium. They pointed out the similarities between this mesodermal tissue and vascular endothelium and found that its permeability to labeled albumin was increased by agents such as histamine, serotonin, dibutyryl cyclic AMP, or theophylline. The authors suggested that a common mechanism could be an increase in cyclic AMP, but offered no additional evidence to support this hypothesis.

C. Kinins and Inflammation

The relation of kinin production to the early stages of inflammation has been explored by many authors (Wilhelm, 1973). Since kinins have potent effects on vascular permeability, and since a multiplicity of factors stimulate their production in blood, they are prime candidates for inflammatory mediators. The role of kinins in disease states and kinins from leukocytes are discussed elsewhere in this volume (see COLMAN and WONG,

p. 593, and GREENBAUM, p. 91), but no chapter on the actions of kinins would be complete without mention of their possible roles in inflammation.

Bradykinin may be a mediator of carrageenin edema, which is a model for testing anti-inflammatory drugs. This type of edema is not readily blocked by antihistaminic or antiserotonergic drugs (LEME et al., 1973). Several studies suggest that kinins are involved. Because prior treatment with 1,10-phenanthroline enhanced the edema formed by carrageenin or cellulose sulfate in the rat paw, CAPASSO and associates (1975) proposed that bradykinin was the endogenous mediator. Phenathroline inhibits kininases in blood (ERDÖS and YANG, 1970) and should enhance kinin-mediated inflammatory changes. However, this agent would also prevent inactivation of complement peptides, particularly C3a anaphylatoxin (BOKISCH and MÜLLER-EBERHARD, 1970; VALLOTA and MÜLLER-EBERHARD, 1973) by kininase I and would presumably also affect metabolism of chemotactic factors. More direct evidence linking kinins with carrageenin edema was provided by the experiments of CRUNKHORN and MEACOCK (1971). They found that treatment of rats with ellagic acid, an activator of Hageman factor, did not interfere with the response to intradermally administered bradykinin, but it markedly reduced the inflammatory response to locally injected carrageenin. Kinins have also been implicated as the mediators of pleurisy in rats caused by instillation of carrageenin into the pleural space (KATORI et al., 1978).

Indirect evidence that kinins are involved in inflammation in the rat paw was provided by the experiments of GECSE et al. (1972). They injected phlogistic agents such as histamine, serotonin, or dextran. Edema formation was accompanied by the appearance of kininogen in the extravascular compartment of the paw and a decrease in kininogen levels in the plasma. This was prevented by treatment with C-phenylglycine-n-heptyl ester, a compound with antihistaminic and antiserotonergic effects.

Several studies suggested that bradykinin was the mediator of thermal edema (LEME et al., 1970, 1973). However, GREEN (1974; 1978) found that the inflammatory edema produced in rat or mouse paws by bradykinin differed from thermal edema in several respects. First, catecholamines supress the development of bradykinin-induced edema but potentiate thermal injury edema (GREEN, 1974). Second, bradykinin does not cause extravasation of erythrocytes, but thermal injury does. Finally, there are differences in the composition of the edema fluid induced by kinin and by heating (GREEN, 1978). Thus, it seems unlikely that bradykinin is the sole mediator of thermal edema.

Prostaglandins influence edema formation in various experimental models. Arachidonic acid, PGE_1, or PGE_2 injected onto the hindpaw of the rat produces edema and extravasation of a circulating dye marker. The permeability enhancing actions of bradykinin were potentiated by prostaglandins E_1 and E_2 but not by arachidonic acid (DAMAS and VOLON, 1976). Since pretreatment of the rats with indomethacin reduced the edema caused by bradykinin, the authors concluded that prostaglandins were involved. However, there is variation in the results obtained from different models. IKEDA et al. (1975) reported that either PGE_2 or arachidonic acid potentiated by 10-fold the increase in vascular permeability caused by injection of bradykinin in rabbit skin. THOMAS and WEST (1974, found that PGE_1, but not PGE_2, potentiated the extravasation of dye in skin of rats injected intradermally with bradykinin. $PFG_{2\alpha}$ inhibited the dye leakage. PGI_2, while devoid of permeability effects alone, potentiated the effects of carrageenin in the rat paw (KOMORIYA et al., 1978) and the effects of intradermal injection of in rabbits (PECK and WILLIAMS, 1978). It was also found that substance P, in a concentration as low as 5×10^{-11} mol, potentiated the extravasation of dye induced by bradykinin in rat skin (CHAHL, 1977). Thus, the potentiating effect of prostaglandins is not unique. Table 1 summarizes some effects of prostaglandins on permeability.

An important issue in the relationship of prostaglandins to kinin effects was raised by WILLIAMS and PECK (1977) who pointed out that vasodilation caused by prostaglandins may be responsible for potentiation of exudation. They studied plasma exudation in rabbit skin by following the appearance of radiolabeled albumin at sites of intradermally injected bradykinin, adenosine, or arachidonic acid. Changes in local blood flow were measured with a xenon tracer. PGE caused a large increase in blood flow with little effect on plasma leakage. Bradykinin increased the vascular permeability but had less potent effects on blood flow. Further, the potentiating effect of PGE_1 on bradykinin-induced extravasation could not be blocked by indomethacin, an observation also made by LEWIS et al. (1975). Other vasodilator substances, including isoproterenol, ADP, and adenosine also potentiated bradykinin effects on vascular permeability (WILLIAMS and PECK, 1977). This raises the possibility that agents such as substance P or PGI_2 (as described above) also influence permeability indirectly by their vasodilator actions. Since some investigators find that arachidonic acid can potentiate edema produced by carrageenin or kaolin but not by bradykinin (LEWIS et al., 1975), these inflammatory states probably involve multiple mediators.

The finding that polymorphonuclear leukocytes contain kinin-forming enzymes (GREENBAUM and KIM, 1967; MOVAT et al., 1973; MELMON and CLINE, 1968) further emphasizes the potentially broad effects of the kinin system in inflammation. Neutrophils contain at least three systems that can generate kinins from plasma substrates: the leukokinin system, the cytoplasmic kinin-generating system, and the kinin-generating lysosomal neutral protease (WINTROUB and AUSTEN, 1976). In addition, a neutrophil-dependent generation of a neutral peptide has been described (WINTROUB et al., 1974). This peptide shares some of the actions of kinins, such as smooth muscle stimulation and enhancement of vascular permeability, but its relation to the kinin system is not yet clear.

D. Kinins in Exercise and Stress

There is no clear association between exercise and changes in the kallikrein-kinin system, but factors such as epinephrine release or hypoxia could easily affect components of the system. Several investigators measured changes in kallikrein and kininogen in relation to exercise. In human volunteers, the excretion of kallikrein and protein in urine increased after strenuous exercise (MURAKAMI et al., 1968; NAKATA, 1971), and in persons undergoing exercise severe enough to be associated with muscle pain, plasma levels of kininogen are elevated (VECCHIET et al., 1976). Others report a decrease in circulating prekallikrein associated with strenuous exercise (FRANCHI et al., 1976). While the mechanism of these changes is not obvious, they may be related to altered tissue oxygenation and metabolism or to changes in circulating hormones.

I. Catecholamines

It is well known that kinins stimulate release of catecholamines from the adrenal medulla and from the superior cervical ganglia (COLLIER, 1970). Epinephrine causes

Table 1. Influence of arachidonic acid and prostaglandins on kinin-induced vascular permeability

Compound	Dose (μg)	Experimental preparation	Effects	References
Arachidonic acid	1	Rabbit skin	Potentiates dye extravasation	Ikeda et al., 1975
			Potentiates plasma exudation	Williams and Peck, 1977
	2–25	Rat paw	No effect on kinin-induced edema	Damas and Volon, 1976
	100		No effect on kinin-induced edema	Lewis et al., 1975
Prostaglandin E_1	0.1–1	Rabbit skin	Potentiates plasma exudation	Williams and Peck, 1977
	0.1	Guinea pig skin	Potentiates dye extravasation	Williams and Morley, 1973
	0.1	Rat skin	Potentiates dye extravasation	Thomas and West, 1974
	0.01–0.1	Rat paw	Potentiates kinin-induced edema	Damas and Volon, 1976
				Lewis et al., 19755
				Thomas and West, 1974
	0.5–5	Rat paw	Potentiates kinin-induced edema	Moncada et al., 1973
Prostaglandin E_2	0.1–1	Rabbit skin	Potentiates dye extravasation	Ikeda et al., 1975
			Potentiates plasma exudation	Williams and Peck, 1977
				Peck and Williams, 1978
	0.1	Guinea pig skin	Potentiates dye extravasation	Williams and Morley, 1973
	0.1	Rat skin	No effect on dye extravasation	Thomas and West, 1974
	0.01–0.1	Rat paw	Potentiates kinin-induced edema	Damas and Volon, 1976
				Lewis et al., 1975
Prostaglandin $F_{2\alpha}$	0.1	Guinea pig skin	Potentiates dye extravasation	Williams and Morley, 1973
	0.5–1	Rat skin	Inhibits dye extravasation	Thomas and West, 1974
	0.25	Rat paw	No effect on kinin-induced edema	Lewis et al., 1975
Prostaglandin I_2	0.1	Rabbit skin	Potentiates plasma exudation	Peck and Williams, 1978

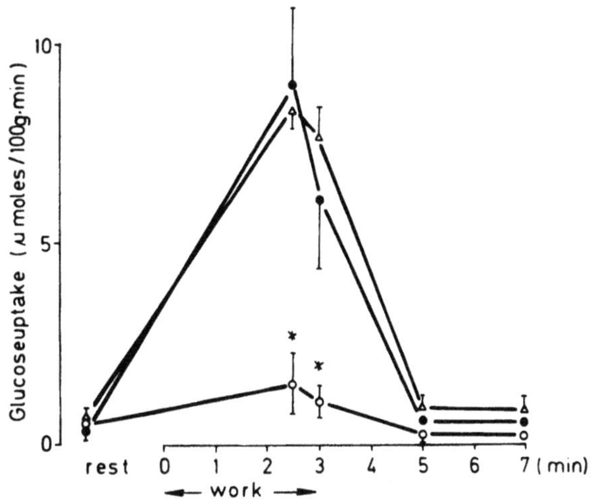

Fig. 5. Glucose uptake in the working human forearm during intravenous infusion of saline (dark circles) or the kallikrein inhibitor, aprotinin, (light circles, and during brachial arterial infusion of bradykinin (open triangles). Values are the mean ±SEM of four volunteers. Asterisks indicate significant ($p<0.025$) difference from controls. (From DIETZE and WICKLMAYR, 1977)

activation of plasma kallikrein, consumption of kininogen, and generation of kinins in rat blood both in vitro and in vivo (CASTANIA and ROTHSCHILD, 1974; ROTHSCHILD et al., 1974; ROTHSCHILD and CASTANIA, 1976). Aspirin (but not indomethacin or sodium salicylate) prevents consumption of kininogen after the intravenous injection of epinephrine (ROTHSCHILD et al., 1975).

II. Hypoxia

Hypoxia may be a physiologic stimulus for kinin formation. Dietze and co-workers (DIETZE and WICKLMAYR, 1977; DIETZE et al., 1977a; 1976b) proposed that kinins are involved in the adaptation of muscle metabolism to exercise or hypoxia. Infusion of the kallikrein inhibitor, aprotinin, into the forearms of human volunteers prevented the enhanced glucose uptake that normally accompanies muscle work. Simultaneous infusion of bradykinin with aprotonin restored the uptake of glucose (DIETZE and WICKLMAYR, 1977). Similarly, in forearms made hypoxic by compression of the brachial artery with a pressure cuff, aprotonin blocked the metabolic response and infusion of bradykinin restored it (DIETZE et al., 1977a; 1977b). These findings are illustrated by Figs. 5 and 6. In addition, oral administration of indomethacin to the subjects prior to experiments partially blocked the effects of bradykinin on glucose uptake, suggesting that this action in muscle may also be mediated by prostaglandins (DIETZE et al., 1978).

Some indirect evidence for the participation of kinins in homeostatic mechanisms in hypoxia was obtained in experiments with human volunteers in a low pressure chamber (HELD, 1977). The subjects were monitored by EEG for signs of cerebral hypoxia and the effect of oral kallikrein was determined. The subjects that received kallikrein had less marked EEG changes than controls, but these effects can not be conclusively related to

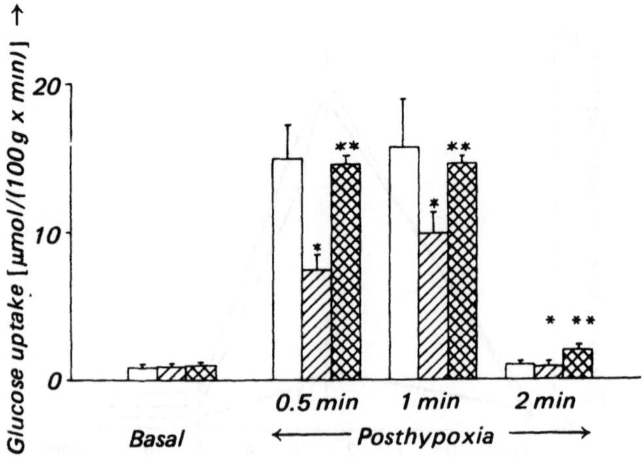

Fig. 6. Uptake of glucose by human forearm after short arrest of perfusion. Glucose uptake was measured during infusion of saline (open columns), aprotinin (cross-hatched columns) or aprotinin plus bradykinin (ckecked columns). Asterisks indicate significant ($p < 0.05$) differences from controls (* compared to saline, iv. ** compared to Trasylol, iv.). (From DIETZE et al., 1977.) Reproduced with permission from the authors

kinin formation since no measurements of kinin system components were made and no inhibitors were used.

Although the effects of orally administered kallikrein have been examined in a number of studies, this route may not be the most efficacious. It is debatable whether a proteolytic enzyme would retain its full activity after contact with the gastric contents. Furthermore, in order to establish hypoxia as a physiological stimulus for kinin generation, rigorous measurements of kinin system components must be made and the formation of free kinin in blood must be shown.

The development of ischemia within tissues can substantially influence the generation of kinins. When local ischemia was produced in the arms of human volunteers, there was a 40% fall in the level of kininogen in the venous blood collected during the period of ischemia (BAVAZZANO et al., 1970). When circulation was restored, the kininogen returned to normal levels. Aprotinin was ineffective in blocking the fall in kininogen during ischemia, suggesting that this effect did not occur by activation of kallikrein. However, either cortisone or taurine inhibited the decrease in kininogen in blood from ischemic tissues.

E. Effects on the Lung

Kinins can influence pulmonary functions both directly and indirectly. The direct actions can be attributed to stimulation of smooth muscle of the blood vessels or the tracheobronchial tree. Indirect effects of kinins result from stimulation of nerves within the respiratory tract or from production of prostaglandins and other mediators.

Some of the observed effects are species specific. For example, bradykinin is a potent constrictor of airway smooth muscle in isolated lungs of guinea pigs but is relatively ineffective in the rat or cat. The puzzling and sometimes paradoxical actions of kinins on the lungs of various animal species were reviewed in a former volume of this series (COLLIER, 1970).

Some of the variations may now be explained by prostaglandin release, but kinins also interact with various humoral factors, and they may also affect airway function by liberation of catecholamines. In addition, some effects of kinins can be attributed to stimulation of nerves within the airways and the pulmonary circulation. DELLA BELLA et al. (1972) found that injection of bradykinin into the jugular vein of guinea pigs stimulates afferent nerves from the lung directly and stimulates vagal efferent pathways indirectly. They proposed that vagal stimulation is mainly responsible for the bronchoconstriction caused by injected bradykinin since vagotomy reduces it.

I. Pulmonary Circulation

Bradykinin does not have striking effects on the pulmonary circulation. The complex and frequently variable actions of kinins on vessels in the lung may be affected by oxygen tension, the tone of the vessels, and the content of endogenous amines. Injection of bradykinin into the pulmonary artery of isolated perfused dog lungs decreases pulmonary vascular resistance (LEVINE et al., 1973). However, in the rabbit or guinea pig bradykinin causes vasoconstriction (COLLIER, 1970). Isolated guinea pig lungs perfused through the pulmonary artery developed increased perfusion pressure in response to an initial injection of bradykinin (25–75 ng), but the vessels became less sensitive to subsequent applications of the peptide (AARSEN and ZEEGERS, 1972).

In man, circulating bradykinin in the presence of an intact mitral valve, causes no change in pulmonary venous pressure but a slight elevation of pulmonary arterial pressure (HARRIS and HEATH, 1977). The pulmonary vascular effects of kinins in experimental animals may be related to prostaglandin production since $PGF_{2\alpha}$ causes constriction of lobar veins in the canine lung and PGE_1 relaxes them (KADOWITZ et al., 1975). Infusion of bradykinin into isolated lungs of guinea pigs releases PGE_2 (PALMER et al., 1973), indicating that prostaglandin release is a concomittant of the pulmonary vascular response to bradykinin.

The action of kinins in the lung may ultimately depend on the intracellular levels of cyclic nucleotides. Stoner et al. (1973) found that a bradykinin concentration of 1–100 μg/ml caused a rapid elevation of both cyclic GMP and cyclic AMP in guinea pig lung slices. KADOWITZ et al. (1975) found that the actions of $PGF_{2\alpha}$ and PGE_1 on canine pulmonary vessels were associated with changes in cyclic nucleotides. $PGF_{2\alpha}$ increased the isometric tension in segments of pulmonary vein and increased intracellular levels of cyclic GMP while cyclic AMP remained unchanged. In contrast, PGE_1 added to vessel segments caused only slight decrease in cyclic GMP and an increase in cyclic AMP in association with relaxation of isometric tension. The results suggest that prostaglandin-induced vasodilation (stimulated by PGE_1 and PGE_2) might be mediated by cyclic AMP and that the vasoconstriction by $PGF_{2\alpha}$ might be mediated by cyclic GMP.

II. Pulmonary Edema

Kinins may contribute to development of interstitial pulmonary edema by their actions on vascular permeability. While small vessels of the pulmonary circulation are resistant to changes in permeability caused by bradykinin and other phlogistic agents, PIETRA et al. (1971) found that subpleural administration of 0.1–100 μg bradykinin in dogs caused a dose-related submucosal and peribronchial accumulation of fluid in the lungs. Examination of the affected lungs by transmission electron microscopy revealed gaps at the endothelial junctions in bronchial venules and accumulation of carbon tracer material in the interstitial spaces and venular walls.

Because high doses of epinephrine activate plasma kallikrein followed by kininogen consumption and kinin release, it was suggested that kinins mediate epinephrine-induced pulmonary edema in rats (ROTHSCHILD et al., 1975; ROTHSCHILD and CASTANIA, 1976). The mechanism of epinephrine-induced edema appears to be complex, since such varied agents as acetylsalicylate, soybean trypsin inhibitor, aprotinin, and carbamylcholine can prevent it. The first three inhibitors prevent not only the edema formation but also the decrease in plasma kininogen, indicating that generation of kinin is blocked. Carbamylcholine did not block consumption of plasma kininogen but it effectively prevented elevation of systolic blood pressure by epinephrine and partially supressed edema formation. Thus, epinephrine-induced pulmonary edema in rats appears to result from a combination of increased hydrostatic pressure and increased vascular permeability. Kinins could contribute to the increase in permeability, but both hydrostatic and permeability changes are required for development of full-blown edema (ROTHSCHILD and CASTANIA, 1976). Kininogen consumption alone, caused by injection of cellulose sulfate into rats, does not cause edema (ROTHSCHILD, 1968; EISEN and LOVEDAY, 1971).

Kinin system components have been identified in the pleural exudates from rats with turpentine-induced pleurisy (DYRUD et al., 1971) and in bronchial washings from normal hamsters (WEESE et al., 1976). In addition, depletion of high molecular weight kininogen in rats by bromelain helps to block pleural fluid exudation caused by carrageenin (KATORI et al., 1978). Thus, kinin formation within the lung itself, as well as within the vascular system, could contribute to inflammation, exudation and pulmonary edema.

III. Airway Smooth Muscle

While bradykinin has a potent constrictor action on the tracheal and bronchiolar smooth muscle of the guinea pig (COLLIER, 1970), other animal species appear to be less sensitive. Since drugs such as aspirin and phenylbutazone can block the bronchoconstrictor effects of kinins in guinea pig lungs, it seems that prostaglandins may mediate this action of bradykinin as well as some of its other effects (COLLIER, 1976). The participation of cyclic nucleotides in the bronchoconstrictor action of bradykinin was also suggested (BERTELLI et al., 1973).

A rapid intravenous injection of bradykinin (1 μg/kg) into normal human volunteers constricts alveolar ducts, as reflected by decreased vital capacity, but does not cause constriction of either large or small airways (NEWBALL and KEISER, 1973). The situation in asthmatic individuals is more complex. ABE et al. (1967) reported that in persons with active, severe bronchial asthma the free kinin in blood is increased. The airways of subjects with bronchial asthma are abnormally sensitive to mediators such as bradykinin and histamine (HERXHEIMER and STRESEMANN, 1961; VARONIER and PANZANI, 1968), but NEWBALL (1974, 1976) found that bradykinin injected intravenously as a bolus (1 μg/kg) into asthmatic subjects decreased airway resistance, indicating dilation of large airways. However, there was no increase in the forced vital capacity, which suggests that bradykinin had an additional, constructive effect distal to the small airways, possibly at the alveolar ducts (NEWBALL, 1976). SIMONSSON et al. (1973) used body plethysmography to measure airway conductance in normal persons and in those with a history of airway obstruction. They found that bradykinin administered by aerosol caused bronchoconstriction in both groups. However, since the bronchoconstriction was blocked by atropine in most of the subjects, they concluded that it was probably due to nonspecific irritation of vagal receptors.

Studies on isolated human bronchi indicate that bradykinin causes contraction, but there is a wide range of sensitivity to the peptide (SIMONSSON et al., 1973). Others report that bradykinin in concentrations of 3–10 μg/ml could both contract and relax in vitro bronchiolar muscle (NEWBALL et al., 1976). The responses of human bronchi to bradykinin are probably due to release or formation of other mediators, such as prostaglandins, although direct effects on the smooth muscle may also be involved. Some investigators propose that bradykinin can relax constricted airways by prostaglandin production (CHAND and EYRE, 1977).

While most studies of kinins in the lung have focused on the role of these peptides in pathologic processes, DAVIS and GOODFRIEND (1969) suggested that kinins control normal airflow within the tracheobronchial tree. This conclusion was based on the observation that guinea pigs sensitized to a complex of bradykinin and albumin had consistently lower pulmonary flow resistance (as measured by total body plethysmography) than controls. The assumption was that antibodies elicited by the complex blocked endogenous bradykinin, but direct evidence for a physiologic role for kinins in airway tone is still lacking.

IV. Secretion

A recent observation suggests that kinins influence lung mucus secretions. Baker and associates (1977) incubated canine tracheal explants in medium containing ^{14}C-labeled D-glucosamine and then isolated labeled macromolecules from the culture medium. They found that kallidin and Met-Lys-bradykinin (but not bradykinin) enhanced incorporation of the labeled material into large molecular weight molecules that may be mucin-type glycoproteins. Since glandular kallikreins release kallidin rather than bradykinin (WEBSTER and PIERCE, 1963) the decapeptide may stimulate formation of respiratory secretions.

A bradykinin-like substance was identified in pulmonary washings from hamsters (WEESE et al., 1976). The kinin, as determined by radioimmunoassay, was present in bronchopulmonary lavage fluids, washings of pooled macrophages and lysates of alveolar macrophages. The capacity for kinin formation and inactivation in these preparations was measured in the presence of hexadimethrine and 1,10-phenanthroline to inhibit the activation of prekallikrein and kininases, but the cellular origin of the material was not determined. The authors speculated that since the major function of alveolar macrophages is phagocytosis, kinins could participate in either chemotaxis or phagocytosis. Kallikrein is a chemotactic agent (KAPLAN et al., 1972), and a kinin-like peptide can be generated from polymorphonuclear neutrophils (WINTROUB and AUSTEN, 1976). Thus, kinin formation within fluids of the airways could contribute to the inflammatory response in the lung.

V. Asthma and Allergic Reactions

Although the underlying causes of asthma and other airway diseases still have to be determined, the major pathophysiologic changes can be mimicked by inflammatory mediators, including kinins. Most experimental work relating kinins to asthma has been done in guinea pigs. These animals are quite sensitive to the bronchoconstrictor effects of kinins, but the parallel of human disease with other animal models is not as good (COLLIER, 1970, 1976). At the present there is no sound experimental evidence to implicate kinins as the cause of asthma or other airway disease in man.

There is experimental evidence, however, to suggest that kinins participate in various allergic diseases, probably in concert with other mediators. WILKENS and BACK (1971) showed that bradykinin or kallidin injected intravenously into dogs (20–100 µg/kg) caused a fall in blood pressure, bronchoconstriction and apena of varying intensity. Similar changes occurred in acute anaphylactic reactions which led these authors to implicate kinins as mediators of anaphylaxis, particularly of hypertension during the later phase. Increased levels of kinin were found in the blood of sensitized guinea pigs following challenge in vivo with antigen, but other mediators also increase under these circumstances (KELLERMYER and SCHWARTZ, 1976). Kinins have been identified in the dermal perfusate of skin wheals in allergic subjects (MICHEL et al., 1968) and in nasal secretions from patients with hay fever (DOLOVICH et al., 1970). Direct evidence, such as kinin formation in sensitized human lung tissue, has not yet been provided, although other mediators are released from the lung by antigen challenge (ORANGE et al., 1971; KALINER et al., 1972). BRISEID et al. (1976) examined plasma from a series of patients with exogenous allergic disease for prekallikrein activator, prekallikrein, and kallikrein inhibitors. They found no difference in these kinin system components between the patient population and normal controls. However, they noted an increased rate of kinin release by hog pancreas kallikrein from plasma of allergic patients.

F. Effects on Gastrointestinal Function

Although stimulation of intestinal smooth muscle in vitro was one of the first recognized actions of the kinins, the contribution of these peptides to normal gastrointestinal function is still not established. While smooth muscle stimulation is a prominent action of kinins in isolated tissues, and the gastrointestinal tract is rich in enzymes both for forming and destroying kinins, evidence linking kinins to gastrointestinal functions is circumstantial. Furthermore, extrapolation of results obtained from in vitro preparations to normal physiologic functions is not entirely satisfactory. Not only is the action of a kinin on a particular organ influenced by neuronal, circulatory and metabolic conditions, but there may be interactions between bradykinin and other mediators at the level of smooth muscle or secretory cell receptors.

Possibly the kinins play a more important role in diseases of the gastrointestinal tract. Some studies suggest that inappropriate formation or metabolism of kinins contributes to the pathogenesis of diseases such as carcinoid (OATES et al., 1966; OATES and BUTLER, 1967), postgastrectomy dumping syndrome (SMITH and ZEITLIN, 1966; WONG et al., 1974; ZEITLIN and SMITH, 1966; CHAIMOFF et al., 1977) and alcoholic liver disease (WONG et al., 1972).

I. Smooth Muscle

Bradykinin stimulates contraction of intestine and most other isolated smooth muscle preparations, but it causes relaxation of rat duodenum (ELLIOT et al., 1960). The isolated jejunum of the cat is particularly sensitive to kinins and contracts in response to bradykinins concentrations as little as 0.1 ng/ml (FERREIRA and VANE, 1967). In some tissues both contraction and relaxation can be observed. For example, AARSEN and VAN CASPEL DE BRUYN (1970) observed that the guinea pig taenia coli had a biphasic response to bradykinin: first decreased and then increased isometric tension. The two phases of the response could be altered independently by changing sodium and calcium concentrations in the medium and by epinephrine, suggesting that there might be more than one receptor for bradykinin. Studies by BONTA and HALL (1973) with isolated guinea pig ileum also suggest different receptors. They found that when the ileum was challenged first with acetylcholine or another spasmogen and then with bradykinin, the relaxation phase was potentiated. The relaxation of the ileum (but not the contraction) in response to bradykinin was blocked by phentolamine, suggesting that adrenergic receptors are involved. However, catecholamine depletion by tyramine or reserpine in vivo did not affect the bradykinin-induced relaxation of rat duodenum and rabbit ileum in vitro (UFKES and VAN DER MEER, 1975). The participation of specific adrenergic or cholinergic components in the smooth muscle response to bradykinin, therefore, is not yet proven. Other investigators found that bradykinin-potentiating peptide, BPP_{5a} (STEWART et al., 1971), could be used to discriminate the contractile and relaxant actions of bradykinin on smooth muscle preparations. This peptide potentiates only the contractile phase in rat intestine (CAMARGO and FERREIRA, 1971; UFKES et al., 1976), and rabbit ileum (UFKES et al., 1976). However, while bradykinin had both stimulatory and inhibitory effects on the guinea pig taenia coli, neither action was potentiated by BPP_{5a} (AARSEN, 1977). Both stimulatory and inhibitory responses to bradykinin are associated with a sodium-dependent depolarization and decrease in membrane resistance. Although BPP_{5a} alone stimulated contraction of the taenia coli, it did not affect membrane potential (AARSEN, 1977).

Many investigators have sought to link kinin-induced contraction or relaxation of smooth muscle in the gastrointestinal tract with changes in cyclic nucleotides (AROLD et al., 1976; PAEGELOW et al., 1975, 1977) since kinins can affect concentrations of cyclic nucleotides in smooth muscle and other tissue (see p. 287). In addition, intracellular ion exchange may be important. Bradykinin increased the intracellular calcium concentration of isolated guinea pig ileum (PAEGELOW et al., 1975, 1977). Finally, kinins may potentiate the actions of other stimuli. For example, STASIEWICZ and co-workers (1977) found that bradykinin not only stimulated contraction of guinea pig isolated gall bladder, but also in low concentrations (1 ng/ml) the peptide potentiated the effects of cholecystokinin and acetylcholine on that preparation.

BARABÉ and co-workers (1975, 1977) concluded that since the effect of the kinin is not altered by anticholinergic, antiadrenergic, or antihistaminic drugs the cat terminal ileum and rat uterus respond specifically to bradykinin. Indomethacin, which would be expected to prevent formation of prostaglandins, was also ineffective. Thus, while many of the actions of kinins, including their effects on blood vessels, probably involve prostaglandins there is as yet no conclusive evidence to link stimulation of other smooth muscles to prostaglandins.

II. Vascular Effects

The contribution of nerves and regional blood flow must also be considered in evaluating the effects of kinins on gastrointestinal functions. Alteration of blood flow by specific vasodilator fibers was proposed by some investigators as a mechanism for regulation of secretion and other functions within the gastrointestinal tract (GAUTVIK et al., 1976).

FASTH and HULTEN (1973) studied the effects of bradykinin and pelvic nerve stimulation on colon motility and blood flow in cats. They found that vasodilation and contraction occurred in response to either nerve stimulation or bradykinin injection, and they concluded that kinin generation might be involved in regulation of colon motility. In a study investigating the role of bradykinin in functional hyperemia of the cat stomach FASTH and MARTINSON (1973) found that intra-arterial injection of bradykinin caused profound relaxation of gastric muscle. This relaxation may be mediated by cholinergic mechanisms, since stimulation of vagal nerves caused a similar effect (FASTH et al., 1975). Figure 7 illustrates this effect. Although the effects of bradykinin on the cat stomach and colon may be due to stimulation of vagal and pelvic nerves, respectively, the reponses are not blocked by hexamethonium, indicating that the kinin does not affect ganglionic cells (FASTH et al., 1975).

RICHARDSON and WITHRINGTON (1977) found that injection of bradykinin into the hepatic artery of anesthetized dogs caused a dose-dependent reduction in hepatic arterial resistance. The kinin was more potent than other agents, such as histamine, serotonin, secretin or PGE_2, and could affect flow at doses as low as 10 pg. The effect was selective since bradykinin did not affect hepatic portal vascular resistance, even at doses 100 times higher than the maximal effective dose for an affect on the hepatic arteries.

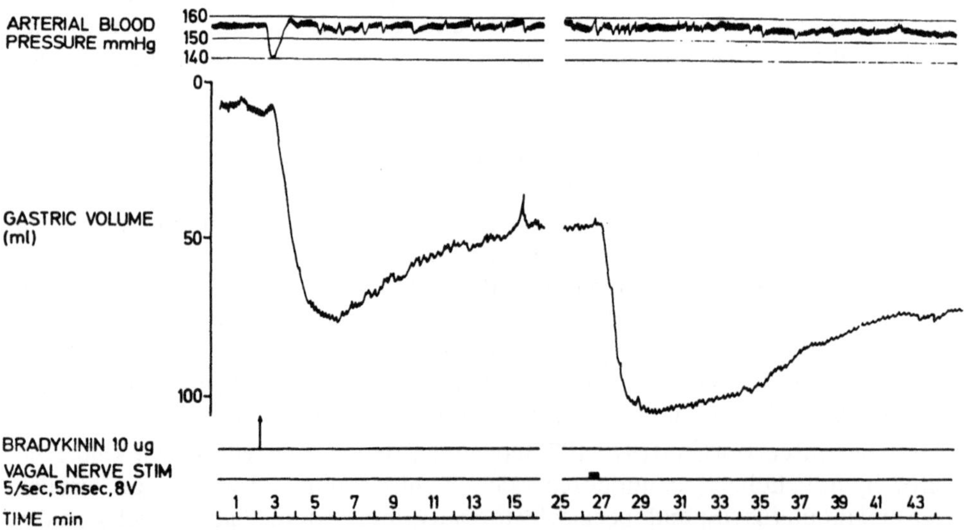

Fig. 7. The effect of intraaortic administration of bradykinin and vagal stimulation on gastric volume and blood pressure in the cat. Bradykinin injection (10 μg) is shown at the left and vagal stimulation at the right. Note that the identical responses are characterized by a rapid relaxation and slow elimination. (From FASTH et al., 1975.) Reproduced with permission from the authors

Under normal circumstances, the circulating levels of bradykinin would be miniscule, due to the rapid inactivation of the peptide in blood. However, under pathologic conditions where there is increased kinin generation (e.g., shock) the highly specific action of kinin on hepatic arteries could evoke alterations in hepatic perfusion and affect distribution of blood flow between arterial and portal circuits.

III. Absorption

In the search for a physiological rôle for pancreatic kallikrein, a number of investigators explored the possibility that kallikrein or kinins might affect intestinal absorption of various nutrients. A glandular type of kallikrein has been isolated from rat intestine (ZEITLIN et al., 1976; MORIWAKI et al., 1977a, b) and it can be released from duodenum by bile salts (FRANKISH and ZEITLIN, 1977). Others have shown that the colon mucosa also contains a kallikrein with properties more like plasma than glomerular kallikrein (SEKI et al., 1971). Since the brush border of the small intestine of man and animals contains kininase II (WARD et al., 1978), kinins may be part of a physiological system for the regulation of uptake of amino acids and other small molecules.

DENNHARDT and HABERICH (1973) studied the influence of kallikrein on the absorption of water, electrolytes and hexoses from rat intestine in vivo. The pancreatic duct was ligated to prevent secretion of endogenous kallikrein. Exogenous kallikrein, introduced through the mucosal side of the intestine, enhanced water and electrolyte absorption from the colon and jejunum. In normal rats (without pancreatic duct ligation), however, kallikrein inhibited water and electrolyte absorption.

MENG and HABERLAND (1973) found that transport of glucose and 3-0-methyl glucose was stimulated by kallikrein (0.01–1.0 U/ml) applied to the mucosal side of everted rat intestine, but that this effect was reversed at higher concentrations of kallikrein. Even though transport of glucose was stimulated by kallikrein, the uptake by intestinal tissue was not changed.

MORIWAKI and associates (1973, 1977b) showed that hog pancreatic kallikrein administered orally to rats can be completely absorbed and that concentrations as low as 10^{-4} U/ml increased valine absorption from the everted intestine. Bradykinin (1 ng/ml) was also effective. Infusion of bradykinin into the superior mesenteric artery also stimulated valine absorption (MORIWAKI et al., 1973). These authors suggested that pancreatic kallikrein releases kinin from intestine and the resulting vasodilation facilitates absorption. However, they noted that ouabain inhibited valine absorption, suggesting that a sodium-dependent transport system is involved. Infusion of kallikrein (10^{-2} U/ml) restored valine absorption (MORIWAKI and FUJIMORI, 1975).

Kallikrein (10^{-3} U/ml) also enhanced transport of methionine and d-glucose from rat jejunum in vivo as determined by recovery of labeled amino acids from the superior mesenteric vein (MORIWAKI and FUJIMORI, 1975), whereas other proteolytic enzymes, such as trypsin and chymotrypsin had no effect. This action of kallikrein was blocked by aprotonin implying that kinin formation is involved in the enhanced transport.

Other investigators failed to find an effect of kallikrein on transport of glucose and valine in the rat intestine (CASPARY and CREUTZFELDT, 1973). However, higher concentrations of kallikrein (1–5 U/ml) were used than in the experiments of MORIWAKI et al., (1973, 1977a and b) and MENG and HABERLAND (1973).

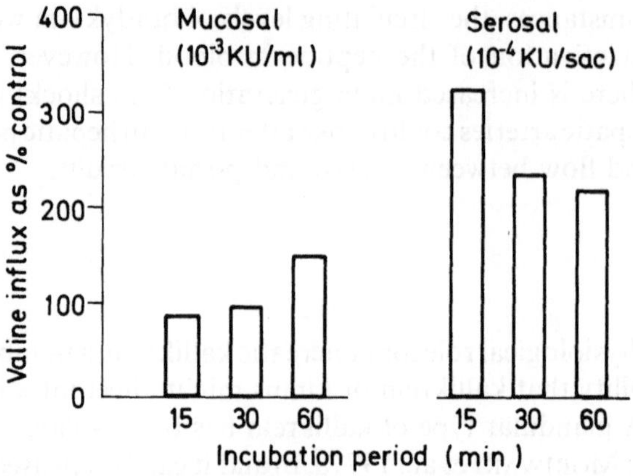

Fig. 8. Enhanced valine transport in everted rat intestine. Kallikrein from rat intestine was applied to the mucosal side (left panel) or to the serosal side (right panel) of everted jejunal sacs and the passage of [^{14}C] valine was measured at the times indicated. (From MORIWAKI et al., 1977). Reproduced with permission of the authors

The site of kinin formation may determine its effects on transportation. For example, kallikrein isolated from rat intestinal mucosa had a more potent effect on valine transport in jejunum when it was added to the serosal side than when it was added to the mucosal side (MORIWAKI et al., 1977a). Figure 8 illustrates this effect. Similarly, bradykinin added to isolated intestinal segments stimulated sodium transport when it was added to the serosal side of the tissue. Application at the mucosal surface alone was ineffective (CROCKER and WILLAVOYS, 1975; MORIWAKI et al., 1977b). CROCKER and WILLAVOYS found that bradykinin had a biphasic effect on transfer of sodium and water from the mucosal side of rat jejunum. When the basal transfer was low, bradykinin (7.0×10^{-2} M) at both serosal and mucosal surfaces caused stimulation of sodium and water transport. When basal transfer rates were high, the same concentration of peptide inhibited it. Since either theophylline or dibutyryl cyclic AMP inhibited the transport, the authors concluded that the inhibitory action of bradykinin may depend on changes in intracellular levels of cyclic AMP.

The work of MORIWAKI and associates (MORIWAKI and FUJIMORI, 1975; MORIWAKI et al., 1977) suggests that the stimulatory effect of bradykinin (or kallikrein) may involve stimulated sodium transport as well. In this regard, it was recently observed that bradykinin increases the potential difference across both the jejunum and the colon of the rat (HARDCASTLE et al., 1978). The effect was reduced by the administration of indomethacin (16 mg/kg), suggesting that in this tissue, as in other organs, prostaglandins may be involved in the kinin response.

IV. Cell Proliferation

The epithelial cells of the gastrointestinal tract have a high rate of turnover, as a result of continuous shedding and replacement. Some investigators have suggested that pancreatic kallikrein is a physiological stimulus for mitotic activity in the gut and that either kallikrein or kinins are required for continual replacement of epithelial cells. ROHEN and PETERHOFF (1973) found that intraluminal application of pancreatic kallikrein in rats stimulated mitoses in the cells of the duodenum and jejunum, but not in the ileum or colon. If the main pancreatic duct in rats was ligated, the number of cells in mitosis decreased in intestinal epithelium, but daily administration of 30 u of kallikrein restored normal mitotic activity. Others showed that either kallikrein or kinin had mitogenic effects on rat thymocytes and bone marrow cells and that these effects may depend on changes in cyclic AMP and calcium during the cell cycle (RIXON et al., 1971; PERRIS and WHITFIELD, 1969; RIXON and WHITFIELD, 1973; BOUCEK and NOBLE, 1973). However, cyclic AMP probably does not affect all cells uniformly and appears to affect only those cells already programmed for division, such as thymocytes (ABELL and MONAHAN, 1973). Thus, it is not yet possible to link kinin formation, cyclic AMP formation, and cell division to a functional role in regeneration of intestinal epithelium.

Kallikrein stimulates proliferation of liver cells in vitro but does not restore tissue after subtotal hepatectomy in rats (RABES, 1975). Possibly the enzyme is metabolized and inactivated during circulation in vivo. If kinin generation occurs locally within damaged tissues, however, it might stimulate proliferation and regeneration in inflammatory or toxic liver damage.

Whatever the mechanism of its mitogenic effect, kallikrein stimulates the proliferation of a wide variety of cells both in vitro and in vivo (SCHUTTE and LINDNER, 1977). This finding may have important implications for the development of tissues and aging, as well as for specific organ-related disease.

V. Kinins and Diseases of the Gastrointestinal Tract

Several observations suggest that abnormal kinin formation or metabolism may be involved in diseases of the gastrointestinal tract, but the experimental evidence is largely indirect. Kinins have been implicated in carcinoid syndrome (OATES and BUTLER, 1967; OATES et al., 1966) and in the post gastrectomy dumping syndrome (WONG et al., 1974; COLMAN et al., 1976). These disease entities are discussed elsewhere in this volume (COLMAN and WONG, see p. 287). ZEITLIN and SMITH (1973) reported increased kallikrein and prekallikrein activities in the mucosal layer of colonic tissue taken from patients with active ulcerative colitis. There was no increase in kallikrein activity of the muscle layers within normal segments of colon, but in damaged portions the enzyme was present in both muscle and mucosal layers. Neither muscle nor mucosal samples from patients with colonic diverticulosis had kallikrein activity.

STEWART et al. (1972) measured kininogen and prekallikrein activity in patients with chronic liver disease to see if a correlation could be made between the formation of kinin and some of the clinical manifestations of cirrhosis, such as vasodilation, hypotension and increased capillary permeability. They found that, while patients with cirrhosis had less plasma kininogen than controls, there were no differences in prekallikrein between the two groups. They concluded that the liver disease probably affected synthesis of kininogen and that the reduced levels did not reflect kinin generation since prekallikrein did not change.

However, other investigators found that prekallikrein levels were diminished in patients with cirrhosis of the liver (WONG et al., 1972, 1977a; FANCIULLACCI et al., 1975; WONG and COLEMAN, p. 287 this volume). Because of the concomittant decrease in prekallikrein and increase in plasma renin activity in patients with hepatorenal syndrome, WONG and associates (1977a) concluded that the relative imbalance between the kallikrein-kinin system and the renin-angiotensin system contributes to this almost uniformly fatal condition.

Additional evidence suggests that the kinin system affects gastric secretion. GEIGER et al. (1977) collected gastric mucus from human subjects and examined it for kininogen. They found that either kallikrein or trypsin liberated kinin activity from the mucus, indicating that both high and low molecular weight kininogens were present. The kinin activity was inactivated by chymotrypsin or by carboxypeptidase B. While kinin was formed in most of the specimens collected, subjects who had undergone vagotomy had no detectable kininogen. Patients with duodenal ulcers had more kininogen than normal subjects. These observations educed the speculation that enhanced kinin formation may be involved in abnormal gastric secretion, but further evidence is required before such a role is established.

G. Effects on Reproduction

Many investigators have sought a role for the kallikrein-kinin system in reproductive functions. Since the factors for kinin generation and degradation are present in secretions of both male and female genital tracts, a functional role for kinins in reproduction seems plausible (PALM and FRITZ, 1975; PALM et al., 1976a, 1976b). While experimental evidence suggests that kinins may be involved in sperm motility and capacitation, the relationship of kinins to female hormonal cycles and the processes of labor and parturition is more tenuous. Possibly as information about the molecular mechanisms of kinin interactions with tissues expands, a more definitive picture will emerge.

I. Influence of Sex Hormones

Circulating sex hormones appear to affect components of the kinin system. Several authors have reported an increase in the levels of plasma kininogen in man (PORTER et al., 1972) and experimental animals during pregnancy (WEIGERSHAUSEN et al., 1968; McCORMICK and SENIOR, 1974a). Figure 9 shows the levels of plasma kininogen in the rat during pregnancy and after parturition. Kininogen levels do not increase in pseudopregnant animals (SENIOR and WHALLEY, 1974a; WIEGERSHAUSEN et al., 1971).

Studies on mature female rats indicate that estrogens have a positive effect on plasma kininogen. McCORMICK and SENIOR (1974a) found that plasma levels of kininogen did not change during estrus cycles, but the onset of estrus in immature animals was associated with an increase in kininogen (McCORMICK and SENIOR, 1974b). Similarly, daily injections of estrogens (stilbesterol, estradiol, or ethinyl estradiol) in doses sufficient to induce estrus caused elevation of plasma kininogen within 5 days of onset of treatment (McCORMICK and SENIOR, 1974a). In contrast, PRASAD et al. (1975) found that plasma kininogen levels in adult goats fluctuated during the estrus cycle, with the highest values at the onset of estrus. Kininogen levels decrease toward the end of estrus in rabbits (WIEGERSHAUSEN et al., 1968) and goats (PRASAD et al., 1975) which suggests that the synthesis of kininogen in the liver is influenced by the falling concentration of estrogen or the increase in progesterone secretion.

Administration of a synthetic progestational agent, norgestrel, to rats also increased kininogen levels (McCORMICK and SENIOR, 1974b), but progesterone in doses as high as 5 mg/kg was ineffective. Androgens had the opposite effect. Administration of either

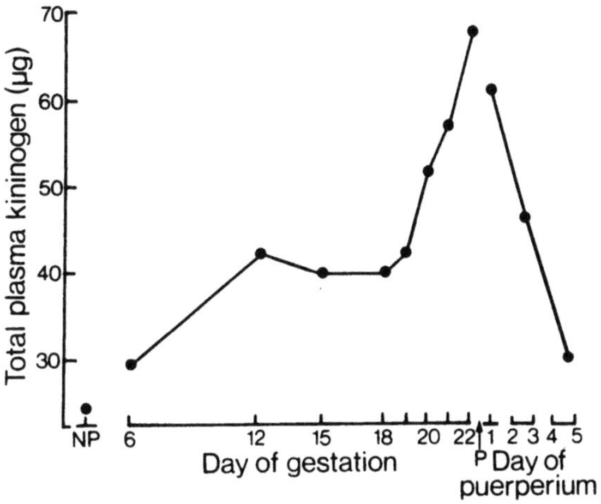

Fig. 9. Influence of pregnancy and the puerperium on total plasma kininogen in rats. NP indicates values in nonpregnant rats, P indicates parturition. (From McCormick and Senior, 1974). Reproduced with permission from the authors

testosterone or norethandrolone to female rats lowers kininogen levels, and male rats have less kininogen than females. Removal of ovaries or testes caused expected changes in plasma kininogen which could be reversed by treatment with exogenous hormones (McCormick and Senior, 1974b; Senior and Whalley, 1975). In addition, adrenalectomy increased plasma kininogen levels in both sexes, but administration of corticosterone had no effect (Senior and Whalley, 1975).

In another study Senior and Whalley (1974b) reported that high doses (10 mg/kg) of progesterone decreased plasma kininogen in rats and that changes in this protein appeared to be related to the ratio of estrogen to progesterone. These provocative studies suggest that the sex hormones influenced the kinin system through an effect on circulating kininogen. However, since other plasma proteins were not measured concomittantly, one can not be sure whether the effect is specific or whether it reflects a general influence on protein synthesis.

The kininase activity in plasma of female rats did not change during the estrus cycle, but decreased in pregnancy with the time of gestation up to the 20th day (McCormick and Senior, 1972). Following parturition, kininase levels increased toward the nonpregnant level and remained stable for at least 14 days postpartum. The changes in kininase activity, as measured by inactivation of bradykinin, may be related to the increase in maternal blood volume during gestation (McCormick and Senior, 1972). However, Erdös and Yang (1970) found that the activity of kininase I increased during pregnancy.

McCormick and Senior (1974a) found that free kinin levels in plasma of nonpregnant rats were low and inconsistent. In spite of the increase in kininogen levels and decrease in kininase activity of plasma during pregnancy, these investigators did not find free kinin in the blood of pregnant rats. Similarly, others found no consistent differences in kinin content of blood from nonpregnant women and those in various stages of gestation (Porter et al., 1972).

II. Parturition

A role for kinins in parturition has been espoused by several investigators. The activity of kinins on regional blood flow, as well as their effects on smooth muscle make them potential participants in the events of labor and parturition. As mentioned earlier, it was proposed that kinins were responsible for the physiological adaptation of the neonatal circulation (Melmon et al., 1968; Heymann et al., 1969). Bradykinin can release norepinephrine from the human placenta, but it is not known whether this response or the related vasoconstriction is involved in parturition (Sherman and Gautieri, 1972). Recently Resnik et al. (1976) showed that bradykinin stimulates uterine blood flow in oophorectomized ewes, and raised the possibility that kinins mediate estrogen effects on uterine circulation. However, infusion of bradykinin at concentrations up to 900 ng/ml into the uterine artery had less effect on blood flow than 17-β-estradiol, PGE_1, or adenosine, and the kinin caused a sustained increase in intrauterine pressure (Still and Greiss, 1978). Thus, it is unlikely that kinins mediate estrogen effects on blood flow.

Depletion of plasma kininogen in pregnant rats by treatment with cellulose sulfate at 19–22 days of pregnancy results in prolongation of the gestation period by several hours, an increase in the duration of preparturient behavior (labor) and a delay in the process of delivery (McCormick and Senior, 1974a). Treatment of pregnant rats with aprotinin at days 19–22 had a similar effect (Senior and Whalley, 1976). Although these experiments indicate that the kinin system may be involved in parturition, direct evidence for kinin formation is lacking.

Branconi and associates (1976) failed to find any change in either plasma prekallikrein or kallikrein inhibitor in blood samples taken from women during the last 3 weeks of pregnancy and at delivery. An increase in the plasma kallikrein activity in women during the second stage of labor was reported (Malofiejew, 1973), but no change was found in kinin concentration of the blood during labor in humans (Porter et al., 1972). The rapid inactivation of kinins in the circulation (see Erdös, p. 427) may preclude measurement of plasma kinin. Free kinin was not consistently detectable in blood of preparturient or nonpregnant rats even after treatment in vivo with dimercaprol, an inhibitor of kininases. Bradykinin plasma levels of approximately 2 ng/ml were measured in samples from parturient rats treated with the inhibitor (McCormick and Senior, 1974a), but this does not suggest a striking activation of the kinin system.

III. Smooth Muscle

The stimulating action of kinins on uterine smooth muscle is well known. Although there is some difference in sensitivity among various animal species, kinins generally stimulate uterine contractions both in vivo and in vitro (Walaszek, 1970). In addition, kallikrein causes contraction of the uterus, possibly by a direct action on smooth muscle (Beraldo et al., 1974).

Other structures of the female reproductive tract are also stimulated by kinins. Bradykinin contracts isolated segments of human Fallopian tubes by a mechanism that appears to be independent of adrenergic stimulation (Senior and Spencer-Gregson, 1969). A kinin-like material was found in fluid from ovarian follicles of humans, rabbits, and cows. The kinin activity was enhanced severalfold after contact with glass beads or when the follicular fluid was combined with cell-free washings of bovine Fallopian tubes

(RAMWELL et al., 1969). Thus, kinin formation within the follicles or tubes could affect tubal motility.

In this regard, STERIN-SPEZIALE and associates (1978) examined the influence of bradykinin and other agents on the motility of ovarian fimbriae and tubo-ovarian ligaments from humans. These structures are involved with the capture and conveyance of oocytes into the tubes at the time of ovulation. Bradykinin enhanced development of tension and increased the frequency of spontaneous contractions in fimbrial strips but had only a slight effect on the tubo-ovarian ligaments. Since the responses were similar in tissues obtained during the follicular phase and those taken after progesterone treatment, the endocrine environment does not appear to affect the response to bradykinin. In contrast, the contractile responses to catecholamines and prostaglandins E_1 and E_2 varied with the hormonal stimulation of the tissues, the estrogen-dominated tissues being more sensitive to the contractile effects of these agents.

As in other tissues, prostaglandin formation and metabolism influence kinin effects on the uterine smooth muscle. The contractile response of myometrial strips in vitro to bradykinin was depressed by treatment with indomethacin, and potentiated by $PGF_{2\alpha}$ (CHIVERS and WHALLEY, 1977).

IV. Lactation

Kinins may affect lactation or milk ejection by their actions on vascular smooth muscle or on the myoepithelial cells in the mammary gland. Injection of kallikrein or bradykinin into lactating cows, sheep, and goats increased blood flow within the mammary glands and caused complex changes in intrammammary pressure (HOUVENAGHEL and PEETERS, 1971, 1972; PEETERS et al., 1972). As little as 0.5–2 ng of bradykinin into lactating cows, sheep, and goats increased blood flow within the mammary glands and caused complex changes in intramammary pressure blood flow through the udder (HOUVENHAGHEL and PEETERS, 1972). Elevation of pressure is presumably related to contraction of perialveolar myoepithelial cells needed for the expulsion of milk. Contraction of myoepithelial cells situated longitudinally along the milk ducts, however, results in dilation of the ducts and increased filling (PEETERS and HOUVENHAGHEL, 1973).

V. Spermatogenesis

While the evidence linking kinin formation with reproductive functions in the female is indirect, there is some indication that kinins facilitate spermatogenesis and sperm motility in man. STUTTGEN (1973) found that kallikrein treatment (DEPOT-PADUTIN) daily for 14 days increased the number of spermatozoa in men with oligospermia. These findings have been substantiated by observations of other investigators (SCHIRREN, 1975; ISHIGAMI and KAMIDONO, 1975; SCHILL, 1975a; SCHILL and HABERLAND, 1974; HOFMANN et al., 1975). The mechanism of enhanced spermatogenesis, however, is not known.

ROHEN and BUSCHHUTER (1975) explored the possibility that kallikrein affected the function of Sertoli cells. In a morphologic study of testes from rats treated with kallikrein, they found an increase in the size of the nuclei in Sertoli cells and speculated that kallikrein might enhance spermatogenesis by facilitating the exchange of

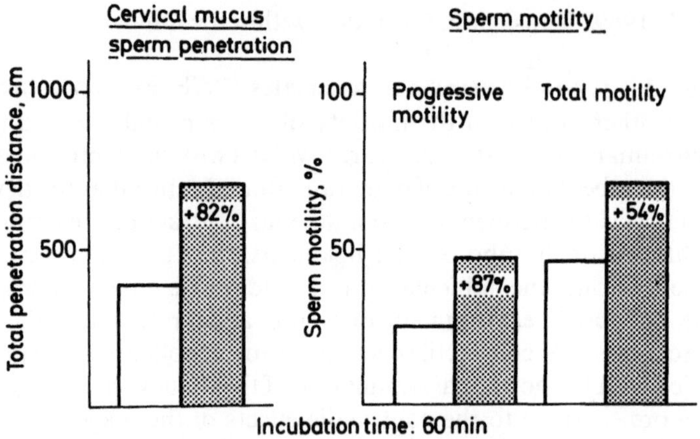

Fig. 10. Correlation between stimulation of sperm motility and cervical mucus penetration. Incubation time was 60 min. Tests were performed independently in two different laboratories on 14 semen samples. The open bars are untreated controls and the stippled bars are semen samples that were treated with 1 KU/ml of kallikrein. (From WALLNER et al., 1975). Reproduced with permission from the authors

substances between Sertoli cells and adjacent spermatids. Other attempts to show an effect of kallikrein on Sertoli cells were less successful (KLEEBERG et al., 1975), and the mechanism through which kallikrein stimulates spermatogenesis remains obscure.

VI. Sperm Motility

The observation that accessory sex glands of the guinea pig contain kininogenase suggested that kinins could be formed during ejaculation to facilitate sperm transport in that species. The enzymatic activity from the coagulation gland was decreased by castration and increased by treatment with testosterone, although the hormone effect did not exactly parallel the increase in the gland weight (MORIWAKI et al., 1975b).

Experiments with human semen showed that kallikrein and kinins added in vitro enhanced sperm motility and migration (LEIDL et al., 1975; SCHILL, 1975a, b; SCHILL and HABERLAND, 1974, 1975; SCHILL et al., 1974; PALM et al., 1976a, b). Addition of carboxypeptidase B to sperm with initially good motility blocked this effect of kallikrein, indicating that the enhanced motility depends on kinin formation and not on a direct effect of kallikrein (SCHILL et al., 1974; SCHILL and HABERLAND, 1975). Others found that porcine kallikrein in concentrations as low as 1 U/ml stimulated motility of bull sperm in vitro (BRATANOV et al., 1978).

WALLNER et al. (1975) showed that kallikrein facilitated sperm penetration through human midcycle cervical mucus in vitro. Penetration distance of sperm into capillary tubes was determined by microscopic observation. Kallikrein (1 U/ml) increased the total penetration distance by 43–82% but bradykinin (1 mg/ml) was without effect. The presence of kininase in the ejaculate (PALM and FRITZ; 1975, ERDÖS, p. 427 this volume) might account for the ineffectiveness of bradykinin. Penetration of sperm into cervical mucus was impaired after addition of carboxypeptidase B or aprotinin to the ejaculate (WALLNER et al., 1975), which supports the supposition that kinin formation is involved in the normal activities of sperm. Figure 10 shows the results of some experiments on sperm motility.

Several speculations about the mechanism of enhanced sperm motility by kallikrein have been advanced. SCHILL et al. (1974) proposed that kinins change the permeability of the sperm membrane to energetically usable substrates and thus stimulate motility. The observation that mefenamate, a potent inhibitor of prostaglandin synthesis, abolishes the effects of kallikrein suggests that prostaglandin formation is involved (GRYGLEWSKI, 1974).

The stimulation of sperm motility by caffeine, an inhibitor of phosphodiesterase, suggested that possibly an increase in the intracellular concentration of cyclic AMP is involved in motility. However, the time course of stimulation by caffeine differed from that for kallikrein, and addition of the two agents together to ejaculates had an additive effect on motility (SCHILL, 1975b). Thus, it is not possible to relate the effect of kallikrein on sperm motility to changes in cyclic AMP.

The provocative finding that acrosin, a protease of the sperm acrosomal cap, is also a kininogenase, suggests that kinin formation plays a role in fertilization (FRITZ et al., 1973; SCHLEUNING et al., 1976). Acrosin has been found in sperm from man and many different animals and appears to be necessary for the penetration of the zona pellucida of the ovum by spermatozoa (FRITZ et al., 1973; SCHILL et al., 1974; PALM et al., 1976). Kininogen is present in human midcycle cervical secretions, and may act as a substrate for acrosin during capacitation (PALM et al., 1976a, b). Proteinase inhibitors have been isolated from both human seminal plasma and from cervical mucus. The inhibitor from semen readily inhibits the enzymatic action of acrosin and is probably the natural inhibitor of this enzyme. The inhibition from cervical mucus has a greater affinity for neutral proteases, such as those from granulocyte lysosomes than for acrosin (SCHIESSLER et al., 1976). Thus, the acrosin is inhibited during transit to the cervix, but during capacitation it must be activated in order to facilitate sperm penetration.

SCHILL and associates (1976) did not find any correlation between the sperm acrosin activity and sperm motility, but they found a correlation between sperm count and the enzyme activity. Men who produce round-headed spermatozoa, which lack the acrosomal cap, are infertile (SCHILL et al., 1976).

Although there are many intriguing indications that the kallikrein–kinin system affects various processes in human reproduction, the exact mechanisms remain to be identified.

H. Epilogue

This chapter described some of the direct and indirect actions of kinins. While some actions of these potent peptides are well known and appear to be involved in pathological states, such as inflammation, kinins still have no generally accepted role in normal physiology. Some exciting ideas are emerging, however. For example, the high concentration of kallikrein–kinin system components in organs of the reproductive system implies that they may affect normal reproduction. The possibility that kinins affect transport within the gastrointestinal tract is another compelling idea. Finally, the interactions of kinins with metabolic functions, such as the uptake of glucose and substrates during exercise or hypoxia, may be of physiological importance. The release of agents such as catecholamines or prostaglandins by kinins to mediate or modulate various physiological and pathological processes is yet another facet of the kinin system.

References

Aarsen, P.: The effects of bradykinin and the bradykinin potentiating peptide BPP_{5a} on the electrical and mechanical responses of the guinea-pig taenia coli. Br. J. Pharmacol. *61*, 523–532 (1977)

Aarsen, P.N., van Caspel de Bruyn, M.: Effect of changes in ionic environment on the action of bradykinin on the guinea-pig taenia coli. Eur. J. Pharmacol. *12*, 348–358 (1970)

Aarsen, P.N., Zeegers, A.: Effects of histamine, 5-hydroxytryptamine and bradykinin on the vascular system of isolated lungs of the guinea-pig and the influenze of phenylbutazone on these effects. Br. J. Pharmakol. *45*, 284–298 (1972)

Abe, K., Watanabe, N., Kumagai, N., Mouri, T., Seki, T., Yoshinaga, K.: Circulating plasma kinin in patients with bronchial asthma. Experientia *23*, 626–627 (1967)

Abell, C.W., Monahan, T.M.: The role of adenosine 3′, 5′-cyclic monophosphate in the regulation of mammalian cell division. J. Cell Biol. *59*, 549–558 (1973)

Ackerman, N.B., Hechmer, P.A.: Effect of pharmacological agents on the microcirculation of tumors implanted in the liver. Bibl. Anat. *15*, 301–303 (1977)

Alexander, W., Gimbrone, M.A.: Stimulation of prostaglandin E synthesis in cultured human umbilical vein smooth muscle cells. Proc. Natl. Acad. Sci. USA *73*, 1617–1620 (1976)

Altura, B.M.: Comparative contractile actions of different kinins on human umbilical arteries and veins. Eur. J. Pharmacol. *19*, 171–179 (1972)

Arold, H., Liebmann, C., Römer, W., Paegelow, I., Reissman, S.: The effect of bradykinin on adenylate cyclase activity in different organs. In: Peptides. Proc. 14th Eur. Pep. Symp. Ed. A. Loffet, pp. 559–564, Editions de l'Universite de Bruxelles, Brussels

Assali, N.S., Johnson, G.H., Brinkman, C.R., Huntsman, D.J.: Effects of bradykinin on the fetal circulation. Am. J. Physiol. *221*, 1375–1382 (1971)

Baker, A.P., Hillegass, L.M., Holden, D.A., Smith, W.J.: Effect of kallidin, substance P and other basic polypeptides on the production of respiratory macromolecules. Am. Rev. Resp. Dis. *115*, 811–817 (1977)

Barabé, J., Drouin, J.-N., Regoli, D., Park, W.K.: Receptors for bradykinin in intestinal and uterine smooth muscle. Can. J. Physiol. Pharmacol. *55*, 1270–1284 (1977)

Barabé, J., Park, W.K., Regoli, D.: Application of drug-receptor theories to the analysis of the myotropic effects of bradykinin. Can. J. Physiol. Pharmacol. *53*, 345–353 (1975)

Bassenge, E., Kucharczyk, M., von Restorff, W., Werle, E.: Effect of bradykinin potentiating peptide on coronary circulation in conscious dogs. Adv. Exp. Med. Biol. *21*, 251–257 (1972)

Bassenge, E., Werle, E., Walter, P., Holtz, J.: Significance of kinins in the coronary circulation. Adv. Exp. Med. Biol. *8*, 141–148 (1970)

Baumgarten, A., Melrose, G.J.H., Vagg, W.J.: Interactions between histamine and bradykinin assessed by continuous recording of increased vascular permeability. J. Physiol. *208*, 669–675 (1970)

Bavazzano, A., Sidell, N., Michelacci, S., Sicuteri, F.: Local ischemia as a kininogen depressant: effect of cortisone, taurine and a kallikrein inhibitor. Adv. Exp. Med. Biol. *8*, 377–383 (1970)

Beraldo, W.T., Lauar, N.S., Siqueira, G., Heneine, I.F., Catanzaro, O.L.: Pecularities of the oxytocic action of rat urinary kallikrein. In: Chemistry and biology of the kallikrein-kinin system in health and disease. Pisano, J.J., Austen, K.F. (eds.), Fogarty International Center Proceeding Vol. 27, pp. 375–378, DHEW Publication No. (NIH) 76–791, U.S. Govt. Printing Office Washington, D.C.

Bertelli, A., Bianchi, C., Beani, L.: Effect of inosine on guinea-pig bronchial muscle. J. Pharm. Pharmacol. *25*, 60–64 (1973)

Blumberg, A.L., Denny, S.E., Marshall, G.R., Needleman, P.: Blood vessel-hormone interactions: angiotensin, bradykinin and prostaglandins. Am. J. Physiol. *232*, H305–310 (1977)

Bobbin, R.P., Guth, P.S.: Venoconstrictive action of bradykinin. J. Pharmacol. Exp. Ther. *160*, 11–21 (1968)

Bokisch, V.A., Müller-Eberhard, H.J.: Anaphylatoxin inactivator of human plasma: its isolation and characterization as a carboxypeptidase. J. Clin. Invest. *49*, 2427–2436 (1970)

Bolam, J. P., Elliot, P.N.C., Ford-Hutchinson, A.W., Smith, M.J.H.: Histamine, 5-hydroxytryptamine, kinins and the anti-inflammatory activity of human plasma fraction in carrageenan-induced paw oedema in the rat. J. Pharm. Pharmacol. *26*, 434–440 (1974)

Bonta, I.L., Hall, D.W.R.: Potentiation of the biphasic bradykinin response of the guinea pig ileum. Br. J. Pharmacol. *49*, 161–162G (1973)
Boucek, R.J., Noble, N.: Histamine, norepinephrine and bradykinin stimulation of fibroblast growth and modification of serotonin response. Proc. Soc. Exp. Biol. Med. *144*, 929–933 (1973)
Branconi, F., Faldi, P., Seravalli, G., Curradi, C., Delbianco, P.L., Sicuteri, F.: Plasmatic prekallikrein and kallikrein inhibitor in pregnancy, labor and in newborn. Adv. Exp. Med. *70*, 261–263 (1976)
Bratanov, K., Somlev, B., Doycheva, M., Tornyov, A., Efremova, V.: Effect of kallikrein on bull sperm motility in vitro. Int. J. Fertil. *23*, 73–75 (1978)
Briseid, K., Qvigstad, E.-K., Engelstad, M., Lagerlov, P., Lange-Nielsen, F.: Assay of factors of the kinin system in plasma from patients with specific exogenous allergies. Acta Allergol. *31*, 297–311 (1976)
Camargo, A., Ferreira, S.H.: Action of bradykinin potentiating factor (BPF) and dimercaprol (BAL) on the responses to bradykinin of isolated preparations of rat intestines. Brit. J. Pharmacol. *42*, 305–307 (1971)
Campbell, A.G.M., Dawes, G.S., Fishman, A.P., Hyman, A.I., Perks, A. M.: Release of a bradykinin-like pulmonary vasodilator substance in foetal and newborn lambs. J. Physiol. (Lond.) *195*, 83–96 (1968)
Capasso, F., Balestrieri, B., di Rosa, M., Persico, P., Sorrentino, L.: Enhancement of carrageein foot oedema by 1, 10 phenanthroline and evidence for the bradykinin as endogenous mediator. Agents Actions *5/4*, 359–363 (1975)
Caspary, W.F., Creutzfeldt, W.: The influence of kallikrein on absorption of sugars and amino acids in rat small intestine in vitro. In: Kininogenases, Haberland, G.L., Rohen, J.W. (eds.), pp. 67–73. Stuttgart, New York: Schattauer 1973
Carter, R.D., Joyner, W.L., Renkin, E.M.: Effect of histamine and some other substances on molecular selectivity of the capillary wall to plasma proteins and dextran. Microvasc. Res. 7, 31–48 (1974)
Castania, A., Rothschild, A.M.: Lowering of kininogen in rat blood by adrenaline and its inhibition by sympatholytic agents, heparin and aspirin. Br. J. Pharmacol. *50*, 375–389 (1974)
Chahl, L.A.: Interactions of substance P with putative mediators of inflammation and ATP. Eur. J. Pharmacol. *44*, 45–49 (1977)
Chaimoff, C., Edery, H., Abraham, S., Gassner, S.: Beneficial effect of alcohol in experimental dumping syndrome in dogs: relation to blood kinins. Isr. J. Med. Sci. *13*, 617–620 (1977)
Chand, N., Eyre, P.: Bradykinin relaxes contracted airways through prostaglandin production. J. Pharm. Pharmacol. *29*, 387–388 (1977)
Chapnick, B.M., Paustian, P.W., Feigen, L.P., Joiner, P.D., Hyman, A.L., Kadowitz, P.J.: Influence of inhibitors of prostaglandin synthesis on renal vascular resistance and on renal vascular responses to vasopressor and vasodilator agents in the cat. Circ. Res. *40*, 348–354 (1977)
Chivers, L., Whalley, E.T.: Action of bradykinin on isolated rat whole uterus and longitudinal myometrial strip. Br. J. Pharmacol. *61*, 506–507P (1977)
Clyman, R.I., Wong, L., Heymann, M.A., Rudolph, A.M.: Responsiveness of the lamb ductus arteriosis to prostaglandins and their metabolites. Prostaglandins *15*, 325–331 (1978)
Collier, H.O.J.: Kinins and ventilation of the lungs. In: Handbook of Experimental Pharmacology. Erdös, E.G. (ed.), Vol. XXV, pp. 409–420. Berlin, Heidelberg, New York: Springer 1970
Collier, H.O.J.: Role of the kallikrein-kinin system in lung diseases. In: Chemistry and biology of the kallikrein-kinin system in health and disease. Fogarty Int. Center Proc. Pisano, J., Austen, K. (eds.), Vol. 27, pp. 495–503, DHEW Publication No. (NIH) 76–791, U.S. Govt. Printing Office, Washington, D.C. 1976
Colman, R.W., Wong, P.Y., Talamo, R.C.: Kallikrein-kinin system in carcinoid and postgastrectomy dumping syndrome. In: Chemistry and biology of the kallikrein-kinin system in health and disease. Pisano, J., Austen, K. (eds.), Fogarty Int. Center Proc., Vol. 27, pp. 487–494, U.S. Govt. Printing Office, Washington, D.C. 1976
Crocker, A.D., Willavoys, S.P.: Effect of bradykinin on transepithelial transfer of sodium and water *in vitro*. J. Physiol. (Lond.) *253*, 401–410 (1975)
Crunkhorn, P., Meacock, S.C.R.: Mediators of the inflammation induced in the rat paw by carrageein. Br. J. Pharmacol. *42*, 392–402 (1971)

Damas, J.: Réactions cardiovasculaires déclenchées par l'introduction de la bradykinine dan les espaces sous-arachnoidiens du chat anesthésié. Archiv. Int. Physiol. Biochem. *82*, 669–677 (1974)
Damas, J.: Sur la stimulation des récepteurs paravasculaires carotidiens par la bradykinine. Arch. Int. Physiol. Biochim. *83*, 111–121 (1975)
Damas, J., Deby, C.: Release of prostaglandins and their precursors by bradykinin. Arch. Int. Physiol. Biochim. *84*, 293–304 (1976)
Damas, J., Mousty, J.C.: Sur l'action hypotensive de la bradykinine chez le Cobaye et le Chat. Comptes rendus des séances de la Société de biologie *170*, 693–697 (1976)
Damas, J., Volon, G.: Sur l'augmentation du pouvoir oedematogene de la bradykinine par les prostaglandines. Bull. Soc. Roy. Sci. Liege. *9–10*, 425–435 (1976)
Davis, T.R.A., Goodfriend, T.L.: Neutralization of airway effects of bradykinin by antibodies. Am. J. Physiol. *217*, 73–77 (1969)
Della Bella, D., Benelli, G., Pajola, E., Valli, P.: Bronchial motility regulation and bradykinin. Advan. Exp. Med. Biol. *21*, 277–283 (1972)
Dennhardt, R., Haberich, F.J.: Effect of kallikrein on the absorption of water electrolytes, and hexoses in the intestine of rats. In: Kininigenases. Haberland, G.L., Rohen, J.W. (eds.), pp. 81–88. Stuttgart, New York: Schattauer 1973
Dietze, G., Wicklmayr, M.: Evidence for a participation of the kallikrein-kinin system in the regulation of muscle metabolism during muscular work. FEBS Letters *74*, 205–208 (1977)
Dietze, G., Wicklmayr, M., Mayer, L.: Evidence for a participation of the kallikrein-kinin system in the physiological regulation of muscular substrate metabolism during muscular work and hypoxia. In: Kininogenases kallikrein 4. Physiological properties and pharmacological rationale. Haberland, G.L., Rohen, J.W., Suzuki, T. (eds.), pp. 291–298. Stuttgart, New York: Schattauer 1977b
Dietze, G., Wicklmayr, M., Mayer, L.: Evidence for a participation of the kallikrein-kinin system in the regulation of muscle metabolism during hypoxia. H. S. Z. Physiol. Chem. *358*, 633–638 (1977a)
Dietze, G., Wicklmayr, M., Mayer, L., Bottger, I., Funcke, H.: Bradykinin and human forearm metabolism: Inhibition of endogenous prostaglandin synthesis. H. S. Z. Physiol. Chem. *359*, 369–378 (1978)
Di Rosa, M., Sorrentino, L.: Some pharmacodynamic properties of carregeenin in the rat. Br. J. Pharmacol. *38*, 214–220 (1970)
Dolovich, J., Back, N., Arbesman, C.E.: Kinin-like activity in nasal secretions of allergic patients. Int. Arch. Allergy Appl. Immunol. *38*, 337–344 (1970)
Dorer, F.E., Ryan, J.W., Stewart, J.M.: Hydrolysis of bradykinin and its higher homologues by angiotensin converting enzyme. Biochem. J. *141*, 915–917 (1974)
Dyer, D.C.: The pharmacology of isolated sheep umbilical cord blood vessels. J. Pharmacol. Exp. Ther. *175*, 565–570 (1970)
Dyer, D.C., Ueland, K., Eng, M.: Responses of isolated monkey umbilical veins to biogenic amines and polypeptides. Arch. Int. Pharmacodyn. Ther. *200*, 213–221 (1972)
Dyrud, O.K., Riesterer, L., Jaques, R.: On the kinin factors in rat pleural exudate. Pharmacology *5*, 264–274 (1971)
Dzizinskii, A.A., Kuimov, A.D.: Blood kinin system in pathogenesis and clinic of ischemic heart desease. Cor. Vasa *14*, 9–15 (1972)
Eisen, V., Loveday, C.: In vivo effects of cellulose sulphate on plasma kininogen, complement and inflammation. Br. J. Pharmacol. *42*, 383–391 (1971)
Elliot, D.F., Horton, E.W., Lewis, G.P.: Actions of pure bradykinin. J. Physiol. (Lond.) *153*, 473–480 (1960)
Erdös, E.G., Yang, H.Y.T.: Kininases. In: Handbook of Experimental Pharmacology. Erdös, E.G. (ed.), pp. 289–323. Berlin, Heidelberg, New York: Springer 1970
Fanciullacci, M., Galli, P., Monetti, M.G., Pela, I., del Bianco, P.L.: Prekallikrein and kallikrein inhibitor in liver cirrhosis and hepatitis. Adv. Exp. Biol. *70*, 201–208 (1975)
Fasth, S., Hulten, L.: Neurohumoral regulation of motility and blood flow in the colon. Experientia *29*, 296–297 (1973)
Fasth, S., Hulten, L., Jahnberg, T., Martinson, J.: Comparative studies on the effects of bradykinin and vagal stimulation on motility in the stomach and colon. Acta Physiol. Scand. *93*, 77–84 (1975)

Fasth, S., Martinson, J.: On the possible role of bradykinin in functional hyperemia of cat's stomach. Acta Physiol. Scand. *89*, 334–341 (1973)

Ferreira, S.H., Vane, J.R.: The detection and estimation of bradykinin in the circulating blood. Brit. J. Pharmacol. Chemother. *29*, 367–377 (1967)

Fonkalsrud, E.W., Sanchez, M., Zerubavel, R., Lassaletta, L., Smeesters, C., Mahoney, A.M.: Arterial endothelial changes after ischemia and perfusion. Surg. Gynecol. *142*, 715–721 (1976)

Franchi, G., Fanciullacci, M., Curradi, C., Nuzzaci, G., Monetti, M.G., Caternolo, M.: Kallikreinogen-kallikrein system during muscular work in patients with intermittant claudication; influence of taurine treatment. Adv. Exp. Med. Biol. *70*, 323–327 (1976)

Frankish, N.H., Zeitlin, I.J.: Kallikrein release from rat duodenum stimulated by bile acids and other factors. J. Physiol. (Lond.) *273*, 60P–61P (1977)

Fritz, H., Schiessler, H., Schleuning, W.D.: Proteinases and proteinase inhibitors in the fertilization process. N. Concepts Control Adv. Biosci. *10*, 271–286 (1973)

Furukawa, S., Hashimoto, K., Kimura, E., Hayakana, H., Ushiyama, S., Miyanaga, Y., Kimura, Y.: Changes in bradykininogen, bradykinin and bradykininase after experimental coronary ligation. Jpn. Circ. J. *33*, 866 (1969)

Gabbiani, G., Badonnel, M.C., Majno, G.: Intra-arterial injections of histamine, serotonin, or bradykinin: A topographic study of vascular leakage. Proc. Soc. Exp. Biol. Med. *135*, 447–452 (1970)

Gabbiani, G., Badonnel, M.C., Gervasoni, C., Portmann, B., Majno, G.: Carbon position in bronchial and pulmonary vessels in response to vasoactive compounds. Proc. Soc. Exp. Biol. Med. *140*, 958–962 (1972)

Gabbiani, G.M., Badonnel, M.C., Rona, G.: Cytoplasmic contractile apparatus in aortic endothelial cells of hypertensive rats. Lab. Invest. **32**, 227–234 (1975)

Garrett, R.L., Brown, J.H.: Bradykinin interaction with 5-hydroxytryptamine norepinephrine and potassium chloride in rabbit aorta. Proc. Soc. Exp. Biol. Med. *139*, 1344–1348 (1972)

Gautvik, K.M., Berg-Oerstadvik, T., Nustad, K.: Role of the kallikrein-kinin system in glandular secretion. In: Chemistry and biology of the kallikrein-kinin system in health and disease. Fogarty Int. Center Proc. Pisano, J.J., Austen, K.F. (eds.), Vol. 27, pp. 335–357, U.S. Govt. Printing Office, Washington, D.C. 1976

Gecse, A., Zsilinszky, E., Lonovics, J., Szekeres, L.: Activation of bradykinin system in acute inflammation induced by endogeneous or exogenous amines. Adv. Exp. Med. Biol. *21*, 391–398 (1972)

Geiger, R., Feifel, G., Haberland, G.: A precursor of kinins in the gastric mucus. H. S. Z. Physiol. Chem. *358*, 931–933 (1977)

Gilbert, R.D., Hessler, J.R., Eitzman, D.V., Cassin, S.: Effect of bradykinin and alterations of blood gases on fetal pulmonary vascular resistance. Am. J. Physiol. *225*, 1486–1489 (1973)

Goldberg, M.R., Chapnick, B.M., Joiner, P.D., Hyman, A.L., Kadowitz, P.J.: Influence of inhibitors of prostaglandin synthesis on venoconstrictor responses to bradykinin. J. Pharmacol. Exp. Ther. *198*, 357–365 (1976)

Green, K.L.: Mechanism of the pro-inflammatory activity of sympathomimetic amines in thermic oedema of the rat paw. Br. J. Pharmacol. *50*, 243–251 (1974)

Green, K.L.: Quantitative studies on the accumulation of serum albumin and erythrocytes in mouse paw oedema induced by bradykinin or thermal injury. Br. J. Exp. Pathol. *59*, 38–47 (1978)

Greenbaum, L.M., Kim, K.S.: The kinin forming and kininase activities of rabbit polymorphonuclear leukocytes. Br. J. Pharmacol. Chemother. *29*, 238–247 (1967)

Gryglewski, R.J.: Prostaglandin synthetase inhibitors. Robinson, H.J., Vane, J.R. (eds.), pp. 33–52. New York: Raven Press 1974

Haddy, F.J., Emerson, T.E., Scott, J.B., Daugherty, R.M.: The effect of kinins on the cardiovascular system. In: Handbook of Experimental Pharmacology. Erdös, E.G. (ed.), Vol. XXV, pp. 362–384. Berlin, Heidelberg, New York: Springer 1970

Hardcastle, J., Hardcastle, P.T., Flower, R.J., Sanford, P.A.: The effect of bradykinin on the electrical activity of rat jejunum. Experienta *34*, 617–618 (1978)

Harris, P., Heath, D.: Pharmacology of the pulmonary circulation. In: The human pulmonary circulation. Its form and function in health and disease, pp. 182–210. Edinbourgh, London, New York: C. Livingstone 1977

Harrison, D.C., Henry, W.L., Paaso, B., Miller, H.A.: Circulatory response to bradykinin before and after autonomic nervous system blockade. Am. J. Physiol. *214*, 1035–1040 (1968)

Hashimoto, K., Hamamoto, H., Honda, Y., Hirose, M., Furukawa, S., Kimura, E.: Changes in components of kinin system and hemodynamics in acute myocardial infarction. Am. Heart J. *95*, 619–626 (1978)
Hashimoto, K., Wanka, J., Kohn, R. N., Wilkens, H. J., Steger, R., Back, N.: The vasopeptide kinin system in acute clinical cardiac diseases. Adv. Exp. Med. Biol. *70*, 245–259 (1976)
Held, HK.: Effect of kallikrein on cerebral capacity and EEG-activity of man during hypoxia. In: Kininogenases, Haberland, G. L., Rohen, J. W., Suzuki, T. (eds.), pp. 345–349. Stuttgart, New York: Schattauer 1977
Herxheimer, H., Stresemann, E.: The effect of bradykinin aerosol in guinea pigs and in man. J. Physiol. (Lond.) *158*, 38P (1961)
Heymann, M. A., Rudolph, A. M., Nies, A. S., Melmon, K. L.: Bradykinin production associated with oxygenation of the fetal lamb. Circ. Res. *25*, 521–523 (1969)
Hofmann, N., Schonberger, A., Gall, H.: Untersuchungen zur Kallikrein-Behandlung männlicher Fertilitätsstörungen. Z. Hautkr. *50*, 1003–1012 (1975)
Houvenaghel, A., Peeters, G.: Action of angiotensin and plasmakinin on blood flow through the mammary artery in unanesthetized lactating goats. Arch. Int. Pharmacodyn. Ther. *192*, 203–204 (1971)
Houvenaghel, A., Peeters, G.: Action of angiotensin and plasmakinins on blood flow through the mammary artery in lactating small ruminants. Arch. Int. Pharmacodyn. Ther. *200*, 320–329 (1972)
Hsueh, W., Isakson, P. D., Needleman, P.: Hormone selective lipase activation in the isolated rabbit heart. Prostaglandins *13*, 1073–1091 (1977)
Hultström, D., Svensjö, E.: Simultaneous fluorescence and electron microscopical detection of bradykinin induced macromolecular leakage. Bibl. Anat. *15*, 466–468 (1977)
Ikeda, K., Tanaka, K., Katori, M.: Potentiation of bradykinin-induced vascular permeability increase by prostaglandin E_2 and arachidonic acid in rabbit skin. Prostaglandins *10*, 747–758 (1975)
Ishigami, J., Kamidono, S.: Clinical experiences with kallikrein in male infertility. In: Kininogenases, kallikrein 2. Haberland, G. L., Rohen, J. W., Schirren, C., Huber, P., (eds.), pp. 155–165. Stuttgart, New York: Schattauer 1975
Ito, H., Matsukawa, H., Takahashi, K., Cho, Y. W.: The effects of catecholamines, acetylcholine and bradykinin on gingival circulation in dogs. Arch. Oral. Biol. *18*, 321–328 (1973)
Johnson, A. R., Erdös, E. G.: Metabolism of vasoactive peptides by human endothelial cells in culture: angiotensin I converting enzyme (kininase II) and angiotensinase. J. Clin. Invest. *59*, 684–695 (1977)
Joyner, W. L., Carter, R. D., Raizes, G. S., Renkin, E. M.: Influence of histamine and some other substances on blood-lymph transport of plasma protein and dextran in the dog paw. Microvasc. Res. 7, 19–30 (1974)
Juan, H., Lembeck, F.: Release of prostaglandins from the isolated perfused rabbit ear by bradykinin and acetylcholine. Agents Actions *6/5*, 642–645 (1976)
Kadowitz, P. J., Joiner, P. D., Hyman, A. L., George, W. J.: Influences of prostaglandins E_1 and F_{2a} on pulmonary vascular resistance, isolated lobar vessels and cyclic nucleotide levels. J. Pharmacol. Exp. Ther. *192*, 677–687 (1975)
Kahn, A., Brachet, E.: The isolated rat mesentery as a model for endothelium. effects of serotonin, bradykinin, dibutyryl-cAMP and theophylline on the passage of ^{125}I-albumin. Arch. Int. Physiol. Biochim. *84*, 343–346 (1976)
Kaliner, M., Orange, R. P., Austen, K. F.: Immunological release of histamine and slow reacting substance of anaphylaxis from human lung. IV. Enhancement by cholinergic and alpha adrenergic stimulation. J. Exp. Med. *136*, 556–567 (1972)
Kaliner, M., Orange, R. P., Austen, K. F.: Immunological release of histamine and slow reacting substance of anaphylaxis from human lung. IV. Enhancement by cholinergic and alpha adrenergic stimulation. J. Exp. Med. *136*, 556–567 (1972)
Kaplan, A. P., Kay, A. B., Austen, K. F.: A prealbumin activator of prekallikrein: III Appearance of chemotactic activity for human neutrophils by the conversion of human prekallikrein to kallikrein. J. Exp. Med. *135*, 81–97 (1972)
Katori, M., Ikeda, K., Harada, Y., Uchida, Y., Tanaka, K., OH-Ishi, S.: A possible role of prostaglandins and bradykinin as a trigger of exudation in carrageenin-induced rat pleurisy. Agents Actions *8*, 108–112 (1978)

Kedra, M., Kleinrok, A., Kolber-Postepska, B., Szurska, G.: Plasma kininogen in patients with myocardinal infarction. Cor. Vasa *15*, 1–8 (1973)
Kellermyer, R.W., Schwartz, H.J.: The kinins: Basic chemistry, biological action, and implication in human asthma. In: Bronchial asthma, mechanisms and therapeutics. Weiss, E.B., Segal, M.S., (eds.) pp. 217–230. Boston: Little, Brown& Co. 1976
Kimura, E., Hashimoto, K., Furukawa, S., Hayakawa, H.: Changes in bradykinin level in coronary sinus blood after the experimental occlusion of a coronary artery. Am. Heart J. *85*, 635–647 (1973)
Kleeberg, S., Prinzen, R., Leidl, W.: Effect of kallikrein on the gonads of premature male rats. In: Kininogenases, kallikrein 2. Haberland, G.L., Rohen, J.W., Schirren, C., Huber, P., (eds.), pp. 99–105. Stuttgart, New York: Schattauer 1975
Komoriya, K., Ohmori, H., Azuma, A., Kurozumi, S., Hashimoto, Y.: Prostaglandin I_2 as a potentiator of acute inflammation in rats. Prostaglandins *15*, 557–564 (1978)
Leidl, W., Prinzen, R., Schill, W.B., Fritz, H.: The effect of kallikrein on motility and metabolism of spermatozoa in vitro. In: Kininogenases, kallikrein 2. Haberland, G. L., Rohen, J.W., Schirren, C., Huber, P., (eds, pp. 33–40. Stuttgart, New York: Schattauer 1975
Leme, J.G., Hamamura, L., Rocha e Silva, M.: Effect of anti-proteases and hexadimethrine bromide on the release of bradykinin-like substance during heating (46 °C) or rat paws. Br. J. Pharmacol. *40*, 294–309 (1970)
Leme, J.G., Hamamura, L., Leite, M.P., Rocha e Silva, M.: Pharmacological analysis of the acute inflammatory process induced in the rat's paw by local injection of carrageenin and by heating. Br. J. Pharmacol. *48*, 88–96 (1973)
Levine, B.W., Talamo, R.C., Kazemi, H.: Action and metabolism of bradykinin in dog lung. J. Appl. Physiol. *34*, 821–826 (1973)
Levy, J.V.: Effect of synthetic bradykinin on contractile tension of human saphenous vein strips. Br. J. Pharmacol. *46*, 517–518 (1972)
Lewis, A.J., Nelson, D.J., Sugrue, M.F.: On the ability of prostaglandin E_1 and arachidonic acid to modulate experimentally induced oedema in the rat paw. Br. J. Pharmacol. *55*, 51–56 (1975)
Limas, C.J.: Selective stimulation of venous prostaglandin E 9-ketoreductase by bradykinin. Biochim. Biophys. Acta *498*, 306–315 (1977)
Ludbrook, J., Vincent, A.H., Walsh, J.A.: The effect of pyridinolcarbamate on the vasodilator action of bradykinin in the human forearm. Aust. J. Exp. Biol. Med. Sci. *51*, 405–409 (1973)
Maciejko, J.J., Marciniak, D.L., Gersabeck, E.F., Grega, G.J.: Effects of locally and systemically infused bradykinin on transvascular fluid and protein transfer in the canine forelimb. J. Pharmacol. Exp. Ther. *205*, 221–235 (1978)
Majno, E., Shea, S.M., Leventhal, M.: Endothelial contraction induced by histamine type mediators: an electron microscopic study. J. Cell Biol. *42*, 647–672 (1969)
Majno, G., Ryan, G.B., Gabbiani, G., Hirschel, B.J., Irle, C., Joris, I.: Contractile events in inflammation and repair. In: Inflammation. Lepow, I.H., Ward, P.A., (eds.), pp. 13–27. New York, London: Academic Press 1972
Malofiejew, M.: Plasma kinin-forming system in labor. Clin. Sci. Mol. Med. *45*, 429–438 (1973)
McCormick, J.T., Senior, J.: The effect of the oestrous cycle, pregnancy and reproductive hormones on the kininase activity of rat blood. J. Reprod. Fertil. *30*, 381–387 (1972)
McCormick, J.T., Senior, J.: Plasma kinin and kininogen levels in the female rat during oestrous cycle, pregnancy, parturition and the puerperium. Br. J. Pharmacol. *50*, 237–241 (1974a)
McCormick, J.T., Senior, J.: Effect of sex hormones on plasma kininogen levels in the rat. Arch. Int. Pharmacodyn. Ther. *210*, 221–231 (1974b)
McGiff, J.C., Terragno, N.A., Malik, K.U., Lonigro, A.J.: Release of a prostaglandin E-like substance from canine kidney by bradykinin. Circ. Res. *31*, 36–43 (1972)
Melmon, K.L., Cline, M.J.: The interaction of leukocytes and the kinin system. Biochem. Pharmacol. [Suppl.] *17*, 271–281 (1968)
Melmon, K.L., Cline, M.J., Hughes, T., Nies, A.S.: Kinins: possible mediators of neonatal circulatory changes in man. J. Clin. Invest. *47*, 1295–1302 (1968)
Meng, K., Haberland, G.L.: Influence of kallikrein on glucose transport in the isolated rat intestine. In: Kininogenases. Haberland, G.L., Rohen, J.W. (eds.), pp. 75–80. Stuttgart, New York: Schattauer 1973

Messina, E.J., Weiner, R., Kaley, G.: Inhibition of bradykinin vasodilation and potentiation of norepinephrine and angiotensin vasoconstriction by inhibitors of prostaglandin synthesis in skeletal muscle of the rat. Circ. Res. *37*, 430–437 (1975)
Michel, B., Russell, T., Winkelmann, R.K., Gleich, G.J.: Release of kinins during wheal and flare allergic skin reactions. J. Clin. Invest. *47*, 68a (1968)
Moncada, S., Ferreida, S.H., Vane, J.R.: Prostaglandins, aspirin-like drugs and the oedema of inflammation. Nature *246*, 217–219 (1973)
Moniuszko-Jakoniuk, J., Wisniewski, K., Ropelewska, J.: The influence of kinins on the metabolic effects of chosen drugs. Biochem. Pharmacol. *25*, 2593–2598 (1976)
Moriwaki, C., Fujimori, H.: Further observations on the influence of the kallikrein-kinin system on the intestinal absorption. In: Kininogenases, Kallikrein 3. Haberland, G.L., Rohen, J.W., Blumel, G., Huber, P., (eds.), pp. 57–62. Stuttgart, New York: Schattauer (1975)
Moriwaki, C., Fujimori, H., Moriya, H., Kizuki, K.: Studies on kallikreins. IV. Enhancement of valine transport across the rat small intestine. Chem. Pharm. Bull. (Tokyo) *25*, 1174–1178 (1977a)
Moriwaki, C., Fujimori, H., Toyono, Y.: Intestinal kallikrein and the influence of kinin on the intestinal transport. In: Kininogenases, kallikrein 4. Haberland, G.L., Rohen, J.W., Suzuki, T., (eds.), pp. 283–290. Stuttgart, New York: Schattauer 1977b
Moriwaki, C., Kizuki, K., Moriya, H.: Kininogenase from the coagulating gland. In: Kininogenases, Kallikrein 2. Haberland, G.L., Rohen, J.W., Schirren, C., Huber, P., (eds.), pp. 23–31. Stuttgart, New York: Schattauer 1975
Moriwaki, C., Moriya, H., Yamaguchi, K., Kizuki, K., Fujimori, H.: Intestinal absorption of pancreatic kallikrein and some aspects of its physiological role. In: Kininogenases, Kallikrein. Haberland, G.L., Rohen, R.W., (eds.), pp. 57–66. Stuttgart, New York: Schattauer 1973
Movat, H.Z., Steinberg, S.G., Habal, F.M., Ranadive, N.S.: Demonstration of kinin-generating enzyme in the lysosomes of human polymorphonuclear leukocytes. Lab. Invest. *29*, 669–684 (1973)
Murakami, N., Hori, S., Masumura, S.: Exercise proteinuria and proteinuria induced by kallikreins. Nature *218*, 481–483 (1968)
Nakata, K.: Synergistic effect of urinary kallikrein and histamine in exercise proteinuria. Mie. Med. J. *21*, 129–139 (1971)
Nakano, J.: Effects of bradykinin, eledoisin, and physalaemin on cardiovascular dynamics. Adv. in Exp. Med. Biol. *8*, 157–170 (1970)
Neto, F.R., Brasil, J.C.F., Antonio, A.: Bradykinin-induced coronary chemo-reflex in the dog. N.S. Arch. Pharmacol. *283*, 135–142 (1974)
Needleman, P.: The synthesis and function of prostaglandins in the heart. Fed. Proc. *35*, 2376–2381 (1976)
Needleman, P., Key, S.L., Denny, S.E., Isakson, P.C., Marshall, G.R.: The mechanism and modification of bradykinin-induced coronary vasodilation. Proc. Natl. Acad. Sci. USA *72*, 2060–2063 (1975)
Newball, H.H.: Response of asthmatic airways to intravenous bradykinin and histamine. Med. Ann. Dist. Col. *43*, 111–114 (1974)
Newball, H.H.: Effects of chemical mediators on asthmatic airways. In: Lung cells in disease. Bouhuys, A., (ed.), pp. 261–264. Elsevier/North Holland, Biomedical Press, Amsterdam 1976
Newball, H.H., Keiser, H.R.: Relative effects of bradykinin and histamine on the respiratory system of man. J. Appl. Physiol. *35*, 552–556 (1973)
Newball, H.H., Keiser, H.R., Webster, M.E., Pisano, J.J.: Effects of bradykinin on human airways. In: Chemistry and biology of the kallikrein-kinin system in health and disease. Pisano, J.J., Austen, K.F., (eds.), pp. 505–511. DHEW Publ. No. (NIH) 76–791, U.S. Govt. Printing Office, Washington, D.C. 1976
Northover, A.M., Northover, B.J.: The effect of histamine, 5-hydroxytryptamine and bradykinin on rat mesenteric blood vessels. J. Pathol. *98*, 265–276 (1969)
Northover, A.M., Northover, B.J.: The effect of vaso-active substances on rat mesenteric blood vessels. J. Pathol. *101*, 99–108 (1970)
Oates, J.A., Butler, T.C.: Pharmacologic and endocrine aspects of carcinoid syndrome. Adv. Pharmacol. *5*, 109–128 (1967)
Oates, J.A., Pettinger, W.A., Doctor, R.B.: Evidence for the release of bradykinin in the carcinoid syndrome. J. Clin. Invest. *45*, 173–178 (1966)

Orange, R.P., Austen, G.W., Austen, K.F.: Immunological release of histamine and slow-reacting substance of anaphylaxis from human lung. I. Modulation by agents influencing cellular levels of cyclic-3',5'-adenosine monophosphate. J. Exp. Med. *134*, 136s–148s (1971)
Oyvin, I.A., Gaponyuk, P.Y., Oyvin, V.I., Tokarev, O.Y.: The mechanism of blood vessel permeability derangement under the influence of histamine, serotonin and bradykinin. Experientia *26*, 843–844 (1970)
Oyvin, I.A., Gaponyuk, P.Y., Volodin, V.M., Oyvin, V.I., Tokaryev, O.Y.: Mechanisms of blood vessel permeability derangement under the influence of permeability factors (histamine, serotonin, kinins) and inflammatory agents. Biochem. Pharmacol. *21*, 89–95 (1972)
Paegelow, I., Reissmann, S., Arold, H.: Charakterisierung der Bradykininwirkung am glatten Muskel unter besonderer Berücksichtigung der Latenzzeit Acta Biol. Med. Germ. *34*, 451–461 (1975)
Paegelow, I., Reissman, S., Vietinghoff, G., Romer, W., Arold, H.: Bradykinin action in the rat duodenum through the cyclic AMP system. Agents Actions 7, 447–451 (1977)
Palm, S., Fritz, H.: Components of the kallikrein-kinin system in human midcycle cervical mucus and seminal plasma. In: Kininogenases, kallikrein 2. Haberland, G.K., Rohen, J.W., Schirren, C., Huber, P., (eds.), pp. 17–21. Stuttgart, New York: Schattauer 1975
Palm, S., Schill, W.B., Wallner, O., Prinzen, R., Fritz, H.: Occurence of components of the kallikrein-kinin system in human genital tract secretions and their possible function in stimulation of sperm motility and migration. Adv. Exp. Med. *70*, 271–279 (1976a)
Palm, S., Schill, W.B., Wallner, O., Prinzen, R., Fritz, H.: Occurrence of components of the kallikrein-kinin system in human genital tract secretions and their possible function in stimulation of sperm motility and migration. In: Kinins: Pharmacodynamics and biological roles. Sicuteri, F., Back, N., Haberland, G.L., (eds.), pp. 271–279. New York: Plenum Press 1976b
Palmer, M.A., Piper, P.J., Vane, J.R.: Release of rabbit aorta contracting substance (RCS) and prostaglandins induced by chemical or mechanical stimulation of guinea pig lungs. Br. J. Pharmacol. *49*, 226–242 (1973)
Peck, M.J., Williams, T.J.: Prostacyclin (PGI_2) potentiates bradykinin-induced plasma exudation in rabbit skin. Br. J. Pharmacol. *62*, 464–465P (1978)
Peeters, G., Houvenaghel, A.: Effets variables de l'ocytocine et des kinines sur la pression intramammaire d'une brebis en lactation. Ann. Biol. Anim., Biochim. Biophys. *13*, 177–185 (1973)
Peeters, G., Houvenaghel, A., Verbeke, R., van Sichem-Reynaert, R.: Effects of bradykinin and kallikrein injected into the udder artery of sheep and goats. Archiv. Int. Pharmacodyn. Ther. *198*, 397–414 (1972)
Perris, A.D., Whitfield, J.F.: The mitogenic action of bradykinin on thymic lymphocytes and its dependence on calcium. Proc. Soc. Exp. Biol. Med. *130*, 1198–1201 (1969)
Pietra, G.G., Szidon, J.P., Leventhal, M.M., Fishman, A.P.: Histamine and interstitial pulmonary edema in the dog. Circ. Res. *29*, 323–337 (1971)
Pitlick, F., Dreyer, B., Mulrow, P., Tan, S.Y., Sweet, P.: PGE_2 synthesis by human cultured cells. Circulation *55/56*, Suppl. III, 121 (1977)
Porter, J.F., Shennan, A.T., Smith, S.: Plasma kinin and kininogen levels in women during pregnancy and labor. J. Reprod. Fert. *30*, 247–254 (1972)
Prasad, S.P., Raviprakash, V., Sabir, M., Bhattacharyya, N.K.: Changes in blood histamine and bradykininogen levels during different periods of the oestrous cycle in goats. J. Reprod. Fertil. *42*, 229–232 (1975)
Rabes, H.: Influence of kallikrein on proliferation of liver cells in vivo and in vitro. In: Kininogenases, kallikrein 3. Haberland, G.L., Rohen, J.W., Blumel, G., Huber, P., (eds.), pp. 137–146. Stuttgart, New York: Schattauer 1975
Ramwell, P.W., Shaw, J.E., Jessup, S.J.: Follicular fluid kinin and its action on fallopian tube. Endocrinology *84*, 931–936 (1969)
Regoli, D., Barabe, J., Theriault, B.: Does indomethacin antagonize the effects of peptides and other agents on the coronary circulation of rabbit isolated hearts? Can. J. Physiol. Pharmacol. *55*, 307–310 (1977a)
Regoli, D., Barabe, J., Park, W.K.: Receptors for bradykinin in rabbit aortae. Can. J. Physiol. Pharmacol. *55*, 855–867 (1977b)

Reis, M.L., Okino, L., Rocha e Silva, M.: Comparative pharmacological actions of bradykinin and related kinins of larger molecular weights. Biochem. Pharmacol. *20*, 2935–2946 (1971)
Reis, M.L., Okino, L., Rocha e Silva, M.: Bradykinin derivatives as permeability factors. Agents Actions *3/5*, 383 (1973)
Resnik, R., Killam, A.P., Barton, M.D., Battaglia, F.C., Makowski, E.L., Meschia, G.: The effect of various vasoactive compounds on the uterine vascular bed. Am. J. Obstet. Gynecol. *125*, 201–206 (1976)
Richardson, P.D.I., Withrington, P.G.: A comparison of the effects of bradykinin, 5-hydroxytryptamine and histamine on the hepatic arterial and portal venous vascular beds of the dog: histamine H_1 and H_2-receptor populations. Br. J. Pharmacol. *60*, 123–133 (1977)
Rixon, R.H., Whitfield, J.F.: Kallikrein, kinin and cell proliferation. In: Kininogenases, kallikrein. Haberland, G.L., Rohen, J.W., (eds.), pp. 131–145. Stuttgart, New York: Schattauer 1973
Rixon, R.H., Whitfield, J.F., Bayliss, J.: The stimulation of mitotic activity in the thymus and bone marrow of rats by kallikrein. Horm. Metab. Res. *3*, 279–284 (1971)
Rocha e Silva, M., Morato, M., de Almeida, A.P., Antonio, A.: Which is the effective agent – bradykinin or prostaglandins – on the isolated mammalian heart. Adv. Exp. Med. Biol. *70*, 117–118 (1976)
Rohen, J.W., Buschhuter, H.: Karyometric measurements on the sertoli cell nuclei in kallikrein-treated albino rats. In: Kininogenases, kallikrein 2. Haberland, G.L., Rohen, J.W., Schirren, C., Huber, P., (eds.), pp. 85–97. Stuttgart, New York: Schattauer 1975
Rohen, J.W., Peterhoff, I.: Stimulation of mitotic activity by kallikrein in the gastrointestinal tract of rats. In: Kininogenases, kallikrein. Haberland, G.L., Rohen, J.W., (eds.), pp. 147–157. Stuttgart, New York: Schattauer 1973
Rothschild, A.M.: Some pharmacodynamic properties of cellulose sulphate, a kininogen-depleting agent in the rat. Br. J. Pharmacol. Chemother. *33*, 501–512 (1968)
Rothschild, A.M., Castania, A.: Contribution of vasopressor and plasma kininogen changes towards acute adrenaline pulmonary edema in the rat. N.S. Archiv. Pharmacol. *295*, 177–181 (1976)
Rothschild, A.M., Castania, A., Cordeiro, R.S.B.: Consumption of kininogen, formation of kinin and activation of arginine ester hydrolase in rat plasma by rat peritoneal fluid cells in the presence of 1-adrenaline. N.S. Arch. Pharmacol. *285*, 243–256 (1974)
Rothschild, A.M., Cordeiro, R.S.B., Castania, A.: Acute pulmonary edema and plasma kininogen consumption in the adrenaline-treated rat: inhibition by acetylsalicylic acid and resistance to salicylate and indomethacin. N.S. Arch. Pharmacol. *288*, 319–321 (1975)
Schiessler, H., Arnhold, M., Ohlsson, K., Fritz, H.: Inhibitors of acrosin and granulocyte proteinases from human genital tract secretions. H.S.Z. Physiol. Chem. *357*, 1251–1260 (1976)
Schill, W.B.: Influences of the kallikrein-kinin system on human sperm motility in vitro. In: Kininogenases, kallikrein 2. Haberland, G.L., Rohen, J.W., Schirren, C., Huber, P., (eds.), pp. 47–57. Schattauer 1975a
Schill, W.B.: Caffeine- and kallikrein-induced stimulation of human sperm motility: A comparative study. Andrologia *7*, 229–236 (1975b)
Schill, W.B., Braun-Falco, O., Haberland, G.L.: The possible role of kinins in sperm motility. Int. J. Fertil. *19*, 163–167 (1974)
Schill, W.B., Haberland, G.: Kinin-induced enhancement of sperm motility. H.S.Z. Physiol. Chem. *355*, 229–231 (1974)
Schill, W.B., Haberland, G.L.: Wirkungen von verschiedenen komponenten des kallikrein-kinin-systems auf die spermatozoen-motilität in vitro. Klin. Wochenschr. *53*, 73–79 (1975)
Schill, W.B., Schleuning, W.D., Fritz, H.: Biochemical and clinical aspects of human sperm acrosin. Excerpta Medica International Congress Series *394*, Biological and Clinical Aspects of Reproduction. Excerpta Medica, Amsterdam, 144–151 (1975)
Schleuning, W.D., Hell, R., Fritz, H.: Multiple forms of human acrosin: Isolation and properties. H.S.Z. Physiol. Chem. *357*, 855–865 (1976)
Schumacher, K.A., Starke, K.: Bradykinin-induced stimulation of cardiac parasympathetic ganglia. Experientia *34*, 223–224 (1978)
Schutte, B., Lindner, J.: Additional aspects of the effect of kallikrein on cell proliferation. In: Kininogenases, kallikrein 4. Haberland, G.L., Rohen, J.W., Suzuki, T., (eds.), pp. 161–177. Stuttgart, New York: Schattauer 1977

Schwartz, M.M., Cotran, R.S.: Vascular leakage in the kidney and lower urinary tract: effects of histamine, serotonin and bradykinin. Proc. Soc. Exp. Biol. Med. *140*, 535–539 (1972)
Sekiya, A., Nakashima, M., Maeda, K., Yamamoto, J., Hirako, I., Oya, H.: Studies on the vascular action of bradykinin. Jpn. J. Pharmacol. *21*, 87–95 (1971)
Seki, T., Nakajima, T., Erdös, E.G.: Colon as possible site of origin of a plasma kallikrein. In: New aspects of trasylol therapy. Brendel, W., Haberland, G.L., (eds.), pp. 17–22. Stuttgart, New York: Schattauer 1971
Senior, J.B., Spencer-Gregson, R.N.: The effects of sympathomimetic drugs and bradykinin on the human fallopian tube in vitro using isometric recording methods. J. Obstet. Gynaecol. Br. Cwlth. *76*, 652–655 (1969)
Senior, J., Whalley, E.T.: The effect of pseudopregnancy and 'pseudoparturition' on the kinin system in the rat. J. Reprod. Fertil. *38*, 165–170 (1974a)
Senior, J., Whalley, E.T.: Variation in the oestrogen-progesterone ratio and its effect on plasma kininogen levels in the rat. J. Reprod. Fertil. *41*, 425–433 (1974b)
Senior, J., Whalley, E.T.: Influence of the adrenals and gonads on plasma kininogen concentrations in male and female rats. J. Pharm. Pharmacol. *27*, 953–955 (1975)
Senior, J., Whalley, E.T.: The influence of drugs on the kinin-forming system in relation to pregnancy and parturition in the rat. J. Reprod. Fertil. *47*, 319–323 (1976)
Sherman, W.T., Gautieri, R.F.: Effect of certain drugs on perfused human placenta X: Norepinephrine release by bradykinin. J. Pharm. Sci. *61*, 878–883 (1972)
Shionoya, S., Nakata, Y., Kamiya, K., Inagaki, A., Yano, T.: Influences of bradykinin on the microcirculation. Angiology *22*, 456–461 (1971)
Sicuteri, F., Antonini, F.M., Del Bianco, P.L., Franchi, G., Curradi, C.: Prekallikrein and kallikrein inhibitor in plasma of patients affected by recent myocardial infraction. Adv. Exp. Med. Biol. *21*, 445–452 (1972)
Simonsson, B.G., Skoogh, B.E., Bergh, N.P., Andersson, R., Svedmyr, N.: In vivo and in vitro effect of bradykinin on bronchial motor tone in normal subjects and patients with airways obstruction. Respiration *30*, 378–388 (1973)
Smith, A.M., Zeitlin, I.J.: The role of bradykinin in vasomotor aspects of the carcinoid and dumping syndromes. Br. J. Surg. *53*, 867–869 (1966)
Staszewska-Barczak, J., Dusting, G.J.: Sympathetic cardiovascular reflex initiated by bradykinin-induced stimulation of cardiac pain receptors in the dog. Clin. Exp. Pharmacol. Physiol. *4*, 443–452 (1977)
Stasiewicz, J., Szalaj, W., Gabryelewicz, A.: Modifying effect of bradykinin on motor activity in the guinea pig gall bladder. Clin. Exp. Pharmacol. Physiol. *4*, 561–654 (1977)
Sterin-Speziale, N., Gimeno, M.F., Zapata, C., Bagnati, P.E., Gimeno, A.L.: The effect of neurotransmitters, bradykinin, prostaglandins and follicular fluid on spontaneous contractile characteristics of human fimbriae and tubo-ovarian ligaments isolated during different stages of the sexual cycle. Int. J. Fertil. *23*, 1–11 (1978)
Stewart, D., Blendis, L.M., Williams, R.: Studies on the prekallikrein-bradykininogen system in liver disease. J. Clin. Pathol. *25*, 410–414 (1972)
Stewart, J.M., Ferreira, S.H., Greene, L.J.: Bradykinin potentiating peptide PCA-Lys-Trp-Ala-Pro. An inhibitor of the pulmonary inactivation of bradykinin and conversion of angiotensin I to II. Biochem. Pharmacol. *20*, 1557–1567 (1971)
Still, J.G., Greiss, F.C.: The effect of prostaglandins and other vasoactive substances on uterine blood flow and myometrial activity. Am. J. Obstet. Gynecol. *130*, 1–8 (1978)
Stoner, J.S., Manganiello, V.C., Vaugham, M.: Effects of bradykinin and indomethacin on cyclic GMP and cyclic AMP in lung slices. Proc. Natl. Acad. Sci. USA *70*, 3830–3833 (1973)
Stuttgen, G.: Clinical substantiation of the effects of kallikrein. In: Kininogenases, kallikrein. Haberland, G.L., Rohen, J.W., (eds.), pp. 189–193. Stuttgart, New York: Schattauer 1973
Svensjö, E., Persson, C.G.A., Rutili, G.: Inhibition of bradykinin induced macromolecular leakage from post-capillary venules by a β_2-adrenoreceptor stimulant, terbutaline. Acta Physiol. Scand. *101*, 504–506 (1977a)
Svensjö, E., Tuma, R.F., Arfors, K.E.: Comparison of arteriolar blood flow in the hamster cheek pouch at two different oxygen tensions. Acta Physiol. Scand. *100*, 404–411 (1977b)
Tallarida, G., Baldoni, F., Peruzzi, G., Semprinin, A., Sangiorgi, M.: Cardiovascular and respiratory reflexes elicited by bradykinin acting on receptor sites (K and P) in the muscular circulatory area. Adv. Exp. Med. Biol. *70*, 301–313 (1976)

Terragno, D.A., Crowshaw, K., Terragno, N.A., McGiff, J.: Prostaglandin synthesis by bovine mesenteric arteries and veins. Circ. Res. *76/80*, 136–137 (1975)
Thomas, G., West, G.B.: Prostaglandins, kinin and inflammation in the rat. Br. J. Pharmacol. *50*, 231–235 (1974)
Toda, N.: Actions of bradykinin on isolated cerebral and peripheral arteries. Am. J. Physiol. *232*, H267–274 (1977)
Tsuru, H., Ishikawa, N., Shigei, T.: Responses of isolated dog veins to bradykinin: distribution and a possible correlation with genesis of the venous system. Jpn. J. Pharmacol. *24*, 931–934 (1974)
Tsuru, H., Ishikawa, N., Shigei, T.: Responsiveness of isolated dog veins to bradykinin and other bioactive peptides: distribution of sensitivity to bradykinin and possible correlation with genesis of the venous system. Blood Vessels *13*, 238–248 (1976)
Uchida, Y., Murao, S.: Bradykinin-induced excitation of afferent cardiac sympathetic nerve fibers. Jpn. Heart J. *15*, 84–91 (1974)
Ufkes, J.G.R., Aarsen, P.N., Van der Meer, C.: The bradykinin potentiating activity of two pentapeptides on various isolated smooth muscle preparations. Eur. J. Pharmacol. *40*, 137–144 (1976)
Ufkes, J.G.R., Van der Meer, C.: The effect of catecholamine depletion on the bradykinin-induced relaxation of isolated smooth muscle. Eur. J. Pharmacol. *33*, 141–144 (1975)
Vallota, E.H., Müller-Eberhard, H.J.: Formation of C3a and C5a anaphylatoxins in whole human serum after inhibition of the anaphylatoxin inactivator. J. Exp. Med. *137*, 1109–1123 (1973)
Varonier, H.S., Panzani, R.: The effect of inhalations of bradykinin on healthy and atopic (asthmatic) children. Int. Arch. Allergy *34*, 293–296 (1968)
Vecchiet, L., Dolce, V., Galleti, R.: Algogenic activity of human plasma following muscular work. Adv. Exp. Med. Biol. *70*, 177–182 (1976)
Walaszek, E.J.: The effect of bradykinin and kallidin on smooth muscle. In: Handbook of Experimental Pharmacology. Erdös, E.G., (ed.), pp. 421–429. Berlin, Heidelberg, New York: Springer 1970
Wallner, O., Schill, W.B., Grosser, A., Fritz, H.: Participation of the kallikrein-kinin-system in sperm penetration through cervical mucus in vitro studies. In: Kininogenases, kallikrein 2. Haberland, G.L., Rohen, J.W., Schirren, C., Huber, P. (eds.), pp. 63–70. Stuttgart, New York: Schattauer 1975
Ward, P.E., Klauser, R.J., Erdös, E.G.: Angiotensin I converting enzyme (peptidyl dipeptidase) in the brush border of human intestinal mucosa. Circulation *58*, II–251 (1978)
Webster, M.E., Pierce, J.V.: The nature of the kallidins released from human plasma by kallikreins and other enzymes. Ann. N.Y. Acad. Sci. *104*, 91–107 (1963)
Weese, W.C., Talamo, R.C., Neyhard, N.L., Kazemi, H.: Presence of a bradykinin-like substance in pulmonary washings. Am. Rev. Resp. Dis. *113*, 81–187 (1976)
Wiegershausen, B., Klausch, B., Hanninghausen, G., Sobat, R.: Der Kininogenspiegel von Ratten und Kaninchen während der Gestation. Experientia *24*, 1128–1129 (1968)
Wiegershausen, B., Paeglow, I., Henninghausen, G.: The kininogen-kinin system during pseudogravity in rabbits. Acta Biol. Med. Germ. *26*, 1251–1253 (1971)
Wilhelm, D.L.: Mechanisms responsible for increased vascular permeability in acute inflammation. Agents Actions *3/5*, 297–306 (1973)
Wilkens, H.J., Back, N.: Bronchonconstriction and apnea in canine anaphylaxis: Possible role of histamine and plasma kinins. Arch. Int. Pharmacol. Ther. *190*, 14–33 (1971)
Wilkins, H., Back, N., Steger, R., Karn, J.: The influence of blood pH on peripheral vascular tone: possible role of proteases and vaso-active polypeptides. In: Shock, Biochemical, pharmacological and clinical aspects. Bertelli, A., Back, N. (eds.), pp. 201–214. New York: Plenum Press 1970
Wilkins, H.J., Steger, R., Back, N.: Effect of protease inhibition on biochemical changes, cardiovascular dynamics and survival in experimental coronary artery occlusion. Circ. Shock *2*, 277–286 (1975)
Williams, T.J., Morley, J.: Prostaglandins as potentiators of increased vascular permeability in inflammation. Nature *246*, 215–217 (1973)
Williams, T.J., Peck, M.J.: Role of prostaglandin-mediated vasodilation in inflammation. Nature *270*, 530–532 (1977)

Wintroub, B.U., Austen, K.F.: Interaction of neutrophil-bound enzymes with plasma protein substrates. In: Immunopathology. Miescher, P.A. (ed.), pp. 251–261. Basel-Stuttgart: Schwabe and Co. 1976
Wintroub, B.U., Goetzl, E.J., Austen, K.F.: A neutrophil-dependent pathway for the generation of a neutral peptide mediator. Partial characterization of components and control by α-1-antitrypsin. J. Exp. Med. *140*, 812–824 (1974)
Wong, P.Y., Colman, R.W., Talamo, R.C., Babior, B.M.: Kallikrein-bradykinin system in chronic alcoholic liver disease. Ann. Int. Med. *77*, 205–209 (1972)
Wong, P.Y., Talamo, R.C., Babior, B.M., Raymond, G.G., Colman, R.W.: Kallikrein-kinin system in postgastrectomy dumping syndrome. Ann. Intern. Med. *80*, 577–581 (1974)
Wong, P.Y., Talamo, R.C., Williams, G.H.: Kallikrein-kinin and renin-angiotensin systems in functional renal failure of cirrhosis of the liver. Gastroenterology *73*, 1114–1118 (1977a)
Wong, P.Y., Terragno, D.A., Terragno, N.A., McGiff, J.C.: Dual effects of bradykinin on prostaglandin metabolism: relationship to the dissimilar vascular actions of kinins. Prostaglandins *13*, 1113–1125 (1977b)
Zeitlin, I.J., Smith, A.M.: 5-Hydroxyindoles and kinins in the carcinoid and dumping syndromes. Lancet November, Vol. 2, part 2, 986–991 (1966)
Zeitlin, I.J., Smith, A.N.: Mobilization of tissue kallikrein in inflammatory disease of the colon. Gut *14*, 133–138 (1973)
Zeitlin, I.J., Singh, Y.N., Lembeck, F., Theiler, M.: The molecular weights of plasma and intestinal kallikrein in rats. N.S. Arch. Pharmacol. *293*, 159–161 (1976)

Release of Vasoactive Substances by Kinins*

N. A. TERRAGNO and A. TERRAGNO

A. Introduction

It has been suggested that kinins participate in a wide range of physiologic and pathologic processes by direct and indirect mechanisms that involve the release of other vasoactive substances. The potential of kinins to activate the prostaglandin synthesizing system in the kidney (TERRAGNO et al., 1972), pregnant uterus (TERRAGNO et al., 1974), and vasculature (TERRAGNO et al., 1975; MESSINA et al., 1975) deserves special attention. This activation of synthesis results in the release of prostaglandins which contribute to the amplification or attenuation of the action of kinins. Thus, mediation of some of the biologic effects of kinins by prostaglandins seems likely. The recognition of a possible contribution of kinins to blood pressure regulation has recently received a great deal of attention (ADETUYIBI and MILLS, 1972; MARIN-GREZ et al., 1972; MARGOLIUS et al., 1971). Kinins are also able to release other tissue hormones, such as histamine, serotonin, catecholamines from the adrenal gland, and antidiuretic hormone from the posterior pituitary. Thereby, they contribute to a number of clinical manifestations of functional disorders.

A full understanding of the interactions of kinins with prostaglandins requires the recognition that bradykinin can not only stimulate the prostaglandin synthetase complex in tissues but may also determine the end products of the enhanced synthesis by stimulation of prostaglandin E (PGE) 9-ketoreductase, the enzyme responsible for the conversion of PGE to PGF (prostaglandin F).

B. Bradykinin-Prostaglandin Interactions

The range of products arising from the prostaglandin synthetase complex (Fig. 1) includes the primary prostaglandins of the E, D, and F series, the prostaglandin endoperoxides, the thromboxanes, as well as other cycloether derivatives such as prostacyclin (PGI_2 or PGX) (TUVEMO et al., 1976; FERREIRA and VANE, 1967; HAMBERG and SAMUELSSON, 1973; PACE-ASCIAK and WOLFFE, 1971; NUGTEREN and HAZELHOF, 1973).

Thromboxane A_2 (TxA_2) and PGI_2 are potent vasoactive substances, with opposite properties on vascular contractility and platelet aggregation, which may be of great significance in the circulatory system. Both substances undergo rapid nonen-

* Supported in part by grants from the National Institutes of Health, United States Public Health Service (HL-HD 22225), the American Heart Association (77894), and Tennessee Heart Association. We thank Mrs. MARY ANN ROBERTS and Mrs. BARBARA LAWRENCE for their assistance and especially Ms. JUDITH EARLY for the bibliographic search and help in the preparation of the manuscript.

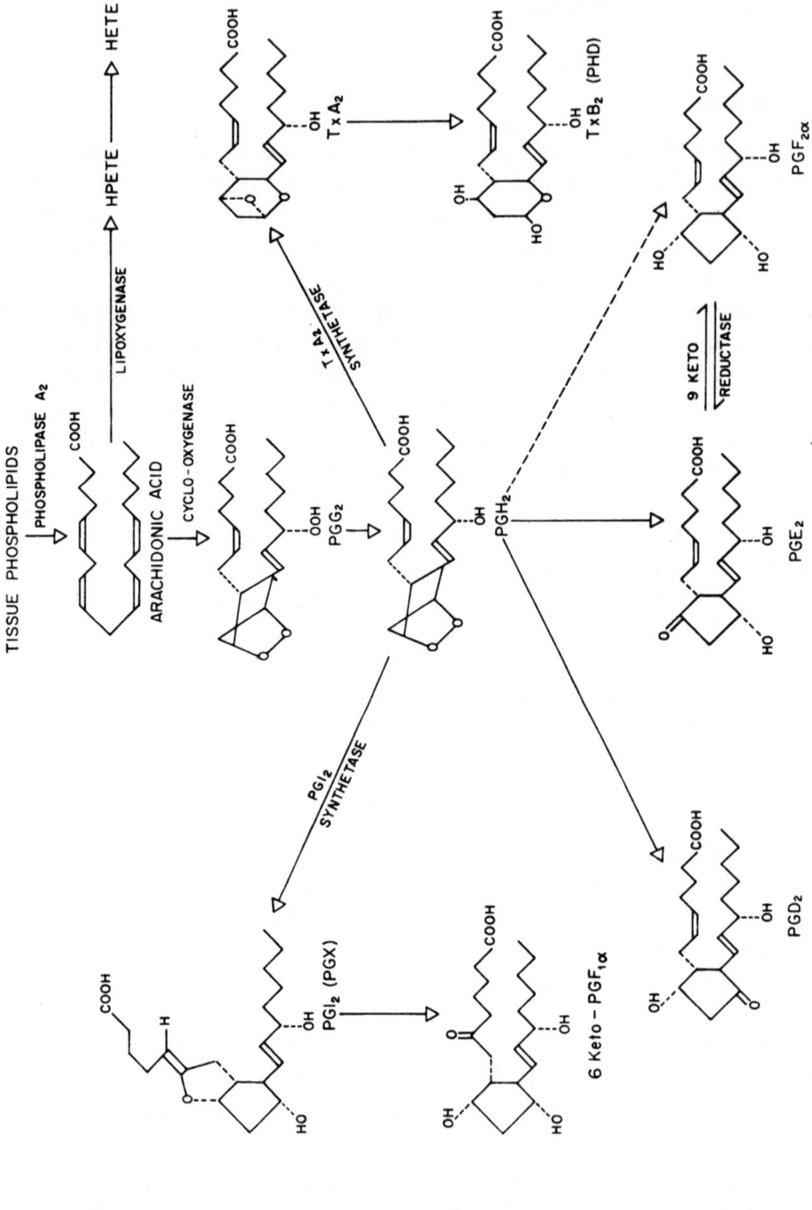

Fig. 1. Major metabolic pathways of arachidonic acid

zymic hydration to stable metabolites under physiologic conditions. TxA_2 is converted to thromboxane B_2 (TxB_2), while PGI_2 is converted to 6 keto-$PGF_{1\alpha}$. In the course of analysis of the products of prostaglandin synthesis by the usual methods of extraction and thin layer chromatography, TxA_2 and PGI_2 are entirely converted to their stable metabolites.

The major studies were devoted to the primary prostaglandins, especially E_2 and $F_{2\alpha}$, and a number of physiologic and pathophysiologic properties have been ascribed to them. Most of these roles need to be reevaluated in the light of newly discovered arachidonate derivatives which could contribute to, or antagonize, the actions of the primary prostaglandins and which we have demonstrated to be present in abundance in fetal and maternal vascular tissues (TERRAGNO et al., 1977b, 1978a).

Most of the prostaglandins, PGE, PGF, 6 keto-$PGF_{1\alpha}$ (the stable metabolite of PGI_2) and TxB_2 (the metabolite of TxA_2), have been identified in the uteroplacental complex and kidney (TUVEMO and WIDE, 1973; TERRAGNO et al., 1974; WILLMAN and COLLINS, 1976; FENWICK et al., 1977; MORRISON et al., 1977). TxB_2 has also been identified in umbilical blood vessels (TUVEMO et al., 1976).

Prostaglandins of the E and F series are removed or inactivated during passage across the lungs (FERREIRA and VANE, 1967; MCGIFF et al., 1969) after release into the circulation from their organ of synthesis. This suggests that they belong to that group of hormones having circumscribed activity, the local or tissue hormones. In addition to the potent vasodilator (PGI_2 and PGE_2) (DUSTING et al., 1977; MCGIFF et al., 1972a) and vasoconstrictor ($PGF_{2\alpha}$ and TxA_2) actions (DUCHARME et al., 1968; NEEDLEMAN et al., 1976), prostaglandins may function as modulators of autonomic nervous activity. Thus, prostaglandins of the E series usually attenuate adrenergic activity (HEDQVIST, 1970) while PGF compounds may have an opposite effect by facilitating adrenergic transmission (KADOWITZ et al., 1972). These properties, together with the ability of prostaglandins of the E series to antagonize the vasoconstrictor effects of pressor stimuli (MCGIFF et al., 1970, 1972a; TERRAGNO et al., 1976; NEGUS et al., 1976) and potentiate the vasodilator effect of bradykinin (MCGIFF et al., 1972b, 1975) suggest that the kallikrein-kinin and prostaglandin systems participate in the regulation of blood pressure and peripheral blood flow.

The idea that prostaglandins are primarily local or tissue hormones (MCGIFF and ITSKOVITZ, 1973), which exert their effects at or near sites of synthesis, has particular significance for the vasculature. The capacity of blood vessels to synthesize prostaglandins intramurally (TERRAGNO et al., 1975) enables them to influence vascular tone and reactively locally through mechanisms involving kinins which enhance prostaglandin synthesis (TERRAGNO et al., 1975). This in turn can affect the vasoconstrictor actions of angiotensin (MCGIFF et al., 1970; TERRAGNO et al., 1976; NEGUS et al., 1976) and catecholamines (MCGIFF et al., 1972a), as well as contribute to the regulation of the release of norepinephrine from adrenergic nerves (HEDQVIST, 1970, 1973).

At the time that most of those studies were performed, existing chromatographic methods did not allow resolution to differentiate between PGE_2 and 6 keto-$PGF_{1\alpha}$ as they chromatograph together in most of the solvent systems previously used to separate the classical prostaglandins. Therefore, when reference is made to previous work in which PGE_2 was not separated from 6 keto-$PGF_{1\alpha}$, we must consider the possibility that a mixture of both vasoactive prostaglandins resulted from the stimulation of prostaglandin synthesis induced by kinins. It is now possible to separate, by chromatography, PGE_2, from PGI_2 using different solvent systems. Further, alkaline treatment, which transforms PGE_2 to PGB_2, or reduction of the 9-carbonyl group of PGE_2 with $NaBH_4$ to an epimeric mixture of $PGF_{2\alpha}$ and $PGF_{2\beta}$, allows individual determination of these substances (TERRAGNO et al., 1977b).

I. Kidney

The vasodilator and diuretic actions of kinins are among their most prominent biologic properties (BARRACLOUGH and MILLS, 1965; WEBSTER and GILMORE, 1964). Sodium deprivation results in increased activity of this system (MARGOLIUS et al., 1974) as indicated by enhanced kallikrein excretion (see WARD and MARGOLIUS, this volume). This would be expected to further decrease extracellular fluid volume and counter those homeostatic mechanisms conserving body fluid, if the effects of kinins were not modified by prostaglandin release.

In the kidney, as well as in other tissues, kinins activate the prostaglandin-synthesizing system (TERRAGNO et al., 1972), which consequently modifies the renal action of kinins. The discovery by VANE (1971) that nonsteroidal anti-inflammatory drugs inhibit prostaglandin biosynthesis was used to examine those components of the renal action of kinins which are amplified, mediated, or attenuated by the release of prostaglandins.

Before considering the interrelationships of prostaglandins and kinins in detail several important points should be explored:

(1) Release of prostaglandins from an organ in response to a stimulus (e.g., administration of angiotensin II) indicates increased prostaglandin synthesis within that organ. This results in the immediate entry of the newly synthesized prostaglandins into the extracellular compartment (ÄNGGÅRD et al., 1972).

(2) The demonstration that kinins induce release of prostaglandins from an organ (i.e., stimulate de novo synthesis of prostaglandins) does not permit the conclusion that kinins directly affect the prostaglandin-synthesizing enzymes. Thus, a direct action of bradykinin on prostaglandin synthesis in the seminal vesicles could not be demonstrated (DAMAS et al., 1973). Further, mepacrine, an antimalarial agent which inhibits phospholipase A_2 and prevents release of the products of prostaglandin synthesis from guinea pig lungs evoked by bradykinin, did not affect the release evoked by arachidonic acid (VARGAFTIG and DAO HAI, 1972). These studies and that of KUNZE and VOGT in 1971 suggest that kinins can activate acylhydrolases such as phospholipase A_2, causing an increase in free fatty acid substrate available to prostaglandin synthetase, thereby increasing synthesis of prostaglandins.

This action, however, cannot explain the differential effect of bradykinin on prostaglandin release from isolated arteries and veins, in which there is a selective increase in production of PGE in the arteries and PGF in the veins (TERRAGNO et al., 1975). This experiment suggests that, in addition to the activation of an acylhydrolase, kinins can alter PGE/PGF ratios by stimulation of PGE 9-ketoreductase, the enzyme responsible for the conversion of PGE to PGF (WONG et al., 1977; LIMAS, 1977).

(3) Formation of prostaglandins of the E and F series has been demonstrated within the renal medulla (CROWSHAW et al., 1970) and very little synthesis has been

previously demonstrated in the renal cortex (CROWSHAW, 1971, 1973). Recent studies performed in our laboratory demonstrate the presence of an active synthesis of prostaglandins E_2, $F_{2\alpha}$, and I_2 by the renal blood vessels. In cortical blood vessels (interlobular and afferent arterioles), as well as renal and arcuate arteries, the most abundant prostaglandin produced is PGI_2, as shown by the presence of its metabolite, 6 keto-$PGF_{1\alpha}$. Figure 2 shows the radiochromatogram scans of the conversion of radiolabeled arachidonic acid to different prostaglandins, by slices of cortex, inner medulla, isolated convoluted tubules, and blood vessels within the cortex. From these experiments, performed in the authors' laboratory, it is clear that prostaglandins are formed in one or more components of the vascular wall (endothelial cells, supporting tissue, and smooth muscle) and released to the interstitial or vascular space.

Cortical blood vessels have a high capacity to synthesize prostaglandins when they are isolated from the surrounding tissues but this capacity is inhibited when these blood vessels are incubated in the supernatant of previously incubated cortical slices (Fig. 3). These studies suggest the presence of an endogenous prostaglandin synthesis inhibitor (EPSI), located in the renal cortex, which controls vascular synthesis of prostaglandins (TERRAGNO et al., 1978b). This is the first demonstration of an endogenous inhibitor of formation of vascular prostaglandins, which could play an important role in the control of prostaglandin synthesis, and suggests that the availability of substrate is not the most important mechanism in the control of the arachidonic acid cascade. Prostaglandins of renal origin are destroyed primarily by the lung (FERREIRA and VANE, 1967). This arrangement allows renal prostaglandins to locally influence the medullary circulation (ITSKOVITZ et al., 1974), in addition to vasomotor tone of the major capacitance vessels (DUCHARME et al., 1968), and thereby affect cardiac output, without having an undesirable effect on the arterial side of the circulation.

The renal action of kinins will now be examined in terms of interrelationships with prostaglandins. We demonstrated that bradykinin release of prostaglandins from the kidney was associated with changes in renal blood flow (TERRAGNO et al., 1972). In other experiments, using the dog isolated blood-perfused kidney to avoid systemic changes in cardiovascular function evoked by vasoactive substances of extrarenal origin (MCGIFF et al., 1975), the effects of bradykinin on renal function were studied before and after inhibition of prostaglandin synthesis by indomethacin. These changes were compared with those produced by another vasodilator polypeptide, eledoisin, which does not release prostaglandins from the kidney. Both polypeptides were infused at rates which produced a similar degree of renal vasodilation. In these experiments, the renal responses to bradykinin before and after administration of indomethacin were compared. After administration of indomethacin, the renal vasodilator action of bradykinin was reduced slightly whereas the vasodilator action of eledoisin was unaffected (MCGIFF et al., 1975).

Although this study clearly showed that the vasodilator action of bradykinin in the canine isolated blood-perfused kidney can be attentuated by diminishing its capacity to generate PGE_2, the most important observation was that the ability of bradykinin to promote excretion of solute-free water is dependent on the generation of a prostaglandin. It is also possible to modify those renal actions of kinins which are mediated through PGE_2 release by accelerating its degradation or by converting

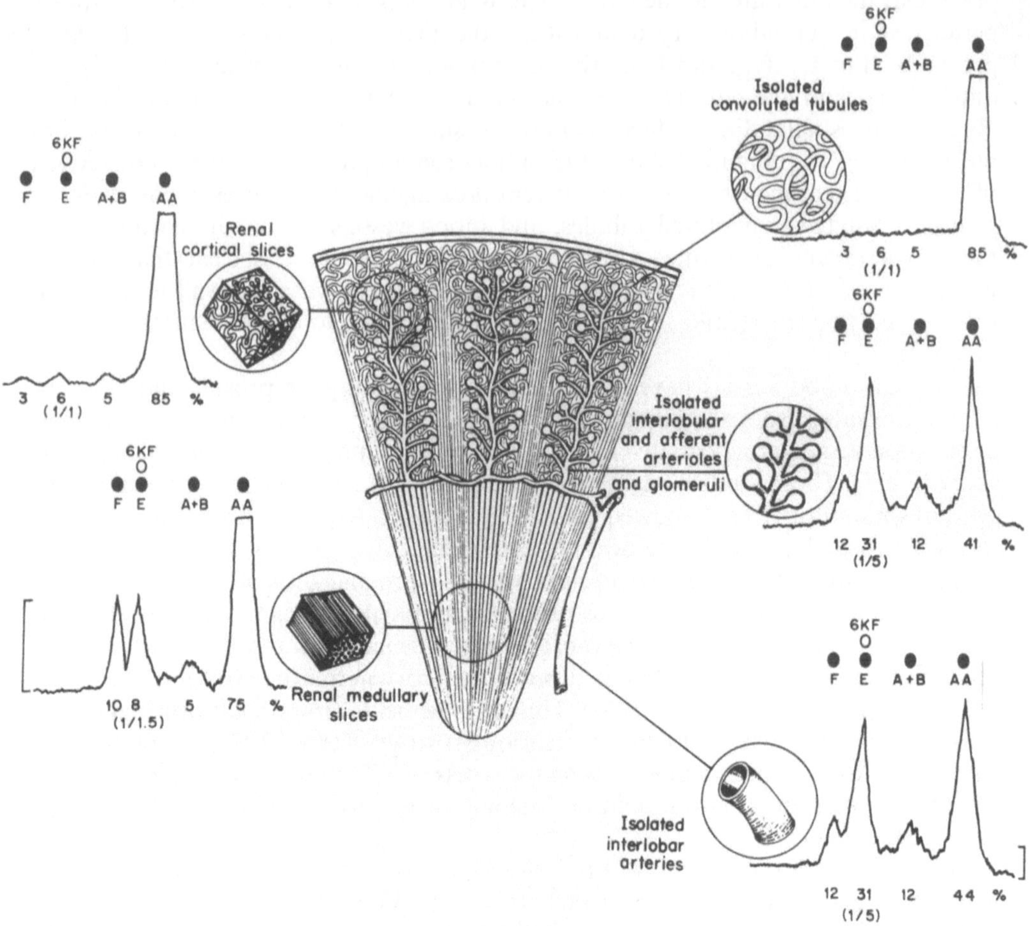

Fig. 2. Schematic representation of different intrarenal structures, showing the radiochromatogram scans of the prostaglandins synthesized from radiolabeled arachidonic acid by slices of different renal structures incubated in Krebs' solution for 3 h at 37 °C without cofactors. After extraction with organic solvents, the radioactive products were chromatographed on silica gel thin-layer plates and developed in chloroform:methanol:acetic acid:water (90:9:1:0.65, v/v). The position of prostaglandin standards on a reference channel developed simultaneously in the same solvent system is displayed above each radiochromatogram scan. The numbers below the scans indicate the percentage of total radioactivity recovered from the incubation fluid. This solvent system does not allow the separation of PGE_2 from 6 keto-$PGF_{1\alpha}$. In order to obtain the PGE/6 keto-PGF ratio the material contained within the area of PGE+6 keto-$PGF_{1\alpha}$ was extracted with organic solvents and rechromatographed in a solvent system consisting of the organic phase of ethyl acetate:iso-octane:acetic acid:water (11:5:2:10, v/v). Numbers in parentheses indicate the ratio of PGE to 6 keto-$PGF_{1\alpha}$. Renal cortical slices did not efficiently convert [1-^{14}C] arachidonic acid to labeled products, despite the fact that interlobular and afferent arterioles isolated from the cortex showed high biosynthetic capacity. The activity of prostaglandin synthetase in cortical blood vessels seems to be under the control of an endogenous prostaglandin synthesis inhibitor (EPSI) released by cortical extravascular tissues. The largest production of prostaglandins in the kidney is associated with the vasculature. F = $PGF_{2\alpha}$; 6 KF = 6 keto-$PGF_{1\alpha}$; E = PGE_2; A + B = PGA_2 + PGB_2; AA = arachidonic acid

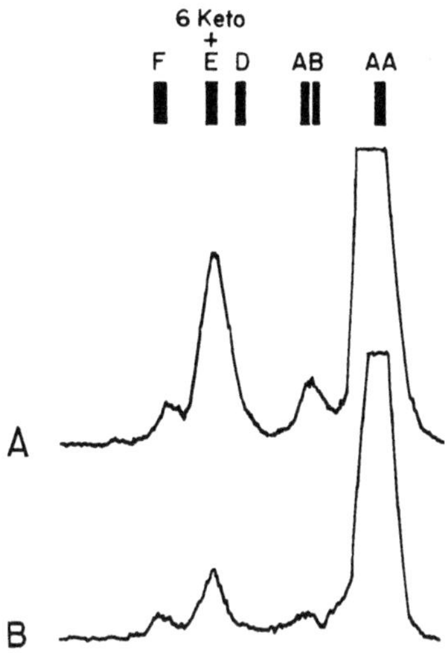

Fig. 3. Radiochromatogram scans of prostaglandins formed from [1-^{14}C] arachidonic acid by renal blood vessels. The arachidonic acid products were extracted from the incubation fluid and chromatographed on silica gel plates developed in chloroform:methanol:acetic acid:water (90:9:1:0.65, v/v). The migration of prostaglandin standards is indicated by the bars above the radiochromatogram scans. *A* Control, 1 g renal arteries incubated in Krebs' solution without cofactors for 3 h at 37 °C, in the presence of 1 µCi [1-^{14}C] arachidonic acid. *B* 1 g renal arteries incubated under the same experimental conditions as the control in Krebs' solution in which cortical slices were previously incubated. The high prostaglandin biosynthetic capacity of the isolated renal blood vessels shown in the control experiments (*A*) is largely inhibited by a factor present in the supernatant of previously incubated renal cortical slices. F = $PGF_{2\alpha}$; 6 keto- = 6 keto-$PGF_1$2; E = PGE_2; A = PGA_2; B = PGB_2; AA = arachidonic acid

it into another compound such as $PGF_{2\alpha}$. The conversion of PGE_2 to $PGF_{2\alpha}$ could be an effective intrarenal mechanism since the latter is less potent intrarenally and does not affect salt and water excretion (TANNENBAUM et al., 1975). Since the enzyme responsible for the conversion (9-ketoreductase) has been demonstrated to be equally distributed in the cortex and medulla (LEE et al., 1975) and bradykinin increases the activity of this enzyme, activation of 9-ketoreductase should be considered as a fine control mechanism for regulating the level of the products of prostaglandin release evoked by kinins (WONG et al., 1977; LIMAS, 1977).

Experiments performed using rabbit isolated kidneys perfused with oxygenated Krebs' solution demonstrated that bradykinin and kininogen increased the efflux of PGE_2 into venous and urinary effluents. Inhibition of kallikrein activity by aprotinin reduced kininogen stimulation of prostaglandin synthesis suggesting that this effect is mediated by an intrarenal increase in kinin generation (NASJLETTI and COLINA-CHOURIO, 1976). Kallikrein synthesized intrarenally could thus act on kininogen to produce kallidin (lysyl-bradykinin) which could easily reach the most active site of prostaglandin synthesis in the kidney, such as vascular tissues. This suggestion is supported by the demonstration of a high note of prostaglandin synthesis in renal blood vessels as compared to other intrarenal structures (TERRAGNO et al., 1978b) (Fig. 2).

Important interactions between mineralocorticoids, kinins, and prostaglandins in the salt-water homeostatic mechanism have been demonstrated by Colina-Chourio et al. (1978). In these experiments, administration of deoxycorticosterone (5 mg) and aldosterone (0.25 mg) to rats for a period of 14 days produced a significant increase in urinary excretion of kallikrein and PGE-like substances which was associated with an increase in urine flow. No changes in sodium excretion or blood pressure were observed. Angiotensin II also stimulates renal production of prostaglandins. However, as mineralocorticoids reduce plasma renin activity and the subsequent angiotensin generation, these studies suggest that the increase in urinary excretion of prostaglandins is independent of changes in the activity of the renin-angiotensin system.

Recent studies of Chapnick et al. (1977), on the influence of prostaglandin synthesis inhibitors on the renal vascular responses to various vasoactive substances, indicate that the administration of indomethacin or meclofenamate produces a progressive increase in renal perfusion pressure and potentiates the vasodilator effect of bradykinin in the cat. These authors conclude that the renal vasodilator effect of bradykinin is not mediated through prostaglandin release. It was assumed that by giving a "prostaglandin synthesis inhibitor" the synthesis of prostaglandins was blocked. In recent studies performed on conscious dogs, we demonstrated that renal blood flow does not change after administration of indomethacin in doses two to five times larger than those known to decrease renal blood flow and inhibit prostaglandin synthesis in the acute anesthetized and laparotomized dog (Terragno et al., 1977a). Measurement of prostaglandin levels in the renal venous blood of conscious dogs shows that prostaglandin synthesis was not inhibited by indomethacin under these experimental conditions. The blockade of bradykinin effects by aspirin and other antiphlogistic acids has been reported to be highly capricious, depending upon the site, species, and circumstances of the study (Collier, 1969).

There remain other alternatives, of which the most important appears to be the undefined role of newly discovered products of renal prostaglandin synthetase, other than PGE_2 and $PGF_{2\alpha}$, which may modify the actions of kinins. Thus, formation of the cyclic endoperoxides PGG_2 and PGH_2, TxA_2, as well as other renal prostaglandins such as PGD_2 and PGI_2, which differ in their potencies and ranges of biologic activities from PGE and PGF compounds, could result from an increase in kallikrein-kinin activity. Further, the possibility that kinins affect the breakdown of the cyclic endoperoxides to either PGE, PGF, PGD, PGI_2, or TxA_2 compounds should be considered.

The physiologic significance of the previous studies performed on the release of prostaglandins by bradykinin in the kidney should be considered provisional until more specific inhibitors of prostaglandins are developed and the metabolic products of arachidonic acid released by bradykinin stimulus under normal and pathologic conditions are identified.

II. Isolated Blood Vessels

Our observations in 1975 that arterial and venous walls from bovine mesenteric blood vessels are able to synthesize prostaglandins and the fact that this synthesis can be increased by addition of bradykinin as well as angiotensin II to the incubation

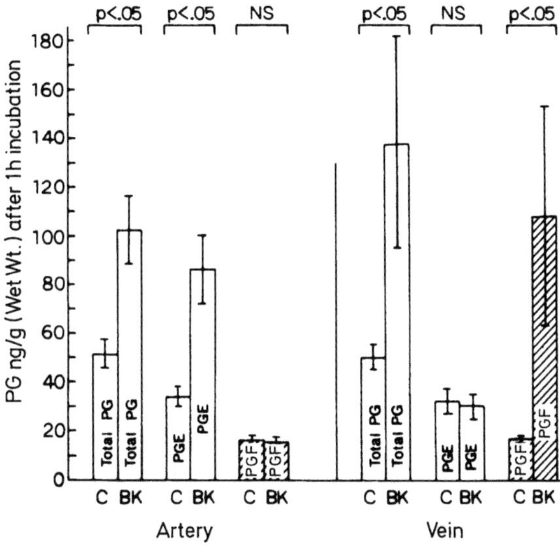

Fig. 4. Differential effects of bradykinin on synthesis of PGE- and PGF-like substances by bovine mesenteric arteries and veins. Blood vessel slices were incubated in Krebs' solution with glutathione for 1 h at 37 °C. The results represent bioassayable material extracted from the incubation medium and expressed as PGE_2 and $PGF_{2\alpha}$ equivalents. NS = no statistical significance; vertical lines = ± standard error of the mean ($n=6$); c = control; Bk = bradykinin. Reprinted from TERRAGNO et al. (1975), by permission of the American Heart Association, Inc.

medium led us to postulate that the vessel wall prostaglandins take part in the control of vascular reactivity. In these experiments (TERRAGNO et al., 1975), we demonstrated that bradykinin in a concentration of 47.6 μ*M* increased the rate of prostaglandin synthesis two- to threefold in both arteries and veins (Fig. 4). However, the pattern of the various prostaglandins produced by bradykinin was different. In arteries, the increase was accounted for mainly by a selective enhancement of the synthesis of a PGE-like substance, whereas in veins the increase was due entirely to enhancement of synthesis of a PGF-like compound.

These differences were unrelated to differences in ratios of PGE to PGF for veins and arteries existing in the control samples. Indeed, control values of prostaglandin production were almost identical for arteries, 50.7 ng/g, and veins, 49.3 ng/g, after 1 h of incubation. The ratio of PGE to PGF was approximately 2:1 for both arteries and veins.

III. Pregnant Uterus

The suggestion that prostaglandins participate in the regulation of uterine vascular reactivity is supported by the following observations: 1) The capacity of the blood vessels to respond to pressor stimuli is higher when basal levels of prostaglandins are low in an organ or after inhibition of prostaglandin synthesis in organs with a high biosynthetic capacity (McGIFF et al., 1970; TERRAGNO et al., 1976) and 2) efflux of a PGE-like compound from the uterus is associated with inhibition of the vasocon-

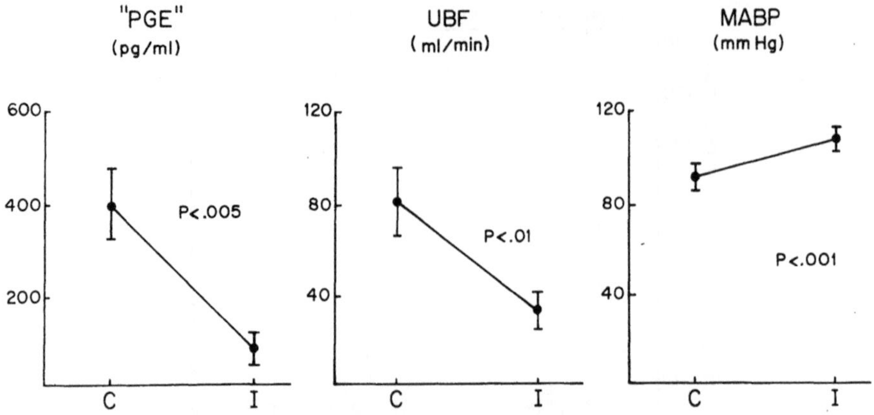

Fig. 5. Effect of intravenous administration of indomethacin (10–25 mg/kg) in morphine-chloralose anesthetized dogs in late pregnancy on the concentration of a prostaglandin E-like material ("PGE"), uterine blood flow of one horn (UBF) and mean aortic blood pressure (MABP). Triangles = mean values; vertical lines = ± standard error of the mean; I = indomethacin; C = control. Reprinted from TERRAGNO et al. (1976), by permission of John Wiley and Sons, Inc.

strictor activity of the pressor stimulus (TERRAGNO et al., 1974). Thus, the capacity of the uterus in late pregnancy to synthesize prostaglandins seems to protect this organ against the vasoconstrictor effect of pressor hormones; in this respect, the uterine vasculature resembles that of the kidney (MCGIFF et al., 1970).

1. Contribution of Prostaglandins to Uterine Blood Flow

As levels of prostaglandins in uterine venous blood increase greatly in late pregnancy, a vasodilator prostaglandin such as a PGE compound may be responsible for maintenance of the high uterine blood flow and the reduced uterine vascular resistance of late pregnancy. Using prostaglandin synthesis inhibitors in late pregnant dogs, with a concomitant measurement of blood levels of prostaglandins, we reproduced three of the major hemodynamic changes of toxemia of pregnancy: increased uterine and renal vascular resistances and elevated systemic blood pressure (Fig. 5) (TERRAGNO et al., 1976).

2. Stimulation of Intrauterine Prostaglandins by Kinins

Experiments performed in our laboratory in late pregnant dogs showed that infusion of bradykinin in doses of 20–100 ng/kg/min into the aorta resulted in a twofold increase in uterine blood flow and increased efflux of PGE and PGF from the uterus, despite high control values for these prostaglandins in uterine venous effluent (Table 1). After indomethacin treatment, the absolute increase in uterine blood flow in response to bradykinin was reduced from a mean of 63 ml/min to one of 34 ml/min, and an increase in the concentration of PGE in uterine venous effluent was not observed during infusion of the kinin. (Control levels of PGE in uterine venous blood had decreased by 70% after indomethacin treatment.) It follows that the release of

Table 1. Effects of bradykinin in late pregnancy

	Mean aortic blood pressure (mm/Hg)	Uterine blood flow (ml/min)	Renal blood flow (ml/min)	Uterine venous „PGE" (ng/ml)	Uterine venous „PGF" (ng/ml)
Control	101±6	54± 8	154±30	0.71±0.07	0.23±0.07
Experimental	95±6	118±21	182±28	1.23±0.12	0.42±0.11
	$P<0.02$	$P<0.01$	$P<0.01$	$P<0.01$	$P<0.05$

prostaglandins by bradykinin from the gravid uterus may contribute to the uterine vasodilator action of the polypeptide, as we have previously reported for the canine kidney (McGIFF et al., 1972b, 1975; TERRAGNO et al., 1972).

The possibility that the gravid uterus may elaborate vasodilator substances with antihypertensive properties deserves special consideration. Substances of uterine origin may prevent hypertension during normal pregnancy, a condition in which both plasma renin activity and extracellular fluid volume are markedly increased (ASSALI, 1972). Conversely, inadequate production of antihypertensive material could condition the development of hypertension and toxemia.

Observations from this laboratory (TERRAGNO et al., 1974, 1976) show that PGE-like substances antagonize angiotensin II responses, potentiate bradykinin vasodilation and attenuate vasoconstrictor responses to norepinephrine. The basal efflux of uterine prostaglandins can be enhanced by vasoactive hormones or inhibited by prostaglandin synthesis inhibitors (TERRAGNO et al., 1974, 1976). In addition, we demonstrated that the capacity to synthesize prostaglandins is significantly decreased in the blood vessels taken from placentas of patients with hypertensive disease of pregnancy (TERRAGNO et al., 1977d). These studies on the vascular synthesis of prostaglandins suggest the possible participation of prostaglandins in the hypertensive disease of pregnancy.

Two major prostaglandin catabolizing enzymes have also been reported to be present in the umbilical blood vessels and placenta (WONG et al., 1977; BLACKWELL and FLOWER, 1976; SCHLEGEL et al., 1974; BRAITHWAITE and JARABAK, 1975; JARABAK, 1972; RÜCKRICH et al., 1976). The enzyme, 15-hydroxydehydrogenase (15-PGDH), which catalyzes the first step in prostaglandin degradation, appears to be under hormonal control (BLACKWELL and FLOWER, 1976); adrenal steroids and thyroid hormones as well as estrogens and progesterone affect the activity of 15-PGDH (THALER-DAO et al., 1976). PGE 9-ketoreductase was shown to be activated by bradykinin in human umbilical blood vessels (WONG et al., 1977). Activation of PGE 9-ketoreductase in some tissues would result primarily in pressor effects by stimulating predominantly the formation of PGF. This demonstrates that reducing changes in prostaglandin production to a simple equation would not work. Thus, increased prostaglandin production does not necesarily decrease vascular reactivity or vice versa that decreased production does not always increase vascular reactivity.

In addition, increased activity of prostaglandin synthetase results in a cascade of vasoactive substances, including prostaglandin endoperoxides, thromboxanes, pros-

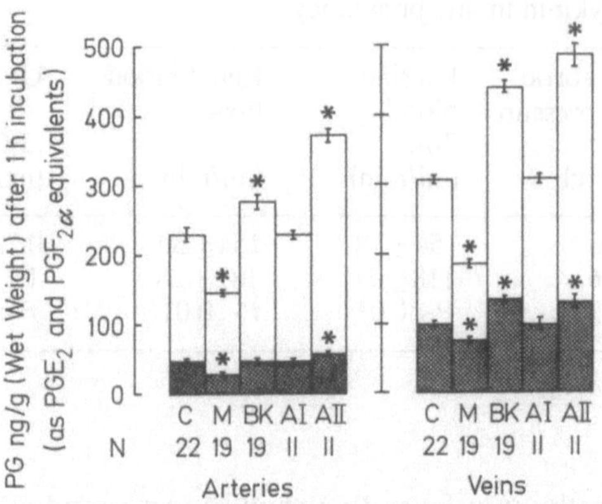

Fig. 6. Synthesis of prostaglandins by slices of human umbilical blood vessels incubated in Krebs' solution with glutathione at 37 °C. C = control; M = meclofenamate (prostaglandin synthetase inhibitor); BK = bradykinin; AI = angiotensin I; AII = angiotensin II; vertical lines = ± standard error of the mean; Bars = prostaglandins released into the incubation medium; white bars = PGE, shaded bars = PGF. * = $p < 0.05$

tacyclin, and their metabolic products, all of which have vascular activity (HAMBERG et al., 1974; RAMWELL et al., 1977). Thus, it seems likely that one or more of the aforementioned products of prostaglandin synthetase will be of greater importance than the primary prostaglandins in regulating blood flow or vascular reactivity in components of the uteroplacental-fetal complex and the vascular responsiveness during pregnancy.

IV. Umbilical Blood Vessels and Ductus Arteriosus

Slices of human umbilical arteries and veins incubated at 37 °C in 0.1 *M* sodium phosphate buffer (pH 8) containing 2 m*M* glutathione released prostaglandins into the incubation medium. Rates of prostaglandin synthesis in human umbilical arteries and veins are two- to threefold greater than those reported from mesenteric blood vessels when studied under identical conditions (TERRAGNO et al., 1975). The addition of meclofenamic acid in a concentration (1.0 m*M*) which decreases prostaglandin synthesis in mesenteric blood vessels by more than 90%, reduced the synthesis in umbilical arteries and veins by 40%. In paired samples obtained from the same umbilical cord, bradykinin increased the synthesis of prostaglandins by 22% in arteries and 43% in veins. Angiotensin II increased the synthesis by about 60% in arteries and veins (Fig. 6).

Studies of the umbilical blood vessels of the calf showed a progressive increase in prostaglandin biosynthetic capacity during pregnancy and a difference in prostaglandin synthesis in the various portions of the umbilical cord. Thus, the highest levels of synthesis were found in those portions of the blood vessels nearest the fetus and the lowest values in those adjacent to the placenta (Table 2) (TERRAGNO et al., 1977c).

The synthesis of prostaglandins by the ductus arteriosus of the calf also increased with maturation of the fetus.

Table 2. Total prostaglandin synthesis in calf umbilical blood vessels and ductus arteriosus at different stages of pregnancy[a]

	<3 months	~5 months	>8 months
Artery	131.0±4	146.7±3	218.0±8
Vein	171.0±6	237.0±3	339.8±9
Ductus arteriosus	157.0±13	141.0±10	210.0±15

[a] Units are ng of prostaglandins per g wet weight of tissue after 1 h incubation. These experiments were performed using all portions of the umbilical blood vessels. $n=5$.

Table 3. Biosynthesis of prostaglandins from [$1-{}^{14}C$]-arachidonic acid[a] by slices of bovine vascular tissues

	Tissues	Phospholipid[b]	$PGF_{2\alpha}$[b]	6 Keto-$PGF_{1\alpha}$[b]	PGE_2[b]	PGA_2+ PGB_2+ Hydroxy FFA[b]	Arachidonic acid[b]
Fetal	Aorta	3.6±1.4	5.5±0.9	23.8±0.7	2.6±0.3	9.3±1.5	52.7±2.8
	Pulmonary artery	3.1±1.2	6.0±0.9	29.8±1.9	3.2±0.5	10.0±1.0	45.4±2.4
	Ductus arteriosus	3.4±1.5	6.3±1.5	20.0±2.2	2.0±0.1	9.2±0.8	56.6±1.3
Maternal	Aorta	1.1±0.1	1.7±0.3	6.8±0.7	1.4±0.1	5.9±1.0	81.6±0.2
	Pulmonary artery	1.5±0.3	2.8±0.2	10.6±0.7	1.6±0.3	6.8±0.5	75.5±1.5
	Mesenteric artery	1.7±0.4	5.8±1.0	20.9±2.0	4.2±0.5	10.1±1.5	54.5±6.6
Non-pregnant	Aorta	2.5±0.2	2.9±0.1	6.1±0.7	1.3±0.1	6.7±0.7	80.0±1.2
	Pulmonary artery	1.8±0.1	2.5±0.2	5.2±0.4	1.3±0.1	5.3±0.9	82.6±0.3
	Mesenteric artery	2.9±0.5	8.6±0.5	19.5±1.3	3.7±0.9	10.7±0.2	51.9±6.5

[a] Percentage of total radioactivity recovered from incubation fluid.
[b] Each value represents the mean with SEM of four experiments.

Most recently, work performed in this laboratory demonstrated that 6 keto-$PGF_{1\alpha}$ is the most abundant prostaglandin synthesized by fetal blood vessels (TERRAGNO et al., 1977b, 1978a). Although in the pregnant and nonpregnant animal, 6 keto-$PGF_{1\alpha}$ is still the most abundant prostaglandin, the capacity in adult animals to synthesize this compound is significantly less than in the fetus (Table 3). In previous studies, we have demonstrated the capacity of blood vessel walls to synthesize the classical or proper PGE and PGF. At that time, the standard solvent system used in thin-layer chromatography or high pressure liquid chromatography did not allow

Table 4. Activation of enzymes or release of prostaglandins and other arachidonic acid derivatives by bradykinin

Organ or tissue	substance released or enzyme activated[a]	Species	Ref.
Isolated lung	RCS	Guinea pig	PIPER and VANE (1969), PICKENS et al. (1972), VARGAFTIG and DAO HAI (1972)
	RCS, PG − LS	Guinea pig	PALMER et al. (1973)
	AA, PGs	Rat	DAMAS et al. (1974a, b)
Kidney	PGE, PGF	Dog	TERRAGNO et al. (1971, 1972), McGIFF et al. (1972b)
Fibroblasts (culture)	PL − A_2 → AA → PGs → cAMP	Man	NEWCOMBE et al. (1977)
	PGE_2, $PGF_{2\alpha}$	Mouse	HONG and LEVINE (1976), HONG et al. (1976)
Isolated mesenteric arteries and veins	PGE − LS, PGF − LS	Cow	TERRAGNO et al. (1975) arteries and veins
Spleen	PG − LS	Dog	MONCADA et al. (1972), FERREIRA et al. (1973a, b)
Isolated heart	PGE − LS	Rabbit	NEEDLEMAN et al. (1975)
Umbilical arteries and veins	PGE, PGF	Man	TERRAGNO et al. (1976)
Isolated perfused ear	PGE − LS, PGE, PGF	Rabbit	JUAN and LEMBECK (1976), LEMBECK et al. (1976)
Isolated kidney	PGE − LS	Rabbit	NASJLETTI and COLINA-CHOURIO (1976)
Isolated hydronephrotic kidney	PG − LS, PGE_2	Rabbit	NISHIKAWA et al. (1977)
Renomedullary interstitial cells (culture)	PGE_2	Rabbit	ZUSMAN et al. (1977a, b)
HSS fraction of mesenteric blood vessels	PGE 9-ketoreductase	Cow	WONG et al. (1977)
		Dog	LIMAS (1977)
Isolated mesenteric blood vessels	PGE − LS	Rabbit	BLUMBERG et al. (1977)
Isolated perfused heart	PL − A_2 → AA → PGs	Rabbit	HSUEH et al. (1977)
Isolated perfused heart and kidney	PL − A_2 → AA	Rabbit	ISAKSON et al. (1977)

[a] PGE = prostaglandin E; PGF = prostaglandin F; PGs = prostaglandins; PG − LS = prostaglandin-like substance; PL − A_2 = Phospholipase A_2; RCS = rabbit aorta contracting substance, identified later as a mixture of thromboxane and endoperoxide (SAMUELSSON, 1976); AA = arachidonic acid; HSS = high speed supernatant.

us to differentiate PGI_2, or its metabolic product 6 keto-$PGF_{1\alpha}$, from PGE_2. This suggests that the increase in PGE-like substances shown in previous work could be a result of stimulation of PGI_2 synthesis by bradykinin (TERRAGNO et al., 1975). The capacities of blood vessel walls to synthesize the various arachidonic acid derivatives are summarized in Table 4.

The presence of prostaglandin synthetase within the wall of blood vessels obviates the need for a circulating prostaglandin to influence peripheral resistance. For those tissues capable of responding to vasoconstrictor or vasodilator hormones by increasing prostaglandin synthesis and, thereby, moderating the effect of these hormones, stimulation of prostaglandin production within the vascular wall may be the most important determinant of the final vascular response.

C. Release of Other Vasoactive Substances

I. Catecholamines

It is well known that many other vasoactive hormones can be released in response to bradykinin. In 1961, LECOMTE et al. demonstrated in the rabbit and rat the participation of catecholamines in the secondary hypertensive response and tachycardia produced by the intravenous infusion of bradykinin. This effect, which could be abolished by bilateral adrenalectomy, suggested the release of medullary catecholamines by the peptide. This finding was later confirmed by other investigators using different experimental conditions in several animal species.

The epinephrine-releasing effect of bradykinin and other peptides was quantitatively studied in the eviscerated cat preparation by measuring the contraction of the denervated nictitating membrane and the rise in blood pressure (FELDBERG and LEWIS, 1963). Under these experimental conditions, intraarterial injection of bradykinin contracted the nictitating membrane and produced changes in blood pressure which matched those produced by intravenous adrenaline. These responses were abolished by adrenalectomy (Table 5).

ROBINSON, in 1967, demonstrated that the secretion of catecholamines by the adrenal medulla depends on the availability of calcium. He also showed that the isolated perfused adrenal gland of the dog was extremely sensitive to angiotensin and bradykinin. These findings do not agree with those of VOGT (1965), who, under the same experimental conditions, showed very little secretory response to angiotensin and bradykinin in organs perfused with Locke's solution.

Intravenous administration of bradykinin in the guinea pig also released catecholamines (mainly epinephrine) in the extracorporeal circulation, as shown by the concomitant relaxation produced in the superfused chick rectum and rat stomach strip used to detect catecholamine release (PIPER et al., 1967).

The release of epinephrine in the cat and dog after intraarterial infusion of kallidin, eledoisin or angiotensin was studied by STASZEWSKA-BARCZAK and VANE in 1967. The capacity of these peptides to release catecholamines was shown to be different; angiotensin was the most powerful substance tested in the cat, followed by kallidin, which was more active than bradykinin. Eledoisin was ineffective. In dogs, kallidin and eledoisin were the most potent peptides, followed by bradykinin and angiotensin.

Bradykinin and kallidin also had a stimulant effect on the superior cervical ganglion of the cat (LEWIS and REIT, 1965; HAEFELY et al., 1966). Bradykinin also showed a weak stimulatory effect on the isolated inferior mesenteric ganglion of the dog (MUSCHOLL and VOGT, 1964). They suggested that the catecholamine released into the effluent fluid is derived from the scattered chromaffin cells of the ganglion.

Table 5. Release of catecholamines by kinins

Kinin administration	Release of change in concentration	Species	Ref.
Intravenous	Catecholamines	Rabbit, rat	LECOMTE et al. (1961, 1964)
Intra-aorta above suprarenals	Adrenaline	Cat	FELDBERG and LEWIS (1963–1965)
Isolated perfused inferior mesenteric ganglion	Catecholamines	Dog	MUSCHOLL and VOGT (1964)
Perfused adrenal medulla	Catecholamines	Dog	VOGT (1965), ROBINSON (1967)
Intra-arterial infusion above arterial supply to adrenal glands	Catecholamines	Dog, cat	STASZEWSKA-BARCZAK and VANE (1965, 1967)
Intravenous	Catecholamines	Guinea pig	COLLIER (1966), PIPER et al. (1967)
Intravenous	Catecholamines	Rat	MIELE and DE NATALE (1966, 1967)
Added to incubation of duodenal tissue	Catecholamines	Rat	MONTGOMERY and KROEGER (1967)
Intra-arterial supply to adrenal gland	No stimulation of catecholamines	Day-old Calf	COMLINE et al. (1968)
	Little or no stimulation of catecholamines	3 and 18 month-old Calf	COMLINE et al. (1968)
	Adrenaline	Cat	COMLINE et al. (1968)
	Catecholamines	Dog	KAYAALP (1968)
	Catecholamines	Cat	DELLA BELLA et al. (1972)
Intra-arterial supply to adrenal gland, intravenous	Catecholamines (indirect-induced by BP changes)	Cat	LANG and PEARSON (1968)
Intravenous	Catecholamines	Rat	YOSHIZAKI (1973)

LANG and PEARSON (1968) demonstrated that the pressor response induced by intracarotid injection of bradykinin is not only produced by catecholamine release from the adrenal gland but also by sympathetically induced vasoconstriction mediated by a central sympathetic mechanism, since it can be reduced by the administration of hexamethonium, as well as by adrenalectomy.

MIELE and DE NATALE (1966) investigated in the rat the effect of guanethidine on the responses of the blood pressure to vasoactive polypeptides; it is known that this procedure depletes catecholamines from the peripheral sympathetic nerve endings without affecting those from the adrenal medulla (CASS et al., 1960; CESSION-FOSSION, 1965; CHANG et al., 1965). Under these conditions, the hypertensive phase was potentiated by guanethidine and/or β-receptor blockers, drugs which enhance the pressor responses to catecholamines.

KROEGER and KRIVOY (1966), using a salivary gland preparation, demonstrated that the polypeptides, by releasing epinephrine, affect salivary gland permeability. MONTGOMERY and KROEGER (1967), using a different tissue, showed that relaxation of the proximal duodenum by bradykinin in the rat is also mediated by catecholamine release, since these effects can be blocked by a combination of α- and β-blocking agents, phenoxybenzamine and propranolol.

In the immature adrenal gland from the day-old calf, administration of bradykinin or angiotensin did not release catecholamines, nor did it potentiate the responses to acetylcholine by the gland (COMLINE et al., 1968). The relative insensitivity to stimulation of the immature adrenal medulla, shown for some time after birth in spite of the gland containing large amounts of epinephrine and norepinephrine (COMLINE and SILVER, 1966), could be an important mechanism contributing to the hemodynamic changes which occur at birth.

DELLA BELLA et al., in 1970, using spleen preparations, in vitro and in vivo, demonstrated that bradykinin simultaneously activates two nervous reflex arcs: a long one relaying at a supraspinal level, and a short one relaying at the level of the coeliac ganglion. The effectors of both reflex arcs are mainly the adrenal medullary cells which release catecholamines into the circulation, which in turn contract the splenic smooth muscle. Histologic studies of the splanchnic area show the presence of sympathetic nervous elements for local reflex activity; this interpretation was also confirmed by the electrophysiologic demonstration of nervous functional correlation (DELLA BELLA et al., 1972).

The existence of the peripheral nervous connections suggests that injected bradykinin can reach the adrenal medulla and directly activate the release of catecholamines. Bradykinin can also provoke stimulation of the afferent sensitive nerve endings and activate local reflex arcs (indirect nervously mediated release). Evidence for the presence of this mechanism was obtained by electrophysiologic and pharmacologic investigations (DELLA BELLA et al., 1972).

From these studies, it appears that the release of bradykinin by catecholamines is an extremely complex process and varies not only with the in vivo or in vitro conditions, but also with the tissues or animal species employed. The finding that bradykinin can influence catecholamine release by a direct or indirect nervous mechanism is of particular relevance and can explain some of the quantitative differences observed in the same animal species. However, a more complex mechanism must be considered to explain the reported insensitivity of immature adrenomedullary cells of the calf.

Analysis of the resulting pressor response to bradykinin indicates that it is in part due to epinephrine release from the adrenal gland since the response is absent after administration of an α-adrenergic blocker (phentolamine) or after adrenalectomy (MIELE and DE NATALE, 1967).

The pressor effect in the adult animal appears to be mediated by sympathetic mechanisms and to involve a central component since the intracarotid injection of the polypeptide can stimulate it.

II. Histamine

A number of vasoactive peptides stimulate histamine release from rat mast cells, rat skin, and granuloma pouches in vitro (GOTH, 1967; ZACHARIAE et al., 1968, 1969; STERN et al., 1962; JOHNSON and ERDÖS, 1973).

STERN et al., in 1962, showed that the histamine-releasing effect of bradykinin injected into granuloma pouches in rats is considerably reduced by pretreatment of the animal with the histamine liberator, compound 48/80. The course of inflammation can be influenced also by bradykinin and an additive effect of histamine and bradykinin was demonstrated in capillary damage. Bradykinin alone produced a weaker inflammatory response than did the combination of both agents. Since bradykinin enhances the inflammatory response provoked by croton oil in the granuloma pouch and the inflammatory reaction to bradykinin was diminished in histamine-depleted skin, STERN et al. (1962) concluded that the effects of bradykinin are in part mediated by histamine release. ZACHARIAE et al. (1968, 1969) also studied the histamine-kinin relationship in the inflammatory process. In these experiments, bradykinin and serotonin were added to human plasma in the presence of Ca^{2+}-EDTA but these mediators did not activate the plasma kallikrein system in vitro. However, under the same experimental conditions, kallikrein is activated presumably by celite, an activator of the Hageman factor. They also investigated the capacity to generate kinins from the rat subcutaneous tissue after subcutaneous injection of different doses of compound 48/80. In all instances, kinin formation was observed. The inactivation of this material by chymotrypsin suggests that it is a kinin. The same investigators, studying the effect of kinins on the histamine content of the skin, found that the mean histamine content of the skin is reduced after local injections of bradykinin. These observations support the idea that plasma kinins participate in histamine release. JOHNSON and ERDÖS (1973) also investigated the capacity of vasoactive peptides to liberate histamine from rat mast cell suspensions in vitro. In these studies, the relative potencies of the peptides were compared with the capacity of compound 48/80 to release histamine. These studies indicated that Polistes kinin was the most potent histamine releaser from mast cells (see PISANO, this volume). It was only slightly less active than compound 48/80, followed in order of potency by substance P, methionyl-lysyl-bradykinin, kallidin, and bradykinin. Eledoisin, angiotensin I, and glucagon did not release histamine; angiotensin II, fibrinopeptide A, and bradykinin tetradecapeptide were only slightly active. The authors clearly demonstrated that histamine-releasing capacity depends on the basic groups of the peptides. The removal of one basic amino acid from bradykinin by carboxypeptidase B renders it inactive as a histamine releaser. It is also suggested that the hypotensive action of the peptide cannot be correlated with histamine release because eledoisin, a potent vasodepressor substance, was unable to release histamine from mast cells.

In a recent study, JOHNSON et al. (1975) demonstrated the capacity of human and porcine serum complements (C3a and C5a) to release histamine from mast cells. In these studies the potencies of C3a and C5a were compared with those of bradykinin and compound 48/80. The complement peptides were more potent histamine liberators than bradykinin but less potent than compound 48/80, at the lower concentrations used. With higher concentrations, bradykinin, and compound 48/80 released 50% and 75% of histamine in contrast to the 25% and 30% liberated by C3a and C5a, respectively. Calcium was demonstrated to influence the histamine release induced by C3a, C5a, and bradykinin, but release by compound 48/80 was not affected by EGTA.

III. Serotonin

A simultaneous increase in serotonin (5-HT) and bradykinin concentration has been reported in several pathologic conditions such as carcinoid and provoked dumping

Table 6. Release of serotonin, histamine or antidiuretic hormone by kinins

Kinin administration	Release or change in concentration	Species	Ref.
Intravenous	5-HT	Man	PELTOLA (1969, 1972)
Injected into lateral ventricle	5-HT increased in the cerebellum, decreased in the midbrain	Rat	BRASZKO and KOŚCIELAK (1975)
Blood platelet incubation	5-HT	Rat	BRASZKO and KOŚCIELAK (1975)
Peritoneal cell incubation	Histamine	Rat	GOTH (1967)
	in skin decreased	Man	ZACHARIAE et al. (1968, 1969)
Peritoneal and pleural cell incubation (6–10% mast cells)	Histamine	Rat	JOHNSON and ERDÖS (1973)
Injected into carotid artery	ADH	Dog	ROCHA E SILVA and MALNIC (1962, 1964)
Intravenous and into carotid artery	ADH	Rat	HARRIS (1970)
Intravenous, injected into carotid artery and injected into vertebral artery	ADH	Cat	ROCHA E SILVA, JR. and HARRIS (1970)

syndromes (OATES et al., 1964; PELTOLA, 1969). Whether the rise in bradykinin level in plasma is secondary to an increase in 5-HT has not been determined. The administration of a serotonin antagonist to clinical subjects suffering from these syndromes is relatively ineffective and does not drastically change the intensity of the attacks. On the other hand, infusion of serotonin does not reproduce the flushing in the carcinoid patient, a finding which suggests the participation of more than one vasoactive substance in the syndrome.

Intravenous administration of bradykinin has been reported by PELTOLA (1969) to reproduce most of the characteristics of a flushing attack. However, aprotinin (a potent inhibitor of kinin formation), used for the treatment of flush, was shown to be relatively ineffective (DOLLINGER and GARDNER, 1966; BACK, 1966; GARDNER et al., 1967; SCHIEVELBEIN, 1968), (Table 6).

A large number of reports indicate that other vasoactive substances produce flushing in these patients; small amounts of epinephrine can also provoke flushing in carcinoid patients (PEART et al., 1961). It is known that kinins can be liberated by epinephrine (HILTON and LEWIS, 1956) and that epinephrine release can be stimulated by kinins (LECOMTE et al., 1961; FELDBERG and LEWIS, 1963). All these reports, therefore, suggest that serotonin release in the carcinoid syndrome is accompanied by the liberation of other vasoactive substances, such as catecholamines, bradykinin and histamine into the circulation (DOLLINGER and GARDNER, 1966).

The serotonin-releasing effect of bradykinin was demonstrated by PELTOLA (1969). This report indicated that infusion of bradykinin to patients in doses of 0.2 and 1 μg/kg/min produced palpitation, dizziness, abdominal cramps, and a fall in blood pressure, concomitant with an increase in urinary excretion of the serotonin metabolite, 5-hydroxyindoleacetic acid (5HIAA). There was a predominant increase in conjugated 5HIAA and small changes in free 5HIAA during the first 2 h period. The author believed that this was a sign of acute serotonin release during the infusion of bradykinin. He suggested that the variation in the excretion of 5HIAA reported by different investigators during the dumping syndrome could be a consequence of estimating free 5HIAA (which remained unchanged after acute intravenous injection of 5-HT) instead of measurement of the excretion of conjugated 5HIAA, which increased remarkably (PELTOLA, 1972).

BRASZKO and KOŚCIELAK (1975) also measured changes in serotonin concentration in the brain under the influence of kallikrein and bradykinin, which were applied into the lateral ventricle. The results showed that the 5-HT concentration in various parts of the brain changed slightly; the only significant differences after bradykinin administration were found in the increased 5-HT concentration in the cerebellum and a decrease in the midbrain. The same authors, studying in vitro the effect of bradykinin on uptake and release of 5-HT from incubated rat blood platelets, found that bradykinin given together with 5-HT to blood platelet suspensions did not significantly affect the uptake. However, bradykinin given 5 min before 5-HT significantly inhibited the uptake of the latter during the first 10 min of incubation. On the other hand, in both cases after 20 min, the release of 5-HT was greater under the influence of the peptide. Addition of bradykinin to the incubation medium markedly increased the release of 5-HT from the platelets.

The mechanism of bradykinin-serotonin interaction and the specific role this interaction plays in different pathologic conditions are still unknown. For the full understanding of the dynamics of this system it is important to study the sequence of events in the interaction of these vasoactive substances. Opposing actions of vasoactive substances with different biologic properties should be considered as part of the body defensive and energy saving mechanism.

IV. Antidiuretic Hormone

Bradykinin has been demonstrated to release antidiuretic hormone (ADH) and affect water diuresis when it is administered to unanesthetized dogs or rats (ROCHA E SILVA and MALNIC, 1962; STÜRMER and BERDE, 1962). The similarity between the antidiuretic effect of administration of bradykinin and that of ADH has been demonstrated by ROCHA E SILVA, JR. and MALNIC (1964) using unanesthetized dogs. In this series of experiments, both peptides produced a long lasting maximal inhibition of diuresis for a similar period of time accompanied by a rise in sodium, chloride and potassium excretion. After maximal antidiuretic effect was achieved the excretion of electrolytes could be independently increased further by higher doses of bradykinin. The creatinine and para-amino-hippuric acid (PAH) clearances were not affected by doses of bradykinin used to demonstrate the antidiuretic effect and changes in the excretion of electrolytes. The authors postulate that the antidiuretic action of bradykinin is mediated by the release of ADH from the hypophysis since a dose of bradykinin which caused antidiuresis when given into the carotid artery was ineffective when administered intravenously or when given to dogs with experimental diabetes insipidus. HARRIS (1970) reported that the antidiuretic effect of bradykinin in the rat was mediated by ADH release and not by the hypotension produced by bradykinin. Hypotension, produced by hemorrhage or isoprenaline, of the same magnitude as that produced by bradykinin caused a smaller and shorter lasting antidiuretic response that did the peptide. This effect was clearer when bradykinin was injected into the cerebral circulation. Under these experimental conditions, injection of bradykinin was followed by a marked antidiuresis without any significant fall in arterial blood pressure. The capacity of bradykinin to directly stimulate the release of ADH was also demonstrated in cats by ROCHA E SILVA, JR. and HARRIS (1970). The authors postulate that bradykinin injected directly into the cerebral circulation stimulates the release of ADH by a mechanism different than hypotension. Increases in ADH levels were observed after intravenous, intracarotid, or intravertebral injections of bradykinin. The release of ADH following intravenous injection of the peptide was demonstrated to be secondary to the hypotensive effect of bradykinin. On the other hand, the release of ADH by the intracerebral injection of bradykinin resulted from direct stimulation of the central nervous system.

References

Adetuyibi, A., Mills, I.H.: Relation between urinary kallikrein and renal function, hypertension, and excretion of sodium and water in man. Lancet *1972 II*, 203–207

Änggård, E., Bohman, S.O., Griffin, J.E. III, Larsson, C., Maunsbach, A.B.: Subcellular localization of the prostaglandin system in the rabbit renal papilla. Acta Physiol. Scand. *84*, 231–246 (1972)

Assali, N.S.: Pathophysiology of gestation. Assali, N. (ed), Vols. I, II, III. London, New York: Academic Press 1972

Barraclough, M.A., Mills, I.H.: Effect of bradykinin on renal function. Clin. Sci. *28*, 69–74 (1965)

Blackwell, G.J., Flower, R.J.: Effects of steroid hormones on tissue levels of prostaglandin 15-hydroxydehydrogenase in the rat. Br. J. Pharmacol. *56*, 343P–344P (1976)

Blumberg, A.L., Denny, S.E., Marshall, G.R., Needleman, P.: Blood vessel-hormone interactions: angiotensin, bradykinin, and prostaglandins. Am. J. Physiol. *232*, H305–H310 (1977)

Braithwaite, S.S., Jarabak, J.: Studies on a 15-hydroxyprostaglandin dehydrogenase from human placenta. J. Biol. Chem. *250*, 2315–2318 (1975)

Braszko, J., Kościelak, M.: Effect of kinins on the central action of serotonin. Pol. J. Pharmacol. Pharm. *27* Suppl., 61–68 (1975)

Cass, R., Kuntzman, R., Brodie, B.B.: Norepinephrine depletion as a possible mechanism of action of guanethidine (SU 5864), a new hypotensive agent. Proc. Soc. Exp. Biol. Med. *103*, 871–872 (1960)

Cession-Fossion, A.: Activités pharmacodynamiques comparées de la guanéthidine, de la béthanidine et du brétylium chez le rat. Arch. Int. Pharmacodyn. Ther. *158*, 45–58 (1965)

Chang, C.C., Costa, E., Brodie, B.B.: Interaction of guanethidine with adrenergic neurons. J. Pharmacol. Exp. Ther. *147*, 303–312 (1965)

Chapnick, B.M., Paustian, P.W., Feigen, L.P., Joiner, P.D., Hyman, A.L., Kadowitz, P.J.: Influence of inhibitors of prostaglandin synthesis on renal vascular resistance and on renal vascular responses to vasopressor and vasodilator agents in the cat. Circ. Res. *40*, 348–354 (1977)

Colina-Chourio, J., McGiff, J.C., Nasjletti, A.: Effects of aldosterone and deoxycorticosterone on the urinary excretion of kallikrein and of prostaglandin E-like substance in the rat. In: Contr. Nephrol. Berlyne, G.M. et al. (eds.), Vol. 12, pp. 126–131. Basel: Karger 1978

Collier, H.O.J.: Self-antagonism of bronchoconstriction induced by bradykinin and angiotensin. In: Hypotensive peptides. Erdös, E.G. (ed.), pp. 305–313. Berlin, Heidelberg, New York: Springer 1966

Collier, H.O.J.: New light on how aspirin works. Nature *223*, 35–37 (1969)

Comline, R.S., Silver, M.: The development of the adrenal medulla of the foetal and new-born calf. J. Physiol. (Lond.) *183*, 305–340 (1966)

Comline, R.S., Silver, M., Sinclair, D.G.: The effects of bradykinin, angiotensin, and acetylcholine on the bovine adrenal medulla. J. Physiol. (Lond.) *196*, 339–350 (1968)

Crowshaw, K.: Prostaglandin biosynthesis from endogenous precursors in rabbit kidney. Nature New Biol. *231*, 240–242 (1971)

Crowshaw, K.: The incorporation of [1-^{14}C] arachidonic acid into the lipids of rabbit renal slices and conversion to prostaglandins E_2 and $F_{2\alpha}$. Prostaglandins *3*, 607–620 (1973)
Crowshaw, K., McGiff, J.C., Strand, J.C., Lonigro, A.J., Terragno, N.A.: Prostaglandins in dog renal medulla. J. Pharm. Pharmacol. *22*, 302–304 (1970)
Damas, J., Bourdon, V., Neuray, J., Deby, C., Lecomte, J.: Bradykinin et biosynthèse des prostaglandines in vitro. C.R. Soc. Biol. (Paris) *167*, 787–790 (1973)
Damas, J., Bourdon, V.: Libération d'acide arachidonique par la bradykinine. C.R. Soc. Biol. (Paris) *168*, 1445–1448 (1974a)
Damas, J., Deby, C., Lecomte, J.: Libération de prostaglandines par la bradykinine chez le rat. C.R. Soc. Biol. (Paris) *168*, 375–378 (1974b)
Della Bella, D., Benelli, G., Gandini, A.: Bradykinin and catecholamines release from the adrenal medulla of the cat: a possible indirect reflex mechanism. In: Advances in experimental medicine and biology. Vol. 8: Bradykinin and related kinins. Sicuteri, F., Rocha e Silva, M., Back, N. (eds.), pp. 601–608. New York, London: Plenum Press 1970
Della Bella, D., Benelli, G., De Paoli, A.M.: Indirect nervous mechanism in some effects of bradykinin. Arch. Int. Pharmacodyn. Ther. *196* Suppl., 50–63 (1972)
Dollinger, M.R., Gardner, B.: Newer aspects of the carcinoid spectrum. Surg. Gynecol. Obstet. *122*, 1335–1347 (1966)
Ducharme, D.W., Weeks, J.R., Montgomery, R.G.: Studies on the mechanism of the hypertensive effect of prostaglandin $F_{2\alpha}$. J. Pharmacol. Exp. Ther. *160*, 1–10 (1968)
Dusting, G.J., Moncada, S., Vane, J.R.: Prostacyclin (PGX) is the endogenous metabolite responsible for relaxation of coronary arteries induced by arachidonic acid. Prostaglandins *13*, 3–15 (1977)
Feldberg, W., Lewis, G.P.: Release of adrenaline from cat's suprarenals by bradykinin and angiotensin. J. Physiol. (Lond.) *167*, 46 P–47 P (1963)
Feldberg, W., Lewis, G.P.: The action of peptides on the adrenal medulla. Release of adrenaline by bradykinin and angiotensin. J. Physiol. (Lond.) *171*, 98–108 (1964)
Feldberg, W., Lewis, G.P.: Further studies on the effects of peptides on the suprarenal medulla of cats. J. Physiol. (Lond.) *178*, 239–251 (1965)
Fenwick, L., Jones, R.L., Naylor, B., Poyser, N.L., Wilson, N.H.: Production of prostaglandins by the pseudopregnant rat uterus, in vitro, and the effect of tamoxifen with the identification of 6-keto-prostaglandin $F_{1\alpha}$ as a major product. Br. J. Pharmacol. *59*, 191–199 (1977)
Ferreira, S.H., Vane, J.R.: Prostaglandins: their disappearance from and release into the circulation. Nature *216*, 868–873 (1967)
Ferreira, S.H., Moncada, S., Vane, J.R.: Prostaglandins and the mechanism of analgesia produced by aspirin-like drugs. Br. J. Pharmacol. *49*, 86–97 (1973a)
Ferreira, S.H., Moncada, S., Vane, J.R.: Further experiments to establish that the analgesic action of aspirin-like drugs depends on the inhibition of prostaglandin biosynthesis. Br. J. Pharmacol. *47*, 629 P–630 P (1973b)
Gardner, B., Dollinger, M., Silen, W., Back, N., O'Reilly, S.: Studies of the carcinoid syndrome: Its relationship to serotonin, bradykinin, and histamine. Surgery *61*, 846–852 (1967)
Goth, A.: Effect of drugs on mast cells. In: Advances in pharmacology, Vol. 5. London, New York: Academic Press 1967
Haefely, W., Hürlimann, A., Thoenen, H.: The effect of bradykinin and angiotensin on ganglionic transmission. In: Hypotensive peptides. Erdös, E.G. (ed.), pp. 314–328. Berlin, Heidelberg, New York: Springer 1966
Hamberg, M., Samuelsson, B.: Detection and isolation of an endoperoxide intermediate in prostaglandin biosynthesis. Proc. Natl. Acad. Sci. USA *70*, 899–903 (1973)
Hamberg, M., Svensson, J., Samuelsson, B.: Prostaglandin endoperoxides. A new concept concerning the mode of action and release of prostaglandins. Proc. Natl. Acad. Sci. USA *71*, 3824–3828 (1974)
Harris, M.C.: Release of the antidiuretic hormone by bradykinin in rats. In: Advances in experimental medicine and biology. Vol. 8: Bradykinin and related kinins. Sicuteri, F., Rocha e Silva, M., Back, N. (eds.), pp. 609–614. New York, London: Plenum Press 1970
Hedqvist, P.: Studies on the effect of prostaglandins E_1 and E_2 on the sympathetic neuromuscular transmission in some animal tissues. Acta Physiol. Scand. *79* Suppl. 345, 1–40 (1970)
Hedqvist, P.: Autonomic neurotransmission. In: The prostaglandins, Vol. 1. New York, London: Plenum Press 1973

Hilton, S.M., Lewis, G.P.: The relationship between glandular activity, bradykinin formation and functional vasodilatation in the submandibular salivary gland. J. Physiol. (Lond.) *134*, 471–483 (1956)
Hong, S.L., Levine, L.: Stimulation of prostaglandin synthesis by bradykinin and thrombin and their mechanisms of action on MC5-5 fibroblasts. J. Biol. Chem. *251*, 5814–5816 (1976)
Hong, S.L., Polsky-Cynkin, R., Levine, L.: Stimulation of prostaglandin biosynthesis by vasoactive substances in methylcholanthrene-transformed mouse BALB/3T3. J. Biol. Chem. *251*, 776–780 (1976)
Hsueh, W., Isakson, P.C., Needleman, P.: Hormone selective lipase activation in the isolated rabbit heart. Prostaglandins *13*, 1073–1091 (1977)
Isakson, P.C., Raz, A., Denny, S.E., Wyche, A., Needleman, P.: Hormonal stimulation of arachidonate release from isolated perfused organs. Relationship to prostaglandin biosynthesis. Prostaglandins *14*, 853–871 (1977)
Itskovitz, H.D., Terragno, N.A., McGiff, J.C.: Effect of a renal prostaglandin on distribution of blood flow in the isolated canine kidney. Circ. Res. *34*, 770–776 (1974)
Jarabak, J.: Human placental 15-hydroxyprostaglandin dehydrogenase. Proc. Natl. Acad. Sci. USA *69*, 533–534 (1972)
Johnson, A.R., Erdös, E.G.: Release of histamine from mast cells by vasoactive peptides. Proc. Soc. Exp. Biol. Med. *142*, 1252–1256 (1973)
Johnson, A.R., Hugli, T.E., Müller-Eberhard, H.J.: Release of histamine from rat mast cells by the complement peptides C3a and C5a. Immunology *28*, 1067–1080 (1975)
Juan, H., Lembeck, F.: Release of prostaglandins from the isolated perfused rabbit ear by bradykinin and acetylcholine. Agents, Actions *6*, 642–645 (1976)
Kadowitz, P.J., Sweet, C.S., Brody, M.J.: Influence of prostaglandins on adrenergic transmission to vascular smooth muscle. Circ. Res. *30, 31* (Suppl. II), II-36–II-50 (1972)
Kayaalp, S.O.: A method for studying the effect of drugs on the catecholamine release from the adrenal medulla in the dog. Ärztl. Forsch. *18*, 84–87 (1968)
Kroeger, D.C., Krivoy, W.: Effect of bradykinin on submandibular salivary gland permeability. In: Hypotensive peptides. Erdös, E.G. (ed.), pp. 289–297. Berlin, Heidelberg, New York: Springer 1966
Kunze, H., Vogt, W.: Significance of phospholipase A for prostaglandin formation. Ann. N.Y. Acad. Sci. *180*, 123–125 (1971)
Lang, W.J., Pearson, L.: Studies on the pressor responses produced by bradykinin and kallidin. Br. J. Pharmacol. *32*, 330–338 (1968)
Lecomte, J., Troquet, J., Dresse, A.: Stimulation médullo-surrénalienne par la bradykinine. Arch. Int. Physiol. Biochim. *69*, 89–91 (1961)
Lecomte, J., Troquet, J., Cession-Fossion, A.: Sur la nature de l'hypertension artérielle provoquée par la bradykinine et la kallidine. Arch. Int. Pharmacodyn. Ther. *147*, 518–524 (1964)
Lee, S.C., Pong, S.S., Katzen, D., Wu, K.Y., Levine, L.: Distribution of prostaglandin E 9-ketoreductase and types I and II 15-hydroxyprostaglandin dehydrogenase in swine kidney medulla and cortex. Biochemistry *14*, 142–145 (1975)
Lembeck, F., Popper, H., Juan, H.: Release of prostaglandins by bradykinin as an intrinsic mechanism of its algesic effect. Naunyn Schmiedebergs Arch. Pharmacol. *294*, 69–73 (1976)
Lewis, G.P., Reit, E.: The action of angiotensin and bradykinin on the superior cervical ganglion of the cat. J. Physiol. (Lond.) *179*, 538–553 (1965)
Limas, C.J.: Selective stimulation of venous prostaglandin E9-ketoreductoase by bradykinin. Biochim. Biophys. Acta *498*, 306–315 (1977)
Margolius, H.S., Geller, R., Pisano, J.J., Sjoerdsma, A.: Altered urinary kallikrein excretion in human hypertension. Lancet *1971 II*, 1063–1065
Margolius, H.S., Horwitz, D., Geller, R.G., Alexander, R.W., Gill, J.R., Jr., Pisano, J.J., Keiser, H.R.: Urinary kallikrein excretion in normal man: relationships to sodium intake and sodium-retaining steroids. Circ. Res. *35*, 812–819 (1974)
Marin-Grez, M., Cottone, P., Carretero, O.A.: Evidence for an involvement of kinins in regulation of sodium excretion. Am. J. Physiol. *223*, 794–796 (1972)
McGiff, J.C., Crowshaw, K., Terragno, N.A., Lonigro, A.J.: Release of a prostaglandin-like substance into renal venous blood in response to angiotensin II. Circ. Res. *26, 27* Suppl. I, I-121–I-130 (1970)

McGiff, J.C., Crowshaw, K., Terragno, N.A., Malik, K.U., Lonigro, A.J.: Differential effect of noradrenaline and renal nerve stimulation on vascular resistance in the dog kidney and the release of a prostaglandin E-like substance. Clin. Sci. *42*, 223–233 (1972)(1972a)

McGiff, J.C., Itskovitz, H.D.: Prostaglandins and the kidney. Circ. Res. *33*, 479–488 (1973)

McGiff, J.C., Itskovitz, H.D., Terragno, N.A.: The actions of bradykinin and eledoisin in the canine isolated kidney: relationships to prostaglandins. Clin. Sci. Mol. Med. *49*, 125–131 (1975)

McGiff, J.C., Terragno, N.A., Malik, K.U., Lonigro, A.J.: Release of a prostaglandin E-like substance from canine kidney by bradykinin: comparison with eledoisin. Circ. Res. *31*, 36–43 (1972b)

McGiff, J.C., Terragno, N.A., Strand, J.C., Lee, J.B., Lonigro, A.J., Ng, K.K.F.: Selective passage of prostaglandins across the lung. Nature *223*, 742–745 (1969)

Messina, E.J., Weiner, R., Kaley, G.: Inhibition of bradykinin vasodilation and potentiation of norepinephrine and angiotensin vasoconstriction by inhibitors of prostaglandin synthesis in skeletal muscle of the rat. Circ. Res. *37*, 430–437 (1975)

Miele, E., De Natale, G.: Modification by guanethidine and nethalide of the pressor effects of bradykinin in the rat. Arch. Int. Pharmacodyn. Ther. *164*, 56–66 (1966)

Miele, E., De Natale, G.: Modification of pressor effects of some vasoactive polypeptides in the rat by guanethidine, propranolol, and related agents. Br. J. Pharmacol. *29*, 8–15 (1967)

Moncada, S., Ferreira, S.H., Vane, J.R.: Does bradykinin cause pain through prostaglandin production? Proc. 5th Int. Congr. Pharmacol., Abstracts of volunteer papers, 160 (1972)

Montgomery, E.H., Kroeger, D.C.: Bradykinin relaxation of duodenum. Fed. Proc. *26*, 465 (Abstract) (1967)

Morrison, A.R., Nishikawa, K., Needleman, P.: Unmasking of thromboxane A_2 synthesis by ureteral obstruction in the rabbit kidney. Nature *267*, 259–260 (1977)

Muscholl, E., Vogt, M.: Secretory responses of extramedullary chromaffin tissue. Br. J. Pharmacol. *22*, 193–203 (1964)

Nasjletti, A., Colina-Chourio, J.: Interaction of mineralocorticoids, renal prostaglandins, and the renal kallikrein-kinin system. Fed. Proc. *35*, 189–193 (1976)

Needleman, P., Key, S.L., Denny, S.E., Isakson, P.C., Marshall, G.R.: Mechanism and modification of bradykinin-induced coronary vasodilation. Proc. Natl. Acad. Sci. USA *72*, 2060–2063 (1975)

Needleman, P., Minkes, M., Raz, A.: Thromboxanes: selective biosynthesis and distinct biological properties. Science *193*, 163–165 (1976)

Negus, P., Tannen, R.L., Dunn, M.J.: Indomethacin potentiates the vasoconstrictor actions of angiotensin II in normal man. Prostaglandins *12*, 175–180 (1976)

Newcombe, D.S., Fahey, J.V., Ishikawa, Y.: Hydrocortisone inhibition of the bradykinin activation of human synovial fibroblasts. Prostaglandins *13*, 235–244 (1977)

Nishikawa, K., Morrison, A., Needleman, P.: Exaggerated prostaglandin biosynthesis and its influence on renal resistance in the isolated hydronephrotic rabbit kidney. J. Clin. Invest. *59*, 1143–1150 (1977)

Nugteren, D.H., Hazelhof, E.: Isolation and properties of intermediates in prostaglandin biosynthesis. Biochim. Biophys. Acta *326*, 448–461 (1973)

Oates, J.A., Melmon, K.L.: Biochemical and physiological studies of the kinins in the carcinoid syndrome. In: Hypotensive peptides. Erdös, E.G. (ed.), pp. 565–578. Berlin, Heidelberg, New York: Springer 1966

Oates, J.A., Melmon, K., Sjoerdsma, A., Gillespie, L., Mason, D.T.: Release of a kinin peptide in the carcinoid syndrome. Lancet *1964 I*, 514–517

Pace-Asciak, C., Wolfe, L.S.: A novel prostaglandin derivative formed from arachidonic acid by rat stomach homogenates. Biochemistry *10*, 3657–3664 (1971)

Palmer, M.A., Piper, P.J., Vane, J.R.: Release of rabbit aorta contracting substance (RCS) and prostaglandins induced by chemical or mechanical stimulation of guinea-pig lungs. Br. J. Pharmacol. *49*, 226–242 (1973)

Peart, W.S., Andrews, T.M., Robertson, J.I.S.: Carcinoid syndrome: Serotonin release induced with intravenous adrenaline or noradrenaline. Lancet *1961 I*, 577–578

Peltola, P.: Release of serotonin during bradykinin infusion. Scand. J. Clin. Lab. Invest. *Suppl. 107*, 81–84 (1969)

Peltola, P.: Bradykinin induced release of serotonin in man. Res. Clin. Stud. Headache *3*, 299–303 (1972)
Pickens, J., West, G.B., Whelan, C.J.: Release by kinin of a substance contracting rabbit aorta (RCS) from guinea-pig lung. Br. J. Pharmacol. *45*, 140P (1972)
Piper, P.J., Vane, J.R.: Release of additional factors in anaphylaxis and its antagonism by anti-inflammatory drugs. Nature *223*, 29–35 (1969)
Piper, P.J., Collier, H.O.J., Vane, J.R.: Release of catecholamines in the guinea-pig by substances involved in anaphylaxis. Nature *213*, 838–840 (1967)
Ramwell, P.W., Leovey, E.M.K., Sintetos, A.L.: Regulation of the arachidonic acid cascade. Biol. Reprod. *16*, 70–87 (1977)
Robinson, R.L.: Stimulation of the catecholamine output of the isolated, perfused adrenal gland of the dog by angiotensin and bradykinin. J. Pharmacol. Exp. Ther. *156*, 252–257 (1967)
Rocha e Silva, M., Jr., Harris, M.C.: The release of vasopressin by a direct central action of bradykinin. In: Advances in experimental medicine and biology. Vol. 8: Bradykinin and related kinins. Sicuteri, F., Rocha e Silva, M., Back, N. (eds.), pp. 561–570. New York, London: Plenum Press 1970
Rocha e Silva, M., Malnic, G.: Antidiuretic action of bradykinin. Pharmacology *7*, 329 (1962)
Rocha e Silva, M., Jr., Malnic, G.: Release of antidiuretic hormone by bradykinin. J. Pharmacol. Exp. Ther. *146*, 24–32 (1964)
Rückrich, M.F., Wendel, A., Schlegel, W., Jackisch, R., Jung, A.: Molecular and kinetic properties of 15-hydroxyprostaglandin dehydrogenase (PG-15-HDH) from human placenta. In: Advances in prostaglandin and thromboxane research, Vol. 1. New York: Raven 1976
Samuelsson, B.: Introduction: New trends in prostaglandin research. In: Advances in prostaglandin and thromboxane research, Vol. 1. New York: Raven 1976
Schievelbein, H.: Carcinoid und Kallikrein-Kinin-System. Hoppe Seylers Z. Physiol. Chem. *349*, 940 (1968)
Schlegel, W., Demers, L.M., Hildebrandt-Stark, H.E., Behrman, H.R., Greep, R.O.: Partial purification of human placental 15-hydroxyprostaglandin dehydrogenase: Kinetic properties. Prostaglandins *5*, 417–433 (1974)
Staszewska-Barczak, J., Vane, J.R.: The release of catecholamines from the adrenal medulla by peptides. J. Physiol. (Lond.) *177*, 57P–58P (1965)
Staszewska-Barczak, J., Vane, J.R.: The release of catecholamines from the adrenal medulla by peptides. Br. J. Pharmacol. *30*, 655–667 (1967)
Stern, P., Nikulin, A., Ferluga, J.: The role of histamine and bradykinin in the inflammatory process. Arch. Int. Pharmacodyn. Ther. *140*, 528–538 (1962)
Stürmer, E., Berde, B.: Kallidin und Bradykinin, vergleichende pharmakologische Untersuchungen. Arch. Exp. Path. Pharmak. *243*, 355–356 (1962)
Tannenbaum, J., Splawinski, J.A., Oates, J.A., Nies, A.S.: Enhanced renal prostaglandin production in the dog. I. Effects on renal function. Circ. Res. *36*, 197–203 (1975)
Terragno, D.A., Crowshaw, K., Terragno, N.A., McGiff, J.C.: Prostaglandin synthesis by bovine mesenteric arteries and veins. Circ. Res. *36*, *37* Suppl. I, I-76–I-80 (1975)
Terragno, D.A., McGiff, J.C., Terragno, N.A.: Prostaglandin synthesis by umbilical blood vessels in toxemia of pregnancy. Fed. Proc. *36*, 547 (Abstract) (1977)
Terragno, N.A., Lonigro, A.J., Malik, K.U., McGiff, J.C.: Bradykinin-induced vasodilation and the release of prostaglandins. Circulation *44* Suppl. II, II-118 (Abstract) (1971)
Terragno, N.A., Lonigro, A.J., Malik, K.U., McGiff, J.C.: The relationship of the renal vasodilator action of bradykinin to the release of a prostaglandin E-like substance. Experientia *28*, 437–439 (1972)
Terragno, N.A., Terragno, D.A., McGiff, J.C.: The role of prostaglandins in the control of uterine blood flow. In: Hypertension in pregnancy. New York: Wiley & Sons 1976
Terragno, N.A., Terragno, D.A., McGiff, J.C.: Contribution of prostaglandins to the renal circulation in conscious, anesthetized, and laparotomized dogs. Circ. Res. *40*, 590–595 (1977a)
Terragno, N.A., Terragno, D.A., McGiff, J.C., Rodriguez, D.J.: Synthesis of prostaglandins by the ductus arteriosus of the bovine fetus. Prostaglandins *14*, 721–727 (1977b)
Terragno, N.A., Terragno, D.A., McGiff, J.C.: Prostaglandin release from human and bovine umbilical blood vessels. Fed. Proc. *36*, 403 (Abstract) (1977c)

Terragno, N.A., Terragno, D.A., Pacholczyk, D., McGiff, J.C.: Prostaglandins and the regulation of uterine blood flow in pregnancy. Nature *249*, 57–58 (1974)
Terragno, N.A., McGiff, J.C., Smigel, M., Terragno, A.: Patterns of prostaglandin production in the bovine fetal and maternal vasculature. Prostaglandins *16*, 847–856 (1978)
Terragno, N.A., Terragno, A., Early, J.A., Roberts, M.A., McGiff, J.C.: Endogenous prostaglandin synthesis inhibitor in the renal cortex. Effects on production of prostacyclin by renal blood vessels. Clin. Sci. Mol. Med. 55, 199s–202s (1978)
Thaler-Dao, H., Saintot, M., Baudin, G., Descomps, B., Crastes de Paulet, A.: Placental 15-hydroxyprostaglandin dehydrogenase binding site requirements. In: Advances in prostaglandin and thromboxane research, Vol. 1. New York: Raven 1976
Tuvemo, T., Strandberg, Kj., Hamberg, M., Samuelsson, B.: Formation and action of prostaglandin endoperoxides in the isolated human umbilical artery. Acta Physiol. Scand. *96*, 145–149 (1976)
Tuvemo, T., Wide, L.: Prostaglandin release from the human umbilical artery in vitro. Prostaglandins *4*, 689–694 (1973)
Vane, J.R.: Inhibition of prostaglandin synthesis as a mechanism of action for aspirin-like drugs. Nature New Biol. *231*, 232–235 (1971)
Vargaftig, B.B., Dao Hai, N.: Selective inhibition by mepacrine of the release of "rabbit aorta contracting substance" evoked by the administration of bradykinin. J. Pharm. Pharmacol. *24*, 159–161 (1972)
Vogt, M.: Release of medullary amines from the isolated perfused adrenal gland of the dog. Br. J. Pharmacol. *24*, 561–565 (1965)
Webster, M.E., Gilmore, J.P.: Influence of kallidin-10 on renal function. Am. J. Physiol. *206*, 714–718 (1964)
Willman, E.A., Collins, W.P.: Distribution of prostaglandins E_2 and $F_{2\alpha}$ within the foetoplacental unit throughout human pregnancy. J. Endocrinol. *69*, 413–419 (1976)
Wong, P.Y.-K., Terragno, D.A., Terragno, N.A., McGiff, J.C.: Dual effects of bradykinin on prostaglandin metabolism: Relationship to the dissimilar vascular actions of kinins. Prostaglandins *13*, 1113–1125 (1977)
Yoshizaki, T.: Effect of histamine, bradykinin, and morphine on adrenaline release from rat adrenal gland. Jpn. J. Pharmacol. *23*, 695–699 (1973)
Zachariae, H., Henningsen, S.J., Søndergaard, J., Wolf-Jürgensen, P.: Plasma kinins in inflammation-relation to other mediators and leukocytes. Scand. J. Clin. Lab. Invest. *Suppl. 107*, 85–94 (1968–1969)
Zusman, R.M., Keiser, H.R.: Prostaglandin E_2 biosynthesis by rabbit renomedullary interstitial cells in tissue culture: Mechanism of stimulation by angiotensin II, bradykinin, and arginine vasopressin. J. Biol. Chem. *252*, 2069–2071 (1977a)
Zusman, R.M., Keiser, H.R.: Prostaglandin biosynthesis by rabbit renomedullary interstitial cells in tissue culture: stimulation by angiotensin II, bradykinin, and arginine vasopressin. J. Clin. Invest. *60*, 215–223 (1977b)

Kininases

E. G. ERDÖS

Since publication of the previous edition of this Handbook in 1970, much new information has been gathered about kininases, the enzymes that inactivate kinins. This chapter provides a survey and update of research on kininases and enzymes that convert longer kinin peptides to the nonapeptide, bradykinin.

Interest in kininases has accelerated rapidly since 1970. Several reasons for this are apparent. First, the best known kininases such as kininase I and II were purified and their properties and distinction from other enzymes were established. Second, in spite of their names, kininases are not substrate (kinin) specific, but they can cleave other peptides with susceptible bonds. Thus, these components of the kallikrein–kinin system can interact with other complex blood-borne systems such as the complement or the renin–angiotensin system. Kininase I also functions as an anaphylatoxin inactivator and kininase II is identical with the angiotensin I converting enzyme. To complicate matters further, it appears that both kininase I and kininase II can be degraded by proteolytic enzymes to lower molecular weight (MW) derivatives, sometimes with an apparent increase in activity. This suggests that plasma kallikrein, in addition to other roles, may cleave and activate kininases (see below).

The finding that the activity of kininases in blood changes in some pathological conditions stimulated interest in measurement of their level as a diagnostic aid.

Further, the synthesis of specific inhibitors of kininase II such as the peptide BPF_{9a}, or SQ 20881, or the orally active inhibitor SQ 14225 (see below and STEWART, this volume) provided useful tools to study the functions of this enzyme. Because inhibition of kininase II decreases the level of circulating angiotensin II and prevents the breakdown of bradykinin, an inhibitor of the enzyme is potentially useful in therapy of hypertension.

Since kininase II also functions as the angiotensin I converting enzyme, many publications deal with the release of angiotensin II by the enzyme. This part of the literature is too extensive for a chapter on kinins, thus the metabolism of kinins rather than the release of angiotensin II will be emphasized. Several reviews on the subject were published, but most deal mainly with the functions of kininase II as angiotensin I converting enzyme (BAKHLE, 1974; BAKHLE and VANE, 1974; ERDÖS, 1975, 1976a, b, 1977; OPARIL, 1976; OPARIL and KATHOLI, 1977; SOFFER, 1976). The many publications on kininases which appeared in Russian are reviewed in this volume by PASKHINA and LEVITSKIY in detail.

A. Kininase I

(Arginine carboxypeptidase, E.C. 3.4.12.7)

Practically all tissue homogenates, biologic fluids, plant and bacterial extracts, and certain purified proteolytic enzyme can cleave kinins. The best known kininases are I and II. The first kininase to be characterized was kininase I. Kininase I is a carboxypeptidase that was discovered in Cohn fraction IV-1 of human plasma (ERDÖS and SLOANE, 1962; ERDÖS, 1962). It was called carboxypeptidase N first to distinguish it from pancreatic carboxypeptidase A and B. The Enzyme Commission named it arginine carboxypeptidase (E.C. 3.4.12.7). The name suggests the biologic function of this enzyme but not its specificity, since actually it cleaves C-terminal lysine faster than arginine in most substrates (OSHIMA et al., 1975). The enzyme is identical with the "anaphylatoxin inactivator" (BOKISCH and MÜLLER-EBERHARD, 1970), or so-called "carboxypeptidase B-type" enzyme of blood mentioned frequently and, alas, erroneously in the literature.

The current surge of interest in kinin metabolism almost two decades after the discovery of kininase I does not make the enzyme an overnight success, but it does pose a potential for renoming of the enzyme with the discovery of each additional substrate.

I. Purification of the Enzyme

Kininase I was partially purified from human plasma by ERDÖS et al. (1967) who reported a 252-fold purification with a 14% yield. BOKISCH, MÜLLER-EBERHARD and associates approached the purification from a different point of view. They found that the anaphylatoxins, C3a, and C5a, released after the activation of the complement system, are very unstable and concluded that plasma contains an inactivator of these peptides. It was observed by the same group of investigators (BOKISCH et al., 1969) that the "anaphylatoxin inactivator" also cleaved kallidin. Characterization of the inactivator as a carboxypeptidase led to the application of ε-NH_2-n-caproic acid during isolation of C3a anaphylatoxin to inhibit its inactivation (VALLOTA and MÜLLER-EBERHARD, 1973). The isolated the anaphylatoxin inactivator was a homogeneous protein of MW 325,000–288,000. Purification was achieved by TEAE-cellulose column chromatography followed by Pevikon block electrophoresis, a step also employed by ERDÖS et al. (1967). Gel filtration on a Sephadex G-200 column yielded the final product. Because the activity of the enzyme was determined only by measuring the inactivation of anaphylatoxin by bioassay, no quantitative data on the purification were given, although the authors estimated a 6% yield. The total amount of kininase I in serum was estimated to be 30–40 μg/ml (BOKISCH and MÜLLER-EBERHARD, 1970).

Complete purification of human plasma enzyme was reported by OSHIMA et al. (1974b, 1975) using hippuryl-argininic acid (Benzoyl or Bz-glycylargininic acid: HLAa) as substrate. The purification consisted mainly of four steps, including chromatography on DEAE-Sephadex, Sepharose 4B-arginine and hydroxyapatite columns. The end result was a homogeneous protein purified 888-fold with a yield of 7.4% (ERDÖS et al., 1976).

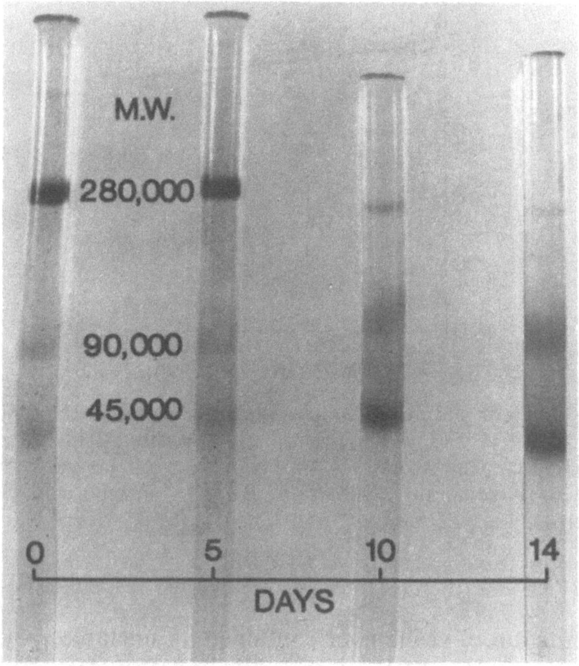

Fig. 1. Dissociation of native kininase I (carboxypeptidase N) to high and low MW subunits in 2 weeks at 4 °C. (OSHIMA et al., 1975)

The freshly purified enzyme had a MW of 280,000 as determined by gel filtration. When the MW of kininase I was determined in disc gel electrophoresis in the presence of sodium dodecyl sulfate, urea and 2-mercaptoethanol, two bands were seen that corresponded to approximately 90,000 and 45,000 MW materials. In disc gel electrophoresis the freshly purified kininase I showed one strongly stained, slowly migrating band and two faint ones. The slow band represented the native enzyme and the two faster migrating ones the 90,000 and 45,000 MW subunits. When the preparation was left standing in buffer, the intensity of staining of the 280,000 MW protein decreased and that of the two lower MW proteins increased (Fig. 1). After 14 days of standing at 4 °C, the 280,000 MW band disappeared and the staining of bands representing the subunits became more intensive. After elution from the gel, the 90,000 MW protein had about 7% of the activity of the native enzyme when measured with the HLAa substrate. The 45,000 MW fraction was also active but was highly unstable. The lower MW dissociated active form of carboxypeptidase can be obtained by gel filtration of the enzyme that was stored for 14 days at 4 °C.

Since previous studies (ERDÖS et al., 1965) of the enzyme in blood of patients indicated that it may originate from the liver, kininase I was also purified from hog liver. Two types of carboxypeptidases were found. The final supernatant of the homogenized liver contained an enzyme which after purification had a MW of 45,000. The substrate specificity was similar to that of human and hog plasma kininase I, but was different from that of hog pancreatic enzyme. In addition, the micro-

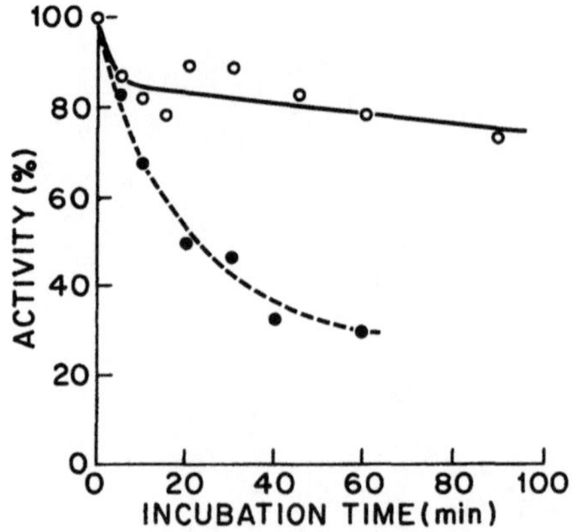

Fig. 2. To show the different stability of native and dissociated carboxypeptidase N during incubation at 37 °C in 0.2 *M* Tris, pH 8. Open circle: Freshly purified carboxypeptidase N. Solid circle: Dissociated enzyme, stored for 30 days. Abscissa: Length of incubation in min. Ordinate: Percent activity remaining. Substrate: Bz-glycyl-arginic acid. Source of enzyme: Human plasma. (OSHIMA et al., 1975)

somal–ribosomal fraction of swine liver contained an unstable enzyme that cleaved HLAa. In gel filtration, the MW of this carboxypeptidase was 280,000. These experiments also support the idea that kininase I originates from the liver.

The importance of the large MW form of the enzyme was established by incubating native enzyme and its dissociated subunits at 37 °C. As shown in Fig. 2, the native enzyme was stable when incubated for 60 min or longer at 37 °C, while the subunits lost 70% of the activity under the same conditions. Thus, complexing of subunits to native enzyme may stabilize it. In addition, the higher MW native enzyme could stay in the circulating blood longer than the subunits since the smaller subunit could be excreted through the kidney.

JEANNERET et al. (1976) reported the purification of kininase I from hog plasma. Their results were similar to those obtained with human plasma except that, in addition to the high and low MW subunits, they detected an even lower MW (30,000) protein fraction released from the native hog plasma enzyme.

They also noted (Table 1) that the activity of the enzyme changed when trypsin was added to either hog or human plasma. The hydrolysis of peptide substrates of carboxypeptidase increased when native plasma was treated with trypsin. Gel filtration indicated that trypsin cleaved kininase I to a lower MW protein, which was approximately half the MW of the native enzyme. The native enzyme is a glycoprotein since it was retained by concanavalin A-Sepharose. It is possible that the activation by trypsin is due to dissociation of the enzyme to active subunits, but an activation of a presumably inactive form of the enzyme present in blood should also be considered.

Recently PLUMMER and HURWITZ (1978) purified kininase I from outdated human plasma. They purified the enzyme essentially by a two step chromatography procedure using a cellulose column first, then a *p*-aminobenzoyl-arginine-Sepharose column for affinity chromatography. Kininase I was selectively eluted from the

Table 1. Effect of trypsin on the activity of carboxypeptidase N (kininase I)
To 30 μl serum or enzyme was added 0.1 mg trypsin; after 90 min at 31 °C the enzyme activity was measured

Sample	Activity (hippuroyllysine)			Activity (hippuroylarginine)		
	No trypsin (U)	Trypsin (U)	Increase (%)	No trypsin (U)	Trypsin (U)	Increase (%)
Rat serum	0.74	1.36	85	0.14	0.19	36
Pig serum	0.71	1.15	62	0.82	1.37	67
Human serum	0.67	1.13	68	0.27	0.40	48
Purified pig enzyme	0.83	1.24	50			
Water		<0.01			<0.01	

Jeanneret et al.: H.S.Z. Physiol. Chem. *357*, 867 (1976).

affinity column with guanidinomethylmercaptosuccinic acid, a potent inhibitor of the enzyme (McKay and Plummer, 1978). The last step alone yielded over a 100-fold purification. The properties of the purified enzyme were similar to those described by Oshima et al. (1974b, 1975). It contained subunits of 83,000, 55,000, and 49,000 MW. The enzyme has 17% carbohydrate and a significant amount of zinc. The carbohydrates were attached to the higher MW subunit (Jeanneret et al., 1976). Because of differences in sialic acid content, Koheil and Forstner (1978) found two forms of kininase I after separating human plasma enzyme by isoelectric focusing.

Kininase I was readily degraded to subunits by plasmin or by trypsin and its peptidase activity increased 20–40% after digestion. Since kininase I was stable after affinity chromatography, the authors suggested that the slow dissociation of kininase I to subunits in storage at 4 °C may result from the action of trace amounts of proteolytic enzyme in the preparation (Plummer and Hurwitz, 1978). They also suggested that the low MW subunit may be enzymatically inactive which is in contrast to the findings of Oshima et al. (1974b, 1975).

Other investigators also separated plasma kininases. Zacest et al. (1974) confirmed the earlier results of Yang and Erdös (1967) by separating two plasma kininases from human blood. They used radiolabeled substrates to measure the activity of kininase I and II (see below). The K_m values for the two enzymes with bradykinin as substrate were 4.1×10^{-7} *M* and 0.93×10^{-7} *M*. The computed velocities at infinite concentrations of the substrate were for kininase I, $V = 2.2 \times 10^{-8}$ *M*/min and for kininase II, 5.7×10^{-9} *M*/min.

Plasma and liver kininase I or carboxypeptidase N are entirely different from pancreatic carboxypeptidase B. It can be estimated from immunologic studies (Geokas et al., 1974) that less than 0.1% of the total carboxypeptidase activity of plasma can be attributed to the pancreatic enzyme. Other differences between the plasma and pancreatic enzyme are summarized in Table 2. The MW of plasma carboxypeptidase of man and hog differs greatly from that of pancreatic enzyme (280,000 vs. 34,000). The plasma enzyme consists of subunits while the pancreatic enzyme has a single chain; the former contains carbohydrate and the latter does not. Furthermore, there are noticeable differences in the rates of cleavage of substrates by

Table 2. Relative rates of hydrolysis of substrates by carboxypeptidase N and by carboxypeptidase B

Substrate	Carboxy-peptidase N	$K_m \times 10^4\ M$[e]	Carboxy-peptidase B	$K_m \times 10^4\ M$[f]	Swine liver
1. Bz-Gly-Lys	1[c]	14	1[d]	77	1
2. Bz-Gly-Arg	0.23	120	4	2	0.3
3. Pro-Phe-Lys	1.9		2.4		
4. Pro-Phe-Gly-Lys	0.3		3		
5. Polylysine	0.2		0.04		
6. Z-Gly-Arg	0.05		1.2		
7. Z-Gly-Gly-Arg	0.04		4.4		
8. Z-Ala-Arg[a]	1.6		3.3		
9. Ac-Phe-Arg[b]	0.05		4		
10. Ac-Phe-Ser-Pro-Phe-Arg[b]	0.2		1.1		0.2
11. Phe-Ser-Pro-Phe-Arg[b]	0.2		1.2		
12. Z-Gly-Orn	0.01		0.07		
13. Bz-Gly-Argininic Acid	5.0	1	12.2	0.4	

[a] C-terminal fragment of anaphylatoxin.
[b] C-terminal fragment of kinins.
[c] 11.6 μmol/min/mg.
[d] 1.21 μmol/min/mg.
[e] Erdös, E.G., and Yang, H.Y.T. (1970) in Handbook of Experimental Pharmacology (Erdös, E.G., ed.), Vol. XXV, pp. 289–323, Springer-Verlag, Heidelberg.
[f] Folk, J.E., Wolff, E.C., and Schirmer, E.W. (1962) J. Biol. Chem. *237*, 3100–3104.
(Sources of enzymes: human plasma, hog pancreas, and hog liver).
Oshima et al., Arch. Biochem. *170*, 132 (1975).

the two enzymes. Pancreatic carboxypeptidase B of either man or hog (Marinkovic et al., 1977; Folk et al., 1960) cleaves peptides bonds of substrates with C-terminal arginine faster than those with a C-terminal lysine. Its esterase activity is accelerated by added cadmium. Kininase I, however, cleaves C-terminal lysine faster than arginine, except in substrates that have alanine in the penultimate position (Oshima et al., 1975), and its esterase activity is inhibited by cadmium. The K_m values of various substrates of carboxypeptidase B and kininase I differ. The C-terminal end of C3a anaphylatoxin is -Ala-Arg-OH (Hugli et al., 1975) and that of C5a is Gly-Arg-OH (Fernandez and Hugli, 1976). This may explain why C3a is much less stable in blood than C5a, since kininase I cleaves Ala-Arg bonds preferentially (Oshima et al., 1975; Erdös et al., 1976).

II. Inhibition

Various inhibitors of kininase I have been described (Erdös and Yang, 1970). Kininase I is not inhibited by the specific inhibitors of kininase II such as BPF_{5a} or BPF_{9a}, SQ 20881 (Igic et al., 1972a; Paskhina et al., 1975). However, the C-terminal pentapeptide of bradykinin, an inhibitor of kininase II, competitively inhibited the hydrolysis of hippuryl-lysine and hippuryl-arginine by human kininase I (Paskhina et al., 1975). Recently McKay and Plummer (1978) indicated that some substituted succinic acid derivatives, which inhibit pancreatic carboxypeptidase B, can also block the activity of kininase I. The prototype inhibitor, guanidino methylmercapto-succinic acid, was used in the purification of the enzyme (PLUMMER and HURWITZ, 1978). It has a K_i of 1×10^{-6} M. The possibility of naturally occurring circulating inhibitors is intriguing. Digested plasma proteins may inhibit kininase I (HAMBERG et al., 1968), because such extracts inhibit pancreatic carboxypeptidase B. KLAUSER and ERDÖS (to be published) found that the C-peptide fragment of human serum albumin, that inhibits kininase II (KLAUSER et al., 1979) also inhibits kininase I, although a higher concentration is required for the inhibition of kininase I; the K_i for kininase II is 1.7×10^{-5} M and for kininase I it is 2.6×10^{-4} M.

NAKAHARA (1972) found that a low MW compound from the lysosomal fraction of homogenized dog skeletal muscle inhibited the cleavage of hippuryl-lysine by kininase I but not the inactivation of bradykinin. In addition, fatty acids inhibit kininase I (ERDÖS and YANG, 1970) in high concentrations and the inhibitory effect increases with the length of the carbon chain (PETAKOVA et al., 1972).

III. Kininase I in Pathological Conditions

Since kininase I is a major enzyme for the inactivation of bradykinin and possibly other blood-borne peptides, changes in its blood level may be important in various disease states. Changes in kininase I activity in plasma under a variety of conditions were described previously (ERDÖS and YANG, 1970) and Table 3 lists some of them.

STREETEN et al. (1972) described a clinical syndrome, which consisted of light-headedness, erythema, orthostatic fall in blood pressure and a rise in heart rate, that resembled the effect of an i. v. injection of bradykinin. The kinin level in plasma was high in these patients and the kinin concentration correlated with a decrease in pulse pressure and increase in heart rate. Kininase activity was somewhat depressed. The low kininase I activity was associated with elevated kinin level in two of the patients investigated but not in two others. Improvement in the condition was seen after the administration of propanolol, fluorocortisone, or cyproheptadine, and the use of an Air Force pressure suit prevented the circulatory changes. The syndrome was attributed to a familial deficiency in kininase I.

CORBIN et al. (1976) used salmine to measure the amount of arginine released by kininase I from this substrate. One unit (U) was defined as 1 nmol of arginine released per minute per ml serum at 37 °C. The mean value for normal human sera was 395 U/ml. Patients in shock after dextran infusion had lower (302 U/ml) activity. Sera of patients with Dengue shock syndrome had a depressed activity with an abnormal mean of 170 U/ml. It was assumed that the decreased inactivation of anaphylatoxin by kininase I may contribute to the development of shock syndrome. A postulated genetic deficiency of kininase I in patients with cystic fibrosis was not confirmed by these authors.

In irradiated rats kininase I activity increased 3 h after treatment then it decreased over the next 4 days to values lower than control. GAPONIUK and UMARCHODGAEV (1969) assumed that the decrease in the enzyme activity would lead to "accumulation of kinins in irradiated animals."

According to NAKAHARA (1973), the activity of dog plasma kininase I decreased in tourniquet shock and corticosteroids and serotonin (10^{-4}, 10^{-5} M) inhibited the

Table 3. Kininase I and II activity in human plasma in various conditions

Condition	Kininase I	Kininase II	Remarks	References
Cirrhosis of the liver	–		Kininase I may originate from the liver	ERDÖS and YANG, 1970 (see also OSHIMA et al., 1974)
Neoplasia	+		Hodgkin's disease	ERDÖS and YANG, 1970
Pregnancy	+			ERDÖS and YANG, 1970
Familial orthostatic hypotension	–		Level of bradykinin is high	STREETEN et al., 1972
Dextran shock	–			CORBIN et al., 1976
Dengue fever	–			CORBIN et al., 1976
Hyperthyroidism	+			ERDÖS and YANG, 1970
Sarcoidosis		+	Increased in lymph nodes	LIEBERMAN, 1975 SILVERSTEIN et al., 1976a, b OPARIL et al., 1976b FANBURG et al., 1976
Gaucher's disease		+	High concentration in spleen cells	LIEBERMAN and BEUTLER, 1976; SILVERSTEIN, FRIEDLAND, 1977
Leprosy		+		LIEBERMAN and REA, 1977
Shock lung		–		OPARIL et al., 1976b
Pulmonary neoplasia		–		ASHUTOSH and KEIGHLEY, 1976
Cesarean section		+	Values higher in maternal blood than in normal delivery. Fetal plasma has normal level	OPARIL et al., 1978
Asthma		–		MUE et al., 1978
Adult respiratory distress syndrome		–		BEDROSSIAN et al., 1978

Activity: + = high; – = low.

enzyme. However, the level of the enzyme did not change in septic shock in patients or in baboons (HIRSCH et al., HERMAN et al., 1974).

The effect of kininase I on edema in the rat paw induced by kaolin was studied by RYBAK et al. (1978). Intraperitoneal application of 20 mg/kg partially purified rat serum kininase I delayed the development of the late phase of edema which was assumed to be caused by kinins.

B. Other Kininases

I. Undifferentiated Kininases

Reports on the presence of various kininases in cells, tissues and body fluids are summarized in Table 4. Most of these enzymes have not been characterized beyond the inactivation of kinin. Some of them undoubtedly will prove to be identical with kininase I or II. It is possible, however, that a new type of kininases will emerge from this group.

Table 4. Undifferentiated kininases. (The activity of the enzymes was usually determined by bio-assay and the exact sites of cleavage of the peptide bonds in kinins were not indicated)

Source of kininase	Remarks	Reference
Human saliva	Increased in periodontal disease	TONZETICH et al., 1969
Human blood	Disulfiram inhibits in vitro erythrocyte kininase; diethyldithiocarbamate inhibits a plasma kininase; no effect on kinin release in vivo	VENNERÖD, 1970 (see also ERDÖS and YANG, 1970)
Human placenta homogenate	One enzyme converts kallidin to bradykinin and another inactivates bradykinin	USZYNSKI and MALOFIEJEW, 1971
Amniotic fluid	No significant increase during pregnancy. Contains kininogen and kinin	WIEGERSHAUSEN et al., 1970; DELHAYE et al., 1969
Human polymorphonuclear leucocytes	$CuSO_4$, $ZnCl_2$ inhibit; EDTA, DFP do not. Enzyme is present in culture medium; *o*-phenanthroline inhibits	MOVAT et al., 1973a, b BIELAWIEC et al., 1974
Human bile, mucous membrane of biliary tract and liver	Metal ions inhibit	NIELSEN, 1969
Human skin	Three different active peaks of kininases were separated by gel filtration	GECSE et al., 1971
Whole blood and plasma (man)	Contradictory results in atherosclerosis, higher activity in hepatitis	DEDICHEN and VYSTYD, 1969 LUKJAN et al., 1972
Human cerebrospinal fluid	Arginine is released; enzyme occurs more frequently in migraine patients than in normal persons	DAMAS, 1969 KANGASNIEMI et al., 1974
Alveolar macrophages (hamster)	*o*-Phenanthroline inhibits	WEESE et al., 1976
Fibroblasts (rodent)	Soluble enzyme, *o*-phenanthroline inhibits	BACK and STEGER, 1976
Whole blood (rat)	Activity decreased during pregnancy or by estrogens	MCCORMICK and SENIOR, 1972
Brain (rat, mouse)	Cerebellar region has highest activity; inhibited differently than plasma enzyme. Activity increased in excited state. Neutral proteinase cleaves most peptide bonds in kinins	IAWATA et al., 1969 MARKS and PIROTTA, 1971
Plasma (rat)	S.c. injection of $CoCl_2$ decreases kininase activity	SMITH and CONTRERA, 1974
Plasma (rhesus monkey)	Increased activity after Plasmodium knowlesi malarial infection	ONABANJO et al., 1970
Plasma (horse)	$CoCl_2$ activates, chelators inhibit	OH-ISHI et al., 1972
Homogenized pig liver, final supernatant	Chymotrypsin (?) type enzyme	DEARNLEY and BAILEY, 1976
Aloe extract	May cleave Gly^4-Phe^5	FUJITA et al., 1975
Clostridia, 9 strains	*o*-Phenanthroline inhibits	MÖSE et al., 1972a, b, c BRANTNER, 1972

Table 4 (continued)

Source of kininase	Remarks	Reference
Plasma (rabbit)	More heat-stable than human kininase, not inhibited by ε-amino-n-caproic acid, pH optimum at 6	DONALDSON, 1973
Kidney, red cells (dog)	Glucagon inhibits the enzyme	OLSEN, 1978
Plasma (guinea pig)	Enzyme, not identical with kininase II, degrades [Phe(αMe)^8]-bradykinin. It is inhibited by SQ 20881	LEDUC et al., 1978
Plasma, red cells (cattle)	Level of enzyme greatly increased after Babesia bovis infection	WRIGHT, 1977

II. Low Molecular Weight Carboxypeptidase-Type Kininases

Several investigators observed the existence of a carboxypeptidase-type kininase which has MW lower than that of the plasma enzyme, but is different from pancreatic carboxypeptidase B. The origin of this kininase is not known. Possibly kininase I releases active subunits either spontaneously or after contact with proteolytic enzymes (OSHIMA et al., 1975; JEANNERET et al., 1976; PLUMMER and HURWITZ, 1978) and these kininases function outside the circulation. Alternatively, tissues may contain a low MW carboxypeptidase which, although not identical with carboxypeptidase B, cleaves the C-terminal arginine of kinins.

The occurrence of such a low MW kininase I was also suggested by experiments in which gel filtration was used to concentrate kininase from amniotic fluid (RYBAK et al., 1971). PETAKOVA et al. (1972) studied kininase I in rat serum and tissues. Purification of rat serum kininase yielded a major peak of activity which contained the higher MW kininase and a minor peak which contained a low MW carboxypeptidase. The same pattern of distribution was obtained with homogenates of rat liver, spleen and lung. The major portion of activity was probably due to kininase I, but the origin of the minor carboxypeptidase-kininase has not been established.

Recently ERDÖS et al. (1978c) separated a carboxypeptidase of about 45,000 MW from homogenized kidney and from human urine. The enzyme did not crossreact with antibody to pure human pancreatic carboxypeptidase B, indicating that the two enzymes are not identical. This carboxypeptidase may originate from the kidney (ERDÖS and YANG, 1966), since the 280,000 MW plasma kininase I would be excluded from the nephron. Its low MW subunits (45,000) however, could be filtered by the glomerulus and be present in active form in the urine.

III. Kininase in the Central Nervous System

In a search for a functional role for kinins in the central nervous system (CNS) numerous investigators studied the metabolism of kinins by extracts of brain (MARKS, 1977; CLARK, this volume). In the rat brain kininase activity was highest in the cerebellar region (IWATA et al., 1969). An increase in kininase activity was associated with CNS excitation in the mouse (IWATA et al., 1970). MARKS and PIROTTA (1971)

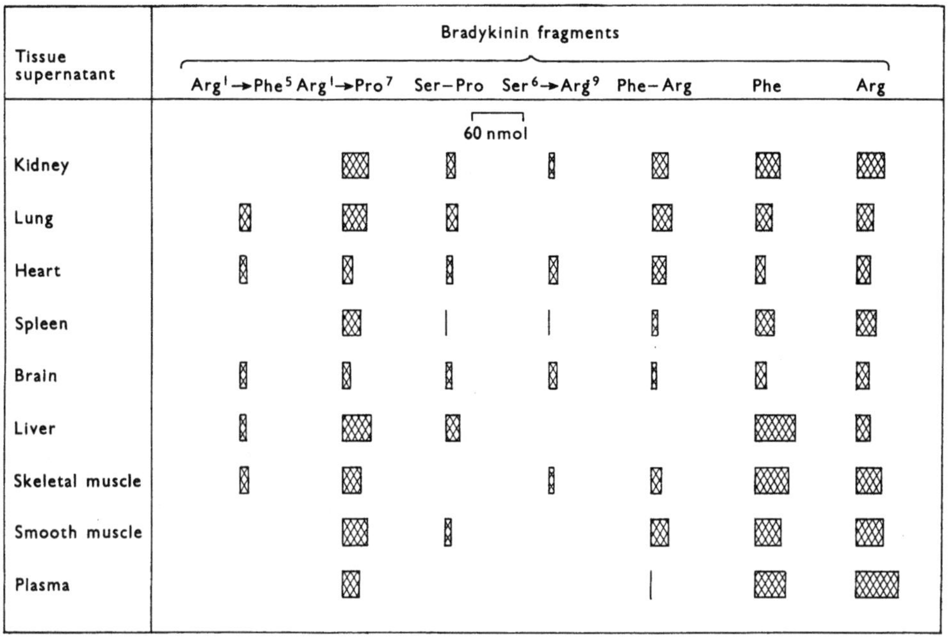

Fig. 3. Hydrolysis of Arg-Pro-Pro-Gly-Phe-Ser-Pro-Phe-Arg (bradykinin) by supernatant fractions derived from rabbit tissue homogenates. The values indicated by the width of the bars are nmol of the peptide or free amino acids recovered after approximately 50% hydrolysis of bradykinin. The enzymic hydrolyzates were prepared as follows: bradykinin (80 nmol) was incubated in 1.0 ml of 0.05 *M* sodium phosphate buffer (pH 7.5)/0.1 *M* NaCl at 35 °C with tissue supernatant fractions. The extent of hydrolysis of bradykinin was determined by bioassay. After 50% of the bradykinin had been hydrolyzed, the reaction was stopped by the addition of 1.2 ml of 30% (v/v) solution of poly(ethylene glycol) in 0.32 *M* sodium citrate buffer containing 0.05 *M* HCl. The hydrolysis products were determined by chromatographic analysis (CICILINI et al., 1977)

attributed the kininase activity of rat brain to a neutral proteinase. The enzyme cleaved several bonds such as Arg^1-Pro^2, Phe^5-Ser^6, Phe^8-Arg^9 in bradykinin. The kininases of the homogenized rabbit brain have been studied systematically by CAMARGO and his colleagues (CAMARGO and GRAEFF, 1969; CAMARGO et al., 1972, 1973; OLIVEIRA et al., 1976a, b; Fig. 3). Two thiol-activated endopeptidases with a pH optimum near 7.5 were purified from the supernatant fraction by the sequential use of ion exchange chromatography, gel filtration, and isoelectric focusing. The first enzyme, kininase A, cleaves the Phe^5-Ser^6 peptide bond in bradykinin and has a MW of 71,000. Brain kininase B hydrolyzes the same Pro^7-Phe^8 bond as does kininase II, but kininase B has a MW of 68,000. It cleaves kinin analogues of bradykinin but not kininogen.

A similar kininase was partially purified from rat brain. After incubating the enzyme with bradykinin, free phenylalanine and arginine were detected (SHIKIMI et al., 1970; SHIKIMI and IWATA, 1970).

In addition, kininase II activity (see below) was localized in various parts of the CNS (YANG and NEFF, 1972, 1973; POTH et al., 1975) including the choroid plexus (IGIC et al., 1977).

IV. Distribution of Kininases

The distribution of kininases in plasma and homogenized tissues of rabbit have been studied systematically by CICILINI et al. (1977; Fig. 3). Tissue homogenates were separately by centrifugation and the kininase content was determined in both the supernatant and the pellet. When plasma was the source of kininase, the heptapeptide, Arg^1-Pro^7-bradykinin, the dipeptide, Phe-Arg, and the free amino acids, Phe and Arg, were detected. More Arg was recovered than Phe, which indicated that kinin was cleaved by both kininase I and II to release Arg and Phe-Arg. The latter dipeptide was then hydrolyzed further by a dipeptidase present. Similar results were obtained with various tissue homogenates, the pattern of cleavage, however, was more complicated. The relative capacity of tissues to inactivate bradykinin varied over a 1200-fold range; kidney and lung had the highest and plasma had the lowest activity. Sensitivity to inhibitors such as EDTA or dithiothreitol also varied greatly.

The kininase activity in the brain was attributed to kininase A and B described by the same group (see above). It is possible, however, that some of the Phe^8 detected did not come from the breakdown of liberated Phe-Arg, but after the cleavage of Arg^9 from bradykinin, a prolylcarboxypeptidase liberated Phe^8 (YANG et al., 1968; ODYA et al., 1978a).

V. Purified Proteases as Kininases

Purified proteases and peptidases from tissues and plants can cleave kinins (Table 5). The most active kininase among the commercially available peptidases is pancreatic carboxypeptidase B (ERDÖS, 1962; ERDÖS and YANG, 1970). Although the hog pancreatic carboxypeptidase B has been used in the past, in vitro and in vivo, to abolish kinin activity, purified human pancreatic carboxypeptidase B (MARINKOVIC et al., 1977) seems to be as active in vitro as the hog enzyme is, when bradykinin is the substrate (unpublished). Interestingly, almost 40% of the activity of a chymotrypsin preparation was attributed to a contamination by 0.4% carboxypeptidase B (SAMPAIO et al., 1976), which also suggests that carboxypeptidase B is much more efficient than chymotrypsin as an inactivator of kinins (ERDÖS, 1962).

OLIVEIRA et al. (1976a, b) purified kininase A and B from rabbit brain and established the bonds cleaved in bradykinin, as shown above. Lamb kidney has an enzyme that cleaves peptide bonds adjacent to proline, including those in bradykinin (KOIDA and WALTER, 1976).

C. Kininase II: Angiotensin I Converting Enzyme

(Peptidyl dipeptidase; E. C. 3.4.15.1)

Many more publications deal with kininase II than with kininase I. The interest in this enzyme is due, in part, to the fact that it also cleaves angiotensin I. Since renin is a crucial factor in the etiology of some forms of hypertension, blockade of the renin system is of considerable importance for clinical diagnosis and treatment of the disease. Because at present there are no renin inhibitors than can be used clinically and the i.v. administration of an angiotensin II antagonist is impractical, many

Table 5. Metabolism of bradykinin by purified proteases and peptidases

Enzyme	Bond cleaved	Remarks	Reference
Chymotrypsin	-Phe^8-Arg^9	40% of hydrolysis is due to 0.4% contamination by carboxypeptidase B	SAMPAIO et al., 1976
Human pancreatic carboxypeptidase B	-Phe^8-Arg^9		MARINKOVIC et al., 1977 JOHNSON, unpublished
Neutral brain endopeptidase (kininase A)	-Phe^5-Ser^6-	Purified from rabbit brain	OLIVEIRA et al., 1976a, b
Kininase B	-Pro^7-Phe^8-	Purified from rabbit brain	OLIVEIRA et al., 1976a, b
Proline hydroxylase rat skin	Hydroxylates Pro^3	Bradykinin is a poor substrate	RHOADS and UDENFRIEND, 1969
Red kidney bean, potato	Several peptide bonds	Aminopeptidase-type metalloenzyme MW is 73,000	HOJIMA et al., 1977
Penicillium janthinellum, acid carboxy-peptidase	-Phe^8-Arg^9 -Pro^7-Phe^8-	MW is 51,000	YOKOYAMA et al., 1975
Stem bromelain	-Phe^5-Ser^6- -Gly^4-Phe^5-		MURACHI and MIYAKE, 1970 MINESHITA and NAGAI, 1977
Post-proline cleaving enzyme	-Pro^3-Gly^4- -Pro^7-Phe^8-	Purified from lamb kidney MW is 115,000	KOIDA and WALTER, 1976
Potato kininase	?	MW 70,000 200-fold purified	HOJIMA et al., 1971a, b

investigators believe that blocking the enzymatic conversion of angiotensin I to II is a valid therapeutic approach. A review of all available information on this subject would exceed the scope of this chapter. Therefore, I will focus primarily on kinin metabolism, and for the sake of a uniform style, I shall refer to this enzyme as kininase II even when the substrate was angiotensin I.

I. Background

Early research on kininase II is summarized in the previous edition of this Handbook (YANG and ERDÖS, 1970). The angiotensin I converting enzyme was discovered in the mid 1950s (SKEGGS et al., 1954, 1956; LENTZ et al., 1956). It was found that horse plasma contains an enzyme which converts angiotensin I (hypertensin I) to angiotensin II. Renin releases the decapeptide, angiotensin I, from angiotensinogen, the substrate of renin, and the decapeptide is in turn converted to the octapeptide angiotensin II by the removal of a histidyl-leucine dipeptide from the C-terminal end. HELMER (1957) also observed that a factor in plasma activated angiotensin in vitro.

Intravenous injections of either angiotensin I or II raise the blood pressure similarly, but angiotensin I is much less active than angiotensin II when applied to isolated tissues in vitro. Thus, angiotensin I must be converted enzymatically to *angiotensin II* before becoming fully active in most biologic systems.

Plasma was originally suspected to be the site of conversion of angiotensin I. VANE and his associate (NG and VANE, 1967, 1968) studied the fate of angiotensin I and II by the use of an isolated, superfused organ bath system (TRAUTSCHOLD, 1970) which distinguished the effects of angiotensin I and II in circulating blood. They found that conversion in plasma was too slow to account for formation of angiotensin II in vivo. However, when they injected angiotensin I i.v. into the dog, they recovered angiotensin II after circulation through the pulmonary vascular bed. Little or no angiotensin II was found in venous blood when angiotensin I was injected into the renal or femoral artery. These authors and BIRON and HUGGINS (1968) concluded that angiotensin I is converted in the pulmonary circulation. Bradykinin was rapidly inactivated during passage through the vascular bed of various organs and the lung was especially active in this respect (KRONEBERG and STOEPEL, 1963; VANE, 1969; FERREIRA and VANE, 1967). Since both bradykinin and angiotensin were metabolized in the lungs, it was tempting to assume that they were substrates for the same or similar enzymes. NG and VANE (1968) indicated that angiotensin I and bradykinin may be cleaved by the same enzyme in lung, but they proposed that carboxypeptidase N (or kininase I) could convert angiotensin I to II, presumably by sequential cleavage of the last two amino acids. BAKHLE (1968) observed that bradykinin potentiating factor of snake venom inhibited the conversion of angiotensin I to angiotensin II by a particulate fraction of the homogenized dog lung, but thought that kininase and converting enzyme activities were due to different enzymes.

It was finally established by YANG et al. (1970a, b, c, 1971) that kininase II is a "dipeptidyl carboxypeptidase" which cleaved both bradykinin and angiotensin I. These investigations were initiated in the early sixties. It was observed that a partially purified collagenase preparation from Clostridium histolyticum inactivated the peptide by cleavage of the Pro^7-Phe^8 bond and released C-terminal Phe^8-Arg^9 (ERDÖS and YANG, 1970). Then, a kininase with similar activity was concentrated from a microsomal fraction of the hog kidney cortex (ERDÖS and YANG, 1966, 1967) and named peptidase P. The same enzyme was also detected in human plasma (YANG and ERDÖS, 1967). To distinguish the second kininase from carboxypeptidase N, it was named kininase II, and carboxypeptidase N was renamed kininase I. When it was found that kininase II cleaves a variety of peptide bonds it was named dipeptidyl carboxypeptidase (YANG et al., 1970a). Unfortunately the name is not entirely correct, but in spite (or maybe because) of this, the term appears frequently in print. The Enzyme Commission named the enzyme peptidyl dipeptide hydrolase or peptidyl dipeptidase.

Initially, the dual activity of the enzyme in metabolism of both bradykinin and angiotensin I was not appreciated. RYAN et al. (1968) studied the mechanism of inactivation of bradykinin in the pulmonary circulation and suggested that the possible site for its inactivation is at or near the vascular endothelium. They perfused the lung with [Pro^2–^{14}C] bradykinin in a Locke-dextran solution at the rate of 2–4 ug/min. The total dose of bradykinin administered was high, 40–80 ug. The peptide fragments collected in the perfusate were separated by electrophoresis and chromatography. The major radioactive peaks contained Pro-Pro and Arg-Pro-Pro-Gly. The only peak found when perfusion fluid contained mercaptoethanol was the N-terminal hexapeptide. The authors concluded: "So far we have identified only one primary cleavage, namely that of the Arg^1-Pro^2 bond." [Inactivation of bradykinin at the N-terminal end by a prolidase (imidopeptidase) was shown previously with erythrocytes (ERDÖS et al., 1963) or kidney as sources of the enzyme (ERDÖS and YANG, 1966).] RYAN et al. (1968) also postulated the cleavage of the C-terminal tripeptide from bradykinin.

The search for an enzyme in lung that would cleave the C-terminal tripeptide of bradykinin was pursued with [Phe^8–^3H]bradykinin and additional kinin fragments, including Phe-Arg, were identified after perfusion (RYAN et al., 1970). When BPF_{5a} and 2-mercaptoethanol were added to the perfusion fluid, the lung released Pro-Phe-Arg. Although in a single circulation time no less than 5 peptide bonds were hydrolyzed in the rat lung, cleavage of only two were considered to be of primary importance, namely Arg^1-Pro^2 and Ser^6-Pro^7 bonds. These authors attributed the release of the C-terminal dipeptide to a secondary hydrolysis of the released Pro^7-Phe^8-Arg^9. In subsequent publications, STEWART et al. (1971), and FREER and STEWART (1975) suggested that the inhibitor BPF_{5a} blocks an enzyme which releases the C-terminal tripeptide in the lung; thus, the hydrolysis of bradykinin and angiotensin I could not be carried out by the same enzyme.

The existence of the enzyme which releases the C-terminal tripeptide was not confirmed by IGIC et al. (1973) who perfused through the rat lung the protected C-terminal tetrapeptide (Ac-Ser-Pro-Phe-Arg) but detected only Phe-Arg and not the tripeptide as product of hydrolysis.

The metabolism of bradykinin and angiotensin I in pulmonary circulation was also studied by BIRON and HUGGINS and associates. BIRON and HUGGINS also noted (1968) that angiotensin I was cleaved by the lung. They, BIRON and CAMPEAU (1971), STANLEY and BIRON (1968) and BIRON et al. (1969) recognized that the pulmonary circulation is not the only site of conversion of angiotensin I, but doubted that kininase activity was due to the action of the angiotensin I converting enzyme (SCHOLZ and BIRON, 1969; HEBERT et al., 1972). The conversion of angiotensin I by the rat lung was not inhibited by 2-mercaptoethanol but bradykinin was at least partially protected by the administration of this compound. ALABASTER and BAKHLE (1972a, b) however, could not inhibit the inactivation of bradykinin by 2-mercapto-ethanol in the perfused lung, but other inhibitors affected the hydrolysis of angio-tensin I and bradykinin similarly.

In contrast to these findings, YANG et al. (1970a, b, c, 1971) tested a partially purified hog plasma enzyme and a microsomal fraction from hog lung and kidney with a variety of substrates and inhibitors in vitro and concluded that kininase II was identical with angiotensin I converting enzyme.

ELISSEEVA et al. (1971) also found that a kidney enzyme, called carboxycathepsin, cleaved both bradykinin and angiotensin I. CUSHMAN and CHEUNG (1971b), using a rabbit lung extract as the enzyme source came to the same conclusion. Final proof was provided by IGIC et al. (1972a, b, c) who obtained a homogeneous hog lung enzyme preparation, which released C-terminal dipeptides from various substrates and inactivated bradykinin and activated angiotensin I.

In the opinion of this reviewer, most of the kininase activity in the lung of many, although not of all species, is due to a peptidyl dipeptidase which cleaves both bradykinin and angiotensin I (see next subheading). This was shown in vitro unequivocally with homogenized tissues and purified enzyme. In studies done in vitro, in the lung in situ and in vivo the replacement of the pentapeptide BPF_{5a}

inhibitor with BPF_{9a} or SQ 20881 simultaneously blocked the conversion of angiotensin I and the inactivation of bradykinin (IGIC et al., 1972a; ENGEL et al., 1972; GREENE et al., 1972). This latter inhibitor is more active than BPF_{5a} in vivo.

In addition, human lung may contain another angiotensin I converting enzyme of higher MW that is similar to tonin, but is not a kininase (OVERTURF et al., 1975; BOAZ et al., 1975). Tonin is a protein of about 30,000 MW originally discovered in submaxillary gland by BOUCHER et al. (1974) which releases angiotensin I from the tetradecapeptide renin substrate. However, bradykinin may be hydrolyzed by other enzymes in the lung such as the imidopeptidase (prolidase; RYAN et al., 1968). The existence of a carboxypeptidase-type enzyme that converts "excessive amounts" of angiotensin I to angiotensin II by stepwise degradation in the rat lung was suggested by BARRETT and SAMBHI (1971).

II. Distribution of Kininase II

Kininase II is widely distributed in the body. It occurs in membrane-bound form in vascular endothelial cells, in epithelial cells of renal tubules and intestinal tract and in soluble form in various body fluids.

The activity of kininase II in crude homogenates of various tissues has been determined. The activity in extracts, even in partially purified extracts, may be influenced by the presence of inhibitors of the enzyme (KLAUSER et al., 1979) and by the solubility of the enzyme. The solubility depends on the mode of homogenization and on the use of detergents. Finally, other enzymes that can cleave the substrates of kininase II may also influence the assay.

Lung homogenates contain high concentrations of kininase II (ROTH et al., 1969), but human lung has much less activity than the lung from 10 other species tested (DEPIERRE and ROTH, 1972).

In the rat the epididymis, testis and lung had the highest activity (CUSHMAN and CHEUNG, 1971a) and liver and gastrocnemius had the lowest. Interestingly, homogenates of rat kidney had little activity, while it was high in intestinal homogenate (ROTH et al., 1969; CUSHMAN and CHEUNG, 1971a, 1972). In other animals the activity in the kidney varied according to the species used; rabbit (CUSHMAN and CHEUNG, 1972) and hog kidney (OSHIMA et al., 1974a) are very active in this respect. A particulate fraction of human kidney has higher activity than the corresponding lung fraction (STEWART, KLAUSER, ERDÖS to be published).

1. Endothelial Cells

The vascular endothelium is particularly rich source of kininase II, as shown by biologic, biochemical and morphologic techniques. The lung has an extensive vascular bed and lung homogenates contained enzymes (FREY et al., 1968; BAKHLE, 1968), which rapidly converted angiotensin I or inactivated bradykinin.

In the perfused dog lung, plasma accounts for 25% of the inactivation of bradykinin and lung tissue for 75%. This inactivation of bradykinin across the lung did not change when the cardiac output was lowered (LEVINE et al., 1973). AIKEN and VANE (1970, 1972) found a higher rate of angiotensin I conversion in the pulmonary artery than in other blood vessels. After centrifugation of the homogenized lung most of the activity was recovered in particulate fractions (BAKHLE, 1968; BAKHLE and REYNARD, 1971; SANDER and HUGGINS, 1971). RYAN and SMITH (1971) used a heavy metal complex to isolate, membrane fraction from homogenized lung that contained membrane-bound 5′-nucleotidase and inactivated bradykinin rapidly. Hog lung kininase II was used to elicit antibodies in the goat. Antibodies were tagged and applied to localize the enzyme in the rat tissues (RYAN et al., 1975) and pig endothelial cells (RYAN et al., 1976a, b). The enzyme was localized on the plasma membrane and in the caveolae of endothelial cells.

Endothelial cells grown in tissue culture contain kininase II activity. The enzyme was identified in cells originating from pulmonary vessels of animals (RYAN et al., 1976a, b) and man (JOHNSON and ERDÖS, 1978) and from human umbilical vein (JOHNSON and ERDÖS, 1975, 1977; HIAL et al., 1976). The enzymatic activity was retained in successive subcultures (JOHNSON and ERDÖS, 1977) but activity was not enhanced by treating the cells with various growth factors (JOHNSON and ERDÖS, 1978; JOHNSON et al., 1979). Endothelial cells isolated from human pulmonary artery, contain more kininase II activity than cells from either pulmonary or umbilical vein (JOHNSON and ERDÖS, 1978). The enzyme is associated with intact monolayers of cultured cells but activity increased when cells were suspended (JOHNSON and BOYDEN, 1977; JOHNSON and ERDÖS, 1977; Fig. 4). The kininase activity of cultured cells was inhibited by antibody to human lung enzyme, indicating that the enzyme was on the cell surface. Fractionation of the cells, however, resulted in release of most of the kininase II activity of the cultured cells into the final supernatant, while in homogenized lung or kidney much of the kininase II activity sedimented with the particulate fraction (SANDER and HUGGINS, 1971; BAKHLE, 1968; OSHIMA et al., 1974a; LANZILLO and FANBURG, 1974). Kininase II in the cultured cells cleaved kallidin and Met-Lys-bradykinin slower than bradykinin (JOHNSON and ERDÖS, 1977) and the lower rate of hydrolysis of longer kinins by endothelial cells may contribute to their more potent hypotensive activity (JOHNSON and ERDÖS, 1977; see also subheading "Properties"). At least one kinin, the 18 amino acid containing polistes kinin, can pass through the pulmonary circulation without being inactivated (RYAN et al., 1970).

In addition to pulmonary endothelial cells, cells in other vascular beds also contain kininase II. This was discovered when the conversion of angiotensin I was studied in experimental animals and in man. Such a conversion in peripheral circulation was already indicated by BIRON and HUGGINS (1968). Others found significant conversion in renal (CARRIERE and BIRON, 1970; DISALVO et al., 1971; HOFBAUER et al., 1973a, b; FRANKLIN et al., 1970), peripheral (KREYE and GROSS, 1971; AIKEN and VANE, 1972; OATES and STOKES, 1974) and splanchnic (DISALVO et al., 1973) vasculature.

Antibody tagged with fluorescein was used to localize kininase II (HALL et al., 1976; CALDWELL et al., 1976a). The enzyme was detected along the small blood vessels of organs such as the liver or kidneys (CALDWELL et al., 1976a) or placenta (WIGGER and STALCUP, 1978). The microvessels of the retina (IGIC et al., 1977; WARD et al., 1978b) and of the brain (ORLOWSKI and WILK, 1978; BRECHER et al., 1978) also contain kininase II. Possibly not every vascular endothelium has high kininase II activity because the endothelium of the glomerulus, isolated or in tissue slices, has very

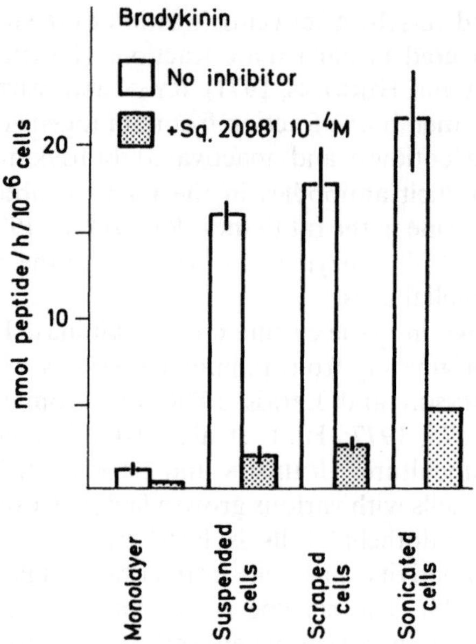

Fig. 4. Inactivation of bradykinin by human endothelial cells. The activity of kininase II (converting enzyme) was measured in endothelial cells. The height of the bars indicates the amount of peptide substrate hydrolyzed per hour per 10^6 cells. Values are means $\pm$S.E.M. of 3–6 experiments. Open bars are enzyme activities without inhibitor; hatched bars are activities after prior incubation with inhibitor. Intact monolayers of cells inactivated bradykinin slowly. This reaction was inhibited by SQ 20881. When the cells were suspended either by treatment with trypsin or by scraping the monolayers with a rubber spatula, kininase II activity increased more than 10-fold. Disruption of the cells by sonication did not result in a further increase in kininase activity, indicating that the enzyme is located on the membrane. (JOHNSON and BOYDEN, 1977)

little activity (WARD et al., 1977; HALL et al., 1976), when measured chemically or with immunofluorescence.

The conversion of angiotensin I outside the lung is much more extensive, especially in man, than first assumed. The estimates for conversion of angiotensin I in the human lung range only from 20 to 40% (SEMPLE, 1977; BIRON and CAMPEAU, 1971; FRIEDLI et al., 1974). The rest of circulating angiotensin I is converted peripherally (COLLIER and ROBINSON, 1974) and is catabolized.

2. Other Types of Cells

Although kininase II was discovered originally in the kidney (ERDÖS and YANG, 1966, 1967), the site of its activity in this organ was localized much later. Experiments with fluorescein-tagged antibody showed that kininase II is localized all along the nephron (HALL et al., 1976) but it was especially concentrated in the cells of the proximal tubules of the hog and rabbit kidney (HALL et al., 1976; CALDWELL et al., 1976a).

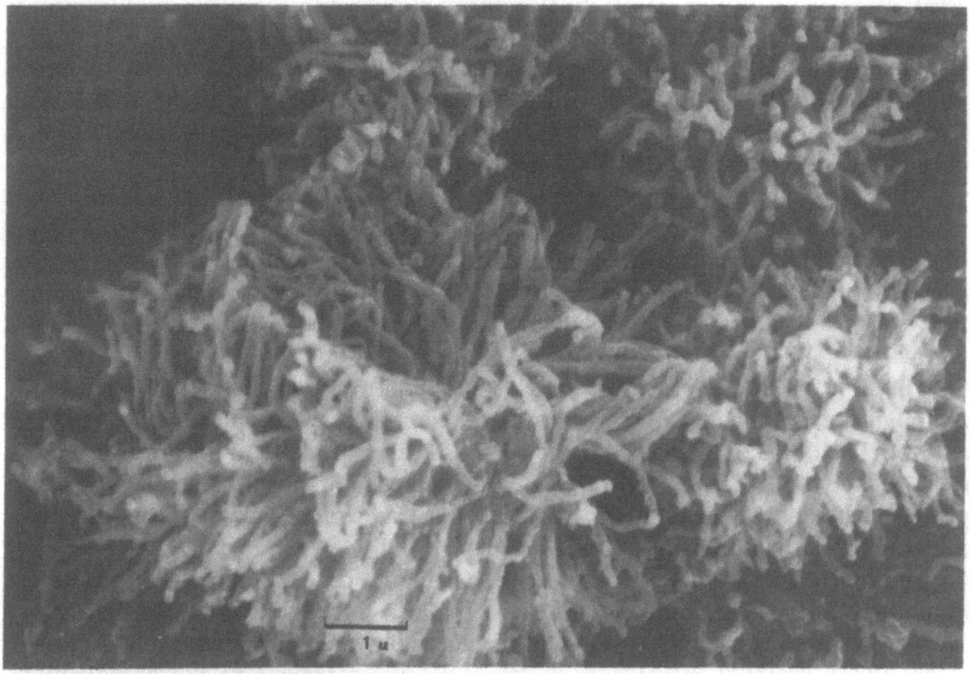

Fig. 5. Scanning electron micrograph of isolated brush border fraction from proximal tubules of the rat kidney. Kininase II activity was 10-fold enriched in the fraction over the crude homogenate. (WARD et al., 1976)

When the brush border of the proximal tubules of the rat was isolated by differential centrifugation, the relative specific activity of kininase II increased 10-fold over the crude homogenate (WARD et al., 1975, 1976). The very high kininase II activity of the microsomal fraction of homogenized kidney (ERDÖS and YANG, 1966, 1967; OSHIMA et al., 1974a) may be explained by the high concentrations of the enzyme on the brush border. Scanning electron micrographs of the isolated fractions show the extensive surface of the brush border where the enzyme is localized (Fig. 5). Scanning electron microscopy and freeze fracture also indicate that the enzyme is membrane-bound since the isolated preparations contain intact surface membrane but core material, microtubules and embedded particles are missing (WARD et al., 1977). In contrast, isolated glomeruli (WARD et al., 1977) or glomeruli in tissue slices (HALL et al., 1976) show much less activity. A high rate of inactivation of bradykinin within the proximal tubules was shown by microinfusing labeled bradykinin (OPARIL et al., 1976a; CARONE et al., 1976). The activity was also high in a tumor originating from the proximal tubules of the rat kidney (HALL et al., 1976). CARONE et al., (1976) found no inactivation of bradykinin in the distal tubules, although immunofluorescent studies indicated the presence of the enzyme (HALL et al., 1976). SCICLI et al. (1978) used a stop-flow technique in dogs and found evidence for some kininase activity in distal tubules. Thus, the portions of bradykinin and angiotensin I that escape cleavage on the endothelial surface of the renal artery may be filtered by the glomerulus and hydrolyzed on the brush border of proximal tubules (WARD et al., 1975, 1976,

1977; Ward and Erdös, 1977). Furthermore, kininase in the distal tubules and in urine can contribute to kinin catabolism (Erdös et al., 1978c).

The lumen of the intestine contains brush border that is similar morphologically and biochemically to the renal brush border (Vannier et al., 1976). In addition, intestinal brush border isolated from human and hog tissues also contains high concentrations of kininase II (Ward et al., 1978a).

Kininase II is present in other cells under certain conditions. For example, lymph nodes contain little enzymatic activity except in sarcoidosis. Non-necrotizing lymph nodes of sarcoid patients contain high concentrations of kininase II (Silverstein et al., 1976a, b). The basal enzymatic activity in rabbit alveolar macrophages or human monocytes in culture is very low but can be increased several-fold by adding a corticosteroid (Friedland et al., 1977, 1978).

The choroid plexus and ciliary body contain active kininase II (Igic et al., 1977), although the cell type which contains the enzyme has not yet been identified. The enzyme is also present in various parts of the brain, especially in the striatum of the rat (Yang and Neff, 1972) or in the caudate nucleus of man (Poth et al., 1975). The posterior lobe of the rat pituitary has over four times more enzymatic activity than the anterior lobe (Yang and Neff, 1972, 1973).

The reproductive organs, such as testicles, contain very high concentrations of kininase II (Cushman and Cheung, 1971a). It may by localized in the epithelial cells of the ducts. The enzyme is also present in the adrenal zona glomerulosa cells (Ackerly et al., 1977), where it might convert des-Asp^1-angiotensin I to the heptapeptide, angiotensin III, which releases aldosterone.

3. Soluble Enzyme

Kininase II is present in plasma (Skeggs et al., 1956; Yang and Erdös, 1967) and other body fluids such as urine (Erdös and Yang, 1970; Kokubu et al., 1978) or renal lymph (Horky et al., 1971). The level of enzymatic activity in plasma varies according to the animal species. For example, it is very high in guinea pig (Yang et al., 1971), but it is low in dog or man. The enzyme in undiluted blood may be inhibited by blood-borne inhibitors, such as albumin, because purified albumin and its fragments inhibit the enzyme in vitro (Klauser et al., 1979). The plasma enzyme seems to be identical with the lung and kidney enzyme. The inhibition pattern of tissue and plasma enzyme is identical (Igic et al., 1972a; Lanzillo and Fanburg, 1976a). Kininase II from hog plasma enzyme is inhibited by antibody elicited against hog kidney enzyme (Oshima et al., 1974a) and rabbit plasma kininase II crossreacts with antibody to the rabbit lung enzyme (Das et al., 1977; see also subheading Antibody). The plasma enzyme also contains sialic acid, as does the kidney enzyme (Oshima et al., 1976), which may be necessary for a prolonged sojourn in the circulation (Das et al., 1977).

Other biologic fluids contain kininase II. Human seminal plasma (Depierre et al. 1978) has a much higher activity than blood plasma. Edema fluid that develops in the perfused blood-free rat lung after antigen antibody reaction and histamine release contains kininase II in higher concentrations than the perfusate (Igic et al., 1973; Erdös et al., 1975).

4. Kininase II in Developing Tissues

Kininase II activity has been studied during development. HEBERT et al., (1972) found the pulmonary conversion of angiotensin I to be twice as high in ewes as in fetal or newborn lamb. The inactivation of bradykinin in the pulmonary circulation of the fetal animals was more pronounced than the conversion of angiotensin I. This was taken as an indication that an additional kininase may inactivate kinins in the prenatal lung. FRIEDLI et al., (1973) found that the ability to inactivate bradykinin in the lung developed late in fetal life of the lamb and at birth the enzyme activity was still lower than in the adult ewes. In embryonic rabbit lungs the activity of kininase II increased up to the time of birth and was approximately doubled by the second day after birth (KOKUBU et al., 1977). In rats and mice the soluble enzyme content of homogenized lung and kidney was much higher in the adult animals than in the newborn. No sex differences were observed by WALLACE et al. (1978).

WIGGER and STALCUP (1978) used immunofluorescence to study the enzyme in fetal rabbits during development. Kininase II was detected after the 17th day of gestation and increased in parallel with vascularization of the lung. In the embryonic kidney, in addition to the proximal tubules and capillaries, the enzyme was detected in the collecting tubules and papillary epithelium. It was also present in the intestinal epithelial cells.

According to OPARIL et al. (1978), there was more kininase II activity in maternal plasma than in plasma taken from the umbilical vein after cesarian section. In contrast, after normal delivery the activity in both fetal and maternal blood was the same and fell within the normal range. The authors suggested that the plasma enzyme may originate from extrapulmonary sources.

III. Specificity of Kininase II

It was first thought that the angiotensin I converting enzyme cleaves only substrates structurally related to the C-terminal end of angiotensin I. Thus substrates such as Bz-Gly-His-Leu (Hippuryl-His-Leu; CUSHMAN and CHEUNG, 1969; 1971b) or Cbz-Pro-Phe-His-Leu, (Cbz or Z = benzyloxycarbonyl; PIQUILLOUD et al., 1968, 1970) were introduced to assay the enzyme. (But kininase II had been shown to cleave Phe-Arg from a protected C-terminal tetrapeptide of bradykinin {ERDÖS and YANG, 1967; YANG and ERDÖS, 1967}).

When the two enzymes were shown to be identical and kininase II was found to cleave peptide bond of a wide variety of amino acids (YANG et al., 1970a, 1971; ELISSEEVA et al., 1971), other substrates were synthesized (Table 6). The simplest are protected tripeptides of glycine such as Bz-Gly-Gly-Gly (Hippuryl-Gly-Gly; YANG et al., 1970a, 1971) or dansyl-Gly-Gly-Gly (IGIC et al., 1972a). Other substrates contain chromophore groups, such as $p(NO_2)$-phenylalanine, as in *t*-Boc-Phe-$p(NO_2)$-Phe-Gly (YANG et al., 1971) or in the Z-Phe-$p(NO_2)$-Gly-Gly (STEVENS et al., 1972; MASSEY and FESSLER, 1976). Bz-Gly-His-Leu and Bz-Gly-Gly-Gly are widely used. These substrates can be employed in the UV spectrophotometer at 254 nm to measure the increase in absorption when hippuric acid is released (FOLK et al., 1960). A modification of this method consists of assaying the released and extracted hippuric acid directly at 228 nm (CUSHMAN and CHEUNG, 1971b) or at the visible range at

Table 6. Short peptide substrates of kininase II used in assays

Representative substrate -R-R_2-R_3-OH ↑	Method	References
Bz-Gly-Gly-Gly	Hippuric acid is determined in UV spectrophotometer or dipeptide in amino acid analyzer. Hippuric acid determined after t.l.c.	YANG et al., 1970a, 1971 DORER et al., 1972 FILIPOVIC et al., 1978
Bz-Gly-His-Leu	As above or fluorometric assay of fluorescent derivative of His-Leu	CUSHMAN and CHEUNG, 1969, 1971b FRIEDLAND and SILVERSTEIN, 1977 HAYAKARI and KONDO, 1977 CONROY and LAI, 1978
^{3}H Bz-Gly-Gly-Gly ^{14}C Bz-Gly-His-Leu	Extracted labeled hippuric acid is assayed in liquid scintillation counter	RYAN et al., 1977 ROHRBACH, 1978
^{14}C Dansyl-Gly-Gly-Gly	Radioactive product assayed after thin-layer chromatography	IGIC et al., 1972a
t-Boc-Phe(NO_2)-Phe-Gly and other NO_2-derivatives	Assay in the UV spectrophotometer	YANG et al., 1971; STEVENS et al., 1972; MASSEY and FESSLER, 1976
αDNP-poly(Pro-Gly-Pro)	Colorimetric, ninhydrin assay for bacterial enzyme	YARON et al., 1972
Z-Pro-Phe-His-Leu	Product determined in fluorometer after coupling with *o*-phthalaldehyde	DEPIERRE and ROTH, 1975 PIQUILLOUD et al., 1968, 1970
2-aminobenzoyl Gly-*p*-(NO_2)-Phe-Pro	Assay of fluorescence $\lambda_{max}=415$ nm	CARMEL and YARON, 1978
p(NO_2)-benzyloxycarbonyl--Gly-Try-Gly	Assay of fluorescence at $\lambda=480$ nm	PERSSON and WILSON, 1977

382 nm after coupling with a suitable reagent (HAYAKARI et al., 1978). The assay is easy, rapid and accurate when purified enzymes are used or when the activity is high enough to eliminate interfering proteins by dilution of an extract. The direct UV method is not practical to use with most crude tissue preparations or with human plasma.

High concentration of Na_2SO_4 (0.6 *M*) accelerates the reaction (DORER et al., 1976) but only with the Bz-Gly-Gly-Gly substrate. Another assay technique is based on coupling the released His-Leu to *o*-phthaldehyde or fluorescamine and measuring the fluorescence of the complex (PIQUILLOUD et al., 1968, 1970; DEPIERRE and ROTH, 1975; CONROY and LAI, 1978; HAYAKARI and KONDO, 1977; FRIEDLAND and SILVERSTEIN, 1977). A complication of this technique may stem from the presence of a dipeptidase in most tissue extracts and plasma which can cleave the product His-Leu. The histidine *o*-phthaldehyde complex is much less fluorescent than the dipeptide complex (FRIEDLAND and SILVERSTEIN, 1977).

Another approach is based on modification of CUSHMAN's technique by using ^3H Bz-Gly-Gly-Gly as substrate. The released labeled hippuric acid is extracted with ethylacetate and the activity of the enzyme is estimated from the radioactivity in the organic phase (RYAN et al., 1977). This technique requires high concentrations of substrate and of Na_2SO_4 to accelerate the reaction. We have also assayed the enzyme by determining the amount of diglycine released from Bz-Gly-Gly-Gly in an automatic amino acid analyzer or by using randomly labeled Bz-Gly-Gly-Gly. A specific inhibitor such as SQ 20881 or SQ 14225 should be used to establish the identity of the enzyme. It is also desirable that the results with protected tripeptide substrates be confirmed by measuring either the inactivation of bradykinin or the release of angiotensin II.

Substrates that promise an improvement in the techniques of assay have been synthetized recently. These substrates, which have a quenched fluorescence become fully fluorescent when the C-terminal dipeptide is released by the enzyme. The activity can be assayed by measuring increase in fluorescence (CARMEL and YARON, 1978; PERSSON and WILSON, 1977). (For data on additional substrates published in Russian literature see PASKHINA and LEVITSKIJ this volume). Table 6 summarized the data on short synthetic substrates used to determine the activity of kininase II.

When longer peptides, are employed as substrates they can be appropriately labeled and the products cleaved can be separated by chromatography or by electrophoresis. Labeled angiotensin I (HUGGINS and THAMPI, 1968; OPARIL et al., 1970; IGIC et al., 1972a), or labeled bradykinin (RYAN et al., 1968; ZACEST et al., 1974) have been used this way. Paper chromatography and thin layer chromatography were also employed to separate the products of enzymatic cleavage of various other peptides (ELISSEEVA et al., 1971).

Tables 6 and 7 show the structure of various substrates. The general structure is R_1-R_2-R_3-OH and the enzyme cleaves between R_1 and R_2. R_1 can be a protected amino acid or a peptide. R_3 should be an amino acid with a free carboxyl terminal but not a dicarboxylic acid such as glutamic acid (ELISSEEVA et al., 1971). R_2 can be any amino acid except proline (YANG et al., 1970a, 1971; ELISSEEVA et al., 1971), because peptides that have proline in the R_2 position are not cleaved. This explains why liberated angiotensin II is not broken down further by the kininase II.

Table 7 lists the biologically active substrates of kininase II. Of these, bradykinin has a much higher affinity for the enzyme than angiotensin I has, as shown by its lower K_m (see below). BLAIR-WEST et al. (1971) suggested first that after the N-terminal amino acid is removed from angiotensin I, angiotensin III can be formed by the converting enzyme (kininase II). Des-Asp^1-angiotensin I is rapidly cleaved to the heptapeptide, angiotensin III (TSAI et al., 1975; CHIU et al., 1976). This hydrolysis is faster than the conversion of angiotensin I to II, thus a dicarboxylic acid, such as aspartic, can slow down the reaction even if it is located at the N-terminal end. (As mentioned above, the enzyme does not cleave substrates with the C-terminal carboxylic acid). The K_m of des-Asp^1-angiotensin I determined with purified rabbit enzyme is about three times lower than that of angiotensin I. Des-Asp^1-angiotensin I has a broader pH optimum than angiotensin I (TSAI and PEACH, 1977).

The K_m values of the shorter optically active substrates, such as hippuryl derivatives, are in the range of about 10^{-3}–10^{-4} M (YANG et al., 1971; OSHIMA et al., 1974a). K_m values for angiotensin I and bradykinin are much lower although they

Table 7. Naturally occurring substrates of kininase II

Peptide	Bond cleaved	Source of enzyme	Reference
Kinins	-Phe-Ser-Pro-Phe-Arg ↑[a] ↑	Kidney, plasma, lung	ERDÖS and YANG, 1966, 1967 YANG and ERDÖS, 1967 YANG et al., 1970a, 1971 ELISSEEVA et al., 1971 CUSHMAN and CHEUNG, 1971b DORER et al., 1974a
Angiotensin I	-Pro-Phe-His-Leu ↑	Kidney, plasma, lung	SKEGGS et al., 1954, 1956 HUGGINS and THAMPI, 1968 DORER et al., 1970 YANG et al., 1970a BARRETT and SAMBHI, 1971 ELISSEEVA et al., 1971 OPARIL et al., 1971
des-Asp[1]-angiotensin I	-Pro-Phe-His-Leu ↑	Lung, plasma	BLAIR-WEST et al., 1971 TSAI et al., 1975 CHIU et al., 1976
Insulin, B chain	-Pro-Lys-Ala ↑	Lung	IGIC et al., 1972a
Leu[5]-enkephalin	Tyr-Gly-Gly-Phe-Leu ↑	Kidney	ERDÖS et al., 1978a, b
Met[5]-enkephalin	Tyr-Gly-Gly-Phe-Met ↑	Kidney	ERDÖS et al., 1978a, b
BPF_{5a} (SQ 20475) (inhibitor pentapeptide)	-Trp-Ala-Pro ↑	Plasma, lung	YANG et al., 1971 CHEUNG and CUSHMAN, 1973

[a] After bradykinin has been completely inactivated by the removal of C-terminal dipeptide.

vary according to the sources of enzyme used. Angiotensin I has a K_m of the order of 10^{-5} M (ANGUS et al., 1973; DORER et al., 1974a). The K_m of bradykinin is 9×10^{-7} M in presence of chloride ions (DORER et al., 1974a) and 4×10^{-6} M in the absence of these ions. A slightly different figure has been obtained with radioimmunoassay using plasma as a source of enzyme; under these conditions the K_m of bradykinin was 10^{-7} M (ZACEST et al., 1974).

OPARIL et al., (1973) demonstrated that angiotensin analogs containing D-amino acid substitutions in position 8–10 were not converted by the dog lung enzyme and analogs containing D-amino acids in positions 5 and 7 were converted but at a slower rate. ERDÖS and YANG (1966) found that the D-Pro^7 derivative of bradykinin was not cleaved by the renal enzyme.

Longer analogs of bradykinin are cleaved more slowly than the nonapeptide. This was observed in vitro (DORER et al., 1974b), when the rates of hydrolysis of bradykinin, kallidin and Met-Lys-bradykinin by purified enzyme were compared. In the absence of Cl^-, bradykinin was cleaved faster than the two other kinins, but at physiological Cl^- concentrations the differences in the rate of hydrolysis was slight. In contrast, kininase II in human endothelial cells cleaved kallidin and Met-Lys-bradykinin slower than bradykinin even in presence of Cl^- (JOHNSON and ERDÖS, 1977). The 18 amino acid containing polistes kinin is not cleaved by the enzyme at all (RYAN et al., 1970).

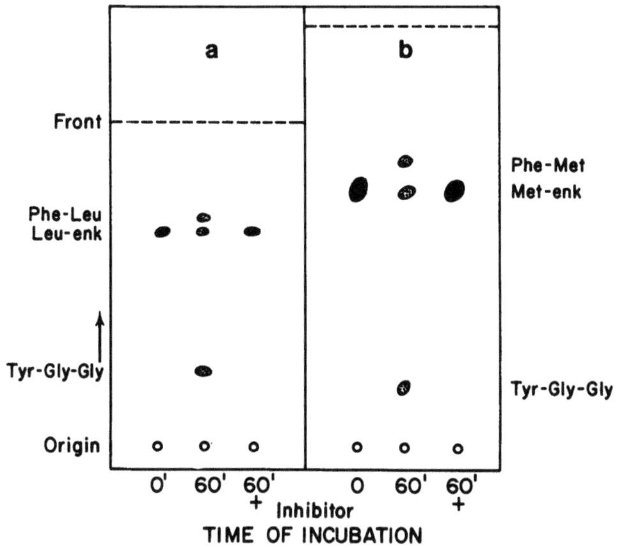

Fig. 6. Hydrolysis of Leu[5]- and Met[5]-enkephalin by purified hog kidney peptidyl dipeptidase (angiotensin I converting enzyme or kininase II) to Tyr-Gly-Gly and Phe-Leu or Phe-Met. The specific inhibitor SQ 14225 (10^{-6} *M*) inhibited the reaction. Peptides were incubated with the enzyme for 60 min in the presence (+) and absence of inhibitor. Panel a: Silica gel t.l.c. plate; solvent: sec-butanol–acetic acid–water (4 : 1 : 5); separation time: 3 h. Panel b: Aluminum oxide t.l.c. plate; solvent: chloroform–methanol–NH_4OH (20 : 20 : 9); separation time: 1.5 h. The plates were sprayed with ninhydrin. (ERDÖS et al., 1978)

When bradykinin was coupled to 500,000 MW soluble dextran it retained 6–29% of its biologic activity and most of its antigenicity, but it was inactivated by kininase II much slower than bradykinin was (ODYA et al., 1978b). Another bradykinin analog, Phe-(α-Me^8)-bradykinin, which had less than 3% of the biologic action of bradykinin was also resistant to purified kininase II (LEDUC et al., 1978). Two other analogs, 8-erythro-β-phenylserine and 8-erythro-α-NH_2-β-phenylbutyric acid bradykinin were also stable to enzymatic degradation (REISSMANN et al., 1975).

Kininase II may have additional important biologic activities by its actions on substrates other than kinins and angiotensin I. In the renin substrate angiotensinogen renin breaks a Leu-Leu bond and thereby releases angiotensin I. Renin releases two products from the synthetic tetradecapeptide substrate, a decapeptide (angiotensin I) and a tetrapeptide. Kininase II cleaves the tetradecapeptide and releases Tyr-Ser, Leu-Val and His-Leu sequentially (DORER et al., 1975) to form the octapeptide, angiotensin II. Kininase II also cleaves the pentapeptide inhibitor BPF_{5a} or SQ 20475 (YANG et al., 1971; CHEUNG and CUSHMAN. 1973) and the B-chain of insulin (IGIC et al., 1972a).

Another important endogenous substrate is enkephalin. Both methionine and leucine enkephalins are cleaved by kininase II (Fig. 6). The rate of hydrolysis approaches that of Bz-Gly-Gly-Gly at the concentration of enkephalin used; (3×10^{-4} *M*; ERDÖS et al., 1978a, b). Thus, cleavage of enkephalins by kininase II in the circulation and in selected areas of the brain may contribute to their short biologic half-life.

IV. Properties of Kininase II

Many of the properties of angiotensin I converting enzyme and kininase II were described in early publications on the basis of studies with crude or partially purified enzyme preparations. Only later were these properties confirmed with the homogeneous enzyme. For example, the requirements for chloride and a metal ion for enzymatic activity were already recognized by SKEGGS et al. (1954, 1956). That kininase II is a membrane-bound protein was observed when the enzyme was detected in the homogenized kidney (ERDÖS and YANG, 1966, 1967). The various purification techniques are summarized on Table 8.

Regardless of the source of the enzyme, kininase II requires a metal ion cofactor and, consequently, it is inhibited by sequestering compounds (ERDÖS and YANG, 1970). As for many other peptidases, Zn^{2+} is the cofactor of the rabbit lung enzyme (DAS and SOFFER, 1975). Zinc probably can be replaced by cobalt or manganese, since after exhaustive dialysis the enzyme can be activated by these ions (YANG et al., 1971; DORER et al., 1970; HUGGINS et al., 1970).

The effect of chloride ions on kininase II depends on the structure of the substrate used (IGIC et al., 1973). The hydrolysis of angiotensin I, Bz-Gly-Gly-Gly and other substrates stops almost entirely in chloride-free medium, but that of bradykinin proceeds at about half of the optimal rate. The cleavage of the pentapeptide inhibitors BPF_{5a} or SQ 20475 (CHEUNG and CUSHMAN, 1973) does not require chloride ions at all. Chloride ion has been described as an allosteric modifier of the enzyme (CHEUNG and CUSHMAN, 1973). Chloride ions lower the K_m and increase the V_{max} of bradykinin with kininase II (DORER et al., 1974a). However, angiotensin I can inhibit the hydrolysis of bradykinin by kininase II even if the medium is low in chloride ions (ALABASTER and BAKHLE, 1973).

When the enzyme is immobilized by coupling it to Sepharose-4B it still cleaves angiotensin I at an appreciable rate in the absence of chloride ions (IGIC et al., 1972a). After studying the UV spectrum of the enzyme in the presence and absence of chloride ions, OSHIMA et al. (1974a) proposed that the enzyme protein could combine with bradykinin in two different configurations, but that it can cleave angiotensin I in only one configuration. Because kininase II is bound to membranes in tissues, we do not know how much its conformation can change in situ.

In addition, the effect of chloride depends on the concentration and on the pH of the incubation mixture (DORER et al., 1976). Chloride ions can be replaced by other monovalent anions, such as acetate or bicarbonate (HUGGINS et al., 1970).

Chloride ions have an additional effect which yet has to be explained. Namely, as mentioned under the subheading of "Specificity", the longer peptide analogs of bradykinin such as Met-Lys-bradykinin or kallidin are hydrolyzed in vitro by kininase II slowery than bradykinin (DORER et al., 1974a) in chloride-free medium.

An interesting observation is that Na_2SO_4 at a very high concentration ($0.6\,M$) accelerates the hydrolysis of Bz-Gly-Gly-Gly. This was attributed to a nonspecific action, to the increase in the dielectric constant of the medium (DORER et al., 1976).

Kininase II contains a carbohydrate moiety. OSHIMA et al. (1974a) estimated an 8% neutral sugar content for the kidney enzyme that was confirmed later by LANZILLO and FANBURG (1976b). SOFFER et al. (1974) estimated the carbohydrate content of the rabbit lung enzyme to be 16%, but this figure was later revised to 26% (DAS and SOFFER, 1975). TSAI and PEACH (1977) estimated 8% hexose content for the

Table 8. Purification of Kininase II

Source of enzyme	Substrate	Purification (-fold)	Specific[a] activity (μmol/min/mg)	Remarks	Reference
Human					
Plasma	Bradykinin	–		Two step purification	ERDÖS and YANG, 1967
Plasma	Labeled angiotensin I	67	0.005	Low purity	LEE et al., 1971d
Plasma	Bz-Gly-His-Leu	101,000	31.4	Hydroxylapatite column gave 187-fold purification because enzyme was not adsorbed	LANZILLO and FANBURG, 1977a
Lung	Labeled angiotensin I	–	–	Ammonium sulfate precipitation and a single gel filtration step used; obtained very high MW product (480,000)	FITZ and OVERTURF, 1972
Lung	Bz-Gly-Gly-Gly	4,560	6.6	The enzyme was solubilized with trypsin	KLAUSER and ERDÖS, to be published
Lung	Bz-Gly-Gly-Gly	–	16.7	Unstable preparation	OSHIMA et al., 1974a
Kidney cortex	Bz-Gly-Gly-Gly	–	11.6	Unstable preparation	OSHIMA et al., 1974a
Lung	Bz-Gly-His-Leu	9,800	13.8	After digestion with trypsin, purification yielded three different MW enzymes. The lowest MW derivative had no mannose and was inhibited differently	NISHIMURA et al., 1977, 1978
Urine	Bz-Gly-His-Leu			Three different MW forms were obtained	KOKUBU et al., 1978
Seminal plasma	Z-Phe-His-Leu	429	0.7	Shows two bands in gel electrophoresis	DEPIERRE et al., 1978
Hog					
Lung, soluble enzyme	Bz-Gly-Gly-Gly	1,380	13.8	Isoelectric point 4.3, after gel filtration detected a dimer of the enzyme	NAKAJIMA et al., 1973

Table 8 (continued)

Source of enzyme	Substrate	Purification (-fold)	Specific activity (μmol/min/mg)	Remarks	Reference
Lung	Bz-Gly-Gly-Gly angiotensin I	1,500	10	The ratio of rates of hydrolysis of the substrates does not change during purification	DORER et al., 1972
Lung, soluble enzyme	Bz-Gly-Gly-Gly	–	–	Homogeneous protein was obtained after prep. electrophoresis which cleaved angiotensin I and bradykinin	IGIC et al., 1972a, c
Plasma	Bz-Gly-Gly-Gly	40	0.05	Partially purified enzyme used as reference	OSHIMA et al., 1974a
Plasma	Labeled angiotensin I	165	0.05	Partial purification	LEE et al., 1971b
Plasma	Angiotensin I	73	0.51	Partial purification	DORER et al., 1970
Kidney cortex, particulate fraction	Bz-Gly-Gly-Gly	161	27	Higher activity than in lung. Isoelectric point 5.2	OSHIMA et al., 1974a
Kidney	Bz-Gly-Gly-Gly	525	31	The enzyme occurs with and without sialic acid	OSHIMA et al., 1976
Bovine					
Kidney cortex		About 1,500		No details of purification given	ELISSEEVA et al., 1971
Kidney cortex	Cbo-Phe-His-Leu	1,600	31	Isoelectric point 4.45	ELISSEEVA et al., 1974a, b
Lung	Cbo-Phe-His-Leu	2,200	29	Activity lower than in renal cortex	ELISSEEVA et al., 1976
Lung, acetone powder of calf lung	Z-Phe(NO_2)-His-Leu	700	1.7	Isoelectric point 4.68, partial purification	STEVENS et al., 1972
Rabbit					
Lung	Bz-Gly-His-Leu	50	1.9	One step purification on a column of coupled substrate	NISHIMURA et al., 1976a
Lung	Bz-Gly-His-Leu		24.3	The enzyme was solubilized with trypsin	NISHIMURA et al., 1976b

Lung, acetone powder	Bz-Gly-His-Leu	22	285	Ratio of rates of angiotensin I and Bz-Gly-His-Leu hydrolysis did not change during purification	CUSHMAN and CHEUNG, 1972
Lung	Bz-Gly-His-Leu	989	89	Contains Zn^{2+}	DAS and SOFFER, 1975
Lung, acetone powder	Bz-Gly-His-Leu	1,302	56	pH optimum with angiotensin I 7.5, with des-Asp[1]-angiotensin I broader (7.5–8.8) MW 180,000	TSAI and PEACH, 1977
Plasma	Angiotensin I	63	8.6 Angiotensin I (μg/h/mg)	Could not separate kininase and converting enzyme activities	UEDA et al., 1971, 1972
Serum	Bz-Gly-His-Leu	57,000	91	Contains three times more sialic acid than lung enzyme. Used antibody affinity column	DAS et al., 1977
Guinea pig					
Lung	Labeled angiotensin I	230	0.01	Partial purification	LEE et al., 1971a
Rat					
Brain	Bz-Gly-His-Leu	100	0.11	Partial purification	BENUCK and MARKS, 1978
Lung, particulate fraction	Bz-Gly-His-Leu	127	17.6	This is essentially a two step purification	LANZILLO and FANBURG, 1974, 1976a
Lung, particulate fraction	Bz-Gly-His-Leu	–	14–21	Homogenate stored for 20 days yielded a low MW (84,000) enzyme	LANZILLO and FANBURG, 1977b
Dog					
Lung	Bz-Gly-His-Leu	1,786	25	Contains 17% carbohydrate	CONROY et al., 1978
Bacteria					
E. coli	α N-DNP-poly--(Pro-Gly-Pro)	1,200	116 (mg/h/mg)	Similar to mammalian enzyme but does not have metal cofactor	YARON et al., 1972
Coryne bacterium equi	Labeled angiotensin I	20	0.04	Has a low MW, 80,000	LEE et al., 1971c

[a] Because of variations in the conditions of assay and substrate concentration, the values can not be compared directly.

rabbit lung enzyme and CONROY et al. (1978) found 17% carbohydrate in the dog lung enzyme. The rabbit lung enzyme also contains fucose, mannose, galactose, N-acetyl-glucosamine, and N-acetylneuraminic acid (DAS and SOFFER, 1975). Rabbit lung and rabbit serum enzyme have similar carbohydrate components except kininase II from serum contains about three times more sialic acid (DAS et al., 1977). The sialic acid content may be necessary to keep the serum kininase in the circulation and prevent its removal by the liver. Kininase II extracted from hog kidney occurs in two forms, with and without sialic acid, but sialic acid can be removed by neuraminidase without affecting catalytic properties (OSHIMA et al., 1976).

The estimates of the MW of kininase II range from 90,000 to 480,000. Initially, in gel filtration kininase II appeared after kininase I was eluted from Sephadex G-200 (YANG and ERDÖS, 1967) indicating a MW lower than that of kininase I, which was later determined to be 280,000 (see above). Because of the high carbohydrate content, kininase II may appear to have a higher MW in gel filtration than determined with other analytical techniques. Values of 300,000 or higher have been reported. Sedimentation studies of partially purified preparations suggested a MW of about 150,000 (LEE et al., 1971a). The MW of the lung and kidney enzyme was estimated to be 195,000–210,000 (OSHIMA et al., 1974a; NAKAJIMA et al., 1973; ERDÖS, 1975) as determined by gel filtration or by electrophoresis in 5% gel.

LANZILLO and FANBURG, however, (1976b) obtained a lower MW in electrophoresis in a higher percentage of polyacrylamide gel. It was also observed by NAKAJIMA et al., (1973) that hog lung enzyme dissociates to subunits after it is denatured under very harsh conditions. LANZILLO and FANBURG (1976b) did not confirm this finding.

DAS and SOFFER (1975) estimated the MW of the rabbit lung enzyme to be 140,000 by electrophoresis in presence of sodium dodecyl sulfate and 129,000 by sedimentation. These authors detected a high and low MW derivative of the enzyme but purified only the low MW variety.

TSAI and PEACH (1977) obtained in gel electrophoresis in 7.5% gel a MW of 180,000 for the rabbit lung enzyme. In the same type of gel the MW of human lung enzyme was estimated to be 200,000 by NISHIMURA et al. (1977).

NAKAJIMA et al. (1973) and OSHIMA et al. (1974a, 1976) purified the low MW derivative of hog lung or kidney enzyme. The high MW complex of the enzyme obtained after gel filtration was probably a dimer which dissociated in urea (NAKAJIMA et al., 1973). Storing rat lung homogenate at 4 °C for a prolonged period (LANZILLO and FANBURG, 1977b) or treating human lung with trypsin (NISHIMURA et al., 1978) yielded the lowest MW enzyme (98,000).

NAKAHARA (1978) found that a fairly high concentration of plasma kallikrein (60 μg) increases kininase II activity in human plasma by 70%. Plasma kallikrein generated two subunits from human plasma kininase II with a MW of 180,000 and 95,000 as estimated by gel filtration. Both subunits were active, they cleaved various substrates. Treatment with other proteolytic enzymes, (trypsin, thrombin or plasmin) inactivated kininase II.

Thus the enzyme extracted with a detergent from tissues and in presence of sodium dodecyl sulfate can have a MW of about 120,000–150,000 (LEE et al., 1971b; DAS and SOFFER, 1975). The MW of the unextracted enzyme and its possible precursor in cells is still not known (FRIEDLAND and SILVERSTEIN, 1978).

V. Antibody to Kininase II

After kininase II was purified to homogeneity it was used to elicit antibodies in rabbits (OSHIMA et al., 1974a). The rabbit antibodies were used to study the identity of the enzyme from different organs and plasma. It was found that the antibody inhibited the hog kininase II of kidney, lung and plasma equally, but not the enzyme from human kidney. Thus, the enzyme appeared to be species but not organ specific. The substrates used to study inhibition by antibody were *t*-Boc-Phe-Phe-Gly, angiotensin I and bradykinin. The cleavage of Bz-Gly-Gly-Gly and Bz-Gly-Gly-His-Leu was inhibited only slightly, less than that of the "bulkier" substrates. It was suggested that the hydrolytic center and the antigenic center in the hog enzyme are different and that the antibodies inhibited by steric interference. The results of the enzyme inhibition experiments were confirmed by immunodiffusion studies. Purified kidney, lung and partially purified plasma kininase II of the hog produced a single precipitin band when reacted with antiserum to hog kidney enzyme. The purified human kidney enzyme did not react with this antiserum. Antibody to human lung enzyme also inhibited the hydrolysis of bradykinin by intact cultured endothelial cells about 50% (JOHNSON and ERDÖS, 1977).

In other studies, as discussed above under the subheading "Distribution of Kininase II", tagged antibodies were used to localize kininase II in endothelial and epithelial cells (RYAN et al., 1976a, b; CALDWELL et al., 1976a; HALL et al., 1976). CONROY et al. (1976) used goat antibody against pure rabbit pulmonary kininase II to discern the homology of enzymes in other species. Immunologically reactive material was found in detergent solubilized extracts of lung particles from rat, guinea pig and dog. No homology was demonstrable with bovine or chicken lung extracts. Antibodies from individual goats varied greatly in extent and specificity of inhibition of heterologous enzyme activity. In experiments done in vitro Bz-Gly-His-Leu was the substrate. The activity of most heterologous enzyme preparations was inhibited 50% or less by 0.5–1 mg IgG fractions. These authors also developed a radioimmunoassay for the enzyme. Then, in experiments done in vivo, antibody was injected into rabbits, where it decreased the hypotensive effect of bradykinin and the hypertensive effect of angiotensin I. Interestingly, all of the animals died in lung injury within 3–6 days after injection (CALDWELL et al., 1976b). In the rabbit, kidney, brain and serum contained kininase II enzymes which were immunologically identical with the lung enzyme. Kininase II in seminal plasma, however, was not completely identical with the lung enzyme immunologically (DAS and SOFFER, 1976). In these experiments an antibody was used which had been purified about 100-fold. The hydrolysis of Bz-Gly-His-Leu was completely inhibited by this protein fraction.

Later it was shown that the degree of homology was much less between the purified rabbit and dog lung enzymes (CONROY et al., 1978), than first estimated with crude extract of dog lung (CONROY et al., 1976). A 65-fold excess of dog enzyme compared to rabbit enzyme was necessary to displace 50% of the radioactive rabbit glycoprotein from its homogeneous immune complex.

VI. Kininase II in Pathological Conditions

Although the level of kininase II is low in normal human plasma, attempts were made to measure changes in enzyme activity in a variety of conditions and to use this parameter as a diagnostic aid (Table 3). However, owing to problems in determining low enzyme activity against a background of high protein concentration and other peptidases, it is difficult to compile absolute values from the literature. The activity of the enzyme in blood increases in sarcoidosis (LIEBERMAN, 1975, 1976; FRIEDLAND and SILVERSTEIN, 1976; FANBURG et al., 1976) but not in some other forms of lung disease, such as tuberculosis. The elevated activity in plasma may originate from the pulmonary lymph nodes of sarcoid patients (SILVERSTEIN et al., 1976a, b). In spite of this, others (FANBURG et al., 1976) doubted that measurement of enzyme level would be useful for establishing or excluding the presence of the disease. In addition, high plasma enzyme activity was reported in leprosy (LIEBERMAN and REA, 1977) and in GAUCHER's disease (LIEBERMAN and BEUTLER, 1976). In GAUCHER's disease the enzyme activity is also elevated in the spleen (SILVERSTEIN and FRIEDLAND, 1977). In these cases, and in sarcoidosis as well, the plasma enzyme is unlikely to originate from endothelial cells, but is probably released by epithelial cells. Kininase II decreased in plasma of chronic asthmatics (MUE et al., 1978). In general, the activity seems to be higher in men than in women (LIEBERMAN, 1975). The enzyme level in blood was reported to decrease in pulmonary neoplasia (ASHUTOSH and KEIGHLEY, 1976) and in patients with shock lung (OPARIL and KATHOLI, 1977) or chronic obstructive pulmonary disease (OPARIL et al., 1976b).

Another condition in which increased enzyme activity was found is hypoxia, which can occur in idiopathic respiratory distress syndrome of the newborn (MATTIOLI et al., 1975) or chronic alveolar hypoxia of experimental animals (MOLTENI et al., 1974). In contrast, BEDROSSIAN et al. (1978) found decreased plasma level in adult respiratory distress syndrome. The activity in arterial and venous blood samples was the same in 12 patients. STALCUP et al. (1978) found a lowered pulmonary clearance of bradykinin in hypoxic dogs, indicating a decreased enzymatic activity. The conversion of angiotensin I also decreased in these animals (LEUENBERGER et al., 1978).

In addition, the release of kininase II was observed when histamine or histamine releasers were perfused through the isolated rat lung (IGIC et al., 1973). The enzyme is also released from the perfused lungs of sensitized rats during anaphylatic shock (ERDÖS et al., 1975). Since the fluid that accumulated within the air space of the lung contained much more activity than the perfusate, presumably kininase II was not released only from vascular endothelial cells but from some other cells in the lung.

VII. Converting Enzymes Which are not Kininases

Several investigators described the existence of different angiotensin I converting enzymes that do not cleave bradykinin. Such enzymes were found in human lung (OVERTURF et al., 1975; BOAZ et al., 1975), guinea pig plasma (GRANDINO and PAIVA, 1974), and in rat submaxillary gland (BOUCHER et al., 1974). The enzyme from the latter source, named tonin, forms angiotensin II from either angiotensin I or from the synthetic tetradecapeptide renin substrate. Tonin has a much lower MW than the peptidyl dipeptidase converting enzyme, or kininase II, and its pH optimum is below neutrality. It is not inhibited by inhibitors of kininase II and it is present in the submaxillary gland and other organs such as the kidney. A tonin-like enzyme occurs in human plasma (DRUILHET et al., 1977). An enzyme that has a higher MW than kininase II has been found in hog and guinea pig plasma; its action becomes apparent only in the presence of added cobalt ions (GRANDINO and PAIVA, 1974). This enzyme releases angiotensin II, but it has no kininase activity. Several forms of another enzyme with properties similar to tonin were obtained from human lung, but its MW was estimated to be an order of magnitude higher (OVERTURF et al., 1975; BOAZ et al., 1975).

VIII. Inhibition in Vitro

Kininase II is inhibited in vitro by numerous compounds (ERDÖS and YANG, 1970; BAKHLE, 1974). Among them are the dipeptides cleaved by the enzyme from angiotensin I or bradykinin such as His-Leu (YANG et al., 1970a, 1971) and Phe-Arg (YANG and ERDÖS, 1967; SANDER et al., 1971) and metal sequestering agents, for example EDTA (SKEGGS et al., 1956) or *o*-phenanthroline (YANG and ERDÖS, 1967; BAKHLE, 1974). Other substrates of kininase II block the conversion of angiotensin I by competing for the enzyme (YANG et al., 1971; SANDER et al., 1971; IGIC et al., 1972a). Structural analogs of angiotensin I modified at various positions in the peptide chain also inhibit the conversion of angiotensin I (NEEDLEMAN et al., 1972), but angiotensin analogs without the N-terminal free carboxyl group are better inhibitors of the enzyme (TSAI and PEACH, 1977). The N-terminal tripeptide portion of bradykinin, Arg-Pro-Pro, is also an inhibitor in vitro (OSHIMA and ERDÖS, 1974). Other peptides that occur naturally in the body can inhibit kininase II. These include angiotensin II (CUSHMAN and CHEUNG, 1971b; ANGUS et al., 1973), angiotensin III (TSAI and PEACH, 1977), insulin, the B chain of insulin (YANG et al., 1971; IGIC et al., 1972a, c; BING et al., 1974; ELISSEEVA et al., 1976), reduced glutathione (IGIC et al., 1972a), and factors in plasma (OSHIMA et al., 1974a; YANG et al., 1971). Kininase II is also inhibited in vitro by the angiotensin II antagonist, Sar^1-Ala^8 angiotensin II (FITZ et al., 1977; CHIU et al., 1976). Some of these compounds inhibit the conversion of angiotensin I in the perfused lung in situ (IGIC et al., 1972a). DAS and SOFFER (1975) studied the inhibition of the enzyme by alanine peptides. The di-, tri- and tetra-alanine peptides inhibit the enzyme competitively to about the same degree. Other peptides, such as those released by collagenase from gelatin, but of known sequence, also inhibit the enzyme in vitro (OSHIMA et al., 1979).

Concanavalin A inhibited guinea pig lung and serum enzyme 35 % at 4×10^{-4} *M* concentration (LANZILLO and FANBURG, 1976a). The mechanism of this inhibition may involve binding to the enzyme at the carbohydrate moiety.

Tranexamic acid and other cyclohexane derivatives inhibit the enzyme but only at a high concentration (SANDER et al., 1972). Phosphates, polycarboxylates and aromatic carboxylates are also inhibitors in 10^{-2} *M* concentration (OSHIMA and NAGASAWA, 1977).

Several substances, including snake venoms (FERREIRA, 1965, 1966), chymotrypsin (EDERY, 1966), and peptides (GLADNER, 1966; HAMBERG et al., 1968) can potentiate the action of bradykinin on isolated organs. Although the mode of action of these potentiators is still not completely understood, much of their activity may be due to inhibition of bradykinin breakdown by kininase II in tissues. (Potentiators and the chemical work leading to the synthesis of potentiators and kininase inhibitors are discussed by STEWART in this volume.) Potentiating peptides extracted from venoms

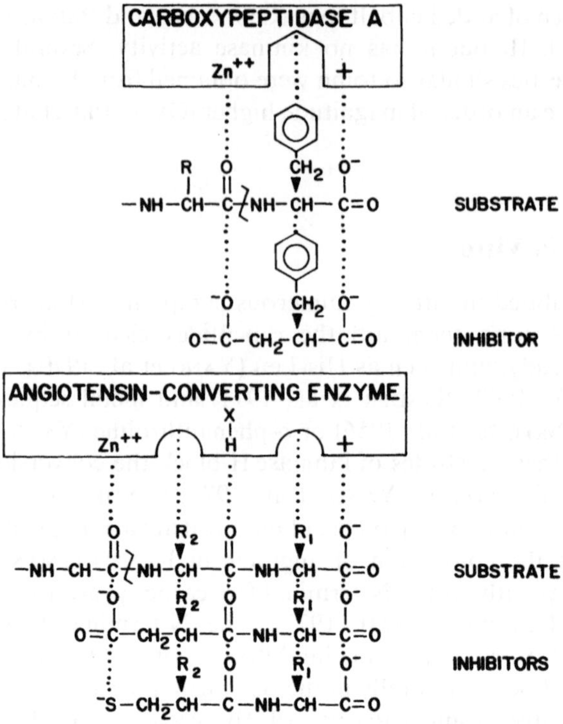

Fig. 7. Diagrammatic model of the active site of carboxypeptidase A and the analogous hypothetical active site of angiotensin-converting enzyme and the proposed binding of substrates and competitive inhibitors. For each enzyme, the known or proposed binding of peptide substrates and competitive inhibitors is indicated. The hexagonal cleft in the model of the active site of carboxypeptidase A represents the hydrophobic pocket of this enzyme; the circular clefts show for angiotensin-converting enzyme represents portions of the active site that interact with substituents R_1 and R_2 of substrates or competitive inhibitors by an undetermined mechanism; X–H represents a hydrogen bonding residue at the active site of angiotensin-converting enzyme. (CUSHMAN et al., 1977)

of Bothrops jararaca and other snakes yielded compounds that inhibited the conversion of angiotensin I as well (BAKHLE, 1968; BAKHLE, 1974; STEWART et al., 1971; FERREIRA et al., 1970; GREENE et al., 1972; KATO and SUZUKI, 1970, 1971). A number of these peptides have been synthesized. The first one was a pentapeptide, BPF_{5a}, SQ 20475 (STEWART et al., 1971; FERREIRA et al., 1970; CUSHMAN et al., 1973) which is a good inhibitor in vitro, but it is also a substrate of the enzyme (YANG et al., 1971; CHEUNG and CUSHMAN, 1973). This peptide is a less effective inhibitor in vivo and has a shorter duration of action than the longer peptide analogs (KRIEGER et al., 1971; ENGEL et al., 1972, 1973; CUSHMAN et al., 1973). The nonapeptide SQ 20881 (BPF_{9a}; teprotide; ONDETTI et al., 1971) and the undecapeptide, "potentiator C", which is constituent of a different type of snake vanom (KATO and SUZUKI, 1971), contain a C-terminal Pro-Pro sequence that is not cleaved by the enzyme. Thus, they inhibit the hydrolysis of bradykinin or angiotensin I without being substrates of the enzyme. The I_{50} values of the peptide inhibitors are low. In concentrations ranging from $10^{-6}\,M$ to $10^{-9}\,M$ (IGIC et al., 1972a; CHEUNG and CUSHMAN, 1973; CUSHMAN et al., 1973), they block 50% of the activity of the enzyme as assayed with short peptide substrates.

Recently ONDETTI et al. (1977) synthesized a compound (SQ 14225, or captopril, 2-thio-3-D-methyl-propanoyl proline) which is the most active inhibitor of kininase II in vitro (CUSHMAN et al., 1977; Fig. 7). This compound is absorbed from the gastrointestinal tract after oral administration. Its K_i is $1.7 \times 10^{-9}\,M$ with Bz-Gly-His-Leu as the substrate. The compound augmented the contractile responses to bradykinin and inhibited those to angiotensin I in the excised ileum (RUBIN et al., 1978). SQ 14225 has a free SH group just as many other inhibitors of kininase II have, including 2-mercaptoethanol, BAL or glutathione (ERDÖS and YANG, 1970; IGIC et al., 1972a). However, this SH group is stable and probably not easily oxidized, even when the drug is given orally. It is linked to proline since peptides with C-terminal proline inhibit kininase II (KATO and SUZUKI, 1970, 1971; CUSHMAN et al., 1973).

The observations that dilution of blood plasma seems to remove an inhibitor of kininase II (YANG et al., 1971) and that the enzyme was inhibited by various endogenous compounds (ERDÖS, 1975, 1976b) led to the search for a blood-borne inhibitor. It was found that albumin inhibits the enzyme in vitro with an $I_{50} = 2 \times 10^{-4}\,M$. Cleaving the albumin molecule and separating 18,000 MW fragment C (sequence 124–298 in human albumin) yielded a more effective noncompetitive inhibitor (KLAUSER et al., 1979). When five of the six bridges were reduced and carboxymethylated, the K_i of this albumin fragment was $3 \times 10^{-6}\,M$. Since concentration of albumin in normal plasma is 5×10^{-4}–$8 \times 10^{-4}\,M$ and albumin is the major protein in various plasma expanders, the inhibition of kininase II by a fragment of albumin is potentially of practical importance. In addition, the albumin fragment inhibits kininase I at a higher concentration than used for kininase II. Inhibition of both kininases may explain some of the hypotensive effect of infused plasma substituents, especially since the preparations may contain bradykinin and prekallikrein activator.

Many investigators have recognized the potential importance of inhibitors such as SQ 20881 or SQ 14227 in the study of kininase II or angiotensin I converting enzyme. Inhibitors have been employed to establish the identity of kininase II with the converting enzyme and to block the conversion of angiotensin I or the inactivation of a kinin. They have been used in laboratory tests to determine whether a substrate is cleaved by kininase II or by contaminating enzyme present in an extract. They have been given to man and to experimental animals to explore the importance of the functions of the enzyme and to specifically block the renin-angiotensin system under a variety of conditions (ERDÖS, 1976b, 1977).

IX. Inhibition of Kininase II in Vivo

Early attempts to inhibit kininases in vivo were summarized in the previous volume (ERDÖS and YANG, 1970). Nine agents, chelators and thio compounds were described as potentiators of the hypotensive effect of kinins in the guinea pig. As mentioned above, guinea pig plasma has the highest level of kininase II and, with hindsight, it can be assumed that this increase in hypotensive effect of kinins after the administration of an inhibitor was due to inhibition of kininase II. (Recently it was suggested that a kininase different from kininase II is inhibited by SQ 20881 in guinea pig plasma in vitro (LEDUC et al., 1978). This enzyme can not be identical with kininase I which is resistant to specific peptide inhibitors of kininase II (IGIC et al., 1972a; PASKHINA et al., 1975).)

It has also been known for quite a while that crude extracts of Bothrops venom potentiated the hypotensive effect of bradykinin in the dog (FERREIRA, 1965, 1966). This finding lead to discovery of potent kininase II inhibitors such as SQ 20881 (see also STEWART this volume).

The first inhibitor from snake venom to be synthetized was the pentapeptide BPF_{5a} or SQ 20475 (STEWART et al., 1971). This compound potentiated the effect of bradykinin, blocked the action of angiotensin I (STEWART et al., 1971), and lowered the increased arterial blood pressure during infusion into rats with renovascular hypertension (KRIEGER et al., 1971). The nonapeptide (teprotide) BPF_{9a} or SQ 20881 had a longer lasting effect than the pentapeptide (ENGEL et al., 1972; BIANCHI et al., 1973; ENGEL et al., 1973; COLLIER et al., 1973) both in man and in experimental animals.

In anesthetized rats, SQ 20881 potentiated the hypotensive effects of bradykinin in a lower dose (less than 0.05 mg/kg, i.v.) than the dose necessary to block the conversion of angiotensin I. The effect on bradykinin metabolism was also longer lasting (ENGEL et al., 1972). SQ 20881 had similar effects in unanesthesized animals (BIANCHI et al., 1973). SQ 20881 has been the prototype inhibitor of kininase II in numerous experiments in vivo. This peptide probably acts by the inhibiting of kininase II present on the surface of the endothelial cells in the pulmonary and in the peripheral vasculature. Experimental evidence for this mechanism was obtained from studies where the nonapeptide (or sometimes the pentapeptide) was given to block the conversion of angiotensin I after i.a. injection in the hind leg (AIKEN and VANE, 1972; BRITTON and DISALVO, 1973), in the renal circulation (DISALVO et al., 1971; BAILIE and BARBOUR, 1975; HOFBAUER et al., 1973a, b), in the isolated perfused lung (IGIC et al., 1972a; BAKHLE, 1971; ALABASTER and BAKHLE, 1972a, b), in the coronary artery (BRITTON and DISALVO, 1973; NEEDLEMAN et al., 1975), and in the splanchnic circulation (TÜRKER and ERCAN, 1975; DISALVO et al., 1973). In addition, it may inhibit the enzyme on the brush border of the proximal tubules and, if administered centrally, it may inhibit kininase II localized in brain nuclei or in the choroid plexus.

Injection of SQ 20881 into anesthetized dogs increased the effect of bradykinin on renal blood flow and prolonged the survival of this kinin during passage through the kidney. The amount of free endogenous kinin increased in the venous blood and in the urine (NASJLETTI et al., 1975). It was assumed that these effects were due to blockage of the inactivation of bradykinin [presumably on the brush border of the proximal tubules (WARD et al., 1976) and on the renal vasular endothelium], although the experiments did not distinguish between the potentiation of the effect of bradykinin and inhibition of the conversion of angiotensin I.

The effect of the inhibitor may depend on the salt intake. In salt-depleted rats, infusion of SQ 20881 resulted in a profound decrease in blood pressure, while producing a negligible effect in salt-loaded animals (THURSTON and LARAGH, 1975). In other studies, a low sodium diet and the administration of the diuretic mercuhydrin reduced the kininase II activity of the dog kidney fourfold (MERRILL et al., 1973).

BAKHLE (1977) used SQ 20881 in the perfused guinea pig and rat lung to establish the contribution of kininase II to bradykinin metabolism. He used bradykinin analogs, 7-homo-Pro- and 8-homo-Phe-bradykinin. The activity of these bradykinin analogs were determined by bioassay. The 8-homo-Phe-bradykinin may be a substrate of lung kininase II in vivo, since its inactivation in the lung was blocked by SQ 20881, although the purified enzyme did not cleave it in vitro (ONDETTI and ENGEL, 1975). BAKHLE suggested that half the activity in guinea pig lung and most of the kininase activity in rat lung is due to enzymes other than kininase II. This supposition is in conflict with the observation of many investigators who found very high kininase II activity in rat lung, although FREER and STEWART (1975) also stated that other kininases were active in the rat lung.

The importance of kininase II and its inhibition of the enzyme was investigated in circulatory shock. SQ 20881, abolished or greatly attenuated the compensatory increase in systemic arterial blood pressure that followed the initial sharp decrease in dogs given endotoxin. In hemorrhagic shock the secondary increase in systemic blood pressure was also significantly lowered by pretreatment with SQ 20881 (ERDÖS et al., 1974). Pretreatment or early postreatment of dogs with SQ 20881 increased the survival rate of the animals in hemorrhagic, but not in endotoxin shock (ERRINGTON and ROCHA E SILVA, Jr., 1976; NEEDLEMAN et al., 1976; MORTON et al., 1977). The beneficial effect of SQ 20881 in shock was attributed to prevention of a severe vasoconstriction in the mesenteric vascular bed that was thought to be responsible for the irreversible hemorrhagic shock. SQ 20881 also blocked intestinal vasoconstriction in cats (MCNEIL, 1974). In these animals vasoconstriction was induced by volume depletion and the effect of vasopressin was abolished by hypophysectomy.

In dogs subjected to hemorrhagic shock the level of angiotensin II in blood rose 20-fold but in the animals pretreated with the inhibitor it rose only twofold. As expected, in the pretreated animals the level of angiotensin I increased as much as 30-fold (MORTON et al., 1977).

Hemorrhagic shock also decreased blood flow to the kidney, possibly by activation of the renin-angiotensin system. Renal angiograms indicated that during hemorrhage the diameter of the main renal artery was reduced by 40% and that the diameters of the intrarenal branches decreased by 70%. Infusion of an inhibitor during decompensation decreased renal vascular resistance and increased the diameter of the renal arteries two to threefold (JAKSCHIK et al., 1974; NEEDLEMAN et al., 1976). YAMASHITA et al. (1977), however, failed to notice any beneficial effects of SQ 20881 on renal perfusion during hemorrhagic shock in dogs.

Possibly the most important application of kininase II inhibitors is in the study of experimental and clinical hypertension. In the dog, acute stenosis of the renal artery increased blood pressure, after the contralateral kidney was excised, and caused renal vasoconstriction. Subsequent administration of SQ 20881 decreased renal vascular resistance and systemic blood pressure (MILLER et al., 1975; AYERS et al., 1974). In chronic experiments in dogs, hypertension was induced by constriction of one renal artery. This form of hypertension was prevented by a constant intravenous infusion of the inhibitor. Single injections of the inhibitor were more effective in the early phase of hypertension than in the later phase, possibly because of the importance of salt and water retention in the maintenance of hypertension (SAMUELS et al., 1976; MILLER et al., 1975). Similar results were obtained in rabbits (ROMERO et al., 1974).

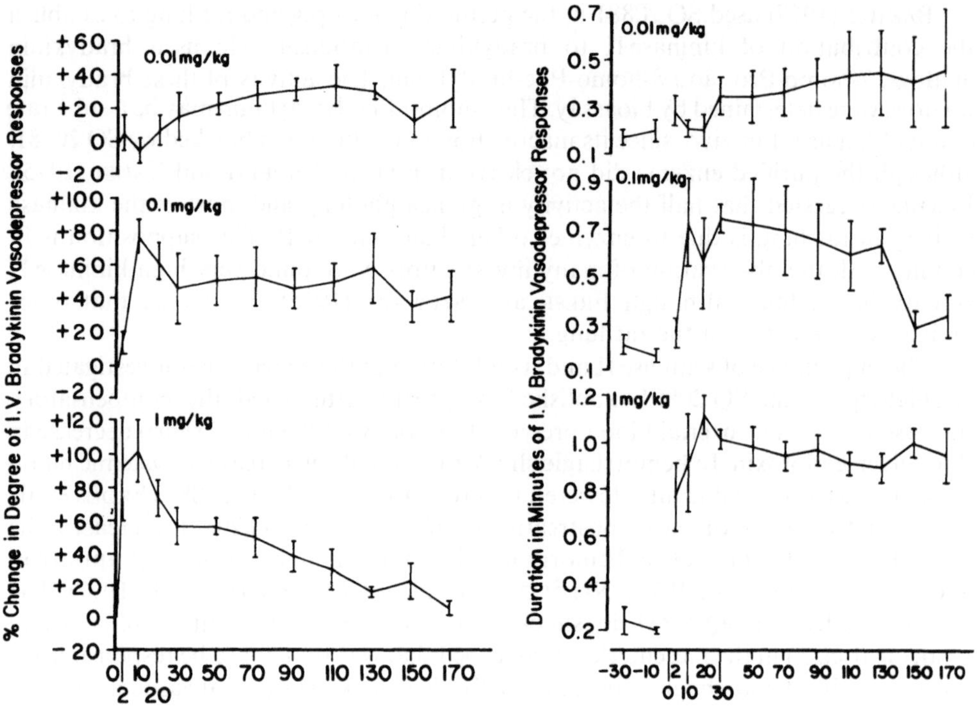

Fig. 8. Changes in degree and duration of i.v. bradykinin (10 µg/kg)-induced vasodepression (decreases in aortic mean blood pressure) by single p.o. doses of SQ 14225 in three groups of four overnight-fasted unanesthetized, normotensive rats. (RUBIN et al., 1978)

Malignant hypertension was also induced in rabbits by unilateral nephrectomy and by clipping the renal artery of the remaining kidney. Long-term administration of SQ 20881 prevented the development of malignant hypertension during the three week duration of the experiments (MUIRHEAD et al., 1974).

In addition to blocking the liberation of angiotensin II, SQ 20881 can inhibit the release of angiotensin III (des-Asp^1-angiotensin II; TSAI et al., 1975). Angiotensinase A removes aspartic acid from the amino terminal end of angiotensin I (KHAIRALLAH and PAGE, 1967). The resulting nonapeptide (des-Asp^1-angiotensin I) can be converted by kininase II to a heptapeptide (angiotensin III) that is biologically active since it can stimulate steroidogenesis in the adrenal cortex (BLAIR-WEST et al., 1971; TSAI et al., 1975).

A more potent inhibitor, SQ 14225 (D-3-mercapto-2-methylpropanoyl-proline or captopril; Fig. 7), was recently tested experimentally and clinically. SQ 14225 blocked the vasopressor effect of angiotensin I in rats (RUBIN et al., 1978) and man (FERGUSON et al., 1977), and prolonged the vasodepressor action of bradykinin (RUBIN et al., 1978; Fig. 8). In the unanesthetized rat, oral SQ 14225 1 mg/kg inhibited the pressor response to angiotensin I 0.3 µg/kg. The compound also potentiated for hours the effect of bradykinin (10 µg/kg) given i.v. in the same type of experiments. SQ 14225 also blocked the hypertensive effects of angiotensin I in dogs, cats and monkeys and in conscious rabbits (MURTHY et al., 1977). Although the inhibitor is active when given orally, it was about eight times more potent when given i.v. SQ 14225 is a more active inhibitor than SQ 20881. SQ 14225, in doses of 3 or 30 mg/kg, lowered the elevated blood pressure of renal hypertensive rats and this effect lasted over 24 h (LAFFAN et al., 1978).

SQ 14225 given per os in experiments lasting 12 days lowered the mean arterial blood pressure in Goldblatt benign and malignant hypertensive rats (BENGIS et al., 1978). The inhibitor increased urinary sodium excretion in both normal and sodium-depleted rats. Two components were observed in the effect of SQ 14225 on the blood pressure. First there is a rapid decrease in the pressure that is proportional to the plasma renin activity in hypertensive rats. Second, in rats with low endogenous renin activity the inhibitor causes a small, but progressive, decrease in blood pressure.

SQ 14225 also lowered the blood pressure in spontaneously hypertensive rats by lowering peripheral vascular resistance. It is assumed that this effect of the inhibitor is exerted through the kinin and not the angiotensin system. The renomedullary system of the kidney could be involved here (MUIRHEAD et al., 1978).

SQ 14225 was also given to conscious sodium-depleted dogs for 14 days (MCCAA et al., 1978). In response to the long-term oral administration (20 mg/kg per day) plasma aldosterone level decreased, plasma renin increased, urinary sodium increased, arterial blood pressure decreased, effective renal plasma flow, glomerular filtration rate and plasma kinin level, and urinary kinin excretion increased while the urinary kallikrein excretion rate dropped (Figs. 9, 10).

MURTHY et al. (1978a) found that SQ 14225 prolonged the hypotensive effect of bradykinin in rabbits less when the kidneys were removed. Indomethacin also decreased the potentiation of bradykinin effect by SQ 14225. These results indicate that part of the prolonged hypotensive effect of bradykinin in the rabbit, after the administration of kininase II inhibitor, is due to renal prostaglandin release by bradykinin.

Possibly the most important application of kininase II inhibitors is in the study of clinical hypertension. After it was established in animals that inhibitors can block the conversion of angiotensin I to II and lower the elevated blood pressure when renin is involved, the clinical investigations began. SQ 20881 was first employed to study the importance of renin in the regulation of normal and elevated blood pressure and to determine the possibility of therapeutic use of the inhibitor. In clinical studies, it was found that the effect of the converting enzyme inhibitor was much longer lasting than that of angiotensin II antagonists such as Sar^1-Ala^8-angiotensin II (GAVRAS et al., 1974; PETTINGER et al., 1975). Unfortunately, both angiotensin antagonists are straight-chained peptides and have to be given intravenously. Since peptides of the MW of SQ 20881 usually have a short half-life in the circulation (min), the long-lasting effect of SQ 20881 may be due to its binding to kininase II. After a single i.v. dose of 4 mg/kg in man the blockade of the enzyme lasted for 16 h. At a dose of 0.5 mg/kg, the effect of inhibitor decreased 50% in 3 h (GAVRAS et al., 1974).

In normotensive subjects, SQ 20881 had no effect on blood pressure. When persons on a normal sodium diet were kept in the supine position, a sudden upright tilting led to renin release (SANCHO et al., 1976). These subjects could compensate for the inhibition of the enzyme, however, without significant hemodynamic changes. In

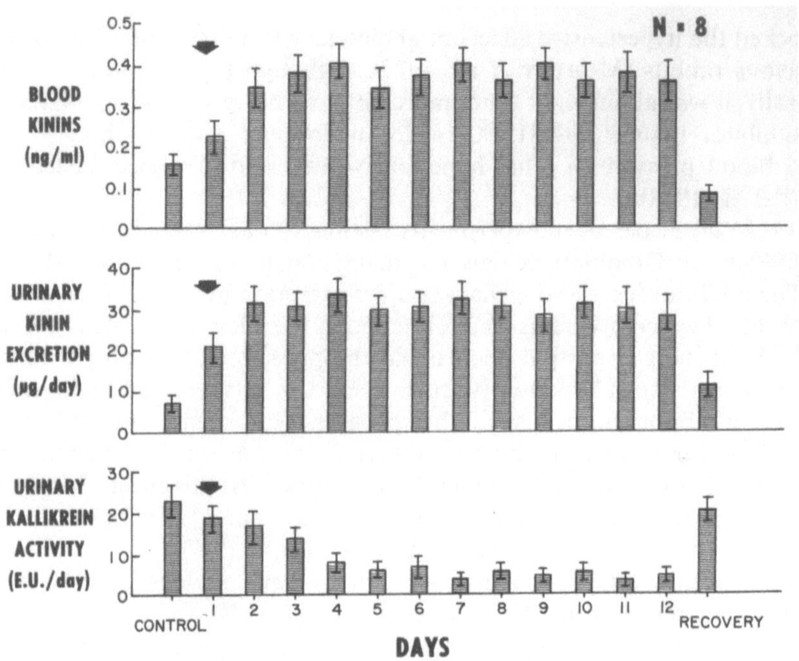

Fig. 9. Response of blood kinins, urinary kinins, and urinary kallikrein activity to long-term oral administration of the inhibitor SQ 14225 at a daily dose of 20 mg/kg in conscious dogs maintained on dietary sodium restriction. Vertical lines indicate ±SE; N indicates number of dogs studied. (According to McCaa et al., 1978)

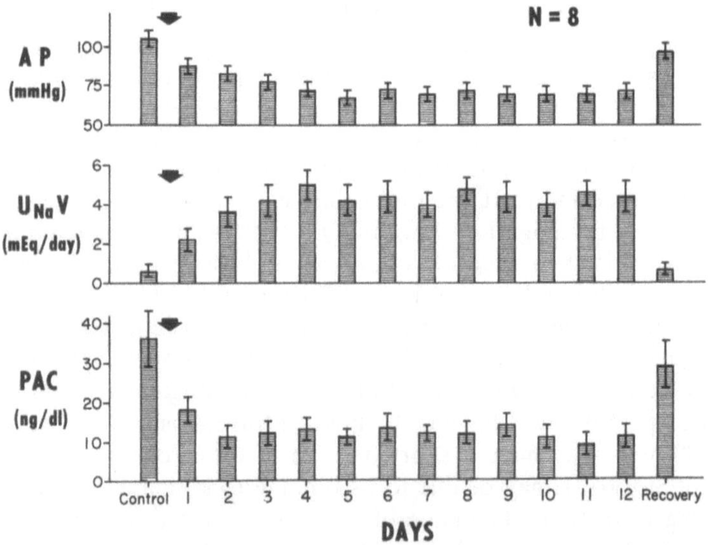

Fig. 10. Response of plasma aldosterone concentration (PAC), urinary sodium excretion ($U_{Na}V$), and arterial blood pressure (AP) to long-term administration of the inhibitor SQ 14225 at a daily dose of 20 mg/kg in conscious dogs maintained on dietary sodium restriction. Vertical lines indicate ±SE; N indicated number of dogs studied. (McCaa, R.E., Hall, J.E., McCaa, C.S., unpublished)

sodium-depleted subjects treated the same way, administration of the inhibitor decreased both the systolic and diastolic blood pressure significantly, whereas the heart rate increased. Four of five subjects in the experiments fainted. The results were taken as an indication that angiotensin II is essential for maintaining the blood pressure in persons depleted of sodium. The inhibitor also blocked the rise in the aldosterone level that accompanied increased renin activity in control subjects.

When the experiments with SQ 20881 were repeated in sodium-depleted individuals with essential hypertension, in contrast to normotensives, only some of the patients developed additional hypotension, when assuming erect position (GAVRAS et al., 1978b).

The effect of SQ 20881 was studied extensively in hypertensive patients. In hypertensive patients with an elevated renin level, SQ 20881 decreased the blood pressure (GAVRAS et al., 1974). The effect was dependent on the dose of inhibitor up to 1 mg/kg administered i.v. Blood pressure was significantly reduced in individuals with renovascular, malignant, and essential hypertension, but not in those with hypertension associated with chronic renal failure. In man, as in rats, the effect of SQ 20881 on the blood pressure was enhanced by sodium depletion. Plasma renin activity increased about threefold and aldosterone decreased to one-third of the preinhibition concentration. SQ 20881 decreased the blood pressure in four of five patients with a normal renin level who had not responded to the administration of the angiotensin II antagonist, Sar^1-Ala^8-angiotensin II.

In another study, SQ 20881 was used as a diagnostic aid in unilateral renal artery stenosis. Because SQ 20881 abolishes the inhibition of renin release by angiotensin II (negative feedback), renin level was higher in the renal venous blood from the afflicted side of patients who received the inhibitor (RE et al., 1978), than in blood from the contralateral side.

GAVRAS et al. (1978a) administered SQ 14225 to 12 patients for 3–24 weeks in oral doses of 400–1000 mg daily. The blood pressure decreased in all patients. Kininase II activity in plasma was reduced to a negligible level. SQ 14225 was effective in this group of patients with essential or renovascular hypertension including subgroups with high, normal, or low plasma renin. At this time SQ 14225 is being tested extensively in several clinical centers.

In clinical as in experimental studies the question arises as to how much of the effect of kininase II inhibitors is due to the blockade of angiotensin II release and how much to inhibition of bradykinin inactivation?

After using SQ 20881 SANCHO et al. (1976) and MILLER et al. (1975) did not find an increase in plasma kinin level in patients or dogs. JAEGER et al. (1978) found no evidence for kinin involvement in normal or spontaneously hypertensive rats after injection of SQ 20881. MURTHY et al. (1978b) took a different position. They assumed that the moderate decrease in arterial blood pressure and the increase in renal blood flow in anesthetized dogs after the administration of SQ 14225 (310 μg/kg, i.v.) may be due either to the loss of endogenous angiotensin II or to an increase in endogenously produced kinin. According to CASE et al. (1976, 1977) the blockade of kinin inactivation by SQ 20881 is not responsible for the effects in hypertensives. WILLIAMS and HOLLENBERG (1977) and WILLIAMS (1977) found that SQ 20881 in normotensives did not raise the plasma level of bradykinin. In hypertensive patients the level of bradykinin rose to 7.4 ng/ml after i.v. administration of SQ 20881 (10 or 30 μg/kg).

They could not determine whether or not some of the changes (such as increase in renal blood flow) were caused by changes in levels of vasoconstrictor or in vasodilator agents.

Recently McCAA et al. (1978) found that the plasma kinin level was elevated after oral administration of SQ 14225 to dogs (Fig. 9). MUIRHEAD et al. (1978) suggested that in the spontaneously hypertensive rats SQ 14225 lowered the blood pressure via kinins.

Because SQ 20881 caused a greater fall in blood pressure in salt-depleted rats than the angiotensin II antagonist, saralasin, it was assumed that potentiation of bradykinin accounts for some of the vasodepressor effects of the inhibitor (THURSTON and SWALES, 1978). GAVRAS et al. (1978c) found that administration of SQ 20881 increased the blood flow in adrenals, brain, kidneys, and heart in dogs with high plasma renin activity. They could not establish whether or not accumulation of bradykinin is the cause of this effect.

Therefore, although kinin levels appear to be elevated after the administration of a kininase II inhibitor to man or experimental animals under certain conditions, it is not possible to accurately assess the contribution of kinins to the overall blood pressure lowering effect.

D. Conversion of Kallidin to Bradykinin

The longer analogs of bradykinin such as kallidin or Met-Lys-bradykinin can be enzymatically converted to bradykinin by the sequential removal of N-terminal amino acids. WEBSTER and PIERCE and ERDÖS et al. found such an enzyme in human plasma in 1963 (for ref. see ERDÖS and YANG, 1970). An enzyme that is probably the same aminopeptidase was purified from human serum by GUIMARAES et al., (1973). This protein, with a MW of 95,000, has a divalent metal ion cofactor and, consequently, it is inhibited by chelating agents. During purification of the enzyme, the aminopeptidase activity increased in parallel with an arylamidase activity. The later was demonstrated with Lys or Arg-β-naphthylamide as substrate. The enzyme was inhibited by *o*-phenanthroline and BAL but not by BPF_{9a} (SQ 20881), the inhibitor of kininase II. The same enzyme was partially purified from human urine (BRANDI et al., 1976). The urinary enzyme as well as the serum and liver enzymes are inhibited by puromycin. The presence of an aminopeptidase that converts kallidin to bradykinin in urine may explain why, although renal and urinary kallikrein release kallidin, urine contains both bradykinin and kallidin (see ERDÖS, 1970, and PISANO, this volume).

A similar aminopeptidase was purified from liver (HOPSU et al., 1966a, b; BORGES et al., 1974) but it is also present in other organs such as kidney or pancreas. This enzyme, which is activated by chloride ions, cleaves Lys^1 from kallidin, but does not hydrolyze the released bradykinin further.

PRADO et al. (1975) studied the conversion of kallidin to bradykinin in the perfused rat liver, where they also observed the inactivation of large amounts of bradykinin. The same organ also converted angiotensin I to II (BORGES et al., 1976).

Others found aminopeptidase activity in oral abscesses and cysts (MÄKINEN and OKSALA, 1973). This enzyme was named aminopeptidase B by HOPSU-HAVU and collaborators (see ERDÖS and YANG, 1970). It cleaves basic N-terminal amino acids, such as Lys[1] in kallidin. The enzyme was found in liver and in erythrocytes (MÄKINEN and MÄKINEN, 1971, 1972) and was purified from rat liver by the same investigators. Very likely both the Brazilian and Finnish groups were studying the same enzyme. A similar aminopeptidase (arylamidase) also occurs in rabbit brain (CAMARGO et al., 1972).

In spite of the presence of aminopeptidase in plasma, probably only a fraction of the circulating kallidin is converted to bradykinin prior to its inactivation by other kininases. Kallidin may be simultaneously a substrate for both the converting aminopeptidase and the inactivating kininases. This idea is supported by the observation that Met-Lys-bradykinin and kallidin injected in vivo act in a quantitatively different manner from bradykinin (see also STEWART this volume). Thus, a complete conversion of kallidin or Met-Lys-bradykinin to bradykinin before acting at a receptor site is unlikely.

E. Functions of Kininases

Kininases, just as other protein components of the kallikrein-kinin system, have functions other than the inactivation of kinins. Although kininase I in blood plasma of man and most animals is the major inactivator of kinins, it also cleaves fibrinopeptides (TEGER-NILSSON, 1968) and anaphylatoxins (BOKISCH and MÜLLER-EBERHARD, 1970). It is tempting to speculate what roles the active subunits of kininase I may have outside the vascular bed, since presumably the higher MW subunit could appear in exudates and the lower one in urine.

There are kininases in brain, but these are different from kininases in other organs. The presence of these inactivators suggests that kinins could have yet unrecognized functions in the CNS.

Kininase II, or the angiotensin I converting enzyme, inactivates kinins and converts angiotensin I to angiotensin II. Thus, the enzyme can inactivate hypotensive kinins and activate hypertensive angiotensin. In addition, it cleaves C-terminal dipeptides from other naturally occurring peptides such as the B chain of insulin and enkephalins. Since the enzyme occurs in many different tissues, it probably has multiple functions which depend on the location in the body and on the animal species. The plasma enzyme probably originates from the endothelial cells of the lung and other vascular beds. Renal lymph contains kininase II which suggests that it is liberated from the kidney. Recent reports on the high level of kininase II in plasma of patients with sarcoidosis indicate that it may also be released by lymph nodes.

Guinea pig plasma has the highest level of kininase II, but dog plasma has only traces of it. This finding suggests a function in the guinea pig. The high level of plasma enzyme may protect guinea pigs from the bronchoconstrictor effect of kinins since this species is particularly sensitive to bronchoconstrictor agents.

The portion of bradykinin released or injected in venous blood which escapes inactivation by plasma kininases (primarily kininase I) is cleaved by kininase II and possibly by some other peptidases present in vascular endothelium of pulmonary blood vessels. Much of the angiotensin I released by venous blood is also converted to angiotensin II by pulmonary endothelium. The portion of angiotensin I that escapes conversion in the lung or angiotensin I released by renin in the arterial blood is cleaved by contact with the vascular endothelial surface in other organs. The same applies to bradykinin, although, in most species, its hydrolysis in circulation is much faster than that of angiotensin owing to the presence of kininase I in blood. Thus, angiotensin is liberated at or close to the sites where it acts, such as the adrenals, hind limb, or kidney. For example the conversion of angiotensin I or des-Asp^1-angiotensin I by the adrenal zona glomerulosa cells releases angiotensin II or III which stimulates biosynthesis of aldosterone in the adrenals (ACKERLY et al., 1977).

The kidney has a very effective system for cleaving angiotensins and kinins that are removed from blood by glomerular filtration. If kinins and angiotensins released intrarenally have important effects on water and sodium metabolism and on prostaglandin release, the kidney must be capable of inactivating these peptides when they enter the nephron from extra-renal sources. Kininase activity in the glomerulus is very low, but kininase II and angiotensinase are highly concentrated on the extensive surface of the brush border of the proximal tubules. This ensures removal of these peptides from the tubular filtrate which eventually reaches the distal tubules. The epithelium of distal tubules and collecting ducts has less enzyme than the proximal tubules, although urine contains kininase activity. At the distal tubule, renal kallikrein interacts with a plasma or tissue kininogen to release renal kinin (see WARD and MARGOLIUS, this volume). The level of kinin at this site can be closely controlled since all traces of extra-renal kinin have been removed. By liberation of kinins within the kidney, kallikrein may alter ion transport and water reabsorption and release prostaglandins in the collecting tubules. Urinary kininases, which include both kininase I and II type enzymes, can inactivate kinins in the distal tubules. Changes in pH of urine could very well influence kinin metabolism, since urinary carboxypeptidase is more effective at an alkaline than at acid pH.

High concentration of kininase II in the brush border of the small intestine suggests additional roles for the enzyme. Bradykinin and angiotensin II may have metabolic functions in the gut, e.g., effects on absorption of glucose, water, and sodium. For example, the enzyme might affect glucose transport negatively and water and sodium transport positively by cleaving kinins and angiotensin I. In addition, digestive enzymes of the pancreas and stomach can release a variety of peptides from ingested proteins. Kininase II can degrade them further to dipeptides. Dipeptidases in the intestinal epithelium could release the single amino acids which are then absorbed. Thus, kininase II could provide substrates for intestinal dipeptidases. This activity may have preceded the metabolism of vasoactive peptides on the evolutionary scale. It will be important to determine whether the chronic oral intake of a kininase II inhibitor affects the metabolic functions of the enzyme. In addition, the intestinal enzyme might bind such an inhibitor and alter its distribution in the body.

The very high activity of kininase II in testicles and in seminal plasma suggests that the enzyme may originate from epithelial cells lining the ducts. Since kallikrein and kallikrein inhibitors are also present in the reproductive system, and since kinins promote sperm motility, the high kininase II in seminal plasma could influence the process of fertilization (see JOHNSON, this volume).

Kininase II in the brain, choroid plexus, and the pituitary gland may release angiotensin II which acts on sympathetic centers and on the drinking reflex (EPSTEIN and SIMPSON, 1974; SEVERS and SUMMY-LONG, 1975). The subfornical body, the site where angiotensin II can elicit drinking, is close to the choroid plexus.

As summarized above kininases have a multiplicity of functions. Their ubiquitous distribution in biologic fluids and tissues implies that they affect numerous biologic activities, in addition to their obvious effects on the circulation.

Support: Some of the experiments described here were supported by NIH, USPHS grant nos. HL 14187, HL 16320, HL 20594 and by a contract from ONR no. N00014-75-C-0807.

Acknowledgements: I am most grateful for the help of Dr. Alice R. JOHNSON, Tess Stewart and Mary Wright. Their collaboration made the writing of this chapter possible.
The figures and tables used in this review were reproduced with the permission of the authors and publishers.

References

Ackerly, J.A., Tsai, B.-S., Peach, M.J.: Role of converting enzyme in the responses of rabbit atria, aortas, and adrenal zona glomerulosa to (des-Asp^1)angiotensin I. Circ. Res. *41*, 231–238 (1977)
Aiken, J.W., Vane, J.R.: The renin-angiotensin system: inhibition of converting enzyme in isolated tissues. Nature *228*, 30–34 (1970)
Aiken, J.W., Vane, J.R.: Inhibition of converting enzyme of the renin-angiotensin system in kidneys and hindlegs of dogs. Circ. Res. *30*, 263–273 (1972)
Alabaster, V.A., Bakhle, Y.S.: Converting enzyme and bradykininase in the lung. Circ. Res. *30/31*, Suppl. II, II-72 – II-84 (1972a)
Alabaster, V.A., Bakhle, Y.S.: The inactivation of bradykinin in the pulmonary circulation of isolated lungs. Br. J. Pharmacol. *45*, 299–310 (1972b)
Alabaster, V.A., Bakhle, Y.S.: The bradykininase activities of extracts of dog lung. Br. J. Pharmacol. *47*, 799–807 (1973)
Angus, C.W., Lee, H.-J., Wilson, I.B.: Substrate specificity of hog plasma angiotensin-converting enzyme. Biochim. Biophys. Acta *309*, 169–174 (1973)
Ashutosh, K., Keighley, J.F.H.: Diagnostic value of serum angiotensin converting enzyme activity in lung diseases. Thorax *31*, 552–557 (1976)
Ayers, C.R., Vaughan, E.D., Yancey, M.R., Bing, K.T., Johnson, C.C., Morton, C.: Effect of 1-sarcosine-8-alanine angiotensin II and converting enzyme inhibitor on renin release in dog acute renovascular hypertension. Circ. Res. *34/35*, Suppl. I, I-27–I-33 (1974)
Back, N., Steger, R.: Kinin-destroying (kininase) activity of cultured rodent fibroblasts L-929. Proc. Soc. Exp. Biol. Med. *153*, 175–179 (1976)
Bailie, M.D., Barbour, J.A.: Effect of inhibition of peptidase activity on distribution of intrarenal blood flow. Am. J. Physiol. *228*, 850–853 (1975)
Bakhle, Y.S.: Conversion of angiotensin I to angiotensin II by cell-free extracts of dog lung. Nature *220*, 919–921 (1968)
Bakhle, Y.S.: Inhibition of angiotensin I converting enzyme by venom peptides. Br. J. Pharmacol. *43*, 252–254 (1971)
Bakhle, Y.S.: Converting enzyme in vitro measurement and properties. In: Handbook of Experimental Pharmacology. Page, I.H., Bumpus, F.M. (eds.), Vol. XXXVII pp. 41–80. Berlin, Heidelberg, New York: Springer 1974
Bakhle, Y.S.: Pulmonary metabolism of bradykinin analogues and the contribution of angiotensin converting enzyme to bradykinin inactivation in isolated lungs. Br. J. Pharmacol. *159*, 123–128 (1977)
Bakhle, Y.S., Reynard, A.M.: Characteristics of the angiotensin I converting enzyme from dog lung. Nature New Biol. *229*, 187–189 (1971)
Bakhle, Y.S., Vane, J.R.: Pharmacokinetic function of the pulmonary circulation. Physiological Rev. *54*, 1007–1045 (1974)
Barrett, J.D., Sambhi, M.P.: Pulmonary activation and degradation of angiotensin I: a dual enzyme system. Res. Commun. Chem. Pathol. Pharmacol. *2*, 128–145 (1971)
Bedrossian, C.W.M., Woo, J., Miller, W.C., Cannon, D.C.: Decreased angiotensin-converting enzyme in the adult respiratory distress syndrome. Am. J. Clin. Pathol. *70*, 244–247 (1978)

Bengis, R.G., Coleman, T.G., Young, D.B., McCaa, R.E.: Long-term blockade of angiotensin formation in various normotensive and hypertensive rat models using converting enzyme inhibitor (SQ 14225). Circ. Res. *43*, Suppl. I, 145–153 (1978)
Benuck, M., Marks, N.: Subcellular localization and partial purification of a chloride dependent angiotensin-I converting enzyme from rat brain. J. Neurochem. *30*, 729–734 (1978)
Bianchi, A., Evans, D.B., Cobb, M., Peschka, M.T., Schaeffer, T.R., Laffan, R.J.: Inhibition by SQ 20881 of vasopressor response to angiotensin I in conscious animals. Eur. J. Pharmacol. *23*, 90–96 (1973)
Bielawiec, M., Bogdanikowa, B., Kiersnowska-Rogowska, B., Lukjan, H.: Studies on the kininogenic system in the supernatant of leukocyte cultures. Arch. Immunol. Ther. Exp. *22*, 369–373 (1974)
Bing, J., Poulsen, K., Markussen, J.: The ability of various insulins and insulin fragments to inhibit the angiotensin I converting enzyme. Acta Pathol. Microbiol. Scand. [A] *82*, 777–782 (1974)
Biron, P., Campeau, L., David, P.: Fate of angiotensin I and II in the human pulmonary circulation. Am. J. Cardiol. *24*, 544–547 (1969)
Biron, P., Campeau, L.: Pulmonary and extrapulmonary fate of angiotensin I. Rev. Can. Biol. *30*, 27–34 (1971)
Biron, P., Huggins, C.G.: Pulmonary activation of synthetic angiotensin I. Life Sci. *7*, 965–970 (1968)
Blair-West, J.R., Coghlan, J.P., Denton, D.A., Funder, J.W., Scoggins, B.A., Wright, R.D.: The effect of the heptapeptide (2–8) and hexapeptide (3–8) fragments of angiotensin II on aldosterone secretion. J. Clin. Endocrinol. Metab. *32*, 575–578 (1971)
Boaz, D., Wyatt, S., Fitz, A.: Angiotensin I (Phe^8-His^9) hydrolase – studies with renin substrates. Biochem. Biophys. Res. Commun. *63*, 490–495 (1975)
Bokisch, V.A., Müller-Eberhard, H.J., Cochrane, C.G.: Isolation of a fragment (C3a) of the third component of human complement containing anaphylatoxin and chemotactic activity and description of an anaphylatoxin inactivator of human serum. J. Exp. Med. *129*, 1109–1130 (1969)
Bokisch, V.A., Müller-Eberhard, H.J.: Anaphylatoxin inactivator of human plasma: its isolation and characterization as a carboxypeptidase. J. Clin. Invest. *49*, 2427–2436 (1970)
Borges, D.R., Prado, J.L., Guimaraes, J.A.: Characterization of a kinin-converting arylamino-peptidase from human liver. N.S. Arch. Pharmacol. *281*, 403–414 (1974)
Borges, D.R., Limaos, E.A., Prado, J.L., Camargo, A.C.M.: Catabolism of vasoactive polypeptides by perfused rat liver. N.S. Arch. Pharmacol. *295*, 33–40 (1976)
Boucher, R., Asselin, J., Genest, J.: A new enzyme leading to the direct formation of angiotensin II. Circ. Res. *34/35*, Suppl. I, I-203–I-209 (1974)
Brandi, C.M., Prado, E.S., Prado, M.J.B.A., Prado, J.L.: Kinin-converting aminopeptidase from human urine partial purification and properties. Int. J. Biochem. *7*, 335–341 (1976)
Brantner, H.: Enzymuntersuchungen an einem onkolytisch wirkenden Clostridium-Stamm (Cl. butyricum-Stamm M_{55}). Zentralbl. Bakteriol. [Orig. A] *220*, 432–434 (1972)
Brecher, P.I., Tercyak, A., Gavras, H., Chobanian, A.V.: Angiotensin-converting enzyme activity in cerebral microvessels. Fed. Proc. *37*, 603 (1978)
Britton, S., Di Salvo, J.: Effects of angiotensin I and angiotensin II on hindlimb and coronary vascular resistance. Am. J. Physiol. *225*, 1226–1231 (1973)
Caldwell, P.R.B., Seegal, B.C., Hsu, K.C., Das, M., Soffer, R.L.: Angiotensin-converting enzyme: vascular endothelial localization. Science *191*, 1050–1051 (1976a)
Caldwell, P.R.B., Wigger, H.J., Das, M., Soffer, R.L.: Angiotensin-converting enzyme: effect of antienzyme antibody in vivo. FEBS Letters *63*, 82–84 (1976b)
Camargo, A.C.M., Graeff, F.G.: Subcellular distribution and properties of the bradykinin inactivation system in rabbit brain homogenates. Biochem. Pharmacol. *18*, 548–549 (1969)
Camargo, A.C.M., Ramalho-Pinto, F.J., Greene, L.J.: Brain peptidases: conversion and inactivation of kinin hormones. J. Neurochem. *19*, 37–49 (1972)
Camargo, A.C.M., Shapanka, R., Greene, L.J.: Preparation, assay, and partial characterization of a neutral endopeptidase from rabbit brain. Biochemistry *12*, 1838–1844 (1973)

Carmel, A., Yaron, A.: An intramolecularly quenched fluorescent tripeptide as a fluorogenic substrate of angiotensin-I-converting enzyme and of bacterial dipeptidyl carboxypeptidase. Eur. J. Biochem. *87*, 265–273 (1978)
Carone, F.A., Pullman, T.N., Oparil, S., Nakamura, S.: Micropuncture evidence of rapid hydrolysis of bradykinin by rat proximal tubule. Am. J. Physiol. *230*, 1420–1424 (1976)
Carriere, S., Biron, P.: Effect of angiotensin I on intrarenal blood flow distribution. Am. J. Physiol. *219*, 1642–1646 (1970)
Case, D.B., Wallace, J.M., Keim, H.J., Weber, M.A., Drayer, J.I.M., White, R.P., Sealey, J.E., Laragh, J.H.: Estimating renin participation in hypertension: superiority of converting enzyme inhibitor over saralasin. Am. J. Med. *61*, 790–796 (1976)
Case, D.B., Wallace, J.M., Keim, H.J., Weber, M.A., Sealey, J.E., Laragh, J.H.: Possible role of renin in hypertension as suggested by renin-sodium profiling and inhibition of converting enzyme. N. Engl. J. Med. *296*, 641–646 (1977)
Cheung, H.S., Cushman, D.W.: Inhibition of homogeneous angiotensin-converting enzyme of rabbit lung by synthetic venom peptides of Bothrops jararaca. Biochim. Biophys. Acta *293*, 451–463 (1973)
Chiu, A.T., Ryan, J.W., Stewart, J.M., Dorer, F.E.: Formation of angiotensin III by angiotensin-converting enzyme. Biochem. J. *155*, 189–192 (1976)
Cicilini, M.A., Caldo, H., Berti, J.D., Camargo, A.C.M.: Rabbit tissue peptidases that hydrolyse the peptide hormone bradykinin. Biochem. J. *163*, 433–439 (1977)
Collier, J.G., Robinson, B.F., Vane, J.R.: Reduction of pressor effects of angiotensin I in man by synthetic nonapeptide (B.P.P.$_{9a}$ or SQ 20,881) which inhibits converting enzyme. Lancet *1*, 72–74 (1973)
Collier, J.G., Robinson, B.F.: Comparison of effects of locally infused angiotensin I and II on hand veins and forearm arteries in man: evidence for converting enzyme activity in limb vessels. Clin. Sci. Mol. Med. *47*, 189–192 (1974)
Conroy, J.M., Hartley, J.L., Soffer, R.L.: Canine pulmonary angiotensin-converting enzyme physicochemical, catalytic and immunological properties. Biochim. Biophys. Acta *524*, 403–412 (1978)
Conroy, J.M., Hoffman, H., Kirk, E. S., Hirzel, H.O., Sonnenblick, E.H., Soffer, R.L.: Pulmonary angiotensin-converting enzyme. Interspecies homology and inhibition by heterologous antibody in vivo. J. Biol. Chem. *251*, 4828–4832 (1976)
Conroy, J.M., Lai, C.Y.: A rapid and sensitive fluorescence assay for angiotensin-converting enzyme. Anal. Biochem. *87*, 556–561 (1978)
Corbin, N.C., Hugli, T.E., Müller-Eberhard, H.J.: Serum carboxypeptidase B: a spectrophotometric assay using protamine as substrate. Anal. Biochem. *73*, 41–51 (1976)
Cushman, D.W., Cheung, H.S.: A simple substrate for assay of dog lung angiotensin converting enzyme. Fed. Proc. *28*, 799 (1969)
Cushman, D.W., Cheung, H.S.: Concentrations of angiotensin-converting enzyme in tissues of the rat. Biochim. Biophys. Acta *250*, 261–265 (1971a)
Cushman, D.W., Cheung, H.S.: Spectrophotometric assay and properties of the angiotensin-converting enzyme of rabbit lung. Biochem. Pharmacol. *20*, 1637–1648 (1971b)
Cushman, D.W., Cheung, H.S.: Studies in vitro of angiotensin-converting enzyme of lung and other tissues. In: Hypertension '72. Genest, J., Koiw, E. (eds.), pp. 532–541. Berlin, Heidelberg, New York: Springer 1972
Cushman, D.W., Pluscec, J., Williams, N.J., Weaver, E.R., Sabo, E.F., Kocy, O., Cheung, H.S., Ondetti, M.A.: Inhibition of angiotensin-converting enzyme by analogs of peptides from Bothrops jararaca venom. Experientia *29*, 1032–1035 (1973)
Cushman, D.W., Cheung, H.S., Sabo, E.F., Ondetti, M.A.: Design of potent competitive inhibitors of angiotensin-converting enzyme. Carboxyalkanoyl and mercaptoalkanoyl amino acids. Biochemistry *16*, 5484–5491 (1977)
Damas, J.: L'activité kininasique du liquide céphalo-rachidien de l'Homme, in vitro. C.R. Soc. Biol. *163*, 2478–2483 (1969)
Das, M., Hartley, J.L., Soffer, R.L.: Serum angiotensin-converting enzyme. Isolation and relationship to the pulmonary enzyme. J. Biol. Chem. *252*, 1316–1319 (1977)
Das, M., Soffer, R.L.: Pulmonary angiotensin-converting enzyme. Structural and catalytic properties. J. Biol. Chem. *250*, 6762–6768 (1975)

Das, M., Soffer, R.L.: Pulmonary angiotensin-converting enzyme antienzyme antibody. Biochemistry *15*, 5088–5094 (1976)
Dearnley, C.N., Bailey, G.S.: Subcellular distribution of kininase activity in pig liver. Biochem. Soc. Transact. *4*, 697–698 (1976)
Dedichen, J., Vystyd, J.: Kininase activity of plasma from patients with arteriosclerosis, diabetes and hepatitis. Scand. J. Clin. Lab. Invest. *107*, 125–127 (1969)
Delhaye, C., Reuse, J.J., Driessche, R.V.: Présence du système bradykininogène – bradykinine – bradykininase dans le liquide amniotique humain. Arch. Int. Pharmacodyn. Ther. *179*, 486–489 (1969)
Depierre, D., Bargetzi, J.-P., Roth, M.: Dipeptidyl carboxypeptidase from human seminal plasma. Biochim. Biophys. Acta. *523*, 469–476 (1978)
Depierre, D., Roth, M.: Activity of a dipeptidyl carboxypeptidase (Angiotensin converting enzyme) in lungs of different animal species. Experientia *28*, 154 (1972)
Depierre, D., Roth, M.: Fluorimetric determination of dipeptidyl carboxypeptidase (angiotensin-I-converting enzyme). Enzyme *19*, 65–70 (1975)
Disalvo, J., Britton, S., Galvas, P., Sanders, T.W.: Effects of angiotensin I and angiotensin II on canine hepatic vascular resistance. Circ. Res. *32*, 85–92 (1973)
Disalvo, J., Peterson, A., Montefusco, C., Menta, M.: Intrarenal conversion of angiotensin I to angiotensin II in the dog. Circ. Res. *29*, 398–406 (1971)
Donaldson, V.H.: Bradykinin inactivation by rabbit serum and butylated hydroxyanisole. J. Appl. Physiol. *35*, 880–883 (1973)
Dorer, F.E., Skeggs, L.T., Kahn, J.R., Lentz, K.E., Levine, M.: Angiotensin converting enzyme: Method of assay and partial purification. Anal. Biochem. *33*, 102–113 (1970)
Dorer, F. E., Kahn, J.R., Lentz, K.E., Levine, M., Skeggs, L.T.: Purification and properties of angiotensin-converting enzyme from hog lung. Circ. Res. *31*, 356–366 (1972)
Dorer, F.E., Kahn, J.R., Lentz, K.E., Levine, M., Skeggs, L.T.: Hydrolysis of bradykinin by angiotensin-converting enzyme. Circ. Res. *34*, 824–827 (1974a)
Dorer, F.E., Kahn, J.R., Lentz, K.E., Levine, M., Skeggs, L.T.: Formation of angiotensin II from tetradecapeptide renin substrate by angiotensin-converting enzyme. Biochem. Pharmacol. *24*, 1137–1139 (1975)
Dorer, F.E., Kahn, J.R., Lentz, K.E., Levine, M., Skeggs, L.T.: Kinetic properties of pulmonary angiotensin-converting enzyme. Hydrolysis of hippurylglycylglycine. Biochim. Biophys. Acta *429*, 220–228 (1976)
Dorer, F.E., Ryan, J.W., Stewart, J.M.: Hydrolysis of bradykinin and its higher homologues by angiotensin-converting enzyme. Biochem. J. *141*, 915–917 (1974b)
Druilhet, R.E., Overturf, M., Kirkendall, W.M.: Action of a human plasma fraction on tetradecapeptide, angiotensin I and angiotensin II. Life Sci. *20*, 1213–1226 (1977)
Edery, H.: Sensitization of smooth muscle to the action of plasma kinins by chymotrypsin. In: Hypotensive peptides. Erdös, E.G., Back, N., Sicuteri, F. (eds.), pp. 341–343. New York: Springer 1966
Elisseeva, Y.E., Orekhovich, V. N., Pavlikhina, L.V., Alexeenko, L.P.: Carboxycathepsin – A key regulatory component of two physiological systems involved in regulation of blood pressure. Clin. Chim. Acta *31*, 413–419 (1971)
Elisseeva, J.J., Orekhovich, V.N., Pavlikhina, L.V.: Properties and specificity of carboxycathepsin (peptidyl-dipeptidase) from bovine kidney. Voprosy Med. Khimii. *22*, 81–89 (1974a)
Elisseeva, Y.E., Orekhovich, V.N., Pavlikhina, L.V.: Isolation and properties of carboxycathepsin (peptidyl-dipeptidase) from bovine lung tissue. Biochemistry (Trans. of Biokhimiya) *41*, 417–422 (1976)
Elisseeva, Y.E., Pavlikhina, L.V., Orekhovich, V.N.: Isolation of carboxycathepsin (peptidyl dipeptidase 3.4.15.1) from beef kidneys. Doklady Akademii Nauk SSSR *217*, 953–956 (1974b)
Engel, S.L., Schaeffer, T.R., Gold, B.I., Rubin, B.: Inhibition of pressor effects of angiotensin I and augmentation of depressor effects of bradykinin by synthetic peptides. Proc. Soc. Exp. Biol. Med. *140*, 240–244 (1972)
Engel, S.L., Schaeffer, T.R., Waugh, M.H., Rubin, B.: Effects of the nonapeptide SQ 20881 on blood pressure of rats with experimental renovascular hypertension. Proc. Soc. Exp. Biol. Med. *143*, 483–487 (1973)

Epstein, A.N., Simpson, J.B.: The dipsogenic action of angiotensin. Acta Physiol. Lat. Am. *24*, 405–409 (1974)
Erdös, E.G.: Enzymes that inactivate polypeptides. In: Metabolic Factors Controlling Duration of Drug Action. Brodie, B.B., Erdös, E.G. (eds.), pp. 159–178. New York: Pergamon Press 1962
Erdös, E.G.: Urinary kinin and colostrokinin. In: Handbook of Experimental Pharmacology. Erdös, E.G. (ed.), Vol. XXV, pp. 579–584. Berlin, Heidelberg, New York: Springer 1970
Erdös, E.G.: Angiotensin I converting enzyme. (Brief review.) Circ. Res. *36*, 247–255 (1975)
Erdös, E.G.: The kinins – A status report. Biochem. Pharmacol. *25*, 1563–1569 (1976a)
Erdös, E.G.: Conversion of angiotensin I to angiotensin II. Am. J. Med. *60*, 749–759 (1976b)
Erdös, E.G.: The angiotensin I converting enzyme. Fed. Proc. *36*, 1760–1768 (1977)
Erdös, E.G., Johnson, A.R., Boyden, N.T.: Inactivation of enkephalins: effect of purified peptidyl dipeptidase and cultured human endothelial cells. "Endorphins". In: Advances in biochemical psychopharmacology. Costa, E., Trabucchi, M. (eds.), Vol. 18, pp. 45–49. New York: Raven Press 1978a
Erdös, E.G., Johnson, A.R., Boyden, N.T.: Hydrolysis of enkephalin by cultured human endothelial cells and by purified peptidyl dipeptidase. Biochem. Pharm. *27*, 843–848 (1978b)
Erdös, E.G., Johnson, A.R., Robinson, C.J.G.: Release of angiotensin I converting enzyme from the shocked rat lung. Circulation *52*, II–88 (1975)
Erdös, E.G., Marinkovic, D.M., Ward, P.E., Mills, I.H.: Characterization of urinary kininase. Fed. Proc. *37*, 657 (1978c)
Erdös, E.G., Massion, W.H., Downs, D.R., Gecse, A.: Effect of angiotensin I converting enzyme inhibitor in shock. Proc. Soc. Exp. Biol. Med. *145*, 948–951 (1974)
Erdös, E.G., Nakajima, T., Oshima, G., Gecse, A., Kato, J.: Kininases and their interaction with other systems. In: Chemistry and Biology of the Kallikrein-kinin System in Health and Disease. Pisano, J.F., Austen, K.F. (eds.). DHEW Publication No. NIH 76-791, pp. 277–285 (1976)
Erdös, E.G., Renfrew, A.G., Sloane, E.M., Wohler, J.R.: Enzymatic studies on bradykinin and similar peptides. Ann. N.Y. Acad. Sci. *104*, 222–234 (1963)
Erdös, E.G., Sloane, E.M.: An enzyme in human blood plasma that inactivates bradykinin and kallidins. Biochem. Pharmacol. *11*, 585–592 (1962)
Erdös, E.G., Wohler, I.M., Levine, M.I., Westerman, M.P.: Carboxypeptidase in blood and other fluids. Values in human blood in normal and pathological conditions. Clin. Chim. Acta. *11*, 39–43 (1965)
Erdös, E.G., Yang, H.Y.T.: Inactivation and potentiation of the effects of bradykinin. In: Hypotensive peptides. Erdös, E.G., Back, B., Sicuteri, F. (eds.), pp. 235–250. Berlin, Heidelberg, New York: Springer 1966
Erdös, E.G., Yang, H.Y.T.: An enzyme in microsomal fraction of kidney that inactivates bradykinin. Life Sci. *6*, 569–574 (1967)
Erdös, E.G., Yang, H.Y.T., Tague, L.L., Manning, N.: Carboxypeptidase in blood and other fluids. III. The esterase activity of the enzyme. Biochem. Pharmacol. *16*, 1287–1297 (1967)
Erdös, E.G., Yang, H.Y.T.: Kininases. In: Handbook of Experimental Pharmacology. Erdös, E.G. (ed.), Vol. XXV, pp. 289–323. Berlin, Heidelberg, New York: Springer 1970
Errington, M.L., Rocha e Silva, M.: On the role of vasopressin and angiotensin in the development of irreversible haemorrhagic shock. J. Physiol. *242*, 119–141 (1974)
Fanburg, B.L., Schoenberger, M.D., Bachus, B., Snider, G.L.: Elevated serum angiotensin I converting enzyme in sarcoidosis. Am. Rev. Resp. Dis. *114*, 525–528 (1976)
Ferguson, R.K., Brunner, H.R., Turini, G.A., Gavras, H., McKinstry, D.N.: A specific orally active inhibitor of angiotensin-converting enzyme in man. Lancet *1*, 775–778 (1977)
Fernandez, H.N., Hugli, T.E.: Partial characterization of human C5a anaphylatoxin. I. Chemical description of the carbohydrate and polypeptide portions of human C5a. J. Immunol. *117*, 1688–1694 (1976)
Ferreira, S.H.: A bradykinin-potentiating factor (BPF) present in the venom of Bothrops jararaca. Br. J. Pharmacol. *24*, 163–169 (1965)
Ferreira, S.H.: Bradykinin-potentiating factor. In: Hypotensive Peptides. Erdös, E.G., Back, N., Sicuteri, F. (eds.), pp. 356–367. New York: Springer 1966

Ferreira, S.H., Bartelt, D.C., Greene, L.J.: Isolation of bradykinin-potentiating peptides from Bothrops jararaca venom. Biochemistry *9*, 2583–2593 (1970)
Ferreira, S.H., Vane, J.R.: The disappearance of bradykinin and eledoisin in the circulation and vascular beds of the cat. Br. J. Pharmacol. Chemother. *30*, 417–424 (1967)
Filipović, N., Mijanovic, M., Igic, R.: A simple spectrophotometric method for estimation of plasma angiotensin I converting enzyme activity. Clin. Chim. Acta *88*, 173–175 (1978)
Fitz, A., Overturf, M.: Molecular weight of human angiotensin I lung converting enzyme. J. Biol. Chem. *247*, 581–584 (1972)
Fitz, A., Wyatt, S., Boaz, D., Fox, B.: Peptide inhibitors of converting enzyme. Life Sci. *21*, 1179–1186 (1977)
Folk, J.E., Piez, K.A., Carroll, W.R., Gladner, J.A.: Carboxypeptidase B. IV. Purification and characterization of the porcine enzyme. J. Biol. Chem. *235*, 2272–2277 (1960)
Franklin, W.G., Peach, M.J., Gilmore, J.P.: Evidence for the renal conversion of angiotensin I in the dog. Circ. Res. *27*, 321–324 (1970)
Freer, R.J., Stewart, J.M.: In vivo pulmonary metabolism of bradykinin, angiotensin I and 5-hydroxytryptamine in the rat. Arch. Int. Pharmacodyn. Ther. *217*, 97–109 (1975)
Frey, E.K., Kraut, H., Werle, E., Vogel, R., Zickgraf-Rüdel, G., Trautschold, I.: Das Kallikrein-Kinin-System und seine Inhibitoren. Stuttgart: Enke 1968
Friedland, J., Silverstein, E.: Similarity in some properties of serum angiotensin converting enzyme from sarcoidosis patients and normal subjects. Biochem. Med. *15*, 178–185 (1976)
Friedland, J., Silverstein, E.: Sensitive fluorimetric assay for serum angiotensin-converting enzyme with the natural substrate angiotensin I. Am. J. Clin. Pathol. *68*, 225–228 (1977)
Friedland, J., Setton, C., Silverstein, E.: Angiotension converting enzyme: induction by steroids in rabbit alveolar macrophages in culture. Science *197*, 64–65 (1977)
Friedland, J., Silverstein, E.: Angiotensin converting enzyme (ACE): apparent identity of rabbit macrophage and lung enzymes and proteolytic processing of predominant large cellular to small extracellular form. Fed. Proc. *37*, 1332 (1978)
Friedland, J., Setton, C., Silverstein, E.: Induction of angiotensin converting enzyme in human monocytes in culture. Biochem. Biophys. Res. Commun. *83*, 843–849 (1978)
Friedli, B., Biron, P., Fouron, J.-C., Davignon, A.: Conversion of angiotensin I in pulmonary and systemic vascular beds of children. Acta Paediatr. Scand. *63*, 17–22 (1974)
Friedli, B., Kent, G., Olley, P.M.: Inactivation of bradykinin in the pulmonary vascular bed of newborn and fetal lambs. Circ. Res. *33*, 421–427 (1973)
Fujita, K., Teradaira, R., Nagatsu, T.: Bradykininase activity of aloe extract. Biochem. Pharmacol. *25*, 205 (1975)
Gaponiuk, P.Ya., Umarchodgaev, E.M.: The changes of plasma kininase activity in irradiated animals. Stud. Biophys. *13*, 225–230 (1969)
Gavras, H., Brunner, H.R., Laragh, J.H., Sealey, J.E., Gavras, I., Vukovich, R.A.: An angiotensin converting-enzyme inhibitor to identify and treat vasoconstrictor and volume factors in hypertensive patients. N. Engl. J. Med. *291*, 817–821 (1974)
Gavras, H., Brunner, H.R., Turini, G.A., Kershaw, G.R., Tifft, C.P., Cuttelod, S., Gavras, I., Vukovich, R.A., McKinstry, D.N.: Antihypertensive effect of the oral angiotensin converting-enzyme inhibitor SQ 14225 in man. N. Engl. J. Med. *298*, 991–995 (1978a)
Gavras, H., Gavras, I., Textor, S., Volicer, L., Brunner, H.R., Rucinska, E.J.: Effect of angiotensin converting enzyme inhibition on blood pressure, plasma renin activity and plasma aldosterone in essential hypertension. J. Clin. Endocrinol. Metabol. *46*, 220–226 (1978b)
Gavras, H., Liang, C-s., Brunner, H.R.: Redistribution of regional blood flow after inhibition of the angiotensin-converting enzyme. Circ. Res. *43*, Supp. I., I-59–I-63 (1978c)
Gecse, A., Lonovics, J., Zsilinszky, E., Szekeres, L.: Characteristics of the human skin bradykinin-destroying enzyme. J. Med. *2*, 129–135 (1971)
Geokas, M.C., Wollesen, F., Rinderknecht, H.: Radioimmunoassay for pancreatic carboxypeptidase B in human serum. J. Lab. Clin. Med. *84*, 574–583 (1974)
Gladner, J.A.: Potentiation of the effect of bradykinin. In: Hypotensive peptides. Erdös, E.G., Back, N., Sicuteri, F. (eds.), pp. 344–355. New York: Springer 1966
Grandino, A., Paiva, A.C.M.: Isolation of angiotensin-converting enzyme without kininase activity from hog and guinea pig plasma. Biochim. Biophys. Acta *364*, 113–119 (1974)

Greene, L.J., Camargo, A.C.M., Krieger, E.M., Stewart, J.M., Ferreira, S.H.: Inhibition of the conversion of angiotensin I to II and potentiation of bradykinin by small peptides present in Bothrops jararaca venom. Circ. Res. *30/31*, Suppl. II, II-62–II-71 (1972)
Guimaraes, J.A., Borges, D.R., Prado, E.S., Prado, J.L.: Kinin-converting aminopeptidase from human serum. Biochem. Pharmacol. *22*, 3157–3172 (1973)
Hall, E.R., Kato, J., Erdös, E.G., Robinson, C.J.G., Oshima, G.: Angiotensin I-converting enzyme in the nephron. Life Sci. *18*, 1299–1303 (1976)
Hamberg, U., Elg, P., Stelwagen, P.: On the mechanism of bradykinin potentiation. In: Advances in Experimental Medicine and Biology. Back, N., Martini, L., Paoletti, R. (eds.), Plenum Press New York, Vol. 2, pp. 626–631, 1968
Hayakari, M., Kondo, Y.: A rapid fluorometric assay of angiotensin-converting enzyme. Tohoku J. Exp. Med. *122*, 313–320 (1977)
Hayakari, M., Kondo, Y., Izumi, H.: A rapid and simple spectrophotometric assay of angiotensin-converting enzyme. Anal. Biochem. *84*, 361–369 (1978)
Hebert, F., Fouron, J.C., Boileau, J.C., Biron, P.: Pulmonary fate of vasoactive peptides in fetal, newborn, and adult sheep. Am. J. Physiol. *223*, 20–23 (1972)
Helmer, O.M.: Differentiation between two forms of angiotensin by means of spirally cut strips of rabbit aorta. Am. J. Physiol. *188*, 571–577 (1957)
Herman, C.M., Oshima, G., Erdös, E.G.: The effect of adrenocorticosteroid pretreatment on the kinin system and coagulation responses to septic shock in the baboon. J. Lab. Clin. Med. *84*, 731–739 (1974)
Hial, V., Gimbrone, Jr., M.A., Wilcox, G., Pisano, J.J.: Human vascular endothelium contains angiotensin I converting enzyme and renin-like activity. Fed. Proc. *35*, 705 (1976)
Hirsch, E.F., Nakajima, T., Oshima, G., Erdös, E.G., Herman, C.M.: Kinin system responses in sepsis following trauma in man. J. Surg. Res. *17*, 147–153 (1974)
Hofbauer, K.G., Zschiedrich, H., Rauh, W., Gross, F.: Conversion of angiotensin I into angiotensin II in the isolated perfused rat kidney. Clin. Sci. *44*, 447–456 (1973a)
Hofbauer, K.G., Zschiedrich, H., Rauh, W., Orth, H., Gross, F.: Reaction of endogenous renin with exogenous renin substrate within the isolated perfused rat kidney. Proc. Soc. Exp. Biol. Med. *142*, 796–799 (1973b)
Hojima, Y., Moriya, H., Moriwaki, C.: Bradykinin inactivating enzymes from red kidney beans (Phaseolus vulgaris) and potatoes (Solanum tuberosum). Agric. Biol. Chem. *41*, 559–565 (1977)
Hojima, Y., Tanaka, M., Moriya, H., Moriwaki, C.: Kinin-inactivating-enzymes from plants I. Partial purification of bradykinin-inactivating-enzyme from potatoes. Allergy *20*, 755–762 (1971a)
Hojima, Y., Tanaka, M., Moriya, H., Moriwaki, C.: Kinin-inactivating-enzymes from plants II. Some properties of bradykinin-inactivating-enzyme from potatoes. Allergy *20*, 763–769 (1971b)
Hopsu, V.K., Mäkinen, K.K., Glenner, G.G.: A peptidase (aminopeptidase B) from cat and guinea pig liver selective for N-terminal arginine and lysine residues. I. Purification and substrate specificity. Acta Chem. Scand. *20*, 1225–1230 (1966a)
Hopsu, V.K., Mäkinen, K.K., Glenner, G.G.: A peptidase (aminopeptidase B) from cat and guinea pig liver selective for N-terminal arginine and lysine residues. II. Modifier characteristics and kinetic studies. Acta Chem. Scand. *20*, 1231–1239 (1966b)
Horky, K., Rojo-Ortega, J.M., Rodriguez, J., Boucher, R., Genest, J.: Renin, renin substrate, and angiotensin I-converting enzyme in the lymph of rats. Am. J. Physiol. *220*, 307–311 (1971)
Huggins, C.G., Corcoran, R.J., Gordon, J.S., Henry, H.W., John, J.P.: Kinetics of the plasma and lung angiotensin I converting enzymes. Circ. Res. *26*/27, Suppl. I, I-93–I-108 (1970)
Huggins, C.G., Thampi, N.S.: A simple method for the determination of angiotensin I converting enzyme. Life Sci. 7, 633–639 (1968)
Hugli, T.E., Vallota, E.H., Müller-Eberhard, H.J.: Purification and partial characterization of human and porcine C3a anaphylatoxin. J. Biol. Chem. *250*, 1472–1478 (1975)
Igic, R., Erdös, E.G., Yeh, H.S.J., Sorrells, K., Nakajima, T.: The angiotensin I converting enzyme of the lung. Circ. Res. *31*, II-51–II-61 (1972a)
Igic, R., Nakajima, T., Yeh, H.S.J., Sorrells, K., Erdös, E.G.: Kininases. In: Pharmacology and the future of man. Acheson, G.H. (ed.), Vol. 5, pp. 307–319. Basel: Karger 1973

Igic, R., Robinson, C.J.G., Erdös, E.G.: Antiotensin I converting enzyme activity in the choroid plexus and in the retina. In: Central actions of angiotensin and related hormones. Buckley, J.P., Ferrario, C.M. (eds.), pp. 23–27. New York: Pergamon Press 1977
Igic, R., Sorrells, K., Yeh, H.S.J., Erdös, E.G.: Identity of kininase II with an angiotensin I converting enzyme. In: Vasopeptides: Chemistry, pharmacology and pathophysiology. Back, N., Sicuteri, F. (eds.), pp. 149–153. New York: Plenum Press 1972b
Igic, R., Yeh, H.S.J., Sorrells, K., Erdös, E.G.: Cleavage of active peptides by a lung enzyme. Experientia *28*, 135–136 (1972c)
Iwata, H., Shimiki, T., Oka, T.: Pharmacological significances of peptidase and proteinase in the brain (Report 1)-enzymatic inactivation of bradykinin in rat brain. Biochem. Pharmacol. *18*, 119–128 (1969)
Iwata, H., Shikimi, T., Iida, M., Miichi, H.: Pharmacological significances of peptidase and proteinase in the brain. Report 4: effect of bradykinin on the central nervous system and role of the enzyme inactivating bradykinin in mouse brain. Jpn. J. Pharmacol. *20*, 80–86 (1970)
Jaeger, P., Ferguson, R.K., Brunner, H.R., Kirchertz, E.J., Gavras, H.: Mechanism of blood pressure reduction by teprotide (SQ 20881) in rats. Kidney Int. *13*, 289–296 (1978)
Jakschik, B.A., McKnight, R.C., Marshall, G.R., Feldhaus, R.A., Needleman, P.: Renal vascular changes during hemorrhagic shock and the pharmacologic modification by angiotensin and catecholamine antagonists. Circ. Shock. *1*, 231–237 (1974)
Jeanneret, L., Roth, M., Bargetzi, J.-P.: Carboxypeptidase N from pig serum. H.-S. Z. Physiol. Chem. *357*, 867–872 (1976)
Johnson, A.R., Boyden, N.T.: Proteases in cultured human endothelial cells. In: Kininogenases, kallikrein. Haberland, G.L., Rohen, J.W., Suzuki, T. (eds.), pp. 113–118. Stuttgart, New York: Schattauer 1977
Johnson, A.R., Boyden, N.T., Wilson, C.M.: The growth-promoting actions of extracts from mouse submaxillary glands on human endothelial cells in culture. Submitted (1979)
Johnson, A.R., Erdös, E.G.: Angiotensin I converting enzyme in human endothelial cells. Circulation *52*, II-59 (1975)
Johnson, A.R., Erdös, E.G.: Metabolism of vasoactive peptides by human endothelial cells in culture: angiotensin I converting enzyme (kininase II) and angiotensinase. J. Clin. Invest. *59*, 684–695 (1977)
Johnson, A.R., Erdös, E.G.: Activities of enzymes in human pulmonary endothelial cells in culture. Circulation *58*, II-108 (1978)
Kangasniemi, P., Riekkinen, P., Penttinen, R., Ivaska, K., Rinne, U.K.: Enzyme changes in the cerebrospinal fluid and serum and their correlation to the breakdown of bradykinin during different stages of headache attacks of migraine patients. Headache *14*, 139–148 (1974)
Kato, H., Suzuki, T.: Amino acid sequence of bradykinin-potentiating peptide isolated from the venom of Agkistrodon halys blomhoffii. Proc. Jpn. Acad. *46*, 176–181 (1970)
Kato, H., Suzuki, T.: Bradykinin-potentiating peptides from the venom of Agkistrodon halys blomhoffii. Isolation of five bradykinin potentiators and the amino acid sequences of two of them, potentiators B and C. Biochemistry *10*, 972–980 (1971)
Khairallah, P.A., Page, I.H.: Plasma angiotensinases. Biochem. Med. *1*, 1–8 (1967)
Klauser, R.J., Robinson, C.J.G., Erdös, E.G.: Inhibition of human peptidyl dipeptidase (angiotensin I converting enzyme; kininase II) by serum albumin and its fragments. Hypertension in press (1979)
Koheil, A., Forstner, G.: Isoelectric focusing of carboxypeptidase N. Biochim. Biophys. Acta *524*, 156–161 (1978)
Koida, M., Walter, R.: Post-proline cleaving enzyme. Purification of this endopeptidase by affinity chromatography. J. Biol. Chem. *297*, 7593–7599 (1976)
Kokubu, T., Kato, I., Nishimura, K., Yoshida, N., Hiwada, K., Ueda, E.: Angiotensin I-converting enzyme in human urine. Clin. Chim. Acta *89*, 375–379 (1978)
Kokubu, T., Ueda, E., Nishimura, K., Yoshida, N.: Angiotensin I converting enzyme activity in pulmonary tissue of fetal and newborn rabbits. Experientia *33*, 1137–1138 (1977)
Kreye, V.A.W., Gross, F.: Conversion of angiotensin I to angiotensin II in peripheral vascular beds of the rat. Am. J. Physiol. *220*, 1294–1296 (1971)
Krieger, E.M., Salgado, H.C., Assan, C.J., Greene, L.L.J., Ferreira, S.H.: Potential screening test for detection of overactivity of renin-angiotensin system. Lancet *1*, 269–271 (1971)

Kroneberg, G., Stoepel, K.: Vergleichende Untersuchungen über die Kreislaufwirkung von Kallikrein (Padutin), Kallidin, und Bradykinin. Arch. Exp. Pathol. Pharmakol. *245*, 284–285 (1963)
Laffan, R.J., Goldberg, M.E., High, J.P., Schaeffer, T.R., Waugh, M.H., Rubin, B.: Antihypertensive activity in rats of SQ 14225, an orally active inhibitor of angiotensin I-converting enzyme. J. Pharmacol. Exp. Ther. *204*, 281–288 (1978)
Lanzillo, J.J., Fanburg, B.L.: Membrane-bound angiotensin-converting enzyme from rat lung. J. Biol. Chem. *249*, 2312–2318 (1974)
Lanzillo, J.J., Fanburg, B.L.: Angiotensin I-converting enzyme from guinea pig lung and serum. A comparison of some kinetic and inhibition properties. Biochim. Biophys. Acta *445*, 161–168 (1976a)
Lanzillo, J.J., Fanburg, B.L.: The estimation and comparison of molecular weight of angiotensin I converting enzyme by sodium dodecyl sulfate-polyacrylamide gel electrophoresis. Biochim. Biophys. Acta *439*, 125–132 (1976b)
Lanzillo, J.J., Fanburg, B.L.: Angiotensin I converting enzyme from human plasma. Biochemistry *16*, 5491–5495 (1977a)
Lanzillo, J.J., Fanburg, B.L.: Low molecular weight angiotensin I converting enzyme from rat lung. Biochim. Biophys. Acta *491*, 339–344 (1977b)
Lee, H.-J., Larue, J.N., Wilson, I.B.: Angiotensin-converting enzyme from guinea pig and hog lung. Biochim. Biophys. Acta *250*, 549–557 (1971a)
Lee, H.-J., Larue, J.N., Wilson, I.B.: Angiotensin-converting enzyme from porcine plasma. Biochim. Biophys. Acta *235*, 521–528 (1971b)
Lee, H.-J., Larue, J.N., Wilson, I.B.: Dipeptidyl carboxypeptidase from *Coryne bacterium equi.* Biochim. Biophys. Acta *250*, 608–613 (1971c)
Lee, H.-J., Larue, J.N., Wilson, I.B.: Human plasma converting enzyme. Arch. Biochem. Biophys. *142*, 548–551 (1971d)
LeDuc, L.E., Marshall, G.R., Needleman, P.: Differentiation of bradykinin receptors and of kininases with conformational analogues of bradykinin. Mol. Pharmacol. *14*, 413–421 (1978)
Lentz, K.E., Skeggs, L.T., Woods, K.R., Kahn, J.R., Shumway, N.P.: The amino acid composition of hypertensin II and its biochemical relationship to hypertension I. J. Exp. Med. *104*, 183–191 (1956)
Leuenberger, P.J., Stalcup, S.A., Mellins, R.B., Greenbaum, L.M., Turino, G.M.: Decrease in angiotensin I conversion by acute hypoxia in dogs. Proc. Soc. Exp. Biol. Med. *158*, 586–589 (1978)
Levine, B.W., Talamo, R.C., Kazemi, H.: Action and metabolism of bradykinin in dog lung. J. Appl. Physiol. *34*, 821–826 (1973)
Lieberman, J.: Elevation of serum angiotensin-converting-enzyme (ACE) level in sarcoidosis. Am. J. Med. *59*, 365–372 (1975)
Lieberman, J.: The specificity and nature of serum-angiotensin-converting enzyme (serum ACE) elevation in sarcoidosis. Ann. N.Y. Acad. Sci. *278*, 488–497 (1976)
Lieberman, J., Beutler, E.: Elevation of serum angiotensin-converting enzyme in Gaucher's disease. N. Engl. J. Med. *294*, 1442–1444 (1976)
Lieberman, J., Rea, T.H.: Serum angiotensin-converting enzyme in leprosy and coccidioidomycosis. Ann. Int. Med. *87*, 422–425 (1977)
Lukjan, H., Bielawic, M., Kiersnowska, B., Korfel, B., Dowzyk, W.: Kininogenase and kininase activity of the blood in arteriosclerosis. Atherosclerosis *16*, 61–66 (1972)
Mäkinen, P.L., Mäkinen, K.K.: Fractionation and properties of aminopeptidase B during purification and storage. Int. J. Pept. Prot. Res. *4*, 241–255 (1972)
Mäkinen, K.K., Mäkinen, P.-L.: Evidence of erythrocyte aminopeptidase B. Int. J. Prot. Res. *III*, 41–47 (1971)
Mäkinen, K.K., Oksala, E.: Evidence on the involvement in inflammation of an enzyme resembling aminopeptidase B. Clin. Chim. Acta *49*, 301–309 (1973)
Marinkovic, D.V., Marinkovic, J.N., Robinson, C.J.G., Erdös, E.G.: Purification of two forms of carboxypeptidase B from human pancreas. Biochem. J. *163*, 253–260 (1977)
Marks, N.: Exopeptidases of the nervous system. Int. Rev. Neurobiol. *11*, 57–97 (1968)
Marks, N.: Conversion and Inactivation of neuropeptides. In: Peptides in neurobiology. Sainer, H. (ed.), pp. 221–258. New York: Plenum Press 1977

Marks, N., Pirotta, M.: Breakdown of bradykinin and its analogs by rat brain neutral proteinase. Brain Res. *33*, 565–567 (1971)

Massey, T.H., Fessler, D.C.: Substrate binding properties of converting enzyme using a series of *p*-nitrophenylalanyl derivatives of angiotensin I. Biochemistry *15*, 4906–4912 (1976)

Mattioli, L., Zakheim, R.M., Mullis, K., Molteni, A.: Angiotensin-I-converting enzyme activity in idiopathic respiratory distress syndrome of the newborn infant and in experimental alveolar hypoxia in mice. J. Pediatr. *87*, 97–101 (1975)

McCaa, R.E., Hall, J.E., McCaa, C.S.: The effects of angiotensin I-converting enzyme inhibitors on arterial blood pressure and urinary sodium excretion. Role of the renal renin-angiotensin and kallikrein-kinin systems. Circ. Res. *43*, Suppl. I, I-32–I-39 (1978)

McCormick, J.T., Senior, J.: The effect of the oestrous cycle, pregnancy and reproductive hormones on the kininase activity of rat blood. J. Reprod. Fertil. *30*, 381–387 (1972)

McKay, T.J., Plummer, T.H.: By-product analogues for bovine carboxypeptidase B. Biochemistry *17*, 401–405 (1978)

McNeill, J.R.: Intestinal vasoconstriction following diuretic-induced volume depletion: role of angiotensin and vasopressin. Can. J. Physiol. Pharmacol. *52*, 829–839 (1974)

Merrill, J.E., Peach, M.J., Gilmore, J.P.: Angiotensin I conversion in the kidney and its modulation by sodium balance. Am. J. Physiol. *224*, 1104–1108 (1973)

Miller, Jr., E.D., Samuels, A.I., Haber, E., Barger, A.C.: Inhibition of angiotensin conversion and prevention of renal hypertension. Am. J. Physiol. *228*, 448–453 (1975)

Mineshita, S., Nagai, Y.: Hydrolysis of bradykinin by stem bromelain. Jpn. J. Pharmacol. *27*, 170–172 (1977)

Molteni, A., Zakheim, R.M., Mullis, K.B., Mattioli, L.: The effect of chronic alveolar hypoxia on lung and serum angiotensin I converting enzyme activity. Proc. Soc. Exp. Biol. Med. *147*, 263–265 (1974)

Morton, J.J., Semple, P.F., Ledingham, I.McA., Stuart, B., Tehrani, M.A., Garcia, A.R., McGarrity, G.: Effect of angiotensin-converting enzyme inhibitor (SQ 20881) on the plasma concentration of angiotensin I, angiotensin II, and arginine vasopressin in the dog during hemorrhagic shock. Circ. Res. *41*, 301–308 (1977)

Möse, J.R., Fischer, G., Briefs, C.: Die Wirkung von Clostridium butyricum (Stamm M 55) auf menschliches Kininogen und ihre Bedeutung für den Onkolyseprozeß. Zentralbl. Bakteriol. [I] *221*, 474–491 (1972a)

Möse, J.R., Fischer, G., Mobascherie, T.B.: Über Bakterienkininasen und deren physiologische Bedeutung 2. Mitteilung: Untersuchungen an Colistämmen. Zentralbl. Bakteriol. [I] *219*, 465–472 (1972b)

Möse, J.R., Fischer, G., Mobascherie, T.B.: Über Bakterienkininasen und deren physiologische Bedeutung 1. Mitteilung: Untersuchungen an Clostridienstämmen. Zentralbl. Bakteriol. [I] *219*, 530–541 (1972c)

Movat, H.Z., Steinberg, S.G., Habal, F.M., Ranadive, N.S.: Demonstration of a kinin-generating enzyme in the lysosomes of human polymorphonuclear leukocytes. Lab. Invest. *29*, 669–684 (1973a)

Movat, H.Z., Steinberg, S.G., Habal, F.M., Ranadive, N.S.: Kinin-forming and kinin-inactivating enzymes in human neutrophil leukocytes. Agents Actions *3/5*, 284–291 (1973b)

Mue, S., Takahashi, M., Ohmi, T., Shibahara, S., Yamauchi, K., Fujimoto, S., Okayama, H., Takishima, T.: Serum angiotensin converting enzyme level in bronchial asthma. Ann. Allergy *40*, 51–57 (1978)

Muirhead, E.E., Brooks, B., Arora, K.K.: Prevention of malignant hypertension by the synthetic peptide SQ 20881. Lab. Invest. *30*, 129–135 (1974)

Muirhead, E.E., Prewitt, R.L., Brooks, B., Brosius, W.L.: Antihypertensive action of the orally active converting enzyme inhibitor (SQ 14225) in spontaneously hypertensive rats. Circ. Res. *43*, Suppl. I, I-53–I-59 (1978)

Murachi, T., Miyake, T.: Action of stem bromelian on bovine bradykininogen II and bradykinin. Physiol. Chem. Phys. *2*, 97–104 (1970)

Murthy, V.S., Waldon, T.L., Goldberg, M. E., Vollmer, R.R.: Inhibition of angiotensin converting enzyme by SQ 14225 in conscious rabbits. Eur. J. Pharmacol. *46*, 207–212 (1977)

Murthy, V.S., Waldron, T.L., Goldberg, M.E.: Inhibition of angiotensin-converting enzyme by SQ 14225 in anesthetized dogs: hemodynamic and renal vascular effects. Proc. Soc. Exp. Biol. Med. *157*, 121–124 (1978a)

Murthy, V.S., Waldron, T.L., Goldberg, M.E.: The mechanism of bradykinin potentiation after inhibition of angiotensin-converting enzyme by SQ 14225 in conscious rabbits. Circ. Res. Suppl. I, I-40–I-45 (1978b)
Nakahara, N.: Plasma hippuryl-L-lysine hydrolase inhibition by low molecular weight substance in lysosomes of skeletal muscle. Biochem. Pharmacol. *21*, 2635–2641 (1972)
Nakahara, M.: Plasma hippuryl-L-lysine hydrolase in tourniquet shock. Experientia *29*, 999–1000 (1973)
Nakahara, M.: Subunits of human plasma kininase II generated by plasma kallikrein. Biochem. Pharmacol. *27*, 1651–1657 (1978)
Nakajima, T., Oshima, G., Yeh, H.S.J., Igic, R.P., Erdös, E.G.: Purification of the angiotensin I converting enzyme of the lung. Biochim. Biophys. Acta *315*, 430–438 (1973)
Nasjletti, A., Colina-Chourio, J., McGiff, J.C.: Disappearance of bradykinin in the renal circulation of dogs. Effects of kininase inhibition. Circ. Res. *37*, 59–65 (1975)
Needleman, P., Douglas, Jr. J.R., Jakschik, B.B., Blumberg, A.L., Isakson, P.C., Marshall, G.R.: Angiotensin antagonists as pharmacological tools. Fed. Proc. *35*, 2488–2493 (1976)
Needleman, P., Johnson, Jr., E.M., Vine, W., Flanigan, E., Marshall, G.R.: Pharmacology of antagonists of angiotensin I and II. Circ. Res. *31*, 862–867 (1972)
Needleman, P., Marshall, G.R., Sobel, B.E.: Hormone interactions in the isolated rabbit heart. Synthesis and coronary vasomotor effects of prostaglandins, angiotensin, and bradykinin. Circ. Res. *37*, 802–808 (1975)
Ng, K.K.F., Vane, J.R.: Conversion of angiotensin I to angiotensin II. Nature *216*, 762–766 (1967)
Ng, K.K.F., Vane, J.R.: Fate of angiotensin I in the circulation. Nature *218*, 144–150 (1968)
Nielsen, H.M.: Kinin forming and destroying activities in human bile and mucous membranes of the biliary tract. Br. J. Pharmacol. *37*, 172–177 (1969)
Nishimura, K., Hiwada, K., Ueda, E., Kokubu, T.: Affinity chromatography of angiotensin I-converting enzyme from rabbit lung using hippurylhistidylleucyl-OH. Biochim. Biophys. Acta *445*, 158–160 (1976a)
Nishimura, K., Hiwada, K., Ueda, E., Kokubu, T.: Solubilization of angiotensin I converting enzyme from rabbit lung using trypsin treatment. Biochim. Biophys. Acta *452*, 144–150 (1976b)
Nishimura, K., Yoshida, N., Hiwada, K., Ueda, E., Kokubu, T.: Purification of angiotensin I-converting enzyme from human lung. Biochim. Biophys. Acta *483*, 398–408 (1977)
Nishimura, K., Yoshida, N., Hiwada, K., Ueda, E., Kokubu, T.: Properties of three different forms of angiotensin I-converting enzyme from human lung. Biochim. Biophys. Acta *522*, 229–237 (1978)
Oates, H.F., Stokes, G.S.: Role of extrapulmonary conversion of mediating the systemic pressor activity of angiotensin I. J. Exp. Med. *140*, 79–86 (1974)
Odya, C.E., Levin, Y., Erdös, E.G., Robinson, C.J.G.: Soluble dextran complexes of kallikrein, bradykinin and enzyme inhibitors. Biochem. Pharmacol. *27*, 173–179 (1978b)
Odya, C.E., Marinkovic, D., Hammon, K.J., Stewart, T.A., Erdös, E.G.: Purification and properties of prolylcarboxypeptidase (angiotensinase C) from human kidney. J. Biol. Chem. *253*, 5927–5931 (1978a)
Oh-Ishi, S., Sakuma, A., Katori, M.: Kininase activity in equine plasma. Biochem. Pharmacol. *21*, 3078–3082 (1972)
Oliveira, E.B., Martins, A.R., Camargo, A.C.M.: Isolation of brain endopeptidases: influence of size and sequence of substrates structurally related to bradykinin. Biochemistry *15*, 1967–1974 (1976a)
Oliveira, E.B., Martins, A.R., Camargo, A.C.M.: Rabbit brain thiol-activated endopeptidase. Hydrolysis of bradykinin and kininogen. Gen. Pharmac. 7, 159–161 (1976b)
Olsen, U.B.: Kininase inhibition by glucagon. Acta Endocrinol. *87*, 552–556 (1978)
Onabanjo, A.O., Bhabani, A.R., Maegraith, B.G.: The significance of kinin-destroying enzymes activity in Plasmodium knowlesi malarial infection. Br. J. Exp. Pathol. *51*, 534–540 (1970)
Ondetti, M.A., Engel, S.L.: Bradykinin analogs containing β-homoamino acids. J. Med. Chem. *18*, 761–763 (1975)

Ondetti, M.A., Rubin, B., Cushman, D.W.: Design of specific inhibitors of angiotensin-converting enzyme: New class of orally active antihypertensive agents. Science *196*, 441–444 (1977)
Ondetti, M.A., Williams, N.J., Sabo, E.F., Pluscec, J., Weaver, E.R., Kocy, O.: Angiotensin-converting enzyme inhibitors from the venom of Bothrops jararaca. Isolation, elucidation of structure, and synthesis. Biochemistry *10*, 4033–4039 (1971)
Oparil, S.: Angiotensin I conversion. In: Renin. Horrobin, D.F. (ed.), Vol. 1, pp. 56–65. Montreal: Eden Press 1976
Oparil, S., Carone, F.A., Pullman, T.N., Nakamura, S.: Inhibition of proximal tubular hydrolysis and reabsorption of bradykinin by peptides. Am. J. Physiol. *231*, 743–748 (1976a)
Oparil, S., Low, J., Koerner, T.J.: Altered angiotensin I conversion in pulmonary disease. Clin. Sci. Mol. Med. *51*, 537–543 (1976b)
Oparil, S., Katholi, R.: Angiotensin I conversion. In: Renin. Horrobin, D.F. (ed.), Vol. 2, pp. 72–83. Montreal: Eden Press 1977
Oparil, S., Koerner, T.J., Lindheimer, M.D.: Plasma angiotensin converting enzyme activity in mother and fetus. J. Clin. Endocrinol. Metabol. *46*, 434–439 (1978)
Oparil, S., Koerner, T., Tregear, G.W., Barnes, B.A., Haber, E.: Substrate requirements for angiotensin I conversion in vivo and in vitro. Circ. Res. *32*, 415–423 (1973)
Oparil, S., Sanders, C.A., Haber, E.: In-vivo and in-vitro conversion of angiotensin I to angiotensin II in dog blood. Circ. Res. *26*, 591–599 (1970)
Oparil, S., Tregear, G.W., Koerner, T., Barnes, B.A., Haber, E.: Mechanism of pulmonary conversion of angiotensin I to angiotensin II in the dog. Circ. Res. *29*, 682–690 (1971)
Oshima, G., Erdös, E.G.: Inhibition of the angiotensin I converting enzyme of the lung by a peptide fragment of bradykinin. Experientia *30*, 733 (1974)
Oshima, G., Gecse, A., Erdös, E.G.: Angiotensin I converting enzyme of the kidney cortex. Biochim. Biophys. Acta *350*, 26–37 (1974a)
Oshima, G., Kato, J., Erdös, E.G.: Subunits of human plasma carboxypeptidase N (Kininase I; anaphylatoxin inactivator). Biochim. Biophys. Acta *365*, 344–348 (1974b)
Oshima, G., Kato, J., Erdös, E.G.: Plasma carboxypeptidase N, subunits and characteristics. Arch. Biochem. Biophys. *170*, 132–138 (1975)
Oshima, G., Nagasawa, K.: Some enzymatic properties of peptidyl dipeptide hydrolase (angiotensin I-converting enzyme). J. Biochem. *81*, 57–63 (1977)
Oshima, G., Nagasawa, K., Kato, J.: Renal angiotensin I-converting enzyme as a mixture of sialo- and asialo-enzyme, and a rapid purification method. J. Biochem. *80*, 477–483 (1976)
Oshima, G., Shimabukuro, H., Nagasawa, K.: Peptide inhibitors of angiotensin converting enzyme in digests of gelatin by bacterial collagenase Biochim. Biophys. Acta *566*, 128–137 (1979)
Orlowski, M., Wilk, E.: Concentration of angiotensin converting enzyme and angiotensin degrading enzymes in brain microvessels. Fed. Proc. *37*, 602 (1978)
Overturf, M., Wyatt, S., Boaz, D., Fitz, A.: Angiotensin I (Phe^8-His^9) hydrolase and bradykininase from human lung. Life Sci. *16*, 1669–1682 (1975)
Paskhina, T.S., Trapeznikova, S.S., Egopova, T.P., Morozova, N.A.: Effect of bradykinin-potentiating snake venom peptides and C-terminal pentapeptide fragment of bradykinin on carboxypeptidase N and kininase activities of human blood serum. Biokhimiya *40*, 844–853 (1975)
Persson, A., Wilson, I.B.: A fluorogenic substrate or angiotensin-converting enzyme. Anal. Biochem. *83*, 296–303 (1977)
Petakova, M., Simonianova, E., Rybak, M.: Carboxypeptidases N (kininase I) in rat serum lungs, liver and spleen and the inactivation of kinins (Bradykinin). Physiol. Bohemosl. *21*, 287–293 (1972)
Pettinger, W.A., Keeton, K., Tanaka, K.: Radioimmunoassay and pharmacokinetics of saralasin in the rat and hypertensive patients. Clin. Pharmacol. Ther. *17*, 146–158 (1975)
Piquilloud, Y., Reinharz, A., Roth, M.: Action de l'enzyme de conversion (converting enzyme) sur des substrats synthétiques. Helv. Physiol. Pharmacol. Acta *26*, 231–232 (1968)
Piquilloud, Y., Reinharz, A., Roth, M.: Studies on the angiotensin converting enzyme with different substrates. Biochim. Biophys. Acta *206*, 136–142 (1970)
Plummer, T.H., Hurwitz, M.Y.: Human plasma carboxypeptidase N. Isolation and characterization. J. Biol. Chem. *253*, 3907–3912 (1978)

Poth, M.M., Heath, R.G., Ward, M.: Angiotensin-converting enzyme in human brain. J. Neurochem. *25*, 83–85 (1975)
Prado, J.L., Limaos, E.A., Roblero, J., Freitas, J.O., Prado, E.S., Paiva, A.C.M.: Recovery and conversion of kinins in exsanguinated rat preparations. N.S. Arch. Pharmacol. *290*, 191–205 (1975)
Re, R., Novelline, R., Escourrou, M.-T., Athanasoulis, C., Bruton, J., Haber, E.: Inhibition of angiotensin-converting enzyme for diagnosis of renal-artery stenosis. N. Engl. J. Med. *298*, 582–586 (1978)
Reissmann, S., Paegelov, I., Leisner, H., Arold, H.: Stabilität verschiedener Bradykininanaloga gegen Kininase II. Experientia *31*, 1395–1396 (1975)
Rhoads, R.E., Udenfriend, S.: Substrate specificity of collagen proline hydroxylase: Hydroxylation of a specific proline residue in bradykinin. Arch. Biochem. Biophys. *133*, 108–111 (1969)
Rohrbach, M.S.: (Glycine-1-^{14}C) hippuryl-L-Histidyl-L-leucine: A substrate for the radiochemical assay of angiotensin converting enzyme. Anal. Biochem. *84*, 272–276 (1978)
Romero, J.C., Mak, S.W., Hoobler, S.W.: Effect of blockade of angiotensin-I converting enzyme on the blood pressure of renal hypertensive rabbits. Cardiovasc. Res. *8*, 681–687 (1974)
Roth, M., Weitzman, A.F., Piquilloud, Y.: Converting enzyme content of different tissues of the rat. Experientia *25*, 1247 (1969)
Rubin, B., Laffan, R.J., Kotler, D.G., O'Keefe, E.H., Demaio, D.A., Goldberg, M.E.: SQ 14225 (D-3-mercapto-2-methylpropanoyl-L-proline), a novel orally active inhibitor of angiotensin I-converting enzyme. J. Pharmacol. Exp. Ther. *204*, 271–280 (1978)
Ryan, J.W., Chung, A., Ammons, C., Carlton, M.L.: A simple radioassay for angiotensin-converting enzyme. Biochem. J. *167*, 501–504 (1977)
Ryan, J.W., Day, A.R., Schultz, D.R., Ryan, U.S., Chung, A., Marlborough, D.I., Dorer, F.E.: Localization of angiotensin converting enzyme (kininase II). I. Preparation of antibody-hemeoctapeptide conjugates. Tissue Cell *8*, 111–124 (1976a)
Ryan, J.W., Roblero, J., Stewart, J.M.: Inactivation of bradykinin in the pulmonary circulation. Biochem. J. *110*, 795–797 (1968)
Ryan, J.W., Roblero, J., Stewart, J.M.: Inactivation of bradykinin in rat lung. Adv. Exp. Med. *8*, 263–271 (1970)
Ryan, J.W., Ryan, U.S., Schultz, D.R., Whitaker, C., Chung, A., Dorer, F.E.: Subcellular localization of pulmonary angiotensin-converting enzyme (kininase II), Biochem. J. *146*, 497–499 (1975)
Ryan, J.W., Smith, U.: A rapid, simple method for isolating pinocytotic vesicles and plasma membrane of lung. Biochim. Biophys. Acta. *249*, 177–180 (1971)
Ryan, U.S., Ryan, J.W., Whitaker, C., Chiu, A.: Localization of angiotensin converting enzyme (kininase II). II. Immunocytochemistry and immunofluorescence. Tissue Cell *8*, 125–245 (1976b)
Rybak, M., Blazkova, B., Petakova, M.: Occurrence of aminopeptidases (arylaminopeptidases) in human amniotic fluid and their participation on kinin degradation. H. S. Z. Physiol. Chem. *352*, 1611–1616 (1971)
Rybak, M., Mansfeld, V., Grimova, J., Petakova, M.: Effect of carboxypeptidase N, aprotinin and anti-inflammatory drugs of pyrazolidine type on experimental inflammations in rats. Pharmacology *16*, 11–16 (1978)
Sampaio, C.A.M., Nunes, S.T., Mazzacoratti, M.D.G.N., Prado, J.L.: Inactivation of kinins by chymotrypsin. Biochem. Pharmacol. *25*, 2391–2394 (1976)
Samuels, A.I., Miller, E.D., Fray, J.C.S., Haber, E., Barger, A.C.: Renin-angiotensin antagonists and the regulation of blood pressure. Fed. Proc. *35*, 2512–2520 (1976)
Sancho, J., Re, R., Burton, J., Barger, A.C., Haber, E.: The role of the renin-angiotensin-aldosterone system in cardiovascular homeostasis in normal human subjects. Circulation *53*, 400–495 (1976)
Sander, G.E., Huggins, C.G.: Subcellular localization of angiotensin I converting enzyme in rabbit lung. Nature New Biol. *230*, 27–29 (1971)
Sander, G.E., West, D.W., Huggins, C.G.: Peptide inhibitors of pulmonary angiotensin I converting enzyme. Biochim. Biophys. Acta *242*, 662–667 (1971)
Sander, G.E., West, D.W., Huggins, C.G.: Inhibitors of the pulmonary angiotensin I-converting enzyme. Biochim. Biophys. Acta *289*, 392–400 (1972)

Scholz, H.W., Biron, P.: Non-identity between pulmonary bradykininase and converting-enzyme activity. Rev. Can. Biol. *28*, 197–200 (1969)
Scicli, A.G., Gandolfi, R., Carretero, O.A.: Site of formation of kinins in the dog nephron. Am. J. Physiol. *234*, F36–F40 (1978)
Semple, P.F.: The concentration of angiotensins I and II in blood from the pulmonary artery and left ventricle of man. J. Clin. Endocrinol. Metabol. *44*, 915–920 (1977)
Severs, W.B., Summy-Long, J.: The role of angiotensin in thirst. Life Sci. *17*, 1513–1526 (1975)
Shikimi, T., Houki, S., Iwata, H.: Pharmacological significances of peptidase and proteinase in the brain Report 3: Substrate specificity and amino acid composition of partially purified enzyme inactivating bradykinin in rat brain. Jpn. J. Pharmacol. *20*, 169–170 (1970)
Shikimi, T., Iwata, H.: Pharmacological significances of peptidase and proteinase in the brain – II. Purification and properties of a bradykinin inactivating enzyme from rat brain. Biochem. Pharmacol. *19*, 1399–1407 (1970)
Silverstein, E., Friedland, J.: Elevated serum and spleen angiotensin converting enzyme and serum lysozyme in Gaucher's disease. Clin. Chim. Acta *74*, 21–25 (1977)
Silverstein, E., Friedland, J., Lyons, H.A., Gourin, A.: Elevation of angiotensin-converting enzyme in granulomatous lymph nodes and serum in sarcoidosis: Clinical and possible pathogenic significance. Ann. N.Y. Acad. Sci. *278*, 498–513 (1976a)
Silverstein, E., Friedland, J., Lyons, H.A., Gourin, A.: Markedly elevated angiotensin converting enzyme in lymph nodes containing non-necrotizing granulomas in sarcoidosis. Proc. Natl. Acad. Sci. USA *73*, 2137–2141 (1976b)
Skeggs, L.T., Kahn, J.R., Shumway, N.P.: The preparation and function of the hypertensin-converting enzyme. J. Exp. Med. *103*, 295–299 (1956)
Skeggs, L.T., Marsh, W.H., Kahn, J.R., Shumway, N.P.: The existence of two forms of hypertensin. J. Exp. Med. *99*, 275–282 (1954)
Smith, R.J., Contrera, J.F.: Cobalt-induced alterations in plasma proteins, proteases and kinin system of the rat. Biochem. Pharmacol. *23*, 1095–1103 (1974)
Soffer, R.L.: Angiotensin-converting enzyme and the regulation of vasoactive peptides. Ann. Rev. Biochem. *45*, 73–94 (1976)
Soffer, R.L., Reza, R., Caldwell, P.R.B.: Angiotensin-converting enzyme from rabbit pulmonary particles. Proc. Natl. Acad. Sci. USA *71*, 1720–1724 (1974)
Stalcup, S.A., Leuenberger, P.J., Lipset, J.S., Turino, G.M., Mellins, R.B.: Decrease in instantaneous pulmonary clearance of bradykinin by acute hypoxia in dogs. Fed. Proc. *37*, 292 (1978)
Stanley, P., Biron, P.: Pressor response to angiotensin I during cardio-pulmonary bypass. Experientia *15*, 46–47 (1969)
Stevens, R.L., Micalizzi, E.R., Fessler, D.C., Pals, D.T.: Angiotensin I converting enzyme of calf lung. Method of assay and partial purification. Biochemistry *11*, 2999–3007 (1972)
Stewart, J.M., Ferreira, S.H., Greene, L.J.: Bradykinin potentiating peptide PCA-Lys-Trp-Ala-Pro. An inhibitor of the pulmonary inactivation of bradykinin and conversion of angiotensin I to II. Biochem. Pharmacol. *20*, 1557–1567 (1971)
Streeten, D.H.P., Kerr, L.P., Kerr, C.B., Prior, J.C., Dalakos, T.G.: Hyperbradykininism: A new orthostatic syndrome. Lancet *3*, 1048–1053 (1972)
Teger-Nilsson, A.-C.: Degradation of human fibrinopeptides A and B in blood serum in vitro. Acta Chem. Scand. *22*, 3171–3182 (1968)
Thurston, H., Laragh, J.H.: Prior receptor occupancy as a determinant of the pressor activity of infused angiotensin II in the rat. Circ. Res. *36*, 113–117 (1975)
Thurston, H., Swales, J.D.: Converting enzyme inhibitor and saralasin infusion in rats. Evidence for an additional vasodepressor property of converting enzyme inhibitor. Circ. Res. *42*, 588–592 (1978)
Tonzetich, J., Eigen, E., Volpe, A.R., Weiss, S.: Relationship of salivary kininase activity to periodontal status in humans. J. Periodontal. Res. *4*, 118–126 (1969)
Trautschold, I.: Assay method in the kinin system. In: Handbook of Experimental Pharmacology. Erdös, E.G. (ed.), Vol. XXV, pp. 52–81. Berlin, Heidelberg, New York: Springer 1970
Tsai, B.-S., Khosla, M.C., Peach, M.J., Bumpus, F.M.: Synthesis and evaluation of Des-Asp^1-angiotensin I: A precursor for Des-Asp^1-angiotensin II (AIII). J. Med. Chem. *18*, 1180–1183 (1975)

Tsai, B.-S., Peach, M. J.: Angiotensin homologs and analogs as inhibitors of rabbit pulmonary angiotensin-converting enzyme. J. Biol. Chem. *252*, 4674–4681 (1977)
Tuerker, R.K., Ercan, Z.S.: High degree of conversion of angiotensin I to angiotensin II in the mesenteric circulation of the isolated perfused terminal ileum of the cat. Arch. Int. Physiol. Biochim. *83*, 845–853 (1975)
Ueda, E., Akutsu, H., Kokubu, T., Yamamura, Y.: Partial purification and properties of angiotensin I converting enzyme from rabbit plasma. Jpn. Circ. J. *35*, 801–806 (1971)
Ueda, E., Kokubu, T., Akutsu, H., Ito, T.: Angiotensin I converting enzyme and kininase. Jpn. Circ. J. *36*, 583–586 (1972)
Uszynski, M., Malofiejew, M.: Kininase activity in the human placenta. Biochem. Pharmacol. *20*, 3211–3212 (1971)
Vallota, E.H., Müller-Eberhard, H.J.: Formation of C3a and C5a anaphylatoxins in whole human serum after inhibition of the anaphylatoxin inactivator. J. Exp. Med. *137*, 1109–1123 (1973)
Vane, J.R.: The release and fate of vaso-active hormones in the circulation. Br. J. Pharmacol. *35*, 209–242 (1969)
Vannier, Ch., Louvard, D., Maroux, S., Desnuelle, P.: Structural and topological homology between porcine intestinal and renal brush border aminopeptidase. Biochim. Biophys. Acta *445*, 185–199 (1976)
Venneröd, A.M.: Effects of tetraethylthiuram disulphide (disulfiram), diethyldithiocarbamate and ethanol on factors of the kinin system in human blood. Acta Pharmacol. Toxicol. *28*, 454–465 (1970)
Wallace, K.B., Bailie, M.D., Hook, J.B.: Angiotensin-converting enzyme in developing lung and kidney. Am. J. Physiol. *234*, R141–R145 (1978)
Ward, P.E., Erdös, E.G., Gedney, C.D., Dowben, R.M., Reynolds, R.C.: Isolation of membrane-bound renal enzymes that metabolize kinins and angiotensins. Biochem. J. *157*, 642–650 (1976)
Ward, P.E., Erdös, E.G.: Metabolism of kinins and angiotensins in the kidney. In: Kininogenases, kallikrein 4. Haberland, G.L., Rohen, J.W., Suzuku, T. (eds.), pp. 107–110. Stuttgart, New York: Schattauer 1977
Ward, P.E., Gedney, C.D., Dowben, R.M., Erdös, E.G.: Isolation of membrane-bound renal kallikrein and kininase. Biochem. J. *151*, 755–758 (1975)
Ward, P.E., Klauser, R.J., Erdös, E.G.: Angiotensin I converting enzyme (peptidyl dipeptidase) in the brush border of human intestinal mucosa. Circulation *58*, II-251 (1978a)
Ward, P.E., Schultz, W., Reynolds, R.C., Erdös, E.G.: Metabolism of kinins and angiotensins in the isolated glomerulus and brush border of rat kidney. Lab. Invest. *36*, 599–706 (1977)
Ward, P.E., Stewart, T.A., Igic, R.P.: Angiotensin I converting enzyme in retinal blood vessels. Fed. Proc. *37*, 658 (1978b)
Weese, W.C., Talamo, R.C., Neyhard, N.L., Kazemi, H.: Presence of a bradykinin-like substances in pulmonary washings. Am. Rev. Resp. Dis. *113*, 181–187 (1976)
Wiegershausen, B., Klausch, B., Hennighausen, G., Paegelow, I., Raspe, R.: Content of kininogen and activity of kininase in the amniotic fluid in the various periods of pregnancy. Gynecol. Invest. *1*, 234–239 (1970)
Wigger, H.J., Stalcup, S.A.: Distribution and development of angiotensin converting enzyme in the fetal and newborn rabbit. An immunofluorescence study. Lab. Invest. *38*, 581–585 (1978)
Williams, G.H.: Angiotensin-dependent hypertension – potential pitfalls in definition. N. Engl. J. Med. *296*, 684–685 (1977)
Williams, G.H., Hollenberg, N.K.: Accentuated vascular and endocrine response to SQ 20881 in hypertension. N. Engl. J. Med. *297*, 184–188 (1977)
Wright, I.G.: Kinin, kininogen and kininase levels during acute Babesia bovis (= B. argentina) infection of cattle. Br. J. Pharmacol. *61*, 567–572 (1977)
Yamashita, M., Oyama, T., Kudo, T.: Effect of the inhibitor of angiotensin I converting enzyme on endocrine function and renal perfusion in haemorrhagic shock. Can. Anaesth. Soc. J. *24*, 695–701 (1977)
Yang, H.Y.T., Erdös, E.G.: Second kininase in human blood plasma. Nature *215*, 1402–1403 (1967)

Yang, H.Y.T., Erdös, E.G., Chiang, T.S.: New enzymatic route for the inactivation of angiotensin. Nature *218*, 1224–1226 (1968)
Yang, H.Y.T., Erdös, E.G., Jenssen, T.A., Levin, Y.: Characterization of an angiotensin I converting enzyme. Fed. Proc. *29*, 281 (1970)
Yang, H.Y.T., Erdös, E.G., Jenssen, T.A., Levin, Y.: Characterization of an angiotensin I converting enzyme. Fed. Proc. *29*, 281 (1970c)
Yang, H.Y.T., Erdös, E.G., Levin, Y.: A dipeptidyl carboxypeptidase that converts angiotensin I and inactivates bradykinin. Biochim. Biophys. Acta. *214*, 374–376 (1970a)
Yang, H.Y.T., Erdös, E.G., Levin, Y.: Characterization of a dipeptide hydrolase (kininase II: angiotensin I converting enzyme). J. Pharmacol. Exp. Ther. *177*, 291–300 (1971)
Yang, H.Y.T., Jenssen, T.A., Erdös, E.G.: Conversion of angiotensin I by a kininase preparation. Clin. Res. *18*, 88 (1970b)
Yang, H.Y.T., Neff, N.H.: Distribution and properties of angiotensin converting enzyme of rat brain. J. Neurochem. *19*, 2443–2450 (1972)
Yang, H.Y.T., Neff, N.H.: Differential distribution of angiotensin converting enzyme in the anterior and posterior lobe of the rat pituitary. J. Neurochem. *21*, 1035–1036 (1973)
Yaron, A., Mlynar, D., Berger, A.: A dipeptidocarboxypeptidase from E. coli. Biochem. Biophys. Res. Commun. *47*, 897–902 (1972)
Yokoyama, S., Oobayshi, A., Tanabe, O., Ohata, K., Shibata, Y., Ichishima, E.: Kininase and anti-inflammatory activities of acid carboxypeptidase from penicillium janthinellum. Experientia *31*, 1122–1123 (1975)
Zacest, R., Oparil, S., Talamo, R.C.: Studies of plasma bradykinins using radiolabelled substrates. Aust. J. Exp. Biol. Med. Sci. *52*, 601–606 (1974)

Note Added in Proof

The literature dealing with kininase II (peptidyl dipeptidase, angiotensin I converting enzyme) is increasing exponentially. Numerous publications appeared during the few months which elapsed between completing the manuscript and printing the page proofs. Many of them dealt with the conversion of angiotensin I by the enzyme and its inhibition in vivo. Some examples of recent reports on kininase II are the following.

Studies on the active center of kininase II of horse plasma (FERNLEY, 1977) and rabbit lung enzyme (BÜNNING et al., 1978) implicated tyrosine as a functional residue. Arginine, glutamic acid and lysine are also essential components of the active center underscoring the similarities between carboxypeptidase A and kininase II. Studies on the carbohydrate content of the rabbit lung enzyme indicate that digestion by pronase released two glycopeptides (HARTLEY and SOFFER, 1978). In addition to the previously described carbohydrates, the enzyme contains glucose and *N*-acetylgalactosamine. Other studies focused on the synthesis of the enzyme. Endothelial cells cultured from hog aorta released kininase II in the medium when deprived of serum (HAYES et al., 1978). The amount of enzyme found in the medium was an order of magnitude higher than that associated with the cells, indicating synthesis of the enzyme by the cells.

The activity of the enzyme was measured in serum of a large number of clinical cases (STUDDY et al., 1978). It was significantly higher than normal in individuals with sarcoidosis, but steroid treatment reduced its level. The authors concluded that the measurement of the serum enzyme is not a specific test for sarcoidosis but that it is a high value aid in diagnosis. In contrast to previous reports, the enzyme level in serum was normal in leprosy (STUDDY et al., 1978). The activity of kininase II in the nervous system has also been investigated. This is normally high in the corpus striatum of human brain, but was greatly reduced in patients dying with Huntington's disease (ARREGUI et al., 1977). The enzyme present in the substantia nigra of some patients was also reduced (ARREGUI et al., 1978). Chronic morphine treatment of mice induces a peptidase in the particulate fraction of the striatum which cleaves enkephalin (MALFROY et al., 1978). A product of hydrolysis of the pentapeptide enkephalin is Tyr-Gly-Gly, indicating that this enzyme may be identical with kininase II.

Angiotensin III (des-Asp^1-angiotensin II) was formed in vivo from the nonapeptide des-Asp^1-angiotensin I when dogs were injected i.v. with the nonapeptide (FREEMAN et al., 1978). The effects of this peptide on the renal blood flow and the systemic blood pressure of dogs were abolished by injection of SQ 20881. This was taken as an indication that angiotensin III was enzymatically released from des-Asp^1-angiotensin I.

An additional role for kininase II inhibitors was suggested by the application of SQ 20881 or teprotide to patients with congestive heart failure (GAVRAS et al., 1978). Injection of teprotide i.v. improved the cardiac functions in both normotensive and hypertensive patients. This improvement was independent of plasma renin level. Captopril (SQ 14225) also was used successfully in treating hypertensive patients with "normal" plasma renin levels (BRUNNER et al., 1978). The elevated blood pressure returned to normal within 8 weeks in patients with severe hypertension associated with chronic renal failure.

References

Arregui, A., Bennett, J.P., Bird, E.D., Yamamura, H.I., Iversen, L.L., Snyder, S.H.: Ann. Neurol. *2*, 294 (1977)
Arregui, A., Emson, P.C., Spokes, E.G.: Europ. J. Pharmacol. *52*, 121 (1978)
Brunner, H.R., Wauters, J.-P., McKinstry, D., Waeber, B., Turini, G., Gavras, H.: Lancet *1978* II, 704
Bünning, P., Holmquist, B., Riordan, J.F.: Biochem. Biophys. Res. Commun. *83*, 1442 (1978)
Fernley, R.T.: Clin. Exp. Pharmacol. Physiol. *4*, 267 (1977)
Freeman, R.H., Davis, J.O., Khosla, M.C.: Am. J. Physiol. *234*, F 130 (1978)
Gavras, H., Faxon, D.P., Berkoben, J., Brunner, H.R., Ryan, T.J.: Circulation *58*, 770 (1978)
Hartley, J.L., Soffer, R.L.: Biochem. Biophys. Res. Commun. *83*, 1545 (1978)
Hayes, L.W., Goguen, C.A., Ching, S.-F., Slakey, L.L.: Biochem. Biophys. Res. Commun. *82*, 1147 (1978)
Malfroy, B., Swerts, J.P., Guyon, A., Roques, B.P., Schwartz, J.C.: Nature *276*, 523 (1978)
Studdy, P., Bird, R., James, D.G., Sherlock, S.: Lancet *1978* II, 1331

Kallikrein in Exocrine Glands

K. BHOOLA, M. LEMON, and R. MATTHEWS

A. Historical Review

The earliest citations of a hypotensive substance (urohypotensine) resembling kallikrein appeared in the publications of ABELOUS and BARDIER (1908, 1909). Later, similar hypotensive activity was observed by PRIBRAM and HERNHEISER (1920) in urine and by MIGAY and PETROFF (1925) in pancreatic juice. About 50 years ago, attempts by FREY and KRAUT to locate the source of a hypotensive macromolecule (F-Stoff) which they had characterized in urine (FREY and KRAUT, 1928) and in serum (KRAUT et al., 1928) led them to the discovery of a similar substance in a pancreatic cyst (FREY et al., 1930). Mammalian pancreas was subsequently found to contain such large amounts of F-Stoff that it was believed to be the site of origin of the hypotensive activity observed by them in urine and blood. This new substance was called "Kreislaufhormon" because of its marked vascular effects. F-Stoff was renamed "kallikrein," the term being derived from the Greek word *Kallikreas* meaning pancreas. Later experiments indicated that pancreatic kallikrein was primarily released into the pancreatic juice in a precursor form which was readily activated by duodenal enterokinase (FREY and WERLE, 1933; WERLE, 1934). This finding spurred WERLE and colleagues to search for this enzyme in other glandular tissues. Investigation of salivary tissue resulted in the identification of kallikrein in the submandibular glands of a number of mammals.

WERLE et al. (1937) reported that if kallikrein was incubated with serum for a few minutes and the mixture tested on the dog intestine, the resulting contraction had a shorter latency and greater magnitude than could be accounted for by kallikrein alone. The activity in the mixture increased gradually and then disappeared slowly. From these observations WERLE et al. (1937) concluded that a new substance had been formed which was released from an inactive plasma protein. Unlike kallikrein, the new substance was dialysable, thermostable, and contracted isolated guinea-pig ileum. It was called substance DK-„*Darmkontrahierende Stoff aus Kallikrein*" (WERLE and GRUNZ, 1939). It was found to contract the guinea-pig ileum and to possess marked hypotensive activity. Later it was renamed kallidin (WERLE and BEREK, 1948).

B. Tissue Content and Secretory Control

Historically, determination of kallikrein in glandular tissues of different species has depended on the ability of kallikrein to release kallidin from kininogen. This method is valid if it is assumed that kinin release is the physiologically important property of this enzyme. The values for kininogenase activity in exocrine glands have been determined with dog plasma as the source of kininogen and as such may be subject to error (see WEBSTER, 1970). Although dog plasma is an effective source of kininogen for the glandular kallikrein of most species, some anomalies do exist. Horse glandular kallikrein releases kinins from horse but not dog plasma. Furthermore, it is difficult to demonstrate the formation of kinin activity with guinea-pig submandibular kallikrein from heated (56–58 °C, 3 h) dialysed guinea-pig plasma, but not from similarly treated dog, cat or human plasma. JACOBSEN (1966) ascribed this to potent kininases and to the low concentration of kininogen in guinea-pig plasma which is able to act as a substrate for glandular kallikrein. The species differences between kallikreins from exocrine glands have been reviewed in detail by WEBSTER (1970).

The demonstration of kininogenases other than kallikrein in the submandibular gland and in the pancreas requires a clear delineation of the enzymic properties of kallikrein. Trypsin, like kallikrein, releases kinins from kininogens and hydrolyses synthetic esters of arginine; it differs in possessing significant proleolytic activity on casein, haemoglobin, and synthetic amide substrates of arginine. Furthermore, trypsin is very effective in releasing kinin from denatured kininogen whereas kallikrein is not, thereby indicating that the tertiary structure of kininogen is important for the enzymic activity of kallikrein. Measurement of kallikrein activity in tissues clearly requires the determination of values for kininogenase and esterase activities and the inhibition by specific inhibitors of serine proteases. The kininogenase activity should be determined using the specific natural kininogen as substrate. The kinin formed should be assayed for smooth muscle contracting (cat jejunum or guinea-pig ileum) and relaxing (rat duodenum) ability and for hypotensive properties. In addition, pancreatic, and submandibular kallikreins should be assayed against several of the synthetic amino-acid substrates known to be cleaved by kininogenases.

I. Gland Content of Pancreatic Kallikrein

Kallikrein in the pancreas was first characterized by WERLE (1937). It was found to occur in an inactive form (WERLE, 1937; FIEDLER and WERLE, 1967) and was secreted into the duodenum mainly as the proenzyme where it was activated by enterokinase (WERLE and ECKEY, 1934; WERLE and URHAHN, 1940; WERLE et al., 1955). Studies on freeze-dried pancreatic gland tissue revealed that a significant amount of kallikrein was present in situ in an inactive form. The amount of active kallikrein was small and probably arose from the readily activable nature of the parent proenzyme molecule. In this respect, kallikreinogen differs from trypsinogen. The proportion of active kallikrein varied from one species to another and was as follows: cat 15% (10%, E. WERLE personal communication), rabbit 25%, dog 30%, and rat 65% (BHOOLA, 1969). In contrast to trypsin and chymotrypsin, active kallikrein has been reported in the pancreatic juice of the cat (HILTON and JONES, 1968) but with only 3% of its potential activity in the dog (BHOOLA and DOREY, 1971a). Using dog plasma as the source of kininogens, KRAUT et al. (1930), and WERLE (1960) have reported considerable species variation in the amount of kallikrein in the pancreas. Since this pioneering work, no comparable study has been undertaken. The pancreatic content of kallikrein was apparently influenced by the type of diet (WERLE, 1960; FORELL, 1960). It was increased in rats on a high protein diet and markedly decreased in animals on a high fat diet; a similar increase of trypsin but not amylase was also observed.

FORELL (1960) designed experiments to elucidate whether kallikrein was primarily secreted as an endocrine or exocrine moiety. Ligation of the pancreatic duct and the simultaneous reimplantation of the common bile duct into the duodenum resulted in complete atrophy of exocrine pancreas and total loss of kallikrein activity. There was no change in kallikrein content in the pancreas of rats with alloxan-induced diabetes. From these studies it seemed unlikely that kallikrein was a hormone.

II. Control of Pancreatic Kallikrein Secretion

Physiologic control of enzyme secretion from mammalian pancreatic exocrine cells is exerted by the vagus nerve (acetylcholine) and the intestinal hormone, cholecystokinin-pancreozymin (CCK-PZ). In 1960, FORELL reported that kallikrein was secreted into the duodenum in parallel with known exocrine enzymes and in response to the same stimuli (see Table 1). Kallikrein, trypsin, and amylase in pancreatic juice increased and the gland content of these enzymes fell after parenteral administration of prostigmine in the rat. Pancreozymin injected intravenously in man produced a marked secretion of kallikrein as measured by its concentration in the duodenal fluid. In the perfused cat pancreas, pancreozymin clearly increased kallikrein output whereas secretin failed to do so (HILTON and JONES, 1968). Enzyme and bicarbonate secretion in response to vagal stimulation shows species variation (HICKSON, 1970a, b). Vagal stimulation in the pig caused profuse flow of bicarbonate-rich juice with an appreciable enzyme content; atropine blocked enzyme release but did not affect bicarbonate secretion. In contrast, in dog there was a less profuse stimulation of fluid secretion and both constituents were inhibited by atropine. Clearly, species variation in the neural and humoral control of pancreatic kallikrein secretion requires further study.

In isolated guinea-pig pancreatic slices, acetylcholine, CCK-PZ (Fig. 1), and the C-terminal synthetic octapeptide of CCK stimulated the secretion of proenzymes with potential esteroprotease activity (ALBANO et al., 1975). The molecular mechanisms involved in the exocytotic release of secretory proteases (e.g., kallikrein) have only recently received attention. One view is that activation by acetylcholine and CCK-PZ of specific receptors on the plasma membrane of pancreatic cells results in a marked, rapid but transient rise in cyclic CMP which precedes enzyme secretion (Fig. 2). The rise in cyclic GMP and proenzyme release evoked by acetylcholine is completely inhibited by atropine (ALBANO et al., 1976b). The enzyme release evoked by acetylcholine, CCK-PZ, and cyclic 8-bromo-GMP was associated morphologically with a reduction in the number of secretory granules counted with the Quantimet 720D, television microdensitometer (ALBANO et al., 1976a). Even though cyclic nucleotides and calcium seem to be implicated in the control of protease secretion (Fig. 3; ALBANO et al., 1977), the precise sequential steps have still to be elucidated. One possibility is that cyclic GMP, formed as a result of activation of guanylate cyclase through specific receptors on the plasma membrane, activates a cyclic GMP-dependent protein kinase which triggers the release of calcium necessary for the stimulation of enzyme secretion by the pancreatic cells. Once secretion is initiated, it is maintained by continued release of ionized calcium (Fig. 4).

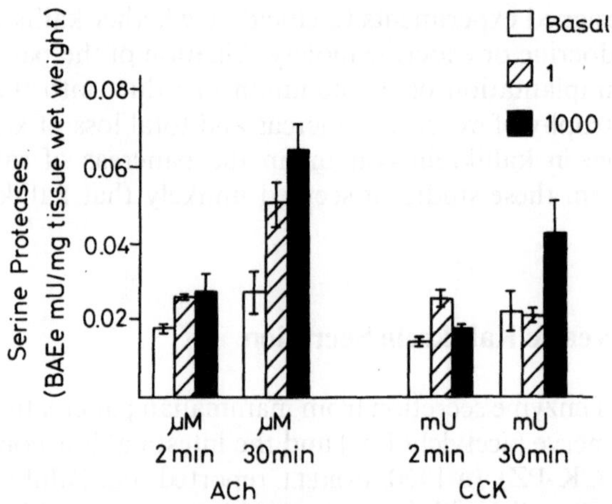

Fig. 1. Dose-dependent stimulation of enzyme secretion from guinea-pig pancreatic slices (ALBANO et al., 1975, 1976a, b.). Tissue was incubated for 2 and 30 min at 37° in a modified Krebs-Ringer bicarbonate buffer (gassed with 95% O_2–5% CO_2), in single Erhlenmeyer flasks placed in a Grant shaking water bath. The cumulative protease (BAEe Δ E_{366} mU/mg wet tissue) secretion into the medium was measured after activation with enterokinase. B = basal; ACh = acetylcholine; CCK = cholecystokinin-pancreozymin (GIR, Karolinska Institute, Stockholm). Bars represent 1 or 2 S.E. of mean, n = 6

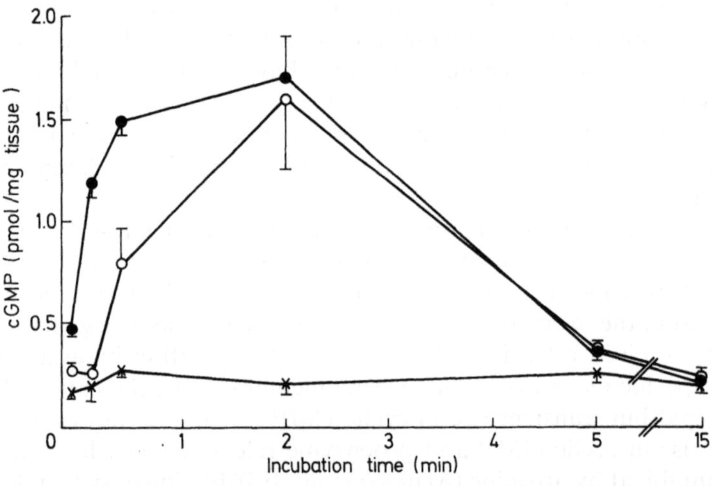

Fig. 2. Time-course of cyclic GMP formation in guinea-pig pancreatic slices (ALBANO et al., 1975, 1976a). Each point represents the mean of three incubations. The tissue cyclic nucleotide content of each incubation sample was measured in triplicate. The cyclic GMP values were calculated as pmol cyclic GMP mg wet weight tissue. X–X = Basal; ●–● = ACH (acetylcholine) 2.5×10^{-3} M; 0–0 = CCK (cholecystokinin-pancreozymin) U/ml. Bar indicates S.E. of mean

III. Gland Content of Salivary Kallikrein

Kallikrein was first demonstrated in the salivary glands of mammals by WERLE and RODEN (1936, 1939). As in the pancreas, kininogenase activity of the various salivary glands of different species was measured using kininogen prepared from dog plasma.

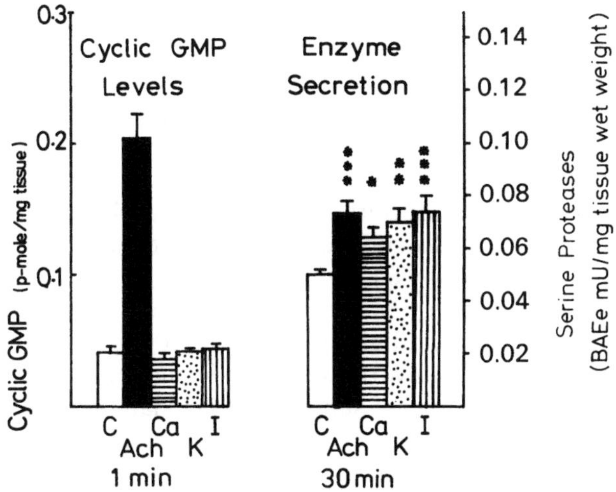

Fig. 3. Effect of acetylcholine, calcium, potassium and ionophore A 28137 on cyclic GMP levels and protease secretion in isolated guinea-pig pancreatic slices (ALBANO et al., 1977). Values represent the mean of three incubinations with determination of cyclic GMP as in Fig. 2 and protease as in Fig. 1. C = control, basal; ACh = acetylcholine, 10^{-6} *M*; Ca = calcium, 10 m*M*; K = potassium, 100 m*M*, I = divalent cation ionophore A 28137, 2 μg/ml (Eli Lilly). Bar represents S.E. of mean. *$p > 0.05$, **$p > 0.01$, ***$p > 0.001$

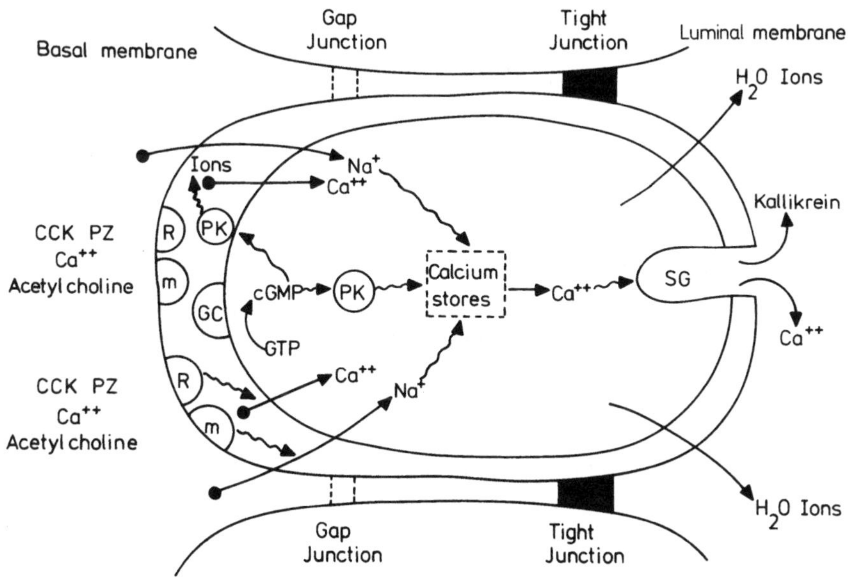

Fig. 4. Molecular model for stimulus-secretion coupling involving cholinergic muscarinic (m) and cholecystokinin-pancreozymin (CCK-PZ; R) receptors in a pancreatic cell. Membrane activation by acetylcholine and CCK-PZ results in the formation of cyclic GMP which may activate membranebound and cytoplasmic protein kinases (PK). The released free calcium is believed to initiate exocytosis of secretory granules (SG). GC, guanylate cyclase

The highest levels were detected in the submandibular rather than in the parotid or lingual gland. Comprehensive studies revealed a wide species variation in the concentration of submandibular kallikrein. With dog kininogen as substrate, the highest kininogenase activity was detected in the mouse and rat (confirming the previous results of WERLE, 1960), moderate levels in the guinea-pig, cat, and hamster, and the least in the dog and rabbit (BHOOLA and DOREY, 1971b; BHOOLA et al., 1974). Very low levels of kallikrein were measured in the submandibular glands of lamb and sheep using sheep kininogen as substrate and even lower amounts in the parotid gland (BEILENSON and SCHACHTER, unpublished).

In addition to kallikrein, a number of esteroproteases have been identified in extracts of mammalian submandibular glands. About 10 years ago, three proteases, characterized by their ability to hydrolyse synthetic and natural substrates of trypsin were isolated and purified from rat submandibular gland (EKFORS et al., 1967; see also FIEDLER in this volume). The first of these enzymes, *salivain*, hydrolysed both the synthetic and natural trypsin substrates readily. Its pH optimum was 9.3 and it was inhibited by aprotinin (Trasylol) but not by ovomucoid or lima bean trypsin inhibitors. The second enzyme, *glandulain*, possessed the same substrate spectrum as *salivain* but its pH optimum was 8.1 and it was inhibited by lima bean and ovomucoid trypsin inhibitors and aprotinin. The third enzyme was called "kallikrein-like peptidase." It consisted of four isoenzymic forms and hydrolysed both esters and amides of N-substituted arginine with a pH optimum of 8.2. This enzyme was relatively ineffective against the natural substrate of trypsin and was only minimally inhibited by trypsin inhibitors and aprotinin. Both *salivain* and kallikrein-like protease, but not *glandulain*, produced a marked fall in blood pressure in rabbits (EKFORS et al., 1967) and a pronounced increase in vascular permeability (EKFORS et al., 1969). Unfortunately, the detailed biochemical studies were not matched by adequate pharmacologic characterization of the kininogenase activity of these enzymes. From the published data, it appears that in addition to kallikrein, *salivain* may possess kininogenase activity. Antibodies to *salivain* apparently cross-reacted with submandibular kallikrein (EKFORS et al., 1969). Recently BRANDTZAEG et al. (1976) purified kallikreins from the rat submandibular gland and characterized them by their hypotensive and oxytocic activity, low caseinolytic property, and immunochemical identity with rat urinary kallikrein. BRANDTZAEG et al. (1976) have suggested that although their purified kallikreins may resemble *salivain*, they clearly differ from the other hypotensive esterases described by EKFORS et al. (1969). Similar trypsin-like esteroproteases have also been isolated from the mouse submandibular gland (EKFORS et al., 1972). The occurrence of trypsin-like enzymes in rodents was confirmed by BHOOLA and DOREY (1971b), who also identified a chymotrypsin-like enzyme in the mouse submandibular gland (BHOOLA et al., 1973, 1974). Experiments with protease inhibitors have revealed differences between kallikreins of various species (VOGEL and WERLE, 1970; BHOOLA and DOREY, 1971b). For example, porcine submandibular kallikrein is inhibited by aprotinin but the enzyme from guinea-pig is not. However, detailed comparisons between the submandibular kininogenases of different species must await complete chemical and pharmacologic characterization of each enzyme.

Ligation of the submandibular duct in mice and dogs resulted in a rapid loss of kallikrein (WERLE, 1960). Similarly BEILENSON et al. (1968) were able to deplete kallikrein in the submandibular gland of the cat and rabbit by ligation of the duct for

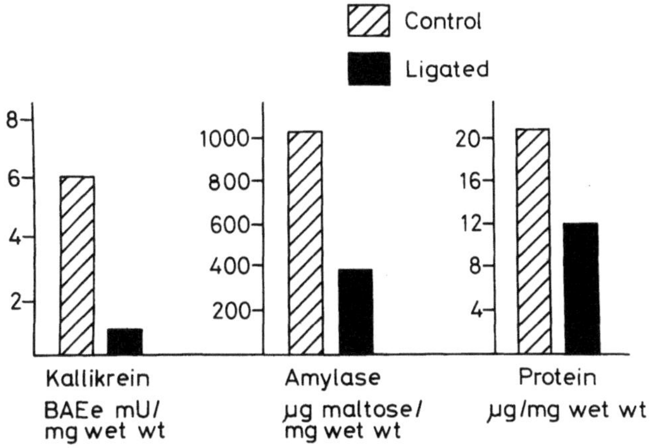

Fig. 5. Effect of duct ligation in guinea-pig submandibular gland (MATTHEWS and BHOOLA, 1977). The left submandibular duct was ligated aseptically. Both the ligated (L) and the control (C) glands of each of six animals were removed 7 days later, washed in saline and homogenized in Tris-HCl buffer (50 m*M*, pH 7.0). The values represent the mean of the measurements performed on six glands. Submandibular kallikrein was determined by BAEe hydrolysis (BAEe Δ E_{366} mU/mg wet gland weight), amylase by the formation of maltose from starch (µg maltose/mg wet gland weight) and protein with bovine serum albumin as a standard (µg/mg wet gland weight)

a period of 3–5 days or in the cat by duct ligation combined with subsequent sympathetic nerve stimulation (see Fig. 12). Recently, MATTHEWS and BHOOLA (1977) have observed a similar reduction in the activity of kallikrein and amylase after duct ligation in the submandibular gland of the guinea-pig (Fig. 5). These observations suggest that submandibular kallikrein is primarily an exocrine enzyme.

IV. Control of Salivary Kallikrein Secretion

Hypotension arising from i.v. injection of extracts of submandibular gland was observed originally by OLIVER and SCHÄFER (1895) and BUSCH (1900). Much later in 1934, Secker again reported a hypotensive agent in saliva which was subsequently shown by FELDBERG and GUIMARAIS (1935) not to be acetylcholine, histamine or an adenosine derivative. Stimulation of the chorda tympani nerve in the cat and dog resulted in secretion of a hypotensive substance in saliva (HILTON and LEWIS, 1955) which was subsequently recognized to be kallikrein. The neural and humoral control of kallikrein secretion by salivary glands is summarized in Table 1. Detailed in vivo studies by BEILENSON et al. (1968) demonstrated that the secretion of kallikrein from the cat submandibular gland was primarily controlled by adrenergic innervation of the gland. Sympathetic nerve stimulation and injection of adrenaline were markedly effective in evoking the secretion of kallikrein-rich saliva, whereas parasympathetic nerve stimulation and injection of pilocarpine produced a relatively low concentration of kallikrein but high concentration of sialotonin. Following such intermittent sympathetic nerve stimulation (20 Hz), the gland was almost completely depleted of kallikrein; the concentration within the gland fell by about 90% within 5 min.

Table 1. Release of Kallikrein (Esteroproteases)

Organ	Species	Stimulus (response)[a]			Reference
		Nerve	Exogenous	Inhibition	
Pancreas	Rat		Pancreozymin (+ +) Prostigmine (+ +)		FORELL (1960)
	Cat		Pancreozymin (+ +) Secretin (−)		HILTON and JONES (1968)
	Guinea-pig		Acetylcholine (+ +) CCK — PZ (+ +) CCK^8 (+ +)	Atropine (+ +)	ALBANO et al. (1975)
			Cyclic 8b–GMP (+ +) Calcium (+ +)		ALBANO et al. (1976b)
Submandibular gland	Cat	Sympathetic (+ +)		Guanethidine (+ +) Tolazoline (−) Phenoxybenzamine (±) Propranolol (±)	BHOOLA et al. (1965)
			Adrenaline (+ +)		BEILENSON et al. (1968)
		Sympathetic (+ +)		Diphentolamine (+ +) Propranolol (−)	KRIZ et al. (1974b)
			Noradrenaline (+) Isoprenaline (−)		
		Prolonged chorda tympani 46 min (+) 60–120 min (+)			BARTON et al. (197?) KRIZ et al. (1974b)
	Dog	Combined sympathetic /chorda tympani (+ +)			BEILENSON et al. (1968)
	Rabbit	Chorda tympani (+)		Atropine (+ +)	BEILENSON et al. (1968)
	Sheep	Chorda tympani (+)		Atropine (+ +)	BEILENSON and SCHACHTER (unpublished)

	Guinea-pig	Sympathetic (+ +)			MATTHEWS and BHOOLA (1977)
		Chorda tympani (+)			
		Combined sympathetic /chorda tympani (+ +)			
			Noradrenaline (+ +)	Propranolol (+)	ALBANO et al. (1976)
				Phentolamine (+)	
				Propranolol/ phentolamine (+ +)	
			Phenylephrine (+ +)		
			Isoprenaline (+ +)		
			Acetylcholine (+ +)	Atropine (+ +)	
			Potassium 75mM(+ +)		
			Calcium 10mM (+ +)		
Salivary glands (mixed saliva)	Human		Unstimulated		WERLE and KORSTEN (1938)
					BHOOLA et al. (1969)
					WOTMAN et al. (1969)
			0.5% Citric acid		BHOOLA et al. (1977)
Submandibular	Human		2% Citric acid		WOTMAN et al. (1969)
Parotid			2% Citrid acid		WOTMAN et al. (1969)
			Ascorbic acid		EICHNER et al. (1976)
			Pilocarpine		

[a] + + = Clear effect. + = Slight effect. − = No effect.
CCK—PZ = Cholecystokinin-pancreozymin. CCK[8] = Cholecystokimnin octapeptide. Cyclic 8b–GMP = Cyclic 8-bromo guanosine monophosphate

BHOOLA et al. (1965) reported that adrenoceptor-mediated salivary secretion in the cat was blocked by guanethidine, unaffected or increased by tolazoline, and unaffected or blocked by phenoxybenzamine and propranolol. Using hydrolysis of BAEe as an indication of kallikrein activity, GAUTVIK et al. (1974b) showed an approximate 40% reduction in the esterase content of cat submandibular gland after sympathetic nerve stimulation. This reduction was completely inhibited by diphentolamine but not altered by propranolol. Close arterial injections of noradrenaline reduced the gland esterase activity by about 25%, whereas isoprenaline was ineffective. Intermittent stimulation of the chorda tympani nerve (10 Hz; actual stimulation time, 40 min) in the cat resulted in either no change or slight increase in the kallikrein content; only stimulation at 20 Hz for 46 min produced a fall approaching 50% (BARTON et al., 1975). GAUTVIK et al. (1974b) demonstrated a 25% reduction in BAEe esterase activity after prolonged stimulation (1–2 h) of the chorda tympani nerve and close arterial infusion of acetylcholine. The fall in BAEe esterase activity was unaffected by atropine. GAUTVIK et al. (1974b) concluded that cholinergic receptors which regulate the secretion of kallikrein (atropine resistant) and those which control secretion of water and electrolytes (atropine sensitive) were not identical. A somewhat similar receptor variation was reported in rat submandibular gland in which salivary secretion in response to chorda tympani nerve stimulation was only partially inhibited by atropine at the higher frequencies of 10 and 20 Hz (THULIN, 1974). In the dog, intermittent sympathetic nerve stimulation was effective in inducing a marked increase in kallikrein secretion only when stimulation of the chorda tympani was superimposed. Kallikrein in rabbit and sheep submandibular saliva was detected both in the spontaneously secreting gland and after parasympathetic nerve stimulation; in both species chorda tympani stimulation was blocked by atropine, whereas the spontaneously evoked flow was not (BEILENSON et al., 1968; BEILENSON and SCHACHTER, unpublished; SMAJE, 1974).

MATTHEWS and BHOOLA (1977) designed experiments to determine the neural control of guinea-pig submandibular kallikrein. A fall in the content of kallikrein and amylase in the gland was observed after intermittent sympathetic or parasympathetic nerve stimulation. The maximum reduction in kallikrein activity (20%) and amylase (40%) was achieved with 10 min intermittent nerve stimulation (8 Hz). Because an increase in protein content of these glands had indicated resynthesis, actinomycin D was injected prior to sympathetic nerve stimulation; this prevented the rise in gland protein and produced a greater loss of kallikrein and amylase. Intermittent parasympathetic nerve stimulation (8 Hz; actual stimulation time, 20 and 40 min) caused a slight rise in gland protein, a small reduction in kallikrein content, and virtually no change in amylase. Combined continuous parasympathetic (20 Hz) and intermittent sympathetic (10 Hz) stimulation for a period of 1 h reduced the gland activity of kallikrein and amylase by about 40%. The secretion of kallikrein from the submandibular gland of the guinea-pig appears to be under dual neural control (Fig. 6).

One of the earliest observations on kallikrein activity in human saliva was made by WERLE and KORSTEN (1938). Three decades later, BHOOLA et al. (1969) examined the kallikrein of whole saliva collected without stimulation over a 30 min period. The kininogenase activity was measured on dog blood pressure, isolated rat uterus (with human kininogen as substrate) and esterase activity with tosyl-L-arginine methyl

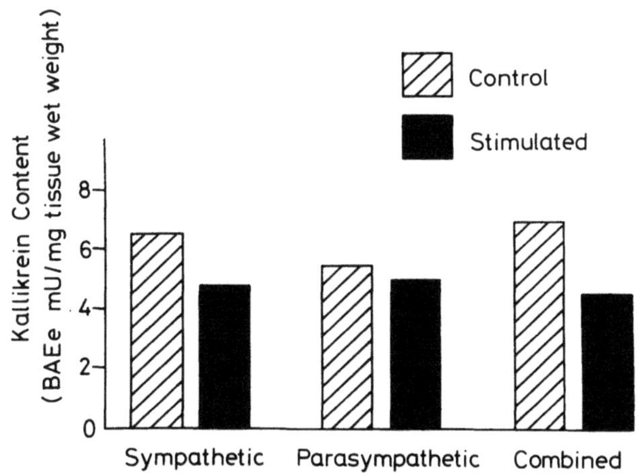

Fig. 6. Neural control of kallikrein secretion in guinea-pig submandibular gland (MATTHEWS and BHOOLA, 1977). Submandibular kallikrein content was measured after intermittent sympathetic (20 s on, 40 s off, at 8Hz and actual stimulation time of 20 min) and parasympathetic (20 s on, 40 s off at 8Hz and actual stimulation time of 40 min) nerve stimulation. For the combined effect the sympathetic nerve was stimulated intermittently (20 s on, 40 s off at 10 Hz and actual stimulation time 10 min) and the parasympathetic continuously for 30 min (20 Hz). Submandibular kallikrein was measured by BAEe hydrolysis BAEe Δ E_{366} mU/mg wet gland weight). The values represent the mean of the measurements performed on control (C, n=6) and stimulated (S, n=6) glands for each of the three groups of experiments

ester (TAMe) as substrate. The agreement between all three methods of determining human salivary kallikrein activity was very good and the correlation coefficients ranged from +0.867 to +0.745. Neither the kininogenase nor the esterase values revealed any sex-linked difference between the samples taken from males and females. WOTMAN et al. (1969) compared the kallikrein activity in whole saliva with that individually collected from the parotid and submandibular glands. Kallikrein was measured by its ability to hydrolyse benzoyl-L-arginine ethyl ester (BAEe) and to release kallidin from dog kininogen (assayed on isolated guinea-pig ileum); both enzymic actions were inhibited by aprotinin. There was little difference in the concentration of kallikrein in parotid and submandibular secretions obtained by reflex stimulation with a 2% citric acid swab. This finding contrasts with the four to fivefold increase in kallikrein tissue levels of submandibular gland reported by WERLE and RODEN (1936). Activity in whole human saliva was much greater than in the parotid or submandibular secretions; WOTMAN et al. (1969) attributed this to the presence of a kallikrein activator in whole saliva. Recently EICHNER et al. (1976) studied the secretion of kallikrein in resting and stimulated human parotid saliva. Parotid secretion was stimulated reflexly by ascorbic acid applied to the tongue or by subcutaneous injection of pilocarpine. Kallikrein was determined using BAEe as substrate. Both ascorbic acid and pilocarpine stimulated a rapid secretion; in the ensuing 20 min after application of the stimulus, the concentration of kallikrein in the parotid saliva fell sharply but the total amount secreted increased substantially. Continuous stimulation resulted in a marked reduction in the capacity of the gland to secrete but the basal rate was restored within 15 min of cessation of the stimulus.

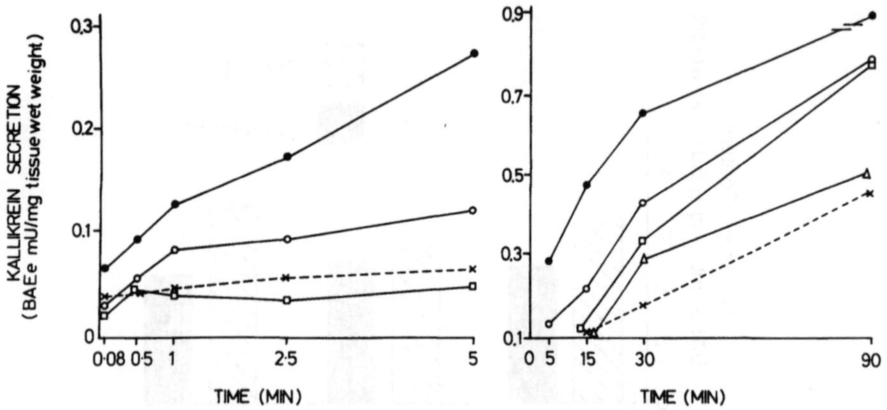

Fig. 7. Time-course of enzyme secretion evoked by noradrenaline, acetylcholine, cyclic AMP and cyclic GMP from guinea-pig submandibular gland slices (ALBANO et al., 1976c). Tissue was incubated as described in Fig. 1. The cumulative submandibular kallikrein (BAEe ΔE_{366} mU/mg wet tissue) secreted into the medium was measured. X–X = Control (basal); ●–● noradrenaline, 40 μ*M*; O–O acetylcholine, 400 μ*M*; □–□ dibutyryl cyclic AMP, 4 m*M*; △–△ dibutyryl cyclic, GMP 4 m*M*. Values represent mean of 3–8 determinations

This finding suggests that human parotid kallikrein is synthesized in cells which have a rapid turnover of protein.

We have recently examined in vitro the role of cyclic nucleotides in the control of kallikrein secretion from isolated slices of guinea-pig submandibular gland (ALBANO et al., 1976c). The cumulative release of kallikrein in response to a number of secretagogues is illustrated in Fig. 7. Noradrenaline increased kallikrein secretion; the initial release of enzyme appeared to be dose-dependent. Isoprenaline (β-adrenoceptor agonist) and phenylephrine (α-adrenoceptor agonist) were almost as potent as noradrenaline in releasing kallikrein. Both propranolol and phentolamine were necessary for the complete inhibition of the noradrenaline-stimulated enzyme secretion. Whereas in the guinea-pig, secretion of submandibular kallikrein in response to noradrenaline involved both β- and α-adrenoceptors (ALBANO et al., 1976), release in the cat was mediated entirely by α-adrenoceptors (GAUTVIK et al., 1974b). In isolated slices of guinea-pig submandibular gland, noradrenaline produced a rise in the intracellular level of cyclic AMP that preceded the stimulated secretion of kallikrein. Of the various adrenergic agents, noradrenaline and isoprenaline were most potent, whereas phenylephrine was significantly less effective in raising basal cyclic AMP values (Fig. 8). Dibutyryl cyclic AMP also stimulated kallikrein secretion. In membrane fragments prepared from homogenates of guinea-pig submandibular gland, noradrenaline activated the adenylate cyclase; this effect was inhibited by propranolol but mainly unaffected by phentolamine (LEMON and BHOOLA, 1975).

The cumulative secretion of kallikrein by the guinea-pig submandibular gland slices evoked by acetylcholine was dose-dependent. The onset of secretion showed a significant time-lag, greater than that observed for noradrenaline. Atropine completely blocked the release of kallikrein by acetylcholine (ALBANO et al., 1976); this contrasts with the observation in the cat where GAUTVIK et al. (1974b) reported

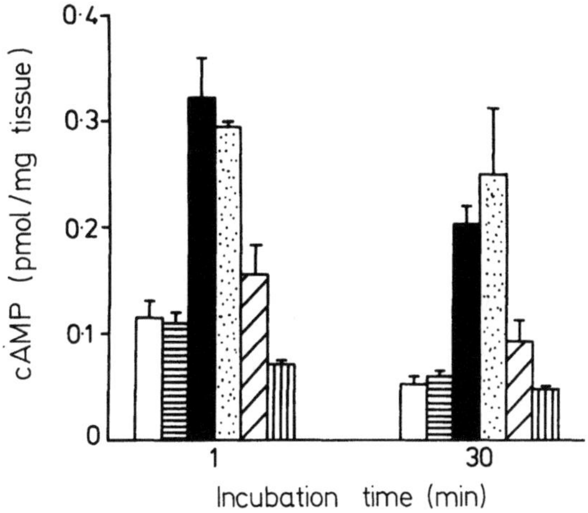

Fig. 8. Comparison of the relative potency of adrenoceptor agonists and acetylcholine in raising cyclic AMP in submandibular gland slices secreting kallikrein. Values for cyclic AMP expressed as pmol/mg wet tissue. Drug concentration 0.4 m*M*. Histograms represent □ basal, ▤ acetylcholine, ■ noradrenaline, ▨ isoprenaline, ▩ phenylephrine and ▥ methoxamine. Bar shows S.E. of mean, n = 3 (each n value was the mean of triplicate cyclic AMP measurements). From ALBANO et al., 1976c

atropine-resistant cholinergic secretion of kallikrein. The failure of acetylcholine and carbachol to stimulate adenylate cyclase (BHOOLA and LEMON, 1973; LEMON and BHOOLA, 1975) and raise the intracellular levels of cyclic AMP (BHOOLA and LEMON, 1974) suggested that the molecular mechanisms controlling the cholinergic secretion of kallikrein were different from those controlling β-adrenoceptor mediated secretion. Acetylcholine raised intracellular levels of cyclic GMP but only when the tissue incubations were performed in the presence of the cyclic nucleotide phosphodiesterase inhibitor, isobutyl-methyl-xanthine. Dibutyryl cyclic GMP caused a transient release of kallikrein which was not maintained (ALBANO et al., 1976c).

A progressive increase in the potassium concentration of the incubating medium bathing the guinea-pig submandibular gland slices resulted in an increase in kallikrein. The peak response was obtained at 75 m*M* K^+, with the threshold between 25 and 75 m*M* K^+. The action of calcium on the stimulation of kallikrein release by neurotransmitters and by cyclic nucleotides was investigated by ALBANO et al. (1976c). The omission of calcium (DOUGLAS, 1968; GAUTVIK and KRIN, 1974), combined with the addition of EGTA to the incubation medium reduced the acetylcholine and dibutyryl cyclic GMP-evoked release of kallikrein to a greater extent than that of noradrenaline, isoprenaline, and dibutyryl cyclic AMP. Increasing concentrations of calcium up to 10 m*M* increased only the acetylcholine and dibutyryl cyclic GMP-stimulated kallikrein secretion (ALBANO et al., 1976c).

The evidence so far indicates a role for cyclic nucleotides in the control of kallikrein secretion from the submandibular gland. Activation of β-adrenoceptors

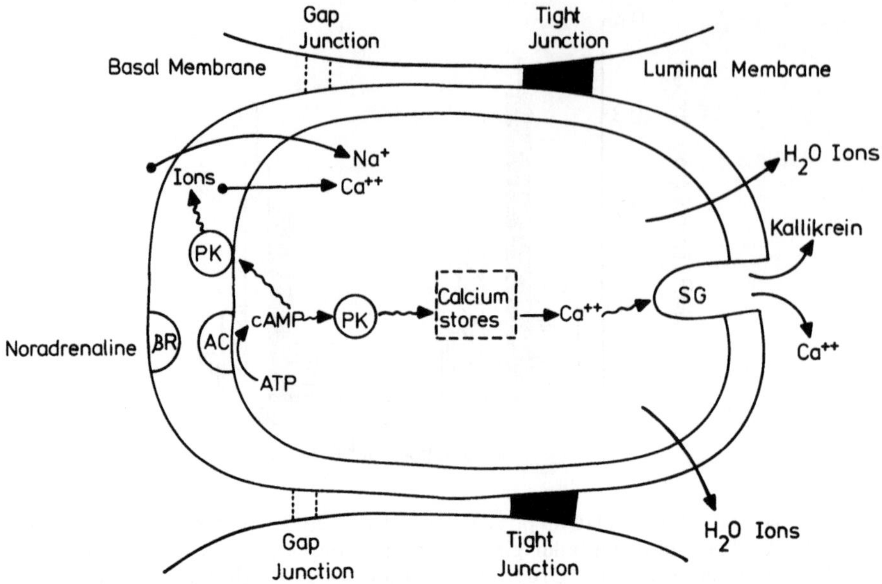

Fig. 9. Molecular model for stimulus-secretion coupling involving β-adrenoceptors in a submandibular gland cell. Noradrenaline combines with the β-adrenoceptor (βR) on the plasma membrane and activates adenylate cyclase (AC). The cyclic AMP formed may activate membrane-bound and cytoplasmic protein kinases (PK) to release free calcium which is thought to initiate exocytosis of secretory granules (SG)

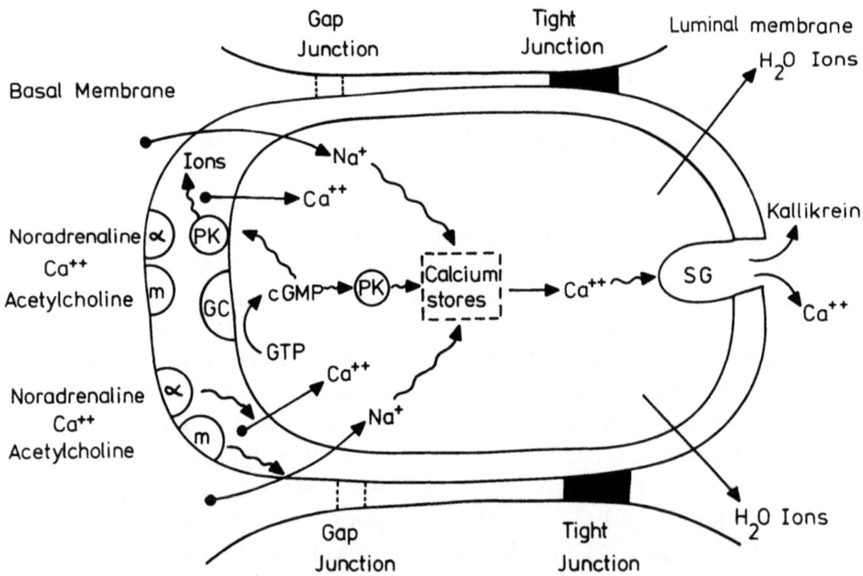

Fig. 10. Molecular model for stimulus-secretion coupling involving cholinergic muscarinic receptors (m) and α-adrenoceptors (α) in a submandibular gland cell. Membrane activation by the transmitters results in the formation of cyclic GMP which may activate menbrane-bound and cytoplasmic protein kinases (PK). The released free calcium is believed to initiate exocytosis of secretory granules (SG). GC, guanylate cyclase; GTP, guanosine triphosphate

induces adenylate cyclase to form cyclic AMP from ATP (Fig. 9); activation of cholinergic muscarinic receptors and α-adrenoceptors stimulates guanylate cyclase to form cyclic GMP from GTP (Fig. 10). Perhaps the cyclic nucleotides so formed combine with specific protein kinases to either phosphorylate or dephosphorylate key membrane proteins and hence alter cation permeability. This could result in an intracellular rise in free calcium and initiate the exocytotic release of kallikrein into the secretory lumen (BHOOLA and COGDELL, 1974; ALBANO et al., 1976c).

C. Subcellular Distribution

I. Subcellular Distribution of Submandibular Kallikrein

In 1962, BHOOLA and OGLE designed experiments to determine the subcellular distribution profile of kallikrein in the submandibular gland of the guinea-pig in the anticipation that such information may be important in determining its functional role in exocrine glands. In these early experiments, about 60% of the kallikrein activity was recovered from fractions sedimented at up to 17,800 × g indicating that it was sequestered in particulate organelles, in contrast to amylase which appeared to be mainly solubilized. The kallikrein-containing organelles were readily lysed by suspension in hypotonic solution. The question whether kallikrein molecules were bound to an intragranular matrix or whether they were in free solution in the organelle could not be resolved. The results (BHOOLA and OGLE, 1966) clearly pointed to a localization of kallikrein in granules with sedimentation properties similar to those described for pancreatic zymogen granules by SIEKEVITZ and PALADE (1958).

After extensive differential centrifugation and sucrose density-gradient experiments, BHOOLA (1968) reported that kallikrein in the guinea-pig submandibular gland was sequestered in particles that equilibrated with 1.7–1.8 M sucrose. These organelles differed distinctly from mitochondria and lysosomes but resembled closely pancreatic zymogen granules in their sedimentation properties. When examined histochemically, the kallikrein-rich granules stained with hemotoxylin-eosin and reacted positively with periodic acid-Schiff (PAS) reagent.

ERDÖS et al. (1968) examined the subcellular distribution profile of kallikrein in rat submandibular gland because it was known to contain the highest amounts of kallikrein (WERLE, 1960). The kallikrein-containing granules were harvested at 480 × g and formed 24% of the total activity of the homogenate. This fraction was subjected to further purification on a discontinuous sucrose density gradient and the kallikrein granules recovered between 1.60 and 1.80 M sucrose. When the kallikrein granules were incubated with Triton X-100 or suspended in hypotonic sucrose solutions (molarity below 0.25), the particle membrane ruptured to release kallikrein. Dissolution of the granules upon addition of Triton X-100 was also visualized under phase-contrast microscopy. Similar to the kallikrein granules isolated from guinea-pig submandibular gland homogenates, the secretory granules from rat were also PAS positive. In order to distinguish kallikrein from the trypsin-like esteroproteases described by EKFORS et al. (1967a, b, 1969), both the kininogenase and esterase activities and the inhibitor profile of particle-associated kallikrein were determined. ERDÖS et al. (1968) also examined the purified kallikrein organelles separated on discontinuous sucrose gradient by electron microscopy and observed that the granules were spherical in shape and about 2 μ in diameter. The morphologic appearance of the granules was similar to the zymogen granules of the pancreas.

In 1964, CARVALHO and DINIZ suggested that renin and kallikrein in the kidney may be located in the same subcellular organelle. Since both kallikrein and renin were known to occur in the submandibular gland of the mouse (WERLE et al., 1957), the subcellular distribution profile of kallikrein and renin was examined by CHIANG et al. (1968). Secretory granules were initially separated by differential centrifugation of the gland homogenate. The washed 480 × *g* pellet contained about 20% of the total renin and kallikrein activities. When subjected to discontinuous sucrose density gradient about 50% of each activity was recovered between 1.60 and 1.84 *M* sucrose. On a continuous sucrose density gradient, the renin and kallikrein showed a similar profile. Only a small percentage of total esterase enzyme was considered to be identical with kallikrein because it possessed kininogenase activity which was diisopropyl-fluorophosphate sensitive. Both the esterase and the kininogenase activities were unaffected by soya bean trypsin inhibitor (SBTI) and aprotinin. Direct identification of the kallikrein granules isolated from guinea-pig, cat, rat, and mouse submandibular glands may now be possible with specific antibodies raised against pure kallikrein prepared from the submandibular gland of each species. Morphologically, the large spherical granules (2 μ in diameter) that contained kallikrein were considered to resemble the pancreatic zymogen granules and the secretory organelles isolated from the submandibular gland of the rat. The small, elliptoid or amorphous organelles were believed to store renin and resembled the granules visualized in the juxtaglomerular apparatus of the kidney. GEIPERT and ERDÖS (1971) extended these studies and examined the sedimentation properties of the secretory granules by rate-zone centrifugation, an experimental procedure which separates subcellular organelles according to their size. Most of the kallikrein granules equilibrated with a higher molarity of sucrose than the renin particles, thereby suggesting that kallikrein and renin were sequestered in different organelles.

BHOOLA and HEAP (1970) designed experiments, using homogenates of guinea-pig submandibular gland, to characterize further kallikrein-containing granules from the various subcellular organelles in order to determine their morphologic properties and to identify chemically the kallikrein sequestered within the secretory organelles. Subcellular particles recovered at 9500 × *g* were layered on a discontinuous sucrose density gradient and centrifuged at 24,500 × *g*. About 85% of the kallikrein-containing organelles were recovered between 1.6 and 1.85 *M* sucrose. This band was recentrifuged on a second discontinuous sucrose density gradient. Each gradient was monitored by means of specific subcellular enzyme markers for mitochondria and lysosomes. Marker enzyme activity and electron micrographs confirmed that a highly purified secretory granule fraction was isolated on the second gradient between 1.80 and 1.85 *M* sucrose. Kallikrein and residual amylase organelles were not separated by this technique. Because proteins similar to kallikrein were known to occur in the rat submandibular gland and may also be sequestered in intracellular particles, we characterized further the properties of membrane-enclosed kallikrein. Neither the kallikrein in the purest granule population nor aqueous extracts of freeze-dried submandibular gland showed any hydrolysis of the trypsin substrate, benzoyl-arginine p-nitroanilide (BANA). Kallikrein from the purest fraction was

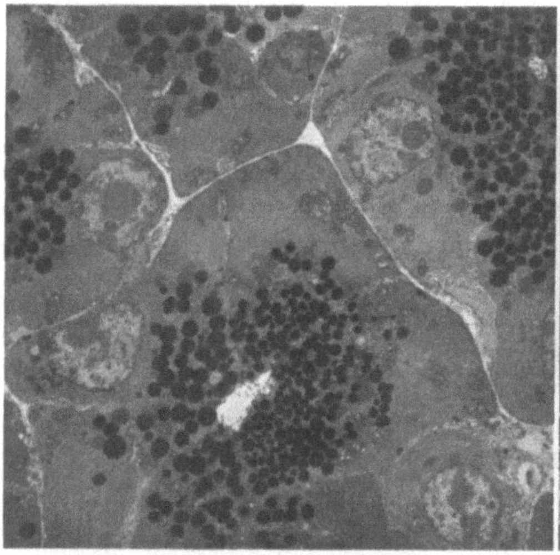

a

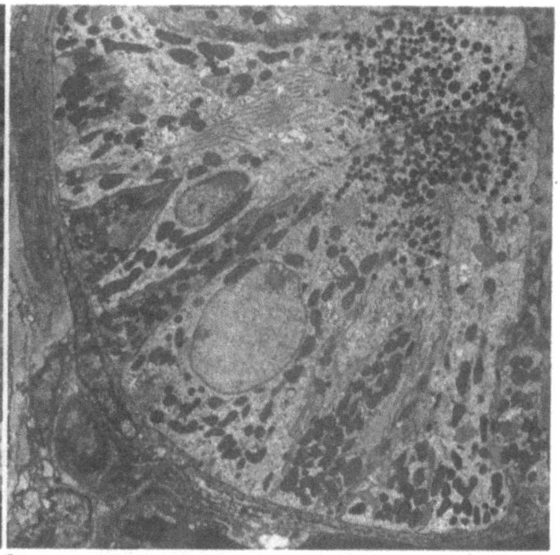

b

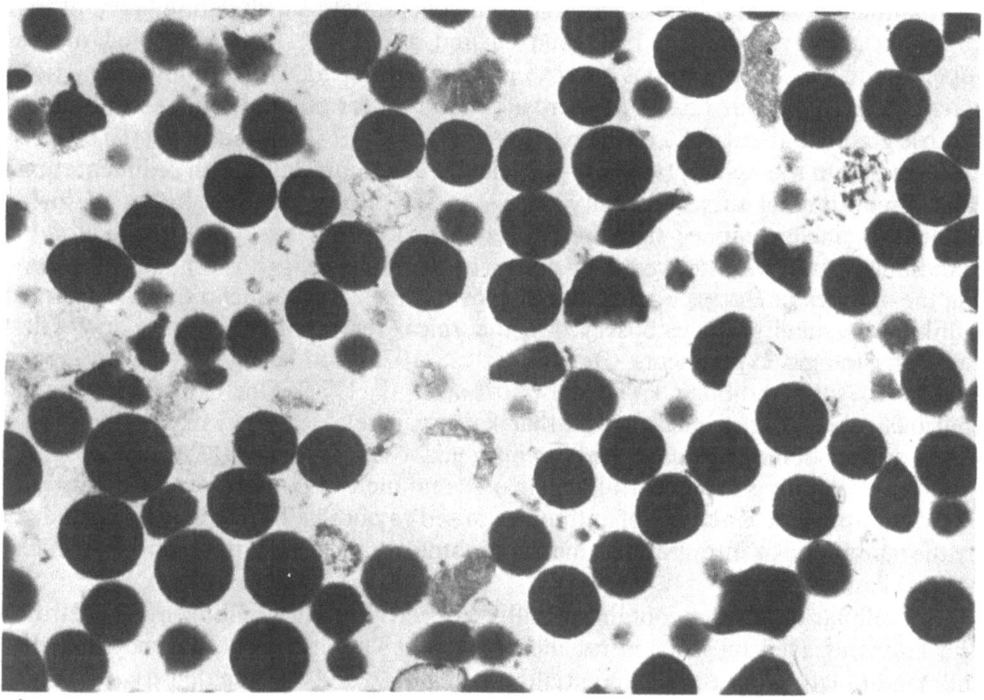

ai

Fig. 11a and b. Acinar and striated duct cells and kallikrein-containing granules isolated from the submandibular gland of the guinea-pig (BHOOLA and HEAP, 1970). **a** Acinar cells with secretory granules. ×1000. (ai) Organelles isolated from homogenates of guinea-pig submandibular gland and separated on a discountinuous sucrose density gradient at 1.8–1.85 *M* sucrose. These organelles stained pink with methylene blue – basic fuschin. ×10,000. **b** Striated duct cells with much smaller granules in the apical area of the cell. ×3000. These particles equilibrated with 1.3 *M* sucrose on discontinuous density gradients. They stained blue with methylene blue – basic fuschin

solubilized with Triton X-100 and subjected to paper electrophoresis; kallikrein migrated to the anode in a similar way to a highly purified preparation of porcine submandibular kallikrein. The biologic activity, indicated by its ability to release kallidin, was determined by assays on guinea-pig ileum, rat duodenum, and dog blood pressure. The organelles which contained the highest kallikrein activity closely resembled, both in ultrastructural appearance and in size, the acinar cells granules (Fig. 11). Bhoola and Heap (1970) concluded that the kallikrein-containing granules separated from homogenates of guinea-pig submandibular gland were derived from the granules in the acinar cells of intact tissue.

The question whether kallikrein in other mammalian species was also sequestered in membrane-enclosed particles was investigated by Bhoola (1969). Differential centrifugation experiments on homogenates prepared from submandibular glands of the cat, dog, rabbit, rat, and guinea-pig showed that 45–60% of the total kallikrein was harvested in granules which sedimented at relatively low g. The subcellular distribution profile of kallikrein in the cat submandibular gland was delineated further (Bhoola and Dorey, 1969). The results showed that kallikrein was stored in cytoplasmic granules, forming a distinct group of particles clearly different from mitochondria and lysosomes. With our differential centrifugation, 44% of the kallikrein activity sedimented at $9500 \times g$ and about 47% was recovered in the supernatant. On discontinuous sucrose gradient about 51% of the low g fraction activity was isolated at 1.5–1.6 M sucrose ($24,500 \times g$ for 60 min); on a second, finer sucrose gradient about 60% of the particles settled at 1.7–1.8 M sucrose ($180,000 \times g$ for 60 min). On the assumption that particle diameter correlated with sedimentation rate, discontinuous sucrose density gradients and ultrastructural studies of these isolated organelles implied that the kallikrein-rich granules isolated from cat submandibular gland were derived from acinar or demilune cells. It is difficult to reconcile the findings of Bhoola and Dorey (1969) with the recent definitive location of kallikrein in small granules observed in the apical region of cat striated duct cells from physiologic experiments (Barton et al., 1975) and using specific antibody against cat submandibular kallikrein (Hojima et al., 1977). One explanation for a spurious subcellular profile may be that kallikrein released from its specific organelles during homogenization had become adsorbed to the large, electron-dense granules originating from central acinar or demilune cells. Alternatively, albeit unlikely, the antigenic reactivity of antibodies raised to pure kallikrein may be occluded by the membrane or intragranular matrix of some organelles but not by others which contain kallikrein.

Subcellular organelles containing kallikrein activity (with kininogen as substrate and kinins assayed on isolated rat uterus) were isolated from homogenates of rat submandibular gland using differential centrifugation and sucrose density gradients (Gautvik and Kriz, 1974), as described by Bhoola and Heap (1970). The kininogenase and the BAEe esterase activities showed a parallel subcellular distribution. The spontaneous lysis of the BAEe esterase-containing organelles was reduced in hyperosmolar solutions, confirming the earlier finding of Erdös et al. (1968). The lysis of granules was reduced at 20 °C and at pH 7.35 when compared with 37 °C and pH 8.0, respectively. The stability of the granules was markedly enhanced by increasing the calcium concentration to 27 mM and to a lesser extent magnesium (25 mM) but was reduced marginally in 60 mM potassium.

BHOOLA and COGDELL (1974) examined the nature of the surface charge on secretory granules isolated from the submandibular gland of the guinea-pig by particle electrophoresis. The granules suspended in morpholenopropane sulphonic acid-KOH buffered sucrose solutions moved to the anode. Increasing the calcium concentrations from 0.04 m*M* to 4.0 m*M* progressively reduced the movement of the granules towards the anode. A similar effect was observed with 4.0 m*M* magnesium. Both the divalent ions seemed to neutralize the net surface of the granules, thereby suggesting that the electrostatic surface charge may be a major factor in controlling the fusion of the secretory granules to the cell membranes, before release of its contents by exocytosis (see MATTHEWS, 1971).

II. Subcellular Distribution of Pancreatic Kallikrein

The concept of membrane-enclosed kallikrein first emerges from the experiments of SIEBERT et al. (1955) who recovered particulate kallikrein by differential centrifugation. Homogenates of hog pancreas were separated into a mitochondrial and a mixed microsomal-cytoplasmic fraction. Significant amounts of kallikrein were located in the mitochondrial fraction.

With the extensive experience gathered in determining the subcellular distribution pattern of kallikrein in mammalian submandibular glands, BHOOLA and DOREY (1969, 1971a) designed experiments to characterize the kallikrein-containing organelles in the cat and dog pancreas. Homogeneity of the subcellular fractions was monitored by following the profile of reference enzymes for mitochondria and microsomes, and using potassium and lactic dehydrogenase as cytoplasmic markers. The kininogenase activity of kallikrein was measured in the presence of SBTI on kininogen from dog plasma and the kinins formed assayed on isolated guinea-pig ileum. Extracts of freeze-dried pancreatic gland indicated that only 15% of cat kallikrein and 30% of dog kallikrein appeared to be in an active form. However, kallikrein in the subcellular fractions was readily released in an active form by a reduction in the tonicity of the homogenizing sucrose solution, with no further activation by incubation with enterokinase. Subcellular distribution patterns after direct measurement or enterokinase activation indicated that kallikrein was located in granules that sedimented mainly at $10{,}000 \times g$. Whereas the subcellular distribution patterns of kallikrein and amylase were very similar, that of trypsinogen was clearly different. Trypsinogen showed two particulate profiles: one resembled kallikrein with a comparable peak in the $10{,}000 \times g$ pellet and the other was clearly different with a peak in the $350{,}000 \times g$ pellet. The secretory granules were subjected to purification on two discontinuous sucrose density gradients.

Subcellular organelles recovered at $16{,}000 \times g$ were layered on a discontinuous sucrose density gradient. The secretory granules containing all three enzymes separated between 1.6 and 1.7 *M* sucrose. This fraction was relayered on a finer second gradient. All three enzymes were once again recovered between 1.7 and 1.775 *M* sucrose. Although the secretory granules were clearly separated from other intracellular particles, the granules containing the individual secretory enzymes possessed similar sedimentation properties. Ultrastructural analysis of the subcellular organelles in the secretory enzyme-containing fraction of the first sucrose gradient revealed two populations; one discrete and electron-dense group and the other pale with a diffuse intragranular structure. The purer granule fraction of the second gradient that possessed the highest kallikrein, trypsin, and amylase activity contained predominantly organelles which in their size, shape, and intragranular appearance were similar to the granules observed in situ in the acinar cells. Parallel studies of kallikrein-containing organelles isolated from homogenates of cat pancreas showed a similar profile on sucrose density gradients and equilibrated with 1.7–1.8 *M* sucrose (BHOOLA, 1969; BHOOLA and DOREY, 1969). However, in view of the findings of SCHACHTER and his colleages (BARTON et al., 1975; HOJIMA et al., 1977) in the cat submandibular gland, the question does arise as to whether the cellular location of pancreatic kallikrein can be inferred from these studies. Until antibodies are raised to cat and dog pancreatic kallikrein and direct localization experiments performed, the conclusions of BHOOLA (1970) on the location of pancreatic kallikrein in acinar cells must remain tentative.

D. Cellular Location

I. Localization of Kallikrein in Rat Submandibular Gland

During the last decade, considerable progress has been made in the isolation and purification of glandular kallikreins. Recently BRANDTZAEG et al. (1976) reported the isolation of three groups of esterases from rat submandibular gland, one of which was resolved into four kallikreins. The three main molecular species are reminiscent of the early isolation studies of EKFORS et al. (1967a, b, see section on Gland Content). The purified kallikreins were differentiated by BRANDTZAEG et al. (1976) from the other two groups of esteroproteases by their ability to release kinin (assayed on isolated rat uterus) from rat kininogen, to produce hypotension in the rat, and by their low caseinolytic activity. All three esteroproteases reacted with the antibody raised in sheep to rat urinary kallikrein. Thus, in order to localize kallikrein immunohistochemically in rat submandibular gland, specificity was achieved by adsorbing the cross-reacting, nonkallikrein esteroproteases to the antibody. For immunofluorescent localization, the antibody was conjugated to tetramethylrodamine isothiocyanate. Specific kallikrein immunofluorescence was observed in the granular tubules, striated ducts and some of the main duct cells of the rat submandibular gland (ÖRSTAVIK et al., 1975; BRANDTZAEG et al., 1976). A similar fluorescent rim was noted in striated ducts of the sublingual glands. No kallikrein was identified in acinar cells, even in submandibular glands stimulated to secrete by close arterial infusion of acetylcholine or adrenaline (see GAUTVIK et al., 1974a). The association of kallikrein with granular tubule cells confirmed the results of ERDÖS et al. (1968) who isolated kallikrein-rich granules identical in morphologic features to zymogen granules which were indistinguishable from the membrane-enclosed organelles observed by DOREY and BHOOLA (1972) in these cells. Kallikrein was also detected in the interstitial tissue and considered by ÖRSTAVIK et al. (1975) to support the view that kallikrein was involved in functional vasodilatation. However, they were unable to exclude the possibility that such a localization may have occurred because of the diffusion of the antigen from intracellular sites during the preparation of the tissue section for immunofluorescent histology. In a subsequent report, no stromal kallikrein was detected (BRANDTZAEG et al., 1976).

Although kallikrein has been identified immunologically in granular tubule and duct cells, there is no evidence at present of a de novo synthesis of kallikrein in these cells. The granular tubule cells contain very small amounts of the cytoplasmic organelles and the endoplasmic reticulum necessary for protein synthesis (SCOTT and PEASE, 1959; MATTHEWS et al., 1971). The view that granular tubule cells sequester, in storage granules, macromolecules synthesized elsewhere (SREEBNY and MAYER, 1964) was investigated by MATTHEWS (1974) using rat submandibular gland. A rapid transfer of tritiated tryptohan was observed from base to apex in autoradiographs of the acinar cells. The time course showed two peaks at the base of the cells, one at 40 min and the other at 120 min. In contrast, in the granular tubule cells there was a single peak at the base of the cells at 60 min, but two peaks at the apex (secretory segment), one at 4 h and the other at 12 h. From these results, MATTHEWS (1974) concluded that protein synthesis occurs in the granular tubule cells but with a much slower turnover time than in the acinar cells. Reinterpretation of the second apical peak observed in the granular tubule cells may suggest that, in addition to synthesizing some new protein, these cells may trap and store luminal macromolecules by emiocytosis. Such an explanation may resolve the paradoxical finding that these cells store very large amounts of secretory protein but contain little of the cytologic components essential for protein synthesis.

II. Localization of Kallikrein in Cat Submandibular Gland

The earliest observations on the histologic changes produced by autonomic nerve stimulation and denervation in acinar, demilunar, and striated duct cells of the cat submandibular gland were made by RAWLINSON (1933, 1935). Recently, such an approach has been used to locate more precisely the cells of the cat submandibular gland which contain kallikrein. In 1975, BARTON et al., reported experiments correlating morphologic changes following autonomic nerve stimulation with the kallikrein content of the gland. Experiments of similar design were performed by GARRETT and KIDD (1975) to determine the neural contribution of striated duct cells to the organic content of saliva.

BARTON et al. (1975) demonstrated that prolonged intermittent, sympathetic nerve stimulation (10–25 min actual stimulation time at 20 Hz) completely depleted the small membrane-bound, electron-dense organelles observed in the apical region of the striated duct cells (Fig. 12), but produced no change in number of the larger granules of the acinar cells. In such stimulated glands, the kallikrein decreased by 90–95%. In the studies of GARRETT and KIDD (1975) sympathetic nerve stimulation was accompanied by loss of intensely staining, diastase-resistant PAS-positive and dimethylaminobenzaldehyde nitrite (DMAB, tryptophan-reactive) positive material. The loss of histochemically reactive substance paralleled the depletion of the small granules in the striated duct cells. In contrast, intermittent chorda tympani nerve stimulation (15–40 min actual stimulation; 5 min on and 5 min off; 10 Hz) resulted in a complete disappearance of acinar cell granules without any fall in the gland content of kallikrein and produced no significant change in the number of striated duct cell granules (BARTON et al., 1975). The changes in acinar cells were reflected by a comparable loss of diastase-resistant, PAS-positive material, whereas the neutral

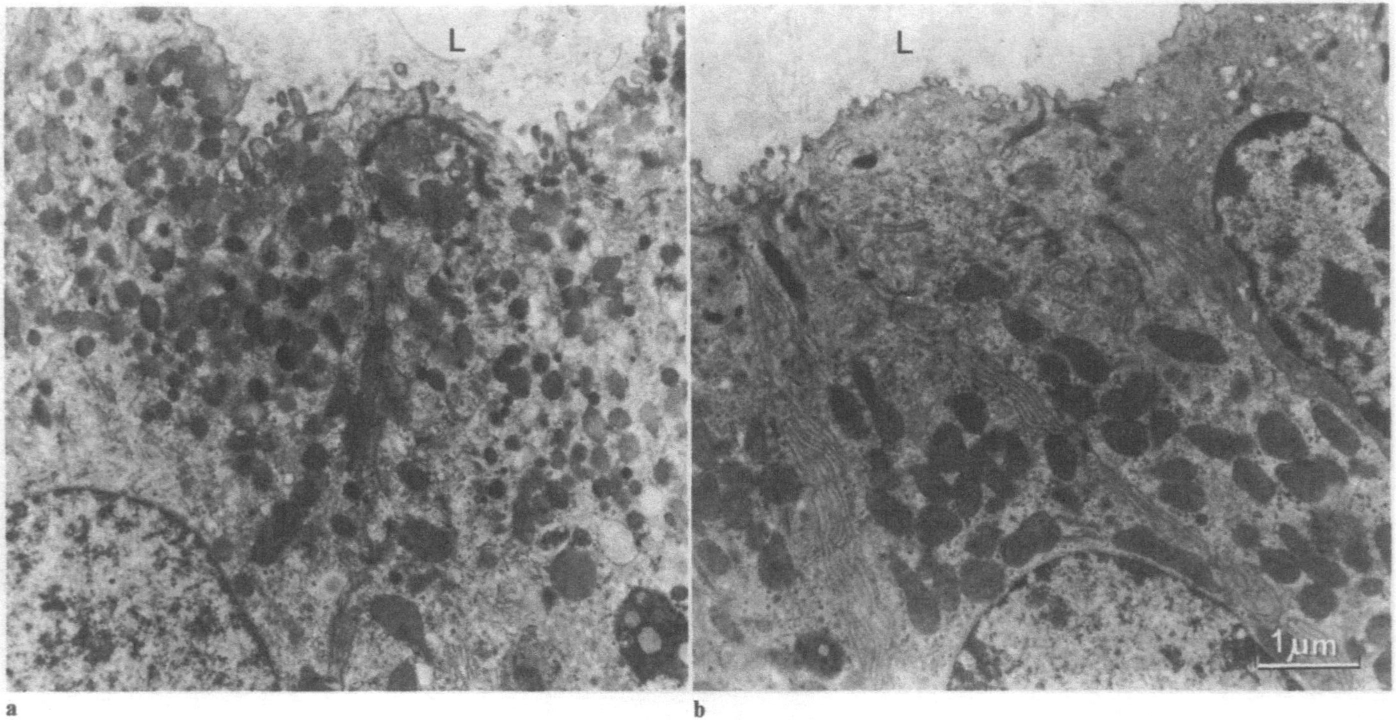

Fig. 12a and b. Effect of duct ligation on secretory granules in striated duct cells of the cat submandibular gland. **a** Normal cat submandibular gland showing numerous small secretory granules in the apical regions of several striated duct cells. **b** Ligated gland 5 days after duct ligation showing absence of apical granules and prominence of mitochondria longitudinally arranged in this region. L = lumen. Bar 1 μM. The small secretory granules seen in the micrograph on the left also disappear after prolonged sympathic nerve stimulation or after degenerative section of the chorda tympani nerve. (From SCHACHTER et al., 1977)

mucins in the duct cells were either unaffected or even increased (GARRETT and KIDD, 1975).

BARTON et al. (1975) reported that stimulation of either nerve did not alter significantly the number of electron-pale organelles in the demilunar cells. But, RAWLINSON (1933) in his light microscopy study showed vacuolization of some demilune cells after sympathetic nerve stimulation. In preliminary experiments following sympathetic nerve stimulation of three cats YOUNG et al. (unpublished), observed that in the demilunar cells membrane-bound organelles with electron-dense inclusion bodies were supplanted by irregular, vesicular organelles of varying size and an active Golgi apparatus.

EMMELIN and HENRIKSSON (1953) found that parasympathetic denervation caused a fall in the kallikrein content of submandibular gland (kininogenase activity was assayed on blood pressure) and was associated with histologic changes in the demilunar cells. Preganglionic parasympathetic nerve denervation of 12–15 days duration was accompanied by almost complete reduction (90%–95%) in the kininogenase content of cat submandibular gland (SCHACHTER and BARTON, 1974); a number of cytoplasmic (lactic dehydrogenase) and membrane-bound (β-glucuronidase) enzymes were relatively unaffected. The kallikrein content was unaltered after long term pre- and postganglionic sympathetic denervation. Histochemically, GARRETT and KIDD (1975) demonstrated that after sectioning of the chorda tympani nerve there was a reduction in neutral mucin and tryptophan-positive material in the apical region of the striated ducts. The small apical granules which contain the neutral mucin were absent in the striated duct cells of the denervated gland (GARRETT and KIDD, (1975). The lack of correlation after chorda nerve stimulation between secretion of kallikrein, gland content of kallikrein, histochemical reactivity of the cells and the number of granules visualized in the demilunar cells and in the apical segment of striated ducts requires further analysis and experimentation. It has been suggested that resynthesis of kallikrein during the stimulation period may account for the lack of correlation. However, present evidence indicates that the turnover of protein in straited duct cells is slow and that they do not possess the capacity to rapidly synthesize protein. Another important and interesting question is the trophic influence of the chorda tympani on the synthesis of kallikrein.

HOJIMA et al. (1977) located kallikrein in the apical part of the striated duct cells of the cat submandibular with a specific, fluorescent antibody. Kallikrein from the cat submandibular gland was purified from aqueous extracts of the gland by acetone precipitation (50–75%), DEAE-Sephadex A-50 chromatography and Sephadex G-75 and G-50 gel filtration (MORIWAKI et al., 1975). The lyophilized purified preparation possessed kininogenase (assayed on dog blood pressure, 1260 U/mg protein) and esterase (24.5 U/mg protein) activities comparable to that of pure hog pancreatic kallikrein. The pure enzyme was only partially (20%) inhibited by aprotinin. The molecular weight was estimated at 50,000 by gel filtration. The pure preparation consisted of several forms (four to six) on isoelectric focusing, but gave a single protein band on disc gel electrophoresis. Antibody to the pure kallikrein was raised in rabbits and immunodiffusion tests gave a single arc in the presence of immune serum.

Light microscopy sections of cat submandibular gland were incubated with immune and nonimmune sera and then reacted with fluorescein isothiocyanate-labeled rabbit anti-IgG. An intense yellow-green fluorescence was visualized at the apical part of the striated duct cell between the nucleus and the luminal border. Some collecting duct cells showed a distinct but narrow fluorescent luminal rim. None of the remaining structures (acinar, demilune, and myoepithelial cells, capillaries or interstitial tissue) showed any significant amount of specific fluorescence. This study clearly demonstrated that kallikrein in the cat submandibular gland was stored in the apical part of the striated duct cells. The question whether kallikrein is synthesized in duct cells, and whether these represent the only site of synthesis in the gland, remains to be answered.

III. Localization of Kallikrein in Guinea-Pig Submandibular Gland

The attempts of BHOOLA and colleagues to ascertain the cellular location of kallikrein through extensive experiments with subcellular organelles in combination with detailed morphologic characterization and through analysis of studies of ontogenic development and hormonal influences, seemed to be an appropriate approach in the early pioneering days of this work. Immunohistochemistry and correlations between nerve stimulation and histologic changes have provided a direct answer.

MATTHEWS and BHOOLA (1976) examined the effect of autonomic nerve stimulation on kallikrein content and on the various secretory granule populations of guinea-pig submandibular gland. Recently, staining thick sections (1 μm) of resin-embedded material using methylene blue and basic fuschin (WILKES, 1976, unpublished) enabled acinar and duct cells granules to be differentiated. The acinar granules stained pink whereas the striated (junctional) duct granules stained blue. Intermittent sympathetic nerve stimulation (8 Hz; total stimulation time 10, 20, and 40 min) produced a marked secretion of kallikrein into the saliva. The secretion was accompanied by reduction of the pink acinar granules. Even after prolonged intermittent stimulation (actual stimulation time, 40 min) when marked changes were observed in acinar cells, the blue, tryptophan-positive granules in the striated (junctional) duct cells showed no obvious reduction in number. Only when combined continuous parasympathetic and intermittent sympathetic nerve stimulation was used was a significant reduction seen in the granule population of substantive numbers of duct cells.

In view of the new histochemical information, BHOOLA and HEAP (unpublished) decided to re-examine the staining properties of the isolated kallikrein-rich granules in the purest subcellular fraction that was processed for electron microscopy in 1969 and retained. The granules in sections from this fraction stained pink with methylene blue-basic fuschin, consistent with the conclusion that the granules were of acinar origin. With this technique, the blue granules were traced to the microsomal fraction which had equilibrated with 1.3 *M* sucrose in the experiments reported by BHOOLA and HEAP in 1970.

BHOOLA et al. (1977) designed experiments to localize kallikrein in guinea-pig submandibular gland by immunofluorescent histochemistry. Kallikrein was extracted by homogenzing ice-cold guinea-pig submandibular glands in 100 m*M* acetic acid. The neutralized supernatant was treated batchwise with DEAE-cellulose slurry and purified, first by gel filtration on Sephadex G-100, and finally by elution with an ammonium acetate gradient from a DEAE-Sephadex A-50 column. The purified enzyme (esterase activity 1.2 μmol BAEe/min/mg dry weight; kininogenase activity: 20 μgeq bradykinin mg dry weight, assayed on isolated guinea-pig ileum with heated dog plasma as the source of kininogen) moved as a single band during electrophoresis on polyacrylamide disc gels. Antibody to the purified enzyme was raised in rabbits and specificity verified by immunodiffusion; a single precipitin arc was obtained. Quantitative inhibition of the antigen was obtained only with the immune serum on rocket immunoelectrophoresis.

Fluorescent staining of guinea-pig submandibular gland sections was performed according to the Coon's "sandwich" technique. Specificity was verified by substituting nonimmune for immune serum in the staining sequence and by blocking the antibody with the enzyme. An intense kallikrein-specific fluorescence was visualized in the acinar and striated (junctional) duct cells. Through further purification (by gel filtration on Sephadex G-100 with 0.1% sodium dodecyl sulphate in 100 mM ammonium acetate) we have separated the guinea-pig submandibular kallikrein used for the immunofluorescent study into two components, one with low and the other with high kininogenase activity. Immunofluorescently, the high activity peak localised mainly in the duct cells and the low activity in both the acini and ducts. The precise cellular storage sites for the guinea-pig submandibular kallikrein remain to be determined, but the site of the kininogenase with a high affinity for BAEE appears to be in the striated (junctional) duct cells. Further experiments are required to determine whether the gland contains multiple kininogenases. The question whether kallikrein is synthesized in duct cells or whether it is captured by emiocytosis remains to be determined. Electron microscopic immunochemistry may resolve the difficult question of whether kallikrein is sequestered in cells in two pools both as a cytoplasmic and as a membrane-enclosed enzyme.

E. Ontogenic Change and Hormonal Influence

Experiments to determine the developmental stage at which synthesis of kallikrein is initiated in exocrine glands was first performed by Werle (1960). Fetal hog, bovine, and dog pancreas contained prekallikrein but the values were about 10% of those found in the adult. Pancreatic levels in neonatal rats (1–10 days old) were lower but those in man and mouse did not differ from adult values. In contrast, fetal human, dog, bovine, and submandibular glands contained little or no kallikrein. Neonatal human, rat, and mouse submandibular glands also differed in having very little kallikrein.

One approach to the cellular location of kallikrein was to follow its postnatal development in rat submandibular gland and to correlate its first appearance with the differentiation of the various cellular elements in the gland (Beraldo et al., 1972). At birth, the gland contained terminal tubules which comprised cells with numerous secretory granules that react with PAS (Jacoby and Leeson, 1959). Intralobular ducts were also present. Submandibular gland from the newborn (12 h old) contained no kallikrein (tested using kininogen from heated rat plasma; kinin formation was assayed on rat uterus). The kallikrein activity was not inhibited by 1-chloro-3-tosylamido-7-amino-2-heptanone (TLCK). The granules visualized in the terminal tubules were therefore considered not to be associated with the synthesis of kallikrein. During the first week, acinar cells began to differentiate from the terminal tubules and correlated with the first appearance of kallikrein in the gland. The increase in kininogenase activity paralleled the maturation of the acini from the first few days after birth to 60–90 days old. From these studies, BERALDO concluded that kallikrein was localized in the acinar cell granules and that the granular tubule and striated duct cells did not participate in the formation of kallikrein.

Contrary results have been obtained by ÖRSTAVIK, BRANDTZAEG, and NUSTAD (see GAUTVIK, 1974a). They followed the development of granular tubules and striated ducts histochemically (the antibody was raised to rat urinary kallikrein). Immunospecificity was tested with purified salivary kallikrein and cross-reactivity with esterase A and B (see BRANDTZAEG et al., 1976). A luminal rim of fluorescence in the intralobular duct cells was observed in the submandibular gland of the 1 week old rat. Cytoplasm of the distal striated ducts also showed fluorescence. The granular tubule cells which began differentiating at 1 month contained fluorescence localized to cytoplasmic particles. At 2 months, the tubules matured and the fluorescent distribution in these cells resembled that of the adult rat. No difference was detected between adult male and female rats even though ERDÖS et al. (1968) reported a higher concentration of kallikrein in the male than in the female. Data on the cellular localization of esterases A and B (BRANDTZAEG et al., 1976) and the sites of synthesis of kallikrein may assist in resolving the opposing results reported by BERALDO and by NUSTAD and GAUTVIK.

Because submandibular glands of newborn mice contained virtually no kallikrein (WERLE, 1960) experiments were designed to examine whether age-related changes in kallikrein levels would correlate with maturation and changes in the number of secretory granules of specific cells in the mouse submandibular gland (BHOOLA et al., 1973). The kininogenase activity (measured by kinin liberation from heated dog plasma and the released kinins assayed in the presence of SBTI and L-cysteine on the cat jejunum) increased 11–20 days postnatally and rose rapidly between 21–30 days. The increase in kallikrein activity coincided with the appearance of organized acinar tissue in both the male and female glands. Although kallikrein activity in the female trailed slightly, it was not significantly different from the activity in the male. A similar observation was reported by TRAUTSCHOLD et al. (1966).

Androgen dependence of proteases and cellular structure in the mouse submandibular gland has been studied extensively. Sex-linked morphologic differences were demonstrated by LACASSAGNE (1940) and CARAMIA (1966a, b). Parallelism between an androgen-dependent increase in proteases and development of granular tubules was indicated by JUNQUEIRA et al. (1949). The biochemical and sexual dimorphism shown by the mouse submandibular gland was considered by BHOOLA et al. (1973) to be of value in determining the cellular localization of the secretory enzymes in the gland. Renin (WERLE, VOGEL and GÖLDEL, 1957; OLIVER and CROSS, 1967; CHIANG et al., 1968) and trypsin-like enzymes were known to be testosterone-dependent (ANGELLETI et al., 1967). BHOOLA et al. (1973) found that chymotrypsin- and trypsin-like enzymes began increasing at 11–20 days and renin at 21–30 days and the increase in enzyme levels was associated with the development of the secretory (granular) tubules. Unlike kallikrein, the changes were observed only in the male. Whereas chymotrypsin, trypsin, and renin activities were abolished in the male within 30 days of castration, there was no reduction in kallikrein activity up to 75 days after castration. The enzyme data correlated with a reduction in the number of secretory tubules and the cells contained fewer granules. In contrast, the acinar cells showed no appreciable change in morphology. Replacement of testosterone in the castrated male produced a parallel return of renin, chymotrypsin, and trypsin activities. Treatment of the female with testosterone was associated with a marked rise in the gland content of the three enzymes and increase in granular tubules. The chymotrypsin- and trypsin-like enzymes and renin showed clear androgen dependence. The question why kallikrein was not induced by testosterone remains unanswered. From the combined study of morphologic changes and enzyme levels, BHOOLA et al. (1973) suggested that kallikrein was synthesized in acinar and intercalated duct cells, and that the chymotrypsin- and trypsin-like proteases and renin were formed in the granular tubules. In view of the recent immunohistochemical localization of kallikrein in the granular tubule cells of the rat, acinar cells of the guinea-pig and in the striated duct cells of the rat, cat, and guinea-pig submandibular glands, one awaits a similar study in the mouse.

The hamster submandibular gland exhibits an oestrogen-dependent biochemical dimorphism. Consequently BHOOLA et al. (1974) studied age- and sex-related effects on both the kallikrein-like esteroproteases and the cellular structure of the gland. Low levels of kallikrein were found in the glands of animals aged 18–22 days. With maturation, the levels rose rapidly 30–35 days after birth, attaining significantly higher values in the female than in the male at 365 days; the sex-related difference became clearly evident about 58–62 days after birth. The ultrastructural organization of acinar granules in the female differed characteristically from that in the male. Following ovariectomy in the female, the fine structure of the acinar granules changed to that of the male and there was a reduction in the esteroprotease activity of the gland. The granules reverted to their original appearance after replacement therapy with oestradial undecylate accompanied by a concomitant rise in the esteroprotease levels of the gland. The evidence suggests regulation of kallikrein activity by the oestrogen group of hormones in the hamster submandibular gland. The cellular location of kallikrein in this species remains to be determined.

Prompted by the experiments in the hamster, BHOOLA et al. (1977) considered that variation in estrogen levels during the menstrual cycle may modulate the synthesis of human kallikrein. Salivary samples from 220 school girls were used to determine the kallikrein content of saliva and to ascertain whether the values changed specifically during the menstrual cycle. Salivary kallikrein activity appeared to alter during the menstrual cycle, the median values showing a distinct premenstrual peak. The question whether changing steroid hormone levels affect the synthesis of human salivary kallikrein merits further study.

F. Recent Views on Functional Role

The pioneering experiments of HEIDENHAIN in 1872 established that salivary secretion but not the vasodilatation that follows stimulation of the chorda tympani nerve to the cat submandibular gland is inhibited by atropine. A functional role for the glandular kallikreins developed from the suggestion by UNGAR and PARROT (1936) that kallikrein was the transmitter for the atropine-resistant vasodilator nerve fibers. HILTON and LEWIS (1955, 1956) reasserted the view that the secretomotor fibers of the chorda tympani released kallikrein from the submandibular gland cells into the interstitial tissue where it formed the vasodilator peptide kallidin from a kininogen substrate; kallidin accounting for the atropine-resistant increase in blood flow. The experiments of HILTON and LEWIS and subsequently those of GAUTVIK established the general view that kallikrein regulated vasodilatation in all glandular organs during secretory activity, in particular in salivary and sweat glands and the pancreas. The evidence for this theory has been reviewed by HILTON (1970), GAUTVIK (1970), and more recently by GAUTVIK et al. (1974a). The generalization and the specific involvement of glandular kallikreins in regulating functional vasodilatation has been questioned by SCHACHTER (1969, 1970, 1974) and by BHOOLA (1968, 1970). The physiologic experiments of SCHACHTER and his colleagues have provided evidence which indicates that kallikrein is not implicated in the vasodilatation produced on stimulation of the chorda tympani nerve.

Evidence for the opposing concepts have been succintly considered in the previous reviews already cited. Clearly, some of the original propositions are no longer tenable. The general view that the glandular kallikreins mediate functional hyperaemia in all glands can no longer be sustained. Specifically, cytochemical work has established that the cholinergic fibers of the chorda tympani nerve innervate blood vessels in the cat submandibular gland (GARRETT, 1966a, b). Physiologic experiments indicate that the innervation is functional. Moreover there is unequivocal evidence that the vasodilatation induced by chorda tympani stimulation is only partially resistant to inhibition by atropine. The time-course of the vasodilatation is influenced by the experimental design, frequency of stimulation, and responsiveness of the blood-flow recording system. Confusion has recently arisen as to precisely which component of the vasodilatation is atropine-resistant. To date, three phases have been described: the first, a rapid initial phase; the second, a maintained or plateau phase, and the third associated with ion transport, in particular with potassium efflux. GAUTVIK (1970) provided evidence for two phases in perfused cat submandibular glands: a rapidly rising one which at the cessation of chorda nerve stimulation continued into a second slowly developing prolonged phase. GAUTVIK believes that the first phase is mediated by cholinergic fibers and the second by the release of kallikrein and the subsequently formed kallidin. DARKE and SMAJE (1972) demonstrated that the nature of the vasodilator response depended on the frequency of stimulation. At frequencies of 1, 2, and 5 Hz, there was an initial high flow rate which subsequently fell to a maintained phase persisting until cessation of stimulation. At frequencies of 10 and 20 Hz, the initial rapid phase gradually increased until a plateau level was attained. Low doses of atropine blocked the initial phase of all frequencies whereas the maintained or plateau response was only affected at low frequencies of stimulation. The general view that chorda tympani stimulates atropine-resistant vasodilatation in the submandibular gland of the cat has arisen from studies in which frequencies of 10 Hz and greater have been used and has resulted in a lack of appreciation of the fact that atropine does partially inhibit the parasympathetically induced increase in blood flow. Using 10 volt pulses of 1 msec duration at a frequency of 25 Hz for the brief stimulation periods of 1–5 secs, POULSEN (1975) uncovered a separate phase. In POULSEN's experiments the first two phases of GAUTVIK and of DARKE and SMAJE were seen as a single event, with a separate subsequent response associated with reuptake of potassium by the gland cells. The first phase was marginally reduced by atropine whereas the subsequent potassium phase was abolished both by atropine and by ouabain.

FERREIRA and SMAJE (1976) described experiments in which stimulation of the chorda lingual nerve to the dog submandibular gland produced salivation, increased blood flow, and released kallidin into the venous effluent. In some glands, the venous output of kinin showed frequency dependence, but in others normal secretory and vascular responses were maintained during the absence of kinin release. After atropine, salivation was abolished and kinin release faded, but the vasodilatation persisted. FERREIRA and SMAJE (1976) concluded that kallikrein can be released into the venous effluent by chorda nerve stimulation and may cause the associated functional vasodilatation. However, they did not consider kallikrein to be the primary mediator of the vasodilatation, nor that it was involved in the causation of the atropine-resistant increase in blood flow in the dog submandibular gland. In contrast, the immunochemical studies of HOJIMA et al. (1977) in the cat and the studies of BRANDTZAEG et al. (1976) in the rat submandibular glands revealed no kallikrein in the interstitial tissue space. SCHACHTER (1977, communication to the Physiological Society) was unable to detect any immunoreactive material in the extracellular space and capillaries of the cat submandibular gland after nerve stimulation. It is therefore desirable that similar studies be performed in the dog submandibular gland, and to follow immunohistochemically the release and movement of kallikrein after nerve stimulation.

The question which remains unanswered since it was first posed over a 100 years ago is the reason for the frequency-dependent, partially atropine-resistant, chorda nerve-induced vasodilatation in the cat submandibular gland. Preoccupation with kallikrein as the essential and significant mediator has inhibited new approaches and fresh attack on this problem. It is possible that there exist separate cholinergic muscarinic receptors with different affinity and binding constants for atropine (BARLOW et al., 1976); these would be analogous to the separate adrenergic and histaminergic receptors, each binding with a specific molecular species of antagonist. Moreover, the assumption that all the fibers in the chorda tympani nerve are cholinergic requires more vigorous testing. The atropine-resistant components may be mediated by purinergic fibers (BURNSTOCK, 1972). Substance P is a potent sialogogue and vasodilator. It is conceivable that in some species in addition to cholinergic fibers, parasympathetic nerves may consist of fibers with purines (ATP) or peptide (substance P) transmitters that augment neural control of secretion and blood flow. Such ideas tested experimentally may assist in elucidating the atropine-resistant functional vasodilatation observed in some secretory glands.

Kallikrein is secreted primarily into the exocrine secretion of the gland and therefore may have an enzymic function in the gastrointestinal tract. Furthermore, because of its location in the striated duct cells of all the species examined so far it may regulate the ionic composition of exocrine secretions. In recent years in particular, analysis of its physiologic actions in the kidney (ADETUYIBI and MILLS, 1972; MARIN-GREZ et al., 1972; PISANO et al., 1974; MILLS and WARD, 1975) has raised the possibility that kallikrein may modulate ion transport across the striated duct cells of exocrine glands. Although this is an attractive proposition, no evidence exists for such an action in the submandibular gland or pancreas. Furthermore, the detailed mechanism and sequential steps involved in such an effect require to be enunciated.

The question whether kallikrein may act directly to alter cell membrane permeability or whether this action is dependent entirely on the release of kallidin remains to be answered. Another interesting new aspects is the effect of the kininogenase-kinin system in the regulation of sperm motility and migration (PALM et al., 1975). The kininogenase acrosin is freed of inhibitors during the *capacitation reaction* in the secretions of the female genital tract. The active acrosin promotes sperm movement, thereby increasing the probability of contact with an ovum. However the precise mode of action and role of kininogenases in the male and female reproductive tracts has to be elucidated. Clearly the different glandular kallikreins may have different but specific physiologic roles.

References

Abelous, J. E., Bardier, E.: Action hypertensive de l'urine humaine normale. C.R. Soc. Biol. (Paris) *64*, 848–849 (1908)

Abelous, J. E., Bardier, E.: Les substances hypotensives de l'urine humaine normale. C.R. Soc. Biol. (Paris) *66*, 511–512 (1909)

Adetuyibi, A., Mills, I. H.: Relationship between urinary kallikrein and renal function, hypertension, and excretion of sodium and water in man. Lancet *1972/II*, 203–207

Albano, Janet, Bhoola, K. D., Croker, M., Harvey, R. F., Heap, P. F.: Stimulus-secretion coupling in the pancreas: role of cyclic GMP in modulating enzyme secretion produced by acetylcholine and cholecystokinin-pancreozymin. J. Physiol. (Lond.) *258*, 87–88 P (1976a)

Albano, Janet, Bhoola, K. D., Harvey, R. F.: Cholecystokinin-pancreozymin and acetylcholine-mediated increase in enzyme secretion and cyclic GMP levels in the pancreas. In: Stimulus-secretion coupling in the gastrointestinal tract. Case, R. M., Goebell, H. (eds.), pp. 227–231. Lancaster: MTP 1975

Albano, Janet, Bhoola, K. D., Harvey, R. F.: Intracellular messenger role of cyclic GMP in exocrine pancreas. Nature (Lond.) *262*, 404–406 (1976b)

Albano, Janet, Bhoola, K. D., Heap, P. F., Lemon, M. J. C.: Stimulus-secretion coupling: Role of cyclic AMP, cyclic GMP, and calcium in mediating enzyme (kallikrein) secretion in the submandibular gland. J. Physiol. (Lond.) *258*, 631–658 (1976c)

Albano, Janet, Bhoola, K. D., Kingsley, Gabrielle: The control of cyclic GMP by calcium, ionophore A 23187, potassium and acetylcholine in enzyme-secreting pancreatic slices. J. Physiol. (Lond.) *267*, 35–36 P (1977)

Angelleti, R. A., Angeletti, P. U., Calissano, P.: Testosterone induction of estro-proteolytic activity in the mouse submaxillary gland. Biochim. Biophys. Acta *139*, 372–381 (1967)

Barlow, R. B., Berry, K. J., Glenton, P. A. M., Nikolaou, N. M., Soh, K. S.: A comparison of affinity constants for muscarine-sensitive acetylcholine receptors in guinea-pig atrial pacemaker cells at 29 °C and in ileum at 29 °C and 37 °C. Br. J. Pharmacol. *58*, 613–620 (1976)

Barton, S., Karpinski, E., Moriwaki, C., Schachter, M.: Sialotonin: Vasopressor substance in saliva and submandibular gland of the cat. J. Physiol. (Lond.) *261*, 523–533 (1976)

Barton, S., Saunders, E. J., Schachter, M., Uddin, M.: Autonomic nerve stimulation, kallikrein content and acinar cell granules of the cat's submandibular gland. J. Physiol. (Lond.) *251*, 363–369 (1975)

Beilenson, S., Schachter, M., Smaje, L. H.: Secretion of kallikrein and its role in vasodilatation in the submaxillary gland. J. Physiol. (Lond.) *199*, 303–317 (1968)

Beraldo, W. T., Siqueira, G., Rodrigues, J. A. A., Machado, C. R. S.: Changes in kallikrein activity of rat submandibular gland during postnatal development. Ad. Exp. Med. Biol. *21*, 239–249 (1972)

Bhoola, K. D.: Intracellular distribution of submaxillary kallikrein. J. Physiol. (Lond.) *196*, 431–445 (1968)

Bhoola, K. D.: Comparative study of the subcellular distribution of submaxillary kallikrein. Biochem. Pharmacol. *18*, 1252–1254 (1969)

Bhoola, K. D.: Kallikrein granules in the submaxillary gland and pancreas. Adv. Exp. Med. Biol. *8*, 615–619 (1970)

Bhoola, K.D., Cogdell, R.: Electrophoresis of isolated secretory granules from the submaxillary gland. Br. J. Pharmacol. *50*, 419–423 (1974)
Bhoola, K.D., Dorey, Gundula: Isolation of kallikrein-containing granules from the pancreas and submaxillary gland of the cat. J. Physiol. (Lond.) *203*, 59–60P (1969)
Bhoola, K.D., Dorey, Gundula: Intracellular localization of kallikrein, trypsin, and amylase in dog pancreas. J. Physiol. (Lond.) *214*, 553–570 (1971a)
Bhoola, K.D., Dorey, Gundula: Kallikrein, trypsin-like proteases, and amylase in mammalian submaxillary glands. Br. J. Pharmacol. *43*, 784–793 (1971b)
Bhoola, K.D., Dorey, Gundula, Jones, C.W.: The influence of androgens on enzymes (chymotrypsin and trypsin-like proteases, renin, kallikrein, and amylase) and on cellular structure of the mouse submaxillary gland. J. Physiol. (Lond.) *235*, 503–522 (1973)
Bhoola, K.D., Dorey, Gundula, Jones, C.W.: The ontogenic development and action of sex hormones on kallikrein and other proteases in the submaxillary gland. In: Chemistry and biology of the kallikrein-kinin system in health and disease. Pisano, J.J., Austen, K.F. (eds.), pp. 365–373. Fogarty Internat. Center Proc. No. 27. Washington: U.S. Gov. Printing Office 1977
Bhoola, K.D., Heap, P.F.: Properties of kallikrein-containing granules isolated from the submaxillary gland of the guinea-pig. J. Physiol. (Lond.) *210*, 421–432 (1970)
Bhoola, K.D., Lemon, M.J.C.: Studies on the activation of adenylate cyclase from the submaxillary gland and pancreas. J. Physiol. (Lond.) *232*, 83–84P (1973)
Bhoola, K.D., Lemon, M.J.C.: Studies on enzyme secretion and cyclic AMP in the submaxillary gland and pancreas. J. Physiol. (Lond.) *245*, 121–122P (1975)
Bhoola, K.D., Lemon, M.J.C., Matthews, R.W.: Immunofluorescent localization of kallikrein in guinea-pig submandibular gland. J. Physiol. (Lond.) *272*, 28–29P (1977)
Bhoola, K.D., Matthews, R.W., Roberts, Fiona: Time-course of changes in salivary kallikrein during the menstrual cycle. J. Physiol. (Lond.) *273*, 36P (1977)
Bhoola, K.D., McNicol, M.W., Oliver, S., Foran, J.: Changes in salivary enzymes in sarcoidosis. N. Engl. J. Med. *281*, 877–879 (1969)
Bhoola, K.D., Morley, J., Schachter, M., Smaje, L.H.: Vasodilatation in the submaxillary gland of the cat. J. Physiol. (Lond.) *179*, 172–184 (1965)
Bhoola, K.D., Ogle, C.W.: Subcellular localisation of kallikrein, amylase, and acetylcholine in the submaxillary gland of the guinea-pig. J. Physiol. (Lond.) *184*, 663–672 (1966)
Brandtzaeg, P., Gautvik, K.M., Nustad, K., Pierce, J.V.: Rat submandibular gland kallikreins: Purification and cellular localization. Br. J. Pharmacol. *56*, 155–167 (1976)
Bunch, J.L.: On the changes in the volume of the submaxillary gland during activity. J. Physiol. (Lond.) *26*, 1–29 (1900)
Burnstock, G.B.: Purinergic nerves. Pharmacol. Rev. *24*, 509–581 (1972)
Caramia, F.: Ultrastructure of mouse submaxillary gland. I. Sexual differences. J. Ultrastruct. Res. *16*, 505–523 (1966a)
Caramia, F.: Ultrastructure of mouse submaxillary gland. II. Effect of castration in the male. J. Ultrastruct. Res. *16*, 524–536 (1966b)
Carvalho, I.F., Diniz, C.R.: Cellular localization of renin and kininogen. Ciencia Cult (Sao Paulo) *16*, 263 (1964)
Chiang, T.S., Erdös, E.G., Miwa, I., Tague, L.L., Coulson, J.J.: Isolation from a salivary gland of granules containing renin and kallikrein. Circulation Res. *23*, 507–517 (1968)
Darke, A.C., Smaje, L.H.: Dependence of functional vasodilation in the cat submaxillary gland upon stimulation frequency. J. Physiol. (Lond.) *226*, 191–203 (1972)
Dorey, Gundula, Bhoola, K.D.: II. Ultrastructure of duct cell granules in mammalian submaxillary glands. Z. Zellforsch. *126*, 335–347 (1972)
Douglas, W.W.: Stimulus-secretion coupling. The concept and clues from chromaffin and other cells. Br. J. Pharmacol. *34*, 451–474 (1968)
Eichner, H., Eichner, V., Fiedler, F., Hochstrasser, K.: Zum Sekretionsverhalten der BAEE-Esterase (Kallikrein) im gesunden menschlichen Parotissekret unter fraktionierter Abnahme bei Ruhe und Reiz. Laryng. Rhinol. *55*, 239–244 (1976)
Ekfors T.O., Hopsu-Havu, V.K., Malmiharju, T.: Increased vascular permeability caused by the trypsin-like enzymes purified from rat submandibular gland. Acta Physiol. Scand. *75*, 157–160 (1969)

Ekfors, T.O., Malmiharju, T., Hopsu-Havu, V.K.: Isolation of six trypsin-like esteropeptidase from the mouse submandibular gland. Enzymologia *43*, 151–165 (1972)
Ekfors, T.O., Malmiharju, T., Riekkinen, P.J., Hopsu-Havu, V.K.: The depressor activity of trypsin-like enzymes purified from rat submandibular gland. Biochem. Pharmacol. *16*, 1634–1639 (1967a)
Ekfors, T.O., Riekkinen, P.J., Malmiharju, T., Hopsu-Havu, V.K.: Four isozymic forms of a peptidase resembling kallikrein purified from the rat submandibular gland. Hoppe Seylers Z. Physiol. Chem. *348*, 111–118 (1967b)
Emmelin, N., Henriksson, K.G.: Depressor activity of saliva after section of the chorda tympani. Acta Physiol. Scand. *30*, 75–82 (1953)
Erdös, E.G., Tague, L.L., Miwa, I.: Kallikrein in granules of the submaxillary gland. Biochem. Pharmacol. *17*, 667–674 (1968)
Feldberg, W., Guimarais, J.A.: Some observations on salivary secretion. J. Physiol. (Lond.) *85*, 15–35 (1935)
Ferreira, S.H., Smaje, L.H.: Bradykinin and functional vasodilatation in the salivary gland. Br. J. Pharmacol. *58*, 201–209 (1976)
Fiedler, F., Werle, E.: Vorkommen zweier Kallikreinogene im Schweinpankreas und Automation der Kallikrein- und Kallikreinogenbestimmung. Hoppe Seylers Z. Physiol. Chem. *348*, 1087–1089 (1967)
Forrell, M.M.: Pancreatic kallikrein in physiological and pathological conditions. In: Polypeptides which affect smooth muscles and blood vessels. Schachter, M. (ed.), pp. 247–252. Oxford: Pergamon Press 1960
Frey, E.K., Kraut, H.: Ein neues Kreislaufhormon und seine Wirkung. Naunyn Schmiedebergs Arch. Pharmak. *133*, 1–56 (1928)
Frey, E.K., Kraut, H., Schultz, F.: Über eine neue innersekretorische Funktion des Pankreas. Naunyn Schmiedebergs Arch. Pharmakol. *158*, 334–347 (1930)
Frey, E.K., Werle, E.: Kallikrein im inneren und äußeren Pankreassekret. Klin. Wochenschr. *12*, 600–601 (1933)
Garrett, J.R.: The innervation of salivary glands. III. The effects of certain experimental procedures on cholinesterase-positive nerves in glands of the cat. J1 R. microsc. Soc. *86*, 1–13 (1966a)
Garrett, J.R.: The innervation of salivary glands. IV. The effects of certain experimental procedures on the ultrastructure of nerves in glands of the cat. J1 R. microsc. Soc. *86*, 15–31 (1966b)
Garrett, J.R., Kidd, A.: Effects of nerve stimulation and denervation on secretory material in submandibular striated duct cells of cats, and the possible role of these cells in the secretion of salivary kallikrein. Cell. Tissue Res. *161*, 71–84 (1975)
Gautvik, K.: Studies on vasodilator mechanisms in the submandibular salivary gland of cats. Universitetsforlaget 1970
Gautvik, K.M., Berg-Oerstadvik, T., Nustad, K.: Role of kallikrein-kinin system in glandular secretion. In: Chemistry and biology of the kallikrein-kinin system in health and disease. Pisano, J.J., Austen, K.F. (eds.), pp. 335–357. Fogarty Internat. Center Proc. No. 27. Washington: U.S. Gov. Printing Office 1977
Gautvik, K.M., Kriz, M.: Release of kallikrein from isolated cellular organelles of the rat submandibular salivary gland. Acta Physiol. Scand. *92*, 95–102 (1974)
Gautvik, K.M., Kriz, M., Lund-Larsen, K., Nustad, K.: Control of kallikrein secretion from salivary glands. In: Secretory mechanisms of exocrine glands. Thorn, N.A., Pettersen, O. (eds.), pp. 168–182. Copenhagen: Munksgaard 1974
Geipert, F., Erdös, E.G.: Properties of granules that contain kallikrein and renin. Experientia *27*, 912–913 (1971)
Heidenhain, R.: Über die Wirkung einiger Gifte auf die Nerven der glandula submaxillaris. Pflügers Arch. *5*, 309–318 (1972)
Hickson, J.C.D.: The secretion of pancreatic juice in response to stimulation of the vagus nerves in the pig. J. Physiol. (Lond.) *206*, 275–297 (1970a)
Hickson, J.C.D.: The secretory and vascular response to nervous and hormonal stimulation in the pancreas of the pig. J. Physiol. (Lond.) *206*, 299–322 (1970b)

Hilton, S.M.: The physiological role of glandular kallikreins. In: Handbook of experimental pharmacology. Vol. XXV: Bradykinin, kallidin, and kallikrein. Erdös, E.G. (ed.), pp. 389–399 Berlin, Heidelberg, New York: Springer 1970
Hilton, S.M., Jones, M.: The role of plasma kinin in functional vasodilatation in the pancreas. J. Physiol. (Lond.) *195*, 521–533 (1968)
Hilton, S.M., Lewis, G.P.: The cause of the vasodilatation accompanying activity in the submandibular gland. J. Physiol. (Lond.) *128*, 235–248 (1955)
Hilton, S.M., Lewis, G.P.: The relationship between glandular activity, bradykinin formation and functional vasodilatation in the submandibular gland. J. Physiol. (Lond.) *134*, 471–483 (1956)
Hojima, Y., Maranda, B., Moriwaki, C., Schachter, M.: Direct evidence for the location of kallikrein in the striated ducts of the cat's submandibular gland by the use of specific antibody. J. Physiol. (Lond.) *268*, 193–801 (1977)
Jacobsen, S.: Substrates for plasma kinin-forming enzymes in rat and guinea-pig plasma. Br. J. Pharmacol. *28*, 64–72 (1966)
Jacoby, F., Leeson, C.R.: The post-natal development of the rat submandibular gland. J. Anat. *93*, 201–216 (1959)
Junqueira, L.C., Fajer, A., Rabinovitch, M., Frankenthal, L.: Biochemical and histochemical observations on the sexual dimorphism of mice submaxillary glands. J. Cell. Comp. Physiol. *34*, 129–135 (1949)
Kraut, H., Frey, E.K., Bauer, E.: Über ein neues Kreislaufhormon. II. Mitteilung. Hoppe Seylers Z. Physiol. Chem. *175*, 97 (1928)
Kraut, H., Frey, E.K., Werle, E.: Der Nachweis eines Kreislaufhormons in der Pankreasdrüse. IV. Mitteilung über dieses Kreislaufhormon. Hoppe Seylers Z. Physiol. Chem. *189*, 97–106 (1930)
Lacassagne, A.: Dimorphisme sexuel de la glande sous-maxillaire chez la souris. C.R. Soc. Biol. (Paris) *133*, 180–181 (1940)
Lemon, M.J.C., Bhoola, K.D.: Excitation-secretion coupling in exocrine glands: Properties of cyclic AMP phosphodiesterase and adenylate cyclase from the submaxillary gland and pancreas. Biochim. Biophys. Acta *385*, 101–113 (1975)
Marin-Grez, M., Cottone, P., Carretero, O.A.: Evidence for an involvement of kinins in regulation of sodium excretion. Am. J. Physiol. *223*, 794–796 (1972)
Matthews, E.K.: The ionogenic nature of the granule surface. In: Subcellular organisation and function in endocrine tissues. Heller, H., Lederis, K. (eds.), pp. 959–968. Cambridge: University Press 1971
Matthews, R.W.: Measurement of protein synthesis in the rat submandibular gland using tritiated tryptophane. Arch. Oral. Biol. *19*, 985–988 (1974)
Matthews, R.W., Beynon, A.D.G., Tonge, C.H.: A preliminary study into the significance of the granular convoluted tubule of the rat submandibular gland. J. Dent. Res. *50*, 677 (1971)
Matthews, R.W., Bhoola, K.D.: Influence of sympathetic nerve stimulation on the kallikrein content and secretory granules in the guinea-pig submandibular gland. J. Dent. Res. *55*, D 123 (1976)
Matthews, R.W., Bhoola, K.D.: Autonomic control of kallikrein and amylase in guinea-pig submandibular glands. J. Dent. Res. *56*, D 130 (1977)
Migay, T.I., Petroff, J.R.: Untersuchungen über die Wirkung des Pancreassaftes auf den Organismus bei parenteraler Einführung. Z. Gesamte Exp. Med. *36*, 457 (1923)
Mills, I.H., Ward, P.E.: The relationship between kallikrein and water excretion and the conditional relationship between kallikrein and sodium excretion. J. Physiol. (Lond.) *246*, 695–707 (1975)
Moriwaki, C., Hojima, Y., Schachter, M.: Purification of kallikrein from cat submaxillary gland. Adv. Exp. Med. Biol. *70*, 151–156 (1975)
Oliver, G., Schäfer, E.A.: On the physiological action of extracts of pituitary body and certain other glandular organs. J. Physiol. *18*, 277 (1895)
Oliver, W.J., Gross, F.: Effect of testerone and duct ligation on submaxillary renin-like principle. Am. J. Physiol. *213*, 341–349 (1967)

Ørstavik, T.B., Brandtzaeg, P., Nustad, K., Halvorsen, K.M.: Cellular localization of kallikreins in rat submandibular and sublingual salivary glands. Immunofluorescent tracing related to histochemical characteristics. Acta Histochem. (Jena) *54*, 183–192 (1975)
Palm, S., Schill, W.B., Wallner, O., Prinzen, R., Fritz, H.: Occurrence of components of the kallikrein-kinin system in human genital tract secretions and their possible function in stimulation of sperm motility and migration. Adv. Exp. Med. Biol. *70*, 271–280 (1975)
Pisano, J.J., Geller, R., Margolius, H.S., Keiser, H.S.: Urinary kallikrein in hypertensive rats. Acta Physiol. Lat. Am. *24*, 73–78 (1974)
Poulsen, J.H.: Two phases of chorda-lingual induced vasodilatation in the cat's submandibular gland during prolonged perfusion with Locke solution. J. Physiol. (Lond.) *253*, 79–94 (1975)
Pribram, H., Hernheiser, G.: Zur Kenntnis der adialysablen Bestandteile des Menschenharnes. Biochem. Z. *111*, 30 (1920)
Rawlinson, H.E.: Cytological changes after autonomic and adrenalin stimulation of the cat's submaxillary gland. Anat. Rec. *57*, 289–296 (1933)
Rawlinson, H.E.: The changes in the cells of the striated ducts of the cat's submaxillary gland after autonomic stimulation and nerve section. Anat. Rec. *63*, 295–313 (1935)
Schachter, M.: Kallikreins and kinins. Physiol. Rev. *49*, 509–547 (1969)
Schachter, M.: Vasodilatation in the submaxillary gland of the cat, rabbit, and sheep. In: Handbook of experimental pharmacology. Vol. XXV: Bradykinin, kallidin, and kallikrein. Erdös, E.G. (ed.), pp. 400–408. Berlin, Heidelberg, New York: Springer 1970
Schachter, M., Barton, S.: Recent observations on salivary, renal, and coagulating gland kininogenases. In: Chemistry and biology of the kallikrein-kinin system in health and disease. Pisano, J.J., Austen, K.F. (eds.), pp. 359–364. Fogarty Internat. Center Proc. No. 27. Washington: U.S. Gov. Printing Office 1977
Schachter, M., Barton, Susanne, Uddin, M., Karpinski, E., Saunders, E.J.: Effect of nerve stimulation, denervation, and duct ligation on kallikrein content and duct cell granules of the cat's submandibular gland. Experientia (1977)
Scott, B.L., Pease, D.C.: Electron microscopy of the salivary and lacrimal glands of the rat. Am. J. Anat. *104*, 115–140 (1959)
Siebert, G., Werle, E., Jung, G., Maier, L.: Intracelluläre Verteilung von Kallikrein und von Bradykininogen in Schweinepankreas. Biochem. Z. *326*, 420–423 (1955)
Siekevitz, P., Palade, G.E.: A cytochemical study on pancreas of the guinea-pig. I. Isolation and enzymic activities of cell fractions. J. Biophys. Biochem. Cytol. *4*, 203–217 (1958)
Smaje, L.H.: Spontaneous secretion in the rabbit submaxillary gland. In: Secretory mechanism of exocrine glands. Alfred Benzon Symposium VII. Thorn, N.A., Peterson, O.H. (eds.), pp. 608–625. Copenhagen: Munksgaard 1974
Sreebny, L.M., Meyer, J.: Hormones, inanition, and salivary glands. In: Salivary glands and their secretions. Sreebny, L.M., Meyer, J. (eds.), pp. 83–102. Oxford: Pergamon Press 1964
Thulin, A.: Motor and secretory effects of autonomic nerves and drugs in the rat submandibular gland. Acta Physiol. Scand. *92*, 217–223 (1974)
Trautschold, I., Werle, E., Schmal, A., Hendrikoff, N.G.: Die hormonelle Beeinflussung des Isorenin-Spiegels der Submandibularisdrüse der weißen Maus und zur Lokalisierung des Enzymes in der Drüse. Hoppe Seylers Z. Physiol. Chem. *344*, 232–243 (1966)
Ungar, G., Parrot, J.L.: Sur la présence de la callicréine dans la salive, et la possibilité de son intervention dans la transmission chimique de l'influx nerveux. C.R. Soc. Biol. (Paris) *122*, 1052–1055 (1936)
Vogel, R., Werle, E.: Kallikrein inhibitors. In: Handbook of experimental pharmacology. Vol. XXV: Bradykinin, kallidin, and kallikrein. Erdös, E.G. (ed.), pp. 213–249. Berlin, Heidelberg, New York: Springer 1970
Webster, Marion E.: Kallikreins in glandular tissues. In: Handbook of experimental pharmacology. Vol. XXV: Bradykinin, kallidin, and kallikrein. Erdös, E.G. (ed.), pp. 131–155. Berlin, Heidelberg, New York: Springer 1970
Werle, E.: Zur Kenntnis des Haushalts des Kallikreins. Biochem. Z. *269*, 415–434 (1934)
Werle, E.: Über die Wirkung des Kallikreins auf den isolierten Darm und über eine neue darmkontrahierende Substanz. Biochem. Z. *281*, 217–233 (1937)
Werle, E.: Kallikrein, kallidin, and related substances. In: Polypeptides which affect smooth muscles and blood vessels. Schachter, M. (ed.), pp. 199–209. Oxford: Pergamon Press 1960

Werle, E., Berek, U.: Zur Kenntnis des Kallikreins. Z. Angew. Chem. *60 A*, 53 (1948)
Werle, E., Eckey, P.: Vergleichende Untersuchung über Kallikrein und Trypsinkonzentration im menschlichen Duodenalsaft. Biochem. Z. *269*, 435–440 (1934)
Werle, E., Forell, M. M., Maier, L.: Zur Kenntnis der blutdrucksenkenden Wirkung des Trypsins. Naunyn Schmiedebergs Arch. Pharmakol. *225*, 369 (1955)
Werle, E., Götze, W., Keppler, A.: Über die Wirkung des Kallikreins auf den isolierten Darm und über eine neue darmkontrahierende Substanz. Biochem. Z. *289*, 217–233 (1937)
Werle, E., Grunz, M.: Zur Kenntnis der darmkontrahierenden uteruserregenden und blutdrucksenkenden Substanz DK. Biochem. Z. *301*, 429–436 (1939)
Werle, E., Korsten, H.: Das Kallikreingehalt des Harns, des Speichels und des Blutes bei Gesunden und Kranken. Z. Gesamte Exp. Med. *10103*, 153 (1938)
Werle, E., Rosen, P.: Über das Vorkommen von Kallikrein in den Speicheldrüsen und im Mundspeichel. Biochem. Z. *286*, 213–219 (1936)
Werle, E., Roden, P.: Über das Vorkommen von Kallikrein in den Speicheldrüsen und im Mundspeichel und über eine blutdrucksteigernde Substanz in der Submaxillarisdrüse des Hundes. Biochem. Z. *301*, 328–337 (1939)
Werle, E., Urhahn, K.: Über den Aktivitätszustand des Kallikreins in der Bauchspeicheldrüse. Biochem. Z. *304*, 387–396 (1940)
Werle, E., Vogel, R., Göldel, L. F.: Über ein blutdrucksteigerndes Prinzip in Extrakten aus der Glandula submaxillaris der weißen Maus. Naunyn Schmiedebergs Arch. Exp. Path. Pharmakol. *230*, 236 (1957)
Wotman, S., Greenbaum, L., Mandel, I.: Studies on human salivary kallikrein. Biochem. Pharmacol. *18*, 1261–1264 (1969)

Renal and Urinary Kallikreins

P. E. Ward and H. S. Margolius

A. Introduction

The serine proteases of the mammalian kidney and urine, known as kallikreins, are generally considered to be glandular kallikreins, distinct from the plasma enzyme and its precursor. (The isolation, purification and behavior of renal and urinary kallikrein have been discussed in detail elsewhere in this volume by Fiedler.) Despite the long continued interest in the properties of these purified glandular kallikreins, there is little information available about the cellular localization, regulation, or role of the enzymes of the entire kallikrein-kinin system within mammalian kidney and urine. However, interest in the kallikrein-kinin system and its relation to kidney function has increased markedly since publication of the previous edition of the Handbook volume on this subject (Erdös, 1970). This interest has been stimulated by studies on the localization of the enzyme and by relating both kallikrein and kinins to specific renal functions, to certain hormones which affect the kidney, or to some common pathologic states.

This chapter will cover some recent advances in the knowledge of renal and urinary kallikrein. Some comments concerning methods of assay and biochemical characteristics will be made, but the reader is referred to other chapters for comprehensive treatment of these subjects. Herein, the origin and location of kallikrein, its relations to renal function, to other hormonal systems, and to disease will be emphasized. A recently published symposium provides an excellent review of developments through late 1975 (McGiff et al., 1976).

B. Methods of Assay

A variety of assay methods have been used to measure kallikrein in kidney and urine. In recent years, traditional bioassay methods have been supplemented with new techniques using radioimmunoassay and radiolabeled synthetic substrates.

I. Bioassay

Renal and urinary kallikrein can be assayed by their ability to release a kinin from plasma kininogen substrate. The liberated kinin is measured by its capacity to induce contractions of isolated smooth muscle preparations, such as guinea pig ileum and rat uterus, or to lower arterial pressure by affecting vascular resistance. Mann et al. (1975) have developed a particularly sensitive kininogenase assay that involves measuring the "diastolic" tone between two sequential contractions of the rat uterus elicited by doses of bradykinin from 0.91 to 1.43 ng. MARIN-GREZ and CARRETERO (1972) described a rapid and sensitive assay of urinary kallikrein which measured the vasodilator effect of the kinin product on the perfused hind limb of the dog. This assay is particularly useful for quickly assaying large numbers of prepared samples. For a detailed review of some classical bioassay preparations, the reader is referred to TRAUTSCHOLD (1970).

The kininogen substrate for the kallikrein assay is usually prepared from heated plasma. Ideally, the kininogen should be prepared from the same species as the kallikrein to be measured. However, for assay of rat renal and urinary kallikrein, the use of rat plasma kininogen is impractical (NUSTAD, 1970a, b). Dog plasma kininogen is a good substrate for both rat and dog kallikrein. Preparation of kininogen from plasma usually involves heat and acid denaturation, ammonium sulfate precipitation, and/or DEAE chromatography to partially purify the substrate and inactivate plasma kallikrein, kininases, and kallikrein inhibitors (AMUNDSEN et al., 1963; JACOBSEN, 1966; NUSTAD, 1970a; MARIN-GREZ et al., 1973; GUIMARAES et al., 1974).

The presence of active kininases in renal extracts makes the measurement of renal kinin production by bioassay particularly difficult unless the kinin-destroying activity can be removed or completely inhibited. NUSTAD (1970a, b) used gel filtration to separate renal kallikrein (MW$\simeq$40,000) from renal kininases (MW$>$100,000) in the rat. However, this procedure cannot be used in human kidney extracts due to the presence of some kininase activity that is associated with a protein of approximately 40,000 daltons, a MW similar to that of kallikrein (ERDÖS et al., 1978). Renal kininase can be inhibited effectively by a combination of the inhibitors, o-phenanthroline, EDTA, and the kininase II inhibitor SQ 20881 (WARD et al., 1975b). There is little urinary kininase activity (ERDÖS et al., 1978) so the assay of kinin generation in urine is less difficult than in kidney extracts. However, kininase inhibitors should still be used.

As an alternative to assaying the rate of kinin generation, rat urinary kallikrein can be determined by measuring its direct oxytocic effect on the isolated rat uterus (PORCELLI and CROXATTO, 1971; BERALDO et al., 1976). Kallikrein levels in whole kidney (or kidney cortex) homogenates are more difficult to assay in this fashion. Presumably this is because kallikrein in the renal homogenate is membrane bound and less concentrated than in urine.

II. Radioimmunoassay

In recent years, kallikrein has been assayed by radioimmunoassay of generated kinin. Radioimmunoassay of kinins has been used to assay plasma kallikrein (TALAMO et al., 1969; BAGDASARIAN et al., 1973) and urinary kallikrein (MACFARLANE et al., 1973; CARRETERO et al., 1976). (Detailed information on the techniques of kinin radioimmunoassay are presented elsewhere in this volume by TALAMO and GOODFRIEND.)

Direct immunoassays of plasma kallikrein (BAGDASARIAN et al., 1974) and human and rat urinary kallikrein (OLE-MOI YOI, O. et al., 1977; OZA et al., 1976a; CARRETERO et al., 1978) have also been developed. The immunoassay of renal and urinary kallikrein eliminates the need to purify kininogen and inactivate kininases. Direct immunoassay of kallikrein may also be more specific than assays measuring kinin generation. However, this point remains to be established by using comparisons of the cross reactivity of kallikrein antibody with enzymes such as plasmin, thrombin, and trypsin.

In recent years, kinin radioimmunoassays have been used to determine endogenous levels of kinin in plasma, urine, and in tissue extracts. It is our opinion that such studies should be approached with extreme caution. Endogenous kinin levels can fluctuate widely with seemingly insignificant changes in methods of sample handling and extraction. The determination and reporting of physiologically accurate endogenous kinin levels may be the exception rather than the rule.

III. Esterase Assay

Synthetic substrates such as α-N-tosyl-L-arginine methyl ester (TAMe), benzoyl-L-arginine ethyl ester (BAEe) and benzyloxycarboxyl-L-arginine ethyl ester (CBZ-AEe) have been widely used to assay the esterase activity of renal and urinary kallikreins. These tritium-labeled substrates make it possible to assay kallikrein rapidly and accurately (BEAVEN et al., 1971). For detailed information on the use of tritiated TAMe and BAEe, the reader is referred to IMANARI et al. (1976).

In some biologic extracts, however, the hydrolysis of synthetic substrates does not necessarily parallel kallikrein activity as determined by bioassay or radioimmunoassay. Total TAMe esterase activity in rat renal homogenates is probably not due entirely to renal kallikrein. However, in purified renal microsomal membranes, TAMe esterase and kallikrein bioassay activities do parallel one another (WARD et al., 1976). In human urine, 95% of the TAMe esterase activity is due to urinary kallikrein but only about 50% of the esterase activity in raw rat urine is due to rat urinary kallikrein (PIERCE and NUSTAD, 1972). Recently, chromogenic substrates, highly specific for glandular kallikrein, have become available (AMUNDSEN et al., 1976; CLAESON et al., 1978). Nevertheless, studies utilizing synthetic substrates should document their results with parallel bioassays or radioimmunoassays.

C. Biochemical Characteristics

Although glandular kallikrein occurs mainly as prekallikrein in the porcine pancreas and this proenzyme has been studied in detail (FIEDLER et al., 1970; FIEDLER, 1976), no such detailed studies are yet available of a renal or urinary prekallikrein. Some earlier work (CARVALHO and DINIZ, 1966) and a recent preliminary report (CORTHORN et al., 1977) indicate that a prekallikrein may exist in kidney and urine. The latter work indicated that the isolated inactive kallikrein is a precursor which can be activated by trypsin or an unidentified activating peptide. In the only study of renal kallikrein synthesis, NUSTAD et al. (1975) isolated from rat kidney slices four newly synthesized kallikreins which were indistinguishable from those found in urine. Although the authors concluded that "kallikreins synthesized and released by the kidney are not changed during their passage through the lower urinary tract," the question of whether newly synthesized prekallikrein could have escaped detection was not considered. Regardless of the conclusions of NUSTAD and co-workers, determination of whether a proenzyme is present in kidney, its localization, and influences which activate it are important topics for future study.

Many investigators agree on the presence of at least two forms of kallikrein in mammalian urine (NUSTAD and PIERCE, 1974; HIAL et al., 1974; FRITZ et al., 1977; SILVA et al., 1974; OZA et al., 1976b; GIUSTI et al., 1976; CHAO and MARGOLIUS, 1977), although others have found only a single form (PORCELLI et al., 1974). Neither the basis nor the significance of this heterogeneity has been fully explained. Whether it lies in differing amino acid compositions or the nature of the glycoprotein moieties is uncertain. Furthermore, the relation of enzyme heterogeneity to enzyme function in situ is not clear.

As is noted elsewhere, FIEDLER et al. (p. 103), there are many natural and synthetic glandular kallikrein inhibitors. Russell's viper venom contains two powerful broad spectrum inhibitors which inactivate all kallikreins and are structurally and functionally similar to aprotinin (TAKAHACHI et al., 1974). A number of novel aromatic tris-amidines have been synthesized recently which have considerable activity against glandular kallikrein (GERATZ et al., 1975, 1976). One of these, alpha^1, alpha^2, alpha^3-tris(4-amidino-2-bromophenoxy)mesitylene (IRT-36), has a K_i value of 2.4×10^{-8} M against porcine pancreatic kallikrein. This inhibitor can also partially inhibit kinin release by human plasma kallikrein at concentrations as low as 1×10^{-10} M (TIDWELL et al., 1976).

We can anticipate that the use of these potent inhibitors both in vivo and in vitro will, in the future, provide valuable information about the physiologic effects of the renal kinin system.

At the present time, little information on the presence of natural kallikrein inhibitors in the kidney is available. However, MANN et al. (1975) have reported isolating fractions, from renal tubules, which strongly inhibited urinary kallikrein activity. This inhibition may be due to a natural kidney inhibitor of low MW (GEIGER and MANN, 1976).

D. Renal Kallikrein

I. Origin

Urinary kallikrein is biochemically different from pancreatic kallikrein (BERALDO et al., 1956) and plasma kallikrein (WEBSTER and PIERCE, 1961, 1963). NUSTAD (1970a) found that kidney and urinary kallikrein in the rat share similar properties. Both enzymes had similar MWs (38,500), were inhibited completely by aprotinin and only marginally by soybean trypsin inhibitor and ovomucoid trypsin inhibitor. Under the conditions of their assay, renal and urinary kallikrein also had similar pH optima (8.5). Using L-[^{3}H]-leucine, NUSTAD et al. (1975) demonstrated that rat kidney slices were capable of synthesizing four radiolabeled kallikreins. The radiolabeled renal kallikreins resembled four urinary kallikreins (NUSTAD and PIERCE, 1974) in their relative amounts, isoelectric points, and electrophoretic mobilities on polyacrylamide disc gels. The authors concluded that the kidney synthesizes four kallikreins which are released into the urine and are not changed by passage through the lower urinary tract.

By perfusing isolated kidneys, ROBLERO et al. (1976a, b) have shown that rat kidneys release renal kallikrein into both the vasculature and into the urine. In these studies, the perfusion medium could not have been the source of enzyme.

Under some circumstances, glandular kallikreins released into blood from a variety of tissues may appear in urine. HILTON and LEWIS (1955) found glandular kallikrein in the venous effluent of the submandibular gland. Active kallikrein, different from normal urinary kallikrein and presumably filtered from the blood, was found in dog urine during acute pancreatitis (OFSTAD, 1970). Nevertheless, it is unlikely that trace levels of glandular kallikrein in blood are normally excreted into urine in an active form since plasma contains inhibitors of glandular kallikreins (HOJIMA et al., 1977) and MILLS et al. (1975) have shown that tracer levels of radiolabeled pancreatic kallikrein infused intravenously are excreted in a degraded form.

While the majority of evidence supports the hypothesis of a renal origin for urinary kallikrein, several questions remain. Total kallikrein activity in 24-h urine collections is approximately eight times the activity found in the corresponding kidneys (NUSTAD, 1970a). In spite of the fact that the kidney kallikrein may have been activated by treatment with deoxycholate (a detergent used during sample preparation), urine was consistently more active than the renal extracts (NUSTAD, 1970a, b). Solubilizing agents and nonionic detergents can activate renal or urinary kallikrein (WILSON et al., 1976; CHAO, 1978). These data imply that the kidney rapidly synthesizes kallikrein, producing its basal level every few hours. However, in the study using L-[^{3}H]-leucine (NUSTAD et al., 1975), the amount of radioactivity incorporated into kallikrein was extremely low. In addition, agents such as aldosterone, thought to induce kallikrein (see Sect. VI), require 2–3 days to alter kallikrein excretion in vivo. However, in vitro, KAIZU and MARGOLIUS (1975) have shown that aldosterone is capable of stimulating isolated renal cells to secrete kallikrein in a matter of hours.

The strongest evidence for rapid renal secretion of kallikrein is provided by the studies of ROBLERO et al. (1976a, b). In perfused rat kidneys, kallikrein appeared in the venous effluent and urine more rapidly than kallikrein activity decreased in the isolated kidney. During approximately 2 h of perfusion, the kallikrein content of the isolated kidney decreased slightly ($\simeq 18\%$) while total kallikrein secretion was 55% of that in the isolated kidney. These data support the hypothesis of rapid synthesis of kallikrein by the kidney. Nevertheless, if the observed loss of activity in the perfused kidney was related to limitations inherent in the technique of kidney isolation and perfusion (NIZET, 1975), the above experiment cannot be considered definitive.

Traditionally, urinary excretion rates of kallikrein have been used as an index of renal kallikrein turnover, although adequately controlled experiments testing this assumption have never been reported. The above experiments cast some doubt on the validity of this practice. Under the experimental conditions mentioned (ROBLERO et al., 1976a, b), kallikrein was secreted in the renal venous effluent much faster than it was excreted in the urine (ROBLERO et al., 1976a). In addition, the proportion of kallikrein, excreted in the urine, compared to that in the venous effluent, may vary under different experimental and pathologic conditions. It appears, therefore, that it would be preferable to measure both renal venous plasma and urinary kallikrein (and kinin) levels to determine the functional state of the renal kallikrein-kinin system. With such studies, the validity of measuring urinary kallikrein alone as an index of renal kallikrein turnover can be determined.

CARVALHO and DINIZ (1964, 1966) and CARVALHO (1971) have shown that renal kallikrein can be activated by low pH and/or hypotonic medium and these observations have recently been confirmed (WARD et al., 1975a). Thus, the previously noted differences between renal and urinary kallikrein activity may be explained not only by rapid renal synthesis but also by activation or release of a membrane-bound renal kallikrein or prekallikrein.

II. Localization

In recent years, several laboratories have directed their attention to determining the cellular and subcellular localization of renal kallikrein. In 1964, CARVALHO and DINIZ reported that rat kidney kallikrein was localized in lysosomes. BAGGIO et al. (1975) also reported a lysosomal localization for renal kallikrein. However, a number of factors make this latter study difficult to evaluate since only synthetic substrate was used to assay kallikrein and no microsomal marker enzymes were assayed. NUSTAD (1970b) and NUSTAD and RUBIN (1970), using both bioassay and BAEe esterolytic assay, found in rats that kallikrein was concentrated in the microsomal fraction. WARD et al. (1975b, 1976) confirmed Nustad's data and fractionated renal microsomes into plasma membrane and endoplasmic reticulum-enriched fractions. Kallikrein was present in both fractions but was particularly enriched in a plasma membrane fraction. The results of CHAO and MARGOLIUS (1978), using intact renal cortical cells, indicate that renal kallikrein is a membrane-bound ectoenzyme with active sites facing the external environment. WARD et al. (1975b, 1976) suggested that after synthesis on endoplasmic reticulum, renal kallikrein is subsequently reoriented to the plasma membrane for activation and release. The association of kallikrein with intermediate structures after synthesis and during reorientation might explain the apparent lysosomal-like localization of renal kallikrein reported by CARVALHO and DINIZ (1964).

At the cellular level, NUSTAD (1970b) showed in rats, and SCICLI et al. (1976) confirmed in dogs, that renal kallikrein was localized predominantly in the cortex. These data, combined with the report that drugs which destroy tubular cells reduced the excretion of kallikrein (WERLE and VOGEL, 1960), led the authors to suggest a proximal tubule localization of renal kallikrein. However, WARD et al. (1975b) found no kallikrein activity in the brush border isolated from rat kidney proximal tubules. In addition, kallikrein was not detected in tumors derived from the pars recta of rat proximal tubules (WARD et al., 1976).

Using stop-flow technique, SCICLI et al. (1976) and CARRETERO and SCICLI (1976) found the highest concentration of dog urinary kallikrein in urine fractions which had the lowest sodium level. These authors concluded that kallikrein is secreted into the urine at the level of the distal tubule by either the tubule itself or by a structure related to this part of the nephron. Kinins were also found in the distal tubule in addition to the collecting duct (SCICLI et al., 1977, 1978). Neither kallikrein nor kinin was detected in the fractions associated with the proximal tubule. ØRSTAVIK et al. (1976) used a fluorescent antibody technique to show that rat renal kallikrein was localized in the segment of the distal tubule reaching from the juxtaglomerular apparatus to the collecting duct. The authors observed a bright luminal rim which may be the previously identified kallikrein-rich plasma membrane (NUSTAD, personal communication).

SCICLI et al. (1976) found little kallikrein activity in purified rat glomeruli and concluded that renal kallikrein was not localized here. However, MANN et al. (1975) did find kallikrein activity and at least partially localized it in microdissected glomeruli. TYLER (1972) reached a similar conclusion in his studies. In an effort to resolve this issue, WARD et al. (1977) isolated glomeruli from rat renal cortex that were free of tubular contamination. Electron microscopy demonstrated that the purified glomeruli were morphologically similar to glomeruli in situ. In addition, the isolated glomeruli had marker enzyme activities that were similar to those in metabolically active glomeruli isolated by others. Since the specific activity of kallikrein in the purified glomeruli was less than that in crude homogenate, the authors concluded that kallikrein is not localized in glomerular corpuscles and that the absence of such activity was not an artifact due to damage of glomeruli during purification. Since few of the isolated glomeruli contained juxtaglomerular cells (less than 1%), no conclusions could be reached as to the possible presence of kallikrein in these renin-containing cells. However, we believe that it may be premature at this time to rule out the possible presence of kallikrein in some component of the juxtaglomerular apparatus. Such a localization could explain much about the relationship seen between urinary kallikrein excretion and renal perfusion pressure. Nevertheless, at present, all available evidence indicates that kallikrein is localized in the cells of distal tubules. It appears to be released into the distal tubular filtrate to generate kinins in the distal nephron and collecting duct filtrates. However, several questions remain unanswered: It is not known whether renal kallikrein acts on a filtered plasma kininogen or on a renal kininogen produced within the kidney. To date, we know of no conclusive data documenting the presence of an endogenous kininogen in normal renal tissue although kininogen has been reported in human urine (PISANO et al., 1978).

The apical localization of kallikrein suggests that it is secreted (ØRSTAVIK et al., 1976) into the filtrate of the distal tubules, but the process by which renal kallikrein enters renal lymph (DE BONO and MILLS, 1974) and the renal venous effluent (ROBLERO et al., 1976a) is unclear. In spite of the extensive relationship between urinary kallikrein excretion and a variety of renal functions, the exact stimuli for renal kallikrein secretion has yet to be established. However, the distal tubular localization of renal kallikrein lends support to the relationship of renal kallikrein with aldosterone as proposed by MARGOLIUS and associates (see Sect. F).

E. Effects of Kallikreins and Kinins on Renal Function

I. Electrolyte and Water Excretion

Whether the renal kallikrein-kinin system participates directly in the control of electrolyte and water excretion and, if so, does it as a natriuretic or as an antinatriuretic system, is uncertain at the present time. Most available evidence indicates that kinins, when injected intravenously or into the renal artery, produce increased diuresis and natriuresis (GILL et al., 1965; WEBSTER and GILMORE, 1964). BARRACLOUGH and MILLS (1965) reported an increase in diuresis despite antidiuretic hormone (ADH) infusion. The similar experiments of WILLIS et al. (1969) indicated that the natriuresis produced by bradykinin is due to the increase in renal blood flow. Although STEIN et al. (1972) found that bradykinin did not affect sodium reabsorption in the proximal tubules of the superficial nephron, these authors suggested that a decrease in reabsorption may occur in deeper nephrons. There is no evidence, to date, that bradykinin has direct inhibitor or stimulatory action on tubular reabsorption of sodium.

Since production of concentrated urine depends on the maintenance of a medullary osmotic gradient, the diuresis associated with kinin infusion into the renal artery may be related to an increased medullary blood flow and thus a "washout" of this gradient. However, MACFARLANE et al. (1972) found little change in blood flow during the diuresis that occurred in response to infusion of kallikrein into the renal artery. In view of the earlier studies of BARRACLOUGH and MILLS (1965) and those of FURTADO (1971), these authors suggested a direct inhibition of ADH by the generated kinins. FURTADO (1971) had earlier demonstrated that bradykinin reversibly inhibits the ADH-induced increase in water permeability of the toad bladder.

In the isolated blood-perfused dog kidney (MCGIFF et al., 1975), intra-arterial injections of bradykinin increased free water clearance without increasing sodium excretion. In this study, there was actually a fall in urinary sodium excretion although these changes were considered insignificant. Interestingly, the subsequent administration of indomethacin increased the fractional sodium excretion produced by bradykinin. MCGIFF et al. (1975) and MCGIFF and NASJLETTI (1976) suggested that a prostaglandin mediates the diuretic action of bradykinin and simultaneously attenuates the actions of the kinin on renal sodium excretion (see Sect. F). In this regard, prostaglandins of the E-series can inhibit the effects of ADH (GRANTHAM and ORLOFF, 1968).

NASJLETTI and COLINA-CHOURIO (1976) altered the activity of kininase II and the renal kallikrein-kinin system with SQ 20881, the kininase II inhibitor, and found augmented diuresis and natriuresis. In these studies of chloralose-anesthetized dogs, intravenous administration of 300 μg SQ 20881/kg body weight increased renal blood flow and decreased mean aortic pressure significantly. Simultaneously, urine flow and sodium excretion were augmented twofold over control values. Both renal venous and urinary kinins were significantly increased and were positively correlated with renal blood flow, sodium excretion, and urine flow. MARIN-GREZ (1974) examined urinary water, sodium, and potassium excretion in anesthetized rats given intravenous saline infusions followed by injections of an antibradykinin serum. The antiserum-treated rats excreted less water and sodium than animals given normal rabbit serum. No differences between groups were observed in the clearances of paraaminohippurate or inulin. The author suggests that the data are not inconsistent with a possible redistribution of renal blood flow between cortical layers as suggested by others (STEIN et al., 1971). Whether this maneuver with antiserum affects renal venous or urinary kinin levels has not yet been determined. Collectively, these data show that kinins alter sodium and water excretion, but do not necessarily prove that kinins per se, either exogenously administered or endogenously released, affect tubular function – since the experiments described may alter the activity of the renin-angiotensin system as well as affect renal blood flow.

II. Renal Hemodynamics

A series of studies in normal human subjects (GILL et al., 1965) and anesthetized dogs (WEBSTER and GILMORE, 1964; STEIN et al., 1972; GOLDBERG et al., 1965; MCNAY and GOLDBERG, 1966; BARRACLOUGH and MILLS, 1965; NAKANO, 1965) have established that either intravenously or intra-arterially administered bradykinin or kallidin cause renal arteriolar vasodilatation; this phenomenon has also been observed in isolated blood-perfused canine kidneys (McGIFF et al., 1975). After the administration of indomethacin, the renal vasodilator action of bradykinin was attenuated in the latter preparation (McGIFF et al., 1975). The fact that pharmacologic doses of kinin, given intravenously or intra-arterially to man, anesthetized animals, or isolated kidneys, produce vasodilatation does not necessarily prove that the renal kallikrein-kinin system performs this function in situ. The question of whether or not the renal kallikrein-kinin system plays a role in the control of renal vascular resistance has not yet been answered. As stated by NASJLETTI and COLINA-CHOURIO (1976):

> Inference of physiological roles on the basis of the aforementioned observations[1] should be regarded with caution, since probably no route of administration of kinins reproduces the effects evoked by release of kinins intrarenally, in terms of either concentrations achieved at their sites of action, localization of activity, or the sequence of vascular elements affected.

Few careful studies have dealt with the intrarenal actions of kinins formed within the kidney, an organ rich in kininase. NASJLETTI and COLINA-CHOURIO (1976) used the kininase II inhibitor, SQ 20881, and showed significant increases in renal blood flow after the administration of SQ 20881, concomitant with a fall in mean aortic pressure. These changes were accompanied by slight, but statistically significant, increases in urinary kinin excretion and renal venous kinin concentration 30 min after intravenous injection of the inhibitor. These investigators ascribed the renal action of the enzyme inhibitor to augmented activity of the kallikrein-kinin system rather than to diminished formation of angiotensin II owing to the inhibition of angiotensin I converting enzyme. The likelihood that diminished angiotensin II formation intrarenally contributed to the observed effects was considered slight because previous studies have shown that an angiotensin II receptor antagonist does not affect renal blood flow in normal dogs (FREEMAN et al., 1973). This may be correct, but correlations between increased endogenous kinin activity and increased renal blood flow and electrolyte excretion may not be indicative of a causal relationship in experiments where both the kallikrein-kinin and renin-angiotensin systems might be altered by a single drug such as SQ 20881 (see also ERDÖS, p. 427). However, confirmatory data have been obtained in conscious sodium-deficient dogs where continuous infusions of SQ 20881 increased plasma and urinary kinins while decreasing urinary kallikrein excretion (McCAA and McCAA, 1977). These authors suggested that the increased circulating and urinary kinins are the result of decreased degradation and may play a role in the hypotensive and natriuretic effects of SQ 20881. In the future, if specific kallikrein and kinin receptor blockers become available, they should help to clarify the basis of these observations.

Other data support a direct correlation between the renal kallikrein-kinin system and renal blood flow. BEVAN et al. (1974) showed that acute unilateral renal artery constriction led to a fall in kallikrein excretion and that release of the constriction was accompanied by rising kallikrein excretion. Statistically significant correlations were found among urinary kallikrein, sodium, and volume. In trained conscious dogs, previously operated to chronically narrow the left renal artery by the method of LUPU et al. (1972) and with bilateral ureterostomies, there was an excellent correlation between the change in renal blood flow produced by the ligature and the decrease in kallikrein excretion (KEISER et al., 1976). Urine volume and potassium

[1] Results of infusions of kinins intravenously or into the renal artery.

excretion were also reduced on the stenotic side. In both studies, the changes in renal blood flow were due to the ligature on the renal artery. Therefore, the changes noted in urinary kallikrein excretion were most probably secondary to the changes in renal blood flow rather than causal. In the study of KEISER et al., no correlations could be found among urinary kallikrein, volume, or sodium excretion. In a study of normal and hypertensive men, LEVY et al. (1977) were able to correlate urinary kallikrein excretion with renal blood flow in almost all groups of subjects. Whether the correlations reflect a contribution of the renal-kallikrein-kinin system to the regulation of renal vascular resistance and blood flow still remains to be determined.

F. Endogenous Kallikrein, Kinins, and Renal Function

I. Electrolyte and Water Balance

A body of recently collected data deals with the relationship between excretion of kallikrein, plasma, and urinary kinins, sodium, and water and supports the hypothesis that the system is natriuretic and diuretic. MILLS and co-workers have shown direct correlations between sodium and kallikrein excretion in man (1972), rabbits (1975), and rats on free salt and water intake, but not in rabbits when dietary sodium intake was constant and either high or low (1975). MARIN-GREZ et al. (1972) measured plasma kinins and urinary kallikrein and detected increased levels of both when dogs were given oral saline loads but not when the oral load was water. MARIN-GREZ and CARRETERO (1971) and CROXATTO et al. (1975) observed positive correlations among urinary sodium, water, and kallikrein in rats during periods of low and high sodium intake. ADETUYIBI and MILLS (1972) have also noted a positive correlation between urinary kallikrein and urine volume in normal man.

All of the above pharmacologic studies and measurements of urinary kallikrein appear to associate the renal kallikrein-kinin system with natriuretic and diuretic events. However, a body of data has recently been gathered which appears inconsistent with the notion that the endogenous renal kallikrein-kinin system promotes natriuresis and diuresis. These studies (GELLER et al., 1972; MARGOLIUS et al., 1974a, b; ABE et al., 1976; JOHNSTON et al., 1976; LAWTON and FITZ, 1976; LEVY et al., 1977; VINCI et al., 1977) have shown that the urinary excretion of kallikrein is increased by low dietary sodium intake in man or the rat. In addition, increased potassium intake (HORWITZ et al., 1975), administration of 9-α-fluorohydrocortisone to man, or desoxycorticosterone to rats or dogs also increases urinary kallikrein excretion (ADETUYIBI and MILLS, 1972; GELLER et al., 1972; MARIN-GREZ et al., 1973; MARGOLIUS et al., 1974a, b, c; NASJLETTI and COLINA-CHOURIO, 1976). Furthermore, normal subjects whose kallikrein excretion had been increased by a low sodium diet show a marked decrease in kallikrein during treatment with the specific aldosterone antagonist, spironolactone (MARGOLIUS et al., 1974a, b, c). Similar relations between kallikrein production, aldosterone, and spironolactone, have been observed with isolated renal cortical cells in suspension (KAIZU and MARGOLIUS, 1975).

In clinical studies of a large population of normal adults, MARGOLIUS et al. (1974a) were unable to show any direct correlation between urinary sodium and kallikrein excretion. Neither GRECO et al. (1974) nor SEINO et al. (1975) saw such a relation in hypertensive adults. Over a 5 year period, studies of urinary kallikrein in relation to urinary electrolytes and blood pressure in over 600 normal children, studied on more than one occasion, did not disclose any positive correlation between urinary sodium and kallikrein (ZINNER et al., 1976, 1977). On the contrary, a repeatedly detectable significant negative correlation existed between these variables, whereas a strong positive correlation between urinary kallikrein and potassium was observed.

The positive correlation between urine volume and kallikrein excretion noted by ADETUYIBI and MILLS (1972), CROXATTO et al. (1975), and NEKRASOVA et al. (1977) could not be confirmed in other studies in man (MARGOLIUS et al., 1974a). However, LEVY et al. (1977) have recently seen significant increases in kallikrein excretion in normal men produced by intravenous water loading during prolonged sodium restriction, but not during periods of normal sodium intake. They also reconfirmed increased kallikrein excretion with low sodium intake.

Collectively, these observations suggested to MARGOLIUS et al. (1974a) that kallikrein excretion is determined, at least in part, by the effective level of circulating sodium-retaining steroid hormone, presumably as a consequence of some action of steroids on renal cells (KAIZU and MARGOLIUS, 1975).

Another confirmation of a relation between kallikrein excretion and aldosterone is the result of studies of patients with Bartter's syndrome. In these normotensive patients with markedly elevated plasma renin activity, hyperaldosteronism, hypokalemia, and juxtaglomerular cell hyperplasia, researchers have measured supranormal urinary kallikrein and plasma bradykinin levels, but, interestingly, subnormal urinary kinin excretion (VINCI et al., 1976; LECHI et al., 1976; HALUSHKA et al., 1977).

An alternate explanation for the presence of high levels of urinary kallikrein excretion in patients with Bartter's syndrome is overproduction of renal kallikrein by juxtaglomerular cells undergoing hyperplasia. However, as mentioned previously, no published data have reported renal kallikrein in juxtaglomerular cells. Therefore, the former explanation remains the most reasonable at this time. However, it is presently unclear whether the observed increase in kallikrein excretion is due to a direct stimulation by aldosterone or to an indirect action. For a discussion of this possibility, the reader is referred to Sect. F.II.4 and p. 549 of this volume (MILLS).

Other indirect evidence suggesting some relations between the kallikrein-kinin system and sodium homeostasis come from (a) the demonstration of a *decrease* in plasma kinin levels with saline infusions in normal volunteers (WONG et al., 1975), a result opposite to that seen by MARIN-GREZ et al. (1972) in dogs, and (b) the increase in plasma kinin on the assumption of upright posture (STREETEN et al., 1972; WONG et al., 1975). Recent studies (VINCI et al., 1977) add further perplexity to the relations between the renal kallikrein-kinin system, electrolyte homeostasis, and sodium-retaining steroid activity. In these studies, the relation of urinary kallikrein excretion to adrenal sodium-retaining steroid activity in man was confirmed. In addition, *plasma* kinin levels rose upon standing and were significantly increased with low dietary sodium intake, as has been suggested before (WONG et al., 1975). However, urinary kinin excretion, presumptively a product of renal and urinary kallikrein activity, was unchanged by either prolonged periods of low dietary sodium intake, administration of fludrocortisone or of ACTH, all of which significantly increased the excretion of urinary kallikrein.

An apparent paradox exists concerning the known natriuretic/diuretic effects of exogenous and endogenous kinins and the repeatedly observed increase in kallikrein excretion under conditions when little sodium is being excreted.

It is obvious that, at present, the relation of the renal kallikrein-kinin system to electrolyte homeostasis is unclear. Nevertheless, the recent and impressive findings on the localization of components of the kallikrein-kinin system along the nephron; the availability of methodology to measure substrate, enzyme, product, and inhibitors in both renal tissues and urine; the long observed effects of kinin peptides on renal vascular and excretory function; and the relation between renal kallikrein and the sodium-retaining steroid hormone, aldosterone, suggest intensified investigation of the role of the renal kallikrein-kinin system in relation to water and electrolyte excretion. Exploration of these relations is not only important because of the presence of components of the system within the kidney at sites where electrolyte and water transport is a primary function, but also because of relations between these functions and hypertensive diseases. This area of endeavor is entirely new since the summary of this system's activity was published in the previous volume of the handbook.

II. Relations to Other Enzymes, Hormones, and Drugs

1. Renin and Angiotensin

From much of the foregoing and from discussion in other Chapters in this handbook, the biochemical similarities and connections of the kallikrein-kinin and renin-angiotensin systems can be seen (Fig. 1). CROXATTO and SAN MARTIN (1970) first showed decreased urinary kallikrein in rats with one-kidney renal hypertension, a situation where renin-angiotensin levels are high. This finding has been extended to various animal models (vide infra) as well as humans with renovascular disease. It is uncertain whether the observed inverse relation between urinary kallikrein and plasma renin reflects decreased activity of the kallikrein-kinin system when renin-angiotensin activity is increased. Under some conditions, the suppression of a vasodilator system occurring during the activation of a vasoconstrictor system could work together to maintain or raise blood pressure.

However, not all studies have shown inverse relationships between these two systems. JOHNSTON et al. (1976) have shown a direct, rather than an inverse, correlation between plasma renin activity and urinary kallikrein excretion. WONG et al. (1975) found parallel changes in plasma kinin levels, angiotensin II levels, and renin activity in normal volunteers, after either saline infusions or the assumption of upright posture, which were not accompanied by altered plasma prekallikrein activity. MACFARLANE et al. (1974) observed increased urinary kallikrein excretion in dogs treated with intra-arterial angiotensin II infusions. MILLS et al. (1976) have suggested that under conditions of high renin-angiotensin generation, the renal kallikrein-kinin system may be activated to prevent excessive vasoconstriction of renal vessels.

Other evidence of interrelations between the renin and kallikrein systems can be found in the data on renal function of NASJLETTI and COLINA-CHOURIO (1976) and MCCAA and MCCAA (1977) using SQ 20881. MERSEY et al. (1977) have measured plasma kinin by radioimmunoassay in normal volunteers before and after intrave-

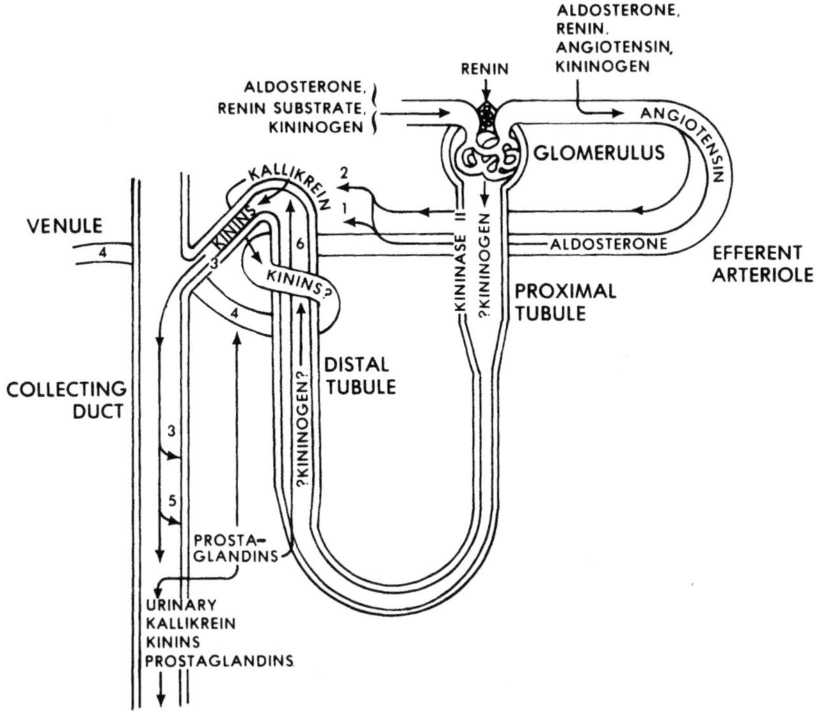

Fig. 1. Localization and possible interactions of the renal kinin-angiotensin-prostaglandin systems. *1* Direct effects of aldosterone on electrolyte transport. *2* Kallikrein induction or activation by aldosterone or angiotensin. *3* Possible sites for direct effects of kinins on transport processes. *4* Possible kinin, angiotensin, and prostaglandin effects on renal vascular resistance. *5* Possible kinin-induced prostaglandin production and subsequent effects on transport or hemodynamic variables. *6* Modulation of kallikrein activity by prostaglandins

nous SQ 20881 and suggested that plasma kinins correlate more closely with acute changes in plasma renin activity and angiotensin I than with angiotensin II or aldosterone. However, CARRETERO et al. (1974) found no correlation between renal tissue kallikrein and plasma renin activity in either two-kidney or one-kidney renal hypertensive rats.

In summary, the evidence available at this time strongly suggests physiologically significant relationships between renal kallikrein and renin. In addition, considering the number of factors known to control or influence renin release, it is not surprising that in the numerous studies, using different experimental approaches, a completely consistent renin-kallikrein interaction has not been found yet. It is quite likely that the interaction of these two renal systems is modulated by several other factors such as electrolyte balance, blood pressure, intravascular volume, adrenal steroids, and the sympathetic nervous system.

2. Catecholamines

Relations between the activity of the sympathetic nervous system or exogenously administered catecholamines and the activity of the renal kallikrein-kinin system are essentially unexplored. However, intra-arterial infusions of dopamine can increase the excretion of kallikrein in urine (MILLS and OBIKA, 1976). BARTON et al. (1975) and ØRSTAVIK and GAUTVIK (1977) have shown that sympathetic nerve stimulation decreased salivary gland kallikrein content in the cat and rat, respectively. The latter authors suggested that α-adrenergic stimulation (and drugs that stimulate the α-adrenergic receptors) was markedly more effective than β-adrenergic or para-sympathetic stimulation. Given the relations of the sympathetic nervous system to the control of systemic vascular resistance and to other parameters of renal and cardiovascular functions, it would seem obligatory to explore interactions between these two systems within the kidney.

3. Prostaglandins

A series of observations have suggested that renal prostaglandins modulate and mediate actions of the renal kallikrein-kinin system (NASJLETTI and COLINA-CHOURIO, 1976). It has been suggested that the intrarenal generation of kinin may set both the basal level and the type of prostaglandin synthesized within the kidney. There is a close anatomic proximity of the two systems, with prostaglandin synthesis occurring in both renal medullary interstitial cells as well as in renal vascular endothelial cells (MCGIFF et al., 1976). In most instances, the prostaglandins seem to modulate the actions of other hormonal systems, e.g., sympathetic nerve stimulation causes prostaglandin E release, which acts presynaptically to decrease the amount of norepinephrine released with nerve stimulation (HEDQVIST, 1972); vasopressin causes prostaglandin E release in the kidney, which decreases the response of the collecting duct to vasopressin (GRANTHAM and ORLOFF, 1968; ZUSMAN et al., 1977). Thus, interactions between the renal kallikrein-kinin system and renal prostaglandins probably contribute to the control of renal blood flow or salt and water homeostasis.

In patients with Bartter's syndrome there is increased urinary prostaglandin E excretion and renomedullary interstitial cell hypertrophy (GILL et al., 1976). As noted above, both urinary kallikrein and plasma bradykinin levels are supranormal, while urinary kinin is subnormal (VINCI et al., 1976; HALUSHKA et al., 1977; LECHI et al., 1976). When these patients are treated with indomethacin or other inhibitors of prostaglandin synthetase, there is a return of all of their physiologically abnormal values to, or toward, normal and the patient remains normotensive (GILL et al., 1976; LECHI et al., 1976; HALUSHKA et al., 1977). Thus, the abnormality in renal prostaglandins appears to be the primary defect in the syndrome from which the other abnormalities result (MCGIFF, 1977). The increase in urinary kallikrein appears to parallel the hyperaldosteronism, while the increase in plasma bradykinin could be related to the increased plasma renin activity, as suggested previously by WONG et al. (1975). The reason for the subnormal urinary kinin excretion is unknown and unexpected in the face of supranormal urinary kallikrein excretion. This finding reinforces the necessity for future measurements of multiple components of the renal kallikrein-kinin system (substrate, kininases, etc.). In any event, this disorder shows vasoactive system interactions which need further investigation. The results also suggest that urinary kallikrein excretion is not the only determinant of urinary kinin levels.

Recent studies of prostaglandin biosynthesis by cultured renomedullary interstitial cells from the rabbit are of interest (ZUSMAN and KEISER, 1977a, b). These cells are stimulated to make predominately prostaglandin E_2 by physiologic doses of bradykinin, angiotensin II, and vasopressin. These agents appear to act by stimulating phospholipase A_2 to make more of the substrate, arachidonic acid, available for prostaglandin biosynthesis. This work is compatible with studies indicating that renal kinins may control and stimulate prostaglandin release (NASJLETTI and COLINA-CHOURIO, 1976; COLINA-CHOURIO et al., 1976; FEIGEN et al., 1978). In these studies, maneuvers known to alter either kallikrein excretion or the activity of the renal kallikrein-kinin system were examined for their effects on kidney prostaglandin E-like substances. Desoxycorticosterone increased significantly both urinary kallikrein and prostaglandin E-like material in the rat. Similar results were obtained with aldosterone. Aprotinin attenuated the increase in urinary prostaglandin E-like material produced by desoxycorticosterone. In isolated perfused rabbit kidneys, both bradykinin and kininogen increased the venous and urinary effluxes of prostaglandin E-like material. Aprotinin reduced the prostaglandin-releasing action of kininogen but not that of bradykinin. Indomethacin, which suppresses the synthesis of prostaglandins, also suppressed the release of prostaglandin evoked by bradykinin or kininogen. Further discussion of kinin-prostaglandin relations can be found on p. 401 (TERRAGNO and TERRAGNO).

4. Aldosterone

A body of data suggests that there are relations between the activity of sodium-retaining steroid hormones and the renal kallikrein-kinin system. Some of these observations were referred to above and include increased kallikrein excretion (a) in patients with primary aldosteronism (MARGOLIUS et al., 1971, 1974a; MIYASHITA, 1971; SEINO et al., 1977); (b) in normal volunteers or patients with essential hypertension on a diet of low sodium or high potassium (MARGOLIUS et al., 1974a; HORWITZ et al., 1975; LEVY et al., 1977; LAWTON and FITZ, 1976); (c) after treatment with 9-α-flurohydrocortisone (ADETUYIBI and MILLS, 1972; MARGOLIUS et al., 1974a); and (d) in Bartter's syndrome (LECHI et al., 1976; HALUSHKA et al., 1977). Patients with Cushing's syndrome have normal urinary kallikrein levels (MIYASHITA, 1971). Kallikrein excretion is reduced markedly in patients with primary aldosteronism or in normal volunteers by treatment with the specific aldosterone antagonist, spironolactone (MARGOLIUS et al., 1974a, b; SEINO et al., 1977). Isolated rat renal cortical cells in suspension produce more kallikrein in response to aldosterone and less in response to spironolactone (KAIZU and MARGOLIUS, 1975). Plasma kinin levels are increased by low dietary sodium intake, exogenously administered mineralocorticoid hormones, or treatment with ACTH (WONG et al., 1975; VINCI et al., 1977). Plasma kininogen levels appear to be reduced during periods of low dietary sodium intake and increased during periods of high dietary sodium intake (NASJLETTI and AZZAM, 1970). Kallikrein activity, both biochemically and immunohistochemically, has been localized in the kidney and in the salivary gland at sites known to be aldosterone-sensitive. The hypothesis that the enzyme kallikrein might be a specific aldosterone-induced protein involved in tubular transport phenomena has been advanced by MARGOLIUS et al. (1976). Whether or not this is true remains to be seen. However, the delineation of the relations among the renal kallikrein-kinin system, steroid hormones, and transport processes in areas where components of the system are localized, could be an important area of study. In this regard, the recent discovery and characterization of a kallikrein in the urinary bladder and skin of the toad, *Bufo marinus*, as well as the observation that this enzyme (and some mammalian urinary kallikreins) can have their biologic and esterase activity inhibited by amiloride (CHAO and MARGOLIUS, 1978) reinforces the possibility that the system plays a fundamentally important role in ion transport across membranes.

5. Miscellaneous

a) Substance P

This undecapeptide, present in nervous tissue, is the most potent natriuretic/diuretic substance known in dogs (MILLS et al., 1974; GULLNER et al., 1977). Low rates of infusion (1–100 ng/min) resulted in dose-dependent increases in the urinary excretion of kallikrein (MILLS et al., 1974) and a drop in renal renin secretion (GULLNER et al., 1977). The mechanisms responsible for the high potency of this peptide may be related to its interaction with the renal kinin and angiotensin systems (GULLNER et al., 1977; WARD and JOHNSON, 1978).

b) Drugs

Spironolactone, the aldosterone antagonist and diuretic, decreases urinary kallikrein excretion in normal volunteers and patients with primary aldosteronism (MARGOLIUS et al., 1974a, b; SEINO et al., 1977). Furosemide, a high-ceiling loop diuretic, appears to increase kallikrein activity in the urine of rats when high doses (5 mg) are given (CROXATTO et al., 1973; ROBLERO et al., 1976b). The relationship of furosemide and kallikrein is less clear in human volunteers (HALUSHKA et al., 1978; SEINO et al., 1978). Acetazolamide, a weakly diuretic catonic anhydrase inhibitor, also increases kallikrein excretion in rats (CROXATTO et al., 1975) as does bumetanide (OLSEN and AHNFELT-RØNNE, 1976), benzoflumethiazide, and hydralazine (NIELSEN and ARRIGONI-MARTELLI, 1977). It has been suggested that the observed changes relate to increases in renal blood flow induced by these drugs (NIELSEN and ARRIGONI-MARTELLI, 1977). Inhibition of the biologic and esterase activity of kallikrein by amiloride was mentioned previously. The significance of these findings is uncertain but indicates that the renal kallikrein-kinin system may be implicated in the mechanism of action of some therapeutic agents at some future time.

III. Kallikrein in Hypertensive Animals

Components of the kallikrein-kinin system have predominantly been measured in the hypertensive rat. The models used include the Okamoto and New Zealand strains of spontaneously hypertensive rat; the Dahl salt-sensitive and salt-resistant rat; a diabetic hypertensive rat model; renovascular hypertensive rat models with either partial renal artery occlusion or aortic coarctation; and desoxycorticosterone-salt hypertensive rats (JOHNSON et al., 1976; MARGOLIUS et al., 1972; GELLER et al., 1975; PORCELLI et al., 1975; CARRETERO et al., 1974, 1976, 1977; ARRIGONI-MARTELLI and NIELSEN, 1975; CROXATTO et al., 1973, 1974; NAMM et al., 1978; RAPP et al., 1978). In the initial study of the Okamoto spontaneously hypertensive rat, urinary kallikrein excretion was found to be higher than that in the NIH Wistar rats used as controls (MARGOLIUS et al., 1972). However, when the study was repeated using the Wistar-Kyoto normotensive control rat, urinary kallikrein excretion was observed to be lower in the spontaneously hypertensive than in the normotensive control (GELLER et al., 1975). Similar observations of lower urinary kallikrein excretion in genetically hypertensive rats has been observed in the Wistar strain of Bianchi (PORCELLI et al., 1975) and perhaps in the New Zealand strain of genetically hypertensive rats (CARRETERO et al., 1977). In addition, salt-sensitive rats excrete significantly less kallikrein than salt-resistant animals (CARRETERO et al., 1977; RAPP et al., 1978). In contrast, another study group, using spontaneously hypertensive Sprague-Dawley rats, reported higher urinary kallikrein excretion in the hypertensive than in the normotensive groups (ARRIGONI-MARTELLI and NIELSEN, 1975). When hypertension was induced in rats, drinking 1% saline, via subcutaneous implementation of desoxycorticosterone acetate (DOCA) pellets, there was a marked increase in urinary kallikrein excretion in the hypertensive animals compared with the control groups not receiving DOCA, but drinking either 1% saline or distilled water (MARGOLIUS et al., 1972). However, it was observed later that desoxycorticosterone alone increased urinary kallikrein excretion in the absence of elevated systemic arterial pressure (GELLER et al., 1972).

Urinary kallikrein excretion has almost universally been observed to be reduced in renal hypertensive rats of either the one-kidney (CROXATTO and SAN MARTIN, 1970; JENNER and CROXATTO, 1973; CARRETERO and OZA, 1973) or the two-kidney type (MARGOLIUS et al., 1972; JENNER and CROXATTO, 1973). Reversal of the renal hypertension by unclamping the renal artery led paradoxically to further decreases in urinary kallikrein excretion (GULATI et al., 1976). In one recent study an increase in urinary kallikrein excretion in the two-kidney renal hypertensive rat and no change in the one-kidney model (JOHNSTON et al., 1976) was reported. This is of interest since kallikrein was measured in these studies by radioimmunoassay of generated kinins, rather than the direct measurement of kallikrein biologic or esterolytic activity used by all other workers. Whether this methodologic difference will lead to additional insight into the activity of urinary kallikrein in renovascular hypertension remains to be seen. In conscious dogs with chronic unilateral renal artery stenosis, KEISER et al. (1976) found markedly reduced kallikrein excretion in the ureter from the compromized kidney versus the normally perfused kidney. This reduced excretion correlated well with the reduced renal blood flow (as measured by para-aminohippurate clearance) produced by the ligature. It remains to be determined whether any other urinary enzymes are influenced by the maneuvers or by the hypertensive state when significant changes in kallikrein excretion are seen.

Tissue kallikrein levels have been measured in the kidneys of spontaneously hypertensive rats of the Bianchi strain (FAVARO et al., 1975) and in renal hypertensive rats (CROXATTO et al., 1974; CARRETERO et al., 1974). In both models, the renal kallikrein content was significantly lower than in normotensive controls. ANTONELLO et al. (1975) showed that renal kallikrein is increased in the remaining kidney after a uninephrectomy in rats and suggest that the change may be related to an increased renal blood flow. Plasma kininogen levels have been measured in a single study in renal hypertensive rats and found to be significantly increased (ALBERTINI et al., 1974).

These studies represent the sum total of experience gathered by measuring components of the kallikrein-kinin system in hypertensive animal models. They do not show that an abnormality in the renal kallikrein-kinin system plays any role in the pathogenesis of the hypertensive diseases associated with these models. None of the cited studies precedes 1970 or includes measurements of multiple components of the renal kinin system. It seems reasonable to expect even greater interest in the role of the system in relation to hypertensive states. This interest is reinforced by findings in human hypertension discussed elsewhere in this volume by MILLS (p. 549).

References

Abe, K., Seino, M., Otsuka, Y., Yoshinaga, K.: Urinary kallikrein excretion and sodium metabolism in human hypertension. In: Chemistry and biology of the kallikrein-kinin system in health and disease. Pisano, J.J., Austen, K.F. (eds.), pp. 411–414. Fogarty Internat. Center Proc. No. 27. Washington: U.S. Gov. Printing Office 1977

Adetuyibi, A., Mills, I.H.: Relation between urinary kallikrein and renal function, hypertension, and excretion of sodium and water in man. Lancet *1972/II*, 203–207

Albertini, R., Roblero, J., Corthorn, J., Croxatto, H.R.: Blood kininogen in uninephrectomized and hypertensive rats. Acta. Physiol. Lat. Am. *24*, 443–447 (1974)

Amundsen, E., Nustad, K., Waaler, B.: A stable substrate for the assay of plasma kinin-forming enzymes. Br. J. Pharmacol. *21*, 500–508 (1963)

Amundsen, E., Svendsen, L., Vennerød, A.M., Laake, K.: Determination of plasma kallikrein with a new chromogenic tripeptide derivative. In: Chemistry and biology of the kallikrein-kinin system in health and disease. Pisano, J.J., Austen, K.F. (eds.), pp. 215–220. Fogarty Internat. Center Proc. No. 27. Washington: U.S. Gov. Printing Office 1977

Antonello, A., Baggio, B., Favaro, S., Zen, A., Sandei, F., Todesco, S., Borsatti, A.: Effect of uninephrectomy on tissue kallikrein concentration of the remaining kidney. Biomedicine *23*, 303–306 (1975)

Arrigoni-Martelli, E., Nielsen, C.K.: Urinary kallikrein excretion in normotensive and spontaneously hypertensive rats. Acta Pharmacol. Toxicol. (Kbh.) *37*, 177–184 (1975)

Bagdasarian, A., Talamo, R.C., Colman, R.W.: Isolation of high molecular weight activators of human plasma prekallikrein. J. Biol. Chem. *248*, 3456–3463 (1973)

Bagdasarian, A., Lahiri, B., Talamo, R.C., Wong, P., Colman, R.W.: Immunochemical studies of plasma kallikrein. J. Clin. Invest. *54*, 1444–1454 (1974)

Baggio, B., Favoro, S., Antonello, A., Zen, A., Zen, F., Borsatti, A.: Subcellular localization of renin and kallikrein in rat kidney. Ital. J. Biochem. *24*, 199–206 (1975)

Barraclough, M.A., Mills, I.H.: Effect of bradykinin on renal function. Clin. Sci. *28*, 69–74 (1965)

Barton, S., Sanders, E.J., Schachter, M., Uddin, M.: Autonomic nerve stimulation, kallikrein content and acinar cell granules of the cat's submandibular gland. J. Physiol. (Lond.) *251*, 363–369 (1975)

Beaven, V., Pierce, J., Pisano, J.: A sensitive isotopic procedure for the assay of esterase activity: Measurement of human urinary kallikrein. Clin. Chim. Acta *32*, 67–73 (1971)

Beraldo, W.T., Feldberg, W., Hilton, S.M.: Experiments on the factor in urine forming substance U. J. Physiol. (Lond.) *133*, 558–565 (1956)

Beraldo, W.T., Lauar, N.S., Siqueira, G., Heneine, I.F., Catanzaro, O.L.: Peculiarities of the oxytocic action of rat urinary kallikrein. In: Chemistry and biology of the kallikrein-kinin system in health and disease. Pisano, J.J., Austen, K.F. (eds.), pp. 375–378. Fogarty Internat. Center Proc. No. 27. Washington: U.S. Gov. Printing Office 1977

Bevan, D.R., Macfarlane, N.A.A., Mills, I.H.: The dependence of urinary kallikrein excretion on renal artery pressure. J. Physiol. (Lond.) *241*, 34P–35P (1974)

Carretero, O.A., Oza, N.B.: Urinary kallikrein, sodium metabolism and hypertension. In: Proceedings of an international workshop conference of mechanisms of hypertension. Sambhi, M. (ed.), pp. 390–399. Amsterdam: Excerpta Medica Foundation 1973

Carretero, O.A., Scicli, A.G.: Renal kallikrein: its localization and possible role in renal function. Fed. Proc. *35*, 194–198 (1976)

Carretero, O.A., Oza, N.B., Scicli, A.G., Schork, A.: Renal tissue kallikrein, plasma renin, and plasma aldosterone in renal hypertension. Acta Physiol. Lat. Am. *24*, 448–452 (1974)
Carretero, O.A., Oza, N.B., Piwonska, A., Ocholik, T., Scicli, A.G.: Measurement of urinary kallikrein activity by kinin radioimmunoassay. Biochem. Pharmacol. *25*, 1–6 (1976)
Carretero, O.A., Scicli, A.G., Piwonska, A., Koch, J.: Urinary kallikrein in rats bred for susceptibility and resistance to the hypertensive effect of salt and in New Zealand genetically hypertensive rats. Mayo Clin. Proc. *52*, 465–467 (1977)
Carretero, O.A., Amin, V.M., Ocholik, T., Scicli, A.G., Koch, J.: Urinary kallikrein in rats bred for their susceptibility and resistance to the hypertensive effect of salt. A new radioimmunoassay for its direct determination. Circ. Res. *42*, 727–731 (1978)
Carvalho, I.F.: Studies on the kinin-forming enzyme (kininogenin) of rat kidney. In: Kidney hormones. Fisher, J.W. (ed.), pp. 585–601. London, New York: Academic Press 1971
Carvalho, I.F., Diniz, C.R.: Kinin forming enzyme (kininogenin) in rat kidney. Ann. N.Y. Acad. Sci. *116*, 912–917 (1964)
Carvalho, I.F., Diniz, C.R.: Kinin forming enzyme (kininogenin) in homogenates of rat kidney. Biochim. Biophys. Acta *128*, 136–148 (1966)
Chao, J.: Activity and structural changes of purified kallikrein with detergent treatment. Arch. Biochem. Biophys. *185*, 549–556 (1978)
Chao, J., Margolius, H.S.: Purification and properties of rat urinary kallikrein isozymes. Fed. Proc. *36*, 1014 (1977)
Chao, J., Margolius, H.S.: Identification of kallikrein in toad urinary bladder and skin and its inhibition by amiloride. Clin. Res. *26*, 63 A (1978)
Chao, J., Margolius, H.S.: Identification of kallikrein on external cell surfaces. Fed. Proc. *37*, 657 (1978)
Claeson, G.: Chromogenic peptide substrates for kallikreins (to be published)
Colina-Chourio, J., McGiff, J.C., Miller, M.P., Nasjletti, A.: Possible influence of intrarenal generation of kinins on prostaglandin release from the rabbit perfused kidney. Br. J. Pharmacol. *58*, 165–172 (1976)
Corthorn, J., Imanari, T., Yoshida, H., Kaizu, T., Pierce, J.V., Pisano, J.J.: Inactive kallikrein in human urine. Fed. Proc. *36*, 893 (1977)
Croxatto, H.R., Albertini, R., Roblero, J., Corthorn, J.: Renal kallikrein (kininogenase activity) in hypertensive rats. Acta Physiol. Lat. Am. *24*, 439–442 (1974)
Croxatto, H.R., Huidobro, F., Rojas, M., Roblero, J., Albertini, R.: The effect of water, sodium overloading and diuretics upon urinary kallikrein. In: Advances in experimental medicine and biology. Vol. 70: Kinins: Pharmacodynamics and biological roles. Sicuteri, F., Back, N., Haberland, G.L. (eds.), pp. 361–373. New York, London: Plenum Press 1975
Croxatto, H.R., San Martin, M.: Kallikrein-like activity in the urine of renal hypertensive rats. Experientia *26*, 1216–1217 (1970)
Croxatto, H.R., Roblero, J.S., Garcia, R.L., Corthorn, J.H., San Martin, M.: Urinary kallikrein under furosemide and plasma kininogen levels in normal and hypertensive rats. Acta Physiol. Lat. Am. *23*, 556–558 (1973)
DeBono, E., Mills, I.H.: Simultaneous increases in kallikrein in renal lymph and urine during saline infusion. J. Physiol. (Lond.) *241*, 127 P–128 P (1974)
Erdös, E. (ed.): Handbook of experimental pharmacology. Vol. XXV: Bradykinin, kallidin, and kallikrein. Berlin, Heidelberg, New York: Springer 1970
Erdös, E.G., Marinkovic, D.M., Ward, P.E., Mills, I.H.: Characterization of urinary kininase. Fed. Proc. *37*, 657 (1978)
Favaro, S., Baggio, B., Antonello, A., Zen, A., Cannella, G., Todesco, S., Borsatti, A.: Renal kallikrein content of spontaneously hypertensive rats. Clin. Sci. Mol. Med. *49*, 69–71 (1975)
Feigen, L.P., Chapnick, B.M., Flemming, J.E., Kadowitz, P.J.: Prostaglandins: renal vascular responses to bradykinin, histamine, and nitroglycerine. Am. J. Physiol. *234*, H496–H502 (1978)
Fiedler, F.: Pig pancreatic kallikrein: structure and catalytic properties. In: Chemistry and biology of the kallikrein-kinin system in health and disease. Pisano, J.J., Austen, K.F. (eds.), pp. 93–95. Fogarty Internat. Center Proc. No. 27. Washington: U.S. Gov. Printing Office 1977
Fiedler, F., Hirschauer, C., Werle, E.: Anreicherung von Präkallikrein B aus Schweinepankreas und Eigenschaften verschiedener Formen des Pankreaskallikreins. Hoppe Seylers Z. Physiol. Chem. *351*, 225–238 (1970)

Freeman, R.H., Davies, J.O., Vitale, S.J., Johnson, J.A.: Intrarenal role of angiotensin II. Circ. Res. *32*, 692–698 (1973)
Fritz, H., Fiedler, F., Dietl, T., Warwas, M., Truscheit, E., Kolb, H.J., Mair, G., Tschesche, H.: On the relationships between porcine pancreatic, submandibular, and urinary kallikreins. In: Kininogenases – kallikrein. Haberland, G.L., Rohen, J.W., Suzuki, T. (eds.), Vol. 4, pp. 15–28. New York: Schattauer 1977
Furtado, M.: Inhibition of the permeability response to vasopressin and oxytocin in the toad bladder: Effects of bradykinin, kallidin, eledoisin, and physalaemin. J. Memb. Biol. *4*, 165–178 (1971)
Geiger, R., Mann, K.: A kallikrein-specific inhibitor in rat kidney tubules. Hoppe Seylers Z. Physiol. Chem. *357*, 553–558 (1976)
Geller, R.G., Margolius, H.S., Pisano, J.J., Keiser, H.R.: Effects of mineralocorticoids, altered sodium intake and adrenalectomy on urinary kallikrein in rats. Circ. Res. *31*, 857–861 (1972)
Geller, R.G., Margolius, H.S., Pisano, J.J., Keiser, H.R.: Urinary kallikrein in spontaneously hypertensive rats. Circ. Res. *36/37* (Suppl. I), 103–106 (1975)
Geratz, J.D., Cheng, M.C.F., Tidwell, R.R.: New aromatic diamidines with central α-oxyalkane or α, ω-dioxyalkane chains. Structure-activity relationships for the inhibition of trypsin, pancreatic kallikrein, and thrombin and for the inhibition of the overall coagulation process. J. Med. Chem. *18*, 477–481 (1975)
Geratz, J.D., Cheng, M.C.F., Tidwell, R.R.: Novel bis(benzamidino) compounds with an aromatic central link. Inhibitors of thrombin, pancreatic kallikrein, trypsin, and complement. J. Med. Chem. *19*, 634–639 (1976)
Gill, J.R., Jr., Melmon, K.L., Gillespie, L., Jr., Bartter, F.C.: Bradykinin and renal function in normal man: effects of adrenergic blockade. Am. J. Physiol. *209*, 844–848 (1965)
Gill, J.R., Jr., Frolich, J.C., Bowden, R.E., Taylor, A.A., Keiser, H.R., Seyberth, H.W., Oates, J.A., Bartter, F.C.: Bartter's syndrome: a disorder characterized by high urinary prostaglandins and a dependence of hyperreninemia on prostaglandin synthesis. Am. J. Med. *61*, 43–51 (1976)
Giusti, E.P., Sampaio, P.A.M., Prado, E.F.: Purification of horse urinary kallikrein by affinity chromatography. In: Kinins 76. An International Symposium (Abs. 43). Rio de Janeiro, Brazil, 1976
Goldberg, L.I., Dollery, C.T., Pentecost, B.L.: Effects of intrarenal infusions of bradykinin and acetylcholine on renal blood flow in man. J. Clin. Invest. *44*, 1052 (1965)
Grantham, J.J., Orloff, J.: Effect of prostaglandin E_1 on the permeability response of the isolated collecting tubule to vasopressin, adenosine 3′,5′-monophosphate, and theophylline. J. Clin. Invest. *47*, 1154–1161 (1968)
Greco, A.V., Porcelli, G., Croxatto, H.R., Fedeli, G., Ghirlanda, G.: Ipertensione arteriosa e callicreina urinaria. Minerva Med. *65*, 3058–3062 (1974)
Gulati, O.P., Carretero, O.A., Morino, T., Oza, N.B.: Urinary kallikrein and plasma renin during the reversal of renovascular hypertension in rats. Clin. Sci. Mol. Med. *51* Suppl. 3, 263 s–266 s (1976)
Guimãraes, J.A., Lu, R.C., Webster, M.E., Pierce, J.V.: Multiple forms of human plasma kininogen. Fed. Proc. *33*, 641 (1974)
Gullner, H.G., Campbell, W.B., Pettinger, W.A.: Substance P: Intrarenal infusion inhibits renin release in the dog. Fed. Proc. *36*, 984 (1977)
Halushka, P.V., Wohltmann, H., Privitera, P.J., Hurwitz, G., Margolius, H.S.: Bartter's syndrome: urinary prostaglandin E-like material and kallikrein; indomethacin effects. Ann. Intern. Med. *87*, 281–286 (1977)
Halushka, P.V., Margolius, H.S., Allen, H., Conradi, E.C.: Effects of furosemide on the urinary excretion of prostaglandin E-like material and kallikrein. Unpublished results.
Hedqvist, P.: Prostaglandin mediated control of sympathetic neuroeffector transmission. In: Advances in the biosciences. International Conference on Prostaglandins. Bergströ, S., Bernhard, S. (eds.), Vol. 9, pp. 461–473 (1972)
Hial, V., Diniz, C.R., Mares-Guia, M.: Purification and properties of human urinary kallikrein (kininogenase). Biochemistry *13*, 4311–4318 (1974)
Hilton, S.M., Lewis, G.P.: The mechanism of the functional hyperaemia in the submandibular salivary gland. J. Physiol. (Lond.) *129*, 253–271 (1955)

Hojima, Y., Isobe, M., Moriya, H.: Kallikrein inhibitors in rat plasma. J. Biochem. *81*, 37–46 (1977)
Horwitz, D., Margolius, H.S., Keiser, H.R.: Effects of potassium intake on urinary kallikrein and aldosterone excretion. Clin. Res. *23*, 221 A (1975)
Imanari, T., Kaizu, T., Yoshida, H., Yates, K., Pierce, J.V., Pisano, J.J.: Radiochemical assays for human urinary salivary and plasma kallikreins. In: Chemistry and biology of the kallikrein-kinin system in health and disease. Pisano, J.J., Austen, K.F. (eds.), pp. 205–213. Fogarty Internat. Proc. No. 27. Washington: U.S. Gov. Printing Office 1977
Jacobsen, S.: Substrates for plasma kinin-forming enzymes in human, dog, and rabbit plasma. Br. J. Pharmacol. *26*, 403–411 (1966)
Jenner, S., Croxatto, H.R.: Urinary kallikrein from normal and hypertensive rats. Experientia *29*, 1359–1361 (1973)
Johnston, C.I., Matthews, P.G., Dax, E.: Effects of dietary sodium, diuretics, and hypertension on renin and kallikrein. In: Systemic effects of antihypertensive agents. Sambhi, M.P. (ed.), pp. 323–338. New York: Stratton Intercontinental 1976
Kaizu, T., Margolius, H.S.: Studies on rat renal cortical cell kallikrein. I. Separation and measurement. Biochim. Biophys. Acta *411*, 305–315 (1975)
Keiser, H.R., Andrews, M.J., Jr., Guyton, R.A., Margolius, H.S., Pisano, J.J.: Urinary kallikrein in dogs with constriction of one renal artery. Proc. Soc. Exp. Biol. *151*, 53–56 (1976)
Lawton, W., Fitz, A.: Normal renin essential hypertension and urinary kallikrein excretion. Clin. Res. *24*, 555 A (1976)
Lechi, A., Covi, G., Lechi, C., Mantero, F., Scuro, L.A.: Urinary kallikrein excretion in Bartter's syndrome. J. Clin. Endocrinol. Metab. *43*, 1175–1178 (1976)
Levy, S.B., Lilley, J.J., Frigon, R.P., Stone, R.A.: Urinary kallikrein and plasma renin activity as determinants of renal blood flow. J. Clin. Invest. *60*, 129–138 (1977)
Lupu, A.N., Maxwell, M.H., Kaufman, J.J., White, F.N.: Experimental unilateral renal artery constriction in the dog. Circ. Res. *30*, 567–574 (1972)
MacFarlane, N.A.A., Mills, I.H., Wraight, E.: The effect of kallikrein infusions on renal function in the dog. J. Endocrinol. *55*, xli–xlii (1972)
MacFarlane, N.A.A., Adetuyibi, A., Mills, I.H.: The radioimmunoassay of bradykinin in the measurement of kallikrein in urine. J. Endocrinol. *58*, xxv (1973)
MacFarlane, N.A.A., Adetuyibi, A., Mills, I.H.: Changes in kallikrein excretion during arterial infusion of angiotensin. J. Endocrinol. *61*, lxxii (1974)
Mann, K., Geiger, R., Werle, E.: A sensitive kinin liberating assay for kininogenase in rat urine, isolated glomeruli and tubules of rat kidney. In: Advances in experimental medicine and biology. Vol. 70: Kinins: pharmacodynamics and biological roles. Sicuteri, F., Back, N., Haberland, G.L. (eds.), pp. 65–73. New York, London: Plenum Press 1975
Margolius, H.S., Geller, R., Pisano, J.J., Sjoerdsma, A.: Altered urinary kallikrein excretion in human hypertension. Lancet *1971/II*, 1063–1065
Margolius, H.S., Geller, R.G., de Jong, W., Pisano, J.J., Sjoerdsma, A.: Urinary kallikrein excretion in hypertension. Circ. Res. *30/31* Suppl. II, 125–131 (1972)
Margolius, H.S., Horwitz, D., Geller, R.G., Alexander, R.W., Gill, J.R., Jr., Pisano, J.J., Keiser, H.R.: Urinary kallikrein excretion in normal man. Relationships to sodium intake and sodium-retaining steroids. Circ. Res. *35*, 812–819 (1974a)
Margolius, H.S., Horwitz, D., Pisano, J.J., Keiser, H.R.: Sodium, water, and kallikrein excretion in man. Acta Physiol. Lat. Am. *24*, 464–468 (1974b)
Margolius, H.S., Horwitz, D., Pisano, J.J., Keiser, H.R.: Urinary kallikrein in hypertension: Relationship to sodium intake and sodium-retaining steroid. Circ. Res. *35*, 820–825 (1974c)
Margolius, H.S., Chao, J., Kaizu, T.: The effects of aldosterone and spironolactone on renal kallikrein. Clin. Sci. Mol. Med. *51* Suppl. 3, 279 s–282 s (1976)
Marin-Grez, M.: The influence of antibodies against bradykinin on isotonic saline diuresis in the rat. Pflügers Arch. *350*, 231–239 (1974)
Marin-Grez, M., Carretero, O.A.: Urinary kallikrein excretion in rats under low and high sodium intake. Physiologist *14*, 189 (1971)
Marin-Grez, M., Carretero, O.A.: A method for measurement of urinary kallikrein. J. Appl. Physiol. *32*, 428–431 (1972)
Marin-Grez, M., Cottone, P., Carretero, O.A.: Evidence for an involvement of kinins in regulation of sodium excretion. Am. J. Physiol. *223*, 794–796 (1972)

Marin-Grez, M., Oza, N.B., Carretero, O.A.: The involvement of urinary kallikrein in the renal escape from the sodium retaining effect of mineralocorticoids. Henry Ford Hospital Med. J. *21*, 85–90 (1973)

McCaa, C.S., McCaa, R.E.: Response of the kallikrein-kinin system to continuous infusion of angiotensin I converting enzyme inhibitor (SQ-20881) into intact conscious dog. Clin. Res. *25*, 61 A (1977)

McGiff, J.C.: Perspective. Bartter's syndrome results from an imbalance of vasoactive hormones. Ann. Intern. Med. *87*, 369–372 (1977)

McGiff, J.C., Nasjletti, A.: Kinins, renal function, and blood pressure regulation. Introduction. Fed. Proc. *35*, 172–174 (1976)

McGiff, J.C., Itskovitz, H.D., Terragno, N.A.: The actions of bradykinin and eledoisin in the canine isolated kidney: relationships to prostaglandins. Clin. Sci. Mol. Med. *49*, 125–131 (1975)

McGiff, J.C., Itskovitz, H.D., Terragno, A., Wong, P., Y.-K.: Modulation and mediation of the action of the renal kallikrein-kinin system by prostaglandins. Fed. Proc. *35*, 175–180 (1976)

McNay, J.L., Goldberg, L.I.: Comparison of the effects of dopamine, isoproterenol, norepinephrine, and bradykinin on canine renal and femoral blood flow. J. Pharmol. Exp. Ther. *151*, 23–31 (1966)

Mersey, J.H., Williams, G.H., Hollenberg, N.K., Dluhy, R.G.: Relationship between aldosterone and bradykinin. Circ. Res. *40* Suppl. 1, 84–88 (1977)

Mills, I.H., Ward, P.E.: The relationship between kallikrein and water excretion and the conditional relationship between kallikrein and sodium excretion. J. Physiol. (Lond.) *246*, 695–707 (1975)

Mills, I.H., Obika, L.F.O.: The effect of adrenergic and dopamine-receptor blockade on the kallikrein and renal response to intra-arterial infusion of dopamine in dogs. J. Physiol. (Lond.) *263*, 150 P–151 P (1976)

Mills, I.H., MacFarlane, N.A.A., Ward, P.E.: Increase in kallikrein excretion during the natriuresis produced by arterial infusion of substance P. Nature *247*, 108–109 (1974)

Mills, I.H., Paterson, C.L., Ward, P.E.: The role of the kidney in the inactivation of injected kallikrein. J. Physiol. (Lond.) *251*, 281–286 (1975)

Mills, I.H., MacFarlane, N.A.A., Ward, P.E., Obika, L.F.O.: The renal kallikrein-kinin system and the regulation of salt and water excretion. Fed. Proc. *35*, 181–188 (1976)

Miyashita, A.: Urinary kallikrein determination and its physiological role in human kidney. Jpn. J. Urol. *62*, 507–518 (1971)

Nakano, J.: Effects of synthetic bradykinin on the cardiovascular system. Arch. Intern. Pharmacodyn. *157*, 1–13 (1965)

Namm, D.H., Squires, J., El-Sayad, S., Wilson, S.J., Parsons, D., Margolius, H.S.: Vascular changes in experimental diabetes mellitus: Development of hypertension and associated changes in arterial metabolism and responsiveness. Unpublished results.

Nasjletti, A., Azzam, M.E.: Variations of plasma kininogen content due to high sodium intake in rats. Experientia *26*, 280–281 (1970)

Nasjletti, A., Colina-Chourio, J.: Interaction of mineralocorticoids, renal prostaglandins, and the renal kallikrein-kinin system. Fed. Proc. *35*, 189–193 (1976)

Nasjletti, A., Colina-Chourio, J., McGiff, J.C.: Disappearance of bradykinin in the renal circulation of dogs. Circ. Res. *37*, 59–65 (1975)

Nekrasova, A.A., Zharova, E.A., Sokolova, R.I.: Role of the kallikrein kinin system of the kidneys in sodium and water transport and its modification by indomethacin. Bull. Exp. Biol. Med. *83*, 456–458 (1977)

Nielsen, K., Arrigoni-Martelli, E.: Effects on rat urinary kallikrein excretion of bumetanide, bendroflumethiazide, and hydralazine. Acta Pharmacol. Toxical. (Kbh.) *40*, 267–272 (1977)

Nizet, A.: The isolated perfused kidney: Possibilities, limitations, and results. Kidney Int. 7, 1–11 (1975)

Nustad, K.: The relationship between kidney and urinary kininogenase. Br. J. Pharmacol. *39*, 73–86 (1970a)

Nustad, K.: Localization of kininogenase in the rat kidney. Br. J. Pharmacol. *39*, 87–98 (1970b)

Nustad, K., Pierce, J.V.: Purification of rat urinary kallikreins and their specific antibody. Biochemistry *13*, 2312–2319 (1974)

Nustad, K., Rubin, I.: Subcellular localization of renin and kininogenase in the rat kidney. Br. J. Pharmacol. *40*, 326–333 (1970)
Nustad, K., Vaaje, K., Pierce, J.V.: Synthesis of kallikreins by rat kidney slices. Br. J. Pharmacol. *53*, 229–234 (1975)
Ofstad, E.: Formation and destruction of plasma kinins during experimental acute hemorrhagic pancreatitis in dogs. Scand. J. Gastroenterol. *5* Suppl. 5, 1–44 (1970)
Ole-Moi Yoi, O., Spragg, J., Halbert, S.P., Austen, K.F.: Immunologic reactivity of purified human urinary kallikrein (urokallikrein) with antiserum directed against human pancreas. J. Immunol. *118*, 667–672 (1977)
Olsen, U.B., Ahnfelt-Rønne, J.: Bumetanide-induced increase of renal blood flow in conscious dogs and its relation to local renal hormones (PGE, kallikrein and renin). Acta Pharmacol. Toxicol. (Kbh.) *38*, 219–228 (1976)
Orstavik, T.B., Gautvik, K.M.: Regulation of salivary kallikrein secretion in the rat sulmand bular gland. Acta Physiol. Scand. *100*, 33–44 (1977)
Orstavik, T.B., Nustad, K., Brandtzaeg, P., Pierce, J.V.: Cellular origin of urinary kallikreins. J. Histochem. Cytochem. *24*, 1037–1039 (1976)
Oza, N.B., Amin, V.M., Gandolfi, R., Yanari, S., Carretero, O.A.: A direct radioimmunoassay for rat urinary kallikrein. Fed. Proc. *35*, 693 (1976a)
Oza, N.B., Amin, V.M., McGregor, R.K., Scicli, A.G., Carretero, O.A.: Isolation of rat urinary kallikrein and properties of its antibodies. Biochem. Pharmacol. *25*, 1607–1612 (1976b)
Pierce, J.V., Nustad, K.: Purification of human and rat urinary kallikrein. Fed. Proc. *31*, 623 (1972)
Pisano, J.J., Yates, K., Pierce, J.V.: Kininogen in human urine. Agents Actions *8*, 153 (1978)
Porcelli, G., Croxatto, H.: Purification of kininogenase from rat urine. Ital. J. Biochem. *20*, 66–88 (1971)
Porcelli, G., Marini-Bertólo, G.B., Croxatto, H.R., di Iorio, M.: Purification and chemical studies on human urinary kallikrein. Ital. J. Biochem. *23*, 44–55 (1974)
Porcelli, G., Bianchi, G., Croxatto, H.: Urinary kallikrein in a spontaneously hypertensive strain of rats. Proc. Soc. Exp. Biol. *149*, 983–986 (1975)
Rapp, J.P., Pan, S.Y., Margolius, H.S.: Plasma renin, adrenocorticoids in urinary kallikrein in salt-sensitive and salt-resistant rats. Endo. Res. Comm. *5*, 35–41 (1978)
Roblero, J.S., Croxatto, H.R., Albertini, R.B.: Release of renal kallikrein to the perfusate by isolated rat kidney. Experientia *32*, 1440–1441 (1976a)
Roblero, J., Croxatto, H., Garcia, R., Corthorn, J., DeVito, E.: Kallikreinlike activity in perfusates and urine of isolated rat kidneys. Am. J. Physiol. *231*, 1383–1389 (1976b)
Scicli, A.G., Carretero, O.A., Oza, N.B., Schork, A.: Distribution of kidney kininogenases. Proc. Soc. Exp. Biol. Med. *151*, 57–60 (1976)
Scicli, A.G., Gandolfi, R., Carretero, O.A.: Site of kinin formation in the dog nephron. Fed. Proc. *36*, 1015 (1977)
Scicli, A.G., Gandolfi, R., Carretero, O.A.: Site of formation of kinins in the dog nephorn. Am. J. Physiol. *234*, F36–F40 (1978)
Silva, E., Diniz, C.R., Mares-Guia, M.: Rat urinary kallikrein: Purification and properties. Biochemistry *13*, 4304–4310 (1974)
Seino, J., Abe, K., Otsuka, Y., Saito, T., Irokawa, N., Yasujima, M., Ciba, S., Yoshinaga, K.: Urinary kallikrein excretion and sodium metabolism in hypertensive patients. Tohoku J. Exp. Med. *116*, 359–367 (1975)
Seino, M., Abe, K., Sakurai, Y., Irokawa, N., Yasujima, M., Chiba, S., Otsuka, Y., Yoshinaga, K.: Effect of spironolactone on urinary kallikrein excretion in patients with essential hypertension and in primary aldosteronism. Tohoku J. Exp. Med. *121*, 111–119 (1977)
Seino, M., Abe, K., Irokawa, N., Ito, T., Yasujima, M., Sakurai, Y., Chiba, S., Saito, K., Ritz, K., Kusaka, T., Miyazaki, S., Yoshinaga, K.: Effect of furosemide on urinary kallikrein excretion in patients with essential hypertension. Tohoku J. Exp. Med. *124*, 197–203 (1978)
Stein, J.H., Ferris, T.F., Huprich, J.E., Smith, T.C., Osgood, R.W.: Effect of renal vasodilation on the distribution of cortical blood flow in the kidney of the dog. J. Clin. Invest. *50*, 1429–1438 (1971)
Stein, J.H., Congbalay, R.C., Karsh, D.L., Osgood, R.W., Ferris, T.F.: The effect of bradykinin on proximal tubular sodium reabsorption in the dog: Evidence for functional nephron heterogeneity. J. Clin. Invest. *51*, 1709–1721 (1972)

Streeten, D.H.P., Kerr, L.P., Kerr, C.B., Prior, J.C., Dalakos, T.G.: Hyperbradykininism: A new orthostatic syndrome. Lancet *1972/II*, 1048–1053
Takahachi, H., Iwanaga, S., Suzuki, T.: Snake venom proteinase inhibitors. I. Isolation and properties of two inhibitors of kallikrein, trypsin, and alpha-kimotrypsin from the venom of Russell's viper (Vipera russelli). J. Biochem. (Tokyo) *76*, 709–713 (1974)
Talamo, R.C., Haber, E., Austen, K.F.: A radioimmunoassay for bradykinin in plasma and synovial fluid. J. Lab. Clin. Med. *74*, 816–827 (1969)
Tidwell, R.R., Fox, L.L., Geratz, J.D.: Aromatic Tris-amidines. A new class of highly active inhibitors of trypsin-like proteases. Biochim. Biophys. Acta *445*, 729–738 (1976)
Trautschold, I.: Assay methods in the kinin system. In: Handbook of experimental pharmacology. Vol. XXV: Bradykinin, kallidin, and kallikrein. Erdös, E.G. (ed.), pp. 52–81. Berlin, Heidelberg, New York: Springer 1970
Tyler, D.W.: The distribution and properties of renal kininogenase. Ph.D. Thesis. University of Alberta, Edmondon, Alberta, 1972
Vinci, J.M., Telles, D.A., Bowden, R.E., Izzo, J.L., Keiser, H.R., Radfar, N., Taylor, A.A., Gill, J.R., Jr., Bartter, F.C.: The kallikrein-kinin system in Bartter's syndrome and its response to prostaglandin synthetase inhibition. Clin. Res. *24*, 414 A (Abstract) (1976)
Vinci, J., Zusman, R., Bowden, R., Horwitz, D., Keiser, H.: Relationship of urinary and plasma kinins to sodium-retaining steroids and plasma renin activity. Clin. Res. *25*, 450 A (Abstract) (1977)
Ward, P.E., Johnson, A.R.: Renal inactivation of substance P in the rat. Biochem. J. *171*, 143–148 (1978)
Ward, P.E., Gedney, C., Dowden, R.M., Erdös, E.G.: Subcellular localization of renal kallikrein. Circulation *52*, 11–14 (1975 a)
Ward, P.E., Gedney, C., Dowden, R.M., Erdös, E.G.: Isolation of membrane-bound renal kallikrein and kininase. Biochem. J. *151*, 755–758 (1975 b)
Ward, P.E., Erdös, E.G., Gedney, C.D., Dowden, R.M., Reynolds, R.C.: Isolation of membrane bound renal enzymes that metabolize kinins and antiotensins. Biochem. J. *157*, 643–650 (1976)
Ward, P.E., Schultz, W., Reynolds, R.C., Erdös, E.G.: Metabolism of kinins and angiotensin in the isolated glomerulus and brush border of rat kidney. Lab. Invest. *36*, 599–606 (1977)
Webster, M.E., Gilmore, J.P.: Influence of kallidin-10 on renal function. Am. J. Physiol. *206*, 714–718 (1964)
Webster, M.E., Pierce, J.V.: Action of the Kallikreins on synthetic ester substrates. Proc. Soc. Exp. Biol. *107*, 186–191 (1961)
Webster, M.E., Pierce, J.V.: The nature of the kallidins released from human plasma by kallikreins and other enzymes. Ann. N.Y. Acad. Sci. *104*, 91–107 (1963)
Werle, E., Vogel, R.: Über die Kallikreinausscheidung im Harn nach experimenteller Nierenschädigung. Archs. Int. Pharmacodyn. Ther. *126*, 171–186 (1960)
Willis, L.R., Ludens, J.H., Hook, J.B., Williamson, H.E.: Mechanism of natriuretic action of bradykinin. Am. J. Physiol. *217*, 1–5 (1969)
Wilson, C.M., Ward, P.E., Erdös, E.G., Gecse, A.: Studies on membrane bound renin in the mouse and rat. Circ. Res. *38*, ii95–ii98 (1976)
Wong, P.Y., Talamo, R.C., Williams, G.H., Coleman, R.W.: Response of the kallikrein-kinin and renin-angiotensin systems to saline infusion and upright posture. J. Clin. Invest. *55*, 691–698 (1975)
Zinner, S.H., Margolius, H.S., Rosner, B., Keiser, H.R., Kass, E.H.: Familial aggregation of urinary kallikrein concentration in childhood. Am. J. Epidemiol. *104*, 124–132 (1976)
Zinner, S.H., Margolius, H.S., Rosner, B., Kass, E.H.: Eight year longitudinal study of blood pressure and urinary kallikrein in childhood. Clin. Res. *25*, 266 A (1977)
Zusman, R.M., Keiser, H.R.: Prostaglandin biosynthesis by rabbit renomedullary interstitial cells in tissue culture: stimulation by vasoactive peptides. J. Clin. Invest. *60*, 215–223 (1977 a)
Zusman, R.M., Keiser, H.R.: Prostaglandin E_2 biosynthesis by rabbit renomedullary interstitial cells in tissue culture. Mechanism of stimulation by angiotensin II, bradykinin, and arginine vasopressin. J. Biol. Chem. *252*, 2069–2071 (1977 b)
Zusman, R.M., Keiser, H.R., Handler, J.F.: Vasopressin-stimulated water permeability in the toad urinary bladder: role of endogenous prostaglandin E biosynthesis. Fed. Proc. *36*, 631 (Abstract) (1977)

Renal Kallikrein and Regulation of Blood Pressure in Man

I. H. MILLS

A. Introduction

The presence of a vasodilator in human urine was first described by ABELOUS and BARDIER in 1909. Subsequently, the presence of kallikrein was described by FREY and KRAUT (1928) in human urine and it was assumed to be the vasodilator of ABELOUS and BARDIER.

A variety of methods have been employed to quantitate human urinary kallikrein and though they give comparable qualitative results, precise quantitative comparisons are sometimes difficult. Early studies utilised direct bioassay for quantitation (FREY et al., 1950; ELLIOT and NUZUM, 1934). More recently, urinary kallikrein has been assayed by its release of kinin which has been quantitated in a variety of ways, e.g., by radioimmunoassay of the kinin released (ADETUYIBI, 1972; MACFARLANE et al., 1973; TALAMO et al., 1969), by bioassay on isolated cat jejunum (CROXATTO et al., 1974) or guinea pig ileum (MARGOLIUS et al., 1974a), or by its vasodilatory action after arterial injection in the hind leg of a dog (MARIN-GREZ and CARRETERO, 1972). Plasma kininogen in various degrees of purity, at pH 8.5, has been used as substrate for kallikrein. Most commonly, kallikrein activity is reported in bradykinin equivalents released per minute of incubation.

The measurement of kallikrein by its esterase activity is now extensively used. The substrate benzoyl-L-arginine-ethyl ester (BAEe) has been used by some (LECHI et al., 1976) but more frequently the substrate has been αN-tosyl-L-arginine-methyl ester (TAMe). The radiochemical esterolytic method of BEAVEN et al. (1971) has been used by a number of workers. Quantitation is by the rate of release of [^{3}H]-methanol which has to be separated from unreacted TAMe. This separation can be achieved by use of a Biorex 70 column as in the original description of the technique or by partition of methanol and the unreacted TAMe between the toluene scintillator and the aqueous phase of the incubation medium (MARGOLIUS et al., 1974a). Assay conditions are varied: pH 8.0 at 30 °C for 30 min (MARGOLIUS et al., 1974a) or pH 8.5 at 37 °C for 60 min (MILLS and WARD, 1975). The esterase unit used has also varied: MARGOLIUS et al. (1974a) defined one esterase unit as the amount of kallikrein hydrolysing one μmol TAMe/min whereas MILLS and WARD defined it as the amount of kallikrein hydrolysing 4.8 μmol TAMe/h. The former definition has been used throughout this volume.

Nonradioactive techniques have also been used to assess the esterolytic activity of kallikrein on TAMe. ADETUYIBI and MILLS (1972) employed a modification of the technique described by ROBERTS (1958). In this technique, the TAMe not hydrolysed by kallikrein is measured and thus the method is relatively inaccurate with low

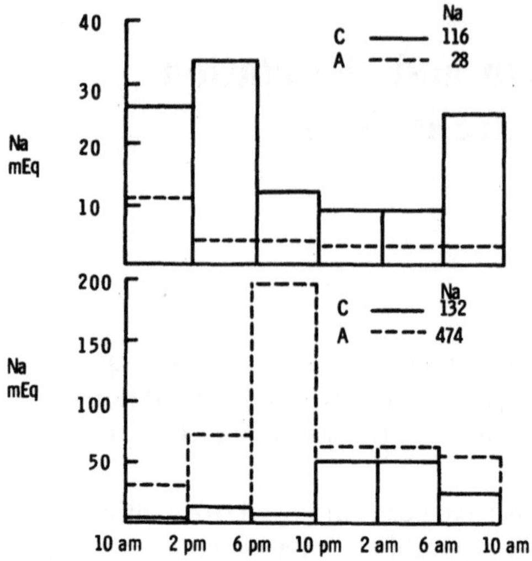

Fig. 1. Sodium excretion in man (mEq./4 h period) before (upper figure) and after (lower figure) administration of 5 mg 9α-fluorohydrocortisone/day for 10 days. Solid lines: Excretion during control infusion of 2.5% dextrose. Dotted lines = Excretion during infusion of angiotensin (2 mg over 24 h in 2.5% dextrose). C— = Total sodium excretion in 24 h of control infusion (mEq.). A--- = Total sodium excretion in 24 h of angiotensin infusion. (From MILLS, 1963)

kallikrein concentrations. MORIYA (1964) described a modification of the technique which involves reaction of the incubated mixture with hydroxylamine and the production of a coloured ferric complex which is measured by colorimetry at 525 nm. MORIYA (1964) defined one esterase unit as being the amount of human kallikrein corresponding to one FREY unit. One of their units hydrolysed 2.6 μmol TAMe/h at 37 ° and the same units were used by SEINO et al. (1975).

MATSUDA et al. (1976) estimated the methanol released from TAMe by a fluorescence technique after converting the alcohol to aldehyde with potassium permanganate. Acetyl acetone was added in ammonium malate and the fluorescence developed at 56 °C. The method is said to be able to detect the hydrolysis of 1 nmol TAMe/min/ml.

B. Acute Hypertension in Man

No direct studies of the effect on kallikrein excretion of producing acute hypertension in man have been reported. However, conclusions may be drawn by considering together two series of experimental studies. In normotensive individuals, infusion of angiotensin at a rate of 1–3 μg/min caused a rise in blood pressure of 15–20 mm Hg, a fall in inulin clearance, and a decrease in sodium excretion (PEART, 1960; MILLS and BARKHAM, 1962). When fludrocortisone was given in a dosage of 5 mg/day to subjects on a normal salt intake until the individuals had escaped from the sodium-retaining effect of the steroids, there was no change in blood pressure. When angiotensin was again infused at the same rate, there was a similar rise in blood pressure but no fall in inulin clearance and a marked natriuresis (Fig. 1) (MILLS, 1963). It is now known that the mechanism of escape from the sodium-retaining effect of fludrocortisone is associated with a marked rise in the excretion of kallikrein (ADETUYIBI and MILLS, 1972; EDWARDS et al., 1973) and patients with primary hyperaldosteronism have high kallikrein excretion (MARGOLIUS et al., 1971). It appears, therefore, that when acute hypertension is produced in man by the infusion of relatively low doses of angiotensin, the response depends upon the kallikrein status of the individual at the outset. On a normal sodium diet, where the kallikrein excretion is relatively low, the response is one of sodium retention. From analogy with the experiments on dogs (MILLS et al., 1976), angiotensin should decrease kallikrein excretion in normotensive subjects. When the same normotensive individuals were in the phase of escape from the sodium-retaining effect of steroids, the kallikrein excretion would be expected to be high (as shown in other patients by EDWARDS et al., 1973). During escape from the sodium-retaining effect of steroids, infusion of the same dose of angiotensin produced a natriuresis in spite of stimulation of aldosterone excretion. From the studies of MILLS et al. (1976) in dogs it would appear that the renal vascular resistance is inversely related to the kallikrein excretion. The same conclusion can be drawn in man from the studies of NEKRASOVA et al. (1970a) and the recent studies of LEVY et al. (1977). It appears, therefore, that high kallikrein production prevents renal artery constriction under the influence of angiotensin and the high blood pressure then effects natriuresis.

In dogs, the infusion of low doses of angiotensin into the renal artery caused a fall in both sodium and kallikrein excretion, though both tended to return towards control values with continued infusion. When acute hypertension was caused by infusion into the renal artery or general circulation of 5–10 μg angiotensin/min, the initial phase of reduced excretion of sodium and kallikrein was short-lived (10 min or less) and was followed by natriuresis associated with a sharp rise in kallikrein excretion (MILLS et al., 1976).

C. Relationship of Kallikrein Excretion to Extracellular Fluid Volume

I. Changes in Sodium Status

1. Changes in Oral Intake

When normal individuals are allowed to choose their own diet and no restriction is placed on the sodium content or the volume of fluid drunk, there is sometimes a relationship between kallikrein excretion and sodium excretion (ADETUYIBI and MILLS, 1972). However, this relationship could not be shown in the normal female control subjects studied by ELEBUTE and MILLS (1976). SEINO et al. (1975) failed to find a correlation between sodium and kallikrein excretion in normal subjects but their results suggest that the relationship might have been significant if the numbers had been greater. MARGOLIUS et al. (1974b) studied 48 normal adults on an uncontrolled sodium diet and found no relationship between sodium and kallikrein excretion.

MILLS and WARD (1975) have suggested in their studies on rabbits that a change in fluid intake with change in sodium intake may be necessary to alter a critical fluid volume in order to change kallikrein excretion. They found a positive correlation between sodium and kallikrein excretion in rabbits, except when the fluid intake was fixed. Intragastric administration of normal (0.9%) saline in dogs was found by MARIN-GREZ et al. (1972) to increase kallikrein excretion. The gut may play some part in influencing sodium excretion after oral ingestion because LENNANE et al. (1975) found that sodium excretion in man was faster after oral loading than after intravenous loading.

2. Changes in Parenteral Intake

MARGOLIUS et al. (1974a) failed to demonstrate an increase in kallikrein excretion in man with intravenous sodium loading at 15 ml 0.9% saline/min. However, their subjects had previously been given approximately 400 ml of water by mouth and 3 ml 5% dextrose/min intravenously until urine flow stabilised after 50 min of infusion. Since they compared the kallikrein excretion during saline infusion with that during water and dextrose loading, any stimulating effect of these on kallikrein excretion might mask an effect of saline infusion in nonhydrated individuals.

WONG et al. (1975) measured the plasma bradykinin by radioimmunoassay and assessed the effect of saline infusion and of a change to upright posture. They found that infusion of 5% glucose at 500 ml/h for 2 h to normal individuals on a 10 mEq. sodium diet had no effect on plasma renin activity, plasma angiotensin II, or plasma bradykinin.

On the other hand, intravenous infusion of 0.9% saline at 500 ml/h to normal individuals on a low salt diet caused approximately a 50% fall in plasma renin activity and plasma angiotensin II and a 60% fall in plasma bradykinin levels in the first hour (Fig. 2). There was no change in plasma prekallikrein levels nor in kallikrein inhibitor levels. In those subjects in which kininase was measured, it also was unchanged.

It seems unlikely, therefore, that the sodium repletion affected plasma bradykinin by a change in plasma kallikrein or its inhibitors or by a change in the activity of plasma kininase. They conclude that a change in glandular kallikrein might account for the changes in plasma bradykinin but note the contrasting veiws of MARGOLIUS et al. (1974a) and ADETUYIBI and MILLS (1972) on the effect of changes in sodium intake on kallikrein excretion in man. It seems unlikely that kinin, released by renal kallikrein and subsequently converted from lysyl-bradykinin (kallidin) to bradykinin by aminopeptidase, would exist long enough to be measured in the general circulation. The release of renal kallikrein into renal venous effluent has been reported by ROBLERO et al. (1976a) in perfused rat kidneys and in perfused rat kidneys treated with furosemide (ROBLERO et al., 1976b). Kallikrein is also released into the renal lymph of dogs during saline infusion (DE BONO and MILLS, 1974) and reaches the circulation in this way. It seems probable that the changes in plasma bradykinin in the studies of WONG et al. (1975) represent changes in the relase of kallikrein into the circulation.

WONG et al. (1975) show clearly in their studies that the changes in plasma bradykinin closely follow those of plasma renin activity and plasma angiotensin II. They do not discuss the relation between these. It was shown by MACFARLANE et al. (1974) that infusion of angiotensin into dog renal artery caused release of kallikrein into the urine. Also, renal artery constriction, which is well known to cause release of

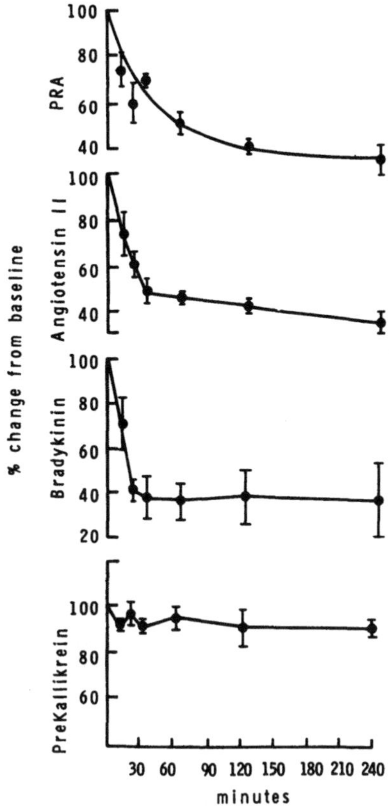

Fig. 2. Response of the kallikrein-bradykinin and renin-angiotensin systems to saline infusion, expressed as percentage of baseline value in normal subjects on a 10 mEq. Na/100 mEq. K diet; normal saline infused at 500 ml/h for 4 h. (From WONG et al., 1975)

renin, caused progressive decrease in renal vascular resistance which was highly correlated with the concentration of kallikrein in the urine (MILLS et al., 1976) though the excretion of kallikrein/min decreased. In the recent studies by LEVY et al. (1977), they demonstrated that renal blood flow is positively correlated with the logarithm of kallikrein excretion and inversely related to plasma renin activity. Their data also show a high correlation between urinary kallikrein excretion and plasma renin activity in the upright posture in individuals on normal or low salt intake, except in black men with hypertension. The fall in plasma bradykinin produced by saline infusion into individuals whose plasma renin is high, as shown by WONG et al. (1975), may, therefore, be due to reduction in plasma renin and reduction of angiotensin-induced kallikrein release.

The effect of change to the upright posture on plasma bradykinin was studied by WONG et al. (1975) in normal individuals on a high salt (200 mEq./day) diet. The upright posture caused a sharp rise in plasma renin activity, plasma angiotensin II, and plasma bradykinin. Here also it seems possible that the angiotensin II generated by release of renin was responsible for the release of renal kallikrein and the generation of bradykinin in the plasma.

3. Escape From the Sodium-Retaining Effects of Steroids

Administration of sodium-retaining steroids to individuals on a normal salt intake leads to escape from continued sodium retention (AUGUST et al., 1958) except under pathological conditions (MILLS, 1962). During development of the escape phenomenon, the excretion of kallikrein rises sharply from the third day onwards (ADETUYIBI and MILLS, 1972; EDWARDS et al., 1973; MARGOLIUS et al., 1974a). Sodium depletion causes a rise in aldosterone production and an increase in kallikrein excretion (MARGOLIUS et al., 1974a). It has been suggested by the latter workers that the factor in common between the escape phenomenon and sodium depletion is a high circulating level of sodium-retaining steroids and that these might stimulate kidney kallikrein release by a direct action. In support of this view is the stimulation in vitro by high concentrations of aldosterone on kallikrein release by kidney cortical cells in suspension (MARGOLIUS et al., 1976). It is difficult to assess this study because the aldosterone concentration used (6.1×10^{-5}–3.1×10^{-4} *M*) was several orders of magnitude above the normal plasma concentration. Similarly, inhibition of kallikrein release by spironolactone was shown but only at highly pharmacological concentrations of spironolactone (4.3×10^{-5}–2.2×10^{-4} *M*).

An alternative explanation of the high kallikrein excretion in the escape phase has been put forward by MILLS et al. (1976). They point out that the increase in kallikrein excretion does not usually occur until the third day of fludrocortisone administration and that appreciable sodium retention has occurred by then. Expansion of the extracellular fluid volume has, therefore, taken place. In studies on six patients EDWARDS et al. (1973) found that during the escape phase (i.e., after the initial sodium retention), kallikrein and sodium excretion were very highly correlated ($P<0.001$). This supported the view that kallikrein excretion rises in relation to the sodium status and facilitates sodium excretion as it does in a wide range of physiological manipulations in animals (MILLS et al., 1976).

It has been pointed out by MILLS et al. (1976) that the hypothesis of MARGOLIUS et al. (1974a) could be tested by administering the sodium-retaining steroids while animals or human subjects were on a low sodium diet. MILLS and his colleagues (1976) quote unpublished data in the rabbit showing no increase in kallikrein excretion when rabbits on a low salt diet were given 2 mg deoxycorticosterone acetate daily intramuscularly.

II. Acute Sodium Deficiency

Acute depletion of sodium can be produced by administration of diuretics while the individuals are on a low salt diet. This has been done by MARGOLIUS et al. (1974a, b). The subjects were on a 9 mEq. sodium diet and given furosemide, 40 mg/day for the first 3 days. The plasma renin activity rose sharply from 3.5 ± 0.9–17.8 ± 2.7 ng angiotensin I/ml/h ($P<0.001$) and kallikrein excretion rose from 12.2 ± 1.1–33.0 ± 2.5 esterase units/day ($P<0.001$). The aldosterone excretion was initially 11.6 ± 1.0 µg/day and rose to 64.6 ± 9.0 µg/day ($P<0.001$) (Table 1).

In two subjects, the administration of spironolactone (400 mg/day) while they were on a low sodium diet caused a sharp fall in kallikrein excretion and a further negative sodium balance of approximately 200 mEq. over 9 days. The authors con-

Table 1. Urinary sodium excretion, plasma renin activity, aldosterone excretion rate, and kallikrein excretion in normal subjects (From MARGOLIUS et al., 1974a).

	Diet		
	Control Na	9 mEq.	259 mEq.
		Na/day	
$U_{Na}V$ (mEq./day)	131 ±13	5 ±2[a]	229 ±10
PRA (ng/ml h^{-1})	3.5± 0.9	17.8±2.7[a]	3.2± 0.7
Aldo (μg/day)	11.6± 1.0	64.6±9.0[a]	6.0± 0.8
Kallikrein (E.U./day)	12.2± 1.1	33.0±2.5[a]	11.2± 0.8

All values are means±S.E. for 13 normal subjects. $U_{Na}V$=urinary sodium excretion, PRA=plasma renin activity. Aldo=aldosterone excretion rate, and kallikrein (E.U./day) =esterase units in a 24 h collection of urine.

[a] Differ from values on control diet (ad libitum sodium or 109 mEq. Na/day) or diet containing 259 mEq. Na/day, $P<0.001$. (From MARGOLIUS et al., 1974a).

cluded that the rise in aldosterone secretion caused the rise in kallikrein secretion and that blocking the action of the steroid caused the fall during spironolactone administration. However, the marked rise in plasma renin activity would be expected to increase angiotensin II stimulation of kallikrein release (MACFARLANE et al., 1974) and this must be at least part of the mechanism causing increased kallikrein excretion. In addition, the diuretic might increase kallikrein excretion by some other mechanism. The very considerable negative sodium balance produced by spironolactone would also be expected to cause further physiological effects. The plasma renin activity rose in one subject from 17–55 and in the other from 37–105 ng angiotensin I/ml/h. No information is given concerning the renal plasma flow and glomerular filtration rate during this natriuresis but it would be surprising if they did not fall. NEKRASOVA et al. (1970a) measured renal blood flow with ^{131}I-labeled hippuran and found it correlated with kallikrein excretion.

Other factors have been shown to decrease kallikrein excretion and may have played a part here. Noradrenaline release increases with decrease in blood volume and, it has been shown, causes constriction of renal vessels when they are resistant to the action of angiotensin (MILLS and WILSON, 1971). The stimulation of kallikrein release by angiotensin depends upon the release of prostaglandin (MILLS et al., 1978). The release of kallikrein by prostaglandin is inhibited by noradrenaline (MILLS and OBIKA, 1977). There are, therefore, alternative possible explanations for the decreased kallikrein excretion during spironolactone administration to subjects on a low salt diet: which of the various possible factors is involved can only be determined by future work.

Further evidence relating to the factors influencing kallikrein excretion in the low sodium state comes from the work of LEVY et al. (1977). Their data show an increase in kallikrein excretion on adaptation to a low sodium diet in both black and white normotensive individuals and in white hypertensives but not in black hypertensives. The plasma renin activity rose with the low salt diet in all groups, including the black hypertensives, both when they were supine and when they were standing (Table 2).

Table 2. 24 h urinary sodium ($U_{Na}V$) and kallikrein and plasma renin activity (PRA) on unrestricted sodium (Un Na) and low sodium diets (Lo Na). (From LEVY et al., 1977)

Group	Diet	$U_{Na}V$	Kallikrein	PRA	
				Supine	Standing
Normotensives					
White	Un Na	149±11	18.7± 3.1	1.6±0.3	6.2±0.9
	Lo Na	18± 5	38.8±12.0	3.7±0.6	10.2±0.9
Black	Un Na	178±20	3.8± 0.9	0.8±0.3	4.3±1.0
	Lo Na	13± 3	20.9± 5.7	1.9±0.7	7.1±1.3
Hypertensives					
White	Un Na	177±20	9.2± 2.3	2.8±1.1	4.6±2.0
	Lo Na	19± 2	30.3± 6.8	8.2±1.4	13.4±3.1
Black	Un Na	165±16	3.0± 1.1	0.7±0.2	1.0±0.4
	Lo Na	19± 3	4.9± 1.9	6.9±2.1	10.7±3.8

Taking together the evidence presented by MACFARLANE et al. (1974), MARGOLIUS et al. (1974a), LEVY et al. (1977), and SEINO et al. (1975), it seems clear that the increased kallikrein excretion on a low salt diet is due to the effect of the renin/angiotensin system in stimulating kallikrein release. In black hypertensives, the elevated plasma renin activity on a low salt diet fails to stimulate kallikrein excretion and this was shown by LEVY et al. (1977) to be associated with a lower renal blood flow than in the white hypertensives and lower than in the same blacks on unrestricted sodium. Since NEKRASOVA et al. (1970a) have shown that lowered renal blood flow is associated with decreased kallikrein excretion, this lowered renal blood flow of the black hypertensives on a low salt diet might explain, at least in part, the failure of their kallikrein excretion to increase during low salt diet.

The positive correlation between increased sodium intake and kallikrein excretion reported in man by ADETUYIBI and MILLS (1972) and in dogs by MARIN-GREZ et al. (1972) seems to be unrelated to the small changes in plasma renin activity associated with sodium loading. The mechanisms at this end of the sodium status scale are presumably related to those which operate with acute sodium loading in animals, as discussed by MILLS et al. (1977).

III. Role of Water Intake

In a number of studies, the excretion of kallikrein in man has been related to urinary volume (ADETUYIBI, 1972; EDWARDS et al., 1973). In studies in animals this relationship has frequently been found and has been discussed at length by MILLS and WARD (1975) and MILLS et al. (1976). Although the kallikrein excretion/min is a function of urine flow rate, the relationship between kallikrein excretion and urine flow rate is often not a direct one, e.g., in the studies of sodium loading by MARIN-GREZ et al. (1972) the increase in kallikrein excretion was more than could be explained by volume changes alone. More impressive is the evidence that there is a negative correlation between kallikrein excretion and urinary osmolality in man

(ELEBUTE and MILLS, 1976; EDWARDS et al., 1973), in rats (WARD, 1974), in rabbits (MILLS and WARD, 1975), and in many studies in dogs (quoted in MILLS et al., 1976).

However, the effect of an increase in water intake on kallikrein excretion is not so clear cut. Since the original report by ADETUYIBI and MILLS (1972) of an increase in kallikrein excretion in normal individuals given an extra liter of water to drink between 08.00 and 08.30 h, no other workers have been able to confirm this in man. MARGOLIUS et al. (1974a) had their subjects on controlled water intake and then added an additional 1–2 liters and found no related increase in kallikrein excretion. However, oral water loading in rats has been found to produce a marked increase in kallikrein excretion (CROXATTO et al., 1976). Oral water loading of anaesthetised dogs by MARIN-GREZ et al. (1972) did not increase kallikrein excretion.

The renal kallikrein/kinin system is related to water excretion and urinary osmolality (see MILLS et al., 1976). Renal kallikrein is released into the distal tubule (SCICLI et al., 1976) and also into the interstitial fluid since it appears in renal lymph at the same rate as it appears in urine during rapid saline infusion (DE BONO and MILLS, 1974). Kininase II is most rich in the brush border of the proximal tubule (WARD et al., 1977). This clearly inactivates the kinins filtered at the glomerulus or passing into the tubular lumen. The kallikrein in the interstitial fluid presumably releases kinin there since the substrate for kallikrein is similar to that of renin and the latter substrate has been demonstrated in renal lymph. How and where the kinins released in the interstitial fluid are inactivated is not yet clear. Such inactivation is of importance if the kinins are to be prevented from releasing prostaglandin E_2 from the renal medulla and so antagonising the action of antidiuretic hormone. Such antagonism of vasopressin has been shown to facilitate water excretion (ORLOFF et al., 1965). Infusion of bradykinin into the renal artery of the dog caused dilution of urine even while vasopressin was infused intravenously (BARRACLOUGH and MILLS, 1965). It would not be surprising, therefore, if water loading increased kallikrein release. In animal studies, stimulation of kallikrein release frequently causes dilution of the urine.

IV. Kallikrein Excretion and Race

A well-marked difference in the excretion of kallikrein has been reported in normotensive black and white individuals in the San Diego area of California (LEVY et al., 1977). This difference was present both when they were on unrestricted sodium intake and when on a low salt diet (see Table 2). A similar difference in kallikrein excretion was shown in hypertensive blacks and whites but in the hypertensives the effect of a low salt diet exaggerated the differences because the black hypertensives had such a small response to the low salt diet (perhaps because of a fall in their renal blood flow).

A study of ZINNER et al. (1976) was carried out on casual urine specimens from 601 children between 5 and 18 years of age and their mothers in 163 families. Since only a casual specimen was obtained, the kallikrein excretion as concentration per ml was all that could be calculated and related to the concentration of other constituents in the urine. When the logarithm of the kallikrein concentration was plotted against frequency among the children an approximation to a normal distribution was found.

The variance within families was significantly less than between families ($P<0.001$) indicating clustering of kallikrein concentration within families. This held for white and black children separately. When adjusted for urinary creatinine concentration, there was still a significant clustering of kallikrein concentrations within families.

The following variables were found to be related to urinary kallikrein concentration with a significance of $P<0.001$: log potassium concentration, log creatinine concentration, mother's kallikrein concentration, and mother's blood pressure.

Racial differences in kallikrein concentration were highly significant with lower values being found among the black children ($r=+0.720$: $P<0.001$).

The mean blood pressures of low kallikrein families were significantly higher than those of high kallikrein families. Of 16 low kallikrein families, 15 were black but of 16 high kallikrein families only five were black ($\chi^2=108$, $P<0.005$).

There was no correlation between kallikrein concentration and sodium concentration on single regression analysis but on multiple regression analysis there was a significant inverse relationship.

Among the 601 children there was no difference in the blood pressure of black and white children.

If these data on kallikrein concentration are reproduced in daily excretion rates, it is possible that the kallikrein/kinin system in the kidney may play some part in determining the onset of hypertension.

V. Bartter's Syndrome

In 1962, BARTTER and his colleagues described a clinical condition characterized by juxtaglomerular hyperplasia, high plasma renin, hyperaldosteronism (resembling the primary type), and normal blood pressure. The response to intravenous infusion of angiotensin II or norepinephrine was subnormal and the fraction of filtered sodium delivered to distal sites was high so that a large excretion of potassium occurred.

LECHI et al. (1976) measured kallikrein excretion in a patient with Bartter's syndrome and found it to be extremely high. They measured the esterase activity using BAEe as substrate and quoted the values in BAEe units (1 unit = amount of kallikrein hydrolyzing 1 μmol BAEe/min). In 40 normal individuals on 155 mEq. sodium diet the kallikrein excretion was 148 ± 10.1 BAEe units/day. In patients with primary hyperaldosteronism the values were 372.6 ± 93.5 BAEe units/day and in the patient with Bartter's syndrome the values were between 1160 and 2155 BAEe units/day while he was on a diet of 155 mEq. sodium.

The plasma renin activity was 15 ng angiotensin I/ml/h and during therapy with propranolol (120 mg/day) and spironolactone (200 mg/day) the level fell to 3.3 (recumbent) and 4.5 ng angiotensin I/ml/h, after ambulation. The kallikrein excretion fell to 514 BAEe units/day. On spironolactone alone (200 mg/day) the kallikrein excretion was 405 BAEe units/day but the plasma renin activity was then 25 ng angiotensin I/ml/h.

LECHI et al. subscribe to the views put forward by MARGOLIUS et al. (1974a) that the high aldosterone is the cause of the high kallikrein excretion and at first sight the data support this view. However, the very high plasma renin level while the patient was on spironolactone alone suggests that the aldosterone antagonist had caused even greater sodium deficiency which had led to the further stimulation of renin release. As pointed out in Sect. C.II, severe sodium depletion may reduce kallikrein excretion by reduction of renal blood flow, as suggested by the data of NEKRASOVA et al. (1970a) (cf. the failure of black hypertensives to raise their kallikrein excretion on a low salt diet when their renal blood flow fell). Also, the increased noradrenaline release with volume depletion would cause the renal vessels to constrict even when they were resistant to the vasoconstricting action of the renin/angiotensin system (MILLS and WILSON, 1971). This would reduce the direct pressure stimulation of kallikrein release because the pressure-sensitive site appears to be distal to the afferent arteriole (BEVAN et al., 1974; MILLS et al., 1976). In addition, noradrenaline inhibits the release of kallikrein which is stimulated by prostaglandin E (MILLS et al., 1977). Prostaglandin is an intermediate in the stimulation of kallikrein excretion by angiotensin (MILLS and OBIKA, 1977). There are, therefore, three mechanisms by which kallikrein excretion could be reduced in Bartter's syndrome by spironolactone, in addition to inhibition of the suggested direct action of aldosterone in stimulating kallikrein excretion. The successful treatment of Bartter's syndrome with indomethacin (GILL et al., 1976) supports the view that a prostaglandin-mediated mechanism is involved in the high kallikrein excretion. In the untreated state, the immunoreactive prostaglandin E excretion in urine was extremely high and so also was the plasma renin activity when the patients were ambulant. Treatment with indomethacin (or, in one case, ibuprofen) to inhibit prostaglandin synthesis led to considerable correction of the abnormalities. Plasma renin activity fell, urinary aldosterone excretion decreased, plasma potassium rose, positive sodium and potassium balance occurred, urinary prostaglandin E excretion fell, and there was appreciable weight gain. Reversal of these occurred with cessation of treatment.

The mechanism by which renin secretion is stimulated by prostaglandin is not clear though recent work of Schnerman (as yet unpublished) suggests that stimulation of the macula densa by chloride ions depends upon prostaglandin for the release of renin. Blocking the synthesis of prostaglandin has been shown to impair the release of renin. In man, lowering of plasma renin activity by depression of prostaglandin synthesis was shown by DONKER et al. (1976) and by RUMPF et al. (1975). The latter workers showed a smaller increase in plasma renin on adopting the upright posture and in response to furosemide. PATAK et al. (1975) showed a smaller rise in plasma renin during furosemide treatment in both normal and hypertensive patients. In animals, indomethacin inhibition of prostaglandin synthesis also decreased kallikrein excretion (OLSEN and AHNFELT-RONNE, 1976; MCGIFF et al., 1976) and prevented the normal renal vascular adaptation to haemorrhage (DATA et al., 1976).

The decrease in plasma renin activity is, therefore, easily explained by inhibition of renal prostaglandin synthesis. The fall in aldosterone excretion would be expected from the lowered release of angiotensin II. This in turn would correct the hypokalaemic alkalosis. Whether these mechanisms alone explain the suppression of the kallikrein excretion is uncertain but it is probable that direct suppression of kallikrein excretion by inhibition of prostaglandin synthesis would also take place because stimulation of kallikrein release by angiotensin appears to be mediated by prostaglandin (MILLS et al., 1978).

D. Renal Kallikrein and Chronic Hypertension

I. Essential Hypertension

The first demonstration of lowered kallikrein excretion in the urine of hypertensive patients was by ELLIOT and NUZUM (1934). Using a bioassay they showed that hypertensive patients excreted approximately 50% of the amount of kallikrein of normotensive individuals. This work was not followed up until 1971 when MARGOLIUS et al. reported that patients with essential hypertension had lower mean kallikrein excretion than normotensive individuals and that patients with an aldosterone-secreting tumour had higher kallikrein excretion than normal.

In 1974, MARGOLIUS et al. (1974b) described measurements of kallikrein excretion in 13 normotensive individuals on either 109 mEq. sodium/day or ad libitum sodium intake and found it to be 12.2±1.1 (mean±S.E.) esterase units/day whereas in nine patients with essential hypertension it was 5.0±0.8 esterase units/day: the difference was highly significant ($P<0.001$). Three patients with primary hyperaldosteronism had urinary kallikrein values of 19.7±6.8 esterase units/day: difference from essential hypertensives, $P<0.05$.

When each group was sodium-depleted by a low salt diet and furosemide (40 mg) daily for 3 days, the kallikrein excretion in normotensives rose to 33.0±2.5 esterase units/day: the rise was highly significant, $P<0.001$. The essential hypertensives also excreted more kallikrein, which rose to 9.4±1.8 esterase units/day ($P<0.001$). This value was still significantly less than that of the normotensives when sodium depleted. The three patients with primary hyperaldosteronism had no significant change in kallikrein excretion.

On an intake of 259 mEq. sodium/day all three groups had kallikrein values similar to their control values. The normotensives did not show any relationship between sodium and kallikrein excretion and neither did the hypertensive group.

This latter observation is contrary to the finding of ADETUYIBI and MILLS (1972): they reported that changing patients with essential hypertension from a normal salt intake to a 10 mEq. sodium diet led to a progressive fall in kallikrein excretion which was correlated with the sodium excretion ($r=0.673$, $P<0.001$). The difference between the studies of MARGOLIUS et al. (1974a, b) and those of ADETUYIBI and MILLS (1972) may be due to the speed and degree of sodium loss. In a later publication MARGOLIUS et al. (1974c) reported that the rise in plasma renin activity in their patients with essential hypertension was significantly less after sodium depletion than in the normotensive group (12.2 ng angiotensin I/ml/h against 18.3±5.9 ng angiotensin I/ml/h; $P<0.005$). PADFIELD et al. (1975) when giving intravenous furosemide found the rise in plasma renin activity 2 h later to be negligible in patients with essential hypertension, whether with low or normal plasma renin activity to start with.

As discussed in Sect. C.II, it is probable that the rise in kallikrein with sodium depletion is due to the stimulating effect of angiotensin on kallikrein release. This has been demonstrated directly by MACFARLANE et al. (1974) in dogs and is strongly supported by the work of LEVY et al. (1977) in man. The transfer of hypertensive patients to a low salt diet without diuretics would be expected to cause less rise in plasma renin activity than when diuretics were given for 3 days on the low salt diet.

Administration of 0.5 mg fludrocortisone daily for 10 days in three patients with essential hypertension studied by MARGOLIUS et al. (1974c) caused a rise in kallikrein excretion from a mean (±S.E.) of 7.1±1.9–17.8±5.5 esterase units/day.

MARGOLIUS et al. (1974c) conclude that they cannot explain the low kallikrein excretion in the patients with essential hypertension but LEVY et al. (1977) show quite clearly that the renal blood flow in their hypertensives was lower than in their normotensive group, both on unrestricted sodium and on low sodium intake. NEKRASOVA et al. (1970a) have shown that reduced renal blood flow is associated with lower urinary kallikrein.

SEINO et al. (1975) found the kallikrein excretion in normotensive patients on a diet of 150 mEq. sodium/day to be (mean±S.E.) 111.3±11.1 esterase units/day (their units are smaller than those of MARGOLIUS et al., 1974a). Patients with essential hypertension had kallikrein excretion values of 75.2±10.0 esterase units/day, which were significantly lower than their normotensive groups; $P<0.02$. The range for the normals was 51–223 and for the hypertensives 10–204 esterase units/day so the overlap between the two groups is large. Similar wide overlap has been found by all other workers.

SEINO et al. studied the effect of reducing the sodium intake from 150–30 mEq./day for 3 days and found a mean (±S.E.) increase in kallikrein excretion from 54.8±7.1 to 80.0±13.0 esterase units/day. Plasma renin rose from 11.3±3.4–21.7±6.3 ng angiotensin I/ml/h. The renin values here were appreciably higher than those of MARGOLIUS et al. (1974b) and are somewhat surprising for only 3 days on a 30 mEq. sodium diet.

SEINO et al. (1975) plotted plasma renin activity against urinary kallikrein excretion and concluded that there was no relationship. Their results, however, show a biphasic relationship. As plasma renin rose from unmeasurable levels up to 10 ng angiotensin I/ml/h, the kallikrein excretion steadily fell. As plasma renin levels rose from 10 ng angiotensin I/ml/h–50 ng angiotensin I/ml/h, kallikrein excretion rose again. These observations are compatible with the conclusions drawn in Sect. C.II.

Lowered kallikrein excretion values in essential hypertension have also been reported by GRECO et al. (1977). For normotensive individuals kallikrein excretion was (mean±S.E.) 24.5±1.7 and in essential hypertension 7.1±1.5 esterase units/day.

Only 'Nekrasova et al. (1970a) report patients with hypertension having higher levels of urinary kallikrein than in their controls but it is not clear whether these patients have essential hypertension or renovascular hypertension. They conclude that the kallikrein excretion is highly correlated with renal blood flow, as measured with radioactive hippuran.

This last observation may be of some importance because although angiotensin stimulates kallikrein excretion in dogs (MACFARLANE et al., 1974), the addition of noradrenaline blocks the effect of prostaglandin on kallikrein release (MILLS et al., 1978). Kallikrein excretion in essential hypertension might, therefore, be the result of a tendency for these patients to have lower plasma renin activity and a greater-than-normal rise in plasma noradrenaline in the upright position (SEVER et al., 1977).

SEINO et al. (1977) found that administration of spironolactone to patients with low renin essential hypertension produced two different patterns of response. In one pattern, the kallikrein fell sharply, natriuresis occurred and plasma renin activity rose. In the other, the kallikrein excretion rose sharply, only slight natriuresis was observed and the rise in plasma renin activity was much smaller. In hypertensives with normal renin the kallikrein excretion did not change significantly.

II. Renovascular Hypertension

Most workers have found that kallikrein excretion in patients with renovascular hypertension is in the same range as in normotensive individuals (GRECO et al., 1977; KEISER et al., 1977; SEINO et al., 1975). KEISER et al. (1977) used bilateral ureteric catheterisation and sometimes found specimens on one side with no kallikrein in them. Since constriction of one renal artery experimentally decreases kallikrein excretion on that side only (BEVAN et al., 1974; KEISER et al., 1976), the mixed urine from both kidneys might well show no difference from normal values. SEINO et al. (1975) found a positive correlation between sodium excretion and kallikrein excretion when they combined their data from both renovascular and primary aldosteronism patients. In rabbits, NEKRASOVA et al. (1970b) found decreased kallikrein excretion from the kidney with clip hypertension and increased kallikrein from the contralateral kidney. They found decreased kallikrein excretion in patients with unilateral or bilateral renal artery stenosis.

1. Impaired Renal Function

Very few data are available concerning the effect of reduction of glomerular filtration rate on kallikrein excretion. ADETUYIBI and MILLS (1972) found that hypertensive patients with severe renal impairment and no oedema had very high kallikrein excretion. They plotted the kallikrein excretion/day against sodium excretion/ml of glomerular filtrate and found that the renal failure patients fell on the same line as the normal individuals. Sodium restriction in renal failure patients led to a very prompt fall in kallikrein excretion.

III. Primary Hyperaldosteronism

All the reports of kallikrein excretion in patients with primary hyperaldosteronism have shown that, on average, the excretion is greater than in normotensive individuals and greater than in essential hypertensive patients (MARGOLIUS et al., 1971; MARGOLIUS et al., 1974c; SEINO et al., 1975). Since treatment with sodium-retaining steroids causes elevation of kallikrein excretion without hypertension (ADETUYIBI and MILLS, 1972; EDWARDS et al., 1973; MARGOLIUS et al., 1974a), it is assumed that the hypertension is not the main factor in the increased kallikrein excretion. Administration of spironolactone to block the effect of aldosterone has been shown to lower kallikrein excretion (MARGOLIUS et al., 1974c; SEINO et al., 1977). Although MARGOLIUS et al. (1974a, c) assumed that the high aldosterone secretion stimulated kallikrein excretion directly, the evidence is not conclusive that this is so. MILLS et al. (1976) suggest that the volume expansion is the effective factor in raising the kallikrein excretion. The patients with primary hyperaldosteronism each had a natriuresis during spironolactone administration and this would have decreased their volume expansion.

IV. Phaeochromocytoma

The excretion of kallikrein by patients with a phaeochromocytoma is, in general, about the same as in normotensive individuals (SEINO et al., 1975). MARGOLIUS et al. (1971) point out that in one patient with this tumour the kallikrein excretion was above normal. The excretion probably depends on the interaction of two factors; one is the direct effect of pressure in increasing kallikrein excretion and the other is the inhibitory effect of noradrenaline on the release of kallikrein by prostaglandin.

E. Kallikrein Excretion in Normal and Hypertensive Pregnancy

There has been one publication on the excretion of kallikrein in the urine during normal and hypertensive human pregnancies (ELEBUTE and MILLS, 1976). They found that normal women (39 collections) in the age group 20–35 years (the same age range as the pregnant patients) excreted 23.9 ± 0.99 esterase units/day (as determined by the residual TAMe technique of ADETUYIBI and MILLS, 1972, but expressed in the esterase units of MILLS and WARD, 1975). They found that in 34 urine collections in early pregnancy (6–14 weeks) the kallikrein excretion was 48.6 ± 2.65 esterase units/day which was highly significantly different from the controls ($P < 0.001$). In mid-pregnancy (15–26 weeks) the kallikrein excretion was 39.7 ± 2.37 esterase units/day and this also was significantly different from the controls ($P < 0.01$). In the last trimester of pregnancy (28–40 weeks) kallikrein excretion had again fallen significantly ($P < 0.01$) to 29.2 ± 2.29 esterase units/day which was not significantly different from the nonpregnant controls (Fig. 3). There was, therefore, a highly significant negative correlation between the kallikrein excretion (esterase units/day) and the stage of pregnancy (in weeks): $r = -0.55$, $P < 0.001$.

In patients developing hypertension during pregnancy (with and without edema and proteinuria), 31 determinations of kallikrein were made from 17 patients. The mean value ($\pm$S.E.) was 12.9 ± 1.7 esterase units/day which was highly significantly different from normal pregnancy values at the same stage of pregnancy ($P < 0.001$) and different from normal nonpregnancy values ($P < 0.001$).

ELEBUTE and MILLS (1976) pointed out that the time of highest kallikrein excretion (first trimester) corresponds to the time when many pregnant women have nocturia. The disappearance of this symptom as pregnancy progresses corresponds with the fall in kallikrein excretion. The cause of the high kallikrein excretion in early pregnancy is not yet known but it was suggested by ELEBUTE and MILLS (1976) that it was unlikely to be due to escape from the sodium-retaining effect of aldosterone because this steroid rises during pregnancy. It might be related to the high plasma renin of early pregnancy (GORDON et al., 1975) but would not correspond to the continued high plasma renin of toxaemic pregnancies. They suggested that a circulating vasodilator would best explain the kallikrein data, the tendency to lower blood pressure in pregnancy, and the increased renal blood flow.

The low kallikrein excretion in hypertension of pregnancy corresponds to that seen in essential hypertension but the mechanism still remains obscure.

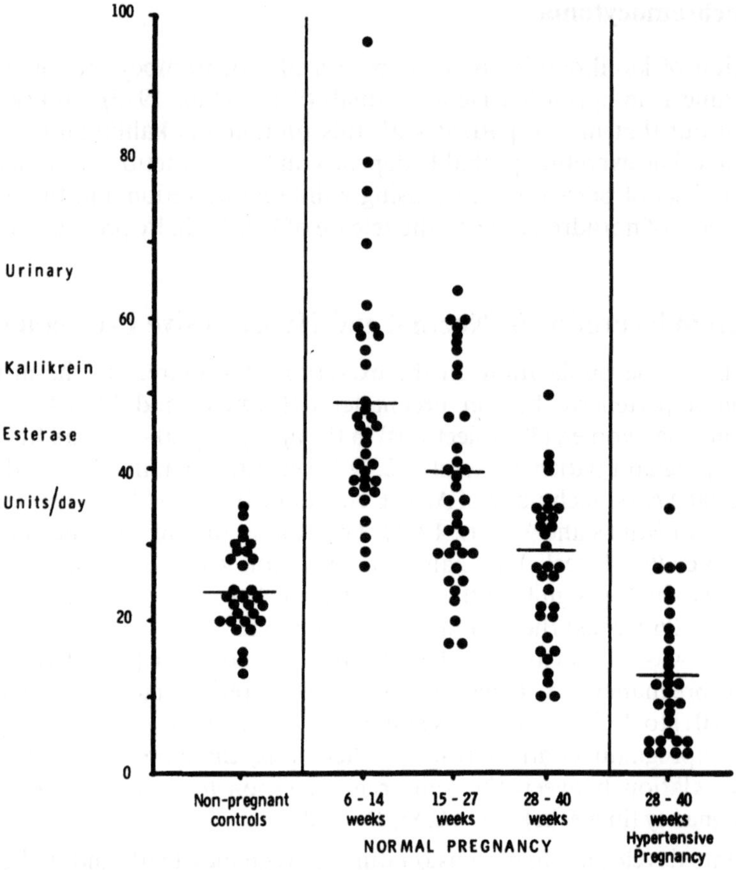

Fig. 3. Urinary kallikrein in control subjects, normal pregnancies for weeks 6–14, 15–27, and 28–40 and hypertensive pregnancies 34–40 weeks. The horizontal bar indicates the mean value in each group. Kallikrein activity is expressed in esterase units (1 unit is the amount of kallikrein hydrolysing 4.8 μmol TAMe/h at 37 °C). (From ELEBUTE and MILLS, 1976)

References

Abelous, J.E., Bardier, E.: Les substances hypotensives de l'urine humaine normale. Comptl. Rend. Soc. Biol. *66*, 511 (1909)

Adetuyibi, A.: Some studies on kallikrein in urine. Ph.D. Thesis. University of Cambridge 1972

Adetuyibi, A., Mills, I.H.: Relation between urinary kallikrein and renal function, hypertension, and excretion of sodium and water in man. Lancet *1972/II*, 203–207

August, J.T., Nelson, D.H., Thorn, G.W.: Response of normal subjects to large amounts of aldosterone. J. Clin. Invest. *38*, 1549–1555 (1958)

Barraclough, M.A., Mills, I.H.: Effect of bradykinin on renal function. Clin. Sci. *28*, 69–74 (1965)

Bartter, F.C., Pronove, P., Gill, J.R., MacCardle, J.C.: Hyperplasia of the juxtaglomerular complex with hyperaldosteronism and hypokalaemic alkalosis. Am. J. Med. *33*, 811–828 (1962)

Beaven, V.H., Pierce, J.V., Pisano, J.J.: A sensitive isotopic procedure for the assay of esterase activity: measurement of human urinary kallikrein. Clin. Chim. Acta *32*, 67–73 (1971)

Bevan, D.R., MacFarlane, N.A.A., Mills, I.H.: The dependence of urinary kallikrein excretion on renal artery pressure. J. Physiol. *241*, 34–35P (1974)

Bono, E. de, Mills, I.H.: Simultaneous increases in kallikrein in renal lymph and urine during saline infusion. J. Physiol. *241*, 127–128P (1974)

Croxatto, H.R., Roblero, J., Albertini, R., Corthorn, J., San Martin, M., Porcelli, G.: The kallikrein-kinin system in renal hypertension. In: Chemistry and biology of the kallikrein-kinin system in health and disease. Pisano, J.J., Austen, K.F. (eds.), pp. 389–397. Fogarty Internat. Center Proc. No. 27. Washington: U.S. Gov. Printing Office 1977
Croxatto, H.R., Albertini, R., Arriagada, R., Roblero, J., Rojas, M., Rosas, R.: Renal urinary kallikrein in normotensive and hypertensive rats during enhanced excretion of water and electrolytes. Clin. Sci. Mol. Med. *51*, 259s–261s (1976)
Data, J.L., Chang, L.C.T., Nies, A.S.: Alteration of canine renal vascular response to hemorrhage by inhibitors of prostaglandin synthesis. Am. J. Physiol. *230*, 940–945 (1976)
Donker, A.J.M., Arisz, L., Brentjens, J.R.H., Van der Hem, G.K., Hollemans, H.J.G.: The effect of indomethacin in kidney function and plasma renin activity in man. Nephron *17*, 288–296 (1976)
Edwards, O.M., Adetuyibi, A., Mills, I.H.: Kallikrein excretion during the 'escape' from the sodium retaining effect of fludrocortisone. J. Endocrinol. *59*, xxxiv (1973)
Elebute, O.A., Mills, I.H.: Urinary kallikrein in normal and hypertensive pregnancies. In: Hypertension in pregnancy. Lindheimer, M.D., Katz, A.I., Zuspan, F.P. (eds.), pp. 329–338. New York: Wiley and Sons 1976
Elliot, R., Nuzum, F.R.: Urinary excretion of a depressor substance (kallikrein of Frey and Kraut) in arterial hypertension. Endocrinology *18*, 462–474 (1934)
Frey, E.K., Kraut, H.: Ein neues Kreislaufhormon und seine Wirkung. Naunyn Schmiedebergs Arch. Exp. Pathol. Pharmacol. *133*, 1 (1928)
Frey, E.K., Kraut, H., Werle, E.: Kallikrein (Padutin). Stuttgart: Enke 1950
Gill, J.R., Jr., Flölich, J.C., Bowden, R.E., Taylor, A.A., Keiser, H.R., Seyberth, H.W., Oates, J.A., Bartter, F.C.: Bartter's syndrome: A disorder characterized by high urinary prostaglandins and a dependence of hyperreninemia on prostaglandin synthesis. Am. J. Med. *61*, 43–51 (1976)
Gordon, R.D., Symonds, E.M., Wilmshurst, E.G., Pawsey, C.G.K.: Plasma renin activity, plasma angiotensin, and plasma and urinary electrolytes in normal and toxaemic pregnancy, including a prospective study. Clin. Sci. Mol. Med. *45*, 115–127 (1975)
Greco, A.V., Porcelli, G., Croxatto, H.R.: Kallikrein excretion in diverse types of hypertension. In: Chemistry and biology of the kallikrein-kinin system in health and disease. Pisano, J.J., Austen, K.F. (eds.), pp. 439–440. Fogarty Internat. Center Proc. No. 27. Washington: U.S. Gov. Printing Office 1977
Keiser, H.R., Margolius, H.S., Brown, R., Rhamey, R., Foster, J.: Urinary kallikrein in patients with renovascular hypertension. In: Chemistry and biology of the kallikrein-kinin system in health and disease. Pisano, J.J., Austen, K.F. (eds.), pp. 423–426. Fogarty Internat. Center Proc. No. 27. Washington: U.S. Gov. Printing Office 1977
Keiser, H.R., Andrews, M.J., Jr., Guyton, R.A., Margolius, H.S., Pisano, J.J.: Urinary kallikrein in dogs with constriction of one renal artery. Proc. Soc. Exp. Biol. Med. *151*, 53–56 (1976)
Lechi, A., Covi, G., Lechi, C., Mantero, F., Scuro, L.A.: Urinary kallikrein excretion in Bartter's syndrome. J. Clin. Endocrinol. Metab. *43*, 1175–1178 (1976)
Lennane, R.J., Carey, R.M., Goodwin, T.J., Peart, W.S.: A comparison of natriuresis after oral and intravenous sodium loading in sodium-depleted man: evidence for a gastrointestinal or portal monitor of sodium intake. Clin. Sci. Mol. Med. *49*, 437–440 (1975)
Levy, S.B., Lilley, J.J., Frigon, R.P., Stone, R.A.: Urinary kallikrein and plasma renin activity as determinants of renal blood flow. The influence of race and dietary sodium intake. J. Clin. Invest. *60*, 129–138 (1977)
MacFarlane, N.A.A., Adetuyibi, A., Mills, I.H.: The radioimmunoassay of bradykinin in the measurement of kallikrein in urine. J. Endocrinol. *58*, xxv (1973)
MacFarlane, N.A.A., Adetuyibi, A., Mills, I.H.: Changes in kallikrein excretion during arterial infusion of angiotensin. J. Endocrinol. *61*, lxxii (1974)
Margolius, H.S., Pisano, J.J., Geller, R., Sjoerdsma, A.: Altered urinary kallikrein excretion in human hypertension. Lancet *1971 II*, 1063–1065
Margolius, H.S., Horwitz, D., Geller, R.G., Alexander, R.W., Gill, J.R., Pisano, J.J., Keiser, H.R.: Urinary kallikrein excretion in normal man. Relationships to sodium intake and sodium-retaining steroids. Circ. Res. *35*, 812–819 (1974a)
Margolius, H.S., Horwitz, D., Pisano, J.J., Keiser, H.R.: Sodium, water, and kallikrein excretion in man. Acta Physiol. Lat. Am. *24*, 464–468 (1974b)

Margolius, H.S., Horwitz, D., Pisano, J.J., Keiser, H.R.: Urinary kallikrein excretion in hypertensive man. Relationships to sodium intake and sodium-retaining steroids. Circ. Res. *35*, 820–825 (1974c)
Margolius, H.S., Chao, J., Kaizu, T.: The effects of aldosterone and spironolactone on renal kallikrein in the rat. Clin. Sci. Mol. Med. *51*, 279s–282s (1976)
Marin-Grez, M., Carretero, O.A.: A method for measurement of urinary kallikrein. J. Appl. Physiol. *32*, 428–431 (1972)
Marin-Grez, M., Cottone, P., Carretero, O.A.: Evidence for an involvement of kinins in regulation of sodium excretion. Am. J. Physiol. *223*, 794–796 (1972)
Matsuda, Y., Moriya, H., Moriwaki, C., Fujimoto, Y., Matsuda, M.: Fluorometric method for assay of kallikrein-like arginine esterases. J. Biochem. *79*, 1197–1200 (1976)
Mills, I.H.: Sodium-retaining steroids in non-oedematous patients. Production of odemea and heart-failure. Lancet *1962 I*, 1264–1267
Mills, I.H.: The non-aldosterone hormonal control of sodium. In: Hormones and the kidney. Williams, P.C. (ed.), pp. 17–24. Memoirs of the Society for Endocrinology No. 13. London, New York: Academic Press 1963
Mills, I.H., Barkham, D.W.: The effect of 9α-fluorohydrocortisone on the response to angiotensin infusions in man. International Congress Series No. 51., Abstract No. 310. Amsterdam: Excerpta Medica 1962
Mills, I.H., Wilson, R.J.: Antagonism by noradrenaline of the changes in renal function associated with development of resistance of the renal vasculature to the arterial infusion of angiotensin. Proc. Int. Union Physiol. Sci. Vol. IX, Abstract No. 1167. Munich: German Physiological Society 1971
Mills, I.H., Ward, P.E.: The relationship between kallikrein and water excretion and the conditional relationship between kallikrein and sodium excretion. J. Physiol. *246*, 695–707 (1975)
Mills, I.H., MacFarlane, N.A.A., Ward, P.E., Obika, L.F.O.: The renal kallikrein-kinin system and the regulation of salt and water excretion. Fed. Proc. *35*, 181–188 (1976)
Mills, I.H., Obika, L.F.O.: A novel effect of intrarenal infusion of a non-vasoconstrictor dose of noradrenaline on renal function: relationship to renal kallikrein and prostaglandin. J. Physiol. *267*, 21–22P (1977)
Mills, I.H., Obika, L.F.O., Newport, P.: Stimulation of the renal kallikrein-kinin system by vasoactive substances and its relationship to the excretion of salt and water. Contributions to Nephrology *12*, 132–144 (1978)
McGiff, J.C., Terragno, N.A., Malik, K.U., Lonigro, A.J.: Release of a prostaglandin E-like substance from canine kidney by bradykinin. Circ. Res. *31*, 36–43 (1972)
McGiff, J.C., Itskovitz, H.D., Terragno, A., Wong, P.Y.-K.: Modulation and mediation of the action of the renal kallikrein-kinin system by prostaglandins. Fed. Proc. *35*, 175–180 (1976)
Moriya, H.: A colorimetric method for the estimation of urinary kallikrein. Jpn. J. Clin. Med. *22*, 2659–2664 (1964)
Nekrasova, A.A., Lantsberg, L.A., Chernova, N.A., Khukharev, V.V.: The kinin system of the kidneys in various physiological states in healthy persons and in patients with essential hypertension. Kardiologiya *10*, 9–15 (1970a)
Nekrasova, A.A., Chernova, N.A., Sharapov, U.B., Kovaleva, N.T.: Kallikrein level in the urine and some indices of kidney function. Urol. Nefrol. (Mosk.) *3*, 12–16 (1970b)
Olsen, U.B., Ahnfelt-Ronne, I.: Bumetanide induced increase of renal blood flow in conscious dogs and its relation to local renal hormones (PGE, kallikrein, and renin). Acta Pharmacol. Toxicol. *38*, 219–228 (1976)
Orloff, J., Handler, J., Bergstrom, S.: The effect of prostaglandin (PGE_1) on the permeability response of toad bladder to vasopressin, theophylline, and adenosine 3′, 5′-monophosphate. Nature (London) *205*, 397 (1965)
Padfield, P.L., Allison, M.E.M., Brown, J.J., Lever, A.F., Luke, R.G., Robertson, C.C., Robertson, J.I.S., Tree, M.: Effect of intravenous frusemide on plasma renin concentration: suppression of response in hypertension. Clin. Sci. Mol. Med. *49*, 353–358 (1975)
Patak, R.V., Mookerjee, B.K., Bentzel, C.J., Hysert, P.E., Babej, M., Lee, J.B.: Antagonism of the effects of furosemide by indomethacin in normal and hypertensive man. Prostaglandins *10(4)*, 649–659 (1975)

Peart, W.S.: Possible relationship between salt metabolism and the angiotensin system. In: Essential hypertension. Bock, K.D., Cottier, P.T. (eds.), pp. 112–120. Berlin, Heidelberg, New York: Springer 1960
Roberts, P.S.: Measurement of the rate of plasmin action on synthetic substrates. J. Biol. Chem. *232*, 285 (1958)
Roblero, J., Croxatto, H.R., Garcia, R., Corthorn, J., de Vitro, R.: Kallikrein-like activity in perfusates and urine of isolated rat kidneys. Am. J. Physiol. *231*, 1383–1389 (1976a)
Roblero, J., Croxatto, H.R., Albertini, R.B.: Release of renal kallikrein to the perfusate by isolated rat kidney. Experientia *32*, 1440–1441 (1976b)
Rumpf, K.W., Frenzel, S., Lowitz, H.D., Scheler, F.: The effect of indomethacin on plasma renin activity in man under normal conditions and after stimulation of the renin angiotensin system. Prostaglandins *10(4)*, 641–648 (1975)
Scicli, A.G., Carretero, O.A., Hampton, A., Cortes, P., Oza, N.B.: Site of kininogenase secretion in the dog nephron. Am. J. Physiol. *230*, 533–536 (1976)
Seino, M., Abe, K., Otsuka, Y., Saito, T., Irokawa, N., Yasujima, M., Chiba, S., Yoshinaga, K.: Urinary kallikrein excretion and sodium metabolism in hypertensive patients. Tohoku J. Exp. Med. *116*, 359–367 (1975)
Seino, M., Abe, K., Sakurai, Y., Irokawa, N., Yasujima, M., Chiba, S., Otsuka, Y., Yoshinaga, K.: Effect of spironolactone on urinary kallikrein excretion in patients with essential hypertension and in primary aldosteronism. Tohoku J. Exp. Med. *121*, 111–119 (1977)
Sever, P.S., Birch, M., Osikowska, B., Tunbridge, R.D.G.: Plasma-noradrenaline in essential hypertension. Lancet *1977 I*, 1078–1081
Talamo, R.C., Haber, E., Austen, K.F.: A radio-immunoassay for bradykinin in plasma and synovial fluid. J. Lab. Clin. Med. *74*, 816–827 (1969)
Ward, P.E.: Studies of the renal kinin systems. Ph.D. Thesis. University of Cambridge 1974
Ward, P.E., Mills, I.H.: Distribution of renal kininases in relation to the kallikrein-bradykinin system and water excretion. J. Endocrinol. *67*, 60P (1975)
Ward, P.E., Schultz, W., Reynolds, R.C., Erdös, E.G.: Metabolism of kinins and angiotensins in the isolated glomerulus and brush border of rat kidney. Lab. Invest. *36*, 599–606 (1977)
Wong, P.Y., Talamo, R.C., Williams, G.H., Colman, R.W.: Response of the kallikrein-kinin and renin-angiotensin systems to saline infusion and upright posture. J. Clin. Invest. *55*, 691–698 (1975)
Zinner, S.H., Margolius, H.S., Rosner, B., Keiser, H.R., Kass, E.H.: Familial aggregation of urinary kallikrein concentration in childhood: relation to blood pressure, race, and urinary electrolytes. Am. J. Epidemiol. *104*, 124–132 (1976)

Kallikrein-Kinin System in Pathologic Conditions

R. W. Colman and P. Y. Wong

A. Deficiency of Proteins Necessary for Kinin Formation

I. Hereditary

1. Factor XII Deficiency (Hageman Trait)

Deficiency of factor XII was first identified by Ratnoff and Colopy (1955) in a patient whose surname, Hageman, has been the eponym for this protein. The prolonged in vitro blood clotting observed in this patient was not associated with an in vivo hemostatic disorder suggesting that an alternative mode of activation of the clotting system must be present in vivo. Several hundred cases of Hageman trait have since been described and reviewed (Ratnoff, 1966). This protein deficiency occurs through an autosomal recessive mode of inheritance (Margolius and Ratnoff, 1956). Thus complete deficiency of factor XII occurs only when two abnormal alleles are present (Kaper et al., 1968). A bimodal distribution of Hageman factor concentrations have been found in study of 50 heterozygotes (Veltkamp et al., 1965) suggesting that at least two normal alleles control production of Hageman factor. The life span in circulation of transfused factor XII is 40–50 h (Fantl et al., 1961).

The lack of participation of this protein in normal hemostasis is underscored by the fact that patients with complete deficiency of factor XII are not protected from thrombotic disorders. At least two individuals with Hageman factor trait have experienced a myocardial infarction (Glueck and Roehill, 1966; Hoak et al., 1966) and the index case, Mr. Hageman, died of a pulmonary embolism (Ratnoff et al., 1968). The assignment of this protein to the coagulation pathway has to do primarily with

Table 1. Glossary of contact activation factors

Name	Synonyms
Factor XII	Hageman factor
XIIa	Activated Hageman factor
XIIf	Hageman factor fragments, prekallikrein activators, large activator
Prekallikrein	Fletcher factor, plasminogen proactivator
Kallikrein	Kininogenase
HMW kininogen	Williams, Fitzgerald, Flaujeac factors, contact activation factor
Factor XI	Plasma thromboplastin antecedent

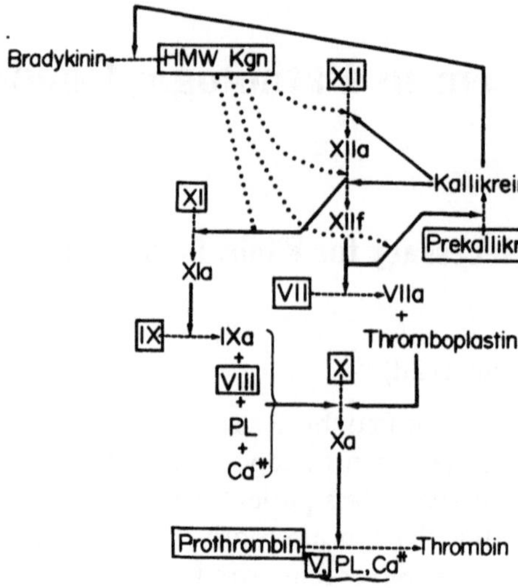

Fig. 1. Participation of components of the kallikrein-kinin system in coagulation and fibrinolysis. *Boxed components* represent precursors. *Dashed arrows* represent transformation of precursor to product. *Solid arrows* are actions of a proteolytic enzyme. *Dotted arrows* are nonproteolytic activation. Kgn = kininogen. .

the method in which the disorder was first detected and the subsequent demonstration that factor XII is necessary for activation of factor XI (RATNOFF et al., 1961).

It is equally important to regard factor XII as the first component in the plasma kallikrein-kinin system (Fig. 1). Addition of kaolin to factor XII-deficient plasma is not followed by either the release of kallikrein or bradykinin (MARGOLIS, 1960; GIREY et al., 1972) even though Hageman trait plasma contains adequate quantities of both precursors (MARGOLIS, 1960; WEBSTER and RATNOFF, 1961; GIGLI et al., 1970). The formation of kinin is initiated by the activation of Hageman factor (MW 80,000–90,000). Recent studies suggest that in the prealbumin anionic components of the human plasma are potent activators of prekallikrein. These prekallikrein activators exhibit a MW of approximately 30,000 (KAPLAN and AUSTEN, 1970; SOLTAY et al., 1971) and arise spontaneously from activated Hageman factor during purification procedures (BAGDASARIAN et al., 1973a), exposure to plasmin (KAPLAN and AUSTEN, 1971; BURROWES et al., 1971), kallikrein (BAGDASARIAN et al., 1973b; COCHRANE et al., 1973), and trypsin (COCHRANE and WUEPPER, 1971). An activator of intermediate molecular weight has been isolated (BAGDASARIAN et al., 1973a, b) which is also a fragment of factor XII produced by limited plasmin digestion. This fragment is resistant to further plasmin digestion and is not an intermediate in the pathway producing prekallikrein activators. The process of transformation of factor XII to the family of prekallikrein activators occurs with a progressive decrease in size, increase in net negative charge, increase in prekallikrein activator potency, and a decrease in clotting activity. No studies are available on factor XII – deficient patients suffering from disease in which the kallikrein-kinin system has been implicated. It would seem likely that no activation would result unless there is another mode of initiation that is not dependent on factor XII.

2. Prekallikrein Deficiency (Fletcher Trait)

In 1965, HATHAWAY et al. (1965) described the existence of a previously unrecognized coagulation protein which they named Fletcher factor after the surname of the affected family. The occurrence in four siblings, the offspring of a consanguineous union, suggested autosomal recessive inheritance. This postulate was confirmed by a later study in the original family (ABILDGAARD and HARRISON, 1974) and three unrelated families (HATTERSLEY and HAYES, 1970). The defect was characterized by a prolonged whole blood clotting time and activated partial thromboplastin time in the presence of normal concentration of all known clotting factors. Similar to individuals with Hageman trait, the affected individuals were entirely asymptomatic without a history of hemostatic disorder. Although the corrective factor in normal plasma was partially purified and shown to behave similar to, though not identical with factor XI on ion exchange chromatography (HATHAWAY and ALSEVER, 1970), it was not until later when WUEPPER (1972) recognized that the missing protein in Fletcher trait was prekallikrein. Furthermore, Fletcher trait plasma had abnormal surface-activated kinin formation, fibrinolysis, and vascular permeability-enhancing activity in diluted plasma, all correctable by purified human prekallikrein (WUEPPER, 1973; WEISS et al., 1974). Both the functional activity and antigenic reactivity of prekallikrein are absent from Fletcher trait plasma (WUEPPER, 1973) and rabbit antiserum prepared against kallikrein inhibits the coagulant (SAITO and RATNOFF, 1974) and kinin-forming (BAGDASARIAN et al., 1974) activity. The relationship of prekallikrein to fibrinolysis is controversial. COLMAN (1969) demonstrated the conversion of plasminogen to plasmin by highly purified kallikrein. Although KAPLAN and AUSTEN (1972) have presented evidence that prekallikrein may be separated from plasminogen proactivator, more recently MANDLE and KAPLAN (1977) agree that the plasminogen proactivator described previously was prekallikrein. They further showed that factor XI also converts plasminogen to plasmin. BOUMA and GRIFFIN (1977) also confirm that kallikrein directly activates plasminogen but were unable to demonstrate plasminogen activating activity associated with factor XI. The absence of plasminogen proactivator from Fletcher trait (prekallikrein deficient) plasma (VENNERÖD and LAAKE, 1976) and the failure to separate these two proteins (LAAKE and VENNERÖD, 1974) is consistent with the evidence (COLMAN, 1969) that kallikrein directly activates plasminogen and renders the existence of plasminogen proactivator as a separate molecular entity unlikely.

One of the most challenging observations (HATHAWAY et al., 1965) concerning prekallikrein is that the abnormally long partial thromboplastin time of patients with Fletcher trait shortens to normal if the plasma is exposed for a prolonged period to a clot-promoting surface such as kaolin before the addition of calcium ions. This finding suggests an indirect or feedback role for kallikrein rather than merely serving as a substrate of factor XII. This postulate was substantiated by the finding that kallikrein can convert unactivated Hageman factor to activated Hageman factor in the fluid phase (BAGDASARIAN et al., 1973b; COCHRANE et al., 1973). The reciprocal activation of Hageman factor and prekallikrein help to clarify the role of these two proteins in the activation of factor VII (Fig. 1). Following the lead of RAPAPORT et al. (1955) who demonstrated shortening of the one stage prothrombin time in glass, GJONNAESS (1972a) found that cold-promoted activation of factor VII depended on the presence of factor XII and kallikrein (GJONNAESS, 1972b).

They postulated that factor XII activated kallikrein which was responsible for the increase of factor VII activity. However, RADCLIFFE et al. (1977) have recently demonstrated that Hageman factor fragments are capable of catalysing a 60-fold increase in factor VII activity while kallikrein has no apparent effect. The role of kallikrein therefore would be to convert unactivated factor XII to fragments which are responsible for the increase in factor VII activity.

In a similar manner to Hageman factor, prekallikrein, a factor needed for in vitro hemostasis, may not be essential in vivo. A patient with this deficiency experienced a myocardial infarction (CURRIMBHOY et al., 1976) again demonstrating the lack of protection for thrombotic disease in individual deficient in this protein.

3. High Molecular Weight Kininogen Deficiency (Williams, Fitzgerald, and Flaujeac Traits)

The extensive studies on the interaction of Hageman factor and prekallikrein in the initiation of plasma proteolysis appeared to have reached a consensus (COLMAN, 1974). However, two disquieting reports suggested that an additional plasma cofactor is required for Hageman factor activation and activity. WEBSTER and PIERCE (1973) suggested that surface-bound factor XII did not activate prekallikrein optimally. SCHIFFMAN and LEE (1974) have shown that purified factor XII did not activate highly purified factor XI. Later studies confirmed that HMW kininogen corrected the deficient activation of prekallikrein (WEBSTER et al., 1976) and the defective activation of factor XI (SCHIFFMAN and LEE, 1975). These latter studies were made possible by the discovery of three individuals with severe defects in the intrinsic coagulation, fibrinolytic, and kinin-forming pathways. Three laboratories recognized a common defect identifying each by their eponym as Williams (COLMAN et al., 1975), Fitzgerald (SAITO et al., 1975), and Flaujeac (LACOMBE et al., 1975) traits. In each case a prolonged activated partial thromboplastin time led to discovery. It was found that the surface-activated fibrinolysis and prekallikrein activation was grossly defective. All patients were entirely asymptomatic. Detailed investigation showed that purified HMW kininogen corrected all the defects (COLMAN et al., 1975; WUEPPER et al., 1975) in Williams and Flaujeac plasmas and this was confirmed in Fitzgerald plasma (DONALDSON et al., 1976; SCHIFFMAN et al., 1975). Two additional patients have recently been described (DONALDSON et al., 1976; LUTCHER, 1976) with deficiency of HMW kininogen. In two families (DONALDSON et al., 1976; LACOMBE, 1975) the defect has been characterized as an autosomal recessive. Most of the patients studied not only lack HMW kininogen but also do not have any detectable LMW kininogen. However, Fitzgerald has 50% of the normal concentration of LMW kininogen. This finding suggests that two separate genes may code for the HMW and LMW kininogens. If human kininogen is similar to bovine kininogen (KATO et al., 1975) then both HMW and LMW kininogen exist as a single polypeptide chain with a large section of common structure. This model is consistant with the finding that antibody against LMW kininogen gives a reaction of complete identity with HMW kininogen. Alternatively two polypeptide chains may be present in HMW kininogen and only one in LMW kininogen similar to the situation in plasma and platelet factor XIII. The possibility that LMW kininogen is a proteolytic breakdown product seem ruled out by the situation in Mr. Fitzgerald. In normal plasma, HMW kininogen makes up 15–

20% of the total kininogen (HABAL et al., 1974). It is the preferred substrate for plasma kallikrein (PIERCE and GUIMARES, 1976). The function of HMW kininogen in contact activation and factor XII activity has been recently reviewed (MEIER et al., 1977a). HMW kininogen enhances the surface-dependant activation of Hageman factor (MEIER et al., 1977b), facilitates the cleavage of Hageman factor by kallikrein (GRIFFIN and COCHRANE, 1976), and increases the initial rate of prekallikrein activation by Hageman factor fragments (LIU et al., 1977) (Fig. 1).

Another interesting linkage between these proteins is the variable prekallikrein levels associated with a deficiency of HMW kininogen. Flaujeac trait has normal prekallikrein concentrations, Williams has 45% prekallikrein, and Fitzgerald has 12% prekallikrein. This observation suggests close genetic linkage between these two proteins. It is important to note that prekallikrein and HMW kininogen circulate in plasma as a complex (MANDLE et al., 1976). Such an association is analogous to that of von Willebrand's protein and factor VIII coagulant protein. Changes in ionic strength during the purification of HMW kininogen and prekallikrein apparently disassociates the complex. The relationship between HMW kininogen and the other proteins of the contact phase needs further definition.

New biologic function for degradation products of HMW kininogen include a peptide which enhances permeability (MATHESON et al., 1976) and a histidine-rich peptide which inhibits factor XII activation (HAN et al., 1975) (see MOVAT elsewhere in this volume). Finally, just as the roles of HMW kininogen are being clarified, evidence has been presented for yet another factor which potentiates prekallikrein activation by factor XII (WEBSTER et al., 1976; CHAN et al., 1977).

II. Acquired

1. Dengue Hemorrhagic Fever

The pathogenesis of the severe and life-threatening manifestations of the serious Asian public health problem, dengue hemorrhagic fever with and without shock, is not completely understood. The complement system has been implicated (BOKISCH et al., 1973). Sequential studies of 18 patients, 11 of whom developed shock, EDELMAN et al. (1975) showed a decrease of C3 and platelet counts on the day of shock with a recovery during convalescence. Although prekallikrein was reduced to 40% of its normal value and factor XII to 60% prior to shock, the values increased progressively even during shock demonstrating that activation of prekallikrein did not occur. Moreover no consistent decrease in kallikrein inhibitory activity occurred and no increase of bradykinin was noted. These changes were therefore more reminiscent of the changes in cirrhosis (see below) with decreased prekallikrein and XII but normal C1 inhibition and low levels of bradykinin. Liver disease has occurred in association with dengue fever (COHEN and HALSTEAD, 1966). Thus it appears that the shock observed is not due to kinin release.

2. Cirrhosis of Liver

In chronic diseases of the liver, the synthesis of many plasma proteins is decreased as reflected in low plasma concentrations. There is abundant evidence that plasma prekallikrein is diminished in patients with cirrhosis of the liver (COLMAN et al., 1969;

Table 2. Hereditary deficiencies in kallikrein-kinin system

Genetic deficiency	Protein missing	Clinical manifestation	References
Hageman trait	Factor XII	Asymptomatic	Ratnoff and Calopy (1955)
Fletcher trait	Prekallikrein	Asymptomatic	Hathaway et al. (1965)
Williams trait	HMW kininogen	Asymptomatic	Colman et al. (1975)
Fitzgerald trait	HMW kininogen	Asymptomatic	Saito et al. (1975)
Flaujeac trait	HMW kininogen	Asymptomatic	Lacombe et al. (1975)
Hereditary angioedema	Cl esterase inhibitor	Edema of skin, subcutaneous tissue, larynx	Landerman et al. (1962)

Wong et al., 1972; Paskhina and Krinskaya, 1974; Fanciullacci et al., 1975; Bagdasarian et al., 1974; Wong et al., in press; Snyder et al., 1974). In a study of 20 patients with alcoholic cirrhosis (Wong et al., 1972), the mean prekallikrein level was significantly depressed when compared to normal control subjects. This depression was found to correlate with severity of alcoholic liver disease; patients with prolonged prothrombin time (>3 s from controls) had significantly lower prekallikrein than those with normal prothrombin time. This finding was in agreement with those reported by others (Paskhina and Krinskaya, 1974; Fanciullacci et al., 1975; Bagdasarian et al., 1974). Fanciullacci et al. (1975) found that prekallikrein level was decreased also in patients hospitalized for acute icteric viral hepatitis. Stewart et al. (1972), however, using the same assay, were unable to confirm this finding. This discrepancy can be explained in part by their patient population which covered a wide variety of chronic liver diseases with varying degrees of severity, and in part from their assay method. Using the same TAMe esterase method as reported by Colman et al. (1969b) their mean plasma prekallikrein in normal subjects was only 16 μmol/ml/h whereas the normal value reported by others varied between 95–98 μmol/ml/h (Colman et al., 1969; Wong et al., 1972; Paskhina and Krinskaya, 1974; Fanciullacci et al., 1975; Bagdasarian et al., 1974; Wong et al., 1977).

All investigators used the TAMe esterase method (Colman et al., 1969b) which depends on the concentration of Hageman factor (Sherry et al., 1966) as well as the prekallikrein level. Decreased functional prekallikrein concentrations may be due to increased consumption of prekallikrein (as in activation of the kallikrein-kinin system), decreased in synthesis of plasma prekallikrein protein or production of nonfunctional (nonproteolytic) kallikrein. It is, therefore, imperative that every component of the kinin cascade be measured before one can deduce the cause of a low prekallikrein value. Hageman factor was measured in 17 of the 20 patients studied (Wong et al., 1972) and was normal in 11 patients. The remaining six patients who had decreased Hageman factor ranged from 25–45%. Colman et al. (1969), however, have shown that a Hageman factor level of 25% or above was adequate for complete conversion of prekallikrein to kallikrein in the assay used. Thus, decreased Hageman factor does not account for the low prekallikrein observed in alcoholic cirrhosis. These same workers (Colman et al., 1969) also showed good evidence that kaolin-activated arginine esterase in the human plasma represented plasma kallikrein activity. Free kallikrein as determined by spontaneous arginine esterase activity was measured by Wong et al. (1972) and Fanciullacci et al. (1975); they failed to detect any increase in the plasma of cirrhotic patients, suggesting that free kallikrein was not released in increased quantities in these patients. The kallikrein inhibitor (C1 esterase inhibitor), because of its stoichiometric combination with free kallikrein, is decreased in conditions where the prekallikrein is activated. In chronic liver disease kallikrein inhibitor was normal (WONG et al., 1972; FANCIULLACCI et al., 1975) suggesting there was no consumption of prekallikrein. The evidence, therefore, suggests that the low prekallikrein in patients with cirrhosis of the liver is caused by a decrease in its synthesis. In support of this concept, plasma prekallikrein levels have been shown to decrease after ablation of the liver by hepatectomy or carbon tetrachloride administration in experimental animals (WERLE et al., 1963). More recently, BAGDASARIAN et al. (1974), employing a radial immunoassay utilizing specific antibody against plasma kallikrein. They found a close correlation between the levels of kallikrein antigen and prekallikrein. The latter was determined by TAMe esterase method measuring functional plasma kallikrein activity (COLMAN et al., 1969b, c) in normal subjects and patients with compensated cirrhosis (normal prothrombin time). However, in severe cirrhotics, the ratio of kallikrein antigen to functional prekallikrein was increased suggesting synthesis of a dysfunctional protein (BAGDASARIAN et al., 1974). The total kininogen in cirrhosis of the liver was decreased also in cirrhosis of the liver (STEWART et al., 1972; DELBIANCO et al., 1972) confirming the suspicion that kininogens were probably synthesized by the liver also. More recently, HMW kininogen measured by a coagulant assay was found to be decreased (SAITO et al., 1976). In viral hepatitis, however, the kininogen was reported as normal (DELBIANCO et al., 1972). The level of plasma bradykinin as measured by bioassay (GALLETTI et al., 1968) or radioimmunoassay (WONG et al., 1972, 1977) decreased when compared to normal. In fact, plasma bradykinin, as determined by radioimmunoassay was not detectable in a large number of patients studied (WONG et al., 1972). However, it was later found that plasma bradykinin was very sensitive to the state of sodium balance which varied in the group of patients studied (WONG et al., 1975, 1976). Subsequently, with the use of a strict metabolic ward diet containing 10 mEq Na, 100 mEq K isocaloric diet, the earlier suspicion that plasma bradykinin was decreased in patients with cirrhosis was confirmed (WONG et al., 1977). The lowest values were observed in patients with functional renal failure (hepatorenal syndrome) of cirrhosis of the liver (WONG et al., 1977). There is now sufficient evidence to suggest that kinin generation in cirrhosis of the liver is diminished as evidenced by low prekallikrein, production of nonfunctional kallikrein, decreased plasma kininogen, and very low plasma bradykinin levels.

In normal individuals, there is a close association between plasma kinin and renin-angiotensin systems (WONG et al., 1975). In cirrhosis of the liver, in addition to the kallikrein-kinin system, the renin-angiotensin system was also abnormal (WONG et al., 1977; SHROEDER et al., 1970; AYERS, 1967; BERKOWITZ et al., 1972; WOLFF et al., 1958; COPPAGE et al., 1962; ROSOFF et al., 1975; SHROEDER et al., 1976). In these patients, the plasma renin activity was almost uniformly increased (WONG et al., 1977; SHROEDER et al., 1970; AYERS, 1965; BERKOWITZ et al., 1972) renin substrate was decreased and the plasma aldosterone (WOLFF et al., 1958; COPPAGE et al., 1962; ROSOFF et al., 1975) was increased. Furthermore, WONG et al. (1977), by the use of radioimmunoassay, found that angiotensin II levels was also increased in cirrhosis, confirming the suspicion by ROSOFF et al. (1975) that the renin-angiotensin system was activated. Since the effector hormones of these two vasoactive systems (kinin and angiotensin II) are potent peptides with opposite effects on the renal vasculature, the question whether these abnormalities could be involved in the pathogenesis of hepatorenal syndrome in cirrhosis of the liver was investigated (WONG et al., 1977). The mean prekallikrein and bradykinin level for the group of cirrhotics with hepatorenal syndrome significantly decreased when compared to those cirrhotics without renal impairment. In contrast, the mean concentration of angiotensin II for the hepatorenal syndrome patients was increased significantly when compared to controls, even though the mean plasma renin activity for the two groups was not statistically different. (The mean plasma renin activity for all 15 patients, however, was increased significantly when compared to normal controls).

Bradykinin has been suggested as a physiologic renal vasodilator (MCGIFF et al., 1972; MCGIFF et al., 1976; GILL et al., 1965; DOLLERY et al., 1965). Its renal vasodilatory effect may be mediated through a prostaglandin E-like substance in the canine kidney (MCGIFF et al., 1972). If this finding holds true in man, then blockade of prostaglandin synthetase in these patients should reproduce a syndrome similar to the hepatorenal syndrome. Indeed, BOYER et al. (in press) could produce a reversible syndrome resembling hepatorenal syndrome by administration of indomethacin to cirrhotic patients with sodium retention. The systemic effect of indomethacin in these patients, however, may be diverse (ROMERO et al., 1976) and the resulting renal failure may be caused by actions completely independent on its effect on the kinin system.

It is difficult to assess whether the renal cortical constriction seen these patients is due to excess angiotensin II or due to decreased kinin formation. However, it is known that angiotensin II infusion in normal man does not lead to renal failure, neither do patients born with congenital absence of kininogen have renal failure. It is possible that combined effects of excess in renal vasoconstrictor hormone (angiotensin II) and the decreased formation of renal vasodilator (bradykinin) may be etiologic in the pathogenesis of hepatorenal syndrome in cirrhosis of the liver. In this discussion, we have not taken into account the potential role of the kinin as an angiotensin cofactor (HASS et al., 1973) and its possible consequence in the systemic and renal circulation in man.

B. Disorders Leading to Increased Kinin Formation

I. Hereditary

1. Hereditary Angioedema

The dramatic picture of a patient with hereditary angioedema suffocating due to edema of the pharyngeal-laryngeal area was first described by Sir William Osler who also recognized the genetic basis of the disease. The clinical picture was well reviewed by LANDERMAN (1962) who culled 414 cases in 155 families. The inheritance was autosomal dominant with almost complete penetrance, 48% of well-studied family members exhibiting the disease. The disease can appear as early as infancy or as late as the middle of the fourth decade. The first symptom usually occurs before the age of 10. Prominent symptoms include recurrent episodes of edema of the gastrointestinal tract manifested by abdominal pain or vomiting and edema of the skin and

Table 3. Acquired disorders of kallikrein-kinin sytem

Pathologic condition	Biochemical changes						References
	Factor XII	Prekallikrein	Kallikrein inhibitor (Cl esterase inhibitor)	Kininogen	Bradykinin	Mechanism	
Dengue fever	Decreased	Decreased	Unchanged	Not determined	Unchanged	Decreased synthesis	EDELMAN et al. (1975)
Cirrhosis of the liver	Decreased	Decreased	Unchanged	Decreased	Decreased	Decreased synthesis	WONG et al. (1972)
Carcinoid syndrome	Not determined	Decreased or unchanged	Decreased or unchanged	Decreased	Increased	1) Release of tissue kallikrein; 2) Activation of plasma kallikrein	OATES et al. (1964) COLMAN et al. (1976)
Postgastrectomy dumping syndrome	Unchanged	Decreased or unchanged	Decreased or unchanged	Decreased	Increased	1) Activation of plasma kallikrein; 2) Release of tissue kallikrein	ZEITLIN et al. (1966) WONG et al. (1974)
Septic shock	Decreased	Decreased	Decreased	Decreased	Increased	Activation of plasma kallikrein	HERMAN et al. (1974); HIRSCH et al. (1974); NIES et al. (1968); MASON et al. (1970)
Hemorrhagic pancreatitis	Unchanged	Unchanged	Decreased	Decreased	Increased	Release of pancreatic kallikrein	BROWN, (1959); RYAN et al. (1965); OFSTAD, (1970)
Myocardial ischema	Decreased	Decreased	Decreased	Decreased	Not determined	Activation of plasma kallikrein	PITT et al. (1969); SICUTERI, (1970)

Table 3.

Pathologic condition	Biochemical changes						References
	Factor XII	Prekallikrein	Kallikrein inhibitor (Cl esterase inhibitor)	Kininogen	Bradykinin	Mechanism	
Disseminated intravascular coagulation							
1) Infection	Decreased	Decreased	Decreased	Not determined	Not determined	Activation of plasma kallikrein	MASON and COLMAN, (1971)
2) Malignancy	Unchanged	Unchanged	Unchanged	Not determined	Not determined	No involvement of system	
Renal allograft rejection (hyperacute)	Decreased	Decreased	Decreased	Not determined	Not determined	Activation of plasma kallikrein	BUSCH et al. (1975a, b)
Hyperlipo-proteinemia							
1) IIa	Unchanged	Decreased	Decreased	Not determined	Not determined	Activation of plasma kallikrein	
2) IV	Unchanged	Unchanged	Unchanged	Not determined	Not determined	No involvement of system	CARVALHO et al. (1977)

Allergic disorders (asthma)	Unchanged	Unchanged	Unchanged	Not determined	Not determined	? Release of tissue kallikrein	BRISEID et al. (1976)
	Not determined	Not determined	Not determined	Decreased	Decreased		LUKJAN, (1972)
Transfusion reactions							
1) Infusion of plasma fractions	Not determined	Decreased	Decreased	Decreased	Not determined	Infusion of activated XII of plasma kallikrein	IZAKA et al. (1975)
2) Isoantibody	Unchanged	Decreased	Decreased	Not determined	Not determined	Activation of plasma kallikrein	LOPAS et al. (1973)
3) Hemodialysis	Decreased	Decreased	Not determined	Decreased	Not determined	Activation of plasma kallikrein	WARDLE and PERCY, (1972)
Cystic fibrosis	Unchanged	Unchanged	Unchanged	Unchanged	Unchanged	No involvement of system	TALAMO et al. (1972) GOLDSMITH et al. (1977)
Typohoid fever	Unchanged	Decreased (complex present)	Decreased (complex present)	Increased	Not determined	Activation of plasma kallikrein	COLMAN et al. (1977)
Nephrotic syndrome	Decreased	Decreased	Decreased	Not determined	Not determined	Activation of plasma kallikrein	LANGE et al. (1974) KALLEN and LEE (1975)

subcutaneous tissues. In a third of the cases the disorder terminates in fatal edema of larynx and upper respiratory tract. LANDERMAN et al. (1962) showed that when diluted serum from a patient with hereditary angioedema was injected intradermally, vascular permeability was enhanced much more than when the diluted plasma was injected into the skin of a normal control. The demonstration of the lack of an inhibitor of plasma kallikrein by LANDERMAN et al. (1962) and $C\bar{1}$ by DONALDSON and EVANS (1963) in hereditary angioedema raised the question of whether excess of either enzyme might be responsible for the symptoms of the disease. Injection of either plasma kallikrein (LANDERMAN et al., 1962) or $C\bar{1}$ (KLEMPERER et al., 1968) intradermally increased vascular permeability, presumably due to the uninhibited action of these enzymes. The complement system is activated during attacks as shown by the appearance of activated $C\bar{1}$, evidenced by increased hydrolysis of its ester substrate ATEe (DONALDSON and ROSEN, 1964). At the same time, one of the protein substrates in the complement system, C2, is present at half its normal concentration even between attacks of angioedema and falls to very low levels at the time of attack (AUSTEN and SHEFFER, 1965). Another substrate of $C\bar{1}$, C4, is split into two components demonstrable by immunoelectrophoresis (DONALDSON and ROSEN, 1964). The catabolism of C4 (CARPENTER et al., 1969) is also increased in vivo. However, the evidence for activation of the plasma kallikrein system is not clear. Parallel changes, such as the appearance of activated kallikrein (LANDERMAN et al., 1962) or the decrease of prekallikrein (COLMAN et al., 1969) have not been documented in an attack. The existence of another kallikrein inhibitor, α_2-macroglobulin, may account for this (HARPEL, 1970). On the other hand, BURDON et al. (1965) have documented decreased kinin-forming ability following an attack in a patient with hereditary angioedema. Since this abnormality could be reversed by a component in serum heated at 61 °C for 30 min, these patients probably had a decrease of kininogen.

The part that both C1 and kallikrein may play in the production of edema has been elucidated by studies of DONALDSON et al. (1969). Patients with a hereditary absence of C2, but not with an acquired absence of C3, develop decreased permeability after intradermal injection of $C\bar{1}$, suggesting the role of this early complement component. A permeability-producing peptide has been isolated from plasma of patients during attacks. It is also formed by incubation in vitro of diluted plasma of patients in remission. The peptide differs from kinin in that it is inactivated by trypsin, possesses mild pressor activity, and behaves differently on electrophoresis and chromatography. The fact that SBTI, which inhibits plasmin and plasma kallikrein but not $C\bar{1}$, blocks the formation of the "permeability peptide" suggests that plasmin or kallikrein may be involved. The observation (DONALDSON, 1968) that Hageman factor can activate $C\bar{1}$ means that kallikrein and $C\bar{1}$ esterase have not only a common inhibitor but a common mechanism of activation. Attempts to disentangle the roles of these two enzymes may be difficult. $C\bar{1}$ inactivator is probably a weak inhibitor of plasmin (RATNOFF et al., 1969). Activation of Hageman factor, converts plasma prekallikrein to kallikrein which in turn activates plasminogen (COLMAN, 1969). The role of plasmin in the generation of this peptide must be considered, since it also may activate $C\bar{1}$. Recent experiments (DONALDSON et al., 1977) indicate that plasmin can release a kinin from the cleavage products of C2 which result from the action of $C\bar{1}$. Trauma, the only well-proven initiator of angioedema, may act through Hageman factor or the fibrinolytic system.

In searching for an effective therapy for angioedema, several approaches have been used based on the pathophysiologic concepts just described. The first and perhaps most obvious approach involves replacement of the missing inhibitor. Infusion of 2 units of plasma abolished attacks in two patients, one with abdominal pain and the other with laryngeal edema (PICKERING et al., 1969). The infusion produced a reasonable rise in inhibitor coupled with a fall in $C\bar{1}$ as well as a rise in C2 and C4. However, the theoretical possibility of feeding fuel (substrate) to the fire (active enzyme) must not be overlooked. Thus, as in treatment of coagulation disorders, a purified preparation of $C\bar{1}$ inhibitor would be valuable. Epsilon aminocaproic acid, an inhibitor of $C\bar{1}$ (SOTER et al., 1975) and plasmin (BROCKWAY and CASTILLINO, 1971) and plasminogen activation has been effective in a double-blind study in decreasing spontaneous attacks (FRANK et al., 1972) and in preventing attacks triggered by surgery (PENCE et al., 1974). These drugs may work by preventing plasmin fragmentation of factor XII or $C\bar{1}$. Anabolic steroids controls the disease by increasing functional $C\bar{1}$ inhibitor protein while retaining normal (α_2-globulin) mobility and normal antigenic reactivity (GADEK et al., 1977). Finally, since heparin increases the total plasma inhibitory activity as measured against purified kallikrein (LAHIRI et al., 1976) by potentiating antithrombin III, it has been suggested (COLMAN, 1976) that heparin may be beneficial in aborting the acute attack.

II. Acquired (Documented)

1. Carcinoid Syndrome

Carcinoid syndrome occurs in only 3% of all carcinoid tumors. These tumors are comparatively rare comprising only 1.5% of all gastrointestinal tumors but the study of these tumors assumes an importance far beyond the number of patients affected by these tumors. Scattered among the digestive and absorptive cells of the intestinal mucosa are cells that have no exocrine or absorptive functions, characterized mainly by their staining characteristics (enterochromaffin, argentaffin or argyrophile cells). Morphologically, these are endocrine cells as indicated by the electron microscopic studies (VASSALIO et al., 1969; FORSMANN et al., 1969) and are classified in the family of APUD (amine precursor uptake and decarboxylation) cells (DAWSON, 1970; BUSSOLATI et al., 1969; CARVALHEIRA et al., 1968). Recently, FORSMANN et al. (1969) have subclassified histochemically these cells into several types, each responsible for formation of specific hormones such as serotonin, catecholamines, and gastrin, etc. Since carcinoid tumors arise from the enterochromaffin cells, study of these tumors provides a unique opportunity for study of the hormone mediators of these cells.

Carcinoid tumors as a rule correspond cytologically to the type of enterochromaffin cells that predominates in the site of origin (BLACK, 1968). Thus, a carcinoid tumor may possess multiple endocrine properties capable of producing a spectrum of clinical conditions rather than a single syndrome. The list of hormones identified with carcinoid tumors now includes serotonin (LEMBECK, 1953), 5-hydroxytryptopham (OATES and SJOERDSMA, 1962), catecholamines (SJOERDSMA and MELMON,

1964), histamine (PENNOW and WALDENSTROM, 1957), insulin (VAN DER SLUYS VEER et al., 1964), adrenocorticotropic hormone (ESCOVITZ and REINGOLD, 1961), and bradykinin (OATES et al., 1964). With the exception of bradykinin and serotonin, none of these agents has been implicated in the genesis of the carcinoid flush. Carcinoid tumors vary widely in their ability to produce or store serotonin; the excessive production of which remains clinically the most characteristic chemical abnormality. Serotonin is eventually oxidized to 5-hydroxy-indoleacetic acid by monoamine oxidase. Most patients with carcinoid syndrome have increased urinary excretion of 5-hydroxy-indoleacetic acid. Although serotonin may mediate the gastrointestinal symptoms of carcinoid syndrome such as diarrhea, intestinal hypermotility and abdominal cramps, the carcinoid flush probably is not caused by excessive serotonin release.

There is abundant evidence implicating kinins in the pathogenesis of carcinoid flush (OATES et al., 1964; ZEITLIN and SMITH, 1966; MELMON et al., 1965; COLMAN et al., 1969; COLMAN et al., 1976; OATES et al., 1966). In normal subjects, infusion of bradykinin mimics carcinoid flushes (ROCHA E SILVA et al., 1960). Moreover, approximately half of the patients with carcinoid syndrome have a significant increase of kinin concentration in hepatic venous blood during catecholamine-induced flushes (OATES et al., 1964). There are at least two mechanisms responsible for the kinin release during carcinoid flush. MELMON et al. (1965) identified an anionic kallikrein in the carcinoid tumor tissue which released lysyl-bradykinin from partially purified human kininogen. However, the kinin released into hepatic venous blood has been determined by chromatographic, electrophoretic, and pharmacologic studies to be bradykinin (OATES et al., 1966). This discrepancy was explained in part by the in vivo conversion of lysyl-bradykinin to bradykinin by an aminopeptidase (OATES et al., 1966). The second possibility (COLMAN et al., 1969; COLMAN et al., 1976), though less frequent, is that release of bradykinin is mediated through the plasma kallikrein. During spontaneous (COLMAN et al., 1969) and epinephrine-induced (COLMAN et al., 1976) carcinoid flushes, several patients had an increase in circulating plasma arginine esterase which had substrate specificity identical to plasma kallikrein. This enzyme activity is inhibited by SBTI (which has no effect on tissue kallikrein). Plasma prekallikrein and kallikrein inhibitor decreased and this is consistent with activation of plasma kallikrein. It is possible that either the tumor tissue releases an activator of plasma prekallikrein *or* that factor XII was activated by the abnormal surfaces in the tumor vessels. The third mechanism for the kinin release in carcinoid flush can be derived from the animal studies of A. M. ROTHSCHILD et al. (1974a, b, 1976). These workers showed that sympathomimetic amines activated the kallikrein system of rat blood, causing up to 50% lowering of kininogen, transient kinin release and transient BAEe hydrolase activity. Moreover, the effect of epinephrine exceed that of nonepinephrine (isoprenaline had no effect) and it is inhibited by either α- or β-adrenergic antagonists – the former being more potent. In the normal man, epinephrine infusion in 1–2 µg doses had no such effect (COLMAN et al., 1976). Since α-adrenergic blockers had been used to reduce the flushing in carcinoid syndrome with some success (OATES et al., 1967), it is possible that in these patients a substance from the tumor is released into the circulation which potentiates the action of epinephrine on the kinin system. Whether this is mediated through a tissue (tumor) or plasma kallikrein is not known.

2. Postgastrectomy Dumping Syndrome

Soon after the advent of gastric surgery, "postgastrectomy dumping syndrome" became a known entity (MIX, 1922). JOHNSON and JESSEPH (1961) showed evidence that this syndrome was mediated by humoral factors. Since then, intensive efforts were made to identify the mediators responsible for this syndrome.

The clinical features of dumping syndrome may be divided into gastrointestinal symptoms such as nausea, vomiting, epigastric fullness, and diarrhea and vasomotor phenomenon. Objective vasomotor changes in this syndrome include increased peripheral blood flow and skin temperature in the face of a decrease in blood volume (BELL, 1965; HINSHAW et al., 1957; DUTHIE et al., 1959; ROBERTS et al., 1954). Although many substances have been postulated as the possible mediator for this syndrome including substance P (PERNOW, 1963), histamine and prostaglandins (LUCAS and READ, 1966), attention soon focused on bradykinin and serotonin as the humoral mediators of this syndrome. Part of the reason was due to the striking similarities of the dumping and carcinoid syndrome as pointed out by ZEITLIN et al. (1966) who were the first to demonstrate the role of kinins in the pathogenesis of dumping symptoms, as assessed by bioassay (BROCKLEHURST and ZEITLIN, 1967).They found elevated plasma kinin and decreased kininogen concentrations in patients with dumping syndrome after they received hypertonic glucose by mouth. This elevation of plasma kinin was not found in normal subjects fed hypertonic glucose or in patients with this syndrome given artifically sweetened water. The mechanism of the kinin release was later studied only in part (ZEITLIN, 1970) by the same workers. These findings were confirmed by others (BLUMEL et al., 1967; CUSCHIERI and ONABANJO, 1971) in humans and MCDONALD et al. (1969) in dogs.

The development of radioimmunoassay for bradykinin (TALAMO et al., 1969) and a biochemical assay for prekallikrein (COLMAN et al., 1969b, c) enabled a detailed examination of the plasma kallikrein-kinin system in the pathogenesis of this syndrome in postgastrectomy patients (WONG et al., 1974). Five patients with characteristic history of dumping syndrome were studied together with five asymptomatic postgastrectomy patients as controls. All patients with dumping syndrome had a drop in mean blood pressure (19%), diarrhea, and headaches, following the test meal consisting of 200 ml 45% glucose. During the symptomatic stage, the kinin concentration rose from normal values to levels exceeding 3 ng/ml. In contrast, none in the control group showed this finding. In two of the five patients with dumping syndrome there was evidence of activation of plasma prekallikrein, as shown by the drop of prekallikrein to 27% and 30% of baseline values together with consumption of kallikrein inhibitor and a five-fold increase in the spontaneous arginine esterase activity. This arginine esterase activity was identified as plasma kallikrein by two criteria. The specificity toward four amino acid substrates was similar to kaolin-activated arginine esterase as well as purified plasma kallikrein (WONG et al., 1974). In addition, incubation of plasma from this patient at the height of symptoms (15 min) released 50 ng/ml of bradykinin from a kininogen substrate compared with 3 ng/ml with buffer. In the remaining three patients, there was no evidence activation of plasma kallikrein-kinin system as was the case in the five control patients. These findings suggest that at least two mechanisms of kinin release exist to account for the vasomotor symptoms. In some patients, formation of plasma kallikrein leads to release of bradykinin in the others, tissue kallikrein apparently causes the increase of bradykinin in plasma. ZEITLIN (1970) presented evidence that exposure of blood-free jejunum to hypertonic glucose resulted in the liberation of kallikrein proportional to the osmolarity. More recently, they (ZEITLIN et al., 1976) were able to isolate kallikrein from the rat intestine by autolytic processes and obtained a single peak of kallikrein activity with a MW of 33,000. This demonstration of mucosal kallikrein activity in the small and large intestine was similar to the findings of others (WERLE, 1960; AMUNDSEN and NUSTAD, 1965) but differs from the work of SEKI et al. (1972) who failed to find any kallikrein activity in the small intestine and showed that colonic kallikrein was essentially similar to that of plasma kallikrein in MW, liberation of bradykinin rather than kallikrein, and susceptibility to proteolytic inhibitors. One possible way to reconcile this discrepancy may be that the mucosa kallikreins isolated by the former workers were purified from rats while the colon kallikrein was isolated from human, dog, and monkey. In addition, a different substrate was used by SEKI et al. (1972). Technically it might be difficult under normal circumstances to isolate the mucosal kallikrein of the gut since these mediators may reside in the APUD cells (as discussed under carcinoid syndrome) which are scattered sparsely in the normal gut mucosal cells. Even though the kinins are capable of causing contractions of the smooth muscle of the gut (SEKI et al., 1972), it is generally believed that in dumping syndrome, they are responsible only for the vasomotor symptoms. The gastrointestinal symptoms of dumping syndrome in the dog usually occur at a later part of the symptom-complex corresponding to the delayed increase in serotonin levels (MACDONALD et al., 1969). Whether this relationship holds true in man remains to be established.

3. Septic Shock

Because of its ability to lower blood pressure in normal man (MASON and MELMON, 1965) and animals (ROCHA E SILVA et al., 1949), bradykinin has been implicated in the pathogenesis of several shock syndrome (e.g., septic, cardiogenic, anaphylactic, etc.). Proper interpretations of many of these studies, however, are not possible due either to poor experimental design or limited number of components of the kallikrein-kinin system measured. The discussion of this section will involve mainly the changes in the kallikrein-kinin system in the pathogenesis of septic shock.

The early peripheral vascular changes accompanying gram-negative bacteremia (MCLEAN et al., 1967) and endotoxin shock (NIES et al., 1968) are similar to that of bradykinin infusion (ELLIOT et al., 1960), including arteriolar dilatation and vascular constriction (PAGE and OLMSTED, 1961; MASON and MELMON, 1965; ROWLEY, 1964).

In experimental works involving Rhesus monkey (NIES et al., 1968), baboons (HERMAN et al., 1974), and dogs (KELLERMEYER and GRAHAM, 1968; SARDESAI and ROSENBERG, 1974), infusion of endotoxin or E. coli led to decrease of plasma kininogen and increase of plasma kinin. In contrast these changes were not found in rabbits (ERDÖS and MIWA, 1968). In rats (MASON et al., 1970; SARDESAI and ROSENBERG, 1974) injection of endotoxin caused a transient decrease in plasma prekallikrein and kallikrein inhibitors. In some of these animal models, cellulose sulfate infusion and prior exposure of plasma to glass beads could partially alleviate the situation. The suggested mechanisms involved were said to be associated with the partial depletion of plasma kininogen by cellulose sulfate and the depletion of factor XII by contact with glass. Unfortunately, the kallikrein-kinin system differ from species to species (GREEN et al., 1974) and the application of these data to man may be hazardous since the kinetics of the kinin forming system in certain laboratory animals (e.g., rabbits, dogs) is very different from man. The changes of this system in man (MASON et al., 1970; HIRSCH et al., 1974; ROBINSON et al., 1975) following gram-negative septicemic shock are similar to those of baboons and monkeys. Early transient appearance of spontaneous arginine esterase occurs (MASON et al., 1970; ROBINSON et al., 1975) with substrate ratio almost identical to purified human kallikrein or kaolin-activated human kallikrein in plasma in some of the patients. By the use of a different method for determining plasma kallikrein (expressed as μg bradykinin released per hour) HIRSCH et al. (1974) did not find any difference in the kallikrein activity in the plasma of shock patients and that of normal controls. However, most studies (MASON et al., 1970; ROBINSON et al., 1975; O'DONNELL et al., 1976) demonstrated a significant decrease in plasma prekallikrein in acute endotoxemia or gram-negative sepsis in man. In some studies (MASON et al., 1970; O'DONNELL et al., 1976) the kallikrein inhibitor was shown to be depleted suggesting the conversion of prekallikrein to kallikrein with subsequent inactivation of the latter in a stoichiometric complex with C1 esterase inhibitor. Another evidence for the activation of plasma kallikrein-kinin system was the depletion of plasma kininogen and the liberation of kinins in plasma (HIRSCH et al., 1974). The mechanism of activation of the plasma kallikrein-kinin system in septic shock in man is probably mediated through Hageman factor since this procoagulant level is decreased in the studied patients (MASON et al., 1970). The biochemical mechanisms of generation of kinin by endotoxin has recently been studied by MILLER et al. (1973). Lately, many workers have shown that plasma kallikrein have other important functions besides the release of plasma kinin (KAPLAN and AUSTEN, 1970; REVAK et al., 1973; WEBSTER and PIERCE, 1973; BAGDASARIAN et al., 1973b). After contact with endotoxin, Hageman factor is converted to plasma prekallikrein activators (KAPLAN and AUSTEN, 1970). The activation of Hageman factor, however, requires a feedback activation by the liberated plasma kallikrein. The measurement of plasma kininogen in septic patients has also prognostic value. In young victims of trauma injuries complicated by sepsis, there was a good correlation between kininogen and the outcome of shock (HIRSCH et al., 1974). A drop in the kininogen substrate of plasma kallikrein to zero or near zero usually indicated a lethal outcome of the shock in hospitalized patients. The kininogen levels rose toward normal in those shock patients who had survived.

The sequence of events in human septic shock may include the following steps: Activation of Hageman factor with resultant decrease in plasma level; conversion of Hageman factor to prekallikrein activators; activation of prekallikrein (as evidenced by drop in plasma value); releae of free kinin into the circulation together with depletion of plasma kininogen. These changes, thus, are part of the systemic response to gram-negative sepsis in man.

The release of plasma kinin, together with the decrease in peripheral vascular resistance, occur early in endotoxemia. However, the appearance and elevated levels of kinin is short-lived (ROBINSON et al., 1975), other mechanisms, possibly initiated by endotoxin are necessary to explain continuation of the hemodynamic changes seen in patients with gram-negative infection. There is increasing clinical evidence that the complement system may be involved in hypotension associated with some bacterial and viral infections (MCCABE, 1973; ROBINSON et al., 1975). The protracted vasodilation seen in the later stages of septic shock may be mediated by the anaphylatoxic activity of C3a and C5a generated by activation of either the classic or alternate pathways.

The role of endotoxin in the activation of plasma kallikrein-kinin system in early stage of septic shock thus appeared well established. This activation is mediated via active Hageman factor which may in turn be released by contact with exposed collagen secondary to endothelial damage. Endotoxin is capable of producing endothelial cell damage by electron microscopy (MCGRATH and STEWART, 1969). Since Hageman factor can also participate in complement activation (RUDDY et al., 1972), the activation of the complement system in these patients in later stages of septic shock could also result from the activation of this procoagulant. In addition to the continued release of endotoxin from the gram-negative bacteremia, there is some evidence that hypotensive episodes from bradykinin could in itself generate endotoxin release from the gut of the animal (CUEVAS and FINE, 1973). Intravenous infusion of bradykinin into the animal for several hours led to the persistence of endotoxemia even after stopping the infusion of bradykinin. This sugests that bradykinin and other vasoactive agents allows endotoxin to enter the circulation from the intestine in an amount sufficient to become a self-sustaining endotoxemia or discontinuation of the infusion. Norepinephrine also participates since sympathetic denervation of a tissue protects it from damage by endotoxin (ZETTERSTROM et al., 1964). WEBSTER and CLARK had shown also that bradykinin by itself could not inflict lasting injury without the participation of endotoxin (WEBSTER and CLARK, 1959). This interrelationship between endotoxin, kinin release, and norepinephrine is rather complex since sympathomimatic amines could active the kinin system (in the rat blood) causing a decrease in kininogen, transient increase in plasma kinin and BAEe hydrolase activity (CASTANIA and ROTHSCHILD, 1974). The exact sequence of events awaits further studies.

4. Hemorrhagic Pancreatitis

One of the most characteristic features of acute hemorrhagic pancreatitis is that of severe hypotension. The main contribution factors leading to shock in these patients are hypovolemia and release of hypotensive substances into the circulation. In dogs with experimentally induced hemorrhagic pancreatitis, the average plasma loss was 31.5% in 4 h (RYAN et al., 1965) and it increased to 39% by 6 h (ANDERSON et al., 1967). Loss of circulating blood volume, however, was not the only reason for shock since in cross-perfusion experiments, healthy recipient dogs infused with blood from dogs with hemorrhagic pancreatitis experienced a fall in blood pressure (NUGENT and ATTENDIO, 1966).

Among the humoral factors suggested as possible cause of shock in hemorrhagic pancreatitis are included prostaglandins, plasma kinins, histamine, myocardial depressant factor and virtually all the pancreatic enzymes. Since none of the animal models resemble human pancreatitis completely, one must use extreme caution in the interpretation of the published data. We will examine the evidence supporting the role of kinins in the pathogenesis of shock in hemorrhagic pancreatitis. By the use of synthetic ester substrates as a measure of kallikrein activity in the plasma, many investigators (COLMAN et al., 1969; BROWN, 1959; MURRAY, 1959; SIEGELMAN et al., 1962; SARDESAI and THAL, 1966; RYAN et al., 1965) have shown an increase of the esterolytic activity during hemorrhagic pancreatitis. This increase in spontaneous arginine esterase did not resemble the activity of any human plasma enzyme including kallikrein, thrombin, plasmin or C1 esterase (COLMAN et al., 1969). This unidentified esterase is probably a tissue kallikrein, possibly human trypsin or pancreatic kallikrein, both of which are able to liberate bradykinin from kininogen. The released kinin may thus lead to shock in pancreatitis in man. During the resolving pancreatitis a decrease of kallikrein inhibitor was noted, but this may be the effect of an unknown protease in plasma rather than consumption of the inhibitor since proteolytic enzymes such as plasmin can also destroy C1 esterase inhibitor (HARPEL, 1970).

In experimental hemorrhagic pancreatitis in the dog, kininogen concentration in the plasma is lowered (RYAN et al., 1965; PROPIERAITIS and THOMPSON, 1969; FORELL, 1955; OFSTAD, 1970). This decrease in plasma kininogen in itself, however, is an uncertain indicator of kinin formation since the decrease can be due to enzymatic destruction without formation of kinins (HABERMANN, 1970), dilution of plasma, general lowering of plasma protein concentration as well as kinin formation. Similarly, the acyl-arginine esters may be split by several proteases (LAAKE and VENNEROD, 1974). Moreover, the complex between kallikrein and α_2-macroglobulin which is without kininogenase activity, retains considerable esterase activity (LAAKE and VENNEROD, 1974). In order to evaluate the pathophysiologic importance of kinins in pancreatitis, it is necessary to measure all the factors of the kinin cascade such as kallikrein activity, kallikrein inhibitor, kininogen content, free kinins, and kininase activities of the circulating plasma, peritoneal fluid, and the arterio-venous differences across the pancreatic bed during pancreatitis. Needless to say, very few studies fulfill such requirements.

OFSTAD (1970) using the canine model of hemorrhagic pancreatitis (by intrapancreatic injection of trypsin) showed that in the exudate that seeps from the pancreas into the peritoneal cavity, there is intense kinin formation, accompanied by a high rate of kinin destruction. Free kallikrein activity could not be demonstrated in the blood, but a moderate increase of free kinin activity was observed in some of the dogs. The kininase activity was high in the circulation and the kininogen content was rather low during the later stages of the pancreatitis. Others using a similar experimental model (PROPIERAITIS and THOMPSON, 1969) have found that the arteriovenous difference in kininogen levels across the pancreatic vascular bed during the induced pancreatitis was 40% suggesting that the kinin release occurs mainly in the pancreas itself. In the exudates from the pancreas (OFSTAD, 1970) the kininogen and inhibitor activity were absent although kallikrein activity was high. In the circulating plasma, however, the free kallikrein activity of these dogs did not change and there was sufficient kallikrein inhibitor activity present. Thus, kinin formation and destruction occurs mainly in the abdominal cavity during hemorrhagic pancreatitis in the dog. This may account for the marked exudation into the peritoneal cavity and the intense abdominal pain associated with this condition. Urine of these dogs contain very high kallikrein activity which was attributed to the pancreatic kallikrein. OFSTAD (1970) postulated the pancreatic kallikrein excreted in urine during hemorrhagic pancreatitis probably resulted from a cleavage of a kallikrein-inhibitor complex in the kidney by renal enzymes.

An inhibitor derived from bovine lung to pancreatic kallikrein has been isolated and shown to be a polypeptide with a molecular weight of 6500 consisting of 58 amino acids (HABERMANN, 1970) and made commercially under the name of Trasylol (aprotinin). Aprotinin inhibits trypsin, chymotrypsin and plasmin (TRAUTSCHOLD et al., 1966; MARX et al., 1959). In experimental animals, aprotinin seemed to reduce the mortality strikingly from induced pancreatitis (RYAN et al., 1965; HAIG and THOMPSON, 1964). Some reports of its human use in pancreatitis were enthusiastic, but this has not been the experience of other investigators (RYAN et al., 1965; HAIG and THOMPSON, 1964). The relative low rate of success in the treatment of hemorrhagic pancreatitis using aprotinin may be explained in part by the difference of the kinin systems in man and dog (GREEN et al., 1974) and that the animal models of pancreatitis may be a poor simulator of human pancreatitis.

III. Acquired (Suspected)

1. Coronary Artery Disease

It has been suggested that the kallikrein-kinin system may take part in the hemodynamic response to myocardial ischemia and the pain associated with decreased perfusion. The final mediator, bradykinin, is a known coronary vasodilator and produces pain. In a study of 11 patients experiencing ischemia with angina or typical ST-segment changes in electrocardiograms during a pacing stress test, seven showed activation of the plasma kallikrein system, with increase of free kallikrein, and with decrease of prekallikrein and kallikrein inhibitor (PITT et al., 1969). Since plasma factor XII activity decreased in patients who experienced ischemia, the changes appeared to be mediated by activation of factor XII. Frequently, this finding represented the first change noted in serial samples. In contrast, in six patients who did not have evidence of ischemia, there were no important changes in factor XII, prekallikrein, kallikrein, or inhibitor as compared to normal controls. At present the mode of activation of factor XII and the hemodynamic factors determining whether activation of plasma kallikrein would occur are unknown. In this disease injection of certain proteolytic enzymes into animals causes cardiovascular shock, with release of kinins and depletion of kininogen. Perhaps ischemic tissue releases prekallikrein activators. Three other groups have confirmed the involvement of the kallikrein-kinin system in coronary artery disease by demonstrating a decrease in kininogen levels in myocardial infarction (SICUTERI et al., 1970; WIEGERSHAUSEN et al., 1970) as well as a fall in prekallikrein and kallikrein inhibitor (SICUTERI et al., 1972). More recently, HASHIMOTO et al. (1975) have demonstrated a marked decrease in prekallikrein in acute myocardial infarction, angina, congestive heart failure, tachyarrythmias, and heart block with an accompanying fall in kininogen in many of these same clinical syndromes. In patients who survived myocardial infarction, the kininase level also dropped but in nonsurvivors the kininase level was normal suggesting that kinin formation may be helpful in reducing the work load of the heart.

2. Intravascular Coagulation

a) Disseminated Intravascular Coagulation (DIC)

Because of the known occurrence of DIC in gram-negative sepsis and the frequent simultaneous occurrence of kallikrein activation (see Sect. II.B.3.) it appeared important to evaluate which of the patients with DIC had changes in the kinin forming system. In 10 patients with DIC (thought to be due to endothelial injury or endotoxinemia including gram-negative sepsis, gram-positive sepsis or viremia), decreased plasma factor XII, prekallikrein, and kallikrein inhibitory activity were documented. This pattern would be expected if factor XII were activated. In contrast, 11 patients with equally severe DIC (due to tissue injury or thromboplastin release including leukemia, carcinoma of the prostate, aortic aneurysm abortion, and cardiac arrest) had no significant changes in the kallikrein system (MASON and COLMAN, 1971; MINNA et al., 1974). Although HARPEL (1970) found a decrease in vivo in C1 inactivator due to the proteolytic digestion of the inhibitor by plasmin, patients with pathologic fibrinolysis in vivo showed no change in free kallikrein, prekallikrein, or $C\bar{1}$ inactivator (COLMAN et al., 1969). Conversely, the formation of kallikrein would be expected to enhance fibrinolysis since purified human kallikrein can directly convert plasminogen to plasmin (COLMAN, 1969).

Activation of the intrinsic coagulation system has also been demonstrated in polycythemia vera (CARVALHO and ELLMAN, 1976). Intravascular coagulation was documented in all of 17 patients by the demonstration of HMW fibrinogen derivatives. In the same patients with polycythemia vera, factor XII was reduced to 55% of normal, prekallikrein to 78% of normal, and kallikrein inhibitor level was decreased in 12 of 17 patients. The pattern suggested occurrence of an initial activation of factor XII with subsequent activation of prekallikrein.

b) Localized Intravascular Coagulation (Renal Allograft Rejection)

Although DIC may occasionally accompany renal allograft rejection, coagulation studies by COLMAN et al. (1969a) in hyperacute and other forms of allograft rejection indicate that localized fibrin formation, platelet aggregates and vasoconstriction are the primary changes leading to ischemia and graft death. COLMAN et al. (1972) studied a patient who was presensitized to all potential donors and was treated with high doses of heparin prior to, during, and following transplantation. The graft survived and no fibrin thrombi were detected in several biopsies. Marked fibrinolysis, manifested by increased fibrin(ogen) products and shortened euglobulin lysis, occurred along with activation of plasma kallikrein, reflected by decreased prekallikrein and kallikrein inhibitory activity. These results have been confirmed and extended in a primate model of hyperacute renal allograft rejection (BUSCH et al., 1975a). Specifically presensitized Macaca speciosa monkeys reject renal allografts in 2 min. High dose heparin prolongs grafts to 105 min (BUSCH et al., 1975b) with increased fibrinolysis (decreased plasma plasminogen) and kallikrein activation (decreased factor XII, prekallikrein, and kallikrein inhibitor). Thus, despite inhibition of thrombin formation and activation by heparin, fibrinolysis occurs probably due to activation of plasminogen by kallikrein. Kallikrein would also be expected to release bradykinin, a potent vasodilator that enhances glomerular filtration and increase renal blood flow. Activation of the kallikrein-kinin system may protect against renal cortical necrosis by opposing the vasoconstriction known to favor it (HOLLENBERG et al., 1968). Independently, MOORE et al. (1974) have also found kallikrein activation, in renal allografts in rats, which did not occur after isografts.

3. Hyperlipoproteinemia

Serious illness and death in patients with the common hyperlipoproteinemias, type II (familial hypercholesterolemia) and type IV (hypertriglyceridemia) are usually from the thrombotic complications of atherosclerosis. Both of these groups of patients have intravascular coagulation characterized by elevation of plasma HMW fibrin(ogen) derivatives (CARVAHLO et al., 1976). However, the mode of activation of the clotting system is not the same. Hyperreactive platelets occur in type II but not type IV individuals (CARVALHO et al., 1974a). Hyperactive platelets may be a cause or a result of the accelerated atherosclerosis in type II patients and may be associated with changes in the vessel lining. Nineteen untreated type II patients had significantly low prekallikrein concentrations (60% of normal) and markedly decreased kallikrein inhibitory activity (50% of normal). Factor XII levels were slightly lower than normal (84%) but not significantly depressed (CARVALHO et al., 1977). These changes suggested the activation of the intrinsic system at the level of Hageman factor may occur with subsequent prekallikrein activation and depleting kallikrein inhibitors. In contrast, no significant changes in factor XII, prekallikrein, or kallikrein inhibitory activity were present in type IV hyperlipoporteinemia. These changes were parallel to platelet function in these two groups. Since platelet hypersensitivity in type II individuals can be partially reversed by clofibrate (CARVALHO et al., 1974b), the efforts of this drug in prekallikrein activation was studied in both types of hyperlipoproteinemia. Clofibrate significantly increased factor XII to 108%, prekallikrein to 88% and kallikrein inhibitory activity to 80% of normal while no appreciable change occurred in these activities in the type IV patients (CARVALHO et al., 1977). The relationship of these changes to the parallel change in platelet function on the drug is uncleàr at present.

4. Thermal Injury

Thermal injury to the skin is associated with cutaneous inflammation which manifests as pain, local vasodilatation, increased capillary permeability, and accumulation of leukocytes. Chemical mediators for the inflammatory process induced by thermal burns has been intensely sought. Histamine (WILHELM and MASON, 1960), serotonin (Leading article, Lancet, 1960), and bradykinin have all been incriminated as possible mediators responsible for the inflammation. Histamine is found locally in the burn area (BROCKLEHURST and ZEITLIN, 1967) yet the administration of antihistamines does not alter the increased permeability induced by controlled burns of guinea pig skin, except for the immediate flush that occurs with very mild burns (SEVITT, 1949). Serotonin is unlikely to work alone as mediator of the inflammation since arterial infusion of serotonin may lead to cutaneous vasoconstriction (EMERSON et al., 1972).

Bradykinin is one of the most potent algogenic (pain-producing) substance in the human skin (KEELE and ARMSTRONG, 1964). The application of bradykinin to a blister base in human skin (KEELE and ARMSTRONG, 1964) or the intra-arterial injections of the peptide causes pain (FOX et al., 1961). This algogenic effect in the human hand is potentiated by prior injection of 5-hydroxytryptamine (serotonin) into the hand vein so that smaller doses of bradykinin are required to produce pain. The vein traumatized by serotonin remains sensitive to bradykinin for days (SICUTERI, 1968). This serotonin-bradykinin interaction may be important in the pathophysiology of pain in thermal injury. The role played by kinin in the regulation of local vasodilatation in thermal injury is not clearly understood. Because of its probable role in the regulation of functional hyperemia in salivary glands (GAUTVIK, 1970a, b, c), it is assumed that kinin release may be important in regulating cutaneous blood flow according to metabolic changes during thermal burns (ROBERTS and MASHFORD, 1972). Kinins are potent substances capable of increasing capillary permeability. On a molar basis, bradykinin is more active than histamine in increasing capillary permeability (ELLIOT et al., 1960). Kinins by themselves are relatively poor chemotactic factors in attracting leucocyte migration. Plasma kallikrein, however, has been shown to possess this property (KAPLAN and AUSTEN, 1972b). Thus, components of the plasma kallikrein-kinin system are capable of producing pain, local vasodilatation, increased capillary permeability and the migration of leucocytes to area of injury in mammals. The tissue elements which accumulate during inflammation included both kinin-forming and kinin-destroying enzymes which are probably different from the corresponding plasma enzymes (GREENBAUM et al., 1970).

By immersing a rat paw in water at 44–45 °C, ROCHA E SILVA and ANTONIO (1960) found that during "thermic edema," bradykinin appeared in the perfusate (from coaxial perfusion of the subcutaneous space). Similarly, the level of bradykinin in venous blood from the human hand has been found to increase by up to 53% when the area is immersed in water at 45 °C. It has been suggested that tissue changes following this kind of mild thermal injury could be mediated entirely by the kinin-releasing system of tissue since the kinin concentration in the blood entering the hand is not increased by this procedure (MASHFORD and ZACEST, 1967).

5. Arthritis

Although sodium urate crystals can activate factor XII (KELLERMEYER, 1964) and kinins can be found in effusions from patients with gouty arthritis (KELLERMEYER and BRECKENRIDGE, 1965; MELMON et al., 1967), subsequent data suggested that kinins do not play a primary role in the pathogenesis of gouty arthritis (KELLERMEYER and NAGG, 1975). The available data, however, do not rule out the possibility that kinins participate in the inflammatory reaction of certain arthitides. In gouty attack, only two components appeared to be absolutely essential – monosodium urate crystals and granulocytic leucocytes (PHELPS and MCCARTY, 1966). Since urate crystals can activate factor XII in vitro, it is important to assess their role in the pathophysiology of acute gout. Although chickens lack factor XII, they were reported to develop gout spontaneously (PETERSON et al., 1971). This kind of gout, however, appeared to be mainly tophaceous. Nevertheless, the data suggest that factor XII is not essential for the inflammation induced by urate crystals. Despite the presence of kinins in the synovial effusions during acute gout, there is no direct data to support their role in the inflammatory process in acuty gouty joints. The simultaneous injection of urate crystals and carboxypeptidase B (a potent kininase) did not result in a diminution of the inflammatory response in the canine stifle joint (PHELPS et al., 1966). TALAMO et al. (1969) using the bradykinin immunoassay, have found kinin levels of less than 3 ng/ml in eight synovial fluids from chronic effusions in patients with osteoarthritis. These levels were comparable to those found in normal human plasma by the same authors. Finally, the direct injection of bradykinin into dog stifle joint produced little inflammation and no pain (VAN ARMAN and BOHIDAR, 1976). The possibility of rapid removal of the injected bradykinin, however, has not been ruled out (ERDÖS, 1969). On the other hand, the same kininases present in the joint fluid may also be present to prevent onset of inflammation in the gouty joint.

6. Allergic Disorders

The chemical mediators of anaphylactic reaction, bronchial asthma, chronic urticaria and other exogenous allergies probably include histamine, kallikrein, kinins, slow-reacting substances, serotonin, catecholamines, complement, neutral proteases, and anaphylotoxin. The mechanism of activation of these factors and their role and interrelations (if any) are still poorly understood.

There is some evidence that kinins may participate in anaphylactic reactions. Raised plasma kinins were reported to occur in animals during anaphylaxis (BERALDO, 1950; BROCKLEHURST and LAHINI, 1962; JONASSON and BECKER, 1966). Antigen-antibody complexes do result in the release of kinins that appears to be dependent on Hageman factor (MOVAT et al., 1966). In addition, these complexes could cause the release of a permeability-enhancing activity that is dependent on $C\bar{1}$, 4, and 3 (DAVIES and LOWE, 1962).

COLLIER et al. (1966) reported that i.v. injection of bradykinin into unsensitized guinea pigs resulted in marked bronchoconstriction. Since then, many investigators have tried to incriminate bradykinin as a major mediator in the pathogenesis of bronchial asthma (LUKJAN et al., 1972; HERXHEIMER and STRESEMAN, 1961). In support of this, LUKJAN et al. (1972) found that during acute asthmatic attack, there was a significant rise in the kallikrein level, a decrease of kininogen, and the appearance of kinins in the plasma. The mean level of kininases in patients with bronchial asthma was significantly lower than that of controls. Others have shown that bradykinin aerosol when given to asthmatic patients resulted in decreased vital capacity, bronchospasm, and wheezing (HERXHEIMER and STRESEMAN, 1961). More recently, these findings have been challenged. BRISEID et al. (1976) in a controlled study found no significant difference in the factor XII, prekallikrein activator, prekallikrein, and kallikrein inhibitors in asthmatic patients and the controls. The discrepancy in findings between the studies of LUKJAN (1972) and BRISEID et al. (1976) could, in part, be explained by different methods of assay since the former used a bioassay and the latter used several established chemical assays.

Recently, there has been scanty evidence suggesting a role of kallikrein-kinin system in urticarial reactions of the skin (DOEGLAS and BLEUMINK, 1975; THUNE et al., 1976; DOEGLAS and BLEUMINK, 1974). Since only one or two components of the kinin pathway were measured, no firm conclusion could be drawn as to the significance of these findings.

7. Transfusion Reactions, Hemodialysis, and Extracorporeal Bypass

The transfusion of a fraction of human plasma containing factor VIII prepared by ether fractionation in glass bottles gave rise to prominent flushing and hypotension resembling the injection of bradykinin (MAYCOCK et al., 1963). Study of this preparation revealed the presence of activated plasma kallikrein which would potentially release large amounts of bradykinin. Ether fractionation is known to remove C$\bar{1}$ inhibitor and glass accelerates the activation of factor XII. Thus, the conversion of prekallikrein to kallikrein arterial hypotension in dogs has been noted in dogs given homologous blood during exchange or bypass (MACKAY et al., 1965) and this can be obviated by avoiding the use of glass. IZAKA et al. (1975) have demonstrated kininogen and kinin-like activity (IZAKA et al., 1974) in plasma fractions isolated using Cohn's cold ethanol fractionation. In addition, MORICHI and IZAKA (1976) found kininase activity and when this enzyme was inhibited with 1.10 phenatholine, a kallikrein-like enzyme was also found. In human patients given these preparations, arterial hypotension has been reported.

An experimental model of transfusion reaction can be produced in Macaca iris monkeys (LOPAS et al., 1973) by infusion of isoantibodies directed against red cells. The monkeys developed severe intravascular hemolysis, DIC (prolonged thrombin time and a fall in platelets, fibrinogen, factors V, VIII, and X). Plasma kallikrein appeared to be activated as evidenced by a fall in prekallikrein to 66% of prefusion level, a fall in kallikrein inhibitor activity to 56% of preinfusion level, and a rise in spontaneous arginine esterase activity to 161% of control levels. In one animal the enzyme was identified as kallikrein. The mechanism of this activation is not clear but may be due to induced endothelial injury by the antibody-antigen complex, plasmin formation or release of activators for white cells or platelets.

In hemodialysis, increased spontaneous enzyme esterase activity (presumptive kallikrein), decreased prekallikrein, and decreased Hageman factor have been observed in the venous effluent in both the Kiil and coil dialysers (WARDLE and PIERCY, 1972) as well as in the systemic venous blood of the patients. Interestingly, platelet factor 4 was also elevated in plasma indicating contact injury to the platelets. Since the lung inactivated 80% of the bradykinin during a single circulation this might not be a major clinical concern. However, during entracorporeal circulation, bypass of the lung might allow accumulation of bradykinin if it were released. Total kininogen is reduced proportional to the time of bypass and kinin was increased during the use of the artificial heart-lung machine (KATORI and NAGAOYA, 1970). However, the kininogen was determined using trypsin and therefore probably did not represent HMW kininogen, the preferred substrate of plasma kallikrein. The inhibition of reduction of kininogen by aprotinin (not a good inhibitor of plasma kallikrein) raises further doubt of the role of plasma kallikrein in this process. Studies are underway in our laboratory using more specific assays to assess the significance of these findings.

8. Cystic Fibrosis

Cystic fibrosis, a disease characterized by abnormally thick mucus secretion and frequent infections, has been attributed to elevated concentrations of macromolecular "factors." These have been postulated to be due to the deficiency of a proteolytic enzyme (RAO and NADLER, 1973) which hydrolyses and inactivates these noxious polypeptides. RAO et al. (1972) found that arginine esterase activity activated by ellagic acid in chloroform-treated plasma from cystic fibrosis patients was about 50% of control plasma and concluded that there was a deficiency in plasma kallikrein activity. These same investigators (RAO and NADLER, 1974), using ion exchange chromatography and iso-electric focusing, demonstrated both quantitative and qualitative abnormalities in arginine esterase activity in patients with cystic fibrosis which they attributed to genetic heterogenity. They further demonstrated a decrease in proteolytic activity using protamine sulfate as a substrate (RAO and NADLER, 1975). However, LIEBERMAN (1974), was unable to confirm any decrease in plasma arginine esterase activity in individuals with cystic fibrosis. Moreover, in a study of five cystic fibrosis patients, TALAMO et al. (1972) demonstrated normal levels of prekallikrein and bradykinin, normal bradykinin-generating ability of plasma, and normal activity of kininases I and II. GOLDSMITH et al. (1977) have extended these studies by showing that plasma kallikrein is not deficient in cystic fibrosis. They demonstrated normal levels of prekallikrein by coagulant and esterase assays as well as by immunochemical determination. The occurrence of a complete deficiency of prekallikrein (Fletcher trait) in asymptomatic individuals (WUEPPER, 1972) apparently eliminates any pathogenetic role for this enzyme is cystic fibrosis. However, these studies do not rule out the deficiency of a yet unrecognized arginine esterase and protease in cystic fibrosis.

9. Typhoid Fever

Unlike gram-negative sepsis, endotoxin has not been detected during typhoid fever although disseminated intravascular coagulation does occur. COLMAN et al. (1978) reported sequential functional and immunochemical assays of six kinin system proteins, three coagulant factors, factor XII (Hageman factor), prekallikrein, HMW kininogen, three protease inhibitors, α_1-antitrypsin, α_2-macroglobulin, and C1 esterase inhibitor in 5 patients with typhoid fever and 5 control individuals who ingested S. typhi but did not contract the disease. The results suggest that the activation of prekallikrein to kallikrein as well as its inhibition through complex formation occurs concomitant with typhoid fever.

Although the time course of the changes in typhoid fever was variable, in a typical course 10 days after ingestion of S. typhi, blood cultures became positive for that organism accompanied by the development of fever. A parallel decrease of platelets, prekallikrein, and kallikrein inhibitory activity occurred in all five patients with a nadir on day 5 of about 50% of the prechallenge level at onset of fever. Thereafter, all of these components returned to baseline by day 9–11 following the fever with development of an overshoot as the fever subsides. No consistent changes occurred in coagulant factor XII or in immunochemical levels of prekallikrein, C1 esterase inhibitor or α_2-macroglobulin. In contrast, α_1-antitrypsin, a known acute phase reactant, rose to a peak value of 145% of prechallenge level on day 7 following fever and then fell to normal during convalescence. HMW kininogen increased to a maximum on day 5–7 and return to normal levels by 13–14 days after fever.

One possible explanation for the decrease in functional kallikrein and its inhibitor, with apparently normal immunochemical levels of both proteins, is the formation of a nonfunctional circulating complex of kallikrein and $C\bar{1}$ esterase inhibitor in which both proteins maintain their antigen identity. Therefore, plasma obtained prior to injection or typhoid and 5–7 days after the onset of fever, were compared in all 5 affected individuals. The results were similar in all five patients: Using immunoelectrophoresis, the existence of a complex displaying the antigenic characteristics of both prekallikrein and C1 esterase inhibitor was demonstrated. In contrast, the precipitin arcs for α_1-antitrypsin and α_2-macroglobulin showed no difference in their position or appearance compared with baseline plasma samples. This kallikrein C1 esterase inhibitor complex was also demonstrable by crossed immunoelectrophoresis using antisera against both proteins.

The failure to detect significant changes in factor XII is not unexpected. Although factor XII must be converted to an active form, the coagulant assay measures both inactive and active but unfragmented factor XII. However, in forming Hageman factor fragment, factor XII loses its coagulant activity and in acute endotoxemic states, factor XII coagulant activity has been decreased although to a lesser extent than prekallikrein (MASON et al., 1970). Factor XII is capable of cleaving more than one molecule of kallikrein and, in the fragmented form, its ability to activate prekallikrein may increase 1000-fold (BAGDASARIAN et al., 1973b). Therefore, only a small number of factor XII molecules must be activated to convert prekallikrein to kallikrein and this may not be detectable with current methods.

The pathogenesis of the changes in HMW kininogen are less clear. Although bovine HMW kininogen loses activity following cleavage by kallikrein (MATHESON et al., 1976), this does not appear to be the case in human preparations (COLMAN et al., 1975). Liberation of all the kinin from human HMW kininogen failed to change its coagulant activity. The variation of this protein in disease is incompletely understood since its vital role in plasma proteolysis has been only recently appreciated. SAITO et al. (1976) have reported a decrease in HMW kininogen in liver disease and disseminated intravascular coagulation. The striking rise of HMW kininogen in typhoid fever may be due to its role as an acute phase reactant. ZEITLIN et al. (1976) have recently reported an elevation in kininogen in rheumatoid arthritis with a decrease with treatment with aspirin and indomethicin.

10. Nephrotic Syndrome

In the past decade it has become evident that abnormalities in the proteins of the intrinsic coagulation system are not uncommon. Low levels of factor XII were first reported in nine of 11 patients and attributed to urinary losses (HONIG and LINDLEY, 1971). However, LANGE et al. (1974) in a detailed study of a patient with nephrotic syndrome and a factor XII of 15% concentration of normal showed that the apparent XII activity in the urine was due to a nonspecific urinary procoagulant. In contrast, the decrease in factor XII appeared to be associated with activation of the intrinsic coagulation system (factor XI of 35%), the kallikrein-kinin system as manifested by prekallikrein of 37% and a concomitant decrease in plasma kallikrein inhibitory activity as well as activation of the fibrinolytic system (elevated fibrin spent products). The activation of the kallikrein-kinin system was confined by KALLEN and SOO-KWANG (1975), who studied 27 nephrotic episodes in 21 children. During the overt nephrotic syndrome prekallikrein was decreased to 58% of normal and kallikrein inhibitor to 35% of normal. With intensive steroid therapy in 14 children the prekallikrein rose to 99% of normal and the inhibitor activity to 84%. Thus, the plasma kinin-generating system may be the host mechanism subserving the increased glomerular capillary permeability.

11. Migraine Syndrome

The early literature has been well summarized by SICUTERI (1970). Perfusates from the tender areas of the scalp and the cerebrospinal fluid of patients with migraine headaches were found by some investigators (OSTFELD et al., 1957; KANGANSNIEMI et al., 1972; CHAPMAN and WOLFF, 1959) to contain kinin-like activities. Intravenous injection of bradykinin in susceptible individuals could produce severe headaches. The changes in the cerebrospinal fluid occur in about 50% of patients with migraine headache (KANGASNIEMI et al., 1972). Recently, BACK et al. (1972) found that increased kinin activity of cerebrospinal fluid is found in 14% of patients with various diseases (excluding migraine), although the cerebrospinal fluid contained none of the components of plasma-kinin system, e.g., kininogen, prekallikrein, and kininase. The significance of these findings await further evaluation.

Acknowledgements. We wish to thank Ms. DELORES LEGARE and Mr. CHARLES USCHMANN for typing this chapter.
The review was supported in part by a grant from the National Institute of Health, HL-16642 and in part by HL-18624.

References

Abildgaard, C.F., Harrison, J.: Fletcher factor deficiency. Blood *43*, 641–644 (1974)
Amundsen, E., Nustad, K.: Kinin-forming and destroying activities of cell homogenates. J. Physiol. (Lond.) *179*, 479–488 (1965)
Anderson, M.C., Schoenfeld, F.B., Iams, W.B., Suwa, M.: Circulatory changes in acute pancreatitis. Surg. Clin. North Am. *47*, 127–140 (1967)
Van Arman, C.G., Bohidar, N.R.: Role of kallikrein kinin system in inflammation. In: Chemistry and biology of the kallikrein-kinin system in health and disease. Pisano, J.J., Austen, K.F. (eds.), pp. 471–481. Fogarty Internat. Center Proc. No. 27. Washington: U.S. Gov. Printing Office 1977
Austen, K.F., Sheffer, A.L.: Detection of hereditary angioneurotic edema by demonstration of reduction of second component of complement. N. Engl. J. Med. *272*, 649–656 (1965)
Ayers, C.R.: Plasma renin activity and renin substrate concentration in patients with liver disease. Circ. Res. *20*, 594–598 (1967)
Back, N., Steger, R., Moscovich, L.L.: Determination of components of the kallikrein-kinin system in the cerebrospinal fluid of patients with various diseases. Res. Clin. Stud. Headaches *3*, 219–226 (1972)
Bagdasarian, A., Talamo, R.C., Colman, R.W.: Isolation of high molecular weight activators of prekallikrein. J. Biol. Chem. *248*, 3456–3463 (1973a)
Bagdasarian, A., Lahiri, B., Colman, R.W.: Origin of the high molecular weight activator of prekallikrein. J. Biol. Chem. *248*, 7742–7747 (1973b)
Bagdasarian, A., Lahiri, B., Talamo, R.C., Wong, P.Y., Colman, R.C.: Immunochemical studies of plasma kallikrein. J. Clin. Invest. *54*, 1444–1454 (1974)
Bell, G.: Peripheral circulation during the dumping syndrome. Br. J. Surg. *52*, 300–303 (1965)
Beraldo, W.T.: Formation of bradykinin in amaphylactic and peptone shock. Am. J. Physiol. *163*, 283–289 (1950)
Berkowitz, H.D., Galvin, C., Miller, L.D.: Significance of altered renin substrate in hepatorenal syndrome. Surg. Forum *23*, 342–343 (1972)

Black, W.C.: Enterochromaffin cell types and corresponding carcinoid tumors. Lab. Invest. *19*, 473 (1968)
Blumel, G., Klauser, G., Neumayr, A., Peschl, L., Rottenbacker-Teubner, H.: Die Bedeutung der Plasmakinine bei der Entstehung des Dumping Syndromes. Med. Welt *46*, 2751–2759 (1967)
Bokisch, V.A., Top, F.H., Jr., Russel, P.K.: The potential pathogenic role of complement in dengue hemorrhagic shock syndrome. N. Engl. J. Med. *289*, 996–1000 (1973)
Bouma, B.N., Griffin, J.H.: Human prekallikrein (plasminogen proactivator): Purification, characterization, and activation by activated factor XII. Proc. of Intl. Cong. on Throm. and Hemo.. Thromb. Hemo *38*, 136 (Abstract) (1977)
Boyer, T.D., Reynolds, T.B.: Prostaglandin insufficiency: A role in hepatorenal syndrome? Gastroenterology (1977)
Briseid, K., Qvigstaid, E.K., Engelstad, M., Kageriov, P., Lange-Nielsen, F.: Assay of factors of the kinin systems in plasma from patients with specific exogenous allergies. Acta Allergol. (Kbh.) *31*, 297–311 (1976)
Brocklehurst, W.E., Lahini, S.C.: Formation and destruction of bradykinin during anaphylaxis. J. Physiol. (Lond.) *165*, 39P (1962)
Brocklehurst, W.E., Zeitlin, I.J.: Determination of plasma kinin and kininogen levels in man. J. Physiol. (Lond.) *191*, 417–426 (1967)
Brockway, W.J., Castellino, F.J.: The mechanism of the inhibition of plasmin activity by E-aminocaproic acid. J. Biol. Chem. *246*, 4641–4647 (1971)
Brown, M.E.: Serum exopeptidase activity in diseases of the pancreas. N. Engl. J. Med. *260*, 331–332 (1959)
Burdon, K.K., Queng, J.T., Thomas, O.C., McGovern, J.P.: Observations on biochemical abnormalities in hereditary angioneurotic edema. J. Allergy *36*, 546–557 (1965)
Burrowes, C.E., Movat, H.V., Soltay, M.J.: The kinin system of human plasma VI. The action of plasmin. Proc. Soc. Exp. Biol. Med. *138*, 959–966 (1971)
Busch, G.J., Martins, A.C.P., Hollenberg, N.K., Wilson, R.E., Colman, R.W.: A primate model of hyperacute renal allograft rejection. Am. J. Pathol. *79*, 31–52 (1975a)
Busch, G.J., Kobayashi, K., Hollenberg, N.K., Birtch, A.G., Colman, R.W.: Hyperacute renal allograft rejection in the primate. Intrarenal effects of heparin and associated net release of factor VIII activity and kallikrein activation. Am. J. Pathol. *80*, 1–17 (1975b)
Bussolati, D., Rost, F.W.D., Pearse, A.G.E.: Fluorescence metachromasia in polypeptide hormone producing cells of the APUD series, and its significance in relation to the structure of the protein precursor. Histochem. J. *1*, 517 (1969)
Carpenter, C.B., Ruddy, S., Shekadeh, I.H., Stechschuste, D.J., Muller-Eberhard, H.J., Merrill, J.P., Austen, K.F.: Complement metabolism in patients with hereditary angioedema. J. Clin. Invest. *48*, 14a (1969)
Carvalheira, A.F., Welsch, U., Pearse, A.G.E.: Cytochemical and ultrastructural observations on the argentaffin and argyrophil cells of the gastrointestinal tract in mammals and their place in the APUD series of polypeptide-secreting cells. Histochemie *14*, 33–46 (1968)
Carvalho, A.C., Ellman, L.: Activation of the coagulation system in polycythemia vera. Blood *47*, 669–678 (1976)
Carvalho, A.C., Colman, R.W., Lees, R.S.: Platelet function in hyperlipoproteinemia. N. Engl. J. Med. *290*, 434–438 (1974a)
Carvalho, A.C., Colman, R.W., Lees, R.S.: Clofibrate reversal of platelet hypersensitivity in hyperlipoproteinemia. Circulation *50*, 570–574 (1974b)
Carvalho, A.C., Lees, R.S., Vaillancourt, R.A., Cabral, R.B., Weinberg, R.M., Colman, R.W.: Intravascular coagulation in hyperlipemia. Thromb. Res. *8*, 843–857 (1976)
Carvalho, A.C., Lees, R.S., Vaillancourt, R.A., Colman, R.W.: Effect of clofibrate on intravascular coagulation in hyperlipoproteinemia. Circulation *56*, 114–118 (1977)
Castania, A., Rothschild, A.M.: Lowering of kininogen in rat blood by adrenalin. Inhibition by sympatholytic agents, heparin, and aspirin. Br. J. Pharmacol. *50*, 375–383 (1974)
Chan, J.Y.C., Burrowes, C.E., Movat, H.Z.: Activation of factor XII (Hageman factor) enhancing effect of a potentiator. Thromb. Res. *10*, 309–314 (1977)
Chapman, L.F., Wolff, H.G.: Studies of proteolytic enzymes in cerobrospinal fluid. Arch. Intern. Med. *103*, 86 (1959)
Cochrane, C.G., Wuepper, K.D.: The first component of the kinin-forming system in human and rabbit plasma. J. Exp. Med. *134*, 986–1004 (1971)

Cochrane, C.G., Revak, S.D., Wuepper, K.D.: Activation of Hageman factor in solid and fluid phases. A critical role of kallikrein. J. Exp. Med. *138*, 1564–1583 (1973)
Cohen, S.H., Halstead, S.B.: Shock associated with dengue infection. I Clinical and physiologic manifestations of dengue hemorrhagic fever in Thailand 1964. J. Pediatr. *68*, 448–456 (1966)
Collier, H.O.J.: Self-antagonism of bronchoconstriction induced by bradykinin and angiotension. In: Hypotensive peptides. Erdös, E.G., Back, N., Sicuteri, F., Wilde, A.F. (eds.), pp. 305–313. Berlin, Heidelberg, New York: Springer 1966
Colman, R.W.: Activation of plasminogen by human plasma kallikrein. Biochem. Biophys. Res. Commun. *35*, 273–279 (1969)
Colman, R.W.: Formation of human plasma kinin. N. Engl. J. Med. *291*, 509–515 (1974)
Colman, R.W.: Hereditary angioedema and heparin therapy. Ann. Intern. Med. *85*, 399 (1976)
Colman, R.W., Braun, W.E., Busch, G.J., Dammin, G.J., Merrill, J.P.: Coagulation studies in hyperacute and other forms of renal allograft rejection. N. Engl. J. Med. *281*, 685–691 (1969a)
Colman, R.W., Mason, J.W., Sherry, S.: The kallikreinogen-kallikrein enzyme system of human plasma. Assay of components and observation in disease states. Ann. Intern. Med. *71*, 763–773 (1969b)
Colman, R.W., Mattler, L., Sherry, S.: Studies on the prekallikrein (kallikreinogen) – kallikrein enzyme system of human plasma II. Evidence relating the kaolin-activated arginine esterase to plasma kallikreins. J. Clin. Invest. *48*, 23–32 (1969c)
Colman, R.W., Girey, G., Galvanek, E.G., Busch, G.J.: Human renal allografts: The protective effects of heparin, kallikrein activation, and fibrinolysis during hyperacture rejection. In: Symposium on coagulation problems in transplanted organs. Kaulla, K. v. (ed.), pp. 87–102. Springfield, Ill.: Thomas 1972
Colman, R.W., Bagdasarian, A., Talama, R.C., Scott, C.F., Seavey, M., Guimaraes, J.A., Pierce, J.V., Kaplan, A.P.: Williams trait. Human kininogen deficiency with diminished levels of plasminogen proactivator and prekallikrein associated with abnormalities of the Hageman factor-dependent pathways. J. Clin. Invest. *56*, 1650–1662 (1975)
Colman, R.W., Wong, P.Y., Talamo, R.C.: Kallikrein-kinin system in carcinoid and postgastrectomy dumping syndrome. In: Chemistry and biology of the kallikrein-kinin system in health and disease. Pisano, J.J., Austen, K.F. (eds.), pp. 487–494. Fogarty Internat. Center Proc. No. 27. Washington: U.S. Gov. Printing Office 1977
Coppage, W.S., Jr., Island, D.P., Cooner, A.E., Liddle, G.W.: The metabolism of aldosterone in normal subjects and in patients with hepatic cirrhosis. J. Clin. Invest. *41*, 1672–1680 (1962)
Cuevas, P., Fine, J.: Production of fatal endotoxin shock by vasoactive substances. Gastroenterology *64*, 285–291 (1973)
Currimbhoy, Z., Vinciguerru, V., Palakavongs, P., Kuslansky, P., Degnan, T.J.: Fletcher factor deficiency and myocardial infarction. Am. J. Clin. Pathol. *65*, 970–974 (1976)
Cuschieri, A., Onabanjo, O.A.: Kinin release after gastric surgery. Br. Med. J. *1971/III*, 565–566
Daugherty, R.M., Jr., Scott, J.B., Emerson, T.E., Jr.: Comparison of IV and IA infusion of vasoactive agents on dog forelimb blood flow. Am. J. Physiol. *214*, 611–619 (1968)
Davies, G.E., Lowe, J.S.: Further studies on permeability factor released from guinea pig serum by antigen-antibody precipitates: relationship to serum complement. Int. Arch. Allergy *20*, 235–250 (1962)
Dawson, I.: The endocrine cells of the gastrointestinal tract. Histochem. J. *2*, 527–549 (1970)
Delbianco, P.L., Fanciullacci, M., Frarchi, G.: Plasmatic kininogen in acute hepatitis and in liver cirrhosis. Adv. Exp. Med. Biol. *21*, 453 (1972)
Doeglas, H.M.G., Bleumink, E.: Familial cold urticaria. Arch. Dermatol. *110*, 382–388 (1974)
Doeglas, H.M.G., Bleumink, E.: Protease inhibitors in plasma of patients with chronic urticaria. Arch. Dermatol. *111*, 979–985 (1975)
Dollery, C.T., Goldberg, L.I., Pentecost, B.L.: Effect of intrarenal infusion of bradykinin and acetylcholine on renal blood flow in man. Clin. Sci. *29*, 433–441 (1965)
Donaldson, V.H.: Mechanism of activation of C'1 esterase in hereditary angioedema plasma in vitro: Role of Hageman factor clot promoting agent. J. Exp. Med. *127*, 411–429 (1968)
Donaldson, V.H., Evans, R.R.: A biochemical abnormality in hereditary angioneurotic edema. Absence of serum inhibitor of C'1 esterase. Am. J. Med. *35*, 35–44 (1963)
Donaldson, V., Rosen, F.S.: Action of complement in hereditary angioneurotic edema: Role of C'1 esterase. J. Clin. Invest. *43*, 2204–2213 (1964)

Donaldson, V.H., Ratnoff, O.D., Dias da Silva, W., Rosen, F.S.: Permeability-increasing activity of hereditary angioneurotic edema. II. Mechanism of formation and partial characterization. J. Clin. Invest. *48*, 642–653 (1969)
Donaldson, V.H., Glueck, H.I., Miller, M.A., Movat, H.Z., Habal, F.: Kininogen deficiency in Fitzgerald trait: Role of high molecular weight kininogen in clotting and fibrinolysis. J. Lab. Clin. Med. *89*, 327–337 (1976)
Donaldson, V.H., Rosen, F.S., Bing, D.H.: Role of the second component of complement (C2) in hereditary angioneurotic edema (HANE) plasma. Clin. Res. *25*, 520A (1977)
Duthie, H.L., Irvine, W.T., Kerr, J.W.: Cardiovascular changes in the postgastrectomy syndrome. Br. J. Surg. *46*, 350–357 (1959)
Edelman, R., Nimmannitya, S., Colman, R.W., Talamo, R.C., Top, F.H.: Evaluation of the plasma kinin system in dengue hemorrhagic fever. J. Lab. Clin. Med. *86*, 410–421 (1975)
Elliot, D.F., Horton, E.W., Lewis, G.P.: Actions of pure bradykinin. J. Physiol. (Lond.) *153*, 473–480 (1960)
Emerson, T.E., Jr., Meier, P.D., Daugherty, R.M., Jr.: Dependence of skeletal muscle vascular response to serotonin upon the level of vascular resistance. Proc. Soc. Exp. Biol. Med. *142*, 1185–1188 (1972)
Erdös, E.G.: The kallikrein-kinin-kininase system. In: Cellular and human mechanisms in anaphylaxic and allergy. Movat, H.Z. (ed.), pp. 233–236. Basel: Karger 1969
Erdös, E.G., Miwa, I.: Effect of endotoxin shock on plasma kallikrein-kinin system of the rabbit. Fed. Proc. *27*, 92–95 (1968)
Escovitz, W.E., Reingold, I.M.: Functioning malignant bronchial carcinoids with Cushing's syndrome and recurrent sinus arrest. Ann. Intern. Med. *54*, 1248–1259 (1961)
Fanciullacci, M., Galli, P., Monetti, P., Pela, I., Delbianco, P.L.: Prekallikrein and kallikrein inhibitor in liver cirrhosis and hepatitis. Adv. Exp. Med. Biol. *70*, 201–308 (1975)
Fantl, P., Morris, K.N., Sawers, R.J.: Repair of cardiac defect in patient with Ehlers-Darlos syndrome and deficiency of Hageman factor. Br. Med. J. *1961/I*, 1202–1204
Forell, M.M.: Zur Frage des Entstehungs-Mechanismus des Kreislaufkollapses bei der akuten Pankreasnekrose. Gastroenterologia (Basel) *84*, 225–251 (1955)
Forsmann, W.G., Orei, L., Pictet, R., Renold, A.E., Roviller, C.: The endocrine cells in the epithelium of the gastrointestinal mucosa of the rat. J. Cell Biol. *40*, 692–715 (1969)
Fox, R.H., Goldsmith, R., Kidd, D.J., Lewis, G.P.: Bradykinin as a vasodilator in man. J. Physiol. (Lond.) *157*, 589–592 (1961)
Frank, M.M., Sergent, J.S., Kane, M.A., Alling, D.W.: Epsilon aminocaprocic acid therapy of hereditary angioedema. A double blind study. N. Engl. J. Med. *281*, 808–812 (1972)
Gadek, J.E., Hosea, S.W., Gelford, S.A., Frank, M.M.: C1 inhibitor phenotypes in hereditary angioedema. Genetic implications of successful Danazol therapy. Clin. Res. *25*, 357a (1977)
Galletti, R., Marra, N., Matassi, L., Vecchiet, L.: Decrease of skin alogogenic reactivity and plasma alogogenic activity in patients with hepatic cirrhosis. Sperimentale *117*, 371 (1967)
Galletti, R., Matassi, L., Chiarini, P., Vecchiet, L., Buzzelli, G., Marra, N.: Plasma kinin activity in cirrhotic subjects. Sperimentale *118*, 253 (1968)
Gantvik, K.: Studies in kinin formation in functional vasodilatation of the submandibular salivary gland of cats. Acta Physiol. Scand. *79*, 174–176 (1970a)
Gantvik, K.: The interaction of two different vasodilator mechanisms in the chorda tympani activated submandibular salivary gland. Acta Physiol. Scand. *79*, 188–192 (1970b)
Gantvik, K.: Parasympathetic neuro-effector transmission and functional vasodilatation in the submandibular salivary gland of cats. Acta Physiol. Scand. *79*, 204–206 (1970c)
Gigli, I., Mason, J.W., Colman, R.W., Austen, K.F.: Interaction of plasma kallikrein with the C1 inhibitor. J. Immunol. *104*, 574–581 (1970)
Gill, J.R., Melmon, K.L., Gillespie, L., Bartter, F.: Bradykinin and renal function in normal man: Effects of adrenergic blockade. Am. J. Physiol. *209*, 844–848 (1965)
Girey, G.J.D., Talamo, R.C., Colman, R.W.: The kinetics of release of bradykinin by kallikrein in normal plasma. J. Lab. Clin. Med. *80*, 465–505 (1972)
Gjonnaess, H.: Cold promoted activation of factor VII: I. Evidence for existance of an activation. Thromb. Diath. Haemorr. *28*, 155–168 (1972a)
Gjonnaess, H.: Cold promoted activation of factor VII. III. Relation to the kallikrein system. Thromb. Diath. Haemorrh. *28*, 182–193 (1972b)

Glueck, H. I., Roehill, W.: Myocardial infarction in a patient with Hageman (factor XII) defect. Ann. Intern. Med. *64*, 390–396 (1966)
Goldsmith, G. H., Stern, R. C., Saito, H., Ratnoff, O. D.: Normal plasma arginine esterase and the Hageman factor (factor XII)-prekallikrein-kininogen system in cystic fibrosis. J. Lab. Clin. Med. *89*, 131–134 (1977)
Green, J., Talamo, R. C., Colman, R. W.: Kinetics of kinin release in canine plasma. Am. J. Physiol. *226*, 784–790 (1974)
Greenbaum, L. M., Chang, J., Freer, R.: Kinin metabolism in normal and malignant leucocytes. In: Bradykinin and related kinins. Sicuteri, F., Rocha e Silva, M., Rothschild, H. A. (eds.), pp. 21–30. New York, London: Plenum Press 1970
Griffin, J. H., Cochrane, C. G.: Mechanisms for the involvement of high molecular weight kininogen in surface dependent reactions of Hageman factor. Proc. Natl. Acad. Sci. U.S.A. *73*, 2554–2558 (1976)
Habal, F. M., Movat, H. Z., Burrowes, C. E.: Isolation of two functionally different kininogens from human plasma. Separation from proteolytic inhibitors and interaction with plasma kallikrein. Biochem. Pharmacol. *23*, 2291–2302 (1974)
Habermann, E.: Kininogens. In: Handbook of experimental pharmacology. Vol. XXV: Bradykinin, kallidin, and kallikrein. Erdös, E. G. (ed.), pp. 250–288. Berlin, Heidelberg, New York: Springer 1970
Haig, T. H. B., Thompson, A. G.: Effect of kallikrein inactivator on experimental acute pancreatitis. Can. J. Surg. *7*, 97–101 (1964)
Han, Y. N., Komiya, M., Iwanaga, S., Suzuki, T.: Studies on the primary structure of bovine highmolecular weight kininogen. Amino acid sequence of a fragment ("Histidine-rich peptide") released by plasma kallikrein. J. Biochem. (Tokyo) *77*, 55–68 (1975)
Harpel, P. C.: C 1 inactivator inhibition by plasmin. J. Clin. Invest. *49*, 568–575 (1970)
Harpel, P. C.: Human plasma alpha-2-macroglobulin. An inhibitor of plasma kallikrein. J. Exp. Med. *132*, 329–352 (1970)
Hashimoto, K., Warka, J., Kohn, R. N., Wilkens, H. J., Steger, R., Back, N.: The vasopeptide kinin system in acute clinical cardiac disease. Adv. Exp. Med. Biol. *70*, 245–261 (1975)
Hass, E., Goldblatt, H., Lewis, L., Gipson, E. C.: Interplay of vasodilators and vasoconstrictor substances in femoral arterial bed. Identification of the angiotensin cofactor. J. Lab. Invest. *28*, 1–7 (1973)
Hathaway, W. E., Alsever, J.: The relation of "Fletcher factor" to factors XI and XII. Br. J. Haematol. *18*, 161–169 (1970)
Hathaway, W. E., Belhanson, L. P., Hathaway, H. S.: Evidence for a new thromboplastin factor: Case report, coagulation studies and physiochemical studies. Blood *26*, 521–532 (1965)
Hattersley, P. G., Hayes, D.: Fletcher factor deficiency; report of three unrelated cases. Br. J. Haematol. *18*, 411–416 (1970)
Herman, C. M., Oshima, G., Erdös, E. G.: The effect of adrenocorticoid pretreatment on kinin system and coagulation response to septic shock in the baboon. J. Lab. Clin. Med. *84*, 731–739 (1974)
Herxheimer, H., Streseman, E.: Effect of bradykinin aerosol in guinea pigs and man. J. Physiol. (Lond.) *158*, 38 P (1961)
Hinshaw, D. B., Joergenson, E. J., Davis, H. A.: Peripheral blood flow and blood volume studies in the dumping syndrome. Arch. Surg. *74*, 686–693 (1957)
Hirsch, E. F., Nagajima, T., Oshima, G., Erdös, E. G., Herman, C. M.: Kinin system responses in sepsis after traume in man. J. Surg. Res. *17*, 147–153 (1974)
Hoak, J. C., Swenson, L. W., Warner, E. D.: Myocardial infarction associated with severe factor XII deficiency. Lancet *1966/II*, 884–886
Hollenberg, N. K., Retik, A. B., Rosen, S. M., Murray, J. E., Merrilim, J. P.: The role of vasoconstriction in the ischemia of renal allograft rejection. Trans. *6*, 59–69 (1968)
Honig, G. R., Lindley, A.: Deficiency of Hageman factor (factor XII) in patients with the nephotic syndrome. J. Pediatr. *78*, 633–637 (1971)
Izaka, K., Tsutsui, E., Mina, Y., Masegawa, E.: A bradykinin-like substance heat treated human plasma protein solution. Trans. *14*, 242–248 (1974)
Izaka, K., Morichi, S., Fujita, Y., Hasegawa, E.: A kininogen-like substance in unheated human plasma proteins. Trans. *15*, 46–53 (1975)

Johnson, L.P., Jesseph, J.E.: Evidence for a humoral etiology of the dumping syndrome. Surg. Forum *12*, 316–317 (1961)
Jonasson, O., Becker, E.L.: Release of kallikrein from guinea pig lung during anaphylaxis. J. Exp. Med. *123*, 509–522 (1966)
Kallen, R.J., Soo-Kwang, L.: A study of the plasma kinin-generating system in children with the minimal lesion, idiopathic nephrotic syndrome. Pediatr. Res. *9*, 705–709 (1975)
Kangasniemi, P., Rickkiner, P., Rinne, U.K.: Kallikrein-like esterase and peptidase activities in CSF during migraine attacks and free intervals. Headache *2*, 66–69 (1972)
Kaper, C.K., Whissell-Buechy, D.Y.E., Aggeler, P.M.: Hageman factor (factor XII) in an affected kindred and normal adults. Br. J. Haematol. *14*, 543–551 (1968)
Kaplan, A.P., Austen, K.F.: A prealbumin activator of prekallikrein. J. Immunol. *105*, 802 (1970)
Kaplan, A.P., Austen, K.F.: A prealbumin activator of prekallikrein II. Derivation of activators of prekallikrein from active Hageman factor by digestion with plasmin. J. Exp. Med. *133*, 696–712 (1971)
Kaplan, A.P., Austen, K.F.: A prealbumin activator of prekallikrein III. Appearance of chemotactic activity by the conversion of prekallikrein to kallikrein. J. Exp. Med. *135*, 81–97 (1972a)
Kaplan, A.P., Austen, K.F.: The fibrinolytic pathway of human plasma. Isolation and characterization of the plasminogen proactivator. J. Exp. Med. *136*, 1378–1393 (1972b)
Kato, H.Y., Han, N., Iwanaga, S., Suzuki, T., Komiya, M.: Bovine plasma HMW and LMW kininogens: Isolation and characterization of the polypeptide fragments produced by plasma and tissue kallikreins. In: Kinins – pharmacodynamics and biological roles. Sicuteri, F., Back, N. (eds.), pp. 135–150. New York, London: Plenum Press 1975
Katori, M., Nagaoka, H.: Significance of the kinin system and inhibition of kinin formation by kallikrein inhibition in extracorporeal circulation in openheart surgery patients. In: Chemistry and biology of the kallikrein-kinin system in health and disease. Pisano, J.L., Austen, K.I. (eds.), pp. 553–556. Fogarty Internat. Center Proc. No. 27. Washington: U.S. Gov. Printing Office 1977
Keele, C.A., Armstrong, D.: Substances producing pain and itch. London: Arnold 1964
Kellermeyer, R.W.: Activation of Hageman factor by sodium urate crystals. In: Proceedings of conference on gout and purine metabolism. Gutman, A.B. (ed.), pp. 741–743. New York: Grune and Stratton 1964
Kellermeyer, R.W., Breckenridge, R.T.: The inflammatory process in acute gouty arthritis. I. Activation of Hageman factor by sodium urate crystals. J. Lab. Clin. Med. *65*, 307–315 (1965)
Kellermeyer, R.W., Graham, R.C.: Kinins-possible physiologic and pathologic roles in the man. N. Engl. J. Med. *279*, 859–866 (1968)
Kellermeyer, R.W., Nagg, G.B.: Chemical mediators of inflammation in acute gouty arthritis. Arthritis Rheum. *18* (Supplement), 765–770 (1975)
Klemperer, M.R., Donaldson, V.H., Rosen, F.S.: Effect of C′1 esterase on vascular permeability in man. J. Clin. Invest. *47*, 604–611 (1968)
Laake, K., Vennerd, A.M.: Factor XII – induced fibrinolysis studies on the separation of prekallikrein, plasminogen proactivator, and factor XI in human plasma. Thromb. Res. *4*, 285–302 (1974)
Lacombe, N.J.: Deficit constitutional en un nouveau facteur de la coagulation intervenant au niveau de contact: le facteur "Flaujeac." C.R. Acad. Sci. [D] (Paris) *280*, 1039–1041 (1975)
Lacombe, M.J., Varet, B., Levy, J.P.: A hitherto underscribed plasma factor acting at the contact phase of blood coagulation (Flaujeac factor): Case report and coagulation studies. Blood *46*, 761–768 (1975)
Lahiri, B., Talamo, R.C., Mitchell, B., Bagdasarian, A., Colman, R.W., Rosenberg, R.: Antithrombin III an inhibitor of human kallikrein. Arch. Biochem. Biophys. *175*, 737–747 (1976)
Landerman, N.S.: Hereditary angioneurotic edema. I. Case reports and review of literature. J. Allerg. *33*, 316–329 (1962)
Landerman, N.S., Webster, M.E., Becker, E.L., Ratcliffe, H.D.: Hereditary angioneurotic edema. II. Deficiency of inhibitor for serum globulin permeability factor and/or plasma kallikrein. J. Allergy *33*, 330–341 (1962)
Lange, L.G., Carvalho, A.C., Bagdasarian, A., Lahiri, B., Colman, R.W.: Activation of Hageman factor in the nephrotic syndrome. Am. J. Med. *56*, 565–569 (1974)

Leading article: Toxaemia of burns. Lancet *1960/I*, 153–155
Lembeck, F.: 5-hydroxytryptamine in carcinoid tumors. Nature (Lond.) *172*, 910–912 (1953)
Lieberman, J.: Plasma arginine esterase activity in cystic fibrosis. Am. Rev. Resp. Dis. *109*, 399–401 (1974)
Liu, C.Y., Scott, C.F., Bagdasarian, A., Pierce, J.V., Kaplan, A.P., Colman, R.W.: Potentiation of the function of Hageman factor fragments by high molecular weight kininogen. J. Clin. Invest. *60* (1977)
Lopas, H., Birndorf, N.I., Bell, C.E., Jr., Robboy, S., Colman, R.W.: Immune hemolytic transfusion in monkeys: Activation of the kallikrein system. Am. J. Physiol. *225*, 372–379 (1973)
Lucas, C.E., Read, R.C.: Vascular hypertoxicity. A mechanism for vasodilation in the dumping syndrome. Surgery *60*, 395–401 (1966)
Lukjan, H., Hofman, J., Kiersnoroska, B., Bielawiec, M., Chyrek-Borowska, S.: The kinin system in allergic states. Allerg. Immunol. Band *18*, 25–30 (1972)
Lutcher, C.L.: Reid trait: A new expression of high molecular weight kininogen (HMW-Kininogen) deficiency. Clin. Res. *24*, 47 (Abstract) (1976)
MacDonald, J.M., Webster, M.M., Jr., Tennyson, C.H., Drapanos, T.: Serotonin and bradykinin in the dumping syndrome. Am. J. Surg. *117*, 204–213 (1969)
Mackay, M.E., Maycock, W., Silk, E., Cambridge, B.S.: Studies on fibrinogen fractions isolated from human plasma by precipitation with cold ether I. Plasma kinin formation by the activation of contaminated plasminogen. Br. J. Haematol. *11*, 563–575 (1965)
Mandle, R., Colman, R.W., Kaplan, A.P.: Identification of prekallikrein and high molecular weight (HMW) kininogen as a circulating complex in human plasma PNAS *73*, 4179–4183 (1976)
Mandle, R., Kaplan, A.P.: Hageman factor substrates II. Human plasma prekallikrein: Mechanism of activation by Hageman factor and participation in Hageman factor dependent proteolysis. J. Biol. Chem. 6097–6103 (1977)
Margolis, S.: The mode of action of Hageman factor in the release of plasma kinin. J. Physiol. (Lond.) *15*, 238–245 (1960)
Margolius, A., Ratnoff, O.D.: Observations on the hereditary nature of Hageman trait. Blood *11*, 565–569 (1956)
Marx, R., Clements, P., Werle, P., Appel, W.: Zum Problem eines Antidoes in der Internen. Thrombotherapie mit Fibrinolytika. Blut *5*, 367–375 (1959)
Masar, D.T., Melmon, K.L.: Effects of bradykinin on forearms venous tone and vascular resistance in man. Circ. Res. *17*, 106–113 (1965)
Mashford, M.L., Zacest, R.: Physiological changes in blood bradykinin levels in man. Aust. J. Exp. Biol. Med. Sci. *45*, 661–664 (1967)
Mason, D.T., Melmon, K.L.: Effects of bradykinin on forearm venous tone and vascular resistance in man. Circ. Res. *17*, 106–113 (1965)
Mason, J.W., Colman, R.W.: The role of Hageman factor in disseminated intravascular coagulation induced by sepsis neoplasia or liver disease. Thromb. Diath. Haemorrh. *26*, 325–331 (1971)
Mason, J.W., Kleeberg, U.R., Dolan, P., Colman, R.W.: Plasma kallikrein and Hageman factor in gram negative bacteremia. Ann. Intern. Med. *73*, 545–551 (1970)
Matheson, R.T., Miller, D.R., Lacombe, M.J., Han, Y.N., Iwanaga, S., Kato, H., Wuepper, K.D.: Reconstitution with highly purified bovine high molecular weight-kininogen and delineation of a new permeability-enhancing peptide released by plasma kallikrein from bovine high molecular weight-kininogen. J. Clin. Invest. *58*, 1395–1406 (1976)
Maycock, W.D.: Further experience with a concentrate containing antihemophilic factor. Br. J. Haematol. *9*, 215–235 (1963)
McCabe, W.R.: Serum complement levels in bacteremia due to gram negative organisms. N. Engl. J. Med. *288*, 21–25 (1973)
McGiff, J.C., Terragno, M.A., Malik, K.U., Lonigro, A.J.: Release of a prostaglandin E-like substance from canine kidney by bradykinin. Comparison with eledoisin. Circ. Res. *31*, 36–43 (1972)
McGiff, J.C., Itskovitz, H.D., Terragno, A., Wong, P.Y.: Modulation and mediation of the action of renal kallikrein-kinin system by prostaglandins. Fed. Proc. *35*, 175–180 (1976)
McGrath, J.M., Stewart, G.J.: The effects of endotoxin on vascular endothelium. J. Exp. Med. *129*, 833–848 (1969)

McLean, L., Mulligan, W.G., MacLean, H.P.H., Duff, J.H.: Patterns of septic shock in man – a detailed study of 56 patients. Ann. Surg. *166*, 533–562 (1967)
Meier, H.K., Webster, M.E., Mandle, R., Colman, R.W., Kaplan, A.P.: Enhancement of the surface dependent Hageman factor activation by high molecular weight kininogen. J. Clin. Invest. *60*, 18–30 (1977a)
Meier, J.L., Scott, C.F., Mandel, R., Jr., Webster, M.E., Pierce, J.V., Colman, R.W., Kaplan, A.P.: Requirements for contact activation of human Hageman factor. Ann. N.Y. Acad. Sci. *283*, 93–103 (1977b)
Melmon, K.L., Lovenberg, W., Sjoerdsma, A.: Characteristics of carcinoid tumor kallikrein: identification of lysyl-bradykinin as a peptide it produces in vitro. Clin. Chim. Acta *12*, 292–297 (1965)
Melmon, K.L., Webster, M.E., Goldfinger, S.E., Seegmiller, J.E.: The presence of a kinin in inflammatory synovial effusion from arthritis of varying etiology. Arthritis Rheum. *10*, 13–20 (1967)
Miller, R.L., Reichgott, M.J., Melmon, K.L.: Biochemical mechanisms of generation of bradykinin by endotoxin. J. Infect. Dis. *125* (suppl.), 144–156 (1973)
Minna, J.D., Robboy, S.J., Colman, R.W.: Disseminated intravascular coagulation in man, pp. 70–76. Illinois: Thomas 1974
Mix, C.L.: "Dumping stomach" following gastrojejunostomy. Surg. Clin. North Am. *2*, 617–622 (1922)
Moore, T.C., Sinclair, M.C., Lemani, C.A.E.: Elevation in plasma kallikrein after rat kidney allografting. Am. J. Surg. *127*, 287–291 (1974)
Morichi, S., Izaka, K.: Some components of the kinin system in Cohn's unheated plasma proteins. Transfusion *16*, 178–181 (1976)
Movat, H.Z., Delorenzo, N.L., Mustard, J.F., Helmel, G.: Activation of Hageman factor and vascular permeability factor in serum by Ag-Ab precipitates. Fed. Proc. *25*, 682 (1966)
Murray, M.: The distribution of fibrinolytic activity in the plasma of patients with various disease entities. Am. J. Clin. Pathol. *31*, 107–111 (1959)
Nies, A.S., Forsyth, R.P., Williams, H.E., Melmon, K.L.: Contribution of kinin to endotoxin shock in unanesthetized Rhesus monkeys. Circ. Res. *22*, 155–164 (1968)
Nugent, F.W., Atendio, W.: Hemorrhagic pancreatitis (aggressive treatment). Postgrad. Med. *40*, 87–94 (1966)
Oates, J.A., Sjoerdsma, A.: A unique syndrome associated with secretion of 5-hydroxytryptophan by metastatic gastric carcinoids. Am. J. Med. *32*, 333–342 (1962)
Oates, J.A., Melmon, K., Sjoerdsma, A., Gillespie, L., Mason, D.T.: Release of a kinin peptide in the carcinoid syndrome. Lancet *1964/I*, 514–518
Oates, J.A., Pettinger, W.A., Doctor, R.B.: Evidence for the release of bradykinin in carcinoid syndrome. J. Clin. Invest. *45*, 173–178 (1966)
O'Donnell, T.F., Clowes, G.H., Jr., Talamo, R.C., Colman, R.W.: Kinin activation in the blood of patients with sepsis. Surg. Gynecol. Obstet. *143*, 539–545 (1976)
Ofstad, E.: Formation and destruction of plasma kinins during experimental acute hemorrhagic pancreatis in dogs. Scand. J. Gastroenterol. *5* (suppl.), 1–44 (1970)
Ostfeld, A.M., Chapman, L.F., Goodell, H., Wolff, H.G.: Studies in headaches: summary of evidence concerning noxious agent active locally during migraine headaches. Psychosom. Med. *19*, 199–208 (1957)
Page, I.H., Olmsted, F.: Hemodynamic effects of angiotension, norepinephrine and bradykinin continuously measured in unanesthetized dog. Am. J. Physiol. *201*, 92–96 (1961)
Paskhina, T.S., Krinskaya, A.V.: Uprochennyimetod opredeleniia kallikreinogena i kallikreinia v syvorotke (plasme) krovi cheloveka v nosme i pri nekotorykh pathologichiecheskikh sostonianiiakh. Vopr. Med. Khim. *20*, (6), 660–663 (1974)
Pence, H.L., Evon, R., Guerney, L.H., Gerhard, R.G.: Prophylactic use of episilon aminocaproic acid for oral surgery in a patient with hereditary angioneurotic edema. J. Allergy Clin. Immunol. *53*, 298–302 (1974)
Pennow, B., Waldenstrom, J.: Determination of 5-hydroxytryptamine, 5-hydroxyindoleacetic acid and histamine in thirty-three cases of carcinoid tumor (Argentaffinoma). Am. J. Med. *23*, 16–21 (1957)
Pernow, B.: Pharmacology of substance P. Ann. N.Y. Acad. Sci. *104*, 393–402 (1963)

Peterson, D.W., Hamilton, W.H., Lilyblade, A.L.: Hereditary susceptability to dietary induction of gout in selected lines of chickens. J. Nutr. *101*, 347–354 (1971)
Phelps, P., McCarty, D.J., Jr.: Crystal induced inflammation in canine joints II. Importance of polymorphonuclear leukocytes. J. Exp. Med. *124*, 115–126 (1966)
Phelps, P., Prockop, D.J., McCarty, D.T.: Crystal-induced inflammation in canine joints. III. Evidence against bradykinin as a mediator of inflammation. J. Lab. Clin. Med. *68*, 433–444 (1966)
Pickering, R.J., Kelly, J.R., Goode, R.A., Gewitz, H.: Replacement therapy in hereditary angioedema: Successful treatment of two patients with fresh frozen plasma. Lancet *1969/I*, 326–330
Pierce, J.V., Guimaraes, J.A.: Further characterization of highly purified human plasma kininogens. In: Chemistry and biology of the kallikrein-kinin system in health and disease. Pisano, J.J., Austen, K.F. (eds.), pp. 121–128. Fogarty Internat. Center Proc. No. 27. Washington: U.S. Gov. Printing Office 1977
Pitt, B., Mason, J., Conti, C.R.: Observations on the plasma kallikrein system during myocardial ischemia. Trans. Assoc. Am. Physicians *82*, 98–108 (1969)
Propieraitis, A.S., Thompson, A.G.: The site of bradykinin release in acute experimental pancreatitis. Arch. Surg. *98*, 73–76 (1969)
Radcliffe, R., Bagdasarian, A., Colman, R.W., Nemerson, Y.: Activation of factor VII by Hageman factor fragments. Blood *50*, 611–618 (1977)
Rao, G.J.S., Nadler, H.L.: Deficiency of trypsin-like activity in saliva of patients with cystic fibrosis. J. Pediatr. *80*, 573–576 (1973)
Rao, G.J.S., Nadler, H.L.: Arginine esterase in cystic fibrosis of the pancreas. Pediatr. Res. *8*, 684–686 (1974)
Rao, G.J.S., Nadler, H.L.: Deficiency of arginine esterase in cystic fibrosis of the pancreas: Demonstration of the proteolytic nature of the activity. Pediatr. Res. *9*, 739–741 (1975)
Rao, G.J.S., Posner, L.A., Nadler, H.L.: Deficiency of kallikrein activity in plasma of patients with cystic fibrosis. Science *177*, 610–611 (1972)
Rapaport, S., Aas, K., Owen, P.A.: Effect of glass upon the activity of various plasma clotting factors. J. Clin. Invest. *34*, 9–19 (1955)
Ratnoff, O.D.: The biology and pathology of the initial coagulation. In: Progress in hematology. Brown, E.B., Moore, C.V. (eds.), Vol. V, pp. 204–245. New York: Grune and Stratton 1966
Ratnoff, O.D., Colopy, J.E.: A familial hemorrhagic trait associated with a deficiency of a clot-promoting fraction of plasma. J. Clin. Invest. *34*, 601–613 (1955)
Ratnoff, O.D., Davie, E.W., Mallet, D.L.: Study on the action of Hageman factor: Evidence that activated Hageman factor in turn activates plasma thromboplastin antecedent. J. Clin. Invest. *40*, 803–819 (1961)
Ratnoff, O.D., Busce, R.J., Sheon, R.P.: The demise of John Hageman. N. Engl. J. Med. *279*, 760–761 (1968)
Ratnoff, O.D., Pensky, J., Ogston, D., Naff, G.B.: The inhibition of plasmin, plasma kallikrein, plasma permeability factor and the C'1r subcomponent of the first component of complement by serum C;1 esterase inhibitor. J. Exp. Med. *129*, 315–331 (1969)
Revak, S.D., Cochrane, C.G., Johnston, A.R.: Structure of Hageman factor in its native and activated forms. Fed. Proc. *32*, 845 (1973)
Roberts, M.L., Mashford, M.L.: Possible physiological and pathological roles of the kallikrein-kinin system. Med. J. Aust. *2*, 887–891 (1972)
Roberts, K.E., Randall, H.T., Farr, H.W.: Cardiovascular and blood volume alterations resulting from intrajejunal administration of hypotonic solutions to gastrectomized patients; the relationship of these changes to the dumping syndrome. Ann. Surg. *140*, 631–640 (1954)
Robinson, J.A., Klodyncky, M.L., Loeb, H.S., Racic, M.R., Gunnar, R.M.: Endotoxin, prekallikrein, complement, and systemic vascular resistance. Sequential measurement in man. Am. J. Med. *59*, 61–67 (1975)
Rocha, E., Silva, M., Antonio, A.: Release of bradykinin and the mechanism of production of a "Thermic" edema (45 °C) in the rat's paw. Med. Exp. (Basel) *3*, 371–375 (1960)
Rocha e Silva, M., Beraldo, W.T., Rosenfeld, G.: Bradykinin, hypotensive, and smooth muscle stimulator released from plasma globulin by snake venoms and by trypsin. Am. J. Physiol. *156*, 261–273 (1949)

Rocha e Silva, M., Corrado, A.P., Ramos, A.O.: Potentiation of duraction of the vasodilator effect of bradykinin by sympatholytic drugs and by reserpine. J. Pharmacol. Exp. Ther. *128*, 217–226 (1960)
Romero, J.C., Dunlop, C.L., Strong, C.G.: The effect of indomethicin and other anti-inflammatory drugs on the renin-angiotension system. J. Clin. Invest. *58*, 282–288 (1976)
Rosoff, L., Jr., Priscilla, A., Reynolds, T.B., Morton, R.: Studies on renin and aldosterone in cirrhotic patients with ascites. Gastroenterology *69*, 698–705 (1975)
Rothschild, A.M., Castania, A., Cordeiro, R.S.B.: Consumption of kininogen, formation of kinin, and activation of arginine ester hydrolase in rat plasma by rat peritoneal fluid cells in the presence of 1-adrenaline. Naunyn Schmiedebergs Arch. Pharmakol. *285*, 243–256 (1974a)
Rothschild, A.M., Cordeiro, R.S.B., Castania, A.: Lowering of kininogen in rat blood by catecholamines. Involvement of non-eosinophil granulocytes and selective inhibition by Trasylol. Naunyn Schmiedebergs Arch. Pharmakol. *282*, 323–327 (1974b)
Rothschild, A.M., Gomes, J.C., Castania, A.: Adrenergic and cholinergic control of the activation of the kallikrein-kinin system in the rat blood. Adv. Exp. Med. Biol. *70*, 197–200 (1976)
Rowley, D.A.: Venous constriction as cause of increased vascular permeability produced by 5-hydroxytryptamine, histamine, bradykinin, and 46/80 in rat. Br. J. Exp. Pathol. *45*, 56–67 (1964)
Ruddy, S., Gigli, I., Austen, K.F.: The complement system of man. N. Engl. J. Med. *287*, 545–548 (1972)
Ryan, J.W., Moffat, J.G., Thompson, A.G.: Role of bradykinin system in acute hemorrhagic pancreatitis. Arch. Surg. *91*, 14–24 (1965)
Saito, H., Ratnoff, O.D.: Inhibition of normal clotting and Fletcher factor activity by rabbit anti-kallikrein antiserum. Nature New Biol. *248*, 597–598 (1974)
Saito, H., Ratnoff, R., Waldmann, Abraham, J.P.: Fitzgerald trait. Deficiency of a hitherto unrecognized agent, Fitzgerald factor, participating in surface mediated reactions of clotting, fibrinolysis, generation of kinins, and the property of diluted plasma enhancing vascular permeability (PF/dil). J. Clin. Invest. *55*, 1082–1089 (1975)
Saito, H., Goldsmith, G., Waldmann: Fitzgerald factor (high molecular weight kininogen) clotting activity in human plasma in health and disease in various animal plasma. Blood *48*, 941–947 (1976)
Sardesai, V.M., Rosenberg, J.C.: Proteolysis and bradykinin turnover in endotoxin shock. J. Trauma *14*, 945–949 (1974)
Sardesai, V.M., Thal, A.P.: The proteolytic process in pancreatic disease. In: Hypotensive peptides. Erdös, E.G., Back, N., Sicuteri, F. (eds.), pp. 463–473. Berlin, Heidelberg, New York: Springer 1966
Schiffman, S., Lee, P.: Preparation, characterization, and activation of a highly purified factor XI: Evidence that a hitherto unrecognized plasma activity participates in the interaction of factors XI and XII. Br. J. Haematol. *27*, 101–114 (1974)
Schiffman, S., Lee, P.: Partial purification and characterization of contact activation cofactor. J. Clin. Invest. *56*, 1082–1092 (1975)
Schiffman, S., Lee, P., Waldman, R.: Identity of contact activation cofactor and Fitzgerald cofactor and Fitzgerald factor. Thromb. Res. *6*, 451–454 (1975)
Schroeder, E.T., Anderson, G.H., Golman, S.H., Streeten, D.: Effect of blockade of angiotension II on blood pressure, renin, and aldosterone in cirrhosis. Kidney International *9*, 511–515 (1976)
Seki, T., Makajime, T., Erdös, E.G.: Colon kallikrein, its relation to the plasma enzyme. Biochem. Pharmacol. *21*, 1227–1235 (1972)
Sevitt, S.: Failure of antihistamine drugs to influence local vascular changes in experimental burns. Br. J. Exp. Pathol. *30*, 540–547 (1949)
Sherry, S., Alkjaersig, N., Fletcher, A.P.: Observations on spontaneous arginine and lysine esterase activity of human plasma and their relation to Hageman factor. Thromb. Diath. Haemorrh. (suppl.) *20*, 243–247 (1966)
Shroeder, E.T., Eich, R.H., Smulejan, H., Gabuzda, G.: Plasma renin level in hepatic cirrhosis: relation to functional renal failure. Am. J. Med. *49*, 186–191 (1970)
Sicuteri, F.: Sensitization of nociceptors by 5-hydroxytryptamine in man. In: Pharmacology of pain. Lim, R.K.S. (ed.), pp. 57–64. Oxford: Pergamon Press 1968

Sicuteri, F.: Bradykinin and intracranial circulation in man. In: Handbook of experimental pharmacology. Vol. XXV: Bradykinin, kallidin, and kallikrein. Erdös, E.G. (ed.), pp. 482–515. Berlin, Heidelberg, New York: Springer 1970
Sicuteri, F., Delbianco, P.L., Fanciullacci, M.: Kinins in the pathogenesis of cardiogenic shock and pain. Adv. Exp. Med. Biol. *9*, 315–322 (1970)
Sicuteri, F., Antonini, F.M., Delbianco, P.L., Franchi, G., Currodi, C.: Prekallikrein and kallikrein inhibitor in plasma of patients affected by recent myocardial infarction. Adv. Exp. Med. Biol. *21*, 445–449 (1972)
Siegelman, A.M., Carlson, A.S., Robertson, T.: Investigation of serum trypsin and related substances. I. The quantitative demonstration of trypsin-like activity in human blood serum by a micromethod. Arch. Biochem. *97*, 159–163 (1962)
Sjoerdsma, A., Melmon, K.: The carcinoid spectrum. Gastroenterology *47*, 104–109 (1964)
Van der Sluys Veer, J., Choufoer, J.C., Querido, A., Van der Heul, R.O., Hollander, C.F., Van Rijssel, T.G.: Metastasizing islet-cell tumour of the pancreas associated with hypoglycemia and carcinoid syndrome. Lancet *1964/1*, 1416–1419
Snyder, A., Hand, M.R., Gewenz, H.: A rapid pH stat assay for plasma prekallikrein and fluctuations in disease. Int. Arch. Allergy *47*, 400–411 (1974)
Soltay, M.J., Movat, H.Z., Ozge-Anwar, A.H.: The kinin system of human plasma. V. The probable derivation of prekallikrein activator from activated Hageman factor (XIIa). Proc. Soc. Exp. Biol. Med. *138*, 952–958 (1971)
Soter, N.A., Austen, K.R., Gigli, I.: Inhibition by episilon amino-caproic acid of the activation of the first component of the complement system. J. Immunol. *114*, 928–932 (1975)
Stewart, D., Blendis, I.M., Williams, R.: Studies on the prekallikrein-bradykinin system in liver disease. J. Clin. Pathol. *25*, 410–414 (1972)
Talamo, R.C., Haber, E., Austen, K.F.: A radioimmunoassay of bradykinin in plasma and synovial fluid. J. Lab. Clin. Med. *74*, 816–827 (1969)
Talamo, R.C., Colman, R.W., Milunsky, A.: The plasma kallikrein-kinin system in cystic fibrosis. Pediatr. Res. *6*, 430 (1972)
Thune, P., Ryan, T.J., Powell, S.M., Ellis, R.J.: The cutaneous reactions to kallikrein, prostaglandin, and thurfyl nicotinate in chronic urticaria and the effect of polyphloretin phosphate. Acta Derm. Venereol. (Stockh.) *56*, 217–221 (1976)
Trautschold, I., Fritz, H., Werle, E.: Kininogenases, kininases, and their inhibitors. In: Hypotensive peptides. Erdös, E.G., Back, N.G., Scicuteri, F. (eds.), pp. 221–235. Berlin, Heidelberg, New York: Springer 1966
Vassalio, G., Solcia, E., Cappella, C.: Light and electronmicroscopic identification of several types of endocrine cells in the gastrointestinal mucosa of the rat. Z. Zellforsch. *98*, 333–336 (1969)
Veltkamp, J.M., Demler, H.C., Locliger, E.A.: Detection of heterozygotes for factor VIII, IX, and XII deficiency. Thromb. Diath. Haemorrh. *13* (suppl.), *17*, 181–189 (1965)
Venneröd, A.M., Laake, K.: Prekallikrein and plasminogen proactivator: Absence of plasminogen proactivator in Fletcher factor deficient plasma. Thromb. Res. *8*, 519–522 (1976)
Wardle, E.N., Piercy, D.A.: Studies on the contact activation in haemodialysis. J. Clin. Pathol. *25*, 1045–1049 (1972)
Webster, M.E., Clark, W.R.: Significance of the callikrein-callidinogen-callidin system in shock. Am. J. Physiol. *197*, 406–412 (1959)
Webster, M.E., Pierce, J.V.: Activators of Hageman factor (Factor XII): Identification and relationship to kallikrein-kinin system. Fed. Proc. *32*, 845 (1973)
Webster, M.E., Ratnoff, O.D.: Role of Hageman factor in the activation of vasodilation activity in human plasma. Nature (Lond.) *192*, 180–181 (1961)
Webster, M.E., Guimaraes, J.A., Kaplan, A.P., Colman, R.W., Pierce, J.V.: Activation of surface bound Hageman factor: Pre-eminent role of high molecular weight kininogen and evidence for a new factor. In: Kinins: pharmacodynamics and biological roles. Sicuteri, F., Back, N., Haberland, G.L. (eds.). New York, London: Plenum Press 1976
Weiss, A.S., Gallin, J.I., Kaplan, A.P.: Fletcher factor deficiency: Abnormalities of coagulation, fibrinolysis, chemotactic activity and kinin generation attributable to the absence of prekallikrein. J. Clin. Invest. *53*, 622–633 (1974)

Werle, E.: Kallikrein, kallidin, and related substances. In: Polypeptides which effect smooth muscle. Schacter, M. (ed.), pp. 199–209. London: Pergamon Press 1960
Werle, E.: Zur Biochemie und Physiologie der Proteinase-Inhibitoren. Arzneim. Forsch. *22*, 41–48 (1968)
Werle, S., Vogel, R., Kaliampetsos, G.: Über das Kallikrein der Darmwand und seine Beziehung zum Blutkallikreingehalt bei Störungen der Darmfunktion. In: Second world congress of gastroenterology. Schmid, E., Tomenius, J., Walkinson, G. (eds.), pp. 788–793. Basel: Karger 1963
Wiegershausen, B., Henninghausen, G., Klausch, B.: Plasma kininogen level in myocardial infarction. Adv. Exp. Med. Biol. *8*, 221–224 (1970)
Wilhelm, D.L., Mason, B.: Vascular permeability changes in inflammation: Role of endogenous permeability factors in mild thermal injury. Br. J. Exp. Pathol. *41*, 487–506 (1960)
Wolff, H.P., Koczorek, K.R., Buchborn, E.: Aldosterone and antidiuretic hormone (adiuretin) in liver disease. Acta Endocrinol. (Kbh.) *27*, 45–49 (1958)
Wong, P.Y., Colman, R.W., Talamo, R.C., Barior, B.M.: Kallikrein-bradykinin system in chronic alcoholic liver disease. Ann. Intern. Med. *77*, 205–209 (1972)
Wong, P.Y., Talamo, R.C., Babior, B.M., Raymond, G.G., Colman, R.W.: Kallikrein-kinin system in postgastrectomy dumping syndrome. Ann. Intern. Med. *80*, 577–581 (1974)
Wong, P.Y., Talamo, R.C., Williams, G.H., Colman, R.W.: Response of the kallikrein-kinin and renin-angiotension systems to saline infusion and up-right posture. J. Clin. Invest. *55*, 691–698 (1975)
Wong, P.Y., Talamo, R.C., Colman, R.W., Williams, G.H.: Dependence of plasma bradykinin on state of sodium balance. In: Chemistry and biology of kallikrein-kinin system in health and disease. Pisano, J.J., Austen, K.F. (eds.), pp. 415–422. Fogarty Internat. Center Proc. No. 27. Washington: U.S. Gov. Printing Office 1977
Wong, P.Y., Talamo, R.C., Williams, G.H.: Kallikrein-kinin and renin-angiotensin systems in functional renal failure in cirrhosis of the liver. (1977)
Wuepper, K.D.: Biochemistry and biology of components of the plasma kinin-forming system. In: Inflammation: mechanisms and control. Lepow, I.N., Ward, P.A. (eds.), pp. 93–117. London, New York: Academic Press 1972
Wuepper, K.D.: Prekallikrein deficiency in man. J. Exp. Med. *138*, 1345–1355 (1973)
Zeitlin, I.J.: Kinin release associated with the gastrointestinal tract. In: Bradykinin and related kinins. Sicuteri, F., Rocha, E.S., Back, N. (eds.), pp. 329–339. New York, London: Plenum Press 1970
Zeitlin, I.J., Smith, A.N.: 5-hydroxyindoles and kinins in the carcinoid and dumping syndrome. Lancet *1966/II*, 986–991
Zeitlin, I.J., Sharma, J.N., Brooks, P.M., Dick, W.C.: An effect of in indomethacin on raised plasma kininogen levels in rheumatoid patients. In: Chemistry and biology of the kallikrein-kinin system in health and disease. Pisano, J.J., Austen, K.F. (eds.), pp. 483–486. Fogarty Internat. Center Proc. No. 27. Washington: U.S. Gov. Printing Office 1977
Zeitlin, I.J., Singh, Y.N., Lembeck, R., Theiller, M.: The molecular weights of plasma and intenstinal kallikreins in rats. Arch. Pharmacol. *293*, 159–161 (1976)
Zetterstrom, B.E.M., Palmerio, C., Fine, J.: Protection of functional and vascular intergrity of the spleen in traumatic shock by denervation. Proc. Soc. Exp. Biol. Med. *117*, 373–376 (1964)

Bradykinin, Kallidin, and Kallikreins

(Publications in Russian)

T. S. PASKHINA and A. P. LEVITSKY

Introduction

This article summarizes the results of investigations of various asepcts of the kallikrein-kinin system of blood plasma and tissues carried out by Soviet scientists. The chemistry, biochemistry, pharmacology, and physiology of kinins; the methods of study and estimation of activity of kinins and main components of the kallikrein-kinin system; as well as the state of this system in healthy subjects and in patients are

---

Glossary of Frequently Used Abbreviations and Terms

AMe	L-Arginine methyl ester	IU	Inhibitor Unit, i.e, amount of inhibitor which inhibits cleanage of 1 μmol substrate
ATEe	acetyl-L-tyrosine ethyl ester	Kininase I, II	See appendix
ATP	adenosine triphosphate	Kininogenase	See appendix
BAA	benzoyl-L-argininamide	K_m	Michaelis constant
BAEe	benzoyl-L-arginine ethyl ester	LBTI	Lima bean trypsin inhibitor
BAL	2,3-dimercaptopropanol	LMW	low molecular weight
BAMe	bezoyl-L-arginine methyl ester	MW	molecular weight
BANA	benzoyl arginine-*p*-nitroanilide	N-terminal	amino terminal
BPP or BPF	bradykinin-potentiating peptides	OMTI	ovomucoid trypsin inhibitor
BPTI	pancreatic trypsin inhibitor, aprotinin, Trasylol	PF/dil	permeability factor
CM	carboxymethyl	SBTI	soybean trypsin inhibitor
CNS	central nervous system	SDS	sodium dodecyl sulfate
CSF	cerebrospinal fluid	Spec. act.	specific activity
C-terminal	carboxyl-terminal	TAMe	N-α-tosyl-L-arginine methyl ester
CTI	colostrum trypsin inhibitor	TCA	trichloroacetic acid
DEAE	diethylaminoethyl	TLCK	1-chloro-3-tosylamido-7-amino-2-heptanone
DFP	diisopropylfluorophosphate	TLMe	N-α-tosyl-L-lysine methyl ester
EACA	ε-amino-n-caproic acid	Tris	tris (hydroxymethyl) aminomethane
EDTA	ethylenediaminetetraacetate	TPCK	α-L-(1-tosylamido-2-phenyl) ethylchloromethyl ketone
FU	Frey Unit for kallikrein	U	Unit of enzyme activity, i.e, amount of enzyme required to catalyze conversion of 1 μmol substrate/min
HF	Hageman factor, factor XII		
HLA	hippuryl-L-arginine		
HLAa	hippuryl-L-argininic acid		
HLL	hippuryl-L-lysine		
HMW	high molecular weight		
I_{50}	concentration of inhibitor that inhibits 50% of enzyme activity		

discussed. The summary deals with papers published in Soviet journals and monographs in the years 1970–1977. Only some of the works published earlier and not mentioned by Dr. TRĈKA in Vol. XXV Handbook of Experimental Pharmacology are referred to.

Since the number of publications on the kinin system, especially on the study of functions of kinins in pathologic conditions, is continuously growing, the authors could not include every paper but refered to the most important ones. We apologize in advance. Data on reviews are given selectively, while abstracts to monographs and materials of conferences are very brief.

A. Methods of Investigation and Estimation of Kinin System Components

This section deals with publications in Russian (1968–1977) on approved (both modified and original) methods for estimation of kinins and some kinin system components. Methods most frequently used for experimental and clinical research are included.

I. Manuals, Approbations, and Modifications

The first manual on methods of estimation of plasma kinins and kinin system components has been compiled by PASKHINA et al. (1968a, b). The first chapter (PASKHINA et al., 1968a) deals with biologic and chromatographic (paper and cellulose thin layer chromatography) methods of separation, determination, and identification of kinins. The second chapter (PASKHINA et al., 1968a) is devoted to enzymatic and biologic assays of kallikrein, kininogen, and carboxypeptidase N (kininase I) in plasma, of TAMe and BAEe esterase activities and of antitrypsin and antikallikrein activities. Analytical procedures, calibration curves, examples of calculations and references are given for each kinin system component on the basis of original papers.

NEKRASOVA et al. (1972a) described a method for kallikrein estimation in human urine developed by TRAUTSCHOLD and WERLE (1961) and the method by ABE (1965) for kinin determination in urine. The authors (NEKRASOVA et al., 1972a) presented data on the specificity of both methods and indicated the excretion values for kallikrein and kinins under conditions of rest and moderate physical load. Considerable individual and diurnal variations in kallikrein and kinin excretion have been found in healthy persons. A healthy person excretes 73 ± 6.6 mU kallikrein during the day and 32 ± 4.0 mU at night, 1 mU of kallikrein is defined as the amount of enzyme required to hydrolyze 1 nmol BAEe/min.

The values for kinin excretion are 1.22 ± 0.08 ng bradykinin · eq/h the daytime and 0.9 ± 0.01 ng bradykinin · eq/h at night. Under physical load the amounts of kallikrein and kinins in the urine of healthy persons increased. This method was used by NEKRASOVA et al. (1970, 1972a, 1973) and CHERNOVA and NEKRASOVA (1971) in the study of the role of kinins in the genesis of essential and renovascular hypertensions.

GOMAZKOV et al. (1972b) suggested the use of BAEe instead of TAMe for assaying the level of contact prekallikrein (COLMAN et al., 1969). Prekallikrein content was equal to hydrolysis of 55±4.4 μmol BAEe/h/ml (540 nm, 25 °C); inhibitor level was 1.07±0.13 U (expressed in the conventional units of COLMAN et al., 1969). Spontaneous BAEe esterase activity was 3.0±0.37 μmol/h. The authors examined both variations of the method and considered their suitability for the evaluation of kinin system states within the first days after myocardial infarction.

The method of FERREIRA and VANE (1967) for estimation of kinins in noncirculating whole blood was used by SUROVIKINA (1971). The author confirmed high selectivity and sensitivity of the upper section of cat jejunum to bradykinin (0.7±0.09 ng/ml) and its almost complete insensitivity to histamine, serotonin, angiotensin, and heparin. The estimation of free kinins by the modified method was carried out in a fresh blood sample (6–10 ml) using siliconization. The blood was collected in a test-tube containing 1–3 heparin units, 8-hydroxyquinoline (1×10^{-3} *M* final concentration) and 100 μg SBTI. Before use, the isolated organ was washed in Krebs solution and the determination was carried out at 35–37 °C. According to SUROVIKINA (1971) the content of free kinins in human venous blood was 3.4±0.31 ng bradykinin · eq/ml, in dog 5.3±0.43, cat (lower vena cava) 2.0±0.38, guinea pig 3.2±0.5, and rat 4.0±0.44. This method was applied by SUROVIKINA (1973), SUROVIKINA et al. (1972, 1974, 1976), and others (OBUKHOV, 1975; ARKATOV et al., 1976) for determination of free kinins and measuring the activity of kininases and kallikrein by bioassay under various pathologic conditions.

BELYAKOV and SYOMUSHKIN (1972, 1976) modified the apparatus and the conditions for estimation of kinins by the superfusion technique of FERREIRA and VANE (1967), and VANE (1969). Using highly sensitive equipment, the authors found that the superfusion technique of kinin determination by bioassay reduces the error in the method as compared to immersion technique from ±20% to ±5% (the test organ was rat uterus or cat jejunum). The "dose-effect" dependence (log–log coordinates) over the range of minor contractions of smooth muscles was highly constant (BELYAKOV and SYOMUSHKIN, 1976).

II. Methods for Kallikrein, Prekallikrein, and "Contact Kallikrein" Estimations in Human Plasma

1. "Chromatographic" Method for Kallikrein and Prekallikrein Estimations

PASKHINA and YAROVAYA (1970a) suggested first the use of "chromatographic" methods for kallikrein determination in human plasma which were further elaborated and supplemented by prekallikrein determination in the same plasma sample (PASKHINA et al., 1973). The analysis may be carried out either by chromatographic column (PASKHINA and YAROVAYA, 1970a; PASKHINA et al., 1973) or in a test tube (PASKHINA and KRINSKAYA, 1974) and requires 0.5 or 0.25 ml serum, respectively. The method is based on the cationic properties of kallikrein and prekallikrein at pH 7.0 which prevents adsorption of these proteins on DEAE-Sephadex A-50 equilibrated with 0.02 *M* Na-phosphate buffer, pH 7.0. After washing of the anionite with this buffer, the activity of kallikrein and content of prekallikrein were determined by measuring the rate of BAEe hydrolysis in the filtrate, i.e., in the fraction of plasma proteins which were not adsorbed on DEAE-Sephadex A-50 under these conditions. Kallikrein was estimated by measuring the spontaneous BAEe-esterase activity of the filtrate (253 nm, 25 °C, light path 1 cm) while prekallikrein was measured after activation of the filtrate by trypsin; trypsin was inactivated by ovomucoid before measuring BAEe hydrolysis. The authors established a close correlation between the values of arginine esterase activity of the filtrate, before and after its activation by trypsin, and their respective content of kallikrein and prekallikrein as measured by monitoring the kininogenase activity (PASKHINA et al., 1973; PASKHINA and KRINSKAYA, 1974). Kallikrein and prekallikrein activity are expressed in mU of enzyme per ml blood serum or plasma; 1 mU is defined as the amount of enzyme required to hydrolyze 1 nmol BAEe/min. No free kallikrein was found by this method in normal human plasma or serum; values of 10–15 mU/ml were within the limit of instrumental error (PASKHINA and KRINSKAYA, 1974). Prekallikrein activity measured by means of the "test tube" modification was 369 ± 59 mU/1 ml serum and 318 ± 57 mU/ml plasma (PASKHINA and KRINSKAYA, 1974); the "column" modification of the method yielded 250–400 mU/ml prekallikrein serum (PASKHINA et al., 1973). Kininogenase activity of donor DEAE-Sephadex A-S0 filtrate after activation by trypsin corresponded to the formation of 4.88 ± 1.23 ng bradykinin · eq by one BAEe esteras mU/min. Prekallikrein content determined by this method decreased considerably in liver deseases (PASKHINA et al., 1975c) and burn shock (PASKHINA et al., 1976) and increased in some kidney diseases (PASKHINA et al., 1977b).

Appearance of free kallikrein in DEAE-Sephadex filtrates from serum or plasma in pathologic conditions such as burns (PASKHINA et al., 1972, 1976), nephrotic syndrome (PASKHINA et al., 1977b), cardiogenic shock (MALAYA et al., 1973a, 1973b; MALAYA and LAZAREVA, 1976) and other diseases attracted considerable interest. Spontaneous BAEe esterase activity of filtrate identified as kallikrein by several criteria was in the range 20–100 mU/ml while its kininogenase activity amounted to 4–5 ng bradykinin/mU. The chromatographic column procedure by PASKHINA and YAROVAYA (1970a) showed that the maximum value of free kallikrein under the cardiogenic shock equals $385 \pm$ mU/ml (MALAYA and LAZAREVA, 1976) and was four times higher than the normal value found by these authors. The source of this kallikrein has not been established so far. It might be assumed (PASKHINA et al., 1977b, c) that under inflammation, stress, and some other pathologic conditions a certain part of the kallikrein is in a weakly bound state, e.g., in the form of a labile complex with one of its inhibitors or with an acid protein. This complex might dissociate due to the contact of threefold diluted plasma or serum with the anioe. PASKHINA and KRINSKAYA studied the specificity and possible limits of the chromatographic test tube procedure. It has been found that 10–20% correction of the error has to be introduced in the calculation of prekallikrein content due to the presence of the second proenzyme. The activity of this proenzyme was inhibited in the presence of LBTI by 10–20% after its activation by trypsin. Prekallikrein, occurring in complexes with other proteins such as HMW kininogen and Hageman factor which decrease its pI value, estimated by this method only partially. Thus the chromatographic method (PASKHINA and YAROVAYA, 1970a; PASKHINA and KRINSKAYA, 1974) may be used for quantitative estimation of both free and loosely bound kallikreins and cationic forms of prekallikrein. The calculation shows that the kinin-generating activity of prekallikrein localized in DEAE-Sephadex filtrates, after activation by trypsin, is 11.2–18.0 μg bradykinin · eq/ml serum which inidcates high potential kinin formation in human plasma.

2. Method of Simultaneous Determination of Prekallikrein, Plasminogen, and Prothrombin

GOMAZKOV and KOMISSAROVA (1976b) further developed the method of COLMAN et al. (1969) and proposed a procedure of simultaneous estimation of prekallikrein, plasminogen, prothrombin as well as their inhibitors in human plasma. Prekallikrein, plasminogen, and prothrombin are activated separately in a plasma samples (0.2–0.4 ml) with kaolin (25 °C), streptokinase or Ca-thromboplastin (37 °C), respectively. The increase of TAMe esterase activity in each sample after 1 min incubation with each activator indicated the formation of the corresponding enzyme from its precursor while the decrease of this activity measured after 5, 30, and 60 min indicated the levels of kallikrein, plasmin, and thrombin inhibitors, respectively. The contents of prekallikrein, plasminogen, and prothrombin were expressed as μmol TAMe/h/ml plasma while the levels of inhibitors were expressed in the conventional units of COLMAN et al. (1969). The rate of TAMe hydrolysis by each enzyme was estimated by the amount of methanol determined colorimetrically after its oxidation to formaldehyde by either chromotropic acid or hydrazone-3-methyl-2-benzotiazolane hydrochloride. The latter reagent considerably increases the sensitivity of the colorimetric assay so that 0.4–0.7 ml plasma can be used for estimation of seven parameters: spontaneous TAMe esterase activity, the content of three precursors of enzymes, and to levels of their three inhibitors. The activation of each proenzyme was sufficiently specific without the involvement of the other two proenzymes in the reaction. This method may be used for determination of three functionally related plasma systems, namely, kininogenesis, fibrinolysis, and coagulation in cardiovascular deseases, especially in myocardial infarction.

3. Determination of Contact Prekallikrein and Kallikrein Inhibitors in Plasma With Protamine as Substrate

VEREMEENKO et al. (1974) used protamine sulfate as substrate in the determination of contact prekallikrein and kallikrein inhibitors in human plasma activated by kaolin under the conditions described by COLMAN et al. (1969). The authors compared the kinetics of the hydrolysis of protamine sulfate and other substrates (TAMe, BAMe) by kaolin-activated plasma, and studied the effect of some kallikrein inhibitors (SBTI, aprotinin), pH of the medium, and other agents on protamine sulfate hydrolysis.

The authors identified the protamine hydrolyzing activity of plasma as kallikrein. There was a close similarity in the kinetics of hydrolysis by kaolin-activated human plasma of protamine sulfate, BAEe, and TAMe (VEREMEENKO et al., 1974). The enzyme hydrolyzing protamine sulfate was completely inactivated if plasma was preincubated with SBTI prior to kaolin treatment. At simultaneous addition of the substrate and SBTI the rate of this reaction decreased by only 60%. The acidification of plasma to pH 2.0 (10 min exposure) prior to kaolin treatment (10 mg/ml) produced changes in the curve which had no specific point of inflection in the first minute due to the loss of acid-labile inhibitors. The curve reached a maximum in the third minute after which the rate remained constant. Kininogenase activity of kaolin-activated human plasma measured in the presence of 8-hydroxyquinoline reached its maximum in 1–3 min (VEREMEENKO et al., 1975; VEREMEENKO, 1977). Kaolin did not activate plasminogen but streptokinase-activated plasma did hydrolyze protamine sulphate (VEREMEENKO et al., 1974).

Estimation of contact prekallikrein as well as rapid and slow inhibitors of kallikrein (VEREMEENKO et al., 1975; VEREMEENKO, 1977) was carried out in the following way: plasma (1.2 ml) was activated by kaolin (10 mg/ml), and after 1, 5, and 30 min the rate of protamine hydrolysis was determined in aliquots from the amount of arginine-containing products soluble in 10% TCA. Contents of prekallikrein and inhibitors were expressed in μmol arginine ($E_{508}^{1\,cm}$) liberated by 100 ml plasma per min. The rapid inhibitor level is determined by the presence of α_2-macroglobulin, while the slow inhibitor level is determined by other kallikrein inhibitors. The values of the four indices in normal plasma were found to be the following: spontaneous protamine hydrolyzing activity – 4.2; prekallikrein – 14.9; rapid inhibitor – 1.77; slow inhibitor – 0.16 μmol Arg/min/100 ml blood plasma. Prekallikrein levels in patients with infectious hepatitis (acute period) went down to 6.6 ± 0.9; rapid inhibitor to 0.7 ± 0.2, and slow inhibitor to 0.1 ± 0.054 μmol Arg/min/100 ml. In the acute phase of pancreatitis the spontaneous protamine hydrolyzing activity increased considerably; prekallikrein levels went down and the general antitrypsin activity increased with a simultaneous decrease in rapid kallikrein inhibitor level (VEREMEENKO et al., 1975).

Refraining from the evaluation of the specificity of every method for estimation of contact prekallikrein we must, however, note that the extensive application of the method described above is restricted due to nonstandard commercial preparations of protamine sulfate.

III. Biologic Assay of Total Kallikrein in Human Plasma

Based on the low specificity of BAEe esterase reaction for kallikrein, SUROVIKINA (1975) suggested the kininogenase reaction to be used with endogenous kininogen for the estimation of two forms of kallikreins in human plasma: the one bound to the inhibitor and the other to the contact-activated form (prekallikrein). The determination was carried out in plasma free of kininases and kallikrein inhibitors because of 3 h exposure at pH 3.0 and 56 °C. The author indicates that neither inactivation of kallikrein nor activation of plasmin occurred under these conditions. The ratio of the two forms of kallikrein was estimated from the amount of kinins liberated spontaneously from endogenous kininogen at pH 7.6 and 37 °C/1 ml plasma. The "bound" form of kininogen was found after 1-h incubation of neutralized plasma (0.5 ml, 37 °C). The "total" form was found in the same aliquot, but after a preliminary 5 min contact with glass. The determination of kinins was carried out in neutralized TCA supernatant by bioassay using the rat uterus or cat jejunum. Human plasma yielded 1.1–1.7 μg bradykinin · eq/h/ml of total kallikrein. In rabbit and guinea pig plasma the values for total kallikrein varied within 1.2–1.6 and 0.05 μg bradykinin · eq/h/ml, respectively. The method was used for the evaluation of the kallikrein-kinin system state in experimental and clinical research (SUROVIKINA, 1973; SUROVIKINA et al., 1974, 1976). This method was also used by other authors.

The laborious procedure of biologic tests limits the application of the method; a disappearance of endogenous kininogen was possible in some cases; partial inactivation of kallikrein at pH 3.0, 56 °C (3 h) may influence the accuracy of the results.

A serious drawback which all the methods discussed in part A here share is the difficulty and sometimes the impossibility of comparing the results which calls for the necessity of unification of methods and of introduction of a unified system for measuring kallikrein activity and prekallikrein content in blood plasma.

IV. Estimation of Carboxypeptidase N Activity (Kininase I) With Chromogenic Substrate

LYUBLINSKAYA et al. (1973) developed a colorimetric method for estimation of kininase I (EC. 3.4.12.7) in human plasma or serum as well as in purified enzyme preparations. This method was based on splitting dipeptide 2,4-DNP-Gly-Gly (2,4-DNP-GG) from the chromogenic 2,4-DNP-Gly-Gly-L-Arg (2,4-DNP-GGA) substrate. The physicochemical properties of this dipeptide differed from the substrate. It was quantitatively extracted from acidified sample by ethylacetate containing 10% ethanol and subsequently transferred by extraction into aqueous solution containing 1% $NaHCO_3$. The 2,4-DNP-GG yield was measured by the optical density of the sample at 360 nm. 2,4-DNP-GG was characterized by a high molar extinction coefficient at 360 nm equal to 15,000 (light path – 1 cm) which allowed high sensitivity and accuracy of the method. The enzymatic reaction was carried out at pH 7.8–8.6 in phosphate or borate buffer solutions containing 1×10^{-4} *M* $CoCl_2$ (4×10^{-4} *M* – optimal substrate concentration). The presence of Co^{2+} increased kininase I activity in blood serum twofold, and in purified enzyme preparations two to threefold. The analysis required 15–20 µl serum diluted 10-fold prior to the determination. Normal human plasma hydrolyzed 0.1 µmol 2,4-DNP-GGA/min/ml.The paper dealt with the synthesis of 2,4-DNP-GGA, the properties and analytical procedures for estimation of kininase I activity in human serum. 2,4 = DNP = GGA may be used for measuring carboxypeptidase B activity.

The rate of 2,4-DNP-GGA hydrolysis by partially purified preparations of kininase I was by one order lower than hydrolysis of hipurryl-L-argininic acid (HLAa) which was accounted for by the greater strength of peptide bond as compared to that of ester bond. This method (LYUBLINSKAYA et al., 1973) is more laborious than spectrophotometric methods where HLL or HLAa were used as substrates, yet it had a number of advantages due to high values of measured optical densities (E_{360}^{1cm}) which allowed a higher degree of accuracy. Besides, the method did not require the use of precision instruments necessary in spectrophotometric measurements at 254 nm. A close correlation has been established in measuring kininase I activity by spectrophotometric (substrate HLAa) and colorimetric (substrate 2,4-DNP-GGA) methods in serum of patients in different periods of burn shock and early burn toxemia (PASKHINA et al., 1972, 1976).

V. Fluorometric Method for Estimation of Carboxycathepsin (Peptidyldipeptidase) in Human Plasma

PAVLIKHINA et al. (1975) developed a method of carboxycathepsin (E.C. 3.4.15.1) determination in human serum on the basis of works by GREGERMAN (1967) and PIQUILLOUD et al. (1970). The dipeptide, His-Leu, was split from the Cbz-Phe-His-Leu substrate and measured fluorometrically in TCA-filtrates after its reaction with o-phthalic aldehyde. Enzymatic reaction was carried out in Tris-HCl buffer (pH 7.4) containing 0.1 M NaCl. The final concentration of the substrate was 2.5×10^{-5} M; on completion of the reaction, serum proteins were precipitated by 5% TCA (final concentration). His-Leu liberated in the reaction was identified chromatographically. The kinetics of Cbz-Phe-His-Leu hydrolysis were studied. The hydrolysis of this substrate by serum was completely inhibited by EDTA (2×10^{-6} M). The method proved to be highly sensitive; the analysis required 0.03 ml serum. The activity of carboxycathepsin in serum of healthy subjects was within 7.5–18 nmol His-Leu/h/mg protein (PAVLIKHINA et al., 1975). The method was used in measuring the carboxycathepsin level under extreme conditions in dog and in hypertension patients (OREKHOVICH et al., 1975, 1976).

VI. Other Methods

KRAYNOVA et al. (1970) suggested a new method of synthesis of the hydrochloride of o-hippuryl-δ-guanidino-L-oxyvalerianic acid (o-hippuryl-L-argininic acid, HLAa) based on the interaction of 2-phenyloxazolinone-5 with the hydrochloride of L-argininic acid.

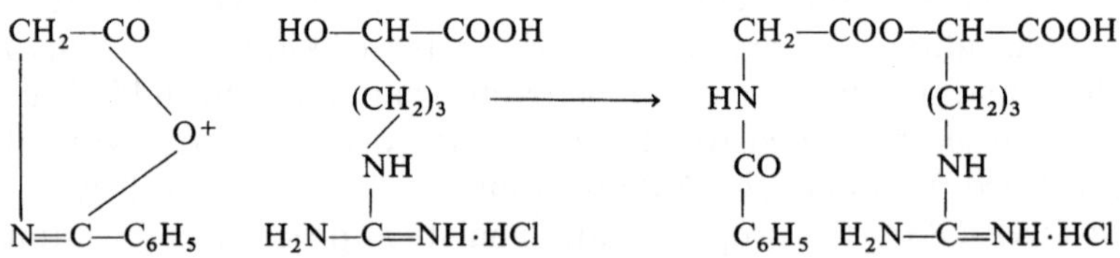

The reaction starts on heating the mixture of components (2:1, w/w) in tert-butanol and achieves completion after addition one more part by weight of oxazolinone. The reaction was controlled chromatographically. HLAa · HCL was extracted from the reaction mixture by transfer into aqueous solution; the crystalline hippuric acid was separated by filtration. The synthesized compound was not different from that described by WOLF et al. (1962) neither in R_f nor in other constants. This HLAa synthesis was considerably simpler than the only one previously described (FOLK and GLADNER, 1959) with the yield being higher (52% and 6%, respectively). Normal human serum hydrolyzed 1 μmol HLAa/min/ml. A comparatively low rate of hydrolysis of the preparation by serum indicates the necessity of additional purification HLAa from initial products. This method of HLAa synthesis was given in detail in the manual edited by OREKHOVICH (1977).

B. New Synthesis of Bradykinin and Its Analogs in Positions 5 and 8

The first bradykinin synthesis in the USSR was carried out by the classical method by SHCHUKINA et al. (1966); the preparation was completely identical in biologic activity to "Sandoz" (Switzerland). A valuable contribution to the problem of increasing bradykinin yield and the simplification of its synthesis was made by VIROVETS et al. (1968) who were the first to use free (unprotected) C-terminal arginine in

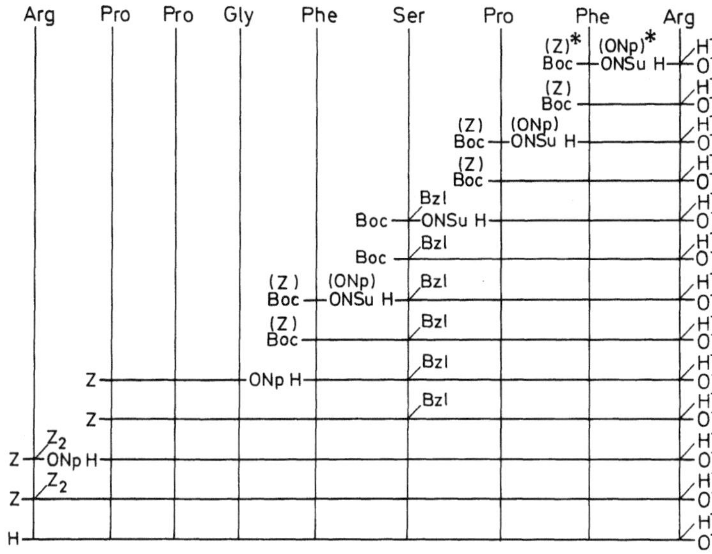

Fig. 1. Scheme of bradykinin synthesis with unprotected arginine (FILATOVA et al., 1975)

the synthesis of 6-glycine-bradykinin; elongation of the polypeptide chain was carried out by the method of p-nitrophenyl esters of Cbz-L-amino acids. The yield of the final product was 40%.

The new synthesis of bradykinin and its peptide and depsipeptide analogs based on the use of unprotected C-arginine was developed by FILATOVA et al. (1975). The synthesis was carried out by stepwise acylation of free arginine with activated esters of appropriate amino acids, peptides and depsipeptides. The method is characterized by simplicity of isolation of intermediate and final products and by high yields at every stage. The following peptides and depsipeptides were synthesized:

1. Bradykinin
2. (5-β-cyclohexyl-L-alanine)-bradykinin: (Cha^5)-bradykinin
3. (8-β-cyclohexyl-L-alanine)-bradykinin: (Cha^8)-bradykinin
4. (5,8-β-cyclohexyl-L-alanine)-bradykinin: ($Cha^{5,8}$)-bradykinin
5. (6-glycolyc acid)-bradykinin: ($Glyc^6$)-bradykinin
6. (6-glycine, 8-phenyllactic acid)-bradykinin: (Gly^6, Phl^8)-bradykinin.

Compounds 5 and 6 have been synthesized earlier (RAVDEL et al., 1967). New bradykinin synthesis was performed according to the scheme given below (Fig. 1) with the total yield of 64%. The same scheme was used in the synthesis of compounds 2–4 (see above), with yields of 54, 60, and 58% respectively. Nonadepsipeptides (compounds 5 and 6) were obtained with yields of 63 and 52%; the intramolecular acyl transfer reaction O→N has been found in the synthesis of these depsipeptides.

Biologic activity of compounds 2–6 listed above was compared to bradykinin by measuring their hypotensive effect in cat and their contractile activity on isolated rat uterus and guinea pig ileum. It was found that only compound 3 was equipotent in biologic activity to bradykinin but did not exceed it as had been found by SCHENCH et al. (1969). Analogs 2 and 4 containing cyclohexyl-L-alanine in positions 5 and 8 instead of Phe were considerably less active than bradykinin which testified the unequality of the "5" and "8" phenyl groups of the bradykinin molecule. The aromatic group in position 5 was evidently especially responsible for the biologic activity of bradykinin. Biologic activity of compounds 5 and 6 were equal to that found earlier by RAVDEL et al. (1967).

KRIT et al. (1976) synthesized another analog of bradykinin modified in position 8, namely (8-N-methyl-L-phenylalanine)-bradykinin. The simplified analogs and a depsipeptide, simplified kallidin analog were also prepared.

7. (8-N-methyl-L-phenylalanine)-bradykinin (Me Phe^8)-bradykinin
8. (6-glycine, 8-N-methyl-L-phenylalanine)-bradykinin: (Gly^6, Me Phe^8)-bradykinin
9. (6-glycine, 8-β-cyclohexyl-L-lactic acid)-bradykinin: [Gly^6, Chl^8)-bradykinin
10. (N-lysil, 6-glycine, 8-β-phenyl-L-lactic acid)-bradykinin: (Lys-, Gly^6, PhLac^8)-bradykinin.

The synthesis was undertaken to obtain analogs more stable to the kininases hydrolyzing peptide bonds of positions 7–8 or 8–9 in the bradykinin molecule.

Synthesis of the bradykinin analogs listed above was carried out by the classical method of stepwise elongation of a peptide chain with unprotected C-terminal arginine (KRIT et al., 1976). Some difficulties were encountered in the synthesis of compound 7 and its simplified analog, 8. The p-nitrobenzyl ester of N^G-nitroarginine has been used as the initial substance in this case. For preparation of the protected C-terminal tripeptide, all protecting groups were discarded by hydrofluoric acid treatment with subsequent hydration. Further elongation of the chain was carried out with unprotected C-terminal arginine.

Biologic activity and the rate of inactivation by tissue kininases of bradykinin analogs modified in position 8 compared to bradykinin were studied by POPKOVA et al. (1976). The authors used carboxypeptidase B (E.C. 3.4.12.3) which did not contain chymotrypsin (Worthington Biochem. Corporation, spec. act. 100 mU/mg), carboxycathepsin (EC. 3.4.15.1) preparation from bovine kidney purified 1500-fold (gift of ELISEEVA, YU. E.) and a lyophilized preparation of dialyzed supernatant of rat uterus homogenate free of particles precipitated at 16,000 *g*. The results are summarized in Table 1.

Table 1 shows that there is a noticeable difference in the biological activity of bradykinin analogs modified in position 8 depending on the test used. An ester bond in positions 7–8 (compound 6), does not effect the contractile activity on isolated rat uterus or guinea pig ileum, but considerably decreases (by 98%) its ability to increase the permeability of capillary membrane and sharply increases (100-fold) its hypotensive action in decerebrated cats. Substitution of phenyl radical Phe^8 for cyclohexyl and introduction of a methyl group into an amide nitrogen (Phe^8) lead to the fall of biologic activity of compounds 7 and 9 in every tests. However, more marked is the decrease in contractile activity in vitro and in the ability to increase permeability of capillary membrane. Decerebrated cats exhibited high sensitivity to i.v. injection of bradykinin and its analogs. The hypotensive effect of depsipeptide analog number 6 in decerebrated cat was considerably more pronounced than the similar effect of this analog in narcotized rats and rabbits as had been shown earlier (RAVDEL et al., 1967).

Table 1. Biologic activity of bradykinin analogs modified in position 8 and their inactivation by kininases (POPKOVA et al., 1976)

Bradykinin and its analogs	Biologic activity (%, bradykinin = 100%)				Kininase activity: nmol hydrolyzed substrate/min/mg protein		
	Constriction		Increase of capillary permeability (rabbit skin)	Hypotensive activity (decerebrated cat)	Carboxypeptidase B	Carboxycathepsin	Homogenate of rat uterus
	rat uterus	guinea pig ileum					
1. Bradykinin	100	100	100	100	956	340	7.5
6. [Gly^6, Phl^8]-bradykinin	100	25	2	10,000	585	220	1.0
3. [Cha^8]-bradykinin	10	10	2	80	58	110	1.4
9. [Gly^6, Chl^8]-bradykinin	5	10	1	170	400	75	1.3
7. [$MePhe^8$]-bradykinin	10	10	—	45	—	—	7.6

Data listed in Table 1 show that the change of peptide bond 7–8 for ester bond, as well as the introduction of a cyclohexyl group instead of the Phe^8 phenyl side group, increased the resistance of the bradykinin analogs to the action of tissue kininases. These data also show that the structure of the side chain in position 8 is essential for the enzymatic activity of both carboxypeptidase B and carboxycathepsin.

POPKOVA et al. (1976) reported that carboxycathepsin exhibited both peptidase and esterase activity. The initial rate of inactivation of bradykinin and its analogs (Table 1) in position 8 by rat uterus homogenate is very low. The analysis of products showed that in rat uterus homogenate there are enzymes of kininase I and II type and also other proteinases hydrolyzing other than 7–8 or 8–9 peptide bonds in the bradykinin molecule or its fragments. Depsipeptide number 6, the most active in the test of isolated rat uterus, was most stable to the action of kininases from rat uterus.

Depsipeptide analogs of the eldoisin fragment have also be prepared. Introduction of an ester group into active octapeptide analog of eledoisin

$(\overset{4}{\text{PyrGlu}}\text{-}\overset{5}{\text{Gly}}\text{-}\overset{6}{\text{Ala}}\text{-}\overset{7}{\text{Phe}}\text{-}\overset{8}{\text{Val}}\text{-}\overset{9}{\text{Gly}}\text{-}\overset{10}{\text{Leu}}\text{-}\overset{11}{\text{Met}}\text{-NH}_2)$, namely

into position 7,L-β-phenyllactic acid, into position 10,-L-α-isocaproic acid, into position 11,-L-α-oxy-γ-methylbutyric acid, decreases biologic activity of the peptides in vitro and in vivo to 0.01–0.1% of original eledoisin ochapeptide fragment activity (ZHUKOVA et al., 1972). These data strongly proved the importance of the amide bonds for manifestation of biologic activity of eledoisin.

C. Biochemistry of the Kinin System

I. Kallikreins of Human and Rabbit Plasma

1. Some Properties and the Effect of Natural Inhibitors

Two kininogenases designated as α- and γ-kininogenases, in accordance with their electrophoretic mobility and chromatographic behaviour, were isolated from human plasma in partially purified form by LAUFER et al. (1969). Both enzymes released bradykinin from heated (61 °C, 3 h) human or guinea pig plasma and had the biologic activity and substrate specificity characteristic of kallikreins. The difference between these two enzymes was quantitative rather than qualitative. γ-Kininogenase was identified as plasma kallikrein on the basis of its physicochemical properties, biologic activity, substrate specificity and relation to some inhibitors (LAUFER et al., 1969). The nature of α-kininogenase was not definitely established; the authors supposed that α-kininogenase was a complex of kallikrein with the α_2-macroglobulin.

Comparison of some properties of human plasma kallikrein and prekallikrein was carried out by PASKHINA et al. (1973). The enzyme and its precursor did not behave differently in polyacrylamide gel electrophoresis at pH 8.6; their MWs were identical and equal to 100,000 (gel filtration on a Sephadex G-150 column). Isoelectric focusing in a sucrose density gradient containing 1% ampholines pH 6–10 (column 110 ml, LKB, Sweden) revealed some microheterogeneity of prekallikrein: some molecular forms of the proenzyme were localized in the protein zone with pI 7.6–8.6.

Table 2. Inhibition of arginine-esterase and kininogenase activities of human and rabbit plasma kallikreins by aprotinin, CTI and SBTI (*Ki* values) (PASKHINA et al., 1975a).

Plasma kallikrein	$K_i \times 10^8 M$					
	Aprotinin		CTI		SBTI	
	BAEE-hydrolysis	Kinin-generation	BAEE-hydrolysis	Kinin-generation	BAEE-hydrolysis	Kinin-generation
Man	0.11	0.048	3.6	3.6	0.47	0.01
Rabbit	0.17	0.170	2.3	2.0	2.30	0.11

DOTSENKO et al. (1977) obtained some evidence that activation of plasma prekallikrein is an autocatalytic process. This process is slow and takes place at 37 °C and pH 8.0 (0.05 *M* Tris-HCl buffer). The authors found that LMW and HMW kininogen obtained from human plasma in partially purified form by the method of HABAL et al. (1974) inhibited the arginine esterase activity of kallikrein and the autoactivation process. The inhibitory effect of HMW kininogen was stronger than that of LMW kininogen. The authors suggested that the inhibitory effect of the HMW type might be apparently explained by the action of one of the kallikrein degradation products of kininogen with the properties of highly basic polypeptide (pI $\geqq$ 10). α_1-Antitrypsin and α_2-macroglobulin have not been found in LMW or HMW kininogen preparations. Data of DOTSENKO et al. (1977) may be of certain interest for understanding the mechanism of prekallikrein activation and regulation of activity of kallikrein in vivo.

ANDREENKO and SUVOROV (1976) obtained proof of the direct activation of rat plasma prekallikrein by a purified preparation of human plasmin (spec. act. 5.3 casein U/mg). The activation was not caused by the presence of HF or HFa in prekallikrein or plasmin preparations.

PASKHINA et al. (1975a) studied the influence of aprotinin (Trasylol, BPTI), trypsin inhibitor from cow colostrum [CTI, component B (D. CECHOVA et al., 1969) the kind gift of Dr. D. Chekhova, CSSR] and SBTI on kininogenase and BAEe esterase activities of partially purified kallikrein from human and rabbit sera. The action of the inhibitors was estimated from values of dissociation constants (K_i) of the enzyme-inhibitor complex determined by the method of GREEN and WORK (1953). Inhibition of both kallikreins by aprotinin, CTI, and SBTI was competitive. Kallikrein – inhibitor complexes obtained dissociated with difficulty. The results are presented in Table 2.

The low order of K_i for aprotinin, SBTI (10^{-10}–10^{-9} *M*) and to a smaller extent for CTI (10^{-8} *M*) indicated that these trypsin inhibitors are potent inhibitors of plasma kallikreins, which suggest similarities in the active center of plasma kallikreins and trypsin. Kininogenase activity of kallikreins is more sensitive to the inhibition by aprotinin and SBTI than is BAEe esterase activity. CTI was similar in primary structure to aprotinin but was less effective as a kallikrein inhibitor than the latter. The effect of CTI on plasma kallikreins was studied for the first time.

Human plasma kallikrein was not inhibited by either TLCK (LAUFER et al., 1969) or by an acid-stable inhibitor of trypsin and chymotrypsin from rabbit serum (NARTIKOVA and PASKHINA, 1969). Rabbit plasma kallikrein was inhibited by TLCK ($I_{50}=2.7\times10^{-4}$ M; the enzyme was preincubated with TLCK for 20 min at 20 °, pH 8.0). Various effect of TLCK on kallikrein of human and rabbit plasma may be due to some species differences in the geometry of the active center of these enzymes (PASKHINA et al., 1968 a).

2. Features of Contact Activation of Kallikrein in Rabbit Plasma

PASKHINA and EGOROVA (1966) noted the stability of kininogen in rabbit plasma on dialysis, dilution or storage of plasma in glass vessels, which indicated the resistance of rabbit prekallikrein to agents normally causing activation. The contact activation of rabbit plasma prekallikrein in vitro and in vivo were studied in detail by PASKHINA and GURTOVENKO (1972a). They found that the kallikrein-kinin system of rabbit as distinct form that of rat and man did not form free kinins on contact with clean glass beads. No decrease in arterial pressure was registered on i.v. administration of 5 ml ellagic acid suspension (2×10^{-4} M) to rabbits; kininogen level was also constant. The same concentration of ellagic acid, a well-known contact activator of HF, caused a stable hypotensive effect in rats which was accompanied by a 30%–40% decrease of kininogen levels. PASKHINA and GURTOVENKO (1972a) assumed that HF did not activate prekallikrein in rabbit plasma. Later, KOMISSAROVA and GOMAZKOV (1976) showed that activation of prekallikrein from rabbit plasma by kaolin was blocked by a certain inhibitor or HF-blocking agent which may be destroyed by treatment of plasma by chloroform for 2 min. This blocking agent also prevented activation of plasminogen in rabbit plasma by streptokinase. KOMISSAROVA and GOMASKOV (1976) interpreted the presence of this blocking agent as another evidence of the functional relation between the kinin system and fibrinolytic systems as HF-dependent systems.

The high content (up to 90%) of "stable" kininogen (LMW) and low content of "labile" (HMW) kininogen may be regarded as a specific feature of the rabbit plasma kallikrein-kinin system (EGOROVA et al., 1975, 1976). In the light of modern understanding of HMW kininogen as the necessary component of contact activation of HF in human plasma (GRIFFIN and COCHRANE, 1976), a considerably lower content of this kininogen in rabbit plasma as compared to man and rat may be one of the causes of slow contact activation of prekallikrein in mammalian species.

II. Prekallikrein Activation in Human and Animal Plasma by Organic Silica

MEGED et al. (1976) studied the influence of high dispersion (200–400 Å) macroporous (300 m^2/g) preparations of silica (aerosil) with chemically grafted surface radicals on the extent and rate of contact activation of prekallikrein in human and animal plasma. It has been established that only hydrophilic gel-forming silicas containing COOH, NH_2, or OH groups possessed a marked ability to activate prekallikrein. Hydrophobic silicas (methylacrosil, butosil, silazanoaerosil) that do not form gels but differed in charge did not activate prekallikrein. Using protamine sulfate as substrate for measuring the amounts of contact kallikrein, MEGED et al. (1976) found that the extent of prekallikrein activation is determined by swelling rather than by charge. The identity of activation curves of human and rat plasma (with the maximum in the first minute and the point of inflection in the fifth) obtained by the use of kaolin (10 mg/ml plasma) and aminoaerosil (5 mg/ml) has been observed. Species and philogenetic features were the cause of slow (3–5 min) and low (50–25%) activation of Hageman factor (HF) by aminoaerosil in dog and rabbit plasma as compared to man. Hen plasma was not subject to contact activation. The data of MEGED et al. (1976) suggest that the hydrophilic character rather than the charge determines the ability of aminoaerosil to activate HF in mamalain plasma. The contradicts the accepted view and needs to be studied further.

III. Low and High Molecular Weight Rabbit Kininogens: Isolation, Properties, and Specificity as Substrates for Different Kallikreins

Systematic studies of rabbit LMW and HMW kininogens and their specificity as kinin-containing substrates for kallikreins of various organs and species were carried out by PASKHINA and coworkers. The properties of highly purified preparations of rabbit LMW kininogen obtained from Cohn plasma fraction IV–I were described earlier (EGOROVA and PASKHINA, 1967). Later studies (EGOROVA et al., 1969, 1975) dealt with determination of amino acid composition, number of S-S bonds, N-terminal amino acid and some other properties, in similar LMW kininogen preparations (Table 3). These investigations showed that LMW rabbit kininogen was similar but not identical to bovine LMW kininogen previously studied detail by Japanese authors (KOMIYA et al., 1974).

EGOROVA et al. (1975, 1976) developed a new method for isolation of LMW and HMW kininogens from one portion of fresh citrated rabbit plasma. At the first step, both forms were strongly adsorbed from dilutied citrate plasma as acid glycoproteins on DEAE-Sephadex, batchwise, (equillibrated with 0.02 M – Na-phosphate buffer pH 7.2, sontaining 0.12 M NaCl and 3×10^{-3} M Na-EDTA) and were separated from main body of plasma proteins (up to 90%) which were not adsorbed under these conditions. Filtrate containing no more than 5%–7% kininogen was discarded and a thick suspension of DEAE-Sephadex A-50 containing both kininogens was transferred on column, where LMW and HMW forms were separated by gradient elution with NaCl of increasing concentrations. Further purification of each kininogen was carried out separately by different chromatographic methods. An interesting feature of HMW kininogen was the increase of its total charge during the purification process. Apparently, as a result of separation of an acid component, HMW kininogen became a weakly-basic protein and could be adsorbed on CM-cellulose at pH 6.5. Under these conditions LMW kininogen was not adsorbed by this exchanger. The yield of the LMW form was only 10%–12% of the total; 15–20 mg LMW kininogen preparation may be obtained from 1 liter of citrated plasma; its spec. act. 18–20 μg bradykinin · eq/mg protein. HMW kininogen yield was 40%–50% of the initial contents of this form in rabbit plasma: its spec. act. was approximately 10 μg bradykinin · eq/mg, i.e., 6–8 mg HMW kininogen may be obtained from 1 liter plasma. The properties of rabbit HMW and LMW kininogens are compared in Table 3. Electrophoresis of purified preparations in polyacrylamide get at pH 8.6

Table 3. The comparison of properties of purified rabbit plasma HMW and LMV kininogen (EGOROVA et al., 1975, 1976).

Properties	LMW	HMW
M.W. (gel-filtration Sephadex G-200)	54,000	140,000
$S^0_{20,w}$	3.6 S	7.6 S
Electrophoretic mobility in PAG (pH 8.6)	α_1-globulin (postalbumin)	α_2-globulin
Isoelectric point	4.6	~ 6.5
Number of S–S bonds per mole	6	14
Kinin content (μg bradykinin · eq/mg protein)	18–20	10
Content in plasma (% from total kininogen)	90	10
Carbohydrate (%)	15.2	16.0
Peptide (%)	82.9	73–75
N-terminal aminoacid	Leucine (?)	Not determined
Treating by 2.5% SDS and 8 *M* urea (37 °C, 72 h)	Did not dissociete into subunits	
Treating by 2-mercaptoethanol and 8 *M* urea (37 °C, 16 h)	Not cleared	Split into two fragments

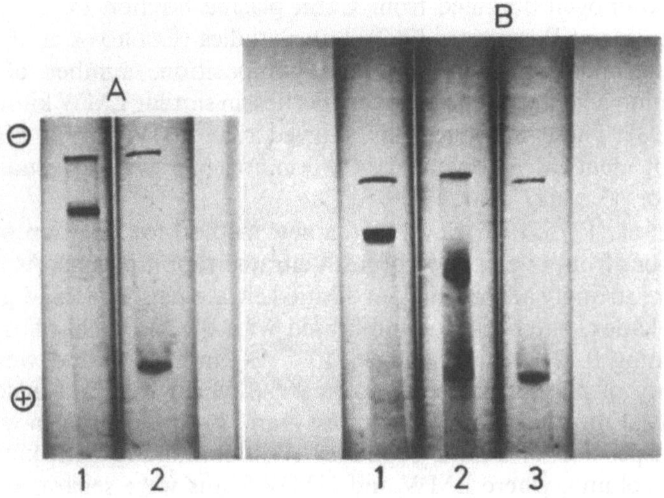

Fig. 2A and B. Polyacrylamide gel electrophoresis of highly purified rabbit HMW and LMW kininogens (from EGOROVA et al., 1976). **A** 7.5% gel; pH 8.3; (1) HMW kininogen (spec. act. 10 μg bradykinin/mg); (2) LMW kininogen (spec. act. 20 μg bradykinin/mg); **B** 7.5% gel; 0.01 M Na-phosphate buffer (pH 7.1), 0.5% SDS; (1) HMW kininogen after treatment with 2.5% SDS and 8 *M* urea (72 h, 37 °C); (2 and 3) HMW kininogen and LMW kininogen after treatment with 0.05 *M* β-mercaptoethanol and 8 *M* urea (20 h, 37 °C)

obtained by this method is shown in Fig. 2A. Treating HMW kininogen with 0.05 *M* 2-mercaptoethanol in the presence of 8 *M* urea (37 °C, 72 h) split HMW kininogen into two fragments with MW 80,000 and 30,000 respectively; the kinin-containing group was localized with the LMW fragment. Under these conditions the LMW forms did not dissociate (Fig. 2B). EGOROVA et al. (1975, 1976) suggested that rabbit HMW and LMW kininogens are different glycoproteins; the HMW com-

Table 4. The rates of kinin release from rabbit LMW and HMW kininogens by kallikreins of various origin and by trypsin.

Rabbit kininogen	Kinin release (μg bradykinin·eq/mg protein/min)			
	Kallikreins (source)			Trypsin
	Human plasma[a]	Human saliva[b]	Pig pancreas[c]	
LMW	0	120–160	~800	5.0
HMW	2.1	16–20	~ 80	5.0

[a] and [b] partially purified preparations and [c] highly purified preparation (isoenzyme B); kind gift of Dr. F. FIEDLER, spec. act. ~200 U/mg; substrate BAEe).

pound being neither, a dimer nor a trimer of the LMW compound. It is not excluded, however, that HMW kininogen is composed of two polypeptide chains. The kinin-containing group in either form did not occupy the C-terminal position.

LMW and HMW rabbit kininogens were functionally different. The LMW was considerably more specific as substrate for glandular kallikreins than the HMW. The latter was more specific for plasma kallikreins (Table 4). The absolute rate of dekinination of LMW kininogen by hog pancreatic and human selivary kallikreins were very high. Trypsin dekininized both substrates equally.

Purified rabbit HMW preparation (EGOROVA et al., 1976) was similar in some of properties to human plasma HMW kininogen isolated by HABAL et al. (1974).

Two functionally different kininogens designated as kininogen I and II were isolated by KAURICHEVA et al. (1971) from horse plasma. The MW of both kininogens was about 60,000. Kininogen I was unstable during storage. Horse plasma kallikrein liberated kinins only from kininogen I. Plasmin and kininogenase from *Bothrops jararaca* venom interacted with both kininogens. The authors suggested that plasmin was the sole kininogenase of plasma which liberated kinins from both "labile" and "stable" substrates.

IV. Mechanism of the Kininogenase Reaction in Model Systems With Purified Components

PASKHINA et al. (1977a) studied the natures of peptide fragments, kinins among them, split from highly purified LMW rabbit kininogen in the process of its dekinination by glandular kininogenases: hog pancreatic kallikrein (component B, gift of Dr. F. FIEDLER) and partially purified kallikrein of human salivary gland (spec. act. 0.55 U/mg; substrate, BAEe). The products of LMW kininogen digestion by both kallikreins were fractionated and identified by use of chromatography on Sephadex G-75 and SP-Sephadex C-25, isoelectrofocusing in polyacrylamide gel, thin-layer chromatography and peptide mapping. Biologic activity of products of digestion was measured on rat uterus and compared to synthetic bradykinin. It has been found that hog pancreatic kallikrein liberated kinins from LMW kininogen at the rate of 800 μg bradykinin · eq/mg preparation and human salivary kallikrein at the rate of 120–160 μg bradykinin · eq/min/mg. The reaction of dekinination of LMW kininogen

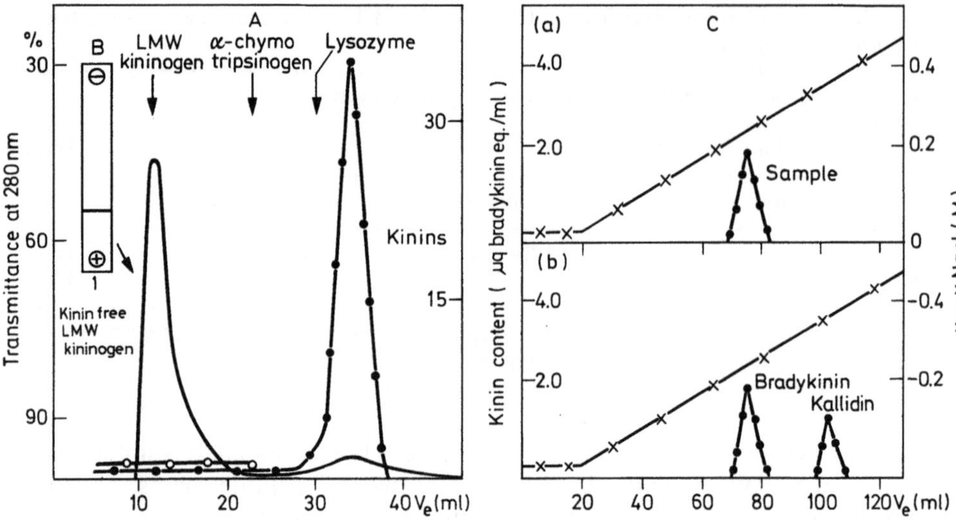

Fig. 3A–C. Fractionation of hog pancreatic kallikrein digest of rabbit plasma LMW kininogen (PASKHINA et al., 1977a). **A** Gel-filtration of LMW kininogen digest (6 mg, 0.2 ml) on a Sephadex G-75 column. Bed dimensions: 0.9 × 60 cm (column K 9/60, Pharmacia, Sweden); eluant: 0.02 *M* Tris-HCl buffer, pH 8.1, 10^{-3} *M* Na_2-EDTA, 10^{-5} *M* Na-oxalate, and 0.1 *M* NaCl; flow rate: 12 ml/h. Kinin activity (isolated rat uterus) before (-●-) and after (-○-) treatment of each fraction with trypsin; (—) transmittance (T^{280} %); arrows above indicate V_e of marker proteins, **B** Isoelectrofocusing of LMW kininogen depleted of kinins pH gradient 3–9; 2% ampholines; 5% gel, **C** Chromatography of kinin fraction on a SP-Sephadex G-25 column. Bed dimensions: 0.9 × 15 cm (column K 9/15, Pharmacia, Sweden); equilibrating buffer: 0.02 *M* Tris-HCl, pH 8.1, 10^{-5} *M* Na-oxalate and 0.02 *M* NaCl; elution: the same buffer with a linear NaCl gradient (0.02–0.50 *M*) flow rate 4 ml/h; 6 °C; (a) aliquots of kinin fraction (Fig. A) containing kinin levels equal to 10 μg bradykinin · eq; (b) mixture of 10 μg bradykinin (Reanal, Hungary) and 10 μg lysyl-bradykinin – (Schering-AG, Germany)

by hog pancreatic kallikrein (pH 8.1; 37 °C, 15 min, weight ratio kallikrein: kininogen = 1:600) was accomponied by hydrolysis of no more than two to three peptide bonds in kininogen since only one HMW component was found in the digest. Its MW is close to that of unhydrolyzed LMW kininogen, i.e., 56,000 (Fig. 3). The only kinin identified by SP-Sephadex C-25 chromatography and by peptide mapping with bradykinin (Fig. 3) was found in the LMW peptide fraction. In contrast to data of KATO et al. (1968) kallidin (lysyl-bradykinin) was not found within the products of LMW kininogen hydrolysis by pancreatic kallikrein. Gradient eluation on SP-Sephadex C-25 column allowed good separation of bradykinin and kallidin. Human salivary kallikrein split kallidin from LMW kininogen under similar conditions. As with hog pancreatic kallikrein this enzyme did not cause extensive fragmentation of the LMW kininogen molecule. These last results were regarded by the authors as preliminary (PASKHINA et al., 1977a).

These studies demonstrated high specificity of the kininogenase reaction as a reaction of limited proteolysis. In the process of dekinination of LMW kininogen by secretory kininogenase only those peptide bonds were hydrolyzed which connected the kinin fragment with the main molecule. It has been shown for the first time that hog pancreatic kallikrein and human salivary kallikrein liberated different kinins

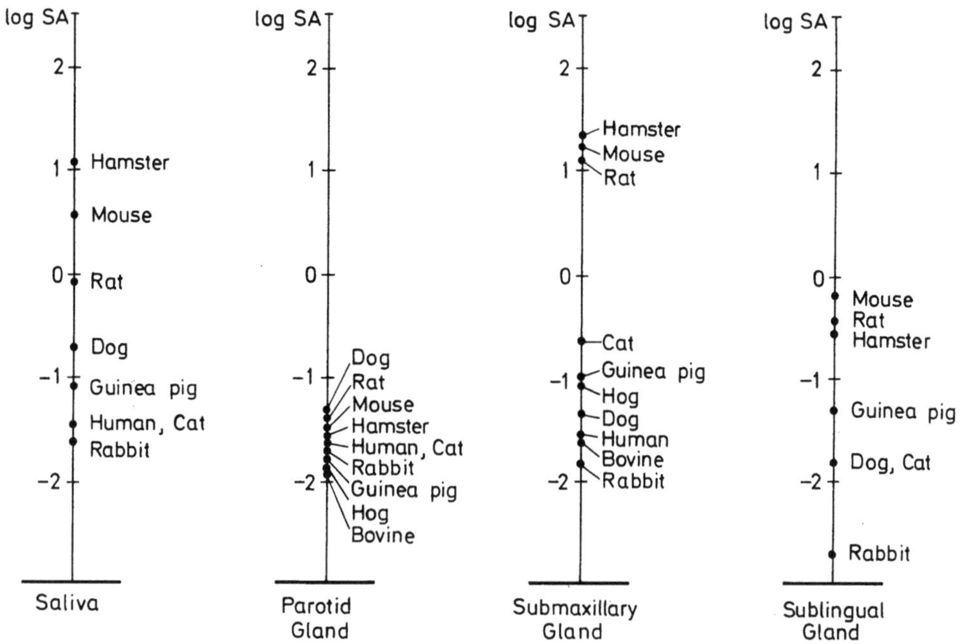

Fig. 4. Kallikrein activity in saliva and salivary glands of men and animals (log of µmol BAEe/min/mg) (LEVITSKY, A.P. unpublished)

from the same LMW kininogen: bradykinin* and kallidin, respectively. The fact that pancreatic kallikrein splits bradykinin from LMW kininogen but not kallidin was consistent with the substrate specificity of hog pancreatic kallikrein (FIEDLER, 1975).

V. Salivary Kallikreins of Man and Mammals

New data on comparative kallikrein content in saliva and salivary glands of man and various animals (mouse, rat, golden hamster, guinea pig, rabbit, cat, dog, swine, cow) have been obtained by LEVITSKIY et al. (1974, 1973). Kallikrein content estimated by BAEe esterase activity was found to vary and to depend on the animal. It was especially high in saliva and submandibulary glands of rodents, golden hamster in particular, where arginine esterase activity was 10 times higher than in rat.

Partially purified kallikrein preparations were obtained from saliva of man, rat, hamster, cat, and dog; their physicochemical and enzymatic properties and biologic activity were investigated by VOVCHUK et al. (1975). Two molecular forms of kallikrein designated by the authors as I and II have been found in mixed as well as parotid and submandibular human saliva. They varied in pI, biologic activity and other properties (VOVCHUK et al., 1975). Molecular form I as distinct from II was not

* *Added in proof.* Unpublished data (MAKEVNINA, L.G., LEVINA, G.O., SCHERSTUCK, S.V. and PASKINA, T.S.) show that pancreatic kallikrein released only kallidin from normal untreated rabbit plasma. Liberation by this enzyme of bradikinin from purified preparation of rabbit LMW kininogen may be the result of some structural transformation of the latter.

Table 5. Hypotensive action of partially purified prepartions of salivary kallikreins of different species (VOVCHUK et al., 1975)

Salivary kallikrein (origin)	Test animal	Hypotensive activity corresponding to 1 arginine esterase unit of each enzyme[a] (in mm Hg)
Rat	Rat	4.8
Hamster	Hamster	10.7
Dog	Dog	179.0
Cat	Cat	447.3
Human kallikrein (molecular form)		
Kallikrein I	Cat	727.0
Kallikrein II	Cat	1212.1

[a] 1 esterase unit of kallikrein is equal to the hydrolysis 1 μmol/BAEe/min.

absorbed on CM-cellulose; it was stable to acetone at −2 °C and had high kininogenase activity (EGOROVA et al., 1976) equal to 50–300 μg bradykinin · eq per arginine esterase unit of the enzyme for preparations of various degrees of purification. Human salivary kallikrein showed a marked affinity for rabbit LMW kininogen; the rate of kinin formation from rabbit HMW kininogen was 5%–10% of that from LMW kininogen (EGOROVA et al., 1976). Preliminary investigations showed that form I split kallidin from LMW kininogen (PASKHINA et al., 1977a).

Acetone-stable kallikrein I apparently corresponded to salivary kallikrein preparations obtained by MORIYA et al. (1966) and FUJIMOTO et al. (1973). The molecular nature kallikrein II, inactivated by acetone, has not been established so far, since its kininogenase activity was not determined and mediators liberated from plasma were nonidentified (VOVCHUK et al., 1975). Kallikrein I and II from human saliva were somewhat different at optimum pH values (9.3 and 9.7, respectively) and K_m values (10^{-3} M and 4×10^{-3} M, BAEe substrate). Kallikrein I and II hydrolysed BAEe faster than protamine sulphate and BANA. Both forms of human salivary kallikrein were not inhibited by SBTI, ovomucoid, p-chloromercuribenzoate, TLCK, and TPCK. Kallikrein I were inhibited by aprotinin.

Human salivary kallikreins sharply decreased the arterial pressure in dog, rat, and rabbit but did not influence the arterial pressure of guinea pig; the hypotensive effect of kallikrein II being four to five times greater than in the case of kallikrein I. Hypotensive effect of partially purified human and animal kallikrein preparations of various kinds relative to arginine esterase units of each enzyme is shown in Table 5. VOVCHUK et al. (1975) assumed that a decrease in arginine esterase and an increase in hypotensive activity of kallikrein preparations studied from rat to man indicated the phylogenetic increase of specific kallikrein function. However, the differences may be accounted for by various physiologic functions of salivary kallikreins in animals of various species in connection with peculiarities of their food and habitation and by the differing sensitivity of these kallikreins to plasma inhibitors. Human salivary kallikreins had low arginine esterase activity and apparently had low sensitivity to kallikrein inhibitors of cat plasma. Besides, one can not exclude the presence of impurities such as additional esterases in enzyme preparations.

VI. Kininogenase From Bovine Spleen

LOKSHINA et al. (1976) have found a neutral proteinase with kininogenase activity in bovine spleen extract. Using rabbit LMW kininogen as substrate, the authors found the activity of maximum purified preparations to be equal to formation of 7.3 μg bradykinin · eq/h/mg (pH 7.5, 37 °C). Spleen kininogenase is evidently a serine proteinase type since the activity of the enzyme was inhibited by DFP (5×10^{-4} *M*); it was also inhibited by aprotinin (1×10^{-5} *M*) but not by SBTI. The MW of the enzyme was approximately 25,000. Kininogenase from spleen tissue did not hydrolize BAEe and BANA. In its properties the enzyme was close to the neutral proteinases from polymorphous nuclear leukocytes of man (MOVAT et al., 1976).

VII. Kininase I: Effect of Bradykinin-Potentiating Peptides and Plasma Inhibitor

PASKHINA et al. (1975b) showed that bradykinin-potentiating peptides – BPP_{5a} (Pyr-Glu-Hys-Trp-Ala-Pro-) and BPP_9 (PyrGly-Gly-Leu-Pro-Arg.Pro-Hys-Ile-Pro-Pro) – identical in structure to peptides isolated from *Bothrops jararaca* and *Agkistrodon halys blomhoffii* venom, did not inhibit peptidase and esterase activities of partially purified preparations of carboxypeptidase-N from human plasma and did not influence kininase activity of human serum in vitro. Thus, the bradykinin-potentiating and prolonging effect of BPP_5 and BPP_9 did not depend on their influence on plasma kininase I. The C-terminal fragment of bradykinin (Phe-Ser-Pro-Phe-Arg) was a competitive inhibitor of kininase I. All the three peptides were synthesized by the classic method of elongation of polypeptide chain by activated p-nitrophenyl esters (RAVDEL et al., 1975).

TRAPEZNIKOVA and MARDASHEV (1975) reported the presence of carboxypeptidase-N inhibitor in human plasma with an apparent polypeptide nature and a MW of about 2000. Its inhibiting effect was considerably more marked under preincubation of the factor with enzyme. The physiologic function and the structure of this inhibitor have not been found so far.

VIII. Carboxycathepsin: Discovery and Properties of Purified Preparations

ELISEEVA and OREKHOVICH (1963) discovered a new enzyme in bovine kidney cortex which they named carboxycathepsin. The enzyme stepwise split dipeptides from C-terminals of polypeptide chain; an unsubstituted C-terminal COOH group was essentially for the enzyme action. Its pH optimum was in the range of pH 7.0–7.3 and it was stable at pH 5–10. Carboxycathepsin was inhibited by EDTA (5×10^{-3} *M*) and by 0.01 *M* cysteine. The enzyme exhibited a wide substrate specificity and hydrolyzed almost any peptide bond formed by the second and third amino acid residues from the C-end of the polypeptide chain with the exception of peptide bonds formed by the iminogroup of proline. Bzn-Gly-Phe-Pro proved to be the best substrate for carboxycathepsin. OREKHOVICH (1968) assumed that the formation of physiologically active peptides, especially the conversion of angiotensin I to angiotensin II, might be one of carboxycathepsin functions. Later OREKHOVICH and co-workers

(ELISEEVA et al., 1970) confirmed this assumption. They demonstrated that highly purified carboxycathepsin preparations from bovine kidney catalyzed the conversion of angiotensin I into angiotensin II and inactivated bradykinin. Both reactions were catalyzed by the same enzyme by splitting the C-terminal dipeptide from both angiotensin I and bradykinin with the formation of His-Leu and Phe-Arg, respectively. Carboxycathepsin did not hydrolyse angiotensin II while bradykinin cleavage went further.

Substrate specificity of carboxycathepsin was studied by using a large number of synthetic and natural peptides (ELISEEVA et al., 1970, 1971, 1974). These and other properties of the purified enzyme (the character of activation by Cl^- ions, inhibition by chelating agents, activation by Co^{2+}, Zn^{2+}, Mn^{2+} etc.) led the authors to conclude that carboxycathepsin was identical to the angiotensin-I-converting enzyme found by SKEGGS et al. (1954) in equine plasma and to the kininase II of human plasma and peptidase P from hog kidney cortex independently found by ERDÖS and YANG and YANG and ERDÖS in 1967.

In the papers cited (ELISEEVA et al., 1970, 1971) and later (OREKHOVICH et al., 1975, 1976) the authors put forward the concept of the key role of carboxycathepsin in the regulation of systemic blood pressure performed by activation of the renin-angiotensin system and inactivation of a powerful hypotensive factor – bradykinin. The concept is now widely accepted.

Highly purified carboxycathepsin preparations from bovine kidney (ELISEEVA et al., 1974, 1976a) and lung (ELISEEVA et al., 1976b) were obtained by modern techniques of preparative enzymology; a highly sensitive fluorometric method (substrate Cbz-Phe-His-Leu) was used for purification and the study of the enzyme properties. The preparation from bovine kidneys had a spec. act. of 31, and that from bovine lung was equal to 29 μmol His-Leu min/mg. The authors reported the identity of carboxycathepsins from these two organs which followed from the comparison of their physicochemical, enzymatic and other properties (ELISEEVA et al., 1976a, b). The enzymes of bovine kidney and lung did not differ in MW (180–190,000 from gel filtration on Sephadex G-200), in optimum pH, or in pI values (4.45 ± 0.15). Both enzymes were activated by chloride ions and inactivated equally by chelating agents. The fact of combining two functions: angiotensin conversion and kinin hydrolysis in the protein obtained from bovine kidney or lung tissue has been confirmed. Carboxycathepsin from bovine kidney and lung was inhibited by its substrates: bradykinin (I_{50} corresponded to 5×10^{-7} *M*) and angiotensin I ($I_{50} = 5 \times 10^{-5}$ *M*) which indicated great affinity of the enzyme for bradykinin (ELISEEVA et al., 1976a, b). Cbz-D-Phe-His-Leu as well as peptides containing proline in the second position from the C-terminal (Gly-Pro-Pro or Gly-Pro-Gly) inhibited carboxycathepsin (ELISEEVA et al., 1976b).

Dry whole venoms of some Central Asia snakes inhibited bovine lung carboxycathepsin (ELISEEVA et al., 1976b). The greatest inhibiting effect was exhibited by venoms of *Echis carinatus* (2.5 μg/ml inhibited lung carboxycathepsin by 35%) and *Naja oxiana Eichiwald* (2.5 μg/ml inhibited the enzyme by 72%). The active component of *Echis carinatus* venom was purified 200 fold; its MW was about 2000.

The influence of bovine kidney carboxycathepsin on the biologic activity of bradykinin was partly reported earlier (ELISEEVA et al., 1970, 1971) and was described in detail by EGOROVA and ELISEEVA (1976).

D. Physiology and Pharmacology of Kinins and the Kallikrein-Kinin System

I. Permeability, Hemo- and Pharmacodynamics

1. Effect of Bradykinin on Capillary Permeability and Hemodynamics

OYVIN et al. (1970) and GAPONYUK and OYVIN (1971b) showed that bradykinin increased vascular permeability in skin sites which did not react to histamine and serotonin in rats, rabbits, and guinea pigs. This indicated that the bradykinin effect on endothelial cells was direct and not influenced by other mediators. Skin vessels in rabbits and rats were 1.5 times more sensitive to bradykinin and Met-Lys-bradykinin than to kallidin (GAPONYUK and OYVIN, 1971a).

No correlation between an increase in permeability of blood microvessels and changes in microcirculation could be found by OYVIN et al. (1970, 1972a) on application of very diluted solutions of bradykinin and histamine on rat mesentery. Increase in capillary permeability under the action of bradykinin, histamine, and serotonin was found to be an active process involving some consumption of energy and dependent on the synthesis of high energy yielding compounds. This finding of the same authors is of significant theoretical importance (OYVIN et al., 1973). No increase in capillary permeability was caused by these mediators under local hypoxia induced by intracutaneous injection of NaCN in concentrations inhibiting tissue respiration (10^{-3}–10^{-2} M). The ability of bradykinin, histamine, and serotonin to increase capillary permeability was restored by administration of ATP (10^{-3}–10^{-2} M) into skin sites locally affected by hypoxia (GAPONYUK and UKLONSKAYA, 1974). These facts confirm the hypothesis of MAJNO and PALADE (1961) and B. ZWEIFACH (1964) developed by OYVIN et al. (1970) that bradykinin, histamine, and serotonin increase the permeability of capillary membrane as a result of active contractility of cell structures of endothelium. However, since increase in permeability of rabbit skin and rat messentery induced by xylol or soft burn was not affected by cyanide in concentrations inhibiting cellular respiration, OYVIN et al. (1970, 1973) doubted the predominant role of bradykinin and histamine as mediators of the early phases of inflammation.

GOMAZKOV and SHIMKOVICH (1974) found that the same bradykinin dose introduced in the aorta was three times more effective than that injected intravenously due to inactivation of bradykinin by lung tissue kininases. The hypotensive effect of bradykinin increased fivefold after i.v. injection of rats by a dose of 40 mg unitiol/kg (bisulphite derivative of 2,3-dimercaptopropanol, the USSR preparation), a kininase inhibitor. This effect was twofold after administration of bradykinin into the aorta. Unitiol did not affect responses to administration of acetylcholine and angiotensin. The hypotensive effect of bradykinin in the case of its simultaneous administration with unitiol and the β-adrenoceptor inhibitor, visken (preparation LB-46; "Sandoz," Switzerland), exceeded the sum of hypotensive responses as compared to bradykinin and one of the above agents separately.

The α-adrenoceptor blocking agent, tropaphen (hydrochloride of torpin series, α-phenyl-β-acetoxyphenylpropionic acid, preparation of USSR), did not affect the hypotensive action of bradykinin (COMAZKOV and SHIMKOVICH, 1974).

The bradykinin-potentiating effect of unitiol was supposed to be due to inhibition of lung kininases while the enhanced effect of β-adrenoceptor blocking agents was determined by their immediate or indirect action on bradykinin receptors in the peripheral vessel bed (GOMAZKOV and SHIMKOVICH, 1974). The same authors showed (GOMAZKOV and SHIMKOVICH, 1975) that bradykinin action in vitro and in vivo was inhibited by ciproheptadin – the serotonin and histamin inhibitor (product of Merck). The ciproheptadin effect was supposed to be based on inhibition of prekallikrein activation and on immediate blocking of the bradykinin receptor.

2. Bradykinin in Angiographic Studies

High sensitivity of human blood vessels to bradykinin was established by selective angiography and by direct measurement of pressure in celiac artery GAPONYUK et al., 1975a). An injection of bradykinin (0.1–10 μg/kg) resulted in a fall of blood pressure, an increase in flow rate and in the diameter of arterial and venous vessels, an increase of arterial-arterial, arterial-venous, and venous-venous anastomosis, and an increase in the number of functioning capillaries. No organ differences in vessel reaction to bradykinin were found. The authors found it expedient to use 5–10 μg/kg doses of bradykinin in angiographic examinations of celiac artery pool and developed a total pharmacoangiographic bradykinin method (GAPONYUK et al., 1975b).

The effects of bradykinin on vessels of healthy tissue and that affected by malignant tumor were completely different in angiographic examinations (STRIGUNOV and GAPONYUK, 1975). The contrast medium was not stored in malignant tumor as was the case in healthy tissue and in nonmalignant tumor; a vessel lumen in malignant tumor contracted in response to bradykinin and did not dilate. The latter observation has been used in the diagnosis of malignant and nonmalignant tumors (STRIGUNOV and GAPONYUK, 1975).

3. Effects of Salivary Kallikreins on Hemodynamics

The effects of partially purified preparations of salivary kallikreins of man, rat, and golden hamster applied on microvessels of rat mesentery and hamster buccal sac were studied by BARABASH et al. (1976b) by the method of life microscopy. Dilatation of arterioles, decrease of venule diameter, and increase in the number of active capillaries have been observed. Species and organ differences of these effects have been found.

II. Possible Mechanism of Bradykinin Action on Smooth Muscle

In experiments with strips of guinea pig muscle *(Taenia coli)*, POGADAEV and TIMIN (1976) and KHODOROV et al. (1976) have obtained new data suggesting the existence of chemoexcitable calcium channels in cellular membrane along with well known electroexcitable calcium channels responsible for the action potential generation. Chemoexcitable channels are activated as a result of interaction of bradykinin with the specific receptor. In physiologic conditions, the low concentration of bradykinin is enough for the critical depolarization of the membrane of the smooth muscle cells. This depolarization activates electroexcitable channels resulting in an action potential which induces muscle fibre contraction. Bradykinin in high concentrations (10^{-5} g/ml) increases the Ca^{2+} influx to such an extent that strong contraction appears even under complete inactivation of electroexcitable channels in high potassium solution. Both chemo- and electroexcitable channels are blocked by verapamil, compound D-600, and Mn^{2+}. The pharmacologic distinction of these two types of calcium channels can be achieved by the use of some local anaesthetics (procain, trimecain, QX-572; all in concentration 10^{-5} g/ml) and papaverine (10^{-6} g/ml) which strongly inhibited the effect of bradykinin. These findings are of great significance in the study of molecular mechanisms of bradykinin action on the excitable membrane.

Bradykinin stimulated the tonus of isolated bronchial fiber of cat and decreased the transmembrane potential of smooth muscle fibers (SHEVCHENKO, 1976). The depolarizing effect of bradykinin was completely depressed by amidopyrine solution (4×10^{-4} g/ml).

The activity of Mg, Na, and K-ATP-ases of brain and kidney microsomes in rat was not affected in vitro by bradykinin over a wide range of concentrations (10^{-12}–10^{-3} *M*); i.v. injection of bradykinin (8 μg/kg rat weight) activated Na, K-ATP-ase by 30–40%; no changes in Mg-ATP-ase activity of brain and kidney microsomes in rat were observed (CHERNUKH et al., 1974a).

III. Antikinin Preparations – Parmidine (Pyridinolcarbamate)

The antiinflammation and antibradykinin effects of parmidine (2,6-pyridinmethan-bis-N-methylcarbamate, pyridinolcarbamate, the USSR analog of Japanese anginin) has been studied. Parmidine doses of 25–50 mg/kg administered to rats per os inhibited exudative inflammation induced by subplanter administration of bradykinin (SHWARTZ et al., 1975). However, parmidine did not decrease the edema of rat paw caused by histamine or dextrane and did not inhibit proliferative inflammation induced by AgCl suspension. Antiexudative effect of parmidine is greater than that of butadione. The authors assumed high antibradykinin selectivity of parmidine. Parmidine concentrations of 10^{-9} g/ml and higher inhibited contraction of guinea pig ileum by bradykinin in vitro; 0.1–0.25 mg/kg completely blocked its bronchoconstrictor effect in guinea pig in vivo. Parmidine was more selective than dimedrol which also exhibited antihistamine, cholinolytic, and antibradykinin effects (SWARTZ and MASHKOVSKIY, 1976). The effect of parmidine on hemostasis in comparison with anginin was studied by MASHKOVSKIY et al. (1976). Inhibition of the platelet aggregation caused by ADP or serotonin and adrenalin, slower blood coagulation, and acceleretion of fibrinolysis were observed in rabbits when parmidine was given orally in doses of 5, 10, and 30 mg/kg. Anginin had the same effect. These latter effects of parmidine may be beneficial in the treatment of arterosclerosis. The existing data on the mechanism of action and pharmacology of pyridinolcarbamate have been considerably developed by the above studies.

IV. Kinin System and Regulation of Some Physiologic Functions

Participation of kidney and plasma kallikrein-kinin system in adaptation to physical load was suggested by LANTSBERG and NEKRASOVA (1972). Examination of healthy persons and sportsmen showed that physical load close to a maximum is accompanied by a decrease in excretion of kallikrein and free kinins in urine and by distinct mobilization of plasma kinin system in physically untrained people. The same load in sportsmen results in an increase of kidney kinin system activity and less marked mobilization of plasma KS.

The importance of kidney kallikrein in regulation of sodium excretionw as established by LANTSBERG et al. (1974). Healthy males aged 18–30 under physical load exhibited an increase in diuresis and sodium excretion along with increased kallikrein excretion. At rest, the decrease in excretion of kallikrein and free kinins did not change diuresis but decreased sodium excretion.

GOMASKOV et al. (1973) and MEERSON et al. (1974) found mobilization of plasma kinin system in rats after hemodynamic adaptation to various physical loads and to altitude hypoxia. The decrease of depressor response to bradykinin in the latter case was accounted for by the increase in the activity of lung kininases.

V. Possible Physiologic Function of Salivary Kallikreins

VOVCHUK et al. (1977) investigated the influence of i.v. injection of partially purified kallikrein from dog submandibular glands on gastric secretion in esophagotomic dogs with fistula in the stomach after simulated feeding. The decrease in gastric secretion and in the concentration and total production of HCl was observed 30 min after i.v. administration of kallikrein. Pepsin activity in gastric juice increased while gastrixin activity remained unchanged. However, the total concentration of secreted pepsin and gastrixin also decreased due to the decrease of gastric secretion. Qualitative and quantitative changes in gastric secretion correlated with doses of 15, 30, 60 µg/kg of preparation. A dose of 160 µg/kg caused sharp inhibition of all the parameters of gastric secretion and 15 µg/kg was close to threshold. The authors assumed that, as with sialogastron, salivary kallikrein produced specific and selective effect on the cell lining of gastric glands.

E. Kallikrein-Kinin System in Pathologic Conditions

I. Cardiovascular Diseases

1. Experimental Research

A thourough study of the kinin system of rat plasma in acute myocardial ischemia was carried out by GOMAZKOV et al. (1972a, 1973). It has been shown that ligation of the left coronary artery in rats resulting in acute myocardial ischemia caused a 30–40% decrease in prekallikrein and labile ("contact") kininogen I levels after 30 min. Kininogen II content determined from the reaction with trypsin remained unchanged. A considerable difference in the arterial-venous level of kininogen I in rat plasma at the developing myocardial infarction was observed (GOMASKOV et al., 1972a). The kinin system in experimental myocardial infarction in dogs was activated in the first minutes of developing ischemia (STUKALOVA et al., 1975). Plasma kallikrein activity in dog determined by the method of PASKHINA and YAROVAYA (1970a) increased sharply after i.v. injection of 1 ml 0.1% adrenalin. The same i.v. adrenalin dose in healthy dogs decreased the kininogen level from 8.22 ± 1.43 to

4.21 ± 0.99 μg bradykinin · eq/ml plasma; hyperglykemia, tachycardia and tremor were simultaneously observed. Kininogen and sugar levels in blood were normalized after 1 h. These results indicated the existence of a close relationship between kinin and sympatathicoadrenal systems in myocardial infarction; the authors considered hyperadrenalinemia to be the trigger in kinin system activation and the development of cardiogenic shock.

2. Experimental Myocarditis

Rabbit kinin system of plasma and of myocardium at the developing allergic myocarditis induced by eightfold immunization by rat cardiac muscle of homogenate containing aluminium hydroxide as ajuvant was studied by SUROVIKINA (1973) and her co-workers (SUROVIKINA and ODINOKOVA, 1974). The level of total kallikrein (SUROVIKINA, 1975), kininogen, and free kinins in plasma increased 2–4 fold in weeks 2–4 of myocarditis while kininase activity decreased. Conversely, kininogen level in rabbit cardiac muscle homogenate decreased by 75% one week after the first antigen administration and by 83% in weeks 4–7 of immunization and correlated with morphologic changes in cardiac muscle. After 10 weeks the kininogen level in myocardium began to increase but remained lower than the normal value for a further 4 months. Anginine, kontrical (BPI-aprotinin) and to a smaller extent aspirin, indomethacin and E-AKK normalized the activity of kinin system components of myocardium and stimulated restoration of the morphologic structure of myocardium (SUROVIKINA et al., 1976). The results were interpreted by authors as a consequence of active involvement of plasma and myocardial kinin system in pathogenesis of allergic myocarditis. High levels of the "acute phase proteins," prekallikrein, and kininogen, at this allergic inflammation are apparently the result of extensive hormonal rearrangement.

3. Clinical Research

Pathogenic and protective-compensatory functions of kinins and the kinin system in clinical myocardial infarction has been investigated by many workers. The data were summarized in a monograph of DZIZINSKIY and GOMAZKOV (1976). The decrease in kininogen level in plasma of patients on the first 1–2 days of acute myocardial infarction was demonstrated by many authors (POPOV et al., 1971; GOMAZKOV et al., 1972b; GOMAZKOV, 1974; MALAYA et al., 1973a, 1973b). A decrease of kininogen level in ischemia with frequent attacks of stenocardia was found by DZIZINSKIY and KUIMOV (1971). 940 patients with myocardial infarction, 134 among them with macrofocal myocardial infarction complicated by cardiogenic shock and collapse, were examined by MALAYA et al. (1973a, 1973b). The kinin system state was monitored by kallikrein activity (chromatographic method by PASKHINA and YAROVAYA, 1970a), kininogen content, kininase I activity (substrate HLAa), and total arginine esterase activity of serum. Changes in the content of main kinin system components were registered from the first days of the desease; kallikrein activity increased up to 175.25 ± 10.03 nmol BAEe/min/ml and kininase I up to 1.26 ± 0.14 μmol HLAa/min/ml while kininogen level decreased to 2.2 ± 0.15 μg bradykinin · eq/ml. The level of these components in healthy persons (control group) was equal to 86.62 ± 7.66, 0.86 ± 0.06, and 4.15 ± 0.37, respectively. The most pronounced changes in kallikrein-kinin system values were found in patients with the most critical clinical cases of acute myocardial infarction with sharp prolonged pain syndrome, dyspnea and progressive insufficiency of the left ventricle of the heart. The activity of kallikrein in cardiogenic shock achieved maximum value (385.8 ± 26 nmol BAEe/min/ml) while kininogen level was represented by the minimal value of 0.7 μg bradykinin · eq/ml (MALAYA and LAZAREVA, 1976). Great importance was attached to the estimation of kallikrein activity as a means of differentiation of collapses and their subsequent treatment. The kallikrein-kinin system activity and blood coagulation were found to be in good agreement (MALAYA et al., 1973a). Corticosteroid therapy in myocardial infarction rendered a normalizing effect on both systems. Kinin system activation in cardiogenic shock was considered to be a pathogenic factor by MALAYA et al. (1973a, b), MALAYA and LAZAREVA (1976).

In myocardial infarction, the kinin system state was estimated by the method of COLMAN et al. (1969), modified by GOMAZKOV et al. (1972b), GOMAZKOV (1974). The greatest changes in values of main components of the kinin system arising in this pathologic state were observed during the first 48 h. The decrease of prekallikrein levels in acute myocardial infarction was regarded by the authors as a more pertinent criterium than the decrease in kininogen level.

The relation between the kallikrein-kinin system and the sympatheticoadrenal system in patients with repeated myocardial infarction complicated by arrhythmia, cardiac asthma, lung edema, and cardiogenic shock was studied by GOLIKOV et al. (1976). Characteristic changes in kallikrein-kinin system component values estimated by the method of GOMAZKOV et al. (1972b) coincided in time of an increase in concentration of adrenalin and norepinephrine in blood plasma.

4. Hypertension

Detailed investigation concerning plasma kallikrein-kinin system in healthy persons as compared to hypertensive patients at rest and when walking were carried out by NEKRASOVA (1973) and by CHERNOVA et al. (1976). Using the method of COLMAN et al. (1969) modified by GOMASKOV et al. (1972b) the authors found a direct and reliable correlation between prekallikrein and kininogen content in plasma. Correlation coefficient values were $r = +0.52$ and $r = +0.47$, respectively ($p < 0.01$). The correlation was broken to a varying degree in hypertensive patients, yet it could be restored in the initial stages of the disease (75% of patients) by the β-adrenoblocking agent, inderal (CHERNOVA et al., 1976).

The results of many years of study of the kinin system in hypertension were summarized by CHERNOVA et al. (1976b) as follows.

Activation of plasma kinin system in healthy persons takes place even under light physical load such as walking. It serves as an indicator of humoral adaptation of the cardiovascular system to changing conditions. There are three symptoms characteristic of a disturbed plasma kinin system state in hypertensive patients, namely; the increase of its activity under rest, the absence of further activation during walking, and the loss of direct correlation between prekallikrein and kininogen levels. Changes in the state of blood kinin system in hypertensive patients may be one of the causes for the formation of a hyperkinetic type of blood circulation.

5. Kidney Kallikrein-Kinin System and Hypertension

Studies of renal kallikrein-kinin system in healthy persons and in hypertensive patients were carried out by NEKRASOVA et al. (1970) and NEKRASOVA and KHUKHAREV (1972). Hypertensive patients, in contrast to healthy subjects, exhibited a decrease of kinin and kallikrein excretion in urine under moderate physical load and not an increase. These values increased when the patients were at rest. NEKRASOVA et al. (1972a) established a direct correlation between the rate of blood flow in kidney and the excretion of kallikrein in patients with cardiovascular disease ($r=0.87$). A correlation was not observed between the value of glomerular filtration and kallikrein excretion ($r=0.33$). The direct dependence between arterial pressure and kallikrein excretion in urine was found in the initial phases of hypertension. In more advanced phases kallikrein excretion decreased and was independent of the value of blood pressure (CHERNOVA and NEKRASOVA, 1971). Kallikrein excretion in renovascular hypertension was due only to the functional state of contralateral kidney and did not correlate with the level of arterial pressure. Changes in diuresis and sodium excretion in hypertension were apparently also connected with changes in activity of renal kallikrein-kinin system (NEKRASOVA and KHUKHAREV, 1972). The authors pointed out the participation of renal and blood kinin system in adaptation of the cardiovascular system and renal function to various external conditions. The interrelation of pressor-depressor systems under physiologic conditions and in arterial hypertensions is evidently performed as negative feedback but through different pathways (SHKHVATSABAYA and NEKRASOVA, 1977).

6. Rheumatism

The state of the kallikrein-kinin system in sera of 59 patients with acute rheumatism has been studied by PASKHINA et al. (1970b); 30 healthy persons made up the control group. The increase of arginine esterase activity and a considerable increase of kallikrein activity, estimated by method PASKHINA and YAROVAYA (1970a) has been established; kininogen content, antitryptic and kininase I activity slightly decreased. It has been assumed that hemodynamic disturbances observed in rheumatism may occur partially due to the activation of the plasma kallikrein-kinin system. Kininogen content in plasma of 85 rheumatic patients with acute common was determined by ZBOROVSKIY and STYAJKOVA (1976). The minimal kininogen content was found in patients with continuously recurring rheumatism; no changes in the activity of the kinin system were found in patients with inactive process.

II. Gastrointestinal Diseases

1. Acute or Chronic Pancreatitis

The activity or level of kinin system components in acute or chronic pancreatitis was studied by many authors. A direct correlation between the decrease of kininogen level in patients with acute pancreatitis and the number of plasma leukocytes and amylase activity in urine was established by ANDRUS (1969). He was the first to show that administration of therapeutic doses of amidopyrine (0.2–0.8 g/day) prevented the decrease of kininogen levels and rendered curative effects: killed pain and helped to normalize hemodynamics in patients with acute pancreatitis. A decrease of kininogen levels from 4.9–1.6 9g bradykinin · eq/ml along with an increase of BAEe esterase and BAPA amidase activities were also observed in acute pancreatitis (GELLER et al., 1972a, b). SUVALSKAYA (1976) found that the levels of kallikrein and plasmin decreased in plasma together with kininogen in acute pancreatitis. BAEe esterase and BAPA amidase activities increased considerably.

VEREMEENKO et al. (1976b) used their modified variant of the method of COLMAN et al. (1969) for estimating the kinin system state in acute pancreatitis (1975). The decrease of prekallikrein level and α_2-macroglobulin in plasma along with the increase of total antitryptic and spontaneous protamine hydrolyzing activities was established.

2. Liver Diseases

The interrelationship of kininogen levels in the plasma of patients with portal cirrhosis as well as with active chronic hepatitis and the decrease of liver protein synthesis in these pathologic states was confirmed by BONDAR et al. (1970).

PASKHINA et al. (1975c) found a considerable decrease in prekallikrein level in patients with different hepatic lesions (cirrhosis of various etiology, fatty hepatitis progressing into cirrhosis, chronic hepatitis in the acute phase). The authors suggested that the decrease of plasma prekallikrein content in patients correlated with the degree of lesion of hepatocytes in each individual case rather than with the character or diagnosis of disease. The authors used to original method of prekallikrein estimation in plasma (PASKHINA and KRINSKAYA, 1974) and suggested that this test was a more sensitive indicator of lesion of the liver function than the methods normally used. A 70% decrease of prekallikrein levels and of rapid and slow reacting kallikrein inhibitors was found in virus hepatitis by VEREMEENKO et al. (1976a). The changes correlated with the severity of the desease. Prekallikrein levels were tested both by the method of VEREMEENKO et al. (1975) and by that of PASHKINA and KRINSKAYA (1974). PASKHINA et al. (1975) and VEREMEENKO et al. (1976a) confirmed that liver is the main site of plasma prekallikrein synthesis.

3. Other Diseases (Stomach and Duodenal Ulcer, Peritonitis, Parodontosis)

GELLER et al. (1972) found a decrease of plasma kininogen levels in patients with stomach and duodenal ulcer, cholecystitis, and colitis. Similar data were obtained in examination of patients with stomach ulcer by STEPANOVA and VISIR (1974). The increased level of free plasma kinins in patients with stomach and duodenal ulcer was found by KOTELNIKOV and PANKOV (1976). The level of kinins increased threefold after perforation. The decrease of the activity and secretion of salivary kallikrein in patients with stomach and duodenal ulcer, especially in the acute phase, was observed by LEVITSKY et al. (1973). The reliable increase of kallikrein and trypsin-like proteinases determined by BAEe hydrolysis in salivary secretion was found by BARABASH et al. (1976a) in examination of a large group of healthy people and patients with paradontosis. The authors established a direct correlation between the secretion of the kallikrein-like enzyme, salivain, with saliva and the degree of age atrophy of periodontal tissue in rats. Consumption of drinking water containing kallikrein preparations causes an active inflammatory-dystrophic process in rat periodontal tissues. Local administration of kallikrein inhibitors (kontrikal, aprotinin, trasylol) inhibited periodontitis both clinically and experimentally.

The decrease of kininogen levels independent of the severity of desease was found in patients with acute suppparative peritonitis by IVASHKEVICH et al. (1976). Kininase activity bioassayed in peritonitis remained almost unchanged.

III. Burn Shock and Early Burn Toxemia

PASKHINA et al. (1972, 1976, 1977c) studied the state of the kinin system in different stages of burn in man and the significance of kinins in pathogenesis of burn shock. Kinin system components, namely, kininogen (the Dinizs method), kallikrein, and kallikreinogen (chromatographic method by PASKHINA and KRINSKAYA, 1974), kininase I (substrate HLAa), BAEe esterase activity, and α_1-antitrypsin levels were determined after short intervals (4, 6, 12 h) in sera of patients with extensive (5–95%) surface (I, II, III up to 60%) and deep (IIIb, IV up to 30%) burns. 64 patients were examined, 56 among them in the shock state. Fibrinolytic activity prior to and after its activation by streptokinase was measured in different phases of shock and during aftershock period in eight patients.

PASKHINA et al. (1972, 1976) found that maximum activation of the kinin system was observed in burn shock in the first 24–36 h after trauma. In acute burn toxemia (days 2–6), kinin system activation was less marked. Prekallikrein content decreased during the first hours after trauma. Kininogen level in burn shock progressively decreased from the first moment of trauma to the end of shock; the decrease in kininogen level 24–36 h after trauma was 50–60% of the initial value. Decrease of total kininogen concentration in blood circulation during the first days after trauma little depended on the changes in protein concentration but correlated with the depth and size of the burn and intensity of shock. The activity of kininase I in the first phase of shock was only 40–50% of the normal; further changes in the activity of this enzyme were phase-dependent (Fig. 5). Antitryptic activity in shock also decreased.

Kallikrein activity was relatively stable 1–6 days after burn. It was always present in supernatant of sera after passage through DEAE-Sephadex A-50 (PASKHINA and YAROVAYA, 1970; PASKHINA and KRINSKAYA, 1974). The authors (PASKHINA et al., 1976) assumed that this kallikrein appears only in pathologic states (PASKHINA et al., 1970, 1972, 1976, 1977c) and is absent in healthy persons; it was released from a labile complex of unknown origin after contact of serum with the anionic surface. In shock the fibrinolytic system was activated simultaneously with the kinin system. Antitryptic activity increased twofold 40–58 h after burn, mainly due to α_1-antitrypsin and was distinctly correlated with the development of burn intoxication. The inclusion of aprotinin (Trasylol) or its USSR analog, ingitril (LAKIN et al., 1972), into the therapy of burn shock and acute toxemia decreased the degree of activation of the kinin system and fibrinolytic system and was noticeably beneficial for patients (PASKHINA et al., 1977c). The dynamics of changes in kinin system components, BAEe esterase activity and α_1-antitrypsin level in the first 6 days of illness under treatment with polyinhibitor and without is shown in Fig. 5.

PASKHINA et al. (1976, 1977c) assumed that several enzymatic systems of plasma are activated after extensive and deep burns and are capable of releasing kinins from

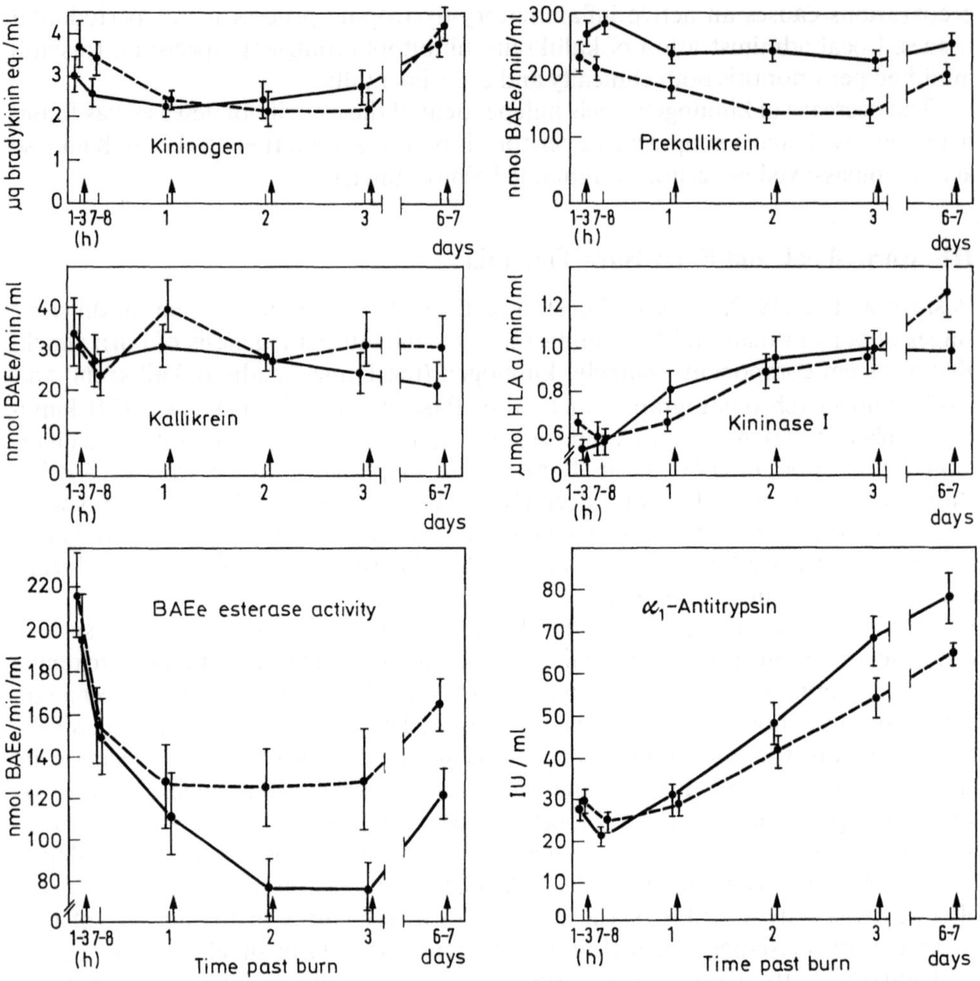

Fig. 5. Activity or content of the main components of the kinin system, BAEe esterase and α_1-antitrypsin, in blood serum of patients with widespread II, III, IIIb and IVth degree burns during shock and early toxemia (PASKHINA et al., 1977c). Abscissa = time intervals after the burn; Ordinate = activity (or content) of each component expressed in corresponding units ±S.E. per ml serum. Solid line = patients treated ($n=20$) and dotted line = patients not treated ($n=16$) by polyvalent proteinase inhibitor. Arrows indicate time of i.v. injection of daily dose of inhibitor (200,000 aprotinin units or 150 inhitril units)

both LMW and HMW kininogen and thus considerable amounts of free kinins are released in circulation and interstitial spaces. These kinins are responsible for hemodynamic disturbances and plasma loss in burn shock, as well as for pain accompanying this trauma together with other mediators of inflammation. The increase of antitryptic activity mostly due to α_1-antitrypsin, indicates the mobilization of the defensive forces of the organism since this inhibitor blocks the proteinases of leukocytes which released the toxic vasoactive substances. The increase of α_1-antitrypsin levels through 36–48 h after burn serves as diagnostic symptom of burn intoxication (PASKHINA et al., 1972, 1976).

The same view of pathogenic function of kinins and their action together with other mediators in the mechanism of homeostatic disturbances in burn shock and early toxemia is also held by OBUKHOV (1975) and ARKATOV et al. (1976). After examination of 123 patients with extensive (5–100% of body surface) and deep (IIIb, IV) burns in the first 3 days after trauma, the authors established that the increase in the concentration of free kinins was two to fourfold. It was below normal only in supercritical thermal injury (ARKATOV et al., 1976). OBUKHOV (1975) found that kinin content in plasma of healthy people was equal to 4–6 ng/ml while in patients it shock was equal to 9–14 ng/ml (the test organ was cat jejenum).

IV. Kinins and Proteinase Inhibitors in Nephrotic Syndrome

Many renal diseases are accompanied by nephrotic syndrome. Pathogenesis of nephrotic syndrome has not been clarified so far. The clinical signs of the disease, including abdominal pains, collapse, and generalized edemas leads to suppose that kinins and the abnormal functions of the most important biologic systems of plasma make considerable contributions to nephrotic syndrome pathogenesis. The state of the kinin system in nephrotic syndrome has not been studied. 59 patients with nephrotic syndrome of various etiology (glomerulonephritis, amyloidosis, systemic lupus erythematosus), 17 patients with latent nephritis and 14 donors have been studied by PASKHINA et al. (1977b). Here the concentration of main kallikrein-kinin system components (kallikreinogen, kallikrein, kininogen, kininase I) and BAEe esterase, activity and the spectra of proteinase inhibitors were studied. The increase in the level of main kallikrein-kinin system components: kallikreinogen, kininogen, kininase I occured in every form of nephropathy. Free kallikrein (chromatographic method) is found only in sera of nephrotic syndrome patients. BAEe esterase activity changes depending on the nephrotic syndrome etiology; it is maximal in amyloidois and decreases in systemic lupus erythematosis. Figure 6 shows the level of the kinin system components, α_1-antitrypsin and α_2-macroglobulin, in patients with acute nephrotic syndrome as compared to those with latent glomerulonephritis.

As seen from Fig. 6, α_1-antitrypsin and α_2-macroglobulin levels in serum increased in patients with latent glomerutonephritis and nephrotic syndrome I with the exception of patients with severe and progressing nephrotic syndrome II. The greatest quantitative shifts in the concentration of kallikrein-kinin system components as well as a marked decrease of antitryptic activity was found in patients with severe nephrotic syndrome with unfavourable development and prognosis. The authors supposed that activation of plasma kallikrein-kinin system and weakening of the pool of proteinase inhibitors aggravates nephrotic syndrome pathogenesis especially in the period of its most acute manifestations.

V. Kinins in the Pathogenesis of Acute Irradiation Injury

GAPONYUK and UMARHODZHAEV (1970) noted a considerable increase of kinin-forming activity of plasma and a decrease in kininogen level and kininase activity in rats irradiated by γ-rays (800 r). The concentration of free kinins in rat blood increased nearly twofold in days 2–4 after irradiation (GAPONYUK et al., 1972a), which coincided in time with gastrointestinal disturbances in irradiated rats. By days 3–4

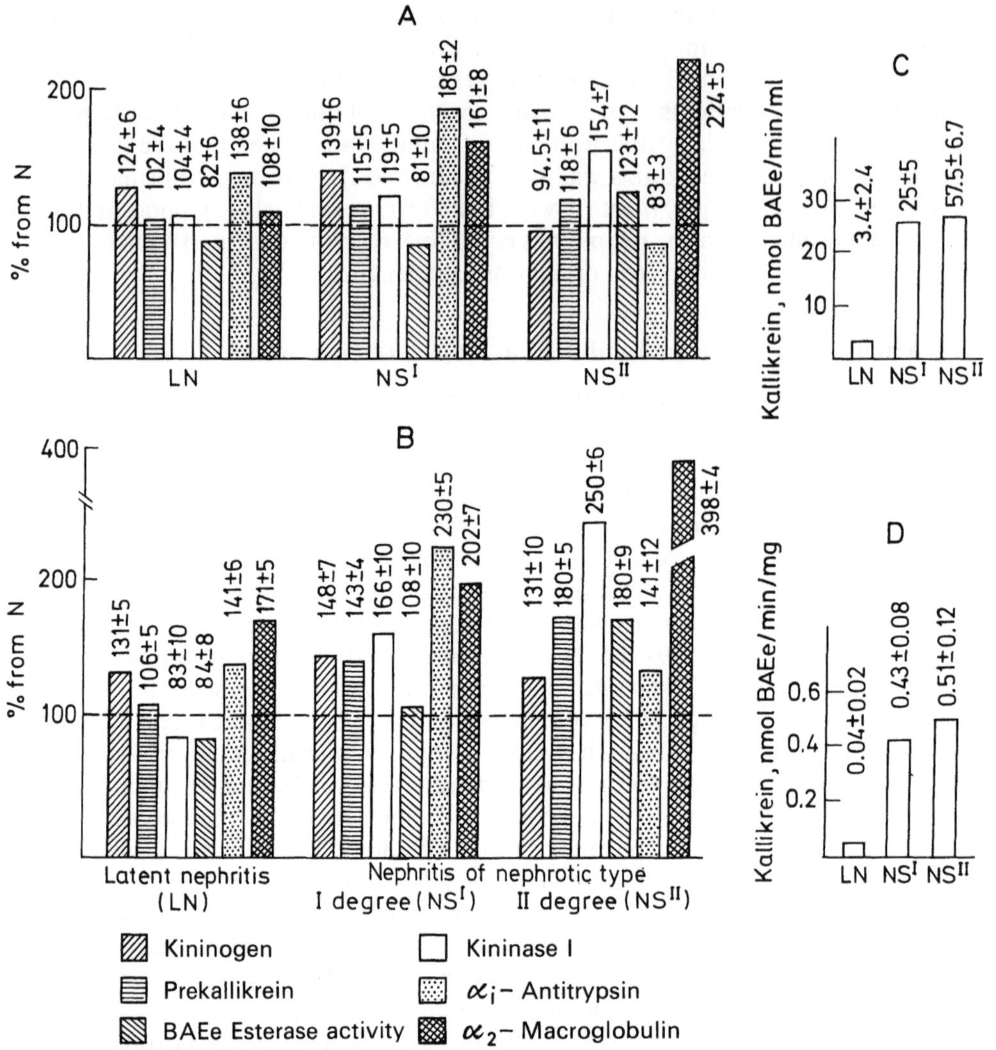

Fig. 6A–D. Kinin system components, α_1-antitrypsin, and α_2-macroglobulin, in blood serum of patients with latent glomerulanephritis (LN) and nephrotic syndrome (NS) of I[st] and IInd degree of activity (in % of mean value of the norm (N) (PASKHINA et al., 1977b). **A** mean value of each component in correspondings units/ml serum ± S.E. **B** the same /mg serum protein, **C** kallikrein activity in µmol BAEe min ml serum ± S.E. (chromatographic method of PASKHINA and KRINSKAYA, 1974), **D** the same in µmol BAEe/min/mg serum protein. NS_I and NS_{II} were diagnosed by the following data: proteinuria 6.7±0.5 g(NS_I); 17.1±0.1 g (NS_{II}) albuminemia 2.6±0.1 g (NS_I); 1.39±0.08 g (NS_{II}); blood cholesterol 318±13 mg% (NS_I); 592±25 mg% (NS_{II}); proteinuria in LN ≦2.0 g

after irradiation, the kinin forming activity of small intestine increased ninefold. This period was also characterized by the lowest plasma kininases activity of small intestine homogenate. Aprotinin and SBTI, administered to animals prior to irradiation, normalized plasma and small intestine kinin system to a certain degree and proved beneficial in acute irradiation desease (GAPONYUK et al., 1972b).

VI. Kallikrein-Kinin System in Other Pathologic States

KHUTSURAULI and TSVERAVA (1974) observed a decrease in the concentration of kininogen and total kininase activity in plasma of patients with myeloblastic leukemia. The changes depended on the degree of leukocytosis and the number of blast cells which were the source of kinin forming and kinin splitting enzymes.

The increase in free kinin levels, kallikrein and kininogen which correlated with the activity of the complement system in patients with acute chronic pneumonia was observed by GAVRILOVA and JURINA (1974). The activity of plasma kininases measured by bioassay decreased considerably.

F. Kinin System in Normal and Pathologic Pregnancy

The significance of kallikrein-kinin system mobilization in a female organism prior to delivery and pathogenetic function of kinins in early and late gestoses has not yet been completely clarified. High kininase activity was observed in placenta and in myometrium of pregnant women (USHINSKIY, 1970) which indicated the protective function of these tissues against the excessive amount of kinins.

GIGINEISHVILI et al. (1973) studied the kininogen content by the DINIZS method and total kininase activity (bioassay) in plasma of a large group of healthy nonpregnant women, healthy pregnant women (3 periods), and pregnant women with early and late toxicosis. The last group included patients with nephropathies of I, II, and III degree and patients with preeclampsia and eclampsia. Data obtained by the authors indicated that changes in kininogen content and plasma kininase activity in normal and pathologic pregnancy went in different directions, i.e., kininogen content and kininase activity increased progressively from the first to the third trimester in the former case and decreased depending on the severity of toxsicosis in the latter. Thus, kininogen levels in normal pregnancy increased threefold as compared to nonpregnant women by the end of the third trimester, it decreased fivefold in nephropathies (third trimester) and tenfold in eclampsia. Kininase activity and kininogen content in plasma increased upon improvement of the clinical state of patients after treatment. These changes may be considered a result of excessive kinin formation in pathologic pregnancy and it is not excluded that such toxicosis symptoms as nausea, vomiting and hypersalivation as well as cramps in eclampsia are accounted for by the toxic action of kinins.

G. Theoretical Considerations, Reviews, Monographs, and Conferences

The first Soviet review on the chemistry, biochemistry, physiology, and pathogenetic significances of kinins and the kallikrein-kinin system of blood plasma and tissues was written by PASKHINA (1966). In subsequent review articles the author considered metabolism of kinins and biochemistry of the kallikrein-kinin system (PASKHINA, 1969, 1972, 1976).

A review by YAROVAYA (1969) deals with interrelationship between the kallikrein-kinin system, blood clotting system and fibrinolysis as well as mechanisms of their regulation. Reviews by PASKHINA (1976), GOMAZKOV and KOMISAROVA (1976a) consider new data on plasma kallikrein as an enzymatic activator of Hageman's factor, on direct and indirect participation of kallikrein in initiation of blood clotting, fibrinolysis, and formation of kinins as well as newer information concerning Hageman's factor.

Basic concepts on the regulatory and pathogenetic role of the kallikrein-kinin system were advanced by GOMAZKOV (1973) and CHERNUKH and GOMAZKOV (1976). The authors consider adjustment of the vascular tone to the biophysical parameters of the circulating blood as a main function of kinins and the kallikrein-kinin system in men and animals. This concept is based on the data which demonstrate an interrelationship between the kinin system, blood clotting systems and fibrinolysis in determining the liquid state of blood and on the distinct effect of bradykinin on vascular tone. CHERNUKH and GOMAZKOV (1976) consider the three systems – kininogenase, blood clotting and fibrinolysis systems – as a single physiologic polysystem. An especially important role of the exogenous and endogenous kinins are regulators of cardiac output was ascribed by the authors. In this connection, the kininases of lungs are considered as locally important and distantly acting regulators of blood circulation. URZAEVA and DUBILEY (1977) discussed nonrespiratory functions of lung and its role in enzymatic inactivation of some vasoactive compounds: bradykinin, histamine, serotonin, angiotensin, prostaglandins. Participation of kinins in regulation of microcirculation is considered in the monograph by CHERNUKH et al. (1974).

Considerable interest was aroused by a concept of interrelationship between physiologic and pathogenetic effects of kinins in the organism. This concept was advanced by CHERNUKH and GOMAZKOV (1976). Considering cardiovascular pathology, with myocardial infarction as an example, the authors showed that activation of the kinin system within the initial periods of the disease tends to compensate for the imbalance of blood circulation in the organism. In other words, activation of kinin system is considered as a compensatory-protective reaction. During the subsequent periods of disease, excessive activation of the kallikrein-kinin system causing uncontrolled production of bradykinin, acquired pathogenetic role.

Role of carboxycathepsin as a key enzyme in regulation of vascular tone and systemic arterial pressure was discussed by OREKHOVICH et al. (1975, 1976).

SHKHVAZABAYA and NEKRASOVA (1977) considered the significance of prostaglandins and kinins in the regulation of blood pressure and in pathogenesis of arterial hypertension. The authors believe that the kinin system of kidney is involved in the rapid response to alterations in homeostasis in the organism under various conditions while the prolonged responses are mediated through prostaglandins. The authors emphasized that prostaglandins mediate many effects of kinins in vivo.

Two mechanisms of increasing vascular permeability in vulgar inflammation – as an active processe requiring the consumption of energy and direct damage (passive process) and their respective therapies were discussed by OYVIN et al. (1973).

Reviews were published on the role of kinins in the pathogenesis of diseases of respiratory organs (SUROVKINA et al., 1972) and of cardiovascular system (SUROVIKINA et al., 1974). Involvement of the blood kallikrein-kinin system in pathogenesis of diseases of the gastrointestinal tract was discussed in the review by MENSHIKOV et al. (1972). The role of investigations of the kallikrein-kinin system in surgery was considered in the review by KUZIN et al. (1974). POLUSHKIN et al. (1972) discussed the role of bradykinin in physiology and pathology of skin.

The first Soviet monograph (DZIZINSKII and GOMAZKOV, 1976) on kinins deals briefly with problems of physiology and biochemistry of the kallikrein-kinin system and contains a detailed discussion of the role of kinins in the physiology and pathology of the cardiovascular system. In an appendix to the monograph, modern biologic, radioimmunoassay and chemical methods for estimation of the main components of the kallikrein-kinin system are described thus providing a valuable supplement to the theoretical considerations.

The monograph by VEREMEENKO (1977) contains concise compilation of data on the kinin system biochemistry of blood plasma and tissues, mechanisms of their regulation, and the pharmacologic activity of kinins. Discussion is presented on the physiologic significance of kinins and their role in the pathogenesis of inflammation and other pathologic processes. Some modern methods used in laboratory practice for estimation of the main components of the kinin system are described.

The first conference on kinins and the kallikrein-kinin system of blood took place in Moscow (December, 1975). The plenary lectures covered the problems of metabolism of kinins and prospects of studies in this field (PASKHINA), pathophysiologic role of the kallikrein-kinin system (CHERNUKH, GOMAZKOV) and role of blood kinins in pathogenesis of allergic diseases (SUROVIKINA). Papers on biochemistry, physiology, pharmacology of kinins and on the alterations in the kallikrein-kinin system under pathologic conditions were presented. Proceedings of the Conference were edited by PASKHINA and MENSHIKOV (1976).

Conclusion

Analysis of the literature, reviewed in the present paper, shows that investigations on various aspects of the kallikrein-kinin system in the USSR have intensified, especially during the last few years. Major theoretical significance in this research may be ascribed to the studies on molecular mechanisms of the effect of kinins on smooth muscles and endothelial cells of capillary membrane, detailed studies of the enzymatic systems participating in the mechanisms of formation and destruction of kinins, studies on the chemical synthesis of bradykinin analogs which are resistant to the inactivating effect of blood plasma, and tissue kininases, as well as to many other lines of research.

Especially interesting problems arise from studies on interactions of the kallikrein-kinin system with other regulatory physiologic systems in the organism (hypophyseal-adrenal system, blood clotting enzyme system, systems of fibrinolysis, complement, or renin-angiotensin) and studies of relationships between the kinins and other transmitters (catecholamines, histamine, serotonin, and prostaglandin). There is a tendency to distinguish the protective-compensatory and pathogenetically essential roles of kinins and the kallikrein-kinin system in some pathologic states which are of practical importance. Considerable practical significance is ascribed also to the possible predominant use of bradykinin (compared with other vasodilators) in angiographic studies, including the studies designed to differentiate malignant and nonmalignant tumors.

Unfortunately, there are still considerable difficulties in evaluating and comparing the results of studies on the kallikrein-kinin system in both experimental and clinical conditions carried out by various authors. These difficulties are due to variability and inadequacy of the existing methods used for estimation of the kallikrein-kinin system components. A revision of the existing methods of estimation of prekallikrein, kallikrein, kininogen, and other kallikrein-kinin system components is probably required. Use of more precise and adequate procedures for their estimation (including immunodiffusion, radioimmunoassay and radioisotopic methods) becomes necessary. Development and general use of these newer research techniques will open new approaches to studies on the biochemistry, physiology and pathology of the kallikrein-kinin system.

Acknowledgements. The authors are grateful to Prof. V. Z. Gorkin and Dr. M. I. Lerman for valuable advice and discussion. We also thank our co-workers T. P. Egorova, A. V. Krinskaya, L. G. Makevnina, V. F. Nartikova, O. G. Ogloblina, R. I. Yakubovskaya for expert technical assistance.

References

Andreyenko, G. V., Suvorov, A. V.: Deystvie plazmina na kallikreinogen. (Effect of plasmin on kallikreinogen.) Biokhimiia *41*, 557–561 (1976)

Andrus, V. N.: Kininy plazmy krovi i patogeneticheskaya terapiya amidopirinom ostrogo pankreatita (Kinins of blood plasma and pathogenetic therapia of acute pancreatitis by amidopyrin). Klin. Khir. No. 5, 52–53 (1969)

Arkatov, V. A., Pekarskiy, D. E., Surovkina, M. S., Obuchov, Yu. E.: Svobodnye kininy i kininazy krovy v patologii ojogovoy bolezni (Free kinins and kininases in the plasma of patients with severe burns). In: Kininy i kininovaya sistema plasmy. Sbornik trudov 1 MMI im. Sechenova. Paskhina, T. S., Menshikov, V. V. (eds.), pp. 34–35. Published by 1 MMI im. Sechenova. Moskva 1976

Barabash, R. D., Levitsky, A. P., Loginova, N. K., Vovchuk, S. V., Genesina, T. I., Konovets, V. M., Volodkina, V. V.: Rol kallikreina slyuny v patogeneze paradontoza (The role of saliva kallikrein in pathogenesis of paradonthosis). Vopr. Med. Khim. *22*, 318–325 (1976 a)

Barabash, R. D., Aleksandrov, P. N., Vovchuk, S. V.: Vliyanie kallikreinov slyuny na micrososudy zashchechnogo meshka khomyakov i bryjeyki krys (The influence of salivary kallikreins upon the microvessels of hamster cheek pouch and rat mesentery). Biul. Eksp. Biol. Med. *81*, 782–785 (1976 b)

Belyakov, N. V., Syomushkin, B. V.: Registratsionnaya apparatura dlya biologicheskikh metodov opredeleniya nekotorykh tkanevykh gormonov (The recording equipment for bioassays of some tissue hormones). Lab. Delo No. 10, 630–632 (1972)

Belyakov, N. V., Syomushkin, B. V.: Superfuziya – apparatura i metod dlya opredeleniya nekotorykh komponentov kininovoy sistemy (Superfusion – the equipment and technique for estimation of some components of kinin system). In: Kininy i kininovaya sistema plasmy. Shornik Trudov 1 MMI im. Sechenova. Paskhina, T. S., Menshikov, V. V. (eds.), pp. 61–62. Moskva 1976 (Published by 1 MMI im Sechenova)

Bondar, Z. A., Paskhina, T. S., Melkumova, I. S.: Soderjanie kininogena v syvorotke krovi bolnykh s zabolevaniami pecheni (The blood serum content of kininogen in patients with hepatic diseases). Lab. Delo No. 4, 237–240 (1970)

Chernova, N. A., Nekrasova, A. A.: Kallikrein mochi pri hipertonicheskoy bolezni i renovaskulyarnoy gipertonii (Urinary kallikrein in hypertensive vascular disease and renovascular hypertension). Kardiologiia *11*, No. 4, 84–89 (1971)

Chernova, N. A., Nekrasova, A. A., Lantsberg, L. A.: Osobennosti izmeneniy kininovoy sistemy krovi pri gipertonicheskoy bolezni (Peculiarities of changes in the kinin system of blood in cases of essential hypertension). Kardiologiia *16*, No. 5, 46–51 (1976)

Chernuch, A. M., Aleksandrov, P. N., Alekseev, O. V.: Microcirculatsiya (Microcirculation). Moskva: Medicina 1974

Chernukh, A. M., Yarovaya, L. M., Glebov, R. N.: Vliyanie bradikinina na aktivnost Na, K-ATF-asy mikrosom pochek i mozga krys (The effect of bradykinin on the activity of Na-K-ATP-ase of microsomes of the kidney and brain of rats). Biul. Eksp. Biol. Med. *78*, No. 8, 50–52 (1974)

Chernukh, A. M., Gomazkov, O. A.: O regulatornoy i patogeneticheskoy roli kallikrein-kininovoy sistemy v organizme (On regulatory and pathogenetic function of kallikrein-kinin system in organism). Patol. Fisiol. Eksp. Ter. No. 1, 5–16 (1976)

Dotsenko, V. L., Yarovaya, G. A., Golosova, N. A., Lebedeva, N. V., Orekhovich, V. N.: Vliyanie kininogena na aktivnost kininogenaznoy sistemy syvorotki krovi cheloveka (Effect of kininogen on the activity of human blood serum kininogenase system). Biokhimiia *42*, 283–286 (1977)

Dzizinsky, A. A., Kuimov, A. D.: Aktivnost kininovoy sistemy krovi pri ishemicheskoy bolezni serdtsa (The activity of the kinin system in cardiac ischemia). Kardiologia *11*, No. 6, 18–22 (1971)

Dzizinsky, A. A., Gomazkov, O. A.: Kininy v fiziologii i patologii serdechno-sosudistoy sistemy (Kinins in physiology and pathology of cardio-vascular system). Novosibirsk: Nauka 1976

Egorova, T. P., Paskhina, T. S.: Ochistka kininogena (bradikininogena) iz plazmy krovi krolika i izuchenie iego svoistv [Purification of kininogen (bradykininogen) from rabbit blood plasma and study its properties]. Biokhimiia *32*, 354–362 (1967)

Egorova, T. P., Makarova, O. V., Paskhina, T. S.: Nekotorye svoystva i substratnaya priroda ochishchenogo kininogena krolika (Some properties and substrate nature of purified rabbit kininogen). Biokhimiia *34*, 610–619 (1969)

Egorova, T. P., Makevnina, L. G., Paskhina, T. S.: Aminokislotny sostav, osobennosti stroeniya i substratnaya specifichnost kininogena plazmy krolika (Amino acid composition, some features of structure and substrate specificity of rabbit plasma kininogen). Biokhimiia *40*, 158–165 (1975)

Egorova, T. P., Eliseeva, Yu. E.: Deystvie karboksikatepsina na biologicheskuyu aktivnost bradikinina (Effect of carboxycathepsin on the biological activity of bradykinin). Vopr. Med. Khim. *22*, 119–122 (1976)

Egorova, T. P., Rossinskaya, E. B., Paskhina, T. S.: Ochistka i svoystva vysokomolekulyarnogo kininogena krolika (Purification and properties of high-molecular weight rabbit kininogen). Biokhimiia *41*, 1052–1060 (1976)

Eliseeva, Yu. E., Orekhovich, V. N.: Vydelenie i izuchenie spetsifichnosti karboxikatepsina (Isolation and investigation of carboxycathepsin specificity). Dokl. Akad. Nauk SSSR *153*, 954–957 (1963)

Eliseeva, Yu. E., Orekhovich, V. N., Pavlikhina, L. V., Alexeenko, L. P.: Karboxikatepsin- klyuchevoy ferment dvukh sistem, regulirujushchikh krovyanoe davlenie (Carboxycathepsin – a key regulatory component of two physiological system involved in regulation of blood pressure). Vopr. Med. Khim. *16*, 646–649 (1970)

Eliseeva, Yu. E., Orekhovich, V. N., Pavlikhina, L. V., Alexeenko, L. P.: Carboxycathepsin – a key regulatory component of two physiological systems involved in regulation of blood pressure. Clin. Chim. Acta *31*, 413–419 (1971)

Eliseeva, Yu. E., Pavlikhina, L. V., Orekhovich, V. N.: Vydelenie karboxikatepsina (peptidil-dipeptidasy, KF. 3.4.15.1) iz pochek byka [Isolation of carboxycathepsin (peptidyl-diepeptidase EC. 3.4.15.1) from bovine kidney]. Dokl. Akad. Nauk SSSR *217*, 953–956 (1974)

Eliseeva, Yu. E., Orekhovich, V. N., Pavlikhina, L. V.: Svoystva i specifichnost karboxikatepsina (peptidil-dipeptidasy) iz pochek byka]Properties and specificity of carboxycathepsin (peptidyl-dipeptidase) from bovine kidney]. Vopr. Med. Khim. *22*, 81–89 (1976 a)

Eliseeva, Yu. E., Orekhovich, V. N., Pavlikhina, L. V.: Vydelenie i svoystva karboxikatepsina (peptidil-dipeptidasy) iz tkaney lyogkieh byka [Isolation and properties of carboxycathepsin (peptidyl-dipeptidase) from bovine lung]. Biokhimiia *41*, 506–512 (1976 b)

Filatova, M. P., Krit, N. A., Shchukina, G. S., Ravdel, G. A., Ivanov, V. T.: Novy sintez bradikinina i ego analogov (A new synthesis of bradykinin and its analogs). Bioorgan. Khim. *1*, 437–446 (1975)

Gaponyuk, P. Ya., Umarkhodjaev, E. M.: Izmenenie kininovoy sistemy krovi pri ostroj luchevoy bolezni (Changes of the blood kinin system in acute radiation injury). Radiobiologiia *10*, 681–684 (1970)

Gaponyuk, P. Ya., Oyvin, V. I.: Sravnitelnoe izuchenie deystviya bradikinina, kallidina, metionil-lizil-bradikinina i eledoizina na pronizaemost sosudov koji (The comparative study of effects of bradykinin, kallidin, methionyl-lysyl-bradykinin and eledoisin on the vascular permeability). Biul. Eksp. Biol. Med. *71*, No. 3, 57–59 (1971 a)
Gaponyuk, P. Ya., Oyvin, V. I.: O neposredstvennom deystvii bradikinina na pronitsaemost sosudov (The direct effect of bradykinin on the vascular permeability). Biul. Eksp. Biol. Med. *71*, No. 6, 23–25 (1971 b)
Gaponyuk, P. Ya., Kalinkina, T. N., Gaponyuk, E. J.: Izmenenie koncentratsii svobodnykh kininov v krovi jivotnykh pri ostroy luchevoy bolezni (Changes of the concentration in the free kinin level in irradiated rats). Radiobiologiia *12*, 735–736 (1972 a)
Gaponyuk, P. Ya., Podsosov, S. P., Rudakov, I. A.: Vliyanie trazilola i soevogo inhibitora tripsina na vyjivaemost obluchennykh jivotnykh (The influence of trasylol and soy-bean inhibitor of trypsin, on the survival of irradiated animals). Radiobiologiia *12*, 927–928 (1972 b)
Gaponyuk, P. Ya., Uklonskaya, L. I.: Energeticheskie aspekty deystviya histamina i bradikinina na pronitsaemost sosudov (Energy aspects of histamine and bradykinin action on vascular permeability). Biul. Eksp. Biol. Med. *78*, No. 10, 18–20 (1974)
Gaponyuk, P. Ya., Tsyb, A. F., Strigunov, V. I., Drozdovsky, B. Ya., Mannanov, I. S.: Vliyanie bradikinina na krovoobrashchenie v basseyne chrevnoy arterii cheloveka (The influence of bradykinin on the blood circulation in the reservoir of the celiac artery in man). Biul. Eksp. Biol. Med. *79*, No. 6, 14–16 (1975 a)
Gapanyuk, P. Ya., Strigunov, V. I., Tsvet, A. Ph., Mannakov, I. S., Drozdovskiy, B. Ja.: Metodika primeneniya bradikinina pri angiograficheskikh issledovaniyakh (The method of bradykinin using of angiographic examinations). Med. Radiobiologia *20*, No. 8, 6–10 (1975 b)
Gavrilova, R. D., Jurina, T. M.: Izmenenie kininovoy sistemy krovi i urovnya komplementa pri khronicheskoy pnevmonii (Changes of the kinin system of the blood and the level of complement in chronic pneumonia). Klin. Med. *52*, No. 12, 75–79 (1974)
Geller, L. I., Amatnyan, A. G., Kobzev, V. S., Romanets, V. A.: Kliniko-farmakologicheskoe izuchenie kininov v gastroeneterologii (Clinical and pharmacological aspects of investigation of kinins in gastroenterology). Vrach. Delo No. 4, 85–88 (1972 a)
Geller, L. I., Ostrovsky, A. B., Kazimirchik, A. P., Amatnyan, A. G.: Svertyvayushchaya, protivossvertyvayushchaya i kininovaya sistema krovi pri obostrenii khronieheskogo pankreatita (Coagulation, anticoagulation and kinin systems of the blood in patients with chronic pancreatitis). Klin. Med. *50*, No. 9, 107–112 (1972 b)
Gigineishvili, M. S., Tsverava, E. N., Jikiya, J. B.: Sistema kininov pri fiziologicheskoy beremennosti (The kinin system in physiological pregnancy). Sabchota Medicine No. 4, 16–18 (1973)
Golikov, A. P., Bobkov, A. I., Ivleva, V. I.: Nekotorye pokazateli kininovoy i simpatiko-adrenalovoy sistem u bolnykh povtornym infarktom miokarda (Some indices of the kinin and sympathoadrenal system in patients with repeated myocardial infarctions). Kardiologia *16*, No. 2, 74–77 (1976)
Gomazkov, O. A., Bolshakova, L. V., Shimkovich, M. V., Komissarova, N. V.: Izmenenie aktivnosti kallikrein-kininovoy sistemy pri ostroy ishemii miokarda v eksperimente (Changes in the activity of the kallikrein-kinin system in experimental acute ischemia of the myocardium). Kardiologia *12*, No. 4, 22–28 (1972 a)
Gomazkov, O. A., Komissarova, N. V., Bolshakova, L. V., Teplova, N. N.: Metodicheskie podkhody k isucheniju kallikrein-kininovoy sistemy pri infarkte miokarda (Methodological approaches to the study of kallikrein-kinin system in myocardial infarction). Kardiologia *12*, No. 6, 25–31 (1972 b)
Gomazkov, O. A.: Kallikrein-kininovaya sistema krovi i regulatciya hemodinamiki. Obzor (Kallikrein-kinine system and regulation of hemodynamics. Review). Kardiologia *13*, No. 7, 130–144 (1973)
Gomazkov, O. A., Komissarova, N. V., Bolshakova, L. V., Shimkovich, M. V.: Aktivatsiya kallikreina i uroven kininogenov v venoznoy i arterialnoy krovi krys pri ostroy ishemii miokarda (Activation of kallikrein and the level of kininogens in the venous and arterial blood of rats in acute myocardial ischemia). Biul. Eksp. Biol. Med. *76*, No. 8, 25–27 (1973)
Gomazkov, O. A.: Das Kallikrein-System bei Myokardischämie und Herzinfarkt. Med. Welt. *25*, 804–807 (1974)

Gomazkov, O.A., Shimkovich, M.V.: Izmenenie depressornyeh otvetov na bradikinin preparatami blokirujushchimi kininazu i adrenoretseptory (Changes of depressor response to bradykinine by using preparations blocking kininase and agrenoreceptors). Kardiologia *14*, No. 7, 57–65 (1974)

Gomazkov, O.A., Shimkovich, M.V.: Tsiprogeptadin kak ingibitor effektov bradikinina (Ciproheptadin as an inhibitor of the bradykinin effects). Biul. Eksp. Biol. Med. *80*, No. 7, 6–9 (1975)

Gomazkov, O.A., Komissarova, N.V.: Obshchie mekhanizmy biokhimicheskoy regulatsii kallikreinovoy, svertyvayushchey i fibrinoliticheskoy sistem krovi (Several mechanisms of biochemical regulation of kallikrein, coagulation and fibrinolytic systems of blood). Usp. Sovrem. Biol. *82*, 356–370 (1976a)

Gomazkov, O.A., Komissarova, N.V.: Metod odnovremennogo opredeleniya predshestvennikov kallikreina, plazmina, trombina i ikh inhibitorov v plazme krovi cheloveka (Method of simultaneous determination of precursors of kallikrein, plasmin, thrombin, and their inhibitors in human blood plasma). Biul. Eksp. Biol. Med. *81*, 632–633 (1976b)

Ivashkevich, G.A., Vuiv, G.P., Khimka, A.S.: Issledovanie nekotorykh komponentov kininovoy sistemy pri ostrykh gnoynykh peritonitakh (The investigation of some components of kinin system in acute suppurative peritonitis). Vestn. Khir. *116*, No. 4, 14–18 (1976)

Kauricheva, N.I., Budnitskaya, P.Z., Bogomolets-Henriques, O.M.: Vydelenie i nekotorye svoystva dvukh kininogenov plasmy krovi loshadi (Isolation and some properties of two kininogens from horse plasma). Vopr. Med. Khim. *17*, 6–12 (1971)

Khodorov, B.I., Timin, E.N., Pogadaev, V.I.: Rol khemovozbudimykh kalcievykh kanalov v mekhanizme deystviya acetilkholina, histamina i bradikinina na depolyarizovannuyu gladkuyu myshtsu (The role of chemoexcitive calcic canals in mechanism of action of acetylcholine, histamine, and bradykinin on depolarized smooth muscle. In: Physiologia and biokhimiya mediatornich processov. Thesis Dokl. Vsesoyuzn. Konf., Posvyashch. 75-letiyu so dnya rojd. Kh. S. Koshtoyantsa. Turpaev, T.M. (ed.), pp. 133–134. Moskva: 1976 (Published by Akad. Sei. USSR)

Khutzurauli, E.Sh., Tsverava, E.N.: Bradikininogen i aktivnost kininaz plazmy krovi pri khronicheskom mieloleykoze (Bradykininogen and kininase activity of blood plasma in patients with chronic myeloleukemia). Sakartvelos SSR. Metsnierebata Akademine moamte, Soobtch. AN Gruz. SSR. *74*, 697–699 (1974)

Komissarova, N.V., Gomazkov, O.A.: Osobennosti kontaktnoy aktivatsii kallikreinovoy i plasminovoy sistem krovi krolika (Some features of contact activation of the kallikreine and plasmin systems of rabbit blood). Biul. Eksp. Biol. Med. *81*, 390–392 (1976)

Kotelnikov, V.P., Pankov, V.I.: Svobodnye kininy krovi u khirurgicheskikh bolnykh (Free blood kinins in surgical patients). Khirurgiia No. 11, 137–140 (1976)

Krit, N.A., Ravdel, G.A., Ivanov, V.T.: Sintez analogow bradikinina, modificirovannykh v polojenii 8 (Synthesis of bradykinin analogs modified in position "8"). Bioorgan. Khim. *2*, 1455–1463 (1976)

Kraynova, B.L., Kiporenko, S.S., Chaman, E.S.: Sintez o-gippuril-δ-guanidino-α-L-oxivalerianovoy kisloty (o-gippuril-L-argininovoy kisloty) [Synthesis o-hippuryl-δ-guonidino-α-L-oxyvalerianic acid (o-hippuryl-L-argininic acid)]. Zh. Obshch. Khim. *40*, 708–709 (1970)

Kuzin, M.I., Menshikov, V.V., Dudnik, V.S., Beljakov, N.V.: Kininovaya sistema i eyo uchastie v patogeneze nekotorykh khirurgicheskikh zabolevaniy (obzor literatury) [Kinin system and its participation in pathogenesis of some surgical diseases (Review)]. Khirurgiia No. 2, 116–120 (1974)

Lakin, K.M., Rachitskaya, N.G., Polonskaya, L.B.: Inhibitor fibrinoliza iz legochnoy tkani – inhitril (Inhitryl – a fibrinolysis inhibitor prepared from the pulmonary tissue). Farmakol. Toksikol. *35*, 320–324 (1972)

Lantsberg, L.A., Nekrasova, A.A.: Ob uchastii kininovoy sistemy pochek i krovi v adaptatsii organisma k fizicheskim nagruzkam (On the participation of the kinin system of kidneys and blood in adaptation of the body to physical stress). Kardiologia *12*, No. 9, 58–63 (1972)

Lantsberg, L.A., Kutyrina, I.M., Nekrasova, A.A., Chernova, N.A.: Rol kininovoy sistemy pochek v regulatsii natriy-uresa (The role of kinin system of kidneys in regulation of sodium excretion). Vestn. Acad. Med. Nauk SSSR No. 10, 51–54 (1974)

Laufer, A.L., Gulikova, O.M., Paskhina, T.S.: O dvukh kininoobrayushchikh fermentakh plazmy krovi cheloveka (Two kinin-producing enzymes of human blood plasma). Biokhimiia *34*, 3–12 (1969)

Levitsky, A.P., Konovets, V.M., Lvov, I.F., Barabash, R.D., Volodkina, V.V.: Kallikrein i nespetcificheskie proteazy v slyune bolnykh yazvennoy boleznyu jeludka i dvenadtsatiperstnoy kishki (Alterations in activities of kallikrein and nonspecific proteases in human saliva in ulcerous disease of stomach and duodenum). Vopr. Med. Khim. *19*, 633–638 (1973)

Levitsky, A.P., Vovchuk, S.V.: Raspredelenie v pishchevaritelnoy sisteme krys proteoliticheskogo fermenta slyuny-salivaina (Distribution of a proteolytic enzyme in the saliva-salivain in the digestive system of rats). Biul. Eksp. Biol. Med. No. 7 12–24 (1973)

Levitsky, A.P., Vovchuk, S.V., Barabash, R.D.: Obnarushenie, vydelenie i svoystva kallikreina slyuny krysy i zolotistogo khomyaka (The detection, purification, and properties of salivary kallikrein in the golden hamster *citellus auratus* and in rats). Zh. Evol. Biokhim. Fisiol. *10*, 510–512 (1974)

Lokshina, L.A., Egorova, T.P., Orekhovich, V.N.: Proteinazy v selezenke byka s kininogenaznoy aktivnostju (Proteinase in bovine spleen with kininogenase activity). Biokhimiia *41*, 2021–2024 (1976)

Lyublinskaya, L.A., Vaganova, T.I., Paskhina, T.S., Stepanov, V.M.: 2,4-dinitrofenil-proizvodnye peptidov – substraty novogo tipa dlya opredeleniya aktivnosti proteoliticheskikh fermentov. Opredelenie aktivnosti karboksipeptidaz (2,4-dinitrophenyl-derivatives of peptides-substrates of a new type for determination of activity of proteolytic enzymes. Determination of carboxypeptidase activity). Biokhimiia *38*, 790–795 (1973)

Malaya, L.T., Berkelieva, S.Ch., Lazareva, S.A.: Aktivnost kininogenazy i kininazy pri infarkte miokarda i kardiogennom shoke (The activity of kininogenase and kininase in myocardial infarction and cardiogenic shock). Vestn. Acad. Med. Nauk SSSR No. 3, 30–40 (1973a)

Malaya, L.T., Lazareva, S.A., Berkelieva, S.Ch.: Aktivnost kininogen-kininovoy sistemy pri ostrom krupnoochagovom infarkte miokarda i ego oslojneniyakh (Kininogen-kinin system in acute macrofocal myocardial infarction and its complications). Klin. Med. *55*, No. 4, 29–36 (1973b)

Malaya, L.T., Lazareva, S.A.: Znachenie aktivatsii kallikrein-kininovoy sistemy dlya diagnostiki infarkta miokarda i naibolee tyajolykh ego oslojneniy (The significance of kallikrein-kinine systeme activation for the diagnostic of myocardial infarction and its severe complications). In: Kinins and kinin systems of blood. Trudy I MMI im. Sechenova. Paskhina, T.S., Menshikov, V.V. (eds.), pp. 68–69. Moskva: 1976 (Published by 1 MMI im Sechenova.)

Mashkovsky, M.D., Lakin, K.M., Ovnatanova, M.S., Schwartz, G.Ya.: Vlijanie parmidina (piridinolkarbamata) na agregatsiyu trombocitov, svertyvanie krovi i fibrinoliz [The effect of parmidine (pyridinolcarbamate) on the platelet aggregation, blood coagulation and fibrinolysis]. Biul. Eksp. Biol. Med. *81*, 322–324 (1976)

Meerson, F.Z., Gomazkov, O.A., Shimkovich, M.V., Bolshakova, L.V.: Znachenie sistemy kininov dlya regulatsii krovoobrashcheniya pri adaptatsii k vysotnoy hipoksii (Significance of the kinin system for regulation of blood circulation during adaptation to high altitude hypoxia). Kardiologia *14*, No. 6, 38–45 (1974)

Meged, N.F., Veremienko, K.M., Pavlof, V.V., Tertykh, V.A.: Activation of blood plasma prekallikrein by high-dispered organic silica. Ukr. Biokhim. Zh. *48*, 370–374 (1976)

Menshikov, V.V., Orlov, V.A., Belyakov, N.V.: Kininovaya sistema krovi v gastroenterologii (biokhimiya i fiziologiya, klinicheskoe znachenie) [Kinin system of blood in gastroenterology (biochemistry, physiology and clinical importance)]. Klin. Med. *50*, No. 1, 12–19 (1972)

Narticova, V.F., Paskhina, T.S.: Ochistka i svoystva kislotostabilnogo ingibitora iz syvorotki krovi krolika (Purification and characteristies of an acid-resistant inhibitor of trypsin from rabbit blood serum). Biokhimiia *34*, 282–292 (1969)

Nekrasova, A.A., Lantsberg, L.A., Chernova, N.A., Khukharev, V.V.: Kininovaya sistema pochek pri razlichnykh fiziologicheskykh sostoyaniyakh u zdorovykh lyudey i pri hipertonicheskoy bolezni (The kinine system of the kidneys in different physiological conditions in healthy persons and in patients with hypertensive vascular disease). Kardiologia *10*, No. 11, 9–25 (1970)

Nekrasova, A.A., Khukharev, V.V.: Kininovaya sistema pochek u bolnykh hipertonicheskoy boleznyu i ego vozmojnaya kompensatornaya rol v regulatsii pochechnogo krovotoka (Renal kinin system in patients with hypertensive disease and its possible compensatory role in the regulation of renal blood flow). Kardioloia *12*, No. 7, 14–19 (1972)

Nekrasova, A.A., Chernova, N.A., Lantsberg, L.A., Khukharev, V.V.: Kininovaya sistema pochek, metody opredeleniya ego osnovnykh komponentov – kallikreina i kininov v moche (Renal kinin system, methods of determination of the main components in urine-kallikrein and kinins). Lab. Delo No. 4, 223–228 (1972)
Nekrasova, A.A., Lantsberg, L.A., Kramer, A.A., Eventov, A.Z.: Sostoyanie kininovoy sistemy krovi u bolnykh hipertonicheskoy boleznyu (Blood kinin system in patients with hypertensive disease). Sov. Med. No. 3, 28–33 (1973)
Obukhov, Yu.E.: Svobodnye kininy krovi v dinamike ojogovoy bolezni (Free plasma kinines in burn). In: Ojogovaya bolezn (Burn disease). Postyanoi, N.F. (ed.), pp. 70–72. Kiev: Zdorovie 1975
Orekhovich, V.N.: Properties, specificity and mechanism of action of the proteolytic enzymes. Ital. J. Biochemistry *17*, 241–256 (1968)
Orekhovich, V.N., Eliseeva, Yu.E., Pavlikhina, L.V., Negovskiy, V.A., Molchanov, L.V.: Fermentativnye osnovy regulyatsii sosudistogo tonusa pri ekstremalnykh sostoyaniyakh (Enzymatic basis of vascular tonus regulation in extrema states). Fisiologiya Cheloveka *1*, 310–316 (1975)
Orekhovich, V.N., Eliseeva, Yu.E., Pavlikhina, L.V.: Enzimologicheskie faktory regulatsii sosudistogo tonusa (Enzymological factors in the vascular tension regulation). Vestn. Aksd. Med. Nauk SSSR *9*, 42–47 (1976)
Orekhovich, V.N.: Sovremennye metody v biokhimii (Modern methods in biochemistry). Orekhovich, V.N. (ed.), Vol. 3. Moskva: Medicina 1977
Oyvin, I.A., Gaponyuk, P.Ya., Oyvin, V.I., Tokarev, O.Yu.: The mechanism of blood vessel permeability derangement under the influence of histamine, serotonin, and bradykinin. Experientia *26*, 843–844 (1970)
Oyvin, I.A., Gaponyuk, P.Ya., Oyvin, V.I., Tokarev, O.Yu., Volodin, V.M.: Mekhanizmy povysheniya pronitsaemosti sosudov pod vliyaniem faktorov pronitsaemosti (histamin, serotonin, bradikinin) i vospalitelnykh razdrajiteley [Mechanisms involved in increasing the vascular permeability under the effect of permeability factors (histamine, serotonin, kinins) and of inflammatory agents]. Patol. Fiziol. Eksp. Ter. No. 4, 19–23 (1972a)
Oyvin, I.A., Gaponyuk, P.Ya., Uklonskaya, L.I.: K mekhanizmu povysheniya pronitaaemosti sosudov kozhi pri mestnov β-obluchenii (On the mechanism of the increased permeability of cutaneous vessels at local β-irradiation of skin). Radiobiologiia *12*, 462–463 (1972b)
Oyvin, I.A., Gaponyuk, P.Ya., Uklonskaya, L.I.: Aktualnye voprosy patogeneza i terapii ostrogo vospaleniya (Obzor) [Important problems of pathogenesis and therapy of accute inflammation (Review)]. Patol. Fiziol. Eksp. Ter. No. 2, 3–10 (1973)
Paskhina, T.S.: Mechanism obrasovaniya, obmen i rol pri sosudistych patologiyach kininov plasmi krovi (The mechanism of formation, methabolism, and role at the cardio-vascular patology). In: Molecularnii osnovi patologii. Orechovich, N. (ed.), pp. 123–178. Moskva: Medicina 1966
Paskhina, T.S., Egorova, T.P.: Ochistka i svoystva kininogena (bradikininagena) iz syvorotki krovi krolika [Purification and properties of kininogen (bradykininogen) of rabbit blood serum]. Biokhimiya *31*, 468–476 (1966)
Paskhina, T.S., Zykova, V.P., Egorova, T.P., Narticova, V.F., Karpova, A.V., Guseva, M.V.: Reactsiya N-α-tozyl-L-lisilkhlormetan s kallikreinom iz plasmy krolika i s kallikreinom iz mochi i slyuny cheloveka (Reaction of N-α-tozyl-L-lysilchlormethane with kallikrein from rabbit plasma and with kallikrein from urine and saliva of man). Biokhimiia *33*, 745–752 (1968a)
Paskhina, T.S., Gulikova, O.M., Egorova, T.P., Surovikina, M.S., Shmyryova, R.K.: Opredeleniye bradikinina pri pomoshchi biologicheskykh i khromatograficheskikh metodov (Estimation of bradykinin by biochemical and chromatographic methods). In: Sovremennye metody v biokhimii (Modern methods in biochemistry). Orekhovich, V.N. (ed.), pp. 205–232. Moskva: Medicina 1968b
Paskhina, T.S., Egorova, T.P., Zykova, V.P., Laufer, A.L., Trapeznikova, S.S., Shimonaeva, E.E.: Khimicheskie i biologicheskie metody opredeleniya osnovnykh komponentov kininovoy sistemy krovi (kininogena, kallikreina, ingibitorov kallikreina, kininasy) [Chemical and biological methods for estimation of main components of kinin system of blood (kininogen, kallikrein, kallikrein inhibitors, kininase)]. In: Sovremennye metody v biokhimii (Modern methods in biochemistry). Orekhovich, V.N. (ed.), Vol. 2, pp. 232–261. Moskva: Medicina 1968c

Paskhina, T.S.: Fermentativny mekhanizm obrazovaniya i raspada kininov plazmy krovi bradikinina i kallidina (Enzymatic mechanism of formation and decomposition of blood plasma kinins – bradikinin and kallidin). In: Chemical factors of enzymatic activity and biosynthesis regulation. Orechovich, V.N. (ed.), pp. 317–359. Moscow: Medicina 1969

Paskhina, T.S., Yarovaya, G.A.: Kallikrein syvorotki krovi cheloveka. Aktivnost fermenta i khromatograficheskiy metod opredeleniya (Kallikrein of the serum of human blood. Enzyme activity and chromatographic method for its determination). Biokhimiia *35*, 1055–1058 (1970a)

Paskhina, T.S., Yarovaya, G.A., Laufer, A.L., Gulikova, O.M., Trapeznikova, S.S., Morozova, N.A., Makarova, O.V., Tikhomirov, I.B., Sysoyev, V.F., Match, E.S.: Soderjanie i aktivnost osnovnykh komponentov kininovoy sistemy v syvorotke krovi bolnykh revmatismom (The content and activity of basic components of kinin system in blood serum of patients with rheumatism). Vopr. Med. Khim. *16*, 152–161 (1970b)

Paskhina, T.S.: Enzymatichesky mekhanism obrazovaniya i raspada kininov (Enzymatic mechanism of formation and destruction of kinins). In: Sovremenniye problemy endocrinologii. Judaev, N.A. (ed.), Vol. 4, pp. 108–122. Moskva: Medicina 1972

Paskhina, T.S., Shrayber, M.I., Yarovaya, G.A., Morozova, N.A., Nartikova, V.F., Trapeznikova, S.S., Docenko, V.L., Makarova, O.V., Maslova, T.M.: Rol kininovoy sistemy v patogeneze ojogovoy bolezny cheloveka. I. Sostoyanie kininovoy sistemy v razlichnye periody ojogovoy bolezny (Role of kinin system in pathogenesis of burn disease. I. State of kinin system in different periods of burn disease). Vopr. Med. Khim. *18*, 137–145 (1972)

Paskhina, T.S., Gurtovenko, V.M.: Vliyanie stekla i ellagovoy kisloty na obrazovanie kininov v plazme krovi krolika (Effects of glass and ellagic acid on formation of kinins in rabbit blood plasma). Vopr. Med. Khim. *27*, 7–15 (1972)

Paskhina, T.S., Dotsenko, V.L., Blinnikova, E.I.: Kallikreinogen syvorotki krovi cheloveka. Metod opredeleniya i nekotorye svoystva (Kallikreinogen in human blood serum; a method of estimation and some properties). Biokhimiia *38*, 420–423 (1973)

Paskhina, T.S., Krinskaya, A.V.: Uproshchenny metod opredeleniya kallikreinogena i kallikreina v syvorotke (plazme) krovi cheloveka v norme i pri nekotorykh patologicheskikh sostoyaniyakh (A simplified method for determination of kallikreinogene and kallikrein in human blood serum in normal and some pathological states). Vopr. Med. Khim. *20*, 660–666 (1974)

Paskhina, T.S., Krinskaya, A.V., Zykova, V.P.: Deystvie ingibitorov tripsina peptidno-belkovoy prirody na kallikreiny syvorotki krovi cheloveka i krolika (Effect of trypsin inhibitor of a peptide-protein nature on kallikreins from human and rabbit blood serum). Biokhimiia *40*, 302–309 (1975a)

Paskhina, T.S., Trapeznikova, S.S., Egorova, T.P., Morozova, N.A.: Vlijanie bradikinin potents iruyushchikh peptidov zmeinogo yada i C-koncevogo pentapeptidnogo fragmenta bradikinina na aktivnost karboksipeptidazy N i kininaznuyu aktivnost syvorotky krovi cheloveka (Effect of bradikinin-potentiating snake venom peptides and C-terminal pentapeptide fragment of bradykinin on carboxypeptidase N and kininase activities of human blood serum). Biokhimiia *40*, 844–852 (1975b)

Paskhina, T.S., Bondar, Z.A., Krinskaya, A.V., Melkumova, I.S., Polikarpova, E.G.: Sostoyanie kallikreinogen-kallikreinovoy sistemy u bolnykh s zabolevaniyami pecheni (State of kallikreinogen-kallikrein system in patients with hepatic diseases). Klin. Med. *53*, No. 8, 9–15 (1975c)

Paskhina, T.S., Menshikov, V.V. (eds.): Kininy i kininovaya sistema krovi (biokhimiya, farmakologiya, patofiziologiya, metody issledovaniya, rol v patologii) [Kinins and kinin system of blood (biochemistry, pharmacology, pathophysiology, methods of assay, role in pathology)]. Moskow: Sbornik trudov 1 MMI imeni Sechenova 1976

Paskhina, T.S.: Kallikrein plazmy krovi – novye funktsii (Plasma kallikrein: new functions). Review. Biokhimiia *41*, 1347–1351 (1976)

Paskhina, T.S., Nartikova, V.F., Docenko, V.L., Maslova, T.M., Morozova, N.A., Trapeznikova, S.S., Yarovaya, L.M.: Sostoyanie kininovoy sistemy pri ojogovom shoke i ranney toksemii (State of kinin system in burn shock and early toxemia). Vopr. Med. Khim. *22*, 696–707 (1976)

Paskhina, T.S., Makevnina, L.G., Egorova, T.P., Levina, G.O.: Identificatsiya kininov osvobozhdaemykh pankreaticheskim kallikreinom svinyi iz nizkomolekulyarnogo kininogena krolika (Identification of kinins released by pig pancreatic kallikrein from low molecular weight rabbit kininogen). Biokhimiia *42*, 1153–1155 (1977 a)
Paskhina, T.S., Polyanceva, L.R., Krinskaya, A.V., Belolipetskaya, Yu.G., Nartikova, V.F., Rossinskaya, E.B., Kargashin, I.A.: Sostoyanie kininovoy sistemy i uroven ingibitorov proteinaz syvorotki krovi pri latentnom nefrite i nefroticheskom sindrome razlichnoy etiologii (State of kinin system and content of proteinase inhibitors in latent nephritis and nephrotic syndrome of various etiology). Vopr. Med. Khim. *23*, 241–251 (1977 b)
Paskhina, T.S., Dolgina, M.I., Nartikova, V.F., Krinskaya, A.V., Morozova, N.A., Rossinskaya, E.B.: Vliyanie polivalentnogo ingibitora proteinaz is lyogkikh byka na sostoyanie kininovoy sistemy pro ozhogovom shoke i ostroy ozhogovoy toksemii (The effect of polyvalent inhibitor of proteinase from bovine lung on the state of kinin in burn shock and acute burn toxemia). Vopr. Med. Khim. *23*, 689–700 (1977 c)
Pavlikhina, L.V., Eliseeva, Ju.E., Pozdnev, B.F., Orekhovich, V.N.: Opredelenie aktivnosti karboxikatepsina (peptidil-di-peptidasy) v syvorotke krovi cheloveka [Estimation of carboxycathepsin activity (peptidyl-dipeptidase) in human blood serum]. Vopr. Med. Khim. *21*, 54–60 (1975)
Pogadaev, V.I., Timin, E.N.: Vlijanie biologicheski aktivnykh veshchestv (acetilkholina, histamina i bradikinina) na depolyarizovannuyu gladkuyu myshtsu taenia coli [Effects of biologically active agents (acetylcholine, histamine and bradykinin) on depolarized smooth muscle of taenia coli]. Biul. Eksp. Biol. Med. *81*, 12–14 (1976)
Polushkin, B.V., Kulaya, V.V., Latysheva, V.V., Ogorodova, T.S.: Bradikinin i ego rol v fiziologii i patologii koji (Bradykinin and its function in dermal physiology and pathology). Vestn. Dermatol. Venerol. No. 10, 19–25 (1972)
Popkova, G.A., Astapova, M.V., Lisunkin, Ju.J., Ravdel, G.A., Krit, N.A.: Sravnitelnoe izuchenie biologicheskoy aktivnosti i ustoychivosti k deystviyu tkanevykh kininaz analogov bradikinina, modificirovannykh v polojenii 8 (A comparative study of biological activity and resistance to tissue kininases of bradykinin analogs modified in position "8"). Bioorgan. Khim. *2*, 1606–1612 (1976)
Popov, V.G., Melkumova, I.S., Sorokin, A.V.: Soderjanie kininogena v syvorotke krovi u bolnykh s koronarnoy nedostatochnostyu (The blood serum content of kininogen in patients with coronary insufficiency). Kardiologiia *11*, No. 8, 30–34 (1971)
Ravdel, G.A., Filatova, M.P., Shchukina, L.A., Paskhina, T.S., Surovicina, M.S., Trapeznikova, S.S., Egorova, T.P.: 6-Glycine-8-phenyllactic acid bradykinin. Its synthesis, biological activity, and splitting by kininase (carboxypeptidase N). J. Med. Chem. *10*, 242–246 (1967)
Ravdel, G.A., Monapova, N.N., Krit, N.A., Filatova, M.P., Lisunkin, Yu.I., Ivanov, V.T.: Sintez i biologicheskie svoystva bradikinin-potentsirujushchikh peptidov iz yada zmey (Synthesis and biological properties of bradykinin-potentiating peptides from snake venom). Khim. Prir. Soed (Uz. SSR) No. 1, 47–56 (1975)
Shchukina, L.A., Ravdel, G.A., Filatova, M.P., Syomkin, B.P., Krasnova, S.M.: Sintez bradikinina (Bradykinin synthesis). Khim. Prirodn. Soed. (Uz.SSR) *No. 2*, 124–130 (1966)
Shevchenko, A.I.: K voprosu o deystvii bradikinina na gladkuyu muskulaturu bronkhov (On the action of bradykinin on smooth muscles of bronchi). In: Kinins and kinin system of blood. Sbornik nauchnykh Trudov 1 MMI im. Sechenova. Paskhina, T.S., Menshikov, V.V. (eds.), p. 48. Moscow: 1976 (Published by 1 MMI im. Sechenova)
Shkhvatsabaya, I.K., Nekrasova, A.A.: Biologichesky aktivnye substancii-prostaglandiny i kininy, ikh rol v regulacii arterialnogo davleniya i razvitii arterialnoy hipertonii (Biologically active substances-prostaglandines and kinins and their function in regulation of arterial blood pressure and development of arterial hypertension). Kardiologiia *17*, No. 2, 136–145 (1977)
Shwartz, G.Ya., Liberman, S.S., Mashkovsky, M.D., Berlgand, E.A.: Eksperimentalnoe izuchenie protivovospalitelnogo deystviya piridinol-karbamata (Experimental investigation of antiphlogistic action of pyridinolcarbamate). Farmakol. Toksikol. *38*, 434–436 (1975)
Shwartz, G.Ya., Mashkovsky, M.D.: (Vliyanie piridinolkarbamata (parmidina) na nekotorye effecty bradikinina [The influence of pyridinolcarbamate (parmidine) on some bradykinin effects]. Farmakol. Toksikol. *39*, 176–179 (1976)

Stepanova, I. V., Vizir, A. D.: Kininovaya sistema krovi u bolnykh yazvennoy boleznyu (Kinine system of the blood in patients with ulcer disease). Vrach. Delo No. 10, 21–22 (1974)
Strigunov, V. I., Gaponyuk, P. Ya.: Primenenie bradikinina dlya differentsialnoy diagnostiki dobrokachestvennykh i zlokachestvennykh novoobrazovaniy (Application of bradykinin for differential diagnostics of benevolent and malignant formations). Med. Radiol. (Mosk.) *20*, No. 8, 11–13 (1975)
Stukalova, T. I., Lazareva, S. A., Ternovaya, L. A.: Aktivnost kallikrein-kininovoy sistemy pri eksperimentalnom infarkte miokarda u sobak i vliyanie na nee katekholaminov (Activity of kallikrein-kinin system in experimental myocardial infarction in dogs and effect on the system of exogenously administered catecholamines). Vopr. Med. Khim. *21*, 88–91 (1975)
Surovikina, M. S.: Specificheskiy biologicheskiy metod opredeleniya svobodnykh kininov v venoznoy krovi cheloveka i jivotnykh (A specific biological method of determination free kinins in the venous blood of man and animals). Biul. Eksp. Biol. Med. *71*, No. 5, 123–125 (1971)
Surovikina, M. S., Paleev, N. R., Gavrilova, R. D.: Kininy plazmy krovi i ikh znachenie v patologii organov dykhaniya (Kinins of blood plasma and their influence on the pathology of respiratory organs). Sov. Med. No. 12, 59–66 (1972)
Surovikina, M. S.: Kininovaya sistema plazmy krovi pri eksperimentalnom allergicheskom miokardite (The kinin system of blood plasma in experimental allergic myocarditis). Kardiologiia *13*, No. 2, 119–123 (1973)
Surovikina, M. S., Odinokova, V. A.: Patogeneticheskaya rol kininov pri allergicheskom povrejdenii miokarda (The pathogenetic role of kinins in allergic damage of the myocardium). Kardiologiia *14*, No. 4, 78–81 (1974)
Surovikina, M. S., Paleev, N. R., Gurevich, M. A., Dokukin, A. V., Yankovskaya, M. O.: Kininy plazmy i serdechno-sosudistaya sistema (Kinins of plasma and cardio-vascular system). Klin. Med. *52*, No. 10, 15–23 (1974)
Surovikina, M. S.: Biologicheskiy metod opredelenia summarnoy aktivnosti kallikreina plasmy cheloveka i laboratornykh jyvotnykh (The biological method of determination total activity of human and of animals plasma kallikrein). Lab. Delo No. 1, 6–9 (1975)
Surovikina, M. S., Odinokova, V. A., Paleev, N. R., Gurevich, M. A., Yankovskaya, M. O.: Izmeneniya kompohentov kininovoy sistemy i struktury miokarda pod vliyaniem antikininovykh preparatov pri allergicheskom miokardite u krolikov (Changes in the components of the kinin system and in the myocardial structure under the effect of antikinin preparation in rabbits with allergic myocarditis). Biul. Eksp. Biol. Med. *81*, 979–981 (1976)
Suvalskaya, L. A.: Kininogenazy i kininogen v plazme krovi bolnykh ostrym pankreatitom (Kininogenases and kininogen in the blood plasma of patients with acute pancreatitis). Klin. Med. *54*, No. 2, 55–57 (1976)
Trapesnikova, S. S., Mardashev, S. R.: Vydelenie, ochistka i svoystva ingibitora karboxipeptidazy N iz syvorotki krovi cheloveka (Isolation, purification, and properties of an inhibitor of carboxypeptidase N from human blood serum). Vopr. Med. Khim. *21*, 417–422 (1975)
Trocka, V.: Summary of the literature published in Czechoslovakian, Polish, and Russian journals. In: Handbook of experimental pharmacology. Vol. XXV: Bradykinin, kallidin, and kallikrein. Erdös, E. G. (ed.), pp. 594–601. Berlin, Heidelberg, New York: Springer 1970
Urzaeva, L. V., Dubley, P. V.: O nekotorykh aspektakh barriernoy functsii lyogkikh po otnosheniyu k ryadu vasoactivnykh veshchestv (On some aspects of barrier function of lung as regards some vasoactive substances). Usp. Sovrem. Biol. *83*, 139–153 (1977)
Ushinsky, M.: Hipotenzionnye polipeptidy (kininy) v rodakh [Hypotensive polypeptides (kinines) in delivery]. Akush. Ginecol. No. 5, 55–58 (1970)
Veremeenko, K. N., Volokhonskaya, L. I., Kizim, A. I., Meged, N. F.: Opredelenie kallikreinogena i ingibitorov kallikreina v plazme krovi (Estimation of kallikreinogen and kallikrein inhibitors in blood plasma). Ukr. Biochim. Zh. *46*, 246–250 (1974)
Veremeenko, K. N., Volokhonskaya, L. I., Kizim, A. I., Meged, N. F.: Metod opredeleniya kontaktnogo prekallikreina i inhibitorov kallikreina v plazme krovi cheloveka (A method for the determination of contact prekallikrein and inhibitors of kallikrein in human blood plasma). Lab. Delo No. 1, 9–12 (1975)
Veremeenko, K. N., Mitchenko, I. K., Gontar, A. M.: Izuchenie prekallikrein-kallikrein sistemy plazmy krovi pri virusnom gepatite (Studies of blood plasma prekallikrein-kallikrein system in virus hepatitis). Vrach. Delo No. 10, 132–134 (1976 a)

Veremeenko, K. N., Verevka, V. S., Meged, N. F.: Issledovanie prekallikrein-kallikrein sistemy plazmy krovi pri ostrom pankreatite (Studies of blood plasma prekallikrein-kallikrein system in acute pancreatitis). Klin, Khir. No. 9, 5–9 (1976b)
Veremeenko, K. N.: Kininovaya sistema (Kinin system). Kiev: Zdorovya 1977
Virovets, S. I., Martynov, V. F., Titov, M. I.: Sintez argininosoderzhashchikh peptidov (Synthesis of arginine-containing peptides). Zh. Obshch. Khim. *38*, 2337 (1968)
Vovchuk, S. V., Barabash, R. D., Levitsky, A. P.: Vydelenie i svoystva dvukh kallikreinov slyuny cheloveka (Purification and properties of two kallikreins of human saliva). Vopr. Med. Khim. *21*, 622–625 (1975)
Vovchuk, S. V., Levitsky, A. P., Osadchy, B. D., Sokolov, S. A.: Vliyanie kallikreina podchelyustnykh jelez sobak na jeludochnuyu sekreciyu (The effects of kallikrein purified from dog submandibular salivary gland upon the gastric secretion). Fiziol. Zh. SSSR *63*, 131–138 (1977)
Yarovaya, G. A.: Obshchye faktory regulatsii kininovoy sistemy, svertyvaniya krovi i fibrinoliza (General factors of regulation of kinin system, blood coagulation, and fibrinolysis). In: Khimicheskie faktory regulatsii aktivnosti i biosintesa fermentov (Chemical factors of regulation of activity and biosynthesis of enzymes). Orekhovich, V. N. (ed.), pp. 275–316. Moscow: Medicina 1969
Zborovsky, A. B., Styajkova, R. A.: Aktivnost kininovoy sistemy krovi u bolnykh revmatizmom (The activity of kinin system in blood of patients with rheumatism). In: Kininy i kininovaya sistema krovi. Paskhina, T. C., Menshilov, V. V. (eds.), pp. 84–85. Sbornik Trudov 1 MMI imeni Sechenova. Moskva: 1976 (Published by 1 MMI im Sechenova)
Zhukova, G. F., Ravdel, G. A., Shchukina, L. A., Paskhina, T. S., Gurtovenko, V. M.: Depsipeptidnye analogi eledoisina. Sintez i biologicheskaya aktivnost (Depsipeptide analogues of eledoisine. Synthesis and biological activity). Sovr. voprosy endokrinologii. Yudaev, N. A. (ed.), Vol. 4, pp. 99–107. Moskva: Medicina 1972

References (Suppl.) *

Abe, K.: Urinary excretion of kinin in man with special reference to its origin. Tohoku J. Exp. Med. *87*, 175–179 (1965)
Cechova, A., Svestkova, V., Keil, B., Sorm, F.: Similarities in primary structures of cow colostrum trypsin inhibitor and bovine pancreatic trypsin inhibitor. FEBS Letters *4*, 155–156 (1969)
Colman, R., Mason, I., Scherry, S.: The kallikreinogen-kallikrein enzyme system of human plasma. Assay of components and observations in disease states. Ann. Intern. Med. *71*, 763–773 (1969)
Erdös, E., Yang, H.: An enzyme in microsomal fraction of kidney that inactivates bradykinin. Life Sci. *6*, 569–574 (1967)
Ferreira, S., Vane, J.: The detection and estimation of bradykinin in the circulating blood. Br. J. Pharmacol. *29*, 367–377 (1967)
Fiedler, F.: Pig pancreatic kallikrein: structure and catalytic properties. Life Sci. *16*, 788–789 (1975)
Folk, J., Gladner, J.: Carboxypeptidase B. III. Specific esterase activity. Biochim. Biophys. Acta *33*, 570–572 (1959)
Fujimoto, Y., Moriya, H., Moriwaki, C.: Studies on human salivary kallikrein. J. Biochem. (Tokyo) *74*, 239–246 (1973)
Green, N., Work, E.: Pancreatic trypsin inhibitor. Biochem. J. *54*, 347–352 (1953)
Gregerman, R.: Identification of His-Leu and other histidyl peptides as normal constituents of human urine. Biochem. Med. *1*, 151–167 (1967)
Griffin, J., Cochrane, C.: The mechanism for the involvement of HMW kininogen in surface-dependent reaction of Hageman factor (blood coagulation, factor XII, prekallikrein, factor XI, fibrinolisis). Proc. Natl. Acad. Sci. U.S.A. *73*, 2554–2558 (1976)
Habal, F. M., Movat, H. Z., Burrowes, C. E.: Isolation of two functionally different kininogens from human plasma. Separation from proteinase inhibitors and interaction with plasma kallikrein. Biochem. Pharmacol. *23*, 2291–2302 (1974)

* List of references of foreign authors cited in this review.

Kato, H., Suzuki, T.: The location and nature of linkage of kinin moiety in bovine kininogen II. Biochem. Biophys. Res. Commun. *32*, 800–805 (1968)

Majno, G., Palade, G. E.: Studies of an inflammation. I. The effect of histamine and serotonin on vascular permeability. An electron microscopic study. J. Biophys. Biochem. Citol. *11*, 571–606 (1961)

Komiya, M., Kato, H., Suzuki, T.: Bovine plasma kininogens. III. Structure comparison of HMW and LMW-kinonogens. J. Biochem. (Tokyo) *76*, 833–845 (1974)

Moriya, H., Moriwaki, Ch., Yamazaki, K., Akimoto, S., Fukushima, H.: Human salivary kallikrein and liberation of colostrokinin. In: Hypotensive peptides. Erdös, E. G., Back, N., Sicuteri, F. (eds.), pp. 161–174. Berlin, Heidelberg, New York: Springer 1966

Movat, H., Habal, F., McMorine, D.: Neutral proteases of human PMN leukocytes with kininogenase activity. Int. Arch. Allergy Appl. Immunol. *50*, 257–281 (1976)

Piquilloud, Y., Reinharz, A., Roth, M.: Studies on the angiotension converting enzyme with different substrates. Biochim. Biophys. Acta *206*, 136–142 (1970)

Schench, F., Oberdorf, A., Schmidt-Kastner, G.: Verfahren zur Herstellung eines Bradykinin homologen Nonapeptides. Ger. Pat. *1*, 298, 997 (1969)

Skeggs, L., March, W., Kahn, J., Shumway, N.: Existence of two forms of hypertensin. J. Exp. Med. *99*, 275–282 (1954)

Trautschold, I., Werle, E.: Spectrophotometrische Bestimmung des Kallikrein und seiner Inaktivatoren. Hoppe Seylers Z. Physiol. Chem. *325*, 48–59 (1961)

Vane, J.: The release and fate of vaso-active hormones in the circulation. Br. J. Pharmacol. *35*, 209–215 (1969)

Wolf, E., Schirmer, E., Folk, J.: The kinetics of carboxypeptidase B activity. I. Kinetic parameters. J. Biol. Chem. *237*, 3094–3099 (1962)

Yang, H., Erdös, E.: Second kininase in human blood plasma. Nature (Lond.) *215*, 1402–1403 (1967)

Zweifach, B. W.: Ismeneniya sostoyanya krowenostnich kapillyarov i ich pronitsaemosti (Changes in blood capillary behavior and their permeability). Patol. Fiziol. Eksp. Ter. No. 2, 6–16 (1964)

Author Index

Page numbers in *italics* refer to bibliography

Subject Index

Handbook of Experimental Pharmacology

Continuation of "Handbuch der experimentellen Pharmakologie"

Springer-Verlag
Berlin
Heidelberg
New York

Handbook of Experimental Pharmacology

Continuation of "Handbuch der experimentellen Pharmakologie"

Volume 25
Bradykinin, Kallidin and Kallikrein

Volume 26
H. Fischer: **Vergleichende Pharmakologie von Überträgersubstanzen in tiersystematischer Darstellung**

Volume 27
Anticoagulantien

Volume 28: Part 1
Concepts in Biochemical Pharmacology I

Part 3
Concepts in Biochemical Pharmacology III

Volume 29
Oral wirksame Antidiabetika

Volume 30
Modern Inhalation Anesthetics

Volume 32: Part 1
Insulin I

Part 2
Insulin II

Volume 34
Secretin, Cholecystokinin, Pancreozymin and Gastrin

Volume 35: Part 1
H. E. Voss, G. Oertel:
Androgene I

Part 2
Androgens II and Antiandrogens/ Androgene II und Antiandrogene

Volume 36
Uranium – Plutonium – Transplutonic Elements

Volume 37
Angiotensin

Volume 38: Part 1
Antineoplastic and Immunosuppressive Agents I

Part 2
Antineoplastic and Immunosuppressive Agents II

Volume 39
Antihypertensive Agents

Volume 40
Organic Nitrates

Volume 41
Hypolipidemic Agents

Volume 42
Neuromuscular Junction

Volume 43
Anabolic-Androgenic Steroids

Volume 44
Heme and Hemoproteins

Volume 45: Part 1
Drug Addiction I

Part 2
Drug Addiction II

Volume 46
Fibrinolytics and Antifibrinolytics

Volume 47
Kinetics of Drug Action

Volume 48
Arthropod Venoms

Volume 49
Ergot Alkaloids and Related Compounds

Volume 50: Part 1
Inflammation

Part 2
Anti-Inflammatory Drugs

Volume 51
Uric Acid

Volume 52
Snake Venoms
(In preparation)

Volume 53
Gangliomic Transmission
(In preparation)

Springer-Verlag
Berlin
Heidelberg
New York

MIX
Papier aus verantwortungsvollen Quellen
Paper from responsible sources
FSC® C105338

If you have any concerns about our products,
you can contact us on
ProductSafety@springernature.com

In case Publisher is established outside the EU,
the EU authorized representative is:
Springer Nature Customer Service Center GmbH
Europaplatz 3, 69115 Heidelberg, Germany

Printed by Libri Plureos GmbH
in Hamburg, Germany